MONOGRAPHS IN CONTACT ALLERGY
Series Editor: Anton C. de Groot

Monographs in Contact Allergy, Volume 1: Non-Fragrance Allergens in Cosmetics
(Part 1 and Part 2)

MONOGRAPHS IN CONTACT ALLERGY
VOLUME 1, PART 2

NON-FRAGRANCE ALLERGENS IN COSMETICS

MONOGRAPHS IN CONTACT ALLERGY
VOLUME 1, PART 2

NON-FRAGRANCE ALLERGENS IN COSMETICS

Anton C. de Groot

With the help of Heleen de Jong in drawing the structural formulas

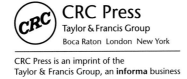

CRC Press
Taylor & Francis Group
Boca Raton London New York

CRC Press is an imprint of the
Taylor & Francis Group, an **informa** business

CRC Press
Taylor & Francis Group
6000 Broken Sound Parkway NW, Suite 300
Boca Raton, FL 33487-2742

© 2018 by Taylor & Francis Group, LLC
CRC Press is an imprint of Taylor & Francis Group, an Informa business

First issued in paperback 2021

No claim to original U.S. Government works

ISBN 13: 978-1-03-207886-1 (pbk)(set)
ISBN 13: 978-1-03-207868-7 (pbk)(part 1)
ISBN 13: 978-1-03-207872-4 (pbk)(part 2)
ISBN 13: 978-1-138-56113-7 (hbk)(set),
ISBN 13: 978-1-138-57325-3 (hbk)(part 1)
ISBN 13: 978-1-138-57338-3 (hbk)(part 2)

Visit the Taylor & Francis Web site at
http://www.taylorandfrancis.com

and the CRC Press Web site at
http://www.crcpress.com

Publisher's Note
The publisher has gone to great lengths to ensure the quality of this reprint but points out that some imperfections in the original copies may be apparent.

Contents

PART 1

PART 1   2.102   CI 12150...282

                2.103   CI 15800...283

                2.104   CI 26100...286

                2.105   CI 45380...288

                2.106   CI 47000...290

                2.107   CI 69825...293

                2.108   CI 75470...294

                2.109   CI 77163...297

                2.110   CI 77288...298

                2.111   CI 77289...299

                2.112   Cinoxate...301

                2.113   CI Pigment red 53:1..304

                2.114   Coal tar..305

                2.115   Cobalt..306

                2.116   Cocamide..307

                2.117   Cocamide DEA..308

                2.118   Cocamidopropylamine oxide...313

                2.119   Cocamidopropyl betaine...315

                2.120   Cocamidopropyl dimethylamine...325

                2.121   Cocamidopropyl hydroxysultaine..328

                2.122   Cocamidopropyl PG-dimonium chloride phosphate..329

                2.123   Coco-betaine..331

                2.124   Coco-glucoside..333

                2.125   Cod liver oil..335

                2.126   Colophonium..336

                2.127   Commiphora mukul resin extract...356

                2.128   Copernicia cerifera (carnauba) wax..358

                2.129   Cucumis sativus (cucumber) extract...359

                2.130   Cyclomethicone..360

                2.131   Cystamine bis-lactamide..361

                2.132   Cysteamine HCl...362

                2.133   DEA-dihydroxypalmityl phosphate..364

                2.134   Decyl glucoside...366

                2.135   Decyl oleate..370

                2.136   2,4-Diaminophenoxyethanol HCl..371

                2.137   Diazolidinyl urea...374

                2.138   4',5-Dibromosalicylanilide..385

                2.139   Dibutyl phthalate..387

                2.140   Dicaprylyl maleate...389

                2.141   Dichlorobenzyl alcohol...391

                2.142   Dichlorodifluoromethane..392

                2.143   Dichlorophene...394

                2.144   Didecyldimonium chloride..398

                2.145   Diethylamino hydroxybenzoyl hexyl benzoate...400

                2.146   Diethylene glycol dimethacrylate..402

                2.147   Diethyl sebacate...404

                2.148   Diethylstilbestrol...405

                2.149   bis-Diglyceryl polyacyladipate-2 406

                2.150   Diglyceryl sebacate/isopalmitate..407

                2.151   Di-HEMA trimethylhexyl dicarbamate..409

                2.152   Dihydroxyacetone...411

                2.153   Diisopropanolamine...413

                2.154   Diisostearyl malate..414

                2.155   Dimethyl oxazolidine...415

                2.156   Dipentaerythrityl hexahydroxystearate/hexastearate/hexarosinate 416

                2.157   Dipotassium glycyrrhizate..417

                2.158   Dipropylene glycol..418

                2.159   Disodium EDTA...419

                2.160   Disodium lauroamphodiacetate..422

2.288   METHOXY PEG-22/DODECYL GLYCOL COPOLYMER

IDENTIFICATION

Description/definition : Methoxy PEG-22/dodecyl glycol copolymer is the polymer that conforms generally to the formula shown below, where x has an average value of 22 and y has an average value of 7

Chemical class(es) : Alkoxylated alcohols; synthetic polymers

Other names : Oxirane, decyl-, polymer with oxirane, monomethyl ether (22 mol EO, 7 mol decyl oxirane, average molar ratios)

CAS registry number (s) : 88507-00-0

Function(s) in cosmetics : EU: emulsion stabilizing; viscosity controlling. USA: dispersing agents – nonsurfactant; emulsion stabilizers; viscosity increasing agents – aqueous; viscosity increasing agents – nonaqueous

Patch testing : 10% pet. (3,4)

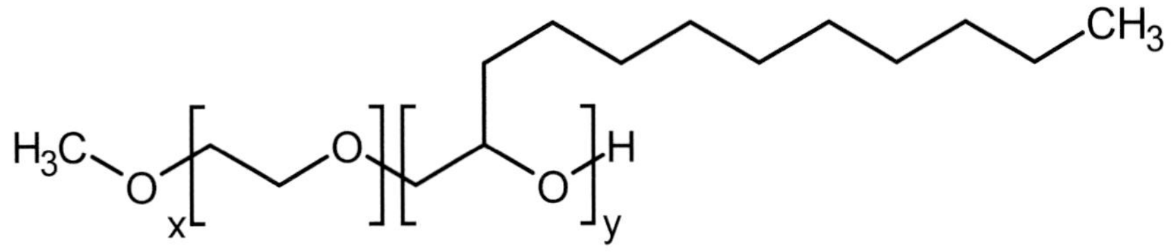

GENERAL

Copolymers are important ingredients in cosmetics, added because of their antistatic, film-forming, binding, suspending, viscosity-increasing, skin-conditioning, and emulsion-stabilizing properties. Copolymers have been underestimated for a long time as to their sensitizing capacities because of their large structures and high molecular weights. Allergic contact dermatitis to copolymers in cosmetics, however, does occur, but the exact nature of the hapten is still unknown. The copolymers are not likely to be haptens themselves in view of their large molecular weights. The sensitizer could be an additive, an impurity, a product that forms during polymerization, a residual monomer, or a degradation product (2).

CONTACT ALLERGY

Case reports and case series

Methoxy PEG-22/dodecyl glycol copolymer was responsible for 4 out of 959 cases of non-fragrance cosmetic allergy where the causal allergen was identified, Belgium, 2000-2010; the copolymer was present in skin care products (1). One or more patients had allergic contact dermatitis from methoxy PEG-22/dodecyl glycol copolymer in a cosmetic cold cream (5).

Contact allergy to methoxy PEG-22/dodecyl glycol copolymer in non-cosmetic products

Methoxy PEG-22/dodecyl glycol copolymer was the allergen or one of the allergens in a tissue accompanying a depilatory wax in 19 patients with contact dermatitis from the wax and/or the tissue (3,4).

Cross-reactions, pseudo-cross-reactions and co-reactions

Methoxy PEG-17/dodecyl glycol copolymer (3,4).

Presence in cosmetic products and chemical analyses

In the USA, in April 2017, methoxy PEG-22/dodecyl glycol copolymer was present in 5 of 56,714 cosmetic products of which the composition is known in FDA's Voluntary Cosmetic Registration Program (VCRP) (data obtained from FDA, May 2017). In March 2017, methoxy PEG-22/dodecyl glycol copolymer was present in 5 of 65,431 cosmetic products of which the composition is known in EWG's Skin Deep Cosmetics Database, USA (http://www.ewg.org/skindeep/). Methoxy PEG-22/dodecyl glycol copolymer was found as an ingredient in 18 moisturizers, 1 sunscreen, 1 foundation, and the tissue accompanying a warm hair removal wax, discussed above (2).

LITERATURE

1   Travassos AR, Claes L, Boey L, Drieghe J, Goossens A. Non-fragrance allergens in specific cosmetic products. Contact Dermatitis 2011;65:276-285

2   Quartier S, Garmyn M, Becart S, Goossens A. Allergic contact dermatitis to copolymers in cosmetics – case report and review of the literature. Contact Dermatitis 2006;55:257-267

3   Goossens A, Armingaud P, Avenel-Audran M, Begon-Bagdassarian I, Constandt L, Giordano-Labadie F, et al. An epidemic of allergic contact dermatitis due to epilating products. Contact Dermatitis 2002;46:67-70

4   Goossens A. An epidemic of allergic contact dermatitis due to epilating products. Contact Dermatitis 2001;45:360

5   Lasek-Duriez A, Castelain MC, Modiano P. Allergic contact dermatitis due to methoxy PEG-22 dodecyl glycol present in a cosmetic cold cream. Ann Dermatol Venereol 2013;140:528-530

2.289   METHYL ACRYLATE*
Not an INCI name

IDENTIFICATION

Description/definition   : Methyl acrylate is the organic compound that conforms to the formula shown below
Chemical class(es)   : Esters
INCI name USA   : Neither in CosIng nor in the Personal Care Products Council Ingredient Database
Chemical/IUPAC name   : Methyl prop-2-enoate
CAS registry number (s)   : 96-33-3
EC number(s)   : 202-500-6
Merck Index monograph   : 7355
Patch testing   : 0.1% pet.
Molecular formula   : $C_4H_6O_2$

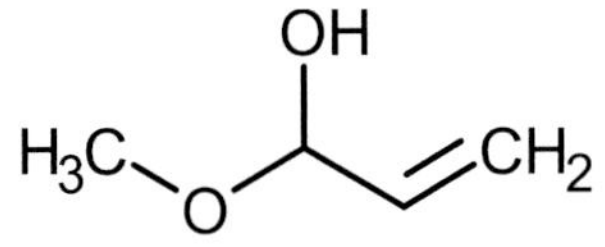

GENERAL

Discussion of contact allergy to (meth)acrylates *from non-cosmetic sources* is considered to fall outside the scope of this book. Therefore, only contact allergy from their presence in cosmetics is presented, which virtually always is from artificial nails. There are many reports of contact allergy to artificial nails, but the specific sensitizers have rarely been identified and – consequently - such publications are not presented in this and other (meth)acrylate mono-graphs. Discussion is limited to publications in which the culprit (meth)acrylates have been identified, e.g., from information found in Material Data Safety Sheets, data obtained from the manufacturer or from chemical analyses.

Patients often react to many (meth)acrylates on patch testing. Primary sensitization to methacrylates may result in both methacrylate and acrylate cross-sensitization. Conversely, patients sensitized to acrylates are unlikely to show cross-sensitization to methacrylates (3).

General aspects of (meth)acrylates are presented in Chapter 2.219 HEMA (hydroxyethyl methacrylate). A discussion of general aspects of artificial nails, contact allergy to these products, the clinical picture of ACD dermatitis and other side effects of such nails can also be found there. A very useful review of contact sensitization to allergens in nail cosmetics, with emphasis on acrylic manicures, was published in 2017 (5).

CONTACT ALLERGY

Patch testing in groups of patients
Studies in which consecutive patients suspected of contact dermatitis have been tested with methyl acrylate (routine testing) and studies testing groups of selected patients are planned to be discussed in a future publication.

Case reports and case series
A cosmetician teaching other cosmeticians how to make artificial nails developed occupational contact dermatitis of the hands and face from contact allergy to methyl acrylate in nail hardener, nail lacquer and UV-curing nail gel (1). Gas chromatography – mass spectrometry (GC-MS) showed that the nail gel contained 0.3% methyl acrylate and the other two products <0.5% (1). One patient had allergic contact dermatitis from a nail polish containing 9% methyl acrylate (2).

OTHER SIDE EFFECTS

Other side effects
Accidental occupational exposure to methyl acrylate has resulted in sensitization (4).

Presence in cosmetic products and chemical analyses
In May 2017, was present in one older product of 66,975 cosmetic products of which the composition is known in EWG's Skin Deep Cosmetics Database, USA (http://www.ewg.org/skindeep/). In the USA, in April 2017, methyl acrylate was present in zero of 56,714 cosmetic products of which the composition is known in FDA's Voluntary Cosmetic Registration Program (VCRP) (data obtained from FDA, May 2017).

LITERATURE

1   Kanerva L, Lauerma A, Estlander T, Alanko K, Henriks-Eckerman M-L, Jolanki RL. Occupational allergic contact dermatitis caused by photobonded sculptured nails and a review of (meth)acrylates in nail cosmetics. Am J Contact Dermatitis 1996;7:109-115

2   Kanerva L, Lauerma A, Jolanki R, Estlander T. Methyl acrylate: a new sensitizer in nail lacquer. Contact Dermatitis 1995;33:203-204

3   Aalto-Korte K, Henriks-Eckerman M-L, Kuuliala O, Jolanki R. Occupational methacrylate and acrylate allergy – cross-reactions and possible screening allergens. Contact Dermatitis 2010;63:301-312

4   Kanerva L, Jolanki R, Estlander T. Accidental occupational sensitization caused by methyl acrylate. Eur J Dermatol 1993;3:195-198

5   Chou M, Dhingra N, Strugar TL. Contact sensitization to allergens in nail cosmetics. Dermatitis 2017;28:231-240

2.290 P-METHYLAMINOPHENOL

IDENTIFICATION

Description/definition   : *p*-Methylaminophenol is the substituted phenol that conforms to the formula shown below

Chemical class(es)   : Amines; color additives – hair; phenols
Chemical/IUPAC name   : 4-(Methylamino)phenol
CAS registry number (s) : 150-75-4
EC number(s)   : 205-768-2
CIR review(s)   : Final report, December 2007 (access: www.cir-safety.org/ingredients)
SCCS opinion(s)   : SCCNFP, 23 June 1999 (2)
Function(s) in cosmetics : EU: hair dyeing. USA: hair colorants
EU cosmetic restrictions : Regulated in Annex III/223 of the Regulation (EC) No. 1223/2009
Patch testing   : 1% pet. (4)
Molecular formula   : C_7H_9NO

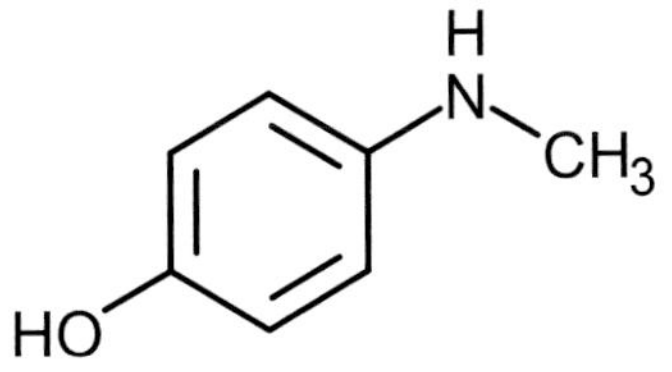

GENERAL

p-Methylaminophenol is used in oxidative hair dying products. The chemistry of oxidative hair dying is discussed in Chapter 2.359 *p*-Phenylenediamine. *p*-Methylaminophenol is used very infrequently (see the section 'Presence in cosmetic products and chemical analyses' below) and, therefore, many positive patch test reactions may be the result of cross-reactivity from sensitization to other para-amino hair dyes.

CONTACT ALLERGY

Patch testing in groups of patients

In 2007-2008, 914 consecutive patients suspected of contact dermatitis were tested (routine testing) with *p*-methylaminophenol 1% pet. and there were 20 (2.2%) positive reactions. Two were considered to be relevant. In the group of 20 positives, 8 patients (40%) co-reacted to other para-amino hair dyes (4).

Case reports and case series

In two patients with positive patch tests to *p*-methylaminophenol, the reactions were considered to explain their current dermatitis (4). Causative products nor clinical data were provided, and therefore, cosmetic allergy has not been verified. However, the most likely explanation of sensitization is – possibly after cross-sensitivity to other hair dyes such as *p*-phenylenediamine or toluene-2,5-diamine - from hair dying.

Cross-reactions, pseudo-cross-reactions and co-reactions

p-Methylaminophenol may cross-react with structurally related chemicals, notably those with a para-structure. Cross-reactivity between para-compounds is discussed in Chapter 2.359 *p*-Phenylenediamine. Possibly there is imme-diate-type cross-reactivity with *p*-aminophenol (1).

Presence in cosmetic products and chemical analyses

In August 2017, *p*-methylaminophenol was present in one older product of 70,366 cosmetic products of which the composition is known in EWG's Skin Deep Cosmetics Database, USA (http://www.ewg.org/skindeep/). In the USA, in April 2017, *p*-methylaminophenol was present in zero of 56,714 cosmetic products of which the composition is known in FDA's Voluntary Cosmetic Registration Program (VCRP) (data obtained from FDA, May 2017).

In southern Germany, in 2013-2014, the labels of 924 permanent oxidative hair dyes were checked for the presence of hair dye components. There were 334 retail products (of seven different brands) and 590 professional products (of six different brands). The 924 products analyzed revealed a total of 58 different hair dye components, with retail products containing 32 and professional products 52. *p*-Methylaminophenol was present in 8 (0.8%) of the 924 products (5). In the USA, in 2012, ingredient labels of 107 different consumer oxidative hair dyes from 10 different companies were assessed in stores across the city of Phoenix, Arizona. *p*-Methylaminophenol (as free base, sulfate, or HCl) was present in one of the products (6).

OTHER SIDE EFFECTS

Immediate-type reactions

One patient developed upper airway stridor and generalized urticaria after using a hair dye on two occasions. He had positive scratch tests to *p*-methylaminophenol, which was present in the cosmetic product, tested 1%, 5% and 10% in water (1).

A review of contact urticaria to cosmetic ingredients has been provided in ref. 3.

LITERATURE

1   Oshima H, Tamaki T, Oh-I T, Koga M. Contact anaphylaxis due to para-aminophenol and para-methylaminophenol in hair dye. Contact Dermatitis 2001;45:359

2   SCCNFP (Scientific Committee on Cosmetics and Non Food Products). Opinion concerning *p*-Methylaminophenol, 23 June 1999. Available at: http://ec.europa.eu/health/scientific_committees/consumer_safety/opinions/sccnfp_opinions_97_04/sccp_out68_en.htm

3   Verhulst L, Goossens A. Cosmetic components causing contact urticaria: a review and update. Contact Dermatitis 2016;75:333-344

4   Søsted H, Rustemeyer T, Gonçalo M, Bruze M, Goossens A, Giménez-Arnau AM, et al. Contact allergy to common ingredients in hair dyes. Contact Dermatitis 2013;69:32-39

5   Kirchlecher S, Hübner A, Uter W. Survey of sensitizing constituents of oxidative hair dyes (retail and professional products) in Germany. J Dtsch Dermatol Ges 2016;14:707-715

6   Hamann D, Yazar K, Hamann CR, Thyssen JP, Lidén C. p-Phenylenediamine and other allergens in hair dye products in the United States: a consumer exposure study. Contact Dermatitis 2014;70:213-218

2.291   4-METHYLBENZYLIDENE CAMPHOR

IDENTIFICATION

Description/definition : 4-Methylbenzylidene camphor is the aromatic organic compound that conforms to the formula shown below

Chemical class(es) : Ketones

Chemical/IUPAC name : (1S,2Z,4R)-4,7,7-Trimethyl-2-[(4-methylphenyl)methylidene]bicyclo[2.2.1]heptan-3-one

Other names : Enzacamene; Eusolex® 6300; 3-(4-methylbenzylidene)camphor

CAS registry number (s) : 36861-47-9; 38102-62-4

EC number(s) : 253-242-6

SCCS opinion(s) : SCCP/1184/08 (45); SCCNFP, January 21, 1998 (46)

Merck Index monograph : 7371

Function(s) in cosmetics : EU: UV-absorber; UV-filter. USA: light stabilizer

EU cosmetic restrictions : Regulated in Annex VI/18 of the Regulation (EC) No. 1223/2009

Patch testing : 10.0% pet. (Chemotechnique, SmartPracticeCanada)

Molecular formula : $C_{18}H_{22}O$

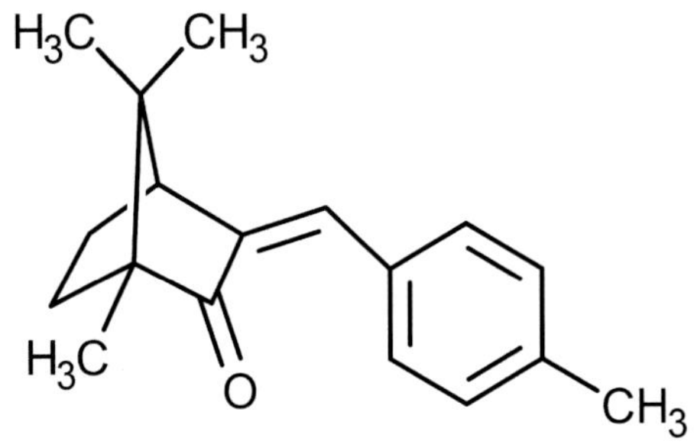

GENERAL

4-Methylbenzylidene camphor is a UVB filter with UV absorbance maximum (λ_{max}) at 300 nm, which has been used in Europe since 1984 (30,53). Most contact allergic reactions to 4-methylbenzylidene camphor have occurred together with contact allergy to isopropyl dibenzoylmethane, with which it was combined in the commercial sunscreen Eusolex® 8021 (6,8,10,17,20,21) (27, photocontact sensitization). After withdrawal of isopropyl dibenzoylmethane in 1993, few reactions to 4-methylbenzylidene camphor have been observed (2). The literature on adverse reactions to sunscreens has been reviewed in several recent and older publications (34-39,61). A review of photocontact allergy to sunscreens was published in 2010 (52).

CONTACT ALLERGY

Patch testing in groups of patients

There are no studies in which 4-methylbenzylidene camphor has been patch tested in consecutive patients suspected of contact dermatitis (routine testing). Results of testing in groups of *selected* patients (e.g., patients suspected of photosensitivity, patients with dermatitis affecting mainly light-exposed skin or with a history of a sunscreen skin reaction) back to 1991 are shown in table 2.291.1. Test concentrations used have been 2% pet., 3% pet., 5% pet. or 10% pet., but the higher test concentrations have not clearly resulted in more positive reactions, the mode of selection probably being the more important determinant.

In 10 studies testing groups of selected patients, frequencies of sensitization have ranged from 0.4% to 8%; in 9 of the 10 studies, rates were 2% or lower. The high frequency of 8% was seen in a German study, where also many patients reacting to isopropyl dibenzoylmethane were observed. Concomitant sensitization to both UV-filters in Eusolex® 8021 may be an explanation for the high rate of sensitization (2). In all but three investigations, the relevance of the positive patch test reactions to 4-methylbenzylidene camphor was either not stated or specified for the UV-filter. In one study, 4 of 6 positive patch tests (67%) were currently relevant (1); in another one, both positive patch test reactions found were considered to be relevant (49). In a study from the USA, finally, all 6 positive patch test reactions were scored as relevant, but this included 'questionable' and 'past' relevance (11).

Case reports and case series

4-Methylbenzylidene camphor was stated to be the (or an) allergen in one patient in a group of 603 individuals suffering from cosmetic dermatitis, seen in the period 2010-2015 in Leuven, Belgium (40). In the period 1996-2013, in a tertiary referral center in Valencia, Spain, 5419 patients were patch tested. Of these, 628 individuals had allergic contact dermatitis to cosmetics. 4-Methylbenzylidene camphor was the responsible allergen in five cases (50, overlap with ref. 47). Five relevant cases of contact allergy or photocontact allergy to 4-methylbenzylidene camphor were seen in one center in Australia in an 18-year period up to 2012 (13). In the period 2000-2007, 202 patients with allergic contact dermatitis caused by cosmetics were seen in Valencia, Spain. In this group, three individuals reacted to 4-methylbenzylidene camphor from its presence in sunscreens (47, overlap with ref. 50). In the period 1978-1991, there were 2 relevant patch test reactions to 4-methylbenzylidene camphor in one center in Leuven, Belgium (23). In the period 1981-1989, 56 patients (43 women, 13 men) were diagnosed with contact allergy or photocontact allergy to UV-filters in one center in Germany. There were 19 contact allergic, 7 photoaggravated contact allergic and 5 photoallergic reactions to 4-methylbenzylidene camphor. All reactions were relevant and all 46 patients who could be (photo)patch tested with their own sunscreens (and a few of them with other cosmetics) had one or more positive (photo)patch tests to these products (55, overlap with refs. 2,8, and 51).

Table 2.291.1 Patch testing in groups of patients: Selected patient groups

Years and Country	Test conc. & vehicle	Number of patients tested | positive (%)		Selection of patients (S); Relevance (R); Comments (C)	Ref.
2011-2013 Colombia	10% pet.	112	2 (1.8%)	S: dermatitis affecting mainly light-exposed skin, a history of a sunscreen or a topical NSAID skin reaction; R: 100%	49
2008-2011 12 European countries	10% pet.	1031	4 (0.4%)	S: patients with exposed site dermatitis or history of a reaction to a sunscreen or topical NSAID; R: not specified	15
2001-2010 Canada		160	2 (1.2%)	S: patients with suspected photosensitivity and patients who developed pruritus or a rash after sunscreen application; R: not stated; C: very weak study: inadequate reading of test results, erythema only was considered to represent a positive patch test reaction	14
2000-2007 USA	10% pet.	922	6 (0.7%)	S: patients tested with a supplemental cosmetic screening series; R: 100%; C: weak study: a. high rate of macular erythema and weak reactions; b. relevance figures included 'questionable' and 'past' relevance	11
2001-2003 Colombia	10% pet.	82	1 (1.2%)	S: patients with a clinical diagnosis of photoallergic contact dermatitis; R: 65% of all reactions in the study were relevant	9
2000-2002 UK, I, NL	10% pet.	1155	6 (0.5%)	S: patients suspected of photosensitivity or reaction to a sunscreen; R: current relevance 4, unknown 2	1
1993-2000 Australia	2% pet.	149	1 (0.7%)	S: patients suspected of photosensitivity; R: of 17 patients who had contact or photocontact reactions to a panel of 10 sunscreens, 10 were considered to have relevant reactions	24
1981-1996 Germany	3%, 5% or 10% pet.	402	32 (8.0%)	S: patients suspected of clinical photosensitivity; R: not stated	2
1990-1994 France	2% or 10% pet.	370	2 (0.5%)	S: patients with suspected photodermatitis; R: not specified, 72% of all reactions in the study were considered relevant	7
1989-1991 UK	2% pet.	99	2 (2%)	S: 45 patients with photosensitivity dermatitis/actinic reticuloid syndrome and 54 with polymorphic light eruption; R: not specified	3

I: Ireland; NL: Netherlands; UK: United Kingdom

In a group of 119 patients with allergic contact dermatitis from cosmetics, investigated in The Netherlands in 1986-1987, two cases were caused by 4-methylbenzylidene camphor in a lipstick with UV-filter (41,42). In a group of 75 patients allergic to cosmetic products, seen in a private practice in The Netherlands in the period 1981-1986, one case was caused by 4-methylbenzylidene camphor in a lipstick with UV-absorber (43, same patient as in ref. 10). Of 10 patients with contact allergy to and allergic contact dermatitis from Eusolex® 8021, all reacted to isopropyl dibenzoylmethane and 5 to 4-methylbenzylidene camphor in sunscreens (n=9, including 5 sunscreen lipsticks) and cosmetic creams (n=1) (10). Five cases of contact allergy to 4-methylbenzylidene camphor were reported from Germany, where also many patients allergic to isopropyl dibenzoylmethane were seen; the positive patch tests were probably relevant from its presence in sunscreens (8); the authors mentioned three more cases (8, note added in proof).

Several authors have presented single case reports of patients allergic to 4-methylbenzylidene camphor in sunscreen products (4,5,6,17,18,19,44,51,54,56,58,59). One patient had allergic contact dermatitis from 4-methylbenzylidene camphor (and from isopropyl dibenzoylmethane), the presence of which was established by chemical analysis (20). Another individual reacted to 4-methylbenzylidene camphor (and isopropyl dibenzoylmethane) in 2 emollient reams (21). A woman had ACD from 4-methylbenzylidene camphor in a skin care product (57). Three patients suffered from allergic contact dermatitis to Eusolex® 8021 in a sunscreen; the 2 components were not tested separately (22,56,60).

Cross-reactions, pseudo-cross-reactions and co-reactions (including photoreactions)
Concomitant sensitization to isopropyl dibenzoylmethane and 4-methylbenzylidene camphor, which were both ingredients of the commercial sunscreen Eusolex® 8021, has been reported repeatedly (6,8,10,17,20,21) (27, photocontact sensitization). It has been suggested that sensitization to the strong allergen isopropyl dibenzoylmethane facilitates and stimulates sensitization to the weaker allergen 4-methylbenzylidene camphor (10)

Presence in cosmetic products and chemical analyses
In June 2017, 4-methylbenzylidene camphor was present in 1 of 68,866 cosmetic products of which the composition is known in EWG's Skin Deep Cosmetics Database, USA (http://www.ewg.org/skindeep/). It should be realized that sunscreen products containing UV-filters are classified as drugs in the USA, not as cosmetics; the number mentioned here, therefore, is that of cosmetics containing the UV-filter, but it does *not* include their presence in sunscreens. In the USA, in April 2017, 4-methylbenzylidene camphor was present in 7 of 56,714 cosmetic products of which the composition is known in FDA's Voluntary Cosmetic Registration Program (VCRP) (data obtained from FDA, May 2017).

In 2012, in Switzerland, 116 cosmetics from seven widely used leave-on product categories (19 lip care products, 8 lipsticks, 29 face creams, 11 liquid makeup foundations, 3 aftershaves, 7 hand creams and 39 sunscreens) were investigated to determine the frequency of occurrence and concentrations of 22 organic UV filters in these products. 4-Methylbenzylidene camphor was found in one product only in a concentration of 4% (48). In a sample of 337 sunscreens marketed in the UK in 2010, 4-methylbenzylidene camphor was present in 1% (33). 4-Methylbenzylidene camphor was present in 5.9% of 4447 cosmetic products collected in Germany, 2006-2009 (16). 4-Methylbenzylidene camphor was present in 17 of 75 (23%) sunscreen creams and lotions from 30 European and US producers purchased in Denmark in 2001 in a concentration range of 0.9-5.7% (26).

OTHER SIDE EFFECTS

Photosensitivity

Photopatch testing in groups of patients
Results of photopatch testing 4-methylbenzylidene camphor in groups of selected patients (e.g., patients suspected of photosensitivity, patients with dermatitis affecting mainly light-exposed skin or with a history of a sunscreen skin reaction) back to 1994 are shown in table 2.291.2. Test concentrations used have been 2% pet., 3% pet, 5% pet and 10% pet., but the higher test concentrations have not clearly resulted in more positive reactions, the mode of selection probably being the more important determinant. In 11 studies, frequencies of photosensitization have ranged from 0.1% to 1.9% (table 2.291.2). In 7/11 studies, positive photoreactions scored 0.7% or lower. In many studies, relevance was either not mentioned or specified for 4-methylbenzylidene camphor, but in the studies that provided relevance data, 0-100% of the positive photopatch tests were considered to be relevant, but this concerned only 1-4 patients per study (1,12,25,28,29).

Case reports
Five relevant cases of contact allergy or photocontact allergy to 4-methylbenzylidene camphor were seen in one center in Australia in an 18-year period up to 2012 (13). Two cases of photocontact allergy to 4-methylbenzylidene camphor were observed in Germany; the positive photopatch tests were probably relevant from its presence in sunscreens (8); the authors mentioned two more cases (8, note added in proof). In a 1-year-period (1996-1997), 3 patients had positive photopatch tests to 4-methylbenzylidene camphor in one center in Italy. One patient had photoallergic contact dermatitis from facial cosmetics, one reaction was of past relevance from sunscreens and in the third patient the relevance was unknown. In two, there was also a positive photopatch test to isopropyl dibenzoylmethane, the other ingredient of Eusolex® 8021 (27). One individual had photoallergic contact dermatitis from 4-methylbenzylidene camphor in various sunscreens (32). In the period 1981-1989, 56 patients (43 women, 13 men) were diagnosed with contact allergy or photocontact allergy to UV-filters in one center in Germany. There were 19 contact allergic, 7 photoaggravated contact allergic and 5 photoallergic reactions to 4-methylbenzylidene camphor. All reactions were relevant and all 46 patients who could be (photo)patch tested with their own sunscreens (and a few of them with other cosmetics) had one or more positive (photo)patch tests to these products (55, overlap with refs. 2,8,51).

Table 2.291.2 Photopatch testing in groups of patients

Years and Country	Test conc. & vehicle	Number of patients tested | positive (%)		Selection of patients (S); Relevance (R); Comments (C)	Ref.
2008-2011 12 European countries	10% pet.	1031	3 (0.3%)	S: patients with exposed site dermatitis or history of a reaction to a sunscreen or topical NSAID; R: 44% current and 11% past relevance for all photoallergens together	15
2000-2011 UK	10% pet.	157	1 (0.6%)	S: children <18 years suspected of photosensitivity; R: the reaction was caused by a sunscreen product	28
2001-2010 Canada		160	1 (0.6%)	S: patients with suspected photosensitivity and patients who developed pruritus or a rash after sunscreen application; R: not stated	14
2003-2007 Portugal	10% pet.	83	1 (1.2%)	S: patients with suspected photoaggravated facial dermatitis or systemic photosensitivity; R: all sunscreen photopatch tests were of current or past relevance	25
2004-2006 Italy	10% pet.	1082	1 (0.1%)	S: patients with histories and clinical features suggestive of photoallergic contact dermatitis; R: none	12
2000-2005 USA	10% pet.	177	3 (1.7%)	S: patients photopatch tested for suspected photodermatitis; R: 1 reaction was relevant	29
2001-2003 Colombia	10% pet.	82	1 (1.2%)	S: patients with a clinical diagnosis of photoallergic contact dermatitis; R: 65% of all reactions in the study were relevant	9
2000-2002 UK, I, NL	10% pet.	1155	4 (0.4%)	S: patients suspected of photosensitivity or reaction to a sunscreen; R: current relevance 2, unknown 2	1
1993-2000 Australia	2% pet.	149	1 (0.7%)	S: patients suspected of photosensitivity; R: of 17 patient who had contact or photocontact reactions to a panel of 10 sunscreens, 10 were considered to have relevant reactions	24
1981-1996 Germany	3%, 5% or 10% pet.	402	5 (1.2%)	S: patients suspected of clinical photosensitivity; R: not stated	2
1990-1994 France	2% or 10% pet.	370	1 (0.3%)	S: patients with suspected photodermatitis; R: not specified, 72% of all reactions in the study were considered relevant	7

I: Ireland; NL: Netherlands; UK: United Kingdom

LITERATURE

1   Bryden A, Moseley H, Ibbotson S, Chowdhury MM, Beck MH, Bourke J, et al. Photopatch testing of 1155 patients: results of the U.K. multicentre photopatch test study group. Brit J Dermatol 2006;155:737-747

2   Schauder S, Ippen H. Contact and photocontact sensitivity. Review of a 15-year experience and of the literature to suncreens. Contact Dermatitis 1997;37:221-232

3   Bilsland D, Ferguson J. Contact allergy to sunscreen chemicals in photosensitivity dermatitis/actinic reticuloid syndrome (PD/AR) and polymorphic light eruption. Contact Dermatitis 1993;29:70-73

4   Hunloh W, Goerz G. Contact dermatitis from Eusolex ® 6300. Contact Dermatitis 1983;9:333-334

5   Helsing P, Austad J. Contact dermatitis mimicking photodermatosis in a 1-year-old child. Contact Dermatitis 1991;24:140-141

6   Marguery MC, Rakotondrazafy J, el Sayed F, Bayle-Lebey P, Journe F, Bazex J. Contact allergy to 3-(4'-methylbenzylidene) camphor and contact and photocontact allergy to 4-isopropyl dibenzoylmethane. Photodermatol Photoimmunol Photomed 1996;11:209-212

7   Journe F, Marguery M-C, Rakotondrazafy J, El Sayed F, Bazex J. Sunscreen sensitization: a 5-year study. Acta Derm Venereol (Stockh) 1999;79:211-213

8   Schauder S, Ippen H. Photoallergic and allergic contact eczema caused by dibenzoylmethane compounds and other sunscreening agents. Hautarzt 1988;39:435-440

9   Rodriguez E, Valbuena M, Rey M, Porras de Quintana L. Causal agents of photoallergic contact dermatitis diagnosed in the national institute of dermatology of Columbia. Photoderm Photoimmunol Photomed 2006;22:189-192

10   De Groot AC, van der Walle HB, Jagtman BA, Weyland JW. Contact allergy to 4-isopropyl-dibenzoylmethane and 3(4-methylbenzylidene) camphor in sunscreen Eusolex 8021. Contact Dermatitis 1987;16:249-254

11   Wetter DA, Yiannias JA, Prakash AV, Davis MD, Farmer SA, el-Azhary RA, et al. Results of patch testing to personal care product allergens in a standard series and a supplemental cosmetic series: an analysis of 945 patients from the Mayo Clinic Contact Dermatitis Group, 2000-2007. J Am Acad Dermatol 2010;63:789-798

12   Pigatto PD, Guzzi G, Schena D, Guarrera M, Foti C, Francalanci S, et al. Photopatch tests: an Italian multicentre study from 2004 to 2006. Contact Dermatitis 2008;59:103-108

13   Nixon RL. Contact dermatitis to sunscreens. Dermatitis 2012;23:140-141

14   Greenspoon J, Ahluwalia R, Juma N, Rosen CF. Allergic and photoallergic contact dermatitis: A 10-year experience. Dermatitis 2013;24:29-32

15 The European Multicentre Photopatch Test Study (EMCPPTS) Taskforce. A European multicentre photopatch test study. Br J Dermatol 2012;166:1002-1009

16 Uter W, Gonçalo M, Yazar K, Kratz E-M, Mildau G, Lidén C. Coupled exposure to ingredients of cosmetic products: III. Ultraviolet filters. Contact Dermatitis 2014;71:162-169

17 Buckley DA, O'Sullivan D, Murphy GM. Contact and photocontact allergy to dibenzoylmethanes and contact allergy to methylbenzylidene camphor. Contact Dermatitis 1993;29:47

18 Goldermann R, Vardarman E, Neumann N, Scharffetter-Kochanek K, Goerz G. Contact dermatitis from UV-A and UV-B filters in a patient with erythropoietic protoporphyria. Contact Dermatitis 1993;28:300-301

19 Hunloh W, Goerz G. Contact dermatitis from Eusolex® 6300. Contact Dermatitis 1983;9:333-334

20 Foussereau J, Cavelier C, Protois JC. Contact dermatitis from Eusolex 8021 elucidated by chemical analysis. Contact Dermatitis 1989;20:311-312

21 Alomar A, Cerda MT. Contact allergy to Eusolex® 8021. Contact Dermatitis 1989;20:74-75

22 Roberts DL. Contact allergy to Eusolex 8021. Contact Dermatitis 1988;18:302-303

23 Theeuwes M, Degreef H, Dooms-Goossens A. Para-aminobenzoic acid (PABA) and sunscreen allergy. Am J Cont Derm 1992;3:206-207

24 Crouch RB, Foley PA, Baker CS. The results of photopatch testing 172 patients to sunscreening agents at the photobiology clinic, St Vincent's Hospital, Melbourne. Australas J Dermatol 2002;43:74

25 Cardoso J, Canelas MM, Gonçalo M, Figueiredo A. Photopatch testing with an extended series of photoallergens: a 5-year study. Contact Dermatitis 2009;60:325-329

26 Rastogi SC. UV filters in sunscreen products – a survey. Contact Dermatitis 2002;46:348-351

27 Ricci C, Pazzaglia M, Tosti A. Photocontact dermatitis from UV filters. Contact Dermatitis 1998;38:343-344

28 Haylett AK, Chiang YZ, Nie Z, Ling TC, Rhodes LE. Sunscreen photopatch testing: a series of 157 children. Br J Dermatol 2014;171:370-375

29 Scalf LA, Davis MDP, Rohlinger AL, Connolly SM. Photopatch testing of 182 patients: A 6-year experience at the Mayo Clinic. Dermatitis 2009;20:44-52

30 Kerr A, Ferguson J. Photoallergic contact dermatitis. Photodermatol Photoimmunol Photomed 2010;26:56-65

31 Wahie S, Lloyd JJ, Farr PM. Sunscreen ingredients and labelling: a survey of products available in the U.K. Clin Exp Dermatol 2007;32:359-364

32 Schmidt T, Ring J, Abeck D. Photoallergic contact dermatitis due to combined UVB (4-methylbenzylidene camphor/octyl methoxycinnamate) and UVA (benzophenone-3/butyl methoxydibenzoylmethane) absorber sensitization. Dermatology 1998;196:354-357

33 Kerr AC. A survey of the availability of sunscreen filters in the U.K. Clin Exp Dermatol 2011;36:541-543

34 Heurung AR, Raju SI, Warshaw EM. Adverse reactions to sunscreen agents: epidemiology, responsible irritants and allergens, clinical characteristics, and management. Dermatitis 2014;25:289-326

35 Heurung AR, Raju SI, Warshaw EM. Contact allergen of the year. Benzophenones. Dermatitis 2014;25:3-10 (contains many mistakes; Erratum in Dermatitis 2014;25:92-95)

36 Avenel-Audran M. Sunscreen products: finding the allergen. Eur J Dermatol 2010;20:161-166

37 Scheuer E, Warshaw E. Sunscreen allergy: a review of epidemiology, clinical characteristics, and responsible allergens. Dermatitis 2006;17:3-11

38 Funk JO, Dromgoole SH, Maibach HI. Sunscreen intolerance: contact sensitization, photocontact sensitization, and irritancy of sunscreen agents. Dermatol Clin 1995;13:473-481

39 Dromgoole SH, Maibach HI. Sunscreening agent intolerance: Contact and photocontact sensitization and contact urticaria. J Am Acad Dermatol 1990;22:1068-1078

40 Goossens A. Cosmetic contact allergens. Cosmetics 2016, 3, 5; doi:10.3390/cosmetics3010005

41 De Groot AC, Bruynzeel DP, Bos JD, van der Meeren HL, van Joost T, Jagtman BA, Weyland JW. The allergens in cosmetics. Arch Dermatol 1988;124:1525-1529

42 De Groot AC. Adverse reactions to cosmetics. PhD Thesis, University of Groningen, The Netherlands: 1988, chapter 3.4, pp.105-113

43 De Groot AC. Contact allergy to cosmetics: Causative ingredients. Contact Dermatitis 1987;17:26-34

44 Haussmann A, Kleinhans D. Allergische Kontaktekzem durch UV-Strahlenfilter in Zonnenschutzcremes – Zwei Fallbeobachtungen. Z Hautkr 1986;61:1654-1656

45 SCCP (Scientific Committee on Consumer Products). Opinion on 4-Methylbenzylidene camphor (4-MBC), 24 June 2008, SCCP/1184/08. Available at: http://ec.europa.eu/health/archive/ph_risk/committees/04_sccp/docs/sccp_o_141.pdf

46 SCCNFP (Scientific Committee on Cosmetics and Non Food Products). Opinion concerning 3-(4'-methylbenzylidene)-d,l camphor, January 21, 1998. Available from: http://ec.europa.eu/health/scientific_committees/consumer_safety/opinions/sccnfp_opinions_97_04/sccp_out27_en.htm

47 Laguna C, de la Cuadra J, Martín-González B, Zaragoza V, Martínez-Casimiro L, Alegre V. Allergic contact dermatitis to cosmetics. Actas Dermosifiliogr 2009;100:53-60

48 Manová E, von Goetz N, Hauri U, Bogdal C, Hungerbühler K. Organic UV filters in personal care products in Switzerland: A survey of occurrence and concentrations. Int J Hyg Environ Health 2013;216:508-514

49 Valbuena Mesa MC, Hoyos Jiménez EV. Photopatch testing in Bogota (Colombia): 2011–2013. Contact Dermatitis 2016;74:11-17

50 Zaragoza-Ninet V, Blasco Encinas R, Vilata-Corell JJ, Pérez-Ferriols A, Sierra-Talamantes C, Esteve-Martínez A, de la Cuadra-Oyanguren J. Allergic contact dermatitis due to cosmetics: A clinical and epidemiological study in a tertiary hospital. Actas Dermosifiliogr 2016;107:329-336

51 Schauder S, Ippen H. Photoallergic and allergic contact dermatitis from dibenzoylmethanes. Photodermatol 1986;3:140-147

52 Shaw T, Simpson B, Wilson B, Oostman H, Rainey D, Storrs F. True photoallergy to sunscreens is rare despite popular belief. Dermatitis 2010;21:185-198

53 Shaath NA. Ultraviolet filters. Photochem Photobiol Sci 2010;9:464-469

54 Rubio-González B, Ortiz-de Frutos FJ. Allergic contact dermatitis to hexyl cinnamaldehyde, cinnamaldehyde, and 3,4 methylbenzylidene camphor in a patient with previous photoallergic contact dermatitis to dexketoprofen. Actas Dermosifiliogr 2015;106:146-148

55 Schauder S. Adverse reactions to sunscreening agents in 58 patients (part 3). Z Hautkr 1991;66:294-318 (article in German)

56 Kimmig W. Allergische Kontaktdermatitis durch Lichtschutzmittel. Z Hautkr 1987;62:73 (article in German) Kleinhans D. Kontaktallergie gegen UV-Filtersubstanzen in Lichtschutzpräparaten. Derm und Kosm 1988;29:28-34 (article in German)

58 Köster W, Juratli A. Verlauf von persistierender Lichtreaktion und aktinischem Retikuloid nach PUVA-Therapie – Eine Kasuistiek. Akt Dermatol 1989;15:167-173 (article in German)

59 Lübben U. Kontaktallergie auf Lichtschutzmittel. Z Hautkr 1987;62:1233 (article in German)

60 Woods B. Dermatitis from Eusolex 8021 sunscreen agent in a cosmetic. Contact Dermatitis 1981;7:168

61 Schauder S. Survey of the literature on adverse reactions to preparations containing UV filters (1947-1989) (Literaturübersicht über Unverträglichkeitsreaktionen auf lichtfilterhaltige Produkte von 1947 bis 1989). Z Hautkr 1990;65:982-998 (article in German)

2.292 METHYLCHLOROISOTHIAZOLINONE (AND) METHYLISOTHISAZOLINONE

IDENTIFICATION

Description/definition
: Methylchloroisothiazolinone (and) methylisothiazolinone is a mixture of methylchloroisothiazolinone and methylisothiazolinone with magnesium chloride and magnesium nitrate

Chemical class(es)
: Heterocyclic compounds

Other names
: 5-Chloro-2-methyl-isothiazol-3(2H)-one and 2-methylisothiazol-3(2H)-one; 5-chloro-2-methyl-4-isothiazolin-3-one and 2-methyl-4-isothiazolin-3-one; MCI/MI; examples of trade names are Kathon® CG, Euxyl® K100 and Microcide® III

CAS registry number (s)
: 55965-84-9; 26172-55-4; 2682-20-4

EC number(s)
: 247-500-7; 220-239-6

CIR review(s)
: J Am Coll Toxicol 1992;11:75-128 (3) (access: www.cir-safety.org/ingredients)

SCCS opinion(s)
: SCCS/1238/09 (104); SCCP/0849/04 (105); SCCNFP/0670/03 (106)

Merck Index monograph
: 7433

Function(s) in cosmetics
: EU: preservative. USA: preservatives

Patch testing
: 0.02% water (Chemotechnique, SmartPracticeCanada); 0.01% water (Chemotechnique, SmartPracticeEurope, SmartPracticeCanada); 0.01% pet. (Chemotechnique)

EU cosmetic restrictions
: Regulated in Annex V/39 of the Regulation (EC) No. 1003/2014; EU legislation: maximum concentration 15 ppm in rinse-off products; not allowed in leave-on products from July 2016 on (45); USA: rinse-off products maximum 15 ppm, stay-on cosmetics maximum 7.5 ppm

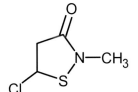

Methylisothiazolinone   Methylchloroisothiazolinone

SEE ALSO CHAPTER 2.299 METHYLISOTHIAZOLINONE

GENERAL

Methylchloroisothiazolinone (and) methylisothiazolinone (MCI/MI) is a preservative system containing a 3:1 mixture of methylchloroisothiazolinone (MCI) and methylisothiazolinone (MI) in water with 23% magnesium chloride and nitrate as stabilizers. It is a broad-spectrum antimicrobial active against both gram-positive and gram-negative bacteria, yeasts, and fungi, and is effective in low concentrations. MCI/MI was introduced in Europe in the mid-1970s and into the United States in the early 1980s (23). This preservative system was soon used extensively in cosmetics, household products (e.g. dishwashing liquids, laundry products and cleaning products) and industrial applications (e.g., metalworking fluids, paints and glues). Examples of reported applications are shown in table 2.292.1.

The best known trade name for this mixture is Kathon, a range of MCI/MI grades with different concentrations and applications. The product intended for cosmetics was Kathon CG (CG = cosmetic grade), containing 1.15% MCI and 0.35% MI. Up to the beginning of the 1990s, but even recently (252,268,278), virtually always the trade name Kathon CG was used in European scientific publications. This can partly be explained by the fact that material for patch testing was often obtained from its manufacturer (Rohm & Haas, USA), that this firm performed analytical investigations for researchers and that ROATs were often performed with a lotion containing Kathon CG 15 ppm active ingredients prepared and made available by the manufacturer. From 1990 on, American (147,160) and European researchers (155,156,157) began to use the INCI names methylchloroisothiazolinone and methylisothiazolinone (MCI/MI) or the chemical names 5-chloro-2-methyl-4-isothiazolin-3-one and 2-methyl-4-isothiazolin-3-one (158) instead.

Table 2.292.1 Reported applications of MCI/MI (examples)

Products	References
Adhesives, glues, tackifiers	43,95,185,207,255,322
Air fresheners	207
Barrier creams	48
Binders	185,209,255,322
Biocides (concentrated MCI/MI solutions)	140,150,192,193,200,201,202,209,229,241,248,255,275,280, 299,322
Biopolymers	207
Black rubber	48
Car care products	322
Carpet shampoos	151,207
Cellulose solutions	203
Cleaning agents	43,95,156,172,174,181,185,298,320,322
Coloring agents	255,322
Construction / building materials	322
Cooling tower water	265
Cosmetics	23,24,26,43,47,48,91,92,93,95,100,116,125,135,136, 140, 147,151,165,185,198,206,211,214,239,253,281,286,295
Curing agents	185
Detergents	43,245,253
Diesel oil	195
Dishwashing liquids	43,174,207
Disinfectant for cooling-tower water	
Disinfectant for swimming-pool water	
Dry shampoo (powder carpet cleaner)	151
Epoxy seaming material	43
Fabric softener	151,173,185,207
Filling agents	95,255,322
Flooring agents	95
Food wrapping paper (moist)	
Fountain solutions	43,180,181
Fungicides	220
Furniture waxes	188
Glass fibre surface protecting products	43
Glues, adhesives, tackifiers	43,95,185,207,255
Grinding dust	46
Gum Arabic	181
Hardeners	95
Hydraulic fluids	207
Impregnating agents	95,322
Inks	207
Ironing water	234,274
Latex emulsions	23
Laundry detergents	174
Liquid laundry products	207
Lubricants	298,322
Medium-density fiber board (MDF)	48
Metal surface treatment remedies	255,322
Metalworking fluids	23,43,115,168,183,207,253
Milk preservative solution	25
Moist toilet paper (hygiene wet wipes)	35,144,199,219,232,238,254,272,279,294,296,315
Mold-resistant tyre coating	48
Oil field water injection	207
Paints and varnishes	43,95,184,185,188,198,215,216,217,226,227,315,322
Paper	217
Paper mills (slime control)	23,150,213,282
Parquet varnish	215

Table 2.292.1 Reported applications of MCI/MI (examples) (*continued*)

Products	References
Pesticides	48,185
Pharmaceutical preparations, topical	163,175
Pharmaceutical skin care products	24
Photographic developing solutions	153,192,193
Pigments	185,207
Plant protection products	217
Plasticine (dough for playing)	211
Polishes	95,185,207,222,253,255,322
Polymer emulsions	203
Pottery glazes	203
Pre-moistened sponges and mops	207
Pre-soaped sponges	290
Preservatives	185
Printing inks	95,185,207,255,322
Products for sanitation	185
Rinse-aid	43
Rubber gloves	48
Seat covers	48
Spin finish oil	218
Surface active agents	255,322
Surface treatment for paper and cardboard	255,322
Synthesis of raw materials	185
Textile processing fluids	207
Thinners	48
Toiletries	see cosmetics
Toners	255,322
Udder cream	206
Ultrasound gel	252
VAC sponge material (polyurethane foam)	275
Vinyl gloves	43
Viscosity changers	322
Waterproofing materials	43
Wet wipes (moist toilet paper)	see moist toilet paper
Wood protection agents	217

The manufacturer of Kathon CG recommended levels of between 0.02% and 0.1% by weight, 3-15 ppm active ingredients (a.i.) in products such as shampoos and hair conditioners, hair and body gels, bubble baths, skin creams and skin lotions (121).

CONTACT ALLERGY

The older literature on MCI/MI allergy has been reviewed in several articles by the author (121,122,143,157). A very useful study has reviewed the literature up to 1999 (207), two more up to 2014 (256,293) and a thesis on the subject of MCI/MI has appeared in 1997 (212). A limited review (with an incorrect title: 'methylchloroisothiazolinone revisited') was published in 2000 (263). An overview of non-cosmetic and unusual cosmetic sources of isothiazolinone derivatives (also MI, benzisothiazolinone, octylisothiazolinone) was published in 2017 (333). Sensitization studies, dose-response studies and exposure studies of MCI/MI have been reviewed in ref. 4.

THE FIRST EPIDEMIC IN THE 1980s

MCI is an extreme to strong sensitizer and MI a strong to moderate sensitizer (17-21) and the sensitizing potential was already known in the first half of the 1980s (110,112,113,119). Nevertheless, in 1982, MCI/MI in a maximum concentration of 50 ppm active ingredients was given provisional clearance for use as a cosmetic and toiletry preservative in the EEC (Council Directive 82/368/EEC, 17 May 1982) (121). In 1986, MCI/MI in a maximum concentration of 30 ppm active ingredients was approved for use as a cosmetic and toiletry preservative in the European Economic Community (Council Directive 86/199/EEC) (130).

   After the first case reports of contact allergy to MCI/MI in cosmetics had appeared 2-3 years later (22,23,129), a sharp increase in contact allergy rates was observed in some European countries, notably Sweden, Finland, The

Netherlands, Italy, Switzerland and Germany, with increasing prevalence rates of 3-8% (table 2.292.2). Lower rates of sensitization were observed in the UK (0.8-1.1% [123,141]), Denmark (0.8% [116]; 1.3% [136]), Belgium (0.7-1.3% [140]), and Czechoslovakia (0.8% [163]). In Austria, the rate of sensitization in the years 1985-1989 was only 0.2% (12/6402 patients patch tested), but when the investigators checked the test material it proved to contain 1.35 ppm MCI/MI instead of 100 ppm. When they started using the proper patch test material in 1990, 28 of 400 patients had positive patch test reactions: 7% (148,149)! Methylchloroisothiazolinone was shown to be the main sensitizer in the preservative mixture (128,145,235). For historical reasons and purposes, the most important studies performed in the 1980s are summarized in table 2.292.2.

Table 2.292.1 Patch testing in groups of patients in the years of the 1980s epidemic in Europe

Years and Country	Test conc. & vehicle	Number of patients tested	positive (%)	Selection of patients (S); Relevance (R); Comments (C)	Ref.
Routine testing					
1990 Austria	0.01% water	400	28 (7.0%)	R: not mentioned; C: in the years before, sensitization rate had been only 0.2%; the cause was that the test material contained 1.35 ppm MCI/MI instead of 100 ppm!	148
1988-90 Switzerland		5768	278 (4.8%)	R: no data available; C: the frequency rose from 3.5% in 1987 to 6.3% in 1988 and 5.6% in 1989-1990	179
1987-90 Netherlands	0.01% water	999	84 (8.4%)	R: 62%	284
1988-89 13 European countries	0.01% water	4713	141 (3.0%)	R: not stated; C: range of positives: 0.4% (UK) to 11.0% (Italy)	161
1988-1989 Spain	0.02% water	626	22 (3.5%)	R: 32%, mostly from cosmetics	154
1987 Switzerland		2491	87 (3.5%)	R: no data; C: personal communication from Dr. Nicole Hunziker to the author, 1988, cited in ref. 143; probably overlap with the data from ref. 146	143
1987 West-Germany	0.01% water	671	23 (3.4%)	R: 52%, cosmetics were the major cause	134
1986-87 Switzerland	0.01% water	1320	47 (3.6%)	R: 1/3, from skin care products; C: probably overlap with the Swiss data cited in ref. 143	146
1986-87 Netherlands	0.01% water	587	36 (6.1%)	R: 27/36 (75%) from using cosmetics containing 12 ppm or less MCI/MI	126
1986-87 Netherlands	0.01% water	3114	155 (5.0%)	R: 70% current relevance; C: in 1985, the prevalence had still been as low as 1.3%	138
1985-1987 Italy	0.01% water	620	52 (8.3%)	R: 42/52 (81%) were relevant, especially from cosmetics	24
1985-1986 Finland	0.01% water	1034	30 (2.9%)	R: 24/35 were relevant, mostly from a moisturizing cream; C: the frequency rose from 0% in 1983 to 0.7% in January-August 1985, to 4.2% in September-December 1985 and to 4.9% in January-March 1986	26
1983-1986 Italy	0.01% water	3744	50 (1.3%)	R: 42/50 (84%) had used creams containing MCI/MI; C: the frequency rose from 0.5% in 1983-1984 to 0.9% in 1985 and to 2.3% in 1986	124
<1986 Germany	0.015% in ?	1894	108 (5.7%)	R: no details known, data cited in ref. 157	133
1985 Sweden	0.025% water	170	10 (5.9%)	R: not found; MCI/MI became the most common sensitizer after nickel	118
1982-1984 Sweden	0.03% water	976	43 (4.4%)		
Testing in groups of selected patients					
1987 UK	0.01% water	37	6 (16%)	S: patients with dermatitis of the face, neck or hands and tested with a 'face series'; R: not found	142
<1987 Germany		49	5 (10%)	S: patients suspected of cosmetic allergy; R: no data available (data cited in ref. 157)	159
<1986 Italy	0.01% water	98	6 (6%)	S: patients with contact dermatitis of the face; R: not stated; no positive patch tests to patients' cosmetics were seen	114
<1986 West-Germany	0.005% water	515	17 (3.3%)	S: women; R: no data available (cited in ref. 157)	158
1984 Netherlands	1% pet.	179	6 (3.4%)	S: patients suspected of cosmetic allergy; R: not stated; C: the patch test material was the commercial product Kathon CG and contained 150 ppm MCI/MI a.i.	22

The European epidemic (143) was not paralleled by an epidemic in the USA. Here, the members of the NACDG found a frequency of positive patch tests of 2.6% in 1984-1985 (tested at 250 ppm) and of 1.7% in 1985-1987 (tested at 100 ppm) in dermatitis patients tested with a 'preservative and vehicle patch test panel' (147). In routine testing with MCI/MI 100 ppm water, the members of the NACDG found a prevalence of 1.9% in 1988-1989 (160) and 1.8% in 1991-1992 (182). Only in a study at the Mayo Clinic, a somewhat higher rate of 3.6% relevant patch test reactions was observed in the period 1983-1986, but this concerned a very small group of 365 patients (135).

Testing in groups of *selected* patients yielded high frequencies of sensitization (6-16%) in patients selected for possible cosmetic allergy (table 2.292.2 [114,142,159).

The products causing allergic contact dermatitis
In nearly all cases, patients were sensitized to leave-on cosmetic products (134,135,309), occupational cases were rare. Many reacted to moisturizing creams or lotions containing 7-15 ppm MCI/MI (23,26,116,126,140), others, notably in Italy, to products containing >30 ppm (24) . Repeated Open Application Tests (ROATs) with creams containing MCI/MI in this concentration range were positive in about half the patients. However, the ROATs lasted for one week only, which we now know is (far) too short, so the observed response rates have been an underestimation (26,118,124). Indeed, when 52 Italian patients sensitized to MCI/MI performed a ROAT with a cream containing only 7 ppm MCI/MI for *two* weeks, all reacted positively (24). The manufacturer tried to convince the dermatological community that a lotion with 15 ppm was safe (127), but this study was heavily criticized because of important (and rather obvious) flaws in study design (126).

Although the majority of cases were related to stay-on products, exacerbations of dermatitis in sensitized individuals were also noted from the use of rinse-off products with only 5-15 ppm MCI/MI (26,160), causing dermatitis of the face and eyelids, sometimes spreading to the body and in single cases even generalizing (136,239,281). Indeed, in a double-blind crossover trial with the use of shampoos containing 15 ppm MCI/MI in allergic individuals, it was convincingly shown that some patients will develop dermatitis from the use of such shampoos, though most patients can use them without problems (190,207). Primary sensitization from the use of rinse-off products containing less than 15 ppm, however, was found to be very unlikely (207).

In the Netherlands, MCI/MI was the most frequent sensitizer (28%) in 119 patients with proven cosmetic allergy (88). In this country, about half the cases of MCI/MI sensitization were from its presence in two very widely used moisturizing creams; another important causative product source were moistened toilet tissues (88,138). In individuals with work-related contact dermatitis, MCI/MI was not an important contact allergen (129). The patients suffering from allergic contact dermatitis caused by MCI/MI usually did not react upon patch testing to the causative products, as their concentrations of <25 ppm and often <15 ppm MCI/MI are nearly always too low to provoke a positive test (false-negative reaction) (26,114). However, patients reacting to the causative cosmetic products have sometimes been observed, though the patch test concentration necessary to elicit a positive reaction is 100-200 ppm in most patients (14,15,24).

In reaction to the European epidemic of contact allergy cases to MCI/MI, in 1989, the allowed use concentrations for MCI/MI in the EU were limited to 15 ppm in both stay-on and rinse-off cosmetic products. In the USA, the Cosmetic Ingredient Review (CIR) panel of the Cosmetic, Toiletry and Fragrance Association (currently: Personal Care Products Council) recommended a concentration limit in leave-on cosmetic products of 7.5 ppm in 1992. After this, MCI/MI contact allergy rates declined, and remained relatively stable, in Denmark and Germany around 2-3% (2,9, 29), and in other European countries and the USA between 1% and 3% (1,7,10,12,13,28,30).

A SECOND – SECONDARY – EPIDEMIC OF MCI/MI ALLERGY
After 2000, the frequency of sensitization appeared to be decreasing in some studies, which was (partly) attributed to replacement of MCI/MI with newer, more popular preservatives, such as methyldibromo glutaronitrile (which was an unlucky choice, see the Chapters Methyldibromo glutaronitrile and Methyldibromo glutaronitrile/phenoxyethanol). The frequency of sensitization to MCI/MI observed by the IVDK (Germany, Austria, Switzerland) was constantly around 2.1% from 1998 to 2009. However, between 2009 and 2011 a sharp increase in the frequency of sensitization to MCI/MI was observed in these countries, rising from 2.3% in 2009 to 3.3% in 2010 and 3.9% in 2011 (11). This was paralleled by an increase in the frequency of allergic reactions to MI in the preservative series from 1.9% in 2009 to 4.4% in 2011 (11) and 4.5% in 2012 (262). The increases were seen especially in female patients, patients with facial dermatitis and patients with suspected cosmetic intolerance. It was concluded that more widespread consumer exposure of methylisothiazolinone (MI), which had been used on a large scale in cosmetics since 2005, had most likely led to an increase in primary sensitization to MI and subsequently to a rise in MCI/MI reactions resulting from cross-reactions (methylchloroisothiazolinone cross-reacting to methylisothiazolinone) and pseudo-cross-reactions (the methylisothiazolinone in the MCI/MI mixture reacting with a positive patch test) (11).

The same trend was observed in the United Kingdom (where MCI/MI allergy had never been a major problem), where in Leeds the frequency of sensitization to MCI/MI (0.02% water) rose from 0.9% in 2008 to 2.9% in 2009, 3.5% in 2010 and 4.9% in 2011 and the first half of 2012 (249). In the same period (except 2008, when MI was not yet tested separately), the frequency of sensitization of MI (0.02%) rose from 0.6% in 2009 to 2.5% in 2012 and the frequencies or reactions to MI 0.2% water (the currently recommended test concentration) even reached 3.8% in 2011 and 4.6% in the first half of 2012. Curiously, the authors did not link the rise of MCI/MI sensitization to the increasing sensitization to MI (249). A similar rise in both MI and MCI/MI sensitization was observed in Spain (176,250,264,278), Finland (27), Belgium (253), Denmark (260), Brazil (292), the UK (44) and in another UK study

(16), where MCI/MI prevalence rose from 4.3% in 2010 to 8.3% in 2013 and MI frequency of sensitization from 1.7% in 2010 to a staggering 11.1% in 2013 (16).

The upward trend was also noticed in the USA by the members of the NACDG. In the 2009-2010 period, the frequency of sensitization to MCI/MI was 2.5% (50). Two years later, it had doubled to 5.0% (49) and further increased to 6.4% in the 2013-2014 NACDG study period (177).

In one of the Spanish studies, the proportion of MI-positive patients among those who reacted to MCI/MI was 13% in 2011, 44% in 2012, and 54% in 2013, which indicates the importance of primary MI sensitization in the rising frequency of MCI/MI allergy (250). Also, the percentage of leave-on products used by the allergic patients that proved to contain MI and/or MCI/MI in one study rose from 7% to 33% two years later (44). This probably was always MI, as MCI/MI was hardly used anymore in leave-on products at that time, as the authors stated. This makes it very likely that that primary sensitization to MI in cosmetic products greatly contributed to the strongly increasing prevalence of MCI/MI sensitization (44). So, since 2009-2010 a new epidemic of MCI/MI allergy was born, mostly from the parallel epidemic of MI allergy caused by its presence in both cosmetic and occupational products.

Finally, in 2014, there was a total ban on the use of MCI/MI in the EU in leave-on products, starting in July 2016 (45).

Patch testing with MCI/MI

In early studies, patch testing was performed with the commercial product Kathon CG in a concentration of 1% in petrolatum, containing 150 ppm MCI/MI (22,23). It was found in 21-day cumulative irritation studies and Draize sensitization studies that a concentration of 0.01% in water (100 ppm) was non-irritant, 200 ppm tended to induce irritant reactions (which was later contradicted by Swedish experience) and 300 ppm induced sensitization (110). Since then, 0.01% MCI/MI in water (100 ppm) became the standard for patch testing and soon became available from commercial suppliers (114). However, already in 1986 it was noted that false-negative reactions to this concentration may occur (26) and are very frequent, up to 50% (117,118). To detect sensitization, the optimal test concentration was suggested to be 250-300 ppm. However, although this did not cause irritant reactions, the authors found an unacceptably high (1%) number of patch test sensitizations (117,118).

In 1987, the members of the International Contact Dermatitis Research Group (ICDRG) and of the European Environmental and Contact Dermatitis Research Group (EECDRG) advised to add MCI/MI 100 ppm in water to the European Standard Series (121), which was implemented in 1988 (152). The material was termed 'Cl + Me-isothiazolinone' to avoid any particular trade name. It was explained that the patch test concentration of 100 ppm water was a compromise, as 200 to 300 ppm would indeed detect 'a few more cases of allergy', but would also produce irritation and active sensitization (152). Soon thereafter, it was confirmed that testing MCI/MI in water was more reliable than testing in petrolatum (with an emulsifier) (155).

In 1991, by testing patients with MCI/MI in two concentrations of 100 ppm and 200 ppm, it was again demonstrated that up to 50% of the cases of sensitization may be missed by testing with 100 ppm water (14) and this was confirmed 18 years (!) later (15,246). In two Spanish studies, 24% of cases of contact allergy to MCI/MI would have been missed by testing with MCI/MI 100 ppm alone (239).

Finally, in 2014, the European Society of Contact Dermatitis and the (EECDRG) decided to increase the test concentration of 0.01% MCI/MI (100 ppm) to 0.02% (200 ppm) in water (251). The decision was partly based on their own investigation, in which patients were tested with both 100 ppm and 200 ppm and where the lower test concentration missed 56% of all sensitizations. Curiously, this investigation had taken place in 2005-2006, 8 years before (257). In 2014, the members of the ICDRG confirmed the superiority of 0.02% over the 0.01% test concentration (327).

Clinical picture of allergic contact dermatitis from MCI/MI

Patients sensitized to MCI/MI are in majority (2/3) women, who most often have dermatitis of the face and/or hands (24,124,126,134,136,140,154,161,264,284). Less frequently, the neck (161), arms (126,264), the perianal region (144,279,284, 294,296) or the axillae (140) are involved, or generalized dermatitis is observed (24,135,136). About half of the patients used the cosmetic products on healthy skin, the others were sensitized by cosmetics used on already damaged skin (atopic dermatitis, irritant dermatitis, ACD, slightly damaged dry skin), especially moisturizers, thereby enhancing the risk of sensitization and aggravating existing dermatitis (26,126,143).

MCI/MI in moist toilet paper causes dermatitis around the anus, on the buttocks and sometimes in the genital area in patients using the product for themselves (35,144,279,294,296), in some cases combined with hand dermatitis (246). Perianal allergic contact dermatitis from MCI/MI in moistened toilet tissues has also caused vesicular dermatitis of both palms as an –id reaction (199) and may sometimes spread (144,238). In few cases, the reaction exacerbated seborrheic dermatitis (167,199) or resembles it (281). In individuals who use the moist papers for the hygiene of others, notably mothers of babies, contact allergy to MCI/MI in the wipes usually causes hand dermatitis (167,232).

Airborne contact dermatitis of the face, the eyelids, and the neck has been reported repeatedly, notably from MCI/MI in paints (184,188,198,215,216,217,227). Some of these patients, who have been presensitized to MCI/MI, also have symptoms of the eyes, nose and airways (188,198,215,217). In rare or single cases, allergic contact dermatitis from MCI/MI manifested as a lupus-like eruption (206), as lymphocytic infiltration of the skin (Jessner) (206), seborrheic dermatitis (206), a photodermatosis (206), atopic dermatitis in case of generalized eruptions (206), generalized urticaria (196), lymphomatoid allergic contact dermatitis (238,254) or follicular contact dermatitis (290) Allergic reactions to MCI/MI in shampoos may resemble seborrheic dermatitis of the scalp (281).

Occupational allergic contact dermatitis from MCI/MI usually manifests as dermatitis of the hands and under-arms, but airborne ACD also occurs (188,198,213,234,248,274). Some individuals have accidental contact with concentrated MCI/MI solutions at work and develop irritant dermatitis or chemical burns followed by sensitization (see below). Systemic contact dermatitis from inhalation of MCI/MI vapors with extensive dermatitis and general symptoms, including malaise, respiratory and gastrointestinal symptoms, has been reported (248).

Contact allergy in the general population and subgroups

There have been several investigations in some European countries in which random samples of the population of certain age groups have been patch tested with MCI/MI (table 2.292.3). The highest prevalence was found in Denmark in 1990: 0.7% (in women 1.1%, men 0.3%) (79). In later years in Denmark, lower frequencies have been observed (78,81). In all these investigations, the patch tests were read only at day 2, which may have resulted in underestima-tion of the actual rate of sensitization. In a study performed in 5 European countries between 2008 and 2011, 0.5% of a population of 3119 individuals from the general population aged 18-74 years proved to be sensitized to MCI/MI (76).

Results of testing MCI/MI in subgroups of the population are shown in table 2.292.3. Sensitization rates of higher than 1% have been found in adult volunteers recruited in Thailand by advertising (82) and in a group of 1141 adults aged 28-78 year with a large percentages (>50%) of atopic individuals in Germany (2.2% in women!) (84,87), which probably resulted from the selection methods. Notably, atopic patients may have run a higher risk of sensitization from MCI/MI from the use of moisturizers on dermatitic or slightly damaged dry skin.

Table 2.292.3   Contact allergy in the general population and subgroups

Year and country	Selection and number tested	Prevalence of contact allergy			Comments	Ref.
		Total	Women	Men		
General population						
2008-11 five Euro-pean countries	general population, random sample, 18-74 years, n=3119	0.5%	0.6%	0.4%		76
2008 Denmark	general population, random sample, 15-41 years, n=469		0.4%	0%	patch tests were read on day 2 only	81
2006 Denmark	general population, random sample, 18-69 years, n=3460	0.2%	0.1%	0.3%	patch tests were read on day 2 only	78
2005 Norway	general population, random sample, 18-69 years, n=1236	0.6%	0.9%	0.4%		80
1990 Denmark	general population, random sample, 18-69 years, n=543	0.7%	1.1%	0.3%	patch tests were read on day 2 only; data from 15-17 years old excluded in the data presented here	79
Subgroups						
2010 Denmark	unselected population of 8th grade schoolchildren in Den-mark, 15 years later; n=442	0.2%	0.4%	0%	follow-up study	77
2005-2006 Thailand	adult volunteers recruited by advertising, 18-55 years, n=1178	1.2%	1.2%	1.2%	patch tests were read on day 2 only; higher prevalence probably from selection by advertising	82
1997-1998 Germany	adults 28-78 years, with a large percentage (>50%) of atopic individuals, n=1141	1.8%	2.2%	1.4%	high prevalence possibly from the use of moisturizers on atopic dermatitis of slightly damaged dry skin in the many atopic patients in this study	84, 87
1995-1996 Denmark	8th grade school children, 12-16 years, n=1146	0%	0%	0%		83, 85
1989 Italy	male soldiers without skin disease, 18-28 years, n=593	0.2%				86

Estimates of the 10-year prevalence of contact allergy to methylchloroisothiazolinone (and) methylisothiazolinone in the general population of Denmark based on the CE-DUR method ranged from 0.31 to 0.42% (74). In a similar study from Germany, the estimated prevalence in the general population in the period 1992-2000 ranged from 0.4-0.9% (75,230).

Patch testing in groups of patients 2000-2015

Results of routine patch testing (testing in consecutive patients suspected of contact dermatitis) back to 2000 are shown in table 2.292.4. Results of testing in groups of *selected* patients (e.g., patients with perianal dermatoses, children with hand eczema, patients suspected of cosmetic reactions, individuals with eyelid dermatitis) back to 1998 are shown in table 2.292.5. It should be realized, that most studies have used a test concentration of 0.01% (100 ppm), but some 0.02% (200 ppm), which makes comparison of these studies difficult. It has recently become evident that between a quarter to – more likely – one half of all sensitizations are missed by the 0.01% test concentration (14, 15,26,117,118,239,246,251,257). This means, that the prevalences found in the studies using this concentration for patch testing, are likely to be an underestimation. It also implies, however, that the increased prevalences found in some recent studies can partly be attributed to the use of this higher test concentration (44,250,276).

Patch testing in consecutive patients suspected of contact dermatitis: routine testing

As MCI/MI is included in the European Baseline Series, the screening tray of the North American Contact Dermatitis Group (NACDG) and most other national series routinely tested in consecutive patients suspected of contact dermatitis, there are many data on MCI/MI contact allergy available, notably from European countries and from the USA + Canada, where the NACDG publishes their patch test results biannually (table 2.292.4).

Table 2.292.4 Patch testing in groups of patients: Routine testing

Years and Country	Test conc. & vehicle	Number of patients tested | positive (%)		Selection of patients (S); Relevance (R); Comments (C)	Ref.
2014-2015 Hungary	0.01% water	314	16 (5.1%)	R: all were relevant, 2 from household products, the other 14 from cosmetic products including a hair dye	277
2014 eight countries [c]	0.01% water	2695	100 (3.7%)	R: not stated; C: range positives: 0-6.8%	327
	0.02% water	2703	152 (5.6%)	R: not stated; C: range positives: 0-8.5%	
2014 nine countries [d]	0.02% water	3865	232 (6.0%)	R: not stated; C: range per center: 0-8.0%	329
2013-14 USA, Canada	0.01% water	4856	309 (6.4%)	R: definite + probable relevance: 52%; C: further increase of sensitization to MCI/MI from primary sensitization to MI; virtually all relevant reactions were caused by cosmetics and wet wipes; the data from ref. 328 are slightly different from those of ref. 177	177, 328
2013-2014 [b] 12 European countries, 46 departments	0.01% water	19,790	(7.4%)	R: not stated; C: results of 6 occupational dermatology clinics and one pediatric clinic not included in these figures; range of positive reactions: 1%-17.9% (0.02% test material) and 3.5%-15.8% (0.02% test material)	317
	0.02% water	9722	(7.7%)		
2012-2014 Sweden	0.02% water	2165	175 (8.1%)	R: not stated; C: contact allergy to MCI/MI and/or MI was significantly associated with formaldehyde allergy and positive reactions to fragrance mix I and/or II	276
2012-2014 USA	0.01% water	719	21 (2.9%)	R: not specified; most relevant products were cosmetics	269, 289
2011-2013 Spain	0.02% water	490	49 (10.0%)	R: 90% were related to cosmetics; C: the prevalence rose from 7.8% in 2011 to 14.3% in 2013 with a concurrent rise of MI sensitization from 1% in 2011 to 7.7% in 2013	250
2011-2013 UK	0.02% water	2315	217 (9.4%)	R: MI and/or MCI was found in shampoos in 22% of the allergic patients, in wipes in 13% and in leave-on products in 20%; there was a steady increase in the number of leave-on products used by the patients, in which MI was found, from 7% in 2011 to 33% in 2013	44
2010-2013 UK	0.02% water, some 0.01%	14,198	794 (5.6%)	R: not stated; C: the prevalence rose from 4.3% in 2010 to 8.3% in 2013; the frequency of MI sensitization rose from 1.7% in 2010 to 11.3% in 2013	16
2005-2013 Spain	True test	863	85 (9.9%)	R: not stated; C: there was a marked increase in sensitiza- from 2010 on to 17.4% in 2012 and 15% in 2013	278
2011-12 USA, Canada	0.01% water	4227	213 (5.0%)	R: definite + probable relevance: 62%	49
2009-2012, 12 European countries [b]	0.01% water	48,720	(3.3%) [a]	R: not stated; C: range per country 1.5-8.6%	308
	0.02% water	17,085	(4.1%) [a]	R: not stated; C: range per country 4.2-8.9%	
2008-2012 UK	0.02% water	2489	91 (3.7%)	R: not stated; the frequency rose from 0.9% in 2008 to 4.9% in 2011 and the first half of 2012; this rise probably resulted	249

Table 2.292.4 Patch testing in groups of patients: Routine testing (*continued*)

Years and Country	Test conc. & vehicle	Number of patients tested | positive (%)	Selection of patients (S); Relevance (R); Comments (C)	Ref.
2009-2011 IVDK	0.01% water	33,118 1048 (3.2%)	(although not suggested as such by the authors) from a steep rise in primary sensitization to MI and (pseudo)-cross-reactivity to MCI/MI R: not stated; C: the frequency of sensitization rose from 2.3% in 2009 to 3.3% in 2010 and 3.9% in 2011; this rise probably resulted from an increase in primary sensitization to MI and (pseudo)-cross-reactivity to MCI/MI	11
2006-2011 Singapore	0.01% water	3150 55 (1.8%)	R: not stated; C: prevalence was 1.2% in men, 2.2% in women	71
2009-10 USA, Canada	0.01% water	4302 108 (2.5%)	R: definite + probable relevance: 55%	50
2007-2010 UK	0.01% water 0.02% water	697 11 (1.6%) 267 10 (3.8%)	R: 52%, sources included moist toilet wipes (7/21), shampoo (4/21), washing-up liquid (2/21), and cosmetics (1/21)	246
2006-2010 USA	0.01% water	3091 (3.4%)	R: 56%	70
2001-2010 Australia	0.01% water	5144 176 (3.4%)	R: 42%	108
1992-2010 IVDK	0.01% water	171,883 (2.3%)	R: not specified; C: the yearly frequencies ranged from 2.0 to 3.1%	2
2009 Sweden	0.02% water	3112 (2.0%)	R: not stated	66
2007-2009 Portugal	0.01% water	629 15 (2.4%)	R: 80% relevant from cosmetics, notably rinse-off products such as shampoos and conditioners	13
1996-2009 IVDK	0.01% water	121,136 2805(2.2%) [a]	R: not stated	9
2007-2008 11 European countries [b]	0.01% water	25,181 591 (2.3%)	R: not stated; range positives 1.2%-4.2%	1
2007-8 USA, Canada	0.01% water	5075 (3.6%)	R: definite + probable relevance 50%	38
2006-2008 Finland	0.01% water	10,821 194 (1.8%)	R: not stated; 50% co-reactivity to methylisothiazolinone	12
2005-6 USA, Canada	0.01% water	4437 (2.8%)	R: definite + probable relevance: 44%	30
2005-6 10 European countries [b]	0.01% water	17,241 448 (2.6%)	R: not stated; C: prevalences in the four regions (Central, West, Northeast and South Europe) ranged from 2.1 to 4.1%	302
1993-2006 Australia	0.01% water	5927 (2.3%)	R: 38%	247
2004-2005 UK	0.01% water	6958 (1.9%)	R: not stated	56
2000-2005 USA	0.01% water	3740 (3.0%)	R: 64%	7
2004, 11 European countries [b]	0.01% water	9349 212 (2.2%) [a]	R: not stated; C: range positives 0.0%- 6.4%	10
2003-4 USA, Canada	0.01% water	5137 112 (2.2%)	R: not stated	39
2000-04 Switzerland		4094 120 (2.9%)	R: not stated	51
1998-2004 Israel	0.01% water	2156 74 (3.4%)	R: not stated	61
1992-2004 Turkey	0.01% water	1038 1 (0.1%)	R: not stated; C: prevalence in women 0.1%, in men 0%	62
2002-2003, 9 European countries [b]	0.01% water	9689 (2.2%)	R: not stated; C: prevalence range per center (n=17) 0.0-9.8%	63
2001-2002 USA	0.01% water	4895 (2.3%)	R: definite + probable relevance: 31%	54
2000-2002 Finland		10,232 (1.3%)	R: not stated	60
1999-2001 Sweden	0.01% water	3790 (2.4%)	R: not stated; C: prevalence in women 2.7%, in men 1.5% (standardized prevalences)	57
1997-2001 Czech Rep.	0.01% water	12,058 174 (1.4%)	R: not stated; C: prevalence in men 1.2%, in women 2.6%	64
2000 United Kingdom	0.01% water	3063 (2.4%)	R: 90% (current and past relevance in one center)	59
1998-2000 USA	0.01% water	5792 (2.7%)	R: definite + probable relevance: 36%	55
1998-2000 USA	0.01% water	1312 (3.1%)	R: not stated	58
1996-2000 Europe	0.01% water	26,210 (2.2%)	R: not stated; C: prevalence in women 2.3%, in men 1.9%; C: ten centers, seven countries, EECDRG study	65

[a] age-standardized and sex-standardized proportions
[b] study of the ESSCA (European Surveillance System on Contact Allergy' network)
[c] members of the ICDRG (International Contact Dermatitis Research Group); participating countries: Japan, Belgium, Sweden, India, Denmark, Singapore, Uruguay, Germany
[d] members of the ICDRG (International Contact Dermatitis Research Group); participating countries: Japan, Belgium, Sweden, India, Denmark, Singapore, United Kingdom, Uruguay, Germany
EECDRG: European Environmental and Contact Dermatitis Research Group
IVDK: Information Network of Dermatological Departments, Germany, Austria, Switzerland

In European countries, from 2000 to 2009-2010, frequencies of positive patch test reactions to MCI/MI have been fairly constant and ranged from 1.3% to 2.9%; most were in the 2-2.5% range. In the NACDG studies and other investigations from the USA, prevalences have consistently been somewhat higher, ranging from 2.2% to 4.3% (table 2.292.4). Data from Australia (108,247), Singapore (71), Israel (61) and Turkey (62) can be found in table 2.292.4.

The scenery drastically changed from 2009-2010 on, when there was a sudden increase in the frequency of sensitization to MCI/MI in European countries, e.g., 7.7% in 12 European countries (up to 17.9% in one center) (317), 8.1% in Sweden (276), 9.4% in the UK (44), 10% in Spain (250) and even 15-17% in 2012 and 2013 in another Spanish study (278). The rise was also noted in the NACDG studies: 2.5% in 2009-2010 (50), a doubling to 5.0% in 2011-2012 (49) and 6.4% in 2013-2014 (177). Had the NACDG members used the test concentration of 0.02%, the frequencies of sensitization would have paralleled those in Europe. This sudden increase can largely be explained by a rise in primary sensitization to MI, which had been used in high concentrations (up to 100 ppm was allowed in the EU) in cosmetics and higher concentrations in occupational products for a number of years, with (pseudo)-cross-reactivity to MCI/MI. This subject is discussed in the section 'A second – secondary – epidemic of MCI/MI allergy' above.

In many studies, no data on relevance of the observed reactions were provided. In those that did, relevance was usually high, ranging from 50 up to 90-100%. Cosmetics were by far the most important source of sensitization and cause of allergic contact dermatitis.

Patch testing in groups of selected patients

Data on patch testing with MCI/MI in groups of selected patients back to 1998 are summarized in table 2.292.5. High frequencies of sensitization were observed in patients with perianal dermatoses (19% [250], 13.7% [330], 10% [271]), patients with pure facial dermatitis (13% [266]), hairdressers suspected of occupational contact dermatitis (10.7% [72]) and adult women with a clinical diagnosis of contact dermatitis of the head and neck region (8.9% [214]). This can easily be explained by the selection procedure in relationship to the profile of patients sensitized to MCI/MI (see the Section 'Clinical picture' above), perianal dermatitis, for example, being caused by wet wipes preserved with MCI/MI. A high rate of sensitization (11.7%) was also observed in children under 16 years of age with hand dermatitis. Many of these probably had atopic dermatitis for which they used moisturizing creams preserved with MCI/MI (173). In other studies in groups of children, no such high prevalences were observed (287,288,311,318), though a 7% score was reported from Italy, 2001-2003. Most of the relevant reactions in this study were also seen in children with hand dermatitis (223). In some investigations, there were relatively high rates of sensitization in hairdressers (72,304), but this was not observed by other authors (73,231,303).

Table 2.292.5 Patch testing in groups of patients: Selected patient groups

Years and Country	Test conc. & vehicle	Number of patients tested | positive (%)		Selection of patients (S); Relevance (R); Comments (C)	Ref.
2004-2016 Spain		124	17 (13.7%)	S: patients with perianal dermatitis; R: 100%; C: causative products were not mentioned	330
2013-2015 USA		1109	47 (4.2%)	S: children 0-18 years suspected of contact dermatitis; R: 74%	318
2005-2015 UK		150	15 (10.0%)	S: patients with perianal dermatoses and/or pruritus ani; R: all were relevant, 13/15 from wet wipes	271
2012-2014 UK	0.02% water	80	10 (13%)	S: patients with pure facial dermatitis; R: not specified, but most reactions were relevant and caused by cosmetics	266
2005-2014 UK	0.01%, later 0.02% water	500	8 (1.6%)	S: children aged 16 years or less; with dermatitis; R: all reactions were considered to be relevant	288
2003-2014 IVDK	0.01% water	5202	(2.2%)	S: patients with stasis dermatitis / chronic leg ulcers; R: not stated; C: percentage of reactions not significantly higher than in a control group of routine testing	312
2002-2013 Italy	0.01% water	2614	83 (3.2%)	S: children aged 1-10 years with dermatitis; R: 48%	287
1996-2013 Netherlands	0.01% water	1000	17 (1.7%)	S: children aged 0-17 years with dermatitis; R: not stated;	311
2007-2012 IVDK	0.01% water	706	39 (6.7%)	S: female hairdressers with current or previous occupational contact dermatitis; R: not stated	304
		1906	43 (2.1%)	S: female patients, clients of hairdressers, in who hair cosmetics were regarded as a cause of dermatitis, and who had never worked as hairdressers; R: not stated	
2001-2012 Spain	0.01% water	37	7 (19%)	S: patients with perianal eczema; R: all were relevant; 4 were caused by moist toilet tissues, 3 were sensitized to other cosmetic products	250
2011 China	0.02% water	201	1 (0.5%)	S: healthy student volunteers 19-30 years; R: not stated	109
2010-2011 Korea	0.01% water	584	32 (5.5%)	S: patients suspected of allergic cosmetic dermatitis; R: not stated	68
2006-2011 IVDK	0.01% water	10,124	304 (3.9%)	S: patients with suspected cosmetic intolerance; R: not stated; C: the prevalence was significantly higher than in a control groups matched for sex and age	291
2002-2011 Denmark		399	7 (1.8%)	S: hairdressers with contact dermatitis; R: not stated	303
2006-2010 USA	0.01% water	100	3 (3%)	S: patients with eyelid dermatitis; R: not stated	41

Table 2.292.5 Patch testing in groups of patients: Selected patient groups (*continued*)

Years and Country	Test conc. & vehicle	Number of patients tested	positive (%)	Selection of patients (S); Relevance (R); Comments (C)	Ref.
2000-2010 IVDK		4388	80 (1.8%)	S: patients with periorbital dermatitis; R: not stated	52
1994-2010 USA, Canada	0.01% water	432	? (?)	S: hairdressers/cosmetologists; R: in the group of 187 patients who had at least one relevant occupationally related reaction, 11 (5.9%) reacted to MCI/MI	305
2005-2009 Spain		111	13 (11.7%)	S: children 0-15 years with hand eczema; R: 12/13 (92%), presumably most or all by cosmetics	173
2002-2008 Italy	0.01% water	321	14 (4.4%)	S: children with dermatitis <3 years; R: present + past relevance in 6 (43%)	37
2000-2007 USA	0.01% water	935	40 (4.3%)	S: patients tested with a supplemental cosmetic screening series; R: 95%; C: weak study: a. high rate of macular erythema and weak reactions; b. relevance figures included 'questionable' and 'past' relevance	6
2003-2006 IVDK	0.01% water	440	(4.1%)	S: female hairdressers with suspected occupational contact dermatitis; R: not stated; C: important allergen in hairdressers versus clients	231
	0.01% water	610	(1.8%)	S: women with suspected reactions to hair cosmetics; R: not stated	231
1994-2004 USA		46	2 (4.3%)	S: patients with allergic contact dermatitis of the eyelids; R: both reactions were relevant, but the causative products were not mentioned	67
2001-2003 Italy	0.01% water	95	7 (7%)	S: children with dermatitis, 5 months-12 years; R: 4 cases; 3 children with hand dermatitis used leave-on moisturizing creams, and 1 child with diaper and facial dermatitis was using wet wipes, all containing MCI/MI	223
1994-2003 Spain		300	(10.7%)	S: hairdressers suspected of occupational contact dermatitis; R: not specified	72
1995-2002 IVDK		884	(3.4%)	S: female hairdressers with present or past occupational contact dermatitis; R: not specified	73
1995-1999 IVDK	0.01% water	933	(1.9%)	S: patients with allergic periorbital contact dermatitis; R: not stated	96
1998 Hong Kong	0.01% water	45	4 (8.9%)	S: adult women with clinical diagnosis of contact dermatitis of the head and neck region; R: all had used cosmetics containing MCI/MI	214
1994-1998 UK	0.01% water	232	4 (1.7%)	S: patients with eyelid dermatitis; R: all were currently relevant	69

IVDK: Information Network of Dermatological Departments, Germany, Austria, Switzerland

Case reports and case series

Case series

Methylchloroisothiazolinone/methylisothiazolinone was stated to be the (or an) allergen in 69 patients in a group of 603 individuals (11.4%) suffering from cosmetic dermatitis, seen in the period 2010-2015 in Leuven, Belgium (53). In the period 1996-2013, in a tertiary referral center in Valencia, Spain, 5419 patients were patch tested. Of these, 628 individuals had allergic contact dermatitis to cosmetics. MCI/MI was the responsible allergen in 172 (27.4%) cases. There was a steep increase in the frequency of reactions to MCI/MI from 2009 on (176, overlap with ref. 107).

MCI/MI was responsible for 54 out of 959 cases (5.6%) of non-fragrance cosmetic allergy where the causal allergen was identified, Belgium, 2000-2010 (5). In the period 2000-2007, 202 patients with allergic contact dermatitis caused by cosmetics were seen in Valencia, Spain. In this group, 55 individuals (27%) reacted to MCI/MI from its presence in gel/soap (n=24), in moisturizing cream (n=14), in shampoo (n=14, of who one was a hairdresser with occupational allergic hand dermatitis), in cleansing wipes (n=6), in aftershave (n=2) and in hair gel (n=1) (107, overlap with ref. 176).

In a group of 2193 patients (1582 women, 611 men) with (presumed) cosmetic allergy, 97 reactions (4%) were caused by MCI/MI in a study of the NACDG, 2001-2004, MCI/MI ranking 16th in the list of most frequent allergens (8). In a group of 119 patients with allergic contact dermatitis from cosmetics, investigated in The Netherlands in 1986-1987, 33 cases (28%) were caused by methylchloroisothiazolinone (and) methylisothiazolinone: 29 in skin care products, one in a hair conditioner, one in mascara, 3 in veterinary creams used as cosmetics, one in a facial makeup product, and one in a sunscreen cream (some patients were allergic to more than one product containing MCI/MI) (88,89). In a group of 75 patients allergic to cosmetic products, seen in a private practice in The Netherlands in the period 1981-1986, eight cases were caused by MCI/MI of which 8 in skin care products and one in a sun milk (90, overlap with ref. 23).

Case reports

Moisturizers

Three patients had ACD around the eyes from MCI/MI in a moisturizing cream (91). Two women had ACD of the face and eyelids from MCI/MI in a moisturizing cream. One of these patients had been sensitized by the cream containing 12 ppm MCI/MI and later had an exacerbation from a baby ointment containing 23 ppm (23). Three individuals reacted to MCI/MI in creams (92). Two patients had relevant positive patch test reactions to moisturizers and to their ingredient MCI/MI (100). A women had ACD from a lotion containing 15 ppm MCI/MI (116). Six patients had ACD from MCI/MI present in cosmetic creams (125). A woman had chronic generalized dermatitis which was linked to allergy to formaldehyde present in clothes. She also reacted to MCI/MI. After stopping the use of a moisturizer containing MCI/MI, the eruption cleared completely, despite continued low-level exposure to formaldehyde (135).

A female patient had ACD of the face from MCI/MI in a cream. Later, she had exacerbations from using a trial size moisturizer found in a hotel room, a sun block, and a soap that she used while hospitalized. These products were unlabeled, as USA legislation did not require labeling (286). Many patients with contact dermatitis from MCI/MI in various cosmetic products including moisturizers are described in an ICDRG study (140). A woman developed ACD from MCI/MI in a moisturizing oil (165). Two patients had photodermatitis-like reactions to MCI/MI in skin care creams (206).

Moist toilet paper / wet wipes

In the period 2011-2014, 79 patients with a positive patch test reaction to an allergen identified with a wet wipe source were identified by the members of the NACDG. MCI/MI was the (or an) allergen in 36% of the cases. Patients with wipe allergy were 15 times more likely to have anal/genital dermatitis compared with those without wipe allergy (310).

Two patients had allergic perianal contact dermatitis from MCI/MI in moist toilet paper (296). A woman had ACD of the vulva and perianal region from the use of moist toilet paper. The cause was claimed to be methylchloro-isothiazolinone (MCI), but this is probably incorrect (and should be MCI/MI), as MCI alone is not used as preservative (294). A 5-year-old girl had ACD of the anogenital area from MCI/MI in moist wipes (279). A woman developed perianal allergic contact dermatitis from MCI/MI in baby wipes, which was later complicated by contact allergy to clotrimazole, probably followed by systemic contact dermatitis from the structurally related fluconazole (272). Two patients had ACD from MCI/MI in baby wipes. The first had dermatitis of the buttock, gluteal cleft, perianal skin, and scrotum; the other individual had used it on a leg amputation stump at the site of a prosthesis. In the latter case, a use test was positive (35).

A man suffered from widespread vesicular fissured eczema of the perianal and genital areas, which had recently spread to the lower limbs, trunk and even the face. The cause was contact allergy to MCI/MI which was present in a concentration of 15 ppm in moist toilet paper he had used for 7 years (144). Three patients had perianal dermatitis from allergy to MCI/MI in moist toilet paper. One also had vesicular hand dermatitis, the second obvious worsening of seborrheic dermatitis of the perianal region, the trunk, face and scalp (167).

Two patients had perianal dermatitis and vesicular dermatitis of both palms. The eruption was caused by contact allergy to MCI/MI in moistened toilet tissues. The vesicular dermatitis was considered to be an -id reaction to the allergic contact dermatitis around the anus, as dermatitis from direct contact with the tissues would (also) affect the fingers and would most likely be asymmetrical (the hand used to wipe the tissues only). In one of these patients, the allergic reaction clearly exacerbated an existing seborrheic dermatitis (199).

Four individuals had ACD from MCI/MI in moistened baby toilet tissues. Two used them for their children, and they had hand eczema. The other two used the wipes for themselves, and they had both hand dermatitis, one of them dermatitis of the scrotum and the other genital pruritus (232). A woman had lymphomatoid allergic contact dermatitis of the buttocks, perineum and the groins, which later spread to the arms, from MCI/MI in baby wipes (238). A man had lymphomatoid dermatitis of the right buttock from MCI/MI in baby wipes (254). Of nine patients with presumed allergic hand dermatitis from baby wipes (moist towelettes), 3 had a positive patch test to MCI/MI. The wipes themselves had not been tested, and it was not ascertained that they actually contained MCI/MI (219).

Four adult patients had severe perianal dermatitis, one of them also genital; all four used moist toilet paper and reacted to MCI/MI. The reactions were ascribed to MCI/MI, and the authors stated that the toilet papers contained the preservative. This is rather curious, as they also provided a list of ingredients, mentioning 'methylisothiazolinone' only (33). In a Letter to the Editor, their mistake was pointed out (34).

Other cosmetics

One individual reacted to MCI/MI in a sunscreen product, another to a cleansing cream; first report of contact allergy to MCI/MI (93). One patient had relevant positive patch test reactions to a sun protection lotion and to its ingredient MCI/MI, another to rouge and MCI/MI contained therein (100). A female patient had dermatitis primarily on the face with eyelid edema, which later spread to the neck and body; she had a positive patch test to MCI/MI. Her dermatitis cleared after discontinuing the use of a shampoo preserved with MCI/MI (136). A similar MCI/MI-allergic patient had primarily facial dermatitis, which later generalized. Her dermatitis also disappeared when she stopped using a shampoo containing MCI/MI (136). Three women had severe periocular dermatitis with a strong edematous component, one of them also had hand dermatitis and another dermatitis of the chest. The cause proved to be MCI/MI present in makeup remover wet wipes. The wipes were labeled to contain phenoxyethanol, not MCI/MI. However, chemical analyses demonstrated the presence of MCI/MI in amounts of 54 to 83 µg/wipe. The Swedish Medical Product Agency was informed and prohibited the sale of the wipes (47).

Three patients had axillary dermatitis from MCI/MI present in deodorants (140). Four women had ACD, notably of the face, from MCI/MI in unspecified cosmetics (147). Many patients with contact dermatitis from MCI/MI in various cosmetic products are described in an ICDRG study (140). Three patients had widespread dermatitis from MCI/MI in a gel, two had hand eczema from hand cleansers and another individual suffered from ACD of the eyelids from MCI in shampoo (239). A woman had seborrheic dermatitis-like eruption on the scalp, that later spread to the neck, trunk and limbs. She was patch test positive to MCI/MI, cocamidopropyl betaine and several shampoos (open test) that contained both chemicals (281). Four women from Hong Kong had facial dermatitis. They had positive patch tests to MCI/MI and cosmetics containing the preservative (2 moisturizing creams, 2 foundation creams, 2 cleansing gels) (214).

Dermatitis of the face and neck, resembling lymphocytic infiltration of the skin, was caused by MCI/MI in a cleansing cream (206). One patient had an eruption on the face resembling lupus erythematosus from MCI/MI in various cosmetics (206). A woman had anogenital lesions from MCI/MI in an intimate hygiene cleansing emulsion (325). Another woman suffered from itching on her head from contact allergy to MCI/MI in a shampoo (325).

Occupational allergic contact dermatitis from MCI/MI in cosmetics

In the period 2010-2012, the members of the Belgian Contact and Environmental Dermatitis Group (6 university clinics, 3 private practices) saw 53 patients with occupational allergic contact dermatitis caused by isothiazolinones (MCI/MI, MI) in both cosmetics (hair care products, soaps, skin care products, hand soap, wipes, 'cosmetics') and non-cosmetic products. Unfortunately, it was not specified which were caused by MCI/MI and which by MI (253). Five hairdressers had occupational contact allergy to MI and/or MCI in shampoos (n=5), in conditioners and hair styling products (n=4) (43). Two beauticians were allergic to MI and/or MCI/MI in skin care products (43). The cases of 63 healthcare workers, 25 beauty workers and 48 hairdressers with occupational allergic contact dermatitis caused by MCI/MI and/or MI in personal care products were reported in the period 1996-2012 to a UK-wide surveillance scheme (EPIDERM) (48).

Two beauticians treating clients with German 'natural' cosmetics developed occupational ACD of the hands and face from MCI/MI present in the natural cosmetics as preservative (26). A hairdresser had occupational ACD from MCI/MI in hair conditioners (24). A shop assistant demonstrating cosmetics preserved with MCI/MI had longstanding (16 years) hand dermatitis. After quitting her job and avoiding products containing MCI/MI, the hand dermatitis cleared completely (136). A physiotherapist had ACD of the hands which was attributed to a massage cream she used at work. She was allergic to the cream itself and to MCI/MI. However, this preservative was not an ingredient of the cream. Later it was found that the cream was adulterated with MCI/MI during the manufacturing of the cosmetic (295). A beautician had become sensitized to MCI/MI from personal and work-related cosmetic products and had to quit her job. Later, she had recurrences of dermatitis from MCI/MI in powder carpet cleaner (dry shampoo) and from fabric softeners preserved with MCI/MI (151). A clerk had occupational OAC of the fingers from MCI/MI in a soap (325).

Contact allergy to MCI/MI in non-cosmetic products

Cases of allergic contact dermatitis from MCI/MI in products other than cosmetics are in the great majority from occupational exposure. They usually manifest as dermatitis of the hands and underarms, but airborne ACD also occurs (188,198,213,234,248,274). Some individuals have accidental contact with concentrated MCI/MI solutions at work and develop irritant dermatitis or chemical burns followed by sensitization (200,201,202,209,229,241,275,280,299). Non-cosmetic products in which MCI/MI may be present or to which concentrated solutions are added for preservation (e.g., as slimicides in paper mills) are summarized in table 2.292.1.

Non-occupational ACD from non-cosmetic sources occurs less frequently. However, airborne allergic contact dermatitis from MCI/MI in paint has been reported quite a few times (184,215,216,217,227). People who have had one or more rooms in their apartments or houses painted (or do the paining themselves) develop contact dermatitis of the face and other exposed areas hours to days after re-entering the painted rooms. They may also have symptoms of the eyes, nose and airways (188,198,215,217). Remarkably, it usually is the (or an) inhabitant of the painted apartment who is affected, not the professional painter. The patients have been sensitized previously by cosmetics (184,215,217) or other products (217) and now develop airborne contact dermatitis from MCI/MI released from the water-based paints applied (215). Thus, it appears that the amounts of MCI/MI released by paint are insufficient to induce sensitization in painters (although paints preserved with methylisothiazolinone *only* certainly can, see Chapter 2.299 Methylisothiazolinone), but are sufficient to elicit ACD in individuals who are already allergic.

Non-occupational ACD from non-cosmetic products
Eight patients had ACD from 'various brands of 'hypoallergenic' pharmaceutical skin care products' containing 17-24 ppm MCI/MI (24). A woman, who had become sensitized to MCI/MI from cosmetic products, had recurrences of dermatitis from MCI/MI in powder carpet cleaner (dry shampoo) and from fabric softeners preserved with MCI/MI (151). A man developed ACD from MCI/MI in a topical minoxidil-containing pharmaceutical preparation to treat androgenic alopecia (163). An 11-year old boy had dermatitis of the right hand from contact allergy to MCI/MI present in beeswax that he used for helping his father in polishing restored old wooden furniture. The manufacturer denied the presence of MCI/MI in the beeswax, but HPLC clearly showed the two peaks of MI and MCI (222). One man had acute ACD from MCI/MI present in ultrasound gel (252). Two patients had non-occupational airborne allergic contact dermatitis from MCI/MI in ironing water (274).

A pre-sensitized man developed ACD of the inner thigh and buttock from a toilet cleaner containing MCI/MI (172). Two young children had ACD of the hands, and one of them of the face, from contact allergy to MCI/MI present in a dough (plasticine) in a concentration of 39 ppm, that they played with. Both also sometimes applied a moisturizing cream containing the preservative (211). A man known to be allergic to MCI/MI experienced a sudden onset of multiple, slightly scaly and pruritic papules, a few millimeters in size, on the periumbilical area, and within days these papules progressively spread, primarily to the back and arms. The cutaneous lesions had a follicular distribution. The eruption was caused by pre-soaped sponges containing 8.3 ppm MCI/MI (290). Dermatitis of the face and neck, resembling lymphocytic infiltration of the skin, was caused by MCI/MI in an udder cream (206).

Airborne contact dermatitis from paints
A woman who had been sensitized by a cosmetic and had experienced ACD from a cream containing 30 ppm MCI/MI previously, developed airborne contact dermatitis of the face and neck from painting her house with a paint containing 30 ppm MCI/MI. The paint itself was also positive when patch tested (184). An otherwise healthy woman had an attack of generalized urticaria twice. The first episode occurred when she was working in a freshly painted office, the second when she was painting her apartment with a water-based wall paint. Patch testing revealed her to be allergic to MCI/MI. A prick test was negative, a patch test for immediate contact reactions was not performed. The authors were convinced of the relevance of the finding, but whether the paints contained MCI/MI was not mentioned (196). Six patients from Germany (5 women, one man) had non-occupational airborne contact dermatitis from MCI/MI in paints. The man had painted the room himself, the women had the paintjobs done by their husband or father. The dermatitis started after 1-3 days, one also had conjunctival irritation. Three patients had previously been sensitized to MCI/MI in cosmetics, the fourth by a massage cream and the other 2 by occupational exposure in their work as nurse and dairy worker (217).

Five women developed non-occupational airborne allergic contact dermatitis of the face, neck and other exposed parts from MCI/MI in wall paint (215). Two also had irritation of the conjunctivae and airways. One had previously reacted to a cosmetic cream containing MCI/MI. Shortly before, their apartments had been painted. All patients reacted to MCI/MI, 2 also to (some of) the paints used, tested undiluted. The materials used for painting from one of the patients was analyzed. In the wall and ceiling paint and in the parquet varnish, MCI/MI was measured at total concentrations ranging from 5 to 28.4 ppm. Emission of MCI/MI from paint was found from wet as well as from dried glass surfaces. Air concentrations of MCI released from paint at the beginning were 80 mg/m^3 and still 5 mg/m^3 after 4 weeks. After application of sodium bisulfite on dried painted surfaces, no emission of MCI/MI was detectable. Quite curiously, the presence of MCI/MI in the paints of 3 patients reacting only to MCI/MI (the paint itself was probably not tested) was not ascertained (215). A man painting his house developed airborne ACD from MCI/MI, starting within 4 hours (216). A boy had airborne ACD of the right arm, neck, upper chest region and face with edematous swelling of the eyelids from contact allergy to MCI/MI in a paint, that had been used to paint the kitchen walls and that contained 30 ppm of the preservative (227). A young boy developed airborne ACD from MI and MCI/MI in paint; he had probably previously become sensitized from the use of wet wipes, which caused dermatitis in the diaper area (315).

In France and Belgium, 44 patients who had suffered from allergic airborne contact dermatitis caused by isothiazolinones (MCI/MI, MI, octylisothiazolinone) in paints, diagnosed in the period beginning of 2012 to January 2016, were collected (319). Eighty per cent of the reactions took place in a private, non-occupational setting and, in nearly half of the cases, the patients had painted the room themselves. There were only 3 painters with occupational allergic contact dermatitis. Most patients developed reactions within 1-3 days (they were already sensitized); in 3 individuals, there was a delay of 13 to 21 days, potentially indicating active (primary) sensitization. Most patients presented with dermatitis limited to non-covered body parts, and ten (23%) also had mucosal symptoms, such as breathing difficulties and/or rhinoconjunctivitis (161). Symptoms were often severe, necessitating repeated consultations (86%), hospitalization (9%), and/or sick leave (20%), and treatment with topical or systemic (27%) corticosteroids. When patch tested, 36 of 44 patients showed positive reactions to MCI/MI and 43/44 to MI. Information on the composition of the incriminated paints could be retrieved in 19 cases, in which MCI/ MI and MI were identified in 10 and 14 cases, respectively (319).

Two patients from Belgium had airborne ACD from MCI/MI (and MI) in paint; they also reacted to other products containing MI (325). A boy with atopic dermatitis developed the clinical picture of superinfection with herpes simplex virus (Kaposi's varicelliform eruption, Kaposi-Juliusberg syndrome), which was, in fact airborne allergic contact dermatitis from MCI/MI (and MI) in paint that had been used to paint the ceiling over his bed (326).

Occupational allergic contact dermatitis from non-cosmetic products

Case series

In the period 2010-2012, the members of the Belgian Contact and Environmental Dermatitis Group (6 university clinics, 3 private practices) saw 53 patients with occupational allergic contact dermatitis caused by isothiazolinones (MCI/MI, MI) in both cosmetics and non-cosmetic products (including paints, detergents, metalworking fluids, polishes). Unfortunately, it was not specified which were caused by MCI/MI and which by MI; it is likely that many (e.g., reactions to paints) were caused by MI, not by MCI/MI (253). Occupational allergic contact dermatitis was caused by MI and/or MCI/MI in liquid soap (n=6), detergents (n=6), hand cleaner (n=5), dishwashing liquid (n=5), metalworking fluid (n=3), paint (n=3), fountain solution additive (n=2), rinse aid, hand wipes, glues/adhesives, waterproofing material, epoxy seaming material, vinyl glove, color, and glass fibre surface protecting product (all n=1) (43).

In the Occupational Dermatology Clinic in Melbourne, Australia, between January 1, 1993 and June 30, 2012, a total of 3404 dermatitis patients underwent patch testing to MCI/MI. There were 49 (1.4%) positive reactions. Nineteen (39% of the patients reacting to MCI/MI) were cooling tower technicians who had occupational ACD from this preservative by pouring MCI/MI solutions in the cooling tower water and testing it (265).

In a survey of occupational dermatoses among present and former employees in a plant producing binders for glues and paints (for which preservatives are needed), allergic contact dermatitis was demonstrated in 13 (17%) individuals. Twelve of these (9 present and 3 former production workers) had an occupational contact allergy to MCI/MI. Four of the present workers had spilled an industrial MCI/MI solution on their skin resulting in chemical burns and allergic contact dermatitis (209). Of 27 workers exposed to metalworking fluids in a plant that manufactured engine parts and who experienced cutaneous problems, 11 (41%) had occupational allergic contact dermatitis from MCI/MI in coolant oil. The hands and arms were most commonly affected, but grinders also had facial involvement, which the other metalworkers did not have. Possibly, more workers had been sensitized, as they were tested with MCI/MI at 50 ppm and 25 ppm, which is (far) too low to detect all cases of sensitization (168). In a period of 2 months, 7 workers in a flax spinning mill developed occupational ACD from MCI/MI in a solution. It was not specified where this was used for (203).

In a nylon mill, 6 out of 40 (15%) workers developed patch test-confirmed allergic contact dermatitis 2 months after MI/MCI was introduced to the manufacturing process. None of these workers had a past history of dermatitis (210). Four machinists working in a jet turbine plant developed occupational ACD of the (dorsal aspects of the) fingers from MCI/MI in metalworking fluids (183). In a group of 9 patients with (previous) occupational allergic contact dermatitis of the hands, 3 were caused by MCI/MI (208). Three milk recorders developed occupational allergic contact dermatitis of the hands from MCI/MI contained in milk preservative solutions they worked with (25). Three male employees of a paint and varnish manufacturer who worked with MCI/MI frequently, developed occupational ACD, despite extensive protective measures (226).

Case reports

A painter developed occupational allergic contact dermatitis from MCI/MI in grinding dust (46). Two mechanics had occupational ACD of the hands and forearms from coolant oils containing MCI/MI. They reacted to both MI and to MCI 300 ppm in petrolatum and to the coolant oil containing 0.1% MCI/MI. One of the investigators in this study became sensitized to the biocide 4 weeks after he commenced working with the commercial product to separate its chemical components. He also reacted to both MI and to MCI (115). An industrial chemist had accidental contact with a 10.1% MCI/MI solution on his skin, which resulted in immediate blistering. One week later, he developed extensive dermatitis while working again with the material. A patch test with MCI/MI 100 ppm in water was strongly positive, indicating that the onetime contact had sensitized this patient (139). A radiographer developed an acute vesicular and bullous dermatitis of one arm which was associated with wheezing. He was sensitized by the use of a technical grade MCI/MI solution added in a high but imprecise concentration to the bath for developing the radiographs (140). Similar cases have been reported by other investigators (192,193).

A technical sales consultant visiting paper mills and coming occasionally in contact with a preservative solution containing MCI/MI used as slimicide, became sensitized to MCI/MI and developed dermatitis from the ventral wrists, anterior thighs and ankles when he was in contact with the biocide (150). A male telecommunications engineer employed by a major UK newspaper on maintenance developed occupational ACD from MCI/MI in a solution of a photographic developing chemical. A film processor had occupational hand dermatitis from MCI/MI, but the causative product was not mentioned (153). A fork-lift truck driver in a chemical firm moved MCI/MI in drums. Although these were apparently sealed, the man became sensitized to the preservative and developed occupational ACD (140). An engine-man applied a cleansing cream containing 10 ppm MCI/MI five times daily and washed it off after 10 seconds. This induced allergic contact dermatitis. A use test was strongly positive, whereas a use test with the same cream, containing another non-isothiazolinone preservative, did not induce dermatitis (156).

A printer developed occupational ACD of his right hand due to allergy to MCI/MI present in a fountain solution (a fountain solution prevents non-image areas of lithographic plates from taking ink) (180). Another printer had also dermatitis from MCI/MI in fountain solutions, but the preservative was also present in a hand cleanser and gum Arabic he had contact with (181). A psychologist, sensitized to MCI/MI probably from cosmetics or fabric softener, had airborne allergic contact dermatitis with malaise, mild conjunctival and nasal symptoms and mild fever from MCI/MI in paint, which had been used to paint her office. She also had minimal itching and skin dryness on the backs of the thighs and buttocks, which were in contact with her chair, caused by MCI/MI present in furniture wax (188). A mechanic working in a bus garage had occupational allergic contact dermatitis of the hands from MCI/MI in diesel oil. When he used a moist toilet paper, an exacerbation was noted. The product proved to contain MCI/MI (195). A waitress had acute dermatitis of the face, neck, forearms, and distal upper arms, together with mild conjunctivitis, one day after returning to work after a holiday. She had previously had ACD of the face from MCI/MI in a moisturizing cream. The walls of the restaurant had been painted a few days before she had returned to work, and the paint manufacturer confirmed that the paints used contained MCI/MI as preservative, explaining this episode of airborne contact dermatitis (198).

A technician in a paper mill developed – despite preventive measures such as a face shield – airborne occupational ACD of the periorbital region from MCI/MI, used in a high concentration as slimicide in the water system of papermaking machinery (213). A woman working at a polyester yarn manufacturing plant had occupational allergic contact dermatitis of the fingers from MCI/MI present in spin finish oil coating yarn, with which she was in frequent contact (218). One (234) and two (274) domestic cleaners had occupational airborne ACD of the face, hands and arms from MCI/MI in ironing water. A female laboratory worker in a latex paint factory had a 4-year history of pruritic, erythematous, blistering eruption of the soles of her feet with secondary eruptions on the neck and arms. Possible contact dermatitis to her work boots was postulated. She had positive patch test reactions to MCI/MI and to her shoes. Her foot dermatitis persisted despite custom work boots without MCI/MI. Through surveillance tapes, the company discovered that a co-worker had been spraying her workplace and shoes with MCI/MI. This case highlights a fascinating incident of maliciously caused contact sensitization (237).

A man had occupational ACD from cleaning large metal elements at high pressure in a washing area, with a detergent to which he added concentrated MCI/MI (245). A worker in a glue factory had to mix glues with concentrated MCI/MI solutions, to which he became allergic. The initial dermatological symptoms were local erythema and burning sensations on the hands, face, and femoral region. These manifestations later developed into a more severe flare-up of the previously affected area, now with a papular vesicular dermatitis pattern, also involving the flexural part of the knees, and general symptoms, including malaise, and respiratory and gastrointestinal symptoms. This was considered to be systemic contact dermatitis from inhalation of MCI/MI vapors (248).

A metal worker received a chemical burn when exposed to an MCI/MI-containing biocide, during an accident at work, and was subsequently sensitized to MCI/MI and MI. He developed persistent contact dermatitis of the lower leg with secondary ulceration. During inpatient wound treatment, a vacuum pump was applied with a polyurethane foam (VAC sponge), which led to deterioration of the skin condition in the wound environment, together with severe itching. Patch tests with the suspected VAC sponge were positive. The manufacturer denied the presence of MCI/MI or MI in the product. However, a chemical analysis with HPLC showed MCI at 754 ppm and MI at 315 ppm in the VAC sponge material (275). A cleaner developed facial allergic contact dermatitis from MCI/MI in a stainless steel cleaner spray (320).

A foreman in a construction company specializing in renovation work had dry cough and rhinitis. A few days following these first symptoms, an eczematous eruption appeared, located on the face, eyelids, chest, the nape of his neck, and the folds of the elbows, resembling atopic dermatitis. Both the respiratory and the dermatological symptoms were caused by airborne exposure to MI in water-based paints and to MI and MCI/MI in pulverized indoor facade renders. The patient reacted to both MCI/MI and MI, and also to the paint and to the indoor facade render (334). Two individuals working in paper mills, who had to add high concentrations of MCI/MI to the mills (whereby their clothes would become contaminated from overflowing) became sensitized to MCI/MI used as a slimicide (282). A vehicle locksmith developed ACD of the dorsal hands favoring the interdigital webs from MCI/MI present in a spray-can lock lubricant and a hand cleanser (298).

There are several reports of workers who have become sensitized from accidental contact with concentrated MCI/MI solutions, often after having developed irritant contact dermatitis or even chemical burns (200,201,202,209,229,241,275,280, and 299).

Miscellaneous case reports

Data on 14 patients allergic to MCI/MI seen in an occupational medicine clinic in Finland with patch test results to MCI/MI, MI, benzisothiazolinone, octylisothiazolinone, occupation, isothiazolinone-related diagnosis, exposures and comments were published in 2017. There were both cases of non-occupational and of occupational allergic contact dermatitis; many cases were caused by cosmetics (especially rinse-off products), others by non-cosmetic products (316).

Cross-reactions, pseudo-cross-reactions and co-reactions

The MCI/MI mixture contains methylisothiazolinone, methylchloroisothiazolinone and a small amount of dichloro-methylisothiazolinone (145). Methylchloroisothiazolinone is the main sensitizer in MCI/MI: in patients allergic to the preservative, all react to methylchloroisothiazolinone and dichloromethylisothiazolinone, but only a few to methyl-isothiazolinone (128,145,235). In patients who have been sensitized to methylisothiazolinone used *per se* as a preservative, co-reactions to MCI/MI are frequent (9,11,12,323,324), in one study 100% with MCI/MI tested at 200 ppm water (250). Whether this is the result of pseudo-cross-reactivity (reaction to methylisothiazolinone in both preparations) or that the co-reaction to MCI/MI can be explained by methylchloroisothiazolinone cross-reacting to methylisothiazolinone, is unknown. Conversely, cross-reactivity of methylisothiazolinone from primary methylchloro-isothiazolinone is unlikely, as all patients allergic to MCI/MI react to methylchloroisothiazolinone, but only very few to methylisothiazolinone (128,145,235). Nevertheless, in a 2014-2015 UK study, 53 of 74 patients (72%) allergic to MCI/MI co-reacted to MI (323).

In some reports, in patients allergic to MCI/MI, there were co-reactions to other isothiazolinones: benzisothia-zolinone and/or octylisothiazolinone (93,170). Whether these chemicals may cross-react is as yet not entirely elucidated. Co-sensitization from occupational exposure may be more likely than cross-sensitization (170). In a larger study population, cross-sensitivity of these chemicals to or from MCI/MI seemed very unlikely (194). No cross-reactions to octylisothiazolinone and dichlorinated octylisothiazolinone were observed in 4 patients allergic to MCI/MI (235). However, in a Belgian study, 15 of 31 patients who were sensitized to MCI/MI and/or MI who co-reacted to octylisothiazolinone without any relevant source, cross-reaction from MI (MCI was not mentioned by the authors) was considered to be likely. In at least 6 of these, the patients were primarily sensitized to MI, not to MCI/MI (253). Indeed, there are strong indications from recent animal experiments that primary sensitization to MI (ergo not to MCI/MI, in which MCI is the sensitizer) may result in cross-reactivity to benzisothiazolinone and octyl-isothiazolinone (169). This subject is discussed in Chapter 2.299 Methylisothiazolinone.

In two UK studies, contact allergies to formaldehyde (240,324), diazolidinyl urea (240), imidazolidinyl urea (240), 2-bromo-2-nitropropane-1,3-diol (240,324) and quaternium-15 (324) were significantly associated with allergy to MCI/MI. This probably results from concomitant or successive sensitization to these chemicals in the same or different products rather than from cross-reactivity (240). In Sweden, allergy to MCI/MI and/or MI was also found to be significantly associated with contact allergy to formaldehyde and to fragrance-mix I and/or II (276). In one report it has been suggested – rather unconvincingly – that metronidazole may cross-react to MCI/MI (297).

Provocation tests

Many investigators have performed ROATs in patients sensitized to MCI/MI to assess the clinical relevance of the reactions and determine which concentrations of MCI/MI are safe in sensitized individuals and which product types and MCI/MI concentrations may elicit ACD from regular use of such products. In older publications, mostly a moisturizing lotion/cream was used for ROATs, containing 15 ppm MCI/MI that had been provided by the manufacturer of the commercial product Kathon CG. Nearly always, the ROATs lasted for only one week. It is now well known that this period is (far) too short for reliable results (228). This implies that the rates of positive ROATs in these studies are an underestimation; more positive reactions would have appeared with longer test periods. Indeed, in Italy, 52 patients sensitized to MCI/MI performed a ROAT with a lotion containing 7 ppm MCI/MI *for 2 weeks,* and all had a positive response after 5-10 days (24). Patients reacting to lower concentrations of MCI/MI in patch tests have significantly more often a positive ROAT than individuals reacting to higher concentrations only (166).

Stay-on products

The results of ROATs with stay-on products are shown in table 2.292.6. Between 31% and 57% of the patients had a positive test to a cream/lotion containing 15 ppm MCI/MI, despite the test period being too short (1 week). With prolonged periods, even preparations containing 2-7.5 ppm MCI/MI gave positive tests (24,26,228), indicating that leave-one preparations containing MCI/MI in these low concentrations may not be safe in sensitized individuals.

Table 2.292.6 Results of Repeated Open Application Tests (ROATs)

Number of patients	Product type	Conc. MCI/MI	Duration of ROAT	Nr. Pos. (%)	Ref.
2	cream	15 ppm	1 week	1 (50%)	26
13	cream	15 ppm	1 week	7 (54%)	118
20	cream	15 ppm	1 week	8 (40%)	124
101	lotion	15 ppm	1 week	31 (31%)	161
7	lotion	15 ppm	1 week	4 (57%)	160
10	lotion	15 ppm	1 week	5 (50%)	160
7	cream	9 ppm	1 week	3 (43%)	160
24	solution	7.5 ppm	4 weeks	14 (56%)	228
52	lotion	7 ppm	2 weeks	52 (100%)	24
10	cream	7 ppm	1 week	5 (50%)	26
25	solution	2 ppm	4 weeks	7 (28%)	228

Conc.: Concentration; Nr.: Number

Twenty-five patients with dermatitis, 18 years of age or older, with a positive reaction to MCI/MI 100 ppm in water, were enrolled in a double-blind, placebo-controlled, dose-response ROAT (228). Ten healthy volunteers who tested negative to 100 ppm water MCI/MI were recruited as control subjects. In the first ROAT period (ROAT 1), test material containing 0.025 mg/cm^2 MCI/MI (concentration 2 ppm) and the vehicle control was applied to the designated skin sites (volar aspect of the forearms). This test period of up to 4 weeks was followed by a wash-out period of 4 weeks when no test material or vehicle control was applied. The wash-out period was followed by application of 0.094 mg/cm^2 MCI/MI (concentration 7.5 ppm) test material and the vehicle control (ROAT 2). In ROAT 1, 7/25 (28%) subjects had a positive ROAT. The average time to a positive reaction was 16.5 days. There were 5 weak, 2 moderate and zero strong reactions. In ROAT 2, 14/24 (56%) subjects had a positive ROAT. The average time to a positive reaction was 12.1 days. There were 7 weak, 6 moderate and one strong reactions. None of the 10 non-allergic control subjects showed any reaction in either ROAT 1 or ROAT 2. The authors concluded, that the elicitation threshold is in the proximity of 0.025 mg/cm^2 (MCI/MI 2 ppm) (228).

Nine patients patch test positive to MCI/MI 100 ppm in water performed a ROAT with a cream containing 100 ppm MI (the maximum allowed concentration in cosmetics in the EU at that time) and 6 (67%) had a positive test (261).

Rinse-off products

In a multicenter study, a randomized, double-blind, 2-period crossover study with 2 shampoos was performed on subjects patch-test-positive to 100 ppm MCI/MI (190). One shampoo was preserved with 15 ppm MCI/MI, the other with 0.3% imidazolidinyl urea (IU). Twenty-seven subjects from 5 European dermatology clinics participated. One individual discontinued use after severe adverse reactions to the MCI/MI shampoo. Another two individuals developed moderate symptoms with the MCI/MI preserved shampoo and discontinued its use, but tolerated the IU-preserved shampoo for the full 2-week period. The majority of subjects had negative findings on the scalp, face, neck, and hands for both shampoos. The physicians' global evaluation data indicated that shampoo with MCI/MI caused fewer skin problems than shampoo with IU. This study showed that most subjects previously sensitized to MCI/MI can successfully use shampoo preserved with MCI/MI. However, since some patients did develop clinical reactions, it would still be prudent for the clinician to advise alternative products not containing MCI/MI, according to the authors (which is of course correct) (190).

In a diagnostic provocative use test, human volunteers who had developed delayed contact hypersensitivity to MCI/MI through exaggerated repeated occlusive exposure, used shampoo, cream rinse hair conditioner, synthetic liquid soap, liquid fabric softener, bath foam, shower foam or a combination of these products preserved with 4-6 ppm of the isothiazolinones mixture for periods of 3 or 6 weeks. None developed allergic contact dermatitis. It was concluded that in their typical use, these products pose at most an extremely small risk of eliciting clinical dermatitis even among consumers who are allergic to the preservative mix (111).

Patch test studies with dilution series

The results of studies performing serial dilution testing in patients reacting to MCI/MI 100 ppm are shown in table 2.292.7. Between 42% and 100% reacted to 50 ppm (median: 64%), 11-47% reacted to 25 ppm and 6-12% had positive patch tests with 10 ppm MCI/MI. This explains why cosmetic products used by patients and causing allergic contact dermatitis are nearly always negative upon patch testing: the concentration of MCI/MI in these cosmetics (<15 ppm, often <10 ppm) is too low to elicit an allergic reaction in the patch test in the great majority of allergic individuals.

Table 2.292.7 Results of serial dilution testing

100 ppm Nr. pos. (%)	50 ppm Nr. pos. (%)	25 ppm Nr. pos. (%)	15 ppm Nr. pos. (%)	10 ppm Nr. pos. (%)	Ref.
9 (100%)	6 (67%)	1 (11%)	0 (0%)	NT	111
18 (100%)	10 (56%)	4 (22%)	NT	1 (6%)	26
26 (100%)	26 (100%)	NT	NT	NT	24
103 (100%)	66 (64%)	30 (29%)	NT	NT	161
24 (100%)	10 (42%)	9 (38%)	NT	NT	190
17 (100%)		8 [a] (47%)	NT	2 (12%)	118

Nr.: number; pos.: positive; NT: Not Tested; [a]: 30 ppm

Thirty-four patients having reacted to MCI/MI 300 ppm or 250 ppm were patch tested with a dilution series of MCI/MI 100 ppm, 30 ppm and 10 ppm in water. Seventeen (50%) reacted to 100 ppm, 8 (23%) to 30 ppm, and 2 (6%) to the 10 ppm patch test (118). It was concluded that, with the generally used test concentration of 100 ppm in water, about half of the sensitized patients are missed (false-negative reactions) (118).

Patch test sensitization

One patient was sensitized by a patch test with 1% Kathon CG, containing 150 ppm MCI/MI (23). One patient became sensitized by a patch test with MCI/MI 200 ppm water (306). Patch testing with 250-300 ppm MCI/MI resulted in approximately 1% patch test sensitizations (117). Indeed, of 976 patients tested with MCI/MI 300 ppm, 8 (0.8%) showed a 'flare-up' reaction, indicating patch test sensitization. Of 170 individuals tested with MCI/MI 250 ppm, 2 (1.2%) were sensitized by the test (118). Of 1396 consecutive patients tested with MCI/MI 0.01% water (100 ppm), one became sensitized by the patch test (136). Of 495 patients tested in the USA with MCI/MI 250 ppm in petrolatum and in water, 3 (0.6%) were actively sensitized (147). One patient was sensitized by a patch test with MCI/MI 200 ppm in water (224, also presented in ref. 225).

Accidental contact with concentrated industrial MCI/MI solutions has resulted in irritant contact dermatitis / chemical burns followed by sensitization in several individuals, notably from occupational exposure (200,201,202,209,229,241,275,280,299).

Presence of MCI/MI in cosmetic products

In May 2017, MCI/MI (by looking for methylchloroisothiazolinone, the INCI name yielded no hits) was present in 2032 of 66,835 cosmetic products of which the composition is known in EWG's Skin Deep Cosmetics Database, USA (http://www.ewg.org/skindeep/). In the USA, in April 2017, methylchloroisothiazolinone (probably as part of MCI/MI) was present in 4662 of 56,714 cosmetic products of which the composition is known in FDA's Voluntary Cosmetic Registration Program (VCRP) (data obtained from FDA, May 2017). MCI/MI was present in 416 of 4737 (8.8%) commonly used cosmetic products of which the full composition was known in 2016 in The Contact Allergen Management Program (CAMP) database of the American Contact Dermatitis Society (313).

MCI/MI was present in 2 (1.1%) of 178 facial wipes for which ingredient information was obtained online and from retail stores, 2016, USA (331). MCI/MI was present in zero of 54 personal hygiene wet wipes for which ingredient information was obtained online and from retail stores, 2016, USA (332). In the USA, in 2015-2016, 63 diaper wipes and 41 topical diaper preparations from a large retailer were screened for the presence of potential sensitizers. MCI/MI was found in 1/63 (2%) disposable diaper wipes and in none of 41 topical diaper preparations (314).

In 2015-2016, 100 USA-made personal care products from different brands were randomly selected and 20 products (20%) were labeled to contain MCI/MI (301). In 2014, in Thailand, the labels of 1000 cosmetic products (593 leave-on, 407 rinse-off products) were examined for the presence of preservatives. These were partly purchased in shops and on markets and partly brought in by patients. MCI/MI was present in 101 products (10%); in the leave-on products, the percentage was 2.5 and in the rinse-off products 21.1 (270). In Switzerland, in 2015, the occurrence of MCI/MI was investigated in 1948 consumer products (1266 cosmetics, 557 detergents, 125 baby products) by checking the labels. MCI/MI was labeled on 3.6% of the cosmetics. Shampoo was the product category with the highest percentage of isothiazolinones (MIC/MI or MI) (34%), followed by shower gel (13%), wet wipes (12%), and make-up remover (12%) (321) . Of 179 emollients available in Poland in 2014, 8 (4.5%) contained MCI/MI (273).

In 2013, 60 cosmetic products manufactured and purchased in Israel (40 stay-on and 20 rinse-off products) were investigated for preservatives. According to the labeling, 14 (23%) cosmetics contained MCI/MI. In the stay-on products (hand and body creams), the percentage was 5, whereas 60% of the 20 shampoos and soaps was preserved with MCI/MI. Analyses showed that the concentration range was 5-15 ppm (267). In 2009, in the USA, the ingredient lists of 657 miscellaneous cosmetics from one company were screened for the presence of MCI/MI. MCI/MI was present in 0% of 195 antiperspirants/deodorants, in 0% of 41 powders, in 0% of 167 shaving products, in 9% of 201 sunblocks, and in 13% of 53 wipes (102). In 2009, in the USA, the ingredient lists of 796 hair products from one company were screened for the presence of MCI/MI. The preservative was present in 52% of 279 shampoos, in 9% of 231 conditioners, and in 8% of 286 styling products (101).

In 2009, in the USA, the ingredient lists of 1591 facial cosmetics from one company were screened for the presence of MCI/MI. The preservative system was present in none of 132 blushers, 38 bronzers, 90 concealers, 174 eyeliners, 304 eyeshadows, 457 foundations, 140 loose and pressed powders, and 256 mascaras (242). In 2009, in the USA, the ingredient lists of 730 lip cosmetics and dental care products from one company were screened for the presence of MCI/MI. This preservative was present in none of 31 lip liners, 429 lipsticks, 92 lip moisturizers, 153 toothpastes, and 25 mouth washes (243). MCI/MI was present in 73/3541 (2.0%) randomly sampled leave-on cosmetic products in Germany, 2006-2009 (31). In Germany, in 2006-2009, the labels of 4680 cosmetic products were screened for the presence of preservatives. MCI/MI was present in 4% of the products, according to labeling information (307).

MCI/MI was present in 22% of 204 cosmetic products (92 shampoos, 61 hair conditioners, 34 liquid soaps, 17 wet tissues) in Sweden, 2008 (32). In 2007, in the USA, MCI/MI was the 10th most frequent preservative in cosmetic products on file with FDA's Voluntary Registration Program, being found in approximately 5% of them (233). Of 276 moisturizers sold in the USA in 2007, 17 (6%) contained MCI/MI (40). Of 23 brands of moist toilet paper marketed in 2006 in Italy, 1 (4%) contained MCI/MI (94).

Methylchloroisothiazolinone (and) methylisothiazolinone was present in 281 of 1774 (15.8%) cosmetics and toiletries in 2002 and in 218 of 1170 (18.6%) such products in 2005 filed in the Danish Product Register Database (PROBAS) (95). In 67 samples of skin creams, randomly selected from retail outlets in Denmark in 1999, 3 (4%) contained methylchloroisothiazolinone (and) methylisothiazolinone in a concentration range of 7.3-12.2 ppm (98). Of 19 brands of moist toilet paper marketed in Spain in 1995, 11 (58%) contained MCI/MI in concentrations ranging from 10 to 15 ppm (191).

In 1992, MCI/MI was present in 550 of about 59,500 products filed in the Danish Product Register Database (PROBAS). The main *cosmetic* categories were hair shampoos (n=81) and skin care products (n=69). Typical use concentrations for shampoos and skin care products were <15 ppm (185). In The Netherlands, approximately 25% of all cosmetic products and toiletries were preserved by the isothiazolinone mixture in 1987 (132). In 1980, 38 of approximately 20,000 cosmetic products on file at the Food and Drug Administration contained MCI/MI (130). Four years later this preservative system had reached a level of 222 uses and already ranked 13th in the list of most frequently employed preservatives (131).

Presence of MCI/MI in non-cosmetic products

MCI/MI was present in 630 of 38,000 active 'substances and materials' registered in PROBAS as active on the Danish market as of March 2014 (322). MCI/MI was most frequently registered in paints and varnishes (n=354), cleaning agents (n=55), and polishing agents (n=38) (322). In 2012, MCI/MI was present in 611 of an unknown number (in 1992: 59,500) products filed in the Danish Product Register Database (PROBAS). Main non-cosmetic product types containing MCI/MI were paints and varnishes (n=363), cleaning/washing agents (n=50), polishing agents (n=32), biocides (n=27), adhesives (n=24), binding agents (n=19) and printing inks (n=13). MCI/MI was registered in concentrations ranging from 0.01 ppm to 14% (the products with high concentrations were commercial neat MCI/MI biocides) (255). In Italy, in 2008, MCI/MI was present in 79% of 43 washing-up liquids, in 35% of 63 laundry detergents, in 43% of 61 fabric conditioners, in 9% of 47 spray cleaners and in 23% of 77 liquid hard surface cleaning products (174).

In 1992, MCI/MI was present in 550 of about 59,500 products filed in the Danish Product Register Database (PROBAS). The main non-cosmetic categories were paints (n=169), cleaning agents (n= 67), printing inks (n=35), preservatives (n=30), polishes (n=21) and pigments (n=12). The concentrations of MCI/MI in 343 products of which concentrations were known were as follows: 36% of the products contained less than 0.001% (10 ppm) MCI/MI, 41% of the products ranged from 0.001% (10 ppm) to less than 0.01% (100 ppm) and 23% of the products contained above or equal to 0.01% (100 ppm) MCI/MI. Typical use concentrations for pigments, cleaning agents and printing inks were <35 ppm and for polishes <25 ppm (185).

Chemical analyses of MCI/MI in cosmetic products

In 2015-2016, 100 USA-made personal care products from different brands were randomly selected. The ingredient labels were examined and the products were analyzed with HPLC for the content of MCI/MI. According to labeling, twenty products (20%) contained MCI/MI. Three products not labeled to contain MCI/MI or MI showed positive results on HPLC (not specified for MCI/MI and MI). Of 35 products labeled to contain MCI/MI or MI, five showed negative results upon HPLC analysis (not specified for MCI/MI and MI). It was concluded that personal care products are an important source of exposure to MCI/MI and that labeling inaccuracies do occur (301).

In 2015, in the USA, 7 cosmetic products (4 shampoos/conditioners, 3 skin care products) labeled as containing MCI, were analysed. They all contained MCI and MI in concentrations ranging from 0.8 to 20 μg/g and 0.7 to 20 μg/g, respectively. The maximum combined concentration was 40 μg/g in a stay-on product, which is well over the in the USA permitted maximum concentration of 7.5 μg/g (ppm) (178). In Switzerland, in 2015, 88 products (69 detergents, 19 cosmetics) labeled to contain isothiazolinones (MCI/MI, MI, benzisothiazolinone, octylisothiazolinone) were analyzed by liquid chromatography–high-resolution mass spectrometry after ultrasonic extraction. The measured concentration ranges of MCI/MI were 4.3-10 ppm in detergents and in cosmetics 4.8 ppm (one product only) (321). Some products sold in the EU between 2008 and 2014 have had too high concentrations of MCI/MI (0.025%-0.36%) (103). In 2011, thirteen rinse-off cosmetics (selection procedure unspecified) were investigated in Spain and 10 (77%) contained MCI/MI in concentrations ranging from <1 to 12 ppm. Two of four stay-on products contained the preservative, both <1 ppm (244).

One hundred moisturizers sold in Sweden were investigated in 1997 using HPLC for the presence of preservatives. Six (6%) were found to contain MCI/MI and, in one of these, MCI/MI was neither declared by the manufacturer / supplier nor stated to be present on the product label. The concentration of MCI/MI was 14.7 ppm in this particular moisturizer, which was higher than in the other moisturizers (205). In 1990, in France, 44 creams were analyzed with liquid chromatography and 8 (18%) proved to contain MCI/MI. Two of these had been responsible for allergic contact dermatitis (285).

In The Netherlands, in 1990, 13 types of moist toilet paper (8 brands) were investigated and 10 (77%) were found to contain MCI/MI in concentrations ranging from 5.9 ppm to 23.4 ppm in the water phase (167). In Denmark, in 1989, MCI/MI was determined by HPLC in 156 of the most commonly used cosmetic products. Forty-two per cent were found to contain MCI/MI; in rinse-off products, the percentage was 48 and in stay-on products it was 31. Twenty-nine products contained <5 ppm MCI/MI, twenty contained 5-10 ppm, fourteen 10-15 ppm and three >15 ppm (162). In Spain in 1988, 23 commonly used cosmetic products were investigated by HPLC and 10 (43%) contained MCI/MI in concentrations ranging from 0.9 to 24.7 ppm. The percentage positives in skin creams and body lotions and in shampoos was 50 (154).

In Denmark, in 1987, 22 commonly used cosmetic products (9 shampoos, 9 skin creams, 3 hair balms and one body lotion) were analyzed with HPLC for the presence of MCI/MI. The preservative system was detected in 11 of the 22 (50%) products investigated (6/9 shampoos, 4/9 skin creams, 1/3 hair balms and 0/1 body lotion) in concentrations ranging from 0.8 to 15 ppm. As the prevalence of sensitization in Denmark at that moment was relatively low, it was suggested that the maximum allowed concentration in the EEC of 30 ppm in leave-on products should be reconsidered (137).

In The Netherlands in 1987, 253 cosmetic products brought in by dermatitis patients *not* allergic to MCI/MI were analyzed by HPLC and 59 (23%) proved to contain MCI/MI. The highest frequencies were in bath/shower foams (64%), all-purpose creams/lotions (43%), body lotions/milks (30%), shampoos (27%) and facial creams (24%) (138). Forty-one cosmetic products brought in by patients reacting to MCI/MI between 1984 and 1987 in Gentofte, Denmark, were analysed. MCI/MI was present in only 4 products in concentrations of 3, 7.7, 8.6 and 15.5 ppm (136). In Sweden, in 1985, 123 cosmetic products, barrier creams, cleaning agents and washing-up liquids were investigated with HPLC for the presence of MCI/MI. The preservative system was found to be present in 38 products (31%) in concentrations ranging from 1 to 15 ppm. Fifteen of 37 (41%) skin creams and lotions were positive, and 12 of 25 (48%) shampoos and hair conditioners contained MCI/MI (36).

Other information

Ten patients who had positive patch test reactions to MCI/MI were retested some years later and in nine (90%), the positive patch test could be reproduced, only 1 having lost the sensitivity (189). There is a high frequency of sensitization to MCI/MI in patients with airborne allergic contact dermatitis, probably from its presence in water-based paints (42).

OTHER SIDE EFFECTS

Irritant contact dermatitis

At industrial strength, MCI/MI biocide is a powerful irritant that can cause burns of the mucosa and skin (110). Such contact has resulted in primary sensitization at various occasions (200,201,202). Two cases of irritant contact dermatitis were reported due to accidental exposure to MCI/MI at a concentration of 2.7%. In the first case, severe erythema over the exposed area subsided after 48 hours, perhaps because the chemical was immediately washed off. In the second case, a man developed painful desquamation over the right gluteal region after sitting on a drum containing the biocide (187). A facilities technician in an electronics plant developed painful irritant dermatitis with erythema and blisters 2 hours after carrying a container of chemicals used for cooling tower water treatment on his right shoulder, which later proved to leak a 1.15% MCI/MI solution. The dermatitis progressed into a mid-dermal burn over the right shoulder and scapular region with a diameter of 10 cm (186, probably also published in ref. 283). In a textile factory worker, the accidental spillage of a small amount of concentrated MCI/MI (concentration not specified) over the pants of his left leg led to a partial-thickness and full-thickness burn and (probably, no patch tests performed) primary sensitization (229).

A process technician and 2 maintenance engineers accidentally spilled a small amount of concentrated MCI/MI on their clothes or skin. After several hours, a painful irritant dermatitis appeared with erythema and vesicles. Two of them subsequently developed allergic contact dermatitis from resp. MCI/MI mist (airborne contact dermatitis) and from the same concentrated material. All three had positive patch tests to MCI/MI; the sensitization had most likely been acquired from the irritant dermatitis/chemical burn (200). Two similar patients were reported from Finland (201) and one from Sweden (202). A patient who was already sensitized to MCI/MI spilled some MCI/MI 13.9% solution over his lower legs and feet, which resulted in acute irritant contact dermatitis followed by allergic contact dermatitis (202). Four workers in a plant producing binders for paints and glues had spilled an industrial MCI/MI solution on their skin resulting in chemical burns followed by allergic contact dermatitis (209).

Immediate-type reactions

Of 50 individuals who had open tests with methylchloroisothiazolinone (and) methylisothiazolinone 0.01% water on the forearm, 3 showed local macular erythema after 45 minutes, termed 'contact urticaria' by the authors (97). In a group of 664 patch tested patients, there were 2 (0.3%) immediate contact reactions to MCI/MI as shown by 'well distinguished erythema' after 30 minutes (99). MCI/MI provoked contact urticaria in one patient; details were not provided, possibly the reaction was observed during patch testing (236).

Other non-eczematous contact reactions

In a report from India, hyperpigmentation of the face, incorrectly termed poikiloderma of Civatte, was – rather unconvincingly – ascribed to contact allergy to MCI/MI in a moisturizing cream (221). In another report, contact allergy to MCI/MI (and fragrances) in a moisturizing cream and various other cosmetics was proposed to be a 'contributory etiology' to poikiloderma of Civatte (171). In a man who regularly added MCI/MI (1.5%) and glutaraldehyde to cooling tower water, spillage of one of these (unknown which) caused a chemical burn, which was followed after 2 weeks by a bullous pemphigoid-like eruption. Rather surprisingly and disappointingly, the investigators did not perform patch tests with these chemicals to elucidate the mechanism of the reaction and try to pinpoint the offending chemical (300).

LITERATURE

1   Uter W, Aberer W, Armario-Hita JC, Fernandez-Vozmediano JM, Ayala F, Balato A, et al. Current patch test results with the European baseline series and extensions to it from the 'European Surveillance System on Contact Allergy' network, 2007-2008. Contact Dermatitis 2012;67:9-19
2   Uter W, Gefeller O, Geier J, Schnuch A. Methylchloroisothiazolinone/methylisothiazolinone contact sensitization: diverging trends in subgroups of IVDK patients in a period of 19 years. Contact Dermatitis 2012;67:125-129
3   Anonymous. Cosmetic Ingredient Review Final report on the safety assessment of methylisothiazolinone and methylchloroisothiazolinone. J Am Coll Toxicol 1992;11:75-128
4   Thyssen JP, Giménez-Arnau E, Lepoittevin J-P, Menné T, Boman A, Schnuch A. The critical review of methodologies and approaches to assess the inherent skin sensitizing potential (skin allergies) of chemicals. Part II. Contact Dermatitis 2012;66 (Suppl. 1):25-52
5   Travassos AR, Claes L, Boey L, Drieghe J, Goossens A. Non-fragrance allergens in specific cosmetic products. Contact Dermatitis 2011;65:276-285
6   Wetter DA, Yiannias JA, Prakash AV, Davis MD, Farmer SA, el-Azhary RA, et al. Results of patch testing to personal care product allergens in a standard series and a supplemental cosmetic series: an analysis of 945 patients from the Mayo Clinic Contact Dermatitis Group, 2000-2007. J Am Acad Dermatol 2010;63:789-798
7   Davis MD, Scalf LA, Yiannias JA, Cheng JF, El-Azhary RA, Rohlinger AL, et al. Changing trends and allergens in the patch test standard series. Arch Dermatol 2008;144:67-72
8   Warshaw EM, Buchholz HJ, Belsito DV et al. Allergic patch test reactions associated with cosmetics: Retrospective analysis of cross-sectional data from the North American Contact Dermatitis Group, 2001-2004. J Am Acad Dermatol 2009;60:23-38

9   Schnuch A, Lessmann H, Geier J, Uter W. Contact allergy to preservatives. Analysis of IVDK data 1996-2009. Br J Dermatol 2011;164:1316-1325

10   ESSCA Writing Group. The European Surveillance System of Contact Allergies (ESSCA): results of patch testing the standard series, 2004. J Eur Acad Dermatol Venereol 2008;22:174-181

11   Geier J, Lessmann H, Schnuch A, Uter W. Recent increase in allergic reactions to methylchloroisothiazolinone/methylisothiazolinone: is methylisothiazolinone the culprit? Contact Dermatitis 2012;67:334-341

12   Ackermann L, Aalto-Korte K, Alanko K, Hasan T, Jolanki R, Lammintausta K, et al. Contact sensitization to methylisothiazolinone in Finland – a multicentre study. Contact Dermatitis 2011;64:49-53

13   Maio P, Carvalho R, Amaro C, Santos R, Cardoso J. Contact allergy to methylchloroisothiazolinone/ methylisothiazolinone (MCI/MI): findings from a contact dermatitis unit. Cutan Ocul Toxicol 2012;31:151-153

14   Färm G, Wahlberg JE. Isothiazolinones (MCI/MI): 200 ppm versus 100 ppm in the standard series. Contact Dermatitis 1991;25:104-107

15   Davies E, Orton D. Identifying the optimal patch test concentration for methylchloroisothiazolinone and methylisothiazolinone. Contact Dermatitis 2009;60:288-289

16   Johnston GA, Contributing Members of the British Society for Cutaneous Allergy (BSCA). The rise in prevalence of contact allergy to methylisothiazolinone in the British Isles. Contact Dermatitis 2014;70:238-240

17   Gerberick GF, Ryan CA, Kern PS, Schlatter H, Dearman RJ, Kimber I, et al. Compilation of historical local lymph node data for evaluation of skin sensitization alternative methods. Dermatitis 2005;16:157-202

18   Basketter DA, Andersen KE, Lidén C, Van Loveren H, Boman A, Kimber I, et al. Evaluation of the skin sensitizing potency of chemicals by using the existing methods and considerations of relevance for elicitation. Contact Dermatitis 2005;52:39-43

19   Kimber I, Basketter DA, Butler M, Gamer A, Garrigue JL, Gerberick GF, et al. Classification of contact allergens according to potency: proposals. Food Chem Toxicol 2003:41:1799-1809

20   Basketter DA, Gilmour NJ, Wright Z, Walters T, Boman A, Lidén C. Biocides: characterization of the allergenic hazard of methylisothiazolinone. Cut Ocul Toxicol 2003;22:187-199

21   Bruze M, Fregert S, Gruvberger B, Persson K. Contact allergy to the active ingredients of Kathon CG in the guinea pig. Acta Derm Venereol 1987;67:315-320

22   De Groot AC, Liem DH, Nater JP, van ketel WG. Patch tests with fragrance materials and preservatives. Contact Dermatitis 1985;12:87-92

23   De Groot AC, Liem DH, Weyland JW. Kathon CG: cosmetic allergy and patch test sensitization. Contact Dermatitis 1985;12:76-80

24   Tosti A. Prevalence and sources of Kathon CG sensitization in Italy. Contact Dermatitis 1988;18:173-174

25   Grattan CEH, Harman RRM, Tan RSH. Milk recorder dermatitis. Contact Dermatitis 1986;14:217-220

26   Hannuksela M. Rapid increase in contact allergy to Kathon® CG in Finland. Contact Dermatitis 1986;15:211-214

27   Lammintausta K, Aalto-Korte K, Ackerman L, Alanko K, Berry P, Hasan T, et al. An epidemic of contact allergy to methylisothiazolinone in Finland. Contact Dermatitis 2014;70:184-185

28   Wilkinson JD, Shaw S, Andersen KE, Brandão FM, Bruynzeel DP. Monitoring levels of preservative sensitivity in Europe. A 10-year overview (1991–2000). Contact Dermatitis 2002;46:207-210

29   Thyssen JP, Engkilde K, Lundov MD, Carlsen BC, Menné T, Johansen JD. Temporal trends of preservative allergy in Denmark (1985–2008). Contact Dermatitis 2010;62:102-108

30   Zug KA, Warshaw EM, Fowler JF Jr, Maibach HI, Belsito DL, Pratt MD, et al. Patch-test results of the North American Contact Dermatitis Group 2005-2006. Dermatitis 2009;20:149-160

31   Schnuch A, Mildau G, Kratz E-M, Uter W. Risk of sensitization to preservatives estimated on the basis of patch test data and exposure, according to a sample of 3541 leave-on products. Contact Dermatitis 2011;65:167-174

32   Yazar K, Johnsson S, Lind M-L, Boman A, Lidén C. Preservatives and fragrances in selected consumer-available cosmetics and detergents. Contact Dermatitis 2011;64:265-272

33   Gardner KH, Davis MD, Richardson DM, Pittelkow MR. The hazards of moist toilet paper: allergy to the preservative methylchloroisothiazolinone/ methylisothiazolinone. Arch Dermatol 2010;146:886-890

34   Garcia-Gavin J, Goossens A. Moist toilet paper: allergy to nonhalogenated derivative methylisothiazolinone preservative alone. Arch Dermatol 2010;146:1186

35   Fields KS, Nelson T, Powell D. Contact dermatitis caused by baby wipes. J Am Acad Dermatol 2006;54:S230-S232

36   Gruvberger B, Persson K, Björkner B, Bruze M, Dahlquist I, Fregert S. Demonstration of Kathon® CG in some commercial products. Contact Dermatitis 1986;15:24-27

37   Fortina AB, Romano I, Peserico A, Eichenfeld LE. Contact sensitization in very young children. J Am Acad Dermatol 2011;65:772-779

38   Fransway AF, Zug KA, Belsito DV, Deleo VA, Fowler JF Jr, Maibach HI, et al. North American Contact Dermatitis Group patch test results for 2007-2008. Dermatitis 2013;24:10-21

39 Warshaw EM, Belsito DV, DeLeo VA, Fowler JF Jr, Maibach HI, Marks JG, et al. North American Contact Dermatitis Group patch-test results, 2003-2004 study period. Dermatitis 2008;19:129-136

40 Zirwas MJ, Stechschulte SA. Moisturizer allergy. Diagnosis and management. J Clin Aesthetic Dermatol 2008;1:38-44

41 Wenk KS, Ehrlich AE. Fragrance series testing in eyelid dermatitis. Dermatitis 2012;23:22-26

42 Breuer K, Uter W, Geier J. Epidemiological data on airborne contact dermatitis – results of the IVDK. Contact Dermattis 2015;73:239-247

43 Vauhkala A-R, Pesonen M, Suomela S, Kuuliala O, Suuronen K, Aalto-Korte K. Occupational contact allergy to methylchloroisothiazolinone/methylisothiazolinone and methylisothiazolinone. Contact Dermatitis 2015;73:150-156

44 Ali FR, Shepherd EL, Yell LC, Buckley DA, Williams JDL. Escalating methylisothiazolinone/methylchloro-isothiazolinone allergy probably attributable to methylisothiazolinone in leave-on body cosmetics. Contact Dermatitis 2014;70:316-317

45 Commission Regulation (EU) No. 1003/2014 of 18 September 2014 amending Annex V to Regulation (EC) No. 1223/2009 of the European Parliament and of the Council on cosmetic products. Off J Eur Union 2014;L 282:1-4. Available at: http://eur-lex.europa.eu/legal-content/EN/TXT/?uri=uriserv:OJ.L_.2014.282.01.0001.01.ENG

46 Isaksson M, Persson L. Occupational contact dermatitis caused by methylchloroisothiazolinone/ methylisothiazolinone through exposure to filler dust containing this preservative and with a positive patch test reaction to the dust. Contact Dermatitis 2015;73:119-120

47 Isaksson M, Persson L. 'Mislabelled' make-up remover wet wipes as a cause of severe, recalcitrant facial eczema. Contact Dermatitis 2015;73:56-59

48 Urwin R, Warburton K, Carder M, Turner S, Agius R, Wilkinson SM. Methylchloroisothiazolinone and methylisothiazolinone contact allergy: an occupational perspective. Contact Dermatitis 2015;72:381-386

49 Warshaw EM, Maibach HI, Taylor JS, Sasseville D, DeKoven JG, Zirwas MJ, et al. North American Contact Dermatitis Group patch test results: 2011-2012. Dermatitis 2015;26:49-59

50 Warshaw EM, Belsito DV, Taylor JS, Sasseville D, DeKoven JG, Zirwas MJ, et al. North American Contact Dermatitis Group patch test results: 2009 to 2010. Dermatitis 2013;24:50-59

51 Janach M, Kühne A, Seifert B, French LE, Ballmer-Weber B, Hofbauer GFL. Changing delayed-type sensitizations to the baseline series allergens over a decade at the Zurich University Hospital. Contact Dermatitis 2010;63:42-48

52 Landeck L, John SM, Geier J. Periorbital dermatitis in 4779 patients – patch test results during a 10-year period. Contact Dermatitis 2014;70:205-212

53 Goossens A. Cosmetic contact allergens. Cosmetics 2016;3:5

54 Pratt MD, Belsito DV, DeLeo VA, Fowler JF Jr, Fransway AF, Maibach HI, et al. North American Contact Dermatitis Group patch-test results, 2001–2002 study period. Dermatitis 2004;15:176-183

55 Marks JG Jr, Belsito DV, DeLeo VA, Fowler JF Jr, Fransway AF, Maibach HI, et al. North American Contact Dermatitis Group patch-test results, 1998–2000. Am J Contact Dermat 2003;14:59-62

56 Jong CT, Statham BN, Green CM, King CM, Gawkrodger DJ, Sansom JE, et al. Contact sensitivity to preservatives in the UK 2004–2005: results of a multicenter study. Contact Dermatitis 2007;57:165-168

57 Lindberg M, Edman B, Fischer T, Stenberg B. Time trends in Swedish patch test data from 1992 to 2000. A multi-centre study based on age- and sex-adjusted results of the Swedish standard series. Contact Dermatitis 2007;56:205-210

58 Wetter DA, Davis MDP, Yiannias JA, Cheng JF, Connolly SM, el-Azhary RA, et al. Patch test results from the Mayo Contact Dermatitis Group, 1998–2000. J Am Acad Dermatol 2005;53:416-421

59 Britton JE, Wilkinson SM, English JSC, Gawkrodger DJ, Ormerod AD, Sansom JE, et al. The British standard series of contact dermatitis allergens: validation in clinical practice and value for clinical governance. Br J Dermatol 2003;148:259-264

60 Hasan T, Rantanen T, Alanko K, Harvima RJ, Jolanki R, Kalimo K, et al. Patch test reactions to cosmetic allergens in 1995–1997 and 2000–2002 in Finland –a multicentre study. Contact Dermatitis 2005;53:40-45

61 Lazarov A. European Standard Series patch test results from a contact dermatitis clinic in Israel during the 7-year period from 1998 to 2004. Contact Dermatitis 2006;55:73-76

62 Akyol A, Boyvat A, Peksari Y, Gurgey E. Contact sensitivity to standard series allergens in 1038 patients with contact dermatitis in Turkey. Contact Dermatitis 2005;52:333-337

63 Uter W, Hegewald J, Aberer W, Ayala F, Bircher AJ, Brasch J, et al. The European standard series in 9 European countries, 2002/2003 –First results of the European Surveillance System on Contact Allergies. Contact Dermatitis 2005;53:136-145

64 Machovcova A, Dastychova E, Kostalova D, et al. Common contact sensitizers in the Czech Republic. Patch test results in 12,058 patients with suspected contact dermatitis. Contact Dermatitis 2005;53:162-166

65 Bruynzeel DP, Diepgen TL, Andersen KE, Brandão FM, Bruze M, Frosch PJ, et al (EECDRG). Monitoring the European Standard Series in 10 centres 1996–2000. Contact Dermatitis 2005;53:146-152

66 Fall S, Bruze M, Isaksson M, Lidén C, Matura M, Stenberg B, Lindberg M. Contact allergy trends in Sweden – a retrospective comparison of patch test data from 1992, 2000, and 2009. Contact Dermatitis 2015;72:297-304

67 Amin KA, Belsito DV. The aetiology of eyelid dermatitis: a 10-year retrospective analysis. Contact Dermatitis 2006;55:280-285

68 Lee SS, Hong DK, Jeong NJ, Lee JH, Choi YS, Lee AY, et al. Multicenter study of preservative sensitivity in patients with suspected cosmetic contact dermatitis in Korea. J Dermatol 2012;39:677-681

69 Cooper SM, Shaw S. Eyelid dermatitis: an evaluation of 232 patch test patients over 5 years. Contact Dermatitis 2000: 42;291-293

70 Wentworth AB, Yiannias JA, Keeling JH, Hall MR, Camilleri MJ, Drage LA, et al. Trends in patch-test results and allergen changes in the standard series: a Mayo Clinic 5-year retrospective review (January 1, 2006, to December 31, 2010). J Am Acad Dermatol 2014;70:269-275

71 Cheng S, Leow YH, Goh CL, Goon A. contact sensitivity to preservatives in Singapore: frequency of sensitization to 11 common preservatives 2006–2011. Dermatitis 2014;25:77-82

72 Valks R, Conde-Salazar L, Malfeito J, Ledo S. Contact dermatitis in hairdressers, 10 years later: patch-test results in 300 hairdressers (1994 to 2003) and comparison with previous study. Dermatitis 2005;16:28-31

73 Uter W, Lessmann H, Geier J, Schnuch A. Contact allergy to ingredients of hair cosmetics in female hairdressers and clients: an 8-year analysis of IVDK data. Contact Dermatitis 2003;49:236-240

74 Thyssen JP, Uter W, Schnuch A, Linneberg A, Johansen JD. 10-year prevalence of contact allergy in the general population in Denmark estimated through the CE-DUR method. Contact Dermatitis 2007;57:265-272

75 Schnuch A, Uter W, Geier J, Gefeller O (for the IVDK study group). Epidemiology of contact allergy: an estimation of morbidity employing the clinical epidemiology and drug-utilization research (CE-DUR) approach. Contact Dermatitis 2002;47:32-39

76 Diepgen TL, Ofenloch RF, Bruze M, Bertuccio P, Cazzaniga S, Coenraads P-J, et al. Prevalence of contact allergy in the general population in different European regions. Br J Dermatol 2016;174:319-329

77 Mortz CG, Bindslev-Jensen C, Andersen KE. Prevalence, incidence rates and persistence of contact allergy and allergic contact dermatitis in The Odense Adolescence Cohort Study: a 15-year follow-up. Brit J Dermatol 2013;168:318-325

78 Thyssen JP, Linneberg A, Menné T, Nielsen NH, Johansen JD. Contact allergy to allergens of the TRUE-test (panels 1 and 2) has decreased modestly in the general population. Br J Dermatol 2009;161:1124-1129

79 Nielsen SH, Menné T. Allergic contact sensitization in an unselected Danish population. The Glostrup Allergy Study, Denmark. Acta Derm Venereol 1992;72:456-460

80 Dotterud LK, Smith-Sivertsen T. Allergic contact sensitization in the general adult population: a population-based study from Northern Norway. Contact Dermatitis 2007;56:10-15

81 Nielsen NH, Linneberg A, Menné T, Madsen F, Frølund L, Dirksen A, et al. Allergic contact sensitization in an adult Danish population: two cross-sectional surveys eight years apart (the Copenhagen Allergy Study). Acta Derm Venereol 2001;81:31-34

82 White JML, Gilmour NJ, Jeffries D, Duangdeeden I, Kullavanijaya P, Basketter DA, et al. A general population from Thailand: incidence of common allergens with emphasis on para-phenylenediamine. Clin Exp Allergy 2007;37:1848-1853

83 Mortz CG, Lauritsen JM, Bindslev-Jensen C, Andersen KE. Contact allergy and allergic contact dermatitis in adolescents: prevalence measures and associations. Acta Derm Venereol 2002;82:352-358

84 Schäfer T, Böhler E, Ruhdorfer S, Weigl L, Wessner D, Filipiak B, et al. Epidemiology of contact allergy in adults. Allergy 2001;56:1192-1196

85 Mortz CG, Lauritsen JM, Bindslev-Jensen C, Andersen KE. Prevalence of atopic dermatitis, asthma, allergic rhinitis, and hand and contact dermatitis in adolescents. The Odense Adolescence Cohort Study on Atopic Diseases and Dermatitis. Br J Dermatol 2001;144:523-532

86 Seidenari S, Manzini BM, Danese P, Motolese A. Patch and prick test study of 593 healthy subjects. Contact Dermatitis 1990; 23:162-167

87 Uter W, Ludwig A, Balda BR, Schnuch A, Pfahlberg A, Schäfer T, Wichmann HE, Ring J. The prevalence of contact allergy differed between population-based data and clinic–based data. J Clin Epidemiol 2004;57:627-632

88 De Groot AC, Bruynzeel DP, Bos JD, van der Meeren HL, van Joost T, Jagtman BA, Weyland JW. The allergens in cosmetics. Arch Dermatol 1988;124:1525-1529

89 De Groot AC. Adverse reactions to cosmetics. PhD Thesis, University of Groningen, The Netherlands: 1988, chapter 3.4, pp.105-113

90 De Groot AC. Contact allergy to cosmetics: Causative ingredients. Contact Dermatitis 1987;17:26-34

91 De Groot AC, Beverdam E, Tjong Ayong C, Coenraads PJ, Nater JP. The role of contact allergy in the spectrum of adverse effects caused by cosmetics and toiletries. Contact Dermatitis 1988;19:195-201

92 Sugai T. Allergic cosmetic dermatitis from Kathon CG. Data presented at the 8th International Symposium on Contact Dermatitis, Cambridge, march 20-22, 1986

93 Foussereau J, Brändle I, Boujnah-Khouadja A. Allergisches Kontaktekzeem durch Isothiazolin-3-on-Derivate. Dermatosen 1984;32:208-211

94 Zoli V, Tosti A, Silvani S, Vincenzi C. Moist toilet papers as possible sensitizers: review of the literature and evaluation of commercial products in Italy. Contact Dermatitis 2006;55:252-254

95 Flyvholm, MA. Preservatives in registered chemical products. Contact Dermatitis 2005;53:27-32

96 Herbst RA, Uter W, Pirker C, Geier J, Frosch PJ. Allergic and non-allergic periorbital dermatitis: patch test results of the Information Network of the Departments of Dermatology during a 5-year period. Contact Dermatitis 2004;51:13-19

97 Emmons WW, Marks JG. Immediate and delayed reactions to cosmetic ingredients. Contact Dermatitis 1985;13:258-265

98 Rastogi SC. Analytical control of preservative labelling on skin creams. Contact Dermatitis 2000;43:339-343

99 Katsarou A, Armenaka M, Ale I, Koufou V, Kalogeromitros, D. Frequency of immediate reactions to the European standard series. Contact Dermatitis 1999;41:276-279

100 Held E, Johansen JD, Agner T, Menné T. Contact allergy to cosmetics: testing with patients' own products. Contact Dermatitis 1999;40:310-315

101 Scheman A, Jacob S, Katta R, Nedorost S, Warshaw E, Zirwas M, et al. Part 2 of a 4 part series. Hair cosmetics: trends and alternatives. Data from the American Contact Alternative Group. J Clin Aesthet Dermatol 2011;4:42-46

102 Scheman A, Jacob S, Katta R, Nedorost S, Warshaw E, Zirwas M, et al. Part 4 of a 4 part series. Miscellaneous products: trends and alternatives in deodorants, antiperspirants, sunblocks, shaving products, powder, and wipes. Data from the American Contact Alternative Group. J Clin Aesthet Dermatol 2011;4:35-39

103 Neza E, Centini M. Microbiologically contaminated and over-preserved cosmetic products according Rapex 2008–2014. Cosmetics 2016, 3, 3; doi:10.3390/cosmetics3010003

104 SCCS (Scientific Committee on Consumer Safety). Opinion on the mixture of 5-chloro-2-methylisothiazolin-3(2H)-one and 2-methylisothiazolin-3(2H)-one, 8 December 2009, SCCS/1238/09. Available from: http://ec.europa.eu/health/scientific_committees/consumer_safety/docs/sccs_o_009.pdf

105 SCCP (Scientific Committee on Consumer Products). Clarification of the SCCNFP Opinion on the Update of Entry n° 39 of Annex VI to Directive 76/768/EEC on Cosmetic Products: Mixture of 5-Chloro-2-Methyl-Isothiazolin-3(2H)-one and 2-Methylisothiazolin-3(2H)-one, 7 December 2004, SCCP/0849/04. Available at: http://ec.europa.eu/health/archive/ph_risk/committees/04_sccp/docs/sccp_o_00a.pdf

106 SCCNFP (Scientific Committee on Cosmetics and Non Food Products). Opinion concerning update of entry n° 39 of annex VI to Directive 76/768/EEC on cosmetic products: mixture of 5-chloro-2-methyl-isothiazolin-3-one and 2-methylisothiazolin-3(2H)-one, 24-25 June 2003, SCCNFP/0670/03. Available at: http://ec.europa.eu/health/archive/ph_risk/committees/sccp/documents/out221_en.pdf

107 Laguna C, de la Cuadra J, Martín-González B, Zaragoza V, Martínez-Casimiro L, Alegre V. Allergic contact dermatitis to cosmetics. Actas Dermosifiliogr 2009;100:53-60

108 Toholka R, Wang Y-S, Tate B, Tam M, Cahill J, Palmer A, Nixon R. The first Australian Baseline Series: Recommendations for patch testing in suspected contact dermatitis. Australas J Dermatol 2015;56:107-115

109 Zhao J, Li LF. Contact sensitization to cosmetic series of allergens in a general population in Beijing. J Cosmet Dermatol 2014;13:68-71

110 Maibach HI. Diagnostic patch test concentration for Kathon CG. Contact Dermatitis 1985;13:242-245

111 Weaver JE, Cardin C, Maibach HI. Dose-response assessments of Kathon® biocide (I). Diagnostic use and diagnostic threshold patch testing with sensitized humans. Contact Dermatitis 1985;12:141-145

112 Kathon CG- Product information sheet 1983. Rohm and Haas, Philadelphia, USA (cited in ref. 23)

113 Chan PK, Baldwin RC, Parsons RD, Moss JN, Stiratelli R, Smith JM, et al. Kathon biocide: manifestation of delayed contact dermatitis in guinea pigs is dependent on the concentration for induction and challenge. J Invest Dermatol 1983;81:409-411

114 Tosti A, Manuzzi P, Padova MP. Contact dermatitis to Kathon CG. Contact Dermatitis 1986;14:326-327

115 Pilger C, Nethercott JR, Weksberg F. Allergic contact dermatitis due to a biocide containing 5-chloro-2-methyl-4-isothiazohn-3-one. Contact Dermatitis 1986;14:201-204

116 Hjorth N, Roed-Petersen J. Patch test sensitivity to Kathon® CG. Contact Dermatitis 1986;14:155-157

117 Björkner B, Bruze M, Dahlquist I, Fregert S, Gruvberger B, Persson K. Contact allergy to the preservative Kathon® CG. Contact Dermatitis 1986;14:199-200

118 Björkner B, Bruze M, Dahlquist I, Fregert S, Gruvberger B, Persson K. Contact allergy to the preservative Kathon® CG. Contact Dermatitis 1986;14:85-90

119 Ping KC, Baldwin RC, Parsons RD, Moss JN, Stiratelli R, Smith JM, Hayes AW. Kathon biocide: manifestation of delayed contact dermatitis in guinea pigs is dependent on the concentration for induction and challenge. J Invest Dermatol 1983;81:409-411

120 Foussereau J, Brändle I, Boujnah-Khouadja A. Allergisches Kontaktekzem durch Isothiazolin-3-on-Derivate. Derm Beruf Umwelt 1984;32:208-211

121 De Groot AC, Bos JD. Preservatives in the European standard Series for epicutaneous testing. Br J Dermatol 1987;116:289-292

122 De Groot AC: Isothiazolinone preservative as important contact allergen in cosmetics. Dermatosen 1987;35:169-173

123 Shuster S, Spiro J. Measurement of risk of sensitisation and its application to Kathon. Contact Dermatitis 1987;17:299-302

124 Meneghini CL, Angelini G, Vena GA. Contact allergy to Kathon® CG. Contact Dermatitis 1987;17:247-249

125 Angelini G, Vena GA, Meneghini CL. Dermatitis da contatto con kathon ® CG. Boll Derm Allerg Profes 1986;1:20-23 (article in Italian)

126 De Groot AC, Bruynzeel DP. Kathon CG. Contact Dermatitis 1987;17:189-190

127 Schwartz SR, Weiss S, Stern E, Morici IJ, Moss JN, Goodman JJ, Scarborough NL. Human safety study of body lotion containing Kathon® CG. Contact Dermatitis 1987;16:203-207

128 Bruze M, Dahlquist I, Fregert S, Gruvberger B, Persson K. Contact allergy to the active ingredients of Kathon® CG. Contact Dermatitis 1987;16:183-188

129 Farm G, Wahlberg JE. Positive test reactions to Kathon® in patients with work-related skin disease. Contact Dermatitis 1987;16:228-229

130 De Groot AC, Weyland JW. Kathon CG. A review. J Am Acad Dermatol 1988;18:350-358

131 Decker RL Jr. Frequency of preservative use in cosmetic formulas as disclosed to FDA--1984. Cosmetics and Toiletries 1985;100:65-68

132 De Groot AC, Barella CGJ, Conemans JMH. Unpublished observations, 1987 (cited in ref. 130)

133 Fuchs T (or Ippen H). Aktuelle Kontaktallergene und ihre Perspektiven. Die Medizinische Welt 1986;37:1305-1307

134 Frosch PJ, Schulze-Dirks A. Kontaktallergie auf Kathon CG. Hautarzt 1987;38:422-425

135 Fransway AF. Sensitivity to Kathon CG: findings in 365 consecutive patients. Contact Dermatitis 1988;19:342-347

136 Menné T, Hjorth N. Kathon® CG reactivity in 1396 consecutively patch tested patients in the Copenhagen area. Contact Dermatitis 1988;19:260-262

137 Rastogi SC. Kathon CG content in cosmetic products. Contact Dermatitis 1988;19:263

138 De Groot AC, Barella CGJ, Conemans JMH. Risk of Sensitization to Kathon CG. Contact Dermatitis 1988;19:210-211

139 O'Driscoll JB, Beck MH. Occupational allergic contact dermatitis from Kathon® WT. Contact Dermatitis 1988;19:63

140 Cronin E, Hannuksela M, Lachapelle JM, Maibach HI, Malten K, Meneghini CL. Frequency of sensitisation to the preservative Kathon® CG. Contact Dermatitis 1988;18:274-279

141 Cox NH, Shuster S. Risk of sensitisation to Kathon. Contact Dermatitis 1988;18:54-55

142 Marston S. Kathon CG in cosmetics. Contact Dermatitis 1988;18:58-59

143 De Groot A, Herxheimer A. Isothiazolinone preservative: Cause of a continuing epidemic of cosmetic dermatitis. Lancet 1989;1:314-316

144 Minet A, Eggers S, Willocx D, Bourlond A, Lachapelle JM. Allergic contact dermatitis from kathon CG™ in moist toilet paper. Contact Dermatitis 1989;21:107-108

145 Bruze M, Dahlquist I, Gruvberger B. Contact allergy to dichlorinated methylisothiazolinone. Contact Dermatitis 1989;20:219-220

146 Pasche F, Hunziker N. Sensitization to Kathon CG in Geneva and Switzerland. Contact Dermatitis 1989;20:115-119

147 Rietschel RL, Nethercott JR, Emmet EA, Maibach HI, Storrs FJ, Larsen WG, et al. Methylchloroisothiazolinone-methylisothiazolinone reactions in patients screened for vehicle and preservative hypersensitivity. J Am Acad Dermatol 1990;22:734-738

148 Aberer W, Retter E, Gailhofer G. Pitfalls in patch testing: problems with rather than from Kathon CG. Contact Dermatitis 1990;23:380-381

149 Aberer W, Philipp T, Ludvan M, Gailhofer G. Sensitization to Kathon CG in Austria: low sensitization rate, no clinical relevance, and controversial literature data. Contact Dermatitis 1990;23:247-248

150 Shehade S, Beck M, Muston H. Industrial sensitization to Kathon WT and organic bromide compounds used as slimicides in the paper industry. Contact Dermatitis 1990;23:247

151 Dooms-Goossens A, Morren M, Dierickx C, Mariën K. A patient bothered by unexpected sources of isothiazolinones. Contact Dermatitis 1990;23:192-193

152 Andersen KE, Burrows D, Cronin E, Dooms-Goossens A, Rycroft RJG, White IR and ICDRG and EECDRG, Recommended changes to standard series. Contact Dermatitis 1988;19:391

153 Brown R. 2 cases of occupational allergy to Kathon 886. Contact Dermatitis 1990;23:116

154 Hasson A, Guimaraens D, Conde-Salazar L. Patch test sensitivity to the preservative Kathon CG in Spain. Contact Dermatitis 1990;22:257-261

155 De Groot AC. Water versus petrolatum as vehicle for patch testing methylisothiazolinone + methylchloroisothiazolinone (Kathon CG). Contact Dermatitis 1990;22:300-301

156 Bruze M, Gruvberger B, Hradil E. Occupational allergic contact dermatitis due to methylisothiazolinones in a cleansing cream. Contact Dermatitis 1990;22:235-237

157 De Groot AC. Methylisothiazolinone/methylchloroisothiazolinone (Kathon CG) allergy: An updated review. Am J Cont Derm 1990;1:151-156

158 Kimmig W, Schulz KH. Aktuelle Kontaktallergene. Dtsch Dermatol 1986;34:662-671 (article in German, data cited in ref. 157)

159 Kleinhans D. Kontaktallergie gegen Isothiazolinone (Kathon ® CG, Euxyl ® K100). In kosmetische Produkten. Derm Kosmet 1987;28:27-33 (article in German, data cited in ref. 157)

160 Marks JG Jr, Moss JN, Parno JR, Fowler JF Jr, Storrs FJ, Belsito DV, et al. Methylchloroisothiazolinone/Methyl-isothiazolinone (Kathon CG) biocide- United States multicenter study of human skin sensitization. Am J Cont Derm 1990;1:157-161

161 Menné, T, Frosch PJ, Veien NK, Hannuksela M, Björkner B, Lachapelle JM, et al. Contact sensitization to 5-chloro-2-methyl-4-isothiazolin-3-one and 2-methyl-4-isothiazolin-3-one (MCI/MI). Contact Dermatitis 1991;24:334-341

162 Rastogi SC. Kathon CG and cosmetic products. Contact Dermatitis 1990;22:155-160

163 Martin-Falero AA, Calderòn Gutierrez MJ, Díaz-Pérez JL. Contact allergy to the preservative Kathon CG. Contact Dermatitis 1990;22:185

164 Macháčková J, Kalenský J, Vocilková A. Patch test sensitivity to Kathon CG in Prague. Contact Dermatitis 1990;22:189-191

165 Zemtsov A. A case of contact allergy to Kathon® CG in the United States. Contact Dermatitis 1991;25:135

166 Menné T. Relationship between use test and threshold patch test concentration in patients sensitive to 5-chloro-2-methyl-4-isothiazolin-3-one and 2-methyl-4-isothiazolin-3-one (MCI/MI). Contact Dermatitis 1991;24:375

167 De Groot AC, Baar TJM, Terpstra H, Weyland JW. Contact allergy to moist toilet paper. Contact Dermatitis 1991;24:135-136

168 Nethercott JR, Rothman N, Holness DL, O'Toole T. Health problems in metalworkers exposed to a coolant oil containing Kathon WT. Am J Cont Derm 1990;1:94-99

169 Schwensen JF, Menné Bonefeld C, Zachariae C, Agerbeck CH, Petersen T, Geisler C, et al. Cross-reactivity between methylisothiazolinone, octylisothiazolinone and benzisothiazolinone using a modified local lymph node assay. Br J Dermatol 2017;176:176-183

170 Schwensen JF, Menné T, Andersen KE, Sommerlund M, Johansen JD. Occupations at risk of developing contact allergy to isothiazolinones in Danish contact dermatitis patients: results from a Danish multicentre study (2009-2012). Contact Dermatitis 2014;71:295-302

171 Khunkhet S, Wattanakrai P. The possible role of contact sensitization to fragrances and preservatives in poikiloderma of civatte. Case Rep Dermatol 2014;6:258-263

172 Lundov MD, Menné T. Airborne exposure to methylchloroisothiazolinone and methylisothiazolinone from a toilet cleaner. Contact Dermatitis 2013;68:252-253

173 Toledo F, García-Bravo B, Fernández-Redondo V, De la Cuadra J, Giménez-Arnau AM, Borrego L, Carrascosa JM, et al. Patch testing in children with hand eczema. A 5-year multicentre study in Spain. Contact Dermatitis 2011;65:213-219

174 Magnano M, Silvani S, Vincenzi C, Nino M, Tosti A. Contact allergens and irritants in household washing and cleaning products. Contact Dermatitis 2009;61:337-341

175 Coloe J, Zirwas MJ. Allergens in corticosteroid vehicles. Dermatitis 2008;19:38-42

176 Zaragoza-Ninet V, Blasco Encinas R, Vilata-Corell JJ, Pérez-Ferriols A, Sierra-Talamantes C, Esteve-Martínez A, de la Cuadra-Oyanguren J. Allergic contact dermatitis due to cosmetics: A clinical and epidemiological study in a tertiary hospital. Actas Dermosifiliogr 2016;107:329-336

177 DeKoven JG, Warshaw EM, Belsito DV, Sasseville D, Maibach HI, Taylor JS, et al. North American Contact Dermatitis Group Patch Test Results: 2013-2014. Dermatitis 2016 Oct 21. [Epub ahead of print]

178 Wittenberg JB, Canas BJ, Zhou W, Wang PG, Rua D, Krynitsky AJ. Determination of methylisothiazolinone and methylchloroisothiazolinone in cosmetic products by ultra high performance liquid chromatography with tandem mass spectrometry. J Sep Sci 2015;38:2983-2988

179 Hunziker N, Pasche F, Bircher A, et al. Sensitization to the isothiazolinone biocide. Report of the Swiss Contact Dermatitis Research Group 1988–1990. Dermatology 1992;184:94-97

180 Rycroft RJG, Neild VS. Allergic contact dermatitis from MCI/MI biocide in a printer. Contact Dermatitis 1992;26:142

181 Reid CM, Rycroft RJG. Allergic contact dermatitis from sources of MCI/MI biocide and formaldehyde in a printer. Contact Dermatitis 1993;28:252-253

182 Marks JG Jr, Moss JN, Parno JR, Adams RM, Belsito DV, DeLeo VA, et al. Methylchloroisothiazolinone/methyl-isothiazolinone (Kathon CG) biocide: Second United States multicenter study of human skin sensitization. Am I Cont Derm 1993;4:87-89

183 Madden SD, Thiboutot DM, Marks JG. Occupationally induced allergic contact dermatitis to methylchloro-isothiazolinone/methylisothiazolinone among machinists. J Am Acad Dermatol 1994;30:272-274

184 Finkbeiner H, Kleinhans D. Airborne allergic contact dermatitis caused by preservatives in home-decorating paints. Contact Dermatitis 1994;31:275-276

185 Nielsen H. Occupational exposure to isothiazolinones. A study based on a product register. Contact Dermatitis 1994;31:18-21

186 Tay P, Ng SK. Delayed skin burns from MCI/MI biocide used in water treatment. Contact Dermatitis 1994;30:54-55

187 Clark EG. Risk of isothiazolinones. J Soc Occup Med 1987;37:30-31

188 De Corrès LF, Navarro JA, Gastaminza G, Del Pozo MD. An unusual case of sensitization to methylchloro- and methylisothiazolinone (MCI/MI). Contact Dermatitis 1995;33:215-216

189 Jacobs M-C, Lachapelle J-M, White IR, McFadden JP. Assessment of continuing sensitivity to MCI/MI (Kathon™ CG). Contact Dermatitis 1995;33:69

190 Frosch PJ, Lahti A, Hannuksela M, Andersen KE, Wilkinson JD, Shaw S, Lachapelle JM. Chloromethylisothiazo-lone/methylisothiazolone (CMI/MI) use test with a shampoo on patch-test-positive subjects Results of a multicentre double-blind crossover trial. Contact Dermatitis 1995;32:210-217

191 Guimaraens D, Condé-Salazar L, Gonzalez MA. Allergic contact dermatitis on the hands from chloromethyliso-thiazolinone in moist toilet paper. Contact Dermatitis 1996;35:254

192 Pazzaglia M, Vincenzi C, Gasparri F, Tosti A. Occupational hypersensitivity to isothiazolinone derivatives in a radiology technician. Contact Dermatitis 1996;34:143-144

193 Bruze M, Gruvberger B, Björkner B. Kathon® CG: an unusual contact sensitizer. In: Menné T, Maibach HI, eds. Exogenous dermatosen: environmental dermatitis. Boston: CRC Press, 1991:283-298

194 Geier J, Schnuch A. No cross-sensitization between MCI/MI, benzisothiazolinone and octylisothiazolinone. Contact Dermatitis 1996;34:148-149

195 Bruynzeel DP, Verburgh CA. Occupational dermatitis from isothiazolinones in diesel oil. Contact Dermatitis 1996;34:64-65

196 Gebhardt M, Looks A, Hipler U C. Urticaria caused by type IV sensitization to isothiazolinones. Contact Dermatitis 1997;36:314

197 Bourke SJ, Convery RP, Stenton SC, Malcolm RM, Hendrick DJ. Occupational asthma in an isothiazolinone manufacturing plant. Thorax 1997;52:746-748

198 Schubert H. Airborne contact dermatitis due to methylchloro- and methylisothiazolinone (MCI/MI). Contact Dermatitis 1997;36:274

199 De Groot AC. Vesicular dermatitis of the hands secondary to perianal allergic contact dermatitis caused by preservatives in moistened toilet tissues. Contact Dermatitis 1997';36:173-174

200 Primka EJ III, Taylor JS. Three cases of contact allergy after chemical burns from methylchloroisothiazolinone/methylisothiazolinone: one with concomitant allergy to methyldibromoglutaronitrile/phenoxyethanol. Am J Cont Derm 1997;8:43-46

201 Kanerva L, Tarvainen K, Pinola A, Leino T, Granlund H, Estlander T, et al. A single accidental exposure may result in a chemical burn, primary sensitization and allergic contact dermatitis. Contact Dermatitis 1994;31:229-235

202 Bruze M, Dahlquist I, Gruvberger B. Chemical burns and allergic contact dermatitis due to Kathon WT. Am J Cont Derm 1990;1:91-93

203 Podmore P. An epidemic of isothiazolinone sensitization in a flax spinning mill. Contact Dermatitis 1998;38:165-166

204 Fewings J, Menné T. An update of the risk assessment for methylchloroisothiazolinone/methylisothiazolinone (MCI/MI) with focus on rinse-off products. Contact Dermatitis 1999;41:1-13

205 Gruvberger B, Bruze M, Tammela M. Preservatives in moisturizers on the Swedish market. Acta Dermato-venereologica (Stockh) 1998;78:52-56

206 Morren MA, Dooms-Goossens A, Delabie J, De Wolf-Peeters C, Mariën K, Degreef H. Contact allergy to isothiazolinone derivatives: unusual clinical presentations. Dermatology 1992;184:260-264

207 Fewings J, Menné T. An update of the risk assessment for methylchloroisothiazolinone/methylisothiazolinone (MCI/MI) with focus on rinse-off products. Contact Dermatitis 1999;41:1-13

208 Fischer T, Bohlin S, Edling C, Rystedt I, Wieslander G. Skin disease and contact sensitivity in house painters using water-based paints. glues and putties. Contact Dermatitis 1995;32:39-45

209 Gruvberger B, Bruze M, Almgren G. Occupational dermatoses in a plant producing binders for paints and glues. Contact Dermatitis 1998;38:71-77

210 Valsecchi R, Leghissa P, Piazzolla S, Cainelli T, Seghizzi P. Occupational dermatitis from isothiazolinones in the nylon production. Dermatology 1993;187:109-111

211 Tosti A, Bassi R, Peluso AM. Contact dermatitis due to a natural plasticine. Contact Dermatitis 1990;22:301-302

212 Gruvberger B. Methylisothiazolinones. Diagnosis and prevention of allergic contact dermatitis. Acta Dermato-venereologica 1997;200:(Suppl,): 1–42

213 Majamaa H, Roto P, Vaalasti A. Airborne occupational hypersensitivity to isothiazolinones in a papermaking technician. Contact Dermatitis 1999;41:220

214 Lee TY, Lam TH. Allergic contact dermatitis due to Kathon® CG in Hong Kong. Contact Dermatitis 1999;41:41-42

215 Bohn S, Niederer M, Brehm K, Bircher AJ. Airborne contact dermatitis from methylchloroisothiazolinone in wall paint. Abolition of symptoms by chemical allergen inactivation. Contact Dermatitis 2000;42:196-201

216 Bentrop I. Aerogenes Kontaktekzem auf (Chlor)Methylisothiazolon in einer Wandfarbe. Allergo J 1999;8:39-40 (article in German)

217 Hausen BM. Aerogene Kontaktdermatitis durch (Chlor)-methylisothiazolinon (Kathon CG) in Wandfarben. Akt Dermatol 1999;25:9-14 (article in German)

218 Podmore P. Occupational allergic contact dermatitis from both 2-bromo-2-nitropropane-1,3-diol and methylchloroisothiazolinone plus methylisothiazolinone in spin finish. Contact Dermatitis 2000;43:45

219 Guin JD, Kincannon J, Church FL. Baby-wipe dermatitis: preservative-induced hand eczema in parents and persons using moist towelettes. Am J Cont Derm 2001;12:189-192

220 Reinhard E, Waeber R, Niederer M, Maurer T, Maly P, Scherer S. Preservation of products with MCI/MI in Switzerland. Contact Dermatitis 2001;45:257-264

221 Sahoo B, Kumar B. Rôle of methylchloroisothiazolinone/methylisothiazolinone (Kathon® CG) in poikiloderma of Civatte. Contact Dermatitis 2001;44:249

222 Corazza M, Mantovani L, Bacilieri S, Virgili A. A child with "occupational" allergic contact dermatitis due to MCI/MI. Contact Dermatitis 2001;44:53

223 Tosti A, Voudouris S, Pazzaglia M. Contact sensitization to 5-chloro-2-methyl-4-isothiazolin-3-one and 2-methyl-4-isothiazolin-3-one in children. Contact Dermatitis 2003;49:215-216

224 Isaksson M, Gruvberger B. Patch test sensitization to methylchloroisothiazolinone + methylisothiazolinone and 4,4'-diaminodiphenylmethane. Contact Dermatitis 2003;48:53-54

225 Isaksson M, Gruvberger B, Bruze M. Occupational contact allergy and dermatitis from methylisothiazolinone after contact with wall covering glue and after a chemical burn from a biocide. Dermatitis 2004;15:201-205

226 Hardcastle NJ, Gawkrodger DJ. Occupational contact dermatitis to 1,2-benzisothiazolin-3-one and 5-chloro-2-methylisothiazolin-3-one/2-methylisothiazolin-3-one in paint manufacturers. Contact Dermatitis 2005;53:115-116

227 Jensen J-M, Harde V, Brasch J. Airborne contact dermatitis to methylchloroisothiazolinone/methylisothiazolinone in a boy. Contact Dermatitis 2006;55:311

228 Zachariae C, Lerbæk A, McNamee PM, Gray JE, Wooder M, Menné T. An evaluation of dose/unit area and time as key factors influencing the elicitation capacity of methylchloroisothiazolinone/methylisothiazolinone (MCI/MI) in MCI/MI-allergic patients. Contact Dermatitis 2006;55:160-166

229 Bayraktar A, Ozcan M. An unusual case: burn following an accidental exposure to methylchloroisothiazolinone/methylisothiazolinone. J Burn Care Res 2007;28:195-197

230 Brasch J, Becker D, Aberer W, Bircher A, Kränke B, Denzer-Fürst S, Schnuch A. Contact Dermatitis. J Dtsch Dermatol Ges 2007;5: 943-951

231 Uter W, Lessmann H, Geier J, Schnuch A. Contact allergy to hairdressing allergens in female hairdressers and clients – current data from the IVDK 2003–2006. J Dtsch Dermatol Ges 2007;5:993-1001

232 Timmermans A, De Hertog S, Gladys K, Vanacker H, Goossens A. 'Dermatologically tested' baby toilet tissues: a cause of allergic contact dermatitis in adults. Contact Dermatitis 2007;57:97-99

233 Steinberg DC. Voluntary registration of cosmetics and 2007 frequency of preservative use. Cosmet Toiletries Mag 2008;123:47-52

234 Hunter KJ, Shelley JC, Haworth AE. Airborne allergic contact dermatitis to methylchloroisothiazolinone/methylisothiazolinone in ironing water. Contact Dermatitis 2008;58:183-184

235 Isaksson M, Bruze M, Gruvberger B. Cross-reactivity between methylchloroisothiazolinone/methylisothiazolinone, methylisothiazolinone, and other isothiazolinones in workers at a plant producing binders for paints and glues. Contact Dermatitis 2008;58:60-62

236 Temesvári E, Pónyai G, Németh I, Hidvégi B, Sas S, Kárpáti S. Periocular dermatitis: a report of 401 patients. JEADV 2009;23:124-128

237 Kwok T, Nethercott JR, Skotnicki-Grant S. Contact dermatitis by proxy: a criminal cause of MCI/MI allergy. Dermatitis 2009;20:224-225

238 Mendese G, Beckford A, Demierre M F. Lymphomatoid contact dermatitis to baby wipes. Arch Dermatol 2010;146:934-935

239 Cuesta L, Silvestre JF, Toledo F, Ballester I, Betlloch I . Delayed hypersensitivity to methylchloroisothiazolinone /methylisothiazolinone not detected by the baseline series of the Spanish group. Contact Dermatitis 2010;62:250-251

240 Statham BN, Smith EV, Bodger OG, Green CM, King CM, Ormerod AD, et al. Concomitant contact allergy to methylchloroisothiazolinone/ methylisothiazolinone and formaldehyde-releasing preservatives. Contact Dermatitis 2010;62:56-57

241 Willi R, Pfab F, Zilker T, Buters J, Schalock P, Huss-Marp J, Todorova A, Ring J, Darsow U. Danger from the workplace: allergic contact dermatitis from the first exposure to isothiazolinones. Contact Dermatitis 2011;64:361-362

242 Scheman A, Jacob S, Katta R, Nedorost S, Warshaw E, Zirwas M, et al. Part 1 of a 4 part series. Facial cosmetics: trends and alternatives. Data from the American Contact Alternative Group. J Clin Aesthet Dermatol 2011;4:25-30

243 Scheman A, Jacob S, Katta R, Nedorost S, Warshaw E, Zirwas M, et al. Part 3 of a 4 part series. Lips and common Dental Care products: trends and alternatives. Data from the American Contact Alternative Group. J Clin Aesthet Dermatol 2011;4:50-53

244 Alvarez-Rivera G, Dagnac T, Lores M, Garcia-Jares C, Sanchez-Prado L, Lamas JP, Llompart M. Determination of isothiazolinone preservatives in cosmetics and household products by matrix solid-phase dispersion followed by high-performance liquid chromatography-tandem mass spectrometry. J Chromatogr A 2012;1270:41-50

245 Friis UF, Menné T, Thyssen JP, Johansen JD. A patient's drawing helped the physician to make the correct diagnosis: occupational contact allergy to isothiazolinone. Contact Dermatitis 2012;67:174-176

246 Higgins E, Kirby B, Rogers S, Collins P. Methylchloroisothiazolinone and methylisothiazolinone allergic contact dermatitis and the effect of patch test concentration. Dermatitis 2013;24:73-76

247 Chow ET, Avolio AM, Lee A, Nixon R. Frequency of positive patch test reactions to preservatives: The Australian experience. Australas J Dermatol 2013;54:31-35

248 Bregnbak D, Lundov MD, Zachariae C, Menné T, Johansen JD. Five cases of severe chronic dermatitis caused by isothiazolinones. Contact Dermatitis 2013;69:57-59

249 Urwin R, Wilkinson M. Methylchloroisothiazolinone and methylisothiazolinone contact allergy: a new 'epidemic'. Contact Dermatitis 2013;68:253-255

250 Leiva-Salinas M, Frances L, Marin-Cabanas I, Bouret AM, Silvestre JF. Methylchloroisothiazolinone/methyl-isothiazolinone and methylisothiazolinone allergies can be detected by 200 ppm of methylchloroisothiazolinone/ methylisothiazolinone patch test concentration. Dermatitis 2014;25:130-134

251 Bruze M, Goossens A, Isaksson M. Recommendation to increase the test concentration of methylchloroiso-thiazolinone/methylisothiazolinone in the European baseline patch test series – on behalf of the European Society of Contact Dermatitis and the European Environmental and Contact Dermatitis Research Group. Contact Dermatitis 2014;71:35-40

252 Verdelli A, Francalanci S, Palleschi GM. Contact allergic dermatitis due to Kathon CG contained in ultrasound gel. Dermatitis 2014;25:35-36

253 Aerts O, Baeck M, Constandt L, Dezfoulian B, Jacobs M-C, Kerre S, et al. The dramatic increase in the rate of methylisothiazolinone contact allergy in Belgium: a multicentre study. Contact Dermatitis 2014;71:41-48

254 Knackstedt TJ, Zug KA. T-cell lymphomatoid contact dermatitis: a challenging case and review of the literature. Contact Dermatitis 2014;72:65-74

255 Fischer Friis U, Menné T, Flyvholm M-A, Ellekilde Bonde JP, Lepoittevin J-P, Le Coz CJ, et al. Isothiazolinones in commercial products at Danish workplaces. Contact Dermatitis 2014;71:65-74

256 Yim E, Baquerizo Nole KL, Tosti A. Contact dermatitis caused by preservatives. Dermatitis 2014;25:215-231

257 Bruze M, Isaksson M, Gruvberger B, Andersen KE, Gonçalo M, Goossens A, et al. Patch testing with methylchloroisothiazolinone/methylisothiazolinone 200 ppm aq. detects significantly more contact allergy than 100 ppm. A multicentre study within the European Environmental and Contact Dermatitis Research Group. Contact Dermatitis 2014;71:31-34

258 Isaksson M, Gruvberger B, Bruze M. Patch testing with serial dilutions of various isothiazolinones in patients hypersensitive to methylchloroisothiazolinone/methylisothiazolinone. Contact Dermatitis 2014;70:270-275

259 González-Pérez R, Sánchez-Martínez L, Piqueres Zubiaurrre T, Urtaran Ibarzábal A, Soloeta Arechavala R. Patch testing in patients with perianal eczema. Actas Dermosifiliogr 2014;105:694-698 (Article in English, Spanish)

260 Madsen JT, Andersen KE. Further evidence of the methylisothiazolinone epidemic. Contact Dermatitis 2014;70:246-247

261 Isaksson M, Gruvberger B, Gonçalo M, Goossens A, Le Coz C-J, Bruze M. Repeated open application test with methylisothiazolinone in individuals sensitive to methylchloroisothiazolinone/methylisothiazolinone.Contact Dermatitis 2014;70:244-246

262 Mahler V, Geier J, Schnuch A. Current trends in patch testing – new data from the German Contact Dermatitis Research Group (DKG) and the Information Network of Departments of Dermatology (IVDK). J Dtsch Dermatol Ges 2014;12:583-592

263 Mowad CM. Methylchloroisothiazolinone revisited. Am J Contact Dermatitis 2000;11:115-118

264 De Unamuno B, Zaragoza Ninet V, Sierra C, de la Cuadra J. Descriptive study of sensitization to methylchloro-isothiazolinone and methylisothiazolinone in a skin allergy unit. Actas Dermosifiliogr 2014;105:854-859

265 Maor D, Nixon R. Allergic contact dermatitis to methylchloroisothiazolinone/methylisothiazolinone in cooling tower technicians. Dermatitis 2015;26:62-64

266 Murad A, Marren P. Prevalence of methylchloroisothiazolinone and methylisothiazolinone contact allergy in facial dermatitis: a single centre Irish study. J Eur Acad Dermatol Venereol 2016;30:60-62

267 Horev L, Isaksson M, Engfeldt M, Persson L, Ingber A, Bruze M. Preservatives in cosmetics in the Israeli market conform well to the EU legislation. J Eur Acad Dermatol Venereol 2015;29:761-766

268 Pirmez R, Fernandes AL, Melo MG. Photoaggravated contact dermatitis to Kathon CG (methylchloroisothia-zolinone /methylisothiazolinone): a novel pattern of involvement in a growing epidemic? Br J Dermatol 2015;173:1343-1344

269 Yu SH, Taylor JS, Murray D, Sood A. Methylisothiazolinone (MI) and methylchloroisothiazolinone/methyl-isothiazolinone (MCI/MI): Three year patch test results from clinical practice. Am J Cont Derm 2016;27:e5

270 Bunyavaree M, Kasemsarn P, Boonchai W. Cosmetic preservative labelling on the Thai market. Contact Dermatitis 2016;74:217-221

271 Abu-Asi MJ, White IR, McFadden JP, White JML. Patch testing is clinically important for patients with peri-anal dermatoses and pruritus ani. Contact Dermatitis 2016;74:298-300

272 Nasir S, Goldsmith P. Anogenital allergic contact dermatitis caused by methylchloroisothiazolinone, methyl-isothiazolinone and topical clotrimazole with subsequent generalized exanthem triggered by oral fluconazole. Contact Dermatitis 2016;74:296-297

273 Osinka K, Karczmarz A, Krauze A, Feleszko W. Contact allergens in cosmetics used in atopic dermatitis: analysis of product composition. Contact Dermatitis 2016;75:241-243

274 Atkar R, Todd P. Four cases of allergic contact dermatitis caused by methylchloroisothiazolinone/methyliso-thiazolinone in ironing water. Contact Dermatitis 2016;75:316-317

275 Schliemann S, Isaksson M, Persson C, Bruze M, Tittelbach J, Elsner P. Allergic contact dermatitis caused by methylchloroisothiazolinone/methylisothiazolinone in a medical device. Contact Dermatitis 2016;75:312-314

276 Pontén A, Bruze M, Engfeldt M, Hauksson I, Isaksson M. Concomitant contact allergies to formaldehyde, methylchloroisothiazolinone/methylisothiazolinone, methylisothiazolinone, and fragrance mixes I and II. Contact Dermatitis 2016;75:285-289

277 Pónyai G, Németh I, Temesvári E. Methylchloroisothiazolinone/methylisothiazolinone and methylisothiazolinone sensitivity in Hungary. Dermatol Res Pract Volume 2016, Article ID 4579071, 5 pages

278 Liuti F, Hernández Hernández Z, Borrego Hernando L. Increased sensitization to Kathon CG (methylchloroiso-thiazolinone plus methylisothiazolinone) in the south of Gran Canaria, Spain. Actas Dermosifiliogr 2014;105:882-883

279 Kazandjieva J, Gergovska M, Darlenski R. Contact dermatitis in a child from methylchloroisothiazolinone and methylisothiazolinone in moist wipes. Pediatr Dermatol 2014;31:225-227

280 Fernandez-Redondo V, Beiras-Fernandez A, Toribio J. Occupational dermatitis in a milk industry worker due to Kathon CG. Dermatitis 2004;15:73-74

281 Brand R, Delaney TA. Allergic contact dermatitis to cocamidopropylbetaine in hair shampoo. Australas J Dermatol 1998;39:121-122

282 Torén K, Brisman J, Meding B. Sensitization and exposure to methylisothiazolinones (Kathon) in the pulp and paper industry--a report of two cases. Am J Ind Med 199731:551-553

283 Ng CK, Tay P. Two case reports of delayed skin burns from methylisothiazolines used in water treatment. Singapore Med J 1996;37:577-578

284 Lucker GP, Hulsmans RF, van der Kley AM, van de Staak WJ. Evaluation of the frequency of contact allergic reactions to Kathon CG in the Maastricht area- 1987-1990. Dermatology 1992;184:90-93

285Vezia V, Renacco E, Castelain PY, Caperan A, Lanza M, Pastor J. Research on Kathon CG in cosmetic and personal hygiene products. Allerg Immunol (Paris) 1990;22:285-286 (Article in French)

286 Larsen WG. Methylchloroisothiazolinone-methylisothiazolinone (Kathon CG). J Am Acad Dermatol 1989;20:703

287 Belloni Fortina A, Fontana E, Peserico A. Contact sensitization in children: a retrospective study of 2,614 children from a single center. Pediatr Dermatol 2016;33:399-404

288 Smith VM, Clark SM, Wilkinson M. Allergic contact dermatitis in children: trends in allergens, 10 years on. A retrospective study of 500 children tested between 2005 and 2014 in one UK centre. Contact Dermatitis 2016;74:37-43

289 Yu SH, Sood A, Taylor JS. Patch testing for methylisothiazolinone and methylchloroisothiazolinone-methylisothiazolinone contact allergy. JAMA Dermatol 2016;152:67-72

290 Concha-Garzón MJ, Solano-López G, Montes A, Fraga J, Sánchez J. Follicular allergic contact dermatitis due to methylchloroisothiazolinone/methylisothiazolinone (MCI/MI) in a rinse-off soap product. Clin Exp Dermatol 2015;40:690-691

291 Dinkloh A, Worm M, Geier J, Schnuch A, Wollenberg A. Contact sensitization in patients with suspected cosmetic intolerance: results of the IVDK 2006-2011. Contact sensitization in patients with suspected cosmetic intolerance: results of the IVDK 2006-2011. J Eur Acad Dermatol Venereol 2015;29:1071-1081

292 Scherrer MA, Rocha VB. Increasing trend of sensitization to methylchloroisothiazolinone/methylisothiazoli- none (MCI/MI). An Bras Dermatol 2014;89:527-528

293 Leiva-Salinas M, Francés L, Silvestre JF. Update on allergic contact dermatitis due to methylchloroisothiazolinone/ methylisothiazolinone and methylisothiazolinone. Actas Dermosifiliogr 2014;105:840-846

294 Foote CA, Brady SP, Brady KL, Clark NS, Mercurio MG. Vulvar dermatitis from allergy to moist flushable wipes. J Low Genit Tract Dis 2014;18:E16-18

295 Cervigón-González I, Conde-Salazar L, Torres-Iglesias LM, Palomo-Arellano A. Contact dermatitis due to methylchloroisothiazolinone/methylisothiazolinone (Kathon CG) as a contaminant in the manufacturing process of a cream. Actas Dermosifiliogr 2013;104:81-82

296 Monroe HR, Hu JC, Chiu MW. Methylchloroisothiazolinone / methylisothiazolinone and moist wipe dermatitis. Dermatol Online J 2010;16(5):14.

297 Wolf R, Orion E, Matz H. Co-existing sensitivity to metronidazole and isothiazolinone. Clin Exp Dermatol 2003;28:506-507

298 Connolly MC, Kirby B, Bhushan M, O'Driscoll JB, Beck MH. Occupational allergic contact dermatitis from methylchloroisothiazolinone and methylisothiazolinone (MCI/MI) in a silicone-emulsion lock lubricant. Contact Dermatitis 2001;44:246-263

299 Kujala V, Niinimäki A. Occupational induction of hypersensitivity after an accidental exposure to chloromethylisothiazolinone and methylisothiazolinone (CMI/MI) in an industrial worker. Occup Med (Lond) 1999;49:51-53

300 Chen DM, Fairley JA. A bullous pemphigoid-like skin eruption after a chemical burn. J Am Acad Dermatol 1998;38(2Pt2):337-340

301 Castanedo-Tardan MP, Engfeldt M, Zug KA, Bruze M. Methylchloroisothiazolinone/methylisothiazolinone (MCI/MI) and methylisothiazolinone (MI) in common personal care products in the American market. Dermatitis 2016;27(6):e11

302 Uter W, Rämsch C, Aberer, W, Ayala F, Balato A, Beliauskiene A, et al. The European baseline series in 10 European Countries, 2005/2006 – Results of the European Surveillance System on Contact Allergies (ESSCA). Contact Dermatitis 2009;61:31-38

303 Schwensen JF, Johansen JD, Veien NK, Funding AT, Avnstorp C, Østerballe M, et al. Occupational contact dermatitis in hairdressers: an analysis of patch test data from the Danish Contact Dermatitis Group, 2002–2011. Contact Dermatitis 2014;70:233-237

304 Uter W, Gefeller O, John SM, Schnuch A, Geier J. Contact allergy to ingredients of hair cosmetics – a comparison of female hairdressers and clients based on IVDK 2007–2012 data. Contact Dermatitis 2014;71:13-20

305 Warshaw EM, Wang MZ, Mathias CGT, Maibach HI, Belsito DV, Zug KA, et al. Occupational contact dermatitis in hairdressers/cosmetologists; retrospective analysis of North American Contact Dermatitis Group data, 1994 to 2010. Dermatitis 2012;23:258-268

306 Kanerva L, Estlander T. Simultaneous active sensitization to multiple chemicals. Contact Dermatitis 1998;38:174-175

307 Uter W, Yazar K, Kratz EM, Mildau G, Lidén C. Coupled exposure to ingredients of cosmetic products: II. Preservatives. Contact Dermatitis 2014;70:219-226

308 Giménez-Arnau AM, Deza G, Bauer A, Johnston GA, Mahler V, Schuttelaar ML, et al. Contact allergy to preservatives: ESSCA* results with the baseline series, 2009-2012. J Eur Acad Dermatol Venereol 2017;31:664-671

309 Kimmig W. Allergische Kontaktdermatitis durch Lichtschutzmittel. Z Hautkr 1987;62:73 (article in German)

310 Warshaw EM, Aschenbeck KA, Zug KA, Belsito DV, Zirwas MJ, Fowler JF Jr, Taylor JS, et al. Wet wipe allergens: Retrospective analysis from the North American Contact Dermatitis Group 2011-2014. Dermatitis 2017;28:64-69

311 Lubbes S, Rustemeyer T, Sillevis Smitt JH, Schuttelaar ML, Middelkamp-Hup MA. Contact sensitization in Dutch children and adolescents with and without atopic dermatitis - a retrospective analysis. Contact Dermatitis 2017;76:151-159

312 Erfurt-Berge C, Geier J, Mahler V. The current spectrum of contact sensitization in patients with chronic leg ulcers or stasis dermatitis - new data from the Information Network of Departments of Dermatology (IVDK). Contact Dermatitis 2017;77:151-158

313 Beene KM, Scheman A, Severson D, Reeder MJ. Prevalence of preservatives across all product types in the Contact Allergen Management Program. Dermatitis 2017;28:81-87

314 Yu J, Treat J, Chaney K, Brod B. Potential allergens in disposable diaper wipes, topical diaper preparations, and disposable diapers: under-recognized etiology of pediatric perineal dermatitis. Dermatitis 2016;27:110-118

315 Andersson AM, Opstrup MS, Zachariae C, Friis UF, Thyssen JP, Johansen JD. The importance of a complete declaration of isothiazolinones in products beyond cosmetics. Contact Dermatitis 2017;77:171-172

316 Aalto-Korte K, Suuronen K. Patterns of concomitant allergic reactions in patients suggest cross-sensitization between octylisothiazolinone and methylisothiazolinone. Contact Dermatitis 2017 Jul 28. doi: 10.1111/cod.12855. [Epub ahead of print]

317 Uter W, Amario-Hita JC, Balato A, Ballmer-Weber B, Bauer A, Belloni Fortina A, et al. European Surveillance System on Contact Allergies (ESSCA): results with the European baseline series, 2013/14. J Eur Acad Dermatol Venereol 2017 Jun 19. doi: 10.1111/jdv.14423. [Epub ahead of print]

318 Goldenberg A, Mousdicas N, Silverberg N, Powell D, Pelletier JL, Silverberg JI, et al. Pediatric Contact Dermatitis Registry inaugural case data. Dermatitis 2016;27:293-302

319 Amsler E, Aerts O, Raison-Peyron N, Debons M, Milpied B, Giordano-Labadie F, et al. and on behalf of the Dermatology Allergy Group (DAG) of the French Society of Dermatology. Airborne allergic contact dermatitis caused by isothiazolinones in water-based paints: a retrospective study of 44 cases. Contact Dermatitis 2017;77:163-170

320 Todberg T, Opstrup MS, Johansen JD, Hald M. Occupational facial contact dermatitis caused by methylchloro-isothiazolinone/methylisothiazolinone in a stainless steel aerosol spray. Contact Dermatitis 2017;77:173–174.

321 Garcia-Hidalgo E, Sottas V, von Goetz N, Hauri U, Bogdal C, Hungerbühler K. Occurrence and concentrations of isothiazolinones in detergents and cosmetics in Switzerland. Contact Dermatitis 2017;76:96-106

322 Schwensen JF, Friis UF, Menné T, Flyvholm MA, Johansen JD. Contact allergy to preservatives in patients with occupational contact dermatitis and exposure analysis of preservatives in registered chemical products for occupational use. Int Arch Occup Environ Health 2017;90:319-333

323 Craig S, Urwin R, Latheef F, Wilkinson M. Patch test clinic experience of potential cross-reactivity of isothiazolinones. Contact Dermatitis 2017;76:299-300

324 Lynch MD, White JM, McFadden JP, Wang Y, White IR, Banerjee P. A dynamic landscape of allergen associations in delayed-type cutaneous hypersensitivity. Br J Dermatol 2017;176:184-196

325 García-Gavín J, Vansina S, Kerre S, Naert A, Goossens A. Methylisothiazolinone, an emerging allergen in cosmetics? Contact Dermatitis 2010;63:96-101

326 Du-Thanh A, Lalande M, Raison-Peyron N, Dereure O. Atypical and severe airborne isothiazolinone contact dermatitis mimicking Kaposi-Juliusberg syndrome. Contact Dermatitis 2017;76:297-298

327 Engfeldt M, Ale I, Andersen KE, Elsner P, Goh CL, Goossens A, Jerajani H, Matsunaga K, Bruze M. Multicenter patch testing with methylchloroisothizoline/methylisothiazolinone in 100 and 200 ppm within the International Contact Dermatitis Research Group. Dermatitis 2017;28:215-218

328 Zirwas MJ, Hamann D, Warshaw EM, Maibach HI, Taylor JS, Sasseville D, et al. Epidemic of isothiazolinone allergy in North America: prevalence data from the North American Contact Dermatitis Group, 2013-2014. Dermatitis 2017;28:204-209

329 Isaksson M, Ale I, Andersen KE, Elsner P, Goh CL, Goossens A, et al. Multicenter patch testing with methylisothiazolinone and methylchloroisothiazolinone/methylisothiazolinone within the International Contact Dermatitis Research Group. Dermatitis 2017;28:210-214

330 Agulló-Pérez AD, Hervella-Garcés M, Oscoz-Jaime S, Azcona-Rodríguez M, Larrea-García M, Yanguas-Bayona JI. Perianal dermatitis. Dermatitis 2017;28:270-275

331 Aschenbeck KA, Warshaw EM. Allergenic ingredients in facial wet wipes. Dermatitis 2017 Mar 23. doi: 10.1097/DER.0000000000000268. [Epub ahead of print]

332 Aschenbeck KA, Warshaw EM. Allergenic ingredients in personal hygiene wet wipes. Dermatitis 2017 Mar 23. doi: 10.1097/DER.0000000000000275. [Epub ahead of print]

333 Aerts O, Goossens A, Lambert J, Lepoittevin JP. Contact allergy caused by isothiazolinone derivatives: an overview of non-cosmetic and unusual cosmetic sources. Eur J Dermatol 2017;27:115-122

334 Herry J, Esquirol Y. Giordano-Labadie F. An intriguing occupational atypical dermatitis with respiratory symptoms. Contact Dermatitis 2016;75:322-323

2.293   METHYLDIBROMO GLUTARONITRILE

IDENTIFICATION

Description/definition   : Methyldibromo glutaronitrile is the brominated methylene glutaronitrile that conforms
                              to the formula shown below
Chemical class(es)   : Halogen compounds
Chemical/IUPAC name   : 2-Bromo-2-(bromomethyl)pentanedinitrile
Other names   : 1,2-Dibromo-2,4-dicyanobutane; bromothalonil; with phenoxyethanol in Euxyl® K 400
CAS registry number (s)   : 35691-65-7
EC number(s)   : 252-681-0
CIR review(s)   : J Am Coll Toxicol 1996;15:140-165 (access: www.cir-safety.org/ingredients)
SCCS opinion(s)   : SCCP/1013/06 (49); SCCP/0863/05 (50); SCCNFP/0806/04 (51); SCCNFP/0585/02 (52)
Function(s) in cosmetics   : EU: formerly used as preservative. USA: preservatives
EU regulations   : Prohibited; delisted in 2008 (stay-on products) and 2010 (rinse-off products)
Patch testing   : 0.5% pet. (Chemotechnique, SmartPracticeCanada); 0.3% pet. (Chemotechnique,
                              SmartPractice Canada, SmartPractice Europe)
Molecular formula   : $C_6H_6Br_2N_2$

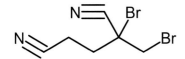

GENERAL

Methyldibromo glutaronitrile (MDBGN) was introduced in 1984 as (ingredient of) Euxyl® K 400 (Schülke & Mayr, Hamburg, Germany, from here on termed methyldibromo glutaronitrile/phenoxyethanol or MDBGN/PE), a combination of MDBGN and phenoxyethanol in a ratio of 1:4. Animal tests showed no or only a weak sensitizing capacity of MDBGN (18,54,69, data summarized in ref. 28). Its popularity grew rapidly, as MDBGN/PE efficiently prevented the growth of microorganisms. It was used both in cosmetics and industrial products. In 1986, the EU Scientific Committee on Cosmetology authorized the use of MDBGN at a maximum concentration of 0.1% in both leave-on and rinse-off cosmetic products. Soon, cases of contact allergy to MDBGN (which is virtually always the sensitizer in MDBGN/PE) were published, and in Germany there was an increase in prevalence of sensitization from 0.7% in 1990 to 2.1% in 1994 (9). In the Netherlands, the prevalence rose from 0.5% in 1991 (62) to 4.0% in 1994 (61) and the European average level of 0.7% positive patch tests in 1991 rose to 3.5% in 2000 (75). During this and the following decade further data were published showing high and increasing rates of sensitization (13,14,80,95,table 2.293.2).

Most reactions were caused by cosmetics, both stay-on and rinse-off products (22,61,67,76,77,88), resulting in hand eczema (77,88,89), facial dermatitis and sometimes generalized dermatitis. In the Netherlands, many patients had perianal dermatitis from using moist toilet tissues preserved with MDBGN/PE (8,24,61,62,79). Both stay-on and rinse-off products were able to induce sensitization as well as elicit ACD in pre-sensitized individuals (77). Stay-on products with 50 ppm MDBGN (0.1% = 1000 ppm was the allowed maximum concentration) caused dermatitis in >60% of patients pre-sensitized to the preservative under experimental conditions (107). As to rinse-off products, it was shown that the presence of detergents in a product lowered the threshold value for elicitation of allergic reactions in MDBGN-sensitized individuals (82).

EU regulations banning methyldibromo glutaronitrile in cosmetics

At that time, it was generally acknowledged that there had been a risk assessment failure concerning MDBGN (101). The preservative was banned from being used in leave-on products in the EU in 2003, brought into force in 2005 (2). A significant decline in sensitization rates ensued, already visible by 2004-2006 (7,15,16,17). In Denmark, for example, the frequency of positive patch tests to MDBGN decreased from 4.6% in 2003 to 2.6% in 2007. The decreasing trend was seen for both men and women. Also, the percentage of current relevant reactions steadily decreased from 51% in 2003 to 29% in 2007 (17).

Following a recommendation of the Scientific Committee on Consumer Products in 2005 (3), MDBGN was banned in rinse-off products in 2007 as well, brought into force in 2008 (4). From an epidemiological point of view, however, rinse-off products appear to have played a minor role in sensitization to MDBGN. Although experimental studies showed that soap containing 0.1% MDBGN (1000 ppm), applied to the forearm twice daily, provoked dermatitis in a number of pre-sensitized individuals (26), it was also shown that MDBGN can probably be used safely in rinse-off cosmetics at concentrations of about 50 ppm, even in individuals already sensitized to MDBGN (19).

Primary sensitization at this low level was considered to be very unlikely (19). Also, already in 2000, a clinical provocation study had shown that the use of a shampoo containing 200 ppm at least three times per week, did not elicit any itching, irritation or dermatitis in MDGN-sensitized individuals during 9-13 weeks of use (71).

Following the total ban, MDBGN is virtually excluded from the cosmetics market (20). The high prevalence of sensitization still observed in some European countries afterwards, is probably due to former exposure and /or to continued occupational (non-cosmetic) exposure (1,7,108). MDBGN can still be present in, for example, paints, cleaning agents, metalworking fluids, glues, wood preservatives, adhesives, color photographic processing solutions, seed disinfectants, paper and paperboard, joint cement, fabric softener concentrates and raw detergents (8,22,68,81).

Situation in the USA
In the United States, the preservative is still used in maximum allowed concentrations of 0.125% MDBGN/PE (0.025% MDBGN) in stay-on and a maximum concentration of 0.3% (containing 0.06% MDBGN) in rinse-off products (28) following the advice of the Cosmetic Ingredient Review Expert Panel (29). Whether this is good policy can be doubted. The patch test data of the North American Contact Dermatitis Group (NACDG) from 2000-2012 show frequencies of sensitization to MDBGN/PE, in which MDBGN is virtually always the sensitizer, ranging from 3.7% to 6.1% (methyldibromo glutaronitrile *per se* is not tested in the USA) (55,56,57,58,59,60). The highest prevalences were found between 2000 and 2008 and the most recent figures were 3.7% and 3.8% between 2009 and 2012. On the other hand, the figures may be less alarming than they look. Possibly, a number of these reactions were irritant, also considering the low relevance rates (20-30% 'definite' + 'probable' relevance) and considering that in a number of patients reacting to MDBGN/PE, there are no positive patch tests to either MDBGN or phenoxyethanol (11,103). Finally, all NACDG members work in tertiary referral centers and, consequently, patients are highly selected, which may push prevalence data upward (55,56,57,58,59,60).
.

Patch testing
Methyldibromo glutaronitrile 0.5% w/w pet. (test preparations with MDBGN in petrolatum were shown to be stable [83]) was added to the European Standard Series in 2005 (86) based on data provided in an EECDRG study (87,91). IVDK data, however, suggest this concentration may not infrequently result in false-positive, irritant patch test reactions (90). This leaves undisputed, that testing with 0.3% or 0.1% will miss clinically relevant sensitizations to MDBGN (91,92,93,100). Sometimes, even a test concentration of 1% is necessary to detect (clinically relevant) sensitization at day 3, lower concentrations (including the 0.5%) resulting in a false-negative reaction (93).

Literature reviews
The literature on contact allergy to methyldibromo glutaronitrile and MDBGN/PE (Euxyl K 400) up to 1996 has been reviewed by the author (22). A very useful review article was published in 2011 (28). Sensitization studies have been briefly summarized in ref. 5. Contact allergy to methyldibromo glutaronitrile specifically from its presence in Euxyl® K 400 (or other brands of this preservative system: MDBGN/PE) is discussed in Chapter 2.294 Methyldibromo glutaronitrile/phenoxyethanol.

CONTACT ALLERGY

General population and subgroups
Estimates of the 10-year prevalence of contact allergy to methyldibromo glutaronitrile in the general population of Denmark based on the CE-DUR method ranged from 0.80-1.08% (41). Patch test studies in (subgroups of) the general population are shown in table 2.293.1. In a small group of Danish 8th grade schoolchildren (follow-up study), 0.5% (0.7% in women, 0% in men) reacted to MDBGN (42). In Germany, a relatively high frequency of sensitization was found in a group of adults 28-78 years (1,7%; 1.2% in women, 2.2% in men). In this group, >50% had atopic dermatitis and sensitization may have occurred from the use of moisturizing preparations (43,44).

Patch testing in groups of patients
Results of studies testing methyldibromo glutaronitrile in consecutive patients suspected of contact dermatitis (routine testing) back to 1991 are shown in table 2.293.2. Results of testing in groups of *selected* patients (e.g., patients suspected of cosmetic dermatitis, patients with leg ulcers / stasis dermatitis, patients with periorbital or anal dermatoses, female hairdressers with occupational contact dermatitis) back to 1992 are shown in table 2.293.3.

Table 2.293.1   Patch testing in the general population and subgroups

Year and country	Selection and number tested	Prevalence of contact allergy			Comments	Ref.
		Total	Women	Men		
Subgroups of the general population						
2010 Denmark	Unselected population of 8th grade schoolchildren in Denmark, 15 years later; n=442	0.5%	0.7%	0%	follow-up study	42
1997-1998 Germany	Adults 28-78 year, with a large percentage (>50%) of atopic individuals, n=1141	1.7%	1.2%	2.2%		43, 44

Patch testing in consecutive patients suspected of contact dermatitis: routine testing

The results of routine testing with methyldibromo glutaronitrile back to 1991 are summarized in table 2.293.2. Many such studies have been published, notably from individual European countries and from multicenter and multi-country studies performed by the ESSCA (European Surveillance System on Contact Allergy Network) with 10-12 participating European countries and most recently 46 departments (124). Patch test concentrations have included 0.05%, 0.1%, 0.2%, 0.25%, 0.3% and 0.5% pet., which makes comparison difficult. It is well known that the 0.5% concentration may cause irritant reactions, whereas concentrations of 0.3% and lower will certainly result in some false-negative reactions. Taking all studies together, the frequencies of sensitization have ranged from 0.5% (test concentration far too low, 0.05% pet. [62]) to 5.3% (21). Frequencies of sensitization began to rise in the early 1990s to high values, especially in Italy, The Netherlands, Denmark and in Germany. In the studies where relevance was mentioned, 50-80% of the positive patch tests were considered to be relevant, mostly from cosmetics, both from stay-on and rinse-off products; in The Netherlands, many reactions were caused by the use of moist toilet paper.

After regulatory intervention in the EU (total ban in 2008), rates of sensitization began to decline, but were still around 2.5% in the 2009-2012 and 2013-2014 studies of the ESSCA (120,124). This cannot be the result of false-positive reactions, as the 0.2% and 0.3% test materials gave about the same results as the 0.5% test substance. The high prevalence of sensitization still observed in some European countries is probably due to former exposure and /or to continued occupational (non-cosmetic) exposure (1,7,108), for example in paints, cleaning agents, metalworking fluids, glues, wood preservatives, adhesives, color photographic processing solutions, seed disinfectants, paper and paperboard, joint cement, fabric softener concentrates and raw detergents (8,22,68,81).

Table 2.293.2 Patch testing in groups of patients: Routine testing

Years and Country	Test conc. & vehicle	Number of patients tested | positive (%)		Selection of patients (S); Relevance (R); Comments (C)	Ref.
2013-2014 12 European countries, 46 departments [b]	0.2% pet. 0.3% pet. 0.5% pet.	5498 13,831 8246	(2.5%) (2.0%) (2.4%)	R: not stated; C: results of 6 occupational dermatology clinics and one pediatric clinic not included in these figures; range of positive reactions: 1.4%-3.7% (0.2% test substance), 0%-6.1% (0.3% test substance) and 0.4%-7.5% (0.5% substance)	124
2009-2012, 12 European countries [b]	0.2% pet. 0.3% pet. 0.5% pet.	13,581 30,984 16,673	(2.8%) [a] (2.7%) [a] (2.5%) [a]	R: not stated; C: range per country 2.0%-3.6% R: not stated; C: range per country 0.6%-6.9% R: not stated; C: range per country 0.9%-3.8%	120
2006-2011 Singapore	0.25% pet.	3170	38 (1.2%)	R: not stated; C: prevalence was 1.1% in men, 1.3% in women	39
2010 IVDK		12,574	(2.5%)	R: not stated; C: it was suggested that few new sensitizations had occurred, as the patient group was relatively old	108
2005-2009 IVDK	0.3% pet. 0.2% pet.	53,545 13,369	2695(4.5%)[a] 371 (2.4%) [a]	R: not stated; C: decrease in prevalence of sensitization R: not stated; C: decrease in prevalence of sensitization	7
2007-2008 four European countries [b]	0.2% pet. 0.3% pet. 0.5% pet.	1900 18,711 3912	(1.9%) [a] (1.8%) [a] (1.8%) [a]	R: not stated; C: frequencies of sensitization ranged from 1.7% to 4.1% R: not stated; C: frequencies of sensitization ranged from 0.3% to 5.7% R: not stated; C: frequencies of sensitization ranged from 0% to 3.1%	1
2003-2007 Denmark 2003 2004 2005 2006 2007	0.3% pet.	19,279 3463 3688 4188 4091 3849	653 (3.4%) 158 (4.6%) 138 (3.7%) 147 (3.5%) 110 (2.7%) 100 (2.6%)	R: the relevance decreased from 51% in 2003 to 29% in 2007; C: the frequency of positive reactions significantly decreased from 4.6% in 2003 to 2.6% in 2007, which was due to EU regulatory intervention banning the use of MDBGN in stay-on cosmetic products; C: some patients were tested with Euxyl K 400 1.5%, containing 0.3% MDBGN	17
2005-6 10 European countries [b]	0.3% pet.	14,499	379 (2.6%)	R: not stated; C: prevalences in the four regions (Central, West, Northeast and South Europe) ranged from 0.1% to 5.6%	115

Table 2.293.2 Patch testing in groups of patients: Routine testing (*continued*)

Years and Country	Test conc. & vehicle	Number of patients tested | positive (%)		Selection of patients (S); Relevance (R); Comments (C)	Ref.
1993-2006 Australia	0.5% pet.	4551	(0.9%)	R: 42%; C: probably routine testing during a certain timeframe in the 1993-2006 period of investigation	123
2004-2005 UK	0.3% pet.	6958	(1.9%)	R: not stated	15
2004, 11 European countries [b]	0.3% pet.	4733	75 (1.5%) [a]	R: not stated; C: range of positives: 0.0%-7.4%	21
	0.2% pet.	405	21 (5.3%) [a]	R: not stated	
2003 Denmark	0.3% pet.	2146	110 (5.0%)	R: 53 (48%), mostly from creams and lotions (31%) and from liquid soaps (23%); C: in one of the 4 clinics, patients were tested with Euxyl K 400 1.5% pet., also containing 0.3% MDBGN	89
2003 Denmark	0.3% pet.	766	40 (5.2%)	R: 80%; 27 had hand eczema, of who 70% cleared after avoidance; in 9 patients with diffuse dermatitis, shampoos were responsible	88
2002 Sweden	0.3% pet.	807	23 (2.9%)	R: of 17 patients with hand dermatitis, 15 healed completely after avoiding cosmetic products containing MDBGN	77
2000-2002 Finland	0.1% pet.	11,786	(1.5%)	R: not stated; C: the authors used MDBGN 0.1% pet. and suggested that the modest rise in rate of sensitization (from 1.0% in 1995-1996 to 1.5% in 2000-2002 may have been related to this (too) low concentration	10
2000 United Kingdom	0.3% pet.	3063	(2.4%)	R: 80% (current and past relevance in one centre)	35
1997-1998 IVDK	0.3% pet.	4343	216 (5.0%)	R: not stated; C: the test concentration of 0.3% pet. was considered to result in many false-positive reactions	14
	0.1% pet.	998	14 (1.4%)		
1995-1996 Finland	0.1% pet.	5218	(1.0%)	R: not stated; C: the authors used MDBGN 0.1% pet. and suggested that the relatively low rate of sensitization may have been related to this (too) low concentration	10
1993-1995 The Netherlands	0.1% pet.	1019	24 (2.4%)	R: 'in most patients, contact with Euxyl K 400 containing products (in particular cosmetics) correlated with exacerbation of dermatitis'; C: 2 men had exacerbation of hand dermatitis from latex paints containing MDBGN	68
1994 France	0.1% pet.	310	6 (1.9%)	R: unknown (article not read), but at least one reacted to creams containing MDBGN; C: 3 patients had to be hospitalized because of generalized dermatitis	125
1994 The Netherlands	0.3%, 0.1% & 0.05% pet.	2943	119 (4.0%)	R: 71% of the reactions were relevant; causative products were cosmetics (2/3) and moist toilet paper (1/3)	61
1993-1994 The Netherlands	0.1% pet.	809	16 (2.0%)	R: 12 reactions were relevant, 11 from moist toilet paper; one woman also had facial dermatitis from a night cream; C: significant rise in prevalence during the 18-month study period	8
1993-1994 Italy	0.5% pet.	919	21 (2.3%)	R: 65% of patients reacting to Euxyl K 400 used cosmetics containing the preservative system; for the subgroup of patients tested with MDBGN, this was not specified	11
1991 The Netherlands	0.05% pet.	1142	6 (0.5%)	R: 4 reactions were relevant, 3 from moist toilet tissues and one beautician had occupational contact dermatitis from cosmetic products containing MDBGN/PE	62

[a] age-standardized and sex-standardized proportions

[b] study of the ESSCA (European Surveillance System on Contact Allergy Network)

IVDK: Information Network of Departments of Dermatology, Germany, Austria, Switzerland

Patch testing in groups of selected patients

Results of testing in groups of selected patients (e.g., patients suspected of cosmetic dermatitis, patients with leg ulcers / stasis dermatitis, patients with periorbital or anal dermatoses, female hairdressers with occupational contact dermatitis) back to 1992 are shown in table 2.293.3. Patch test concentrations have included 0.1%, 0.2%, 0.3% and 0.5% pet., which makes comparison difficult. It is well known that the 0.5% concentration may cause irritant reactions, whereas concentrations of 0.1%, 0.2% and 0.3% will certainly result in some false-negative reactions. The 2% test concentration mentioned in a US study (40) is always certainly a mistake and probably represents methyldibromo glutaronitrile/phenoxyethanol (Euxyl K 400), containing 0.4% MDBGN. In 19 studies, frequencies of sensitization have ranged from 0.6% to 13.6% (table 2.293.2). The highest concentration was found in an IVDK study in a group of 159 female hairdressers, but the relevance of the observed reactions was not mentioned (110). Other high sensitization rates of >5% were found in patients with stasis dermatitis (6.1% [122]), hairdressers with dermatitis of the hands or face (6.0% [12]), adult consecutive patients (i.e., routine testing, but excluding patients of 18 years and younger) from Lithuania (5.5% [109]), and patients with dermatitis possibly caused by hair cosmetics

(5.0% [110]). In 14/19 studies, no relevance data were provided. In the studies that did address the relevancy issue, the rates of relevant reactions were 21% (111), 50% (4 of 8 reactions [98]), 73% (109) and 100% (2 reactions only [37]). Causative products were never mentioned.

Table 2.293.3 Patch testing in groups of patients: Selected patient groups

Years and Country	Test conc. & vehicle	Number of patients tested | positive (%)		Selection of patients (S); Relevance (R); Comments (C)	Ref.
2003-2014 IVDK	0.3% pet.	<5202	(6.1%)	S: patients with stasis dermatitis / chronic leg ulcers; R: not stated; C: percentage of reactions not significantly higher than in a control group of routine testing	122
	0.2% pet.	<5202	(3.8%)		
1996-2013 Nether-lands	0.3% pet.	998	11 (1.1%)	S: children aged 0-17 years; R: not stated	121
2007-2012 IVDK	0.2% pet.	525	14 (3.6%)	S: female hairdressers with current or previous occupational contact dermatitis; R: not stated	117
		1374	24 (1.5%)	S: female patients, clients of hairdressers, in who hair cosmetics were regarded as a cause of dermatitis, and who had never worked as hairdressers; R: not stated	
2003-2012 IVDK		1680	79 (4.7%)	S: nurses with occupational contact dermatitis; R: not stated	30
2011 China	0.5% pet.	201	2 (1.0%)	S: healthy student volunteers 19-30 years; R: not stated	112
2010-2011 Korea	0.5% pet.	584	9 (1.5%)	S: patients suspected of allergic cosmetic dermatitis; R: not stated	38
2006-2011 IVDK	0.2% or 0.3% pet.	10,124	299 (3.2%)	S: patients suspected of cosmetic intolerance; R: not stated	114
2002-2011 Denmark		390	6 (1.5%)	S: hairdressers with contact dermatitis; R: not stated	116
2001-2010 Australia	0.3% pet.	4644	75 (1.6%)	S: not stated; R: 21%	111
2000-2010 IVDK		3125	79 (2.5%)	S: patients with periorbital dermatitis; R: not stated	33
2006-2008 Lithuania	0.3% pet.	816	45 (5.5%)	S: adult consecutive patients; R: 73%	109
2005-2008 IVDK		470	(6.3%)	S: patients with anal dermatoses; R: unknown (article not read), but these IVDK studies rarely mention relevance rates	126
2005-2006 IVDK	0.3% pet.	159	(13.6%)	S: female hairdressers; R: not stated	110
		321	(5.0%)	S: patients with dermatitis possibly caused by hair cosmetics; R: not stated	
2003-2004 USA	2% pet.	268	8 (3.0%)	S: patients with pure eyelid dermatitis; R: this was the number of relevant reactions; C: it is highly likely that the test material was not MDBGN, but Euxyl K 400 2% pet. containing 0.4% MDBGN	40
1994-2004 USA		46	2 (4.3%)	S: patients with allergic contact dermatitis of the eyelids; R: both were relevant, but the causative products were not mentioned	37
1993-2004 Australia		1375	8 (0.6%)	S: patients tested in an occupational dermatology clinic with a cosmetic series; R: 4/8 (50%)	98
1995-1999 IVDK	0.1% pet.	579	(2.1%)	S: patients with allergic periorbital contact dermatitis; R: not stated	46
1990-1994 Germany	0.1% pet.	11,052	196 (1.8%)	S: patients tested with a preservative series; R: not stated	36
1989-1992 The Netherlands	0.5% pet.	103	6 (6.0%)	S: hairdressers with dermatitis of the hands (n=98) or the face; R: not stated	12

IVDK: Information Network of Departments of Dermatology, Germany, Austria, Switzerland

Case reports and case series

Case series

Methyldibromo glutaronitrile (MDBGN) was stated to be the (or an) allergen in 29 patients in a group of 603 individuals suffering from cosmetic dermatitis, seen in the period 2010-2015 in Leuven, Belgium (34). This is surprising and possibly incorrect, as the preservative has been banned from cosmetics since 2005 (leave-on products) resp. 2008 (rinse-off products). In the period 1996-2013, in a tertiary referral center in Valencia, Spain, 5419 patients were patch tested. Of these, 628 individuals had allergic contact dermatitis to cosmetics. Methyldibromo glutaronitrile was the responsible allergen in eight cases (113, overlap with ref. 53). MDBGN was responsible for 8 out of 959 cases of non-fragrance cosmetic allergy where the causal allergen was identified, Belgium, 2000-2010 (6). In the period 2000-2007, 202 patients with allergic contact dermatitis caused by cosmetics were seen in Valencia, Spain. In this group, five individuals reacted to methyldibromo glutaronitrile from its presence in moisturizing cream (n=4) and in cleansing wipes (n=1) (53, overlap with ref. 113).

In a period of 9 months in 2002, sixteen patients were seen in one university clinic in Denmark with hand dermatitis caused by a variety of cosmetic products containing MDBGN, including body lotion (n=7), hand cream (n=4), liquid hand soap (n=4), facial cream (n=3), shampoo (n=2) and rinsing milk (n=1) (77). In a group of 38 patients with positive patch tests to MDBGN seen in 2003 in Denmark, 27 had hand eczema, with a relevant exposure predominantly from wash-off products, either liquid soaps or shampoos, in 24 patients (88). In 53 patients with relevant reactions to MDBGN seen in 2003 in Denmark, creams and lotions were responsible for 31% of the reactions and liquid soaps for 23%; there were also 2 patients whose dermatitis was caused by hair gel or wax (89).

Case reports

Stay-on products
One patient had ACD from MDBGN in an anti-wrinkle lotion (first reported case of contact allergy in cosmetics) (23). MDBGN in a self-made skin care product caused ACD in one individual (25). A young atopic girl developed ACD of the face and extremities from MDBGN in a cosmetic gel (64). A woman had acute ACD of the face and neck from MDBGN in a cosmetic cream (65). Contact allergy to MDBGN in an eye gel caused dermatitis of the face and the periorbital skin in a female patient (66).

A woman suffered from 4 outbreaks of dermatitis. Three times the face was involved and the cause was contact allergy to MDBGN in a cleansing milk and makeup. Hand dermatitis was caused by contact allergy to MDBGN in a body milk (67). Contact allergy to MDBGN in a hair mousse and leave-on hair conditioner resulted in worsening of seborrheic dermatitis in a young female patient (70). A woman had episodes of dermatitis on the arms, legs and her thigh, which sometimes had the form of a hand. She proved to be allergic to Euxyl K 400 and MDBGN. She did not use cosmetics containing MDBGN. Instead, the dermatitis proved to be caused by a hand moisturizer used by her husband (connubial contact dermatitis) (97).

Rinse-off products
One patient had hand dermatitis from MDBGN in liquid soap (93). A nurse had hand dermatitis from MDBGN in a hand cleanser she used at home (98). One patient had dermatitis from MDBGN in a cleansing product (27). A man developed contact dermatitis of the genital skin, groins and perianal skin each time after he had sexual intercourse, from washing these areas afterwards with a liquid soap containing MDBGN (81).

Moist toilet tissues and cleansing wipes
Four patients (24), five individuals (62) and another five patients (8) had perianal allergic contact dermatitis from MDBGN in Euxyl K 400 present in moist toilet tissues. A female patient had acute allergic CD of the face and neck from using make-up removal wipes containing MDBGN (84). One patient had perianal ACD from MDBGN in a moist toilet tissue, present in a concentration of 0.1% (79).

Occupational contact dermatitis
A mechanic had occupational allergic hand dermatitis from MDBGN in liquid soap and shower cream which he used at his work. Later, the eczema relapsed when he used a moisturizer at home, which proved to contain the combination of phenoxyethanol and MDBGN (92). In the same publication, a female kitchen assistant was presented who had hand dermatitis from a moisturizer (92). In both cases, there was incorrect labelling of products; the presence of MDBGN was established or verified by HPLC (92). A maintenance technician developed hand dermatitis from a cosmetic cream to protect the hands, containing MDBGN (94). A mechanic and a machine fitter both had occupational ACD of the hands from MDBGN in a hand cleaner (98).

A car glass installer presented with occupational hand dermatitis from contact allergy to MDBGN in industrial hand degreasing moist toilet paper (99). A female beautician, who reacted to MDBGN, had dermatitis of the face and hands. She also had positive patch test reactions to several cosmetics that she used both for her clients and herself; these proved to contain MDBGN/PE (62). A physiotherapist, who was allergic to MDBGN, developed occupational contact dermatitis of the hands from contact with patients' cosmetics containing MDBGN while massaging (8). A masseur had occupational hand dermatitis from contact allergy to MDBGN present in a massage lotion (first reported case of MDBGN contact allergy in cosmetics) (23). Three nurses had occupational allergic hand dermatitis from MDBGN present in hand washes (76).

Contact allergy to methyldibromo glutaronitrile in non-cosmetic products
Two metalworking machinists had occupational allergic contact dermatitis from MDBGN in metalworking fluids (31). Two patients reacted to MDBGN in an NSAID cream (32). A maintenance mechanic developed dermatitis of the hands and arms from contact allergy to MDBGN in a paste glue (first report of contact allergy to MDBGN) (63). Two patients had ACD from MDBGN after application of gel for ultrasonography containing MDBGN/PE (72,73). Three patients had occupational ACD of the hands and forearms from contact allergy to MDBGN in hand cleansers and

work creams (74). MDBGN itself was not tested, but the patients reacted to MDBGN/PE and the products were stated to contain MDBGN (74). A woman had an recurrent itchy vulvar dermatitis from contact allergy to MDBGN in the adhesive of a sanitary pad she wore during menstruation (98). Two women had severe genital dermatitis from contact allergy to MDBGN in vaginal examination gel (88).

Cross-reactions, pseudo-cross-reactions and co-reactions

Pseudo-cross-reactions may be observed to methyldibromo glutaronitrile/phenoxyethanol (MDBGN/PE, Euxyl K 400), as this is the allergenic ingredient in nearly all cases of sensitization to the preservative mixture.

Repeated open application tests (ROATs)

In 2002, 51 patients with doubtful or positive reactions to at least 1 of 4 simultaneously patch tested preparations with MDBGN in pet. at 1.0% w/w, 0.5%, 0.3% and 0.1%, participated in a ROAT study performed by the EECDRG (91). Eighteen (35%) had a positive ROAT to a moisturizer containing 0.03% MDBGN. This included some patient who had positive patch tests to MDBGN 0.5% but not to 0.3% or 0.1%. The authors concluded that testing with MDBGN 0.1% or 0.3% will result in missing clinically relevant patch tests to it (91). In a nearly identical study performed some years later, 19 (59%) of 32 MDBGN-allergic patients developed a positive ROAT result on the arm on which the moisturizer containing 0.03% MDBGN was applied, whereas no patients with doubtful or negative reactions to MDBGN reacted. Again, some of these patients reacted upon patch testing only to 0.5% pet. or 1.0% pet. The percentage positive ROATs was dependent on the patch test concentration to which the patients reacted, decreasing from 100% in those with positive patch tests to 0.1% MDBGN to 25% in the patients reacting to 1% MDBGN only. Again, the conclusion was, that patch testing with MDBGN at 0.3% and 0.1% will miss clinically relevant patch test reactions to MDBGN (100).

In an IVDK study designed to find a maximum non-eliciting concentration for rinse-off products in MDBGN patch test-positive patients, use-related tests [repeated open application tests (ROAT)] in patients sensitized to MDBGN with a liquid soap containing three concentrations of MDBGN (50, 200, and 400 ppm MDBGN, respectively) were performed. The soap at 50 ppm was used twice daily for 4 weeks. If no reaction of the skin was observed, the product with the next higher concentration was used for another 4 weeks, etc. In total, 32/37 evaluated cases (86%) did not react to any of the preparations. The remaining reacted as follows: 1/37 reacted to 50 ppm, 3/37 to 200 ppm, and 1/37 to 400 ppm. The cumulative non-response to 50 ppm was 97.3%. It was concluded that the majority of subjects sensitized to MDBGN tolerated rinse-off products containing a maximum concentration of 400 ppm. A concentration in rinse-off products in the range of 50 ppm could be regarded as safe for most individuals already sensitized. In addition, it was suggested that these concentrations will presumably prevent induction (sensitization) also (19). ROATs with liquid soap containing 0.1% MDBGN (1000 ppm, at that time the highest permitted concentration in the EU) twice daily for 4 weeks in 19 subjects with contact allergy to MDBGN, provoked contact dermatitis in 7 (37%) (26).

In a study where ROATs and serial dilution patch tests were performed in patients allergic to MDBGN, it was shown that the ROAT response rate in terms of dose per application was significantly higher compared with the same dose in the patch test. This means that even though a certain dose in a patch test is negative, an allergic person might react to this dose (per unit area per application) in a ROAT, or from repeated contact with products containing low amounts of MDBGN. Thus, elicitation is not only dependent on the allergen dose per application, but also on the frequency of exposure (102).

ROATs in individuals known to be sensitized to MDBGN with a hydroalcoholic solution of MDBGN 0.01% applied 4 times daily, had approximately equal capabilities of producing allergic reactions than ROATS with a higher concentration (0.04%), applied one time per day (85). In a Danish study, eighteen volunteers with contact allergy to MDBGN were exposed to repeated open application tests (ROATs) with two moisturizers with a high and a low lipid content, respectively, both containing MDBGN at a concentration of 50 ppm. Ten (56%) developed dermatitis on the test area, of whom seven had a positive reaction already on day 2 or 3. Reactions to the low-lipid moisturizer were the more frequent. Controls all had negative ROATs. It was concluded that even 50 ppm MDBGN cannot be regarded as a safe concentration for use and that the prohibition of MDBGN is scientifically well founded (107).

Use tests

In a provocative use test, 9 of 17 patients (53%) allergic to MDBGN, who washed part of an underarm with liquid soap containing 0.1% MDBGN twice daily for 3 weeks, developed allergic contact dermatitis at the contact site (96). A clinical provocation study in 11 MDBGN-sensitized individuals, with a shampoo containing 200 ppm MDBGN, used at least 3 times per week, elicited no itching, irritation and/or dermatitis during 9-13 weeks of use (71).

Serial dilution testing

Nineteen allergic patients were tested with MDBGN in alc./water 1:1 in concentrations ranging from 0.2% (2000 ppm) to 0.001% (10 ppm); 7 reacted down to the lowest concentration, for four test subjects, 0.2% was the lowest threshold for a positive patch test reaction (26).

Presence in cosmetic products and chemical analyses

In July 2017, methyldibromo glutaronitrile was present in 13 of 69,692 cosmetic products of which the composition is known in EWG's Skin Deep Cosmetics Database, USA (http://www.ewg.org/skindeep/). In the USA, in April 2017, methyldibromo glutaronitrile was present in 73 of 56,714 cosmetic products of which the composition is known in FDA's Voluntary Cosmetic Registration Program (VCRP) (data obtained from FDA, May 2017). In the period 2008-2014, some cosmetic products sold in the EU still contained methyldibromo glutaronitrile (48). In Germany, in 2006-2009, the labels of 4680 cosmetic products were screened for the presence of preservatives. MDBGN was present in 0.7% of the products, according to labelling information (119). MDBGN was present in 2002 in 36 of 1774 (2.0%) cosmetics and in 2005 in 44 of 1170 (3.8%) such products filed in the Danish Product Register Database (PROBAS) (45). In a group of 67 samples of skin creams, randomly selected from retail outlets in Denmark in 1999, 4 (6%) contained methyldibromo glutaronitrile in a concentration range of 0.010-0.017% (47). Investigations of cosmetics on the market in Sweden in 1997 showed MDBGN in 4% of 100 moisturizers in the concentration range 100-290 ppm (78).

In June 1992, cosmetics on the Dutch market were analyzed for MDBGN. It was detected in 11 of 76 (14%) rinse-off products such as shampoos and bath foams, and in seven of 42 (17%) emulsions such as creams, body lotions and sunscreens. The concentration range was 0.004% to 0.03% (8). Three years later, the percentage had risen to 25-35% of cosmetics, among which were some of the bestselling brands in the main product categories (61). In addition, MDBGN was found to be present in 15 of 24 (63%) brands and types of moist toilet paper in The Netherlands (61). In 1990, 13% of cosmetic products sold in The Netherlands was preserved with MDBGN (in the form of Euxyl K 400) (62). Chemical analysis of 12 products causing allergic hand dermatitis in patients with positive patch tests to MDBGN showed that lotions contained 149-390 ppm of MDBGN, liquid hand soap 144-399 ppm, a rinsing cream 293 ppm and shampoos 78-79 ppm (77). In another investigation, chemical analysis showed 11 ppm to 473 ppm MDBGN in products used by patients suffering from ACD caused mainly by rinse-off products (88).

LITERATURE

1   Uter W, Aberer W, Armario-Hita JC, Fernandez-Vozmediano JM, Ayala F, Balato A, et al. Current patch test results with the European baseline series and extensions to it from the 'European Surveillance System on Contact Allergy' network, 2007-2008. Contact Dermatitis 2012;67:9-19
2   Commission of the European Communities. Commission directive 2003/83/EC of 24 September 2003. Official Journal of the European Union 2003;238:23-27
3   Scientific-Committee-on-Consumer-Products. Opinion on methyl dibromoglutaronitrile (sensitisation only) (SCCP/0863/05), 2005. *Available at:*
    http://ec.europa.eu/health/ph_risk/committees/04_sccp/docs/sccp_o_00f.pdf
4   Commission of the European Communities. Commission directive 2007 /17 /EC of 22 March 2007. Official Journal of the European Union 2007;82:27-30
5   Thyssen JP, Giménez-Arnau E, Lepoittevin J-P, Menné T, Boman A, Schnuch A. The critical review of methodologies and approaches to assess the inherent skin sensitizing potential (skin allergies) of chemicals. Part II. Contact Dermatitis 2012;66 (Suppl. 1):25-52
6   Travassos AR, Claes L, Boey L, Drieghe J, Goossens A. Non-fragrance allergens in specific cosmetic products. Contact Dermatitis 2011;65:276-285
7   Schnuch A, Lessmann H, Geier J, Uter W. Contact allergy to preservatives. Analysis of IVDK data 1996-2009. Br J Dermatol 2011;164:1316-1325
8   Van Ginkel CJW, Rundervoort G. Increasing incidence of contact allergy to the new preservative 1,2-dibromo-2,4-dicyanobutane (methyldibromoglutaronitrile). Br J Dermatol 1995;132:918-920
9   Geier J, Schnuch A, Fuchs T. Zunahme der Kontaktallergien gegen Methyldibromoglutaronitril in Deutschland. Allergologie 1996;19:399-402
10 Hasan T, Rantanen T, Alanko K, Harvima RJ, Jolanki R, Kalimo K, et al. Patch test reactions to cosmetic allergens in 1995–1997 and 2000–2002 in Finland – a multicenter study. Contact Dermatitis 2005;53:40-45
11 Tosti A, Vincenzi C, Trevisi P, Guerra L. Euxyl K 400: incidence of sensitization, patch test concentration and vehicle. Contact Dermatitis 1995;33:193-195
12 Van der Walle HB, Brunsveld VM. Dermatitis in hairdressers (I): the experience of the past 4 years. Contact Dermatitis 1994;4:217-221
13 McFadden JP, Ross JS, Jones AB, Rycroft RJ, Smith HR, White IR. Increased rate of patch test reactivity to methyldibromo glutaronitrile. Contact Dermatitis 2000;42:54-55

14 Geier J, Schnuch A, Brasch J, Gefeller O. Patch testing with methyldibromoglutaronitrile. Am J Contact Dermatitis 2000;11:207-212

15 Jong CT, Statham BN, Green CM, King CM, Gawkrodger DJ, Sansom JE, et al. Contact sensitivity to preservatives in the UK, 2004–2005: results of multicentre study. Contact Dermatitis 2007;57:165-168

16 Thyssen JP, Engkilde K, Lundov MD, Carlsen BC, Menné T, Johansen JD. Temporal trends of preservative allergy in Denmark (1985–2008). Contact Dermatitis 2010;62:102-108

17 Johansen JD, Veien N, Laurberg G, Avnstorp C, Kaaber K, Andersen KE, et al. Decreasing trends in methyldibromo glutaronitrile contact allergy – following regulatory intervention. Contact Dermatitis 2008;59:48-51

18 Hausen BM. The sensitizing potency of Euxyl® K 400 and its components 1,2-dibromo-2,4-dicyanobutane and 2-phenoxyethanol. Contact Dermatitis 1993;28:149-153

19 Heratizadeh A, Killig C, Worm M, Soost S, Simon D, Bauer A, et al. Quantitative repeated open application testing with a rinse-off product in methyldibromo glutaronitrile-sensitive patients: results of the IVDK. Contact Dermatitis 2010;62:330-337

20 Mildau G. INCI Labelling of fragrances and preservatives on 5451 randomly selected cosmetic products in Germany, 2006 to 2009. Karlsruhe: Chemisches und Veterinär-Untersuchungsamt, 2010

21 ESSCA Writing Group. The European Surveillance System of Contact Allergies (ESSCA): results of patch testing the standard series, 2004. J Eur Acad Dermatol Venereol 2008;22:174-181

22 De Groot AC, van Ginkel CJW, Weijland JW. Methyldibromoglutaronitrile (Euxyl K 400): An important 'new' allergen in cosmetics. J Am Acad Dermatol 1996;35:743-747

23 Senff H, Exner M, Gortz J, Goos M. Allergic contact dermatitis from Euxyl K 400. Contact Dermatitis 1989;20:381-382 (also published in Dermatosen 1989;37:45-46)

24 Hulsmans R-FHJ, Lucker GPH, van der Kley AMJ, et al. Kathon CG and methyldibromoglutaronitrile: important contact allergens in patients with perianal dermatitis. Aktuelle Koloproktologie 1992;9:275-286

25 Keilig W. Kontaktallergie auf einen neuen Konservierungsstof (Euxyl K 400). Paffumerie Kosmetik 1991;72:167-168

26 Jensen CD, Johansen JD, Menné T, Andersen KE. Methyldibromoglutaronitrile in rinse-off products causes allergic contact dermatitis: an experimental study. Br J Dermatol 2004;150:90-95

27 Goossens A, Baret I, Swevers A. Allergic contact dermatitis caused by tetrahydroxypropyl ethylenediamine in cosmetic products. Contact Dermatitis 2011;64:161-164

28 Aakhus AE, Warshaw EM. Allergy to methyldibromoglutaronitrile/phenoxyethanol (Euxyl K 400): Regulatory issues, epidemiology, clinical characteristics, and management. Dermatitis 2011;22:127-140

29 Cosmetic Ingredient Review Expert Panel. Final report on the safety assessment of methyldibromo glutaronitrile. J Am Coll Toxicol 1996;15:140-165

30 Molin S, Bauer A, Schnuch A, Geier J. Occupational contact allergy in nurses: results from the Information Network of Departments of Dermatology 2003–2012. Contact Dermatitis 2015;72:164-171

31 Suuronen K, Aalto-Korte K, Piipari R, Tuomi T, Jolanki R. Occupational dermatitis and allergic respiratory diseases in Finnish metalworking machinists. Occup Med 2007;57:277-283

32 Amaro C, Cravo M, Fernandes C, Santos R, Gonçalo M. Undisclosed methyldibromo glutaronitrile causing allergic contact dermatitis in a NSAID cream. Contact Dermatitis 2012;67:173-174

33 Landeck L, John SM, Geier J. Periorbital dermatitis in 4779 patients – patch test results during a 10-year period. Contact Dermatitis 2014;70:205-212

34 Goossens A. Cosmetic contact allergens. Cosmetics 2016;3. doi: 10.3390/cosmetics3010005

35 Britton JE, Wilkinson SM, English JSC, Gawkrodger DJ, Ormerod AD, Sansom JE, et al. The British standard series of contact dermatitis allergens: validation in clinical practice and value for clinical governance. Br J Dermatol 2003;148:259-264

36 Schnuch A, Geier J, Uter W, Frosch PJ. Patch testing with preservatives, antimicrobials and industrial biocides. Results from a multicentre study. Br J Dermatol 1998;138:467-476

37 Amin KA, Belsito DV. The aetiology of eyelid dermatitis: a 10-year retrospective analysis. Contact Dermatitis 2006;55:280-285

38 Lee SS, Hong DK, Jeong NJ, Lee JH, Choi YS, Lee AY, et al. Multicenter study of preservative sensitivity in patients with suspected cosmetic contact dermatitis in Korea. J Dermatol 2012;39:677-681

39 Cheng S, Leow YH, Goh CL, Goon A. contact sensitivity to preservatives in Singapore: frequency of sensitization to 11 common preservatives 2006–2011. Dermatitis 2014;25:77-82

40 Rietschel RL, Warshaw EM, Sasseville D, Fowler JF Jr, DeLeo VA. Belsito DV, et al. Common contact allergens associated with eyelid dermatitis: data from the North American Contact Dermatitis Group 2003-2004 study period. Dermatitis 2007;18:78-81

41 Thyssen JP, Uter W, Schnuch A, Linneberg A, Johansen JD. 10-year prevalence of contact allergy in the general population in Denmark estimated through the CE-DUR method. Contact Dermatitis 2007;57:265-272

42 Mortz CG, Bindslev-Jensen C, Andersen KE. Prevalence, incidence rates and persistence of contact allergy and allergic contact dermatitis in The Odense Adolescence Cohort Study: a 15-year follow-up. Brit J Dermatol 2013;168:318-325

43 Schäfer T, Böhler E, Ruhdorfer S, Weigl L, Wessner D, Filipiak B, et al. Epidemiology of contact allergy in adults. Allergy 2001;56:1192-1196

44 Uter W, Ludwig A, Balda BR, Schnuch A, Pfahlberg A, Schäfer T, Wichmann HE, Ring J. The prevalence of contact allergy differed between population-based data and clinic–based data. J Clin Epidemiol 2004;57:627-632

45 Flyvholm, MA. Preservatives in registered chemical products. Contact Dermatitis 2005;53:27-32

46 Herbst RA, Uter W, Pirker C, Geier J, Frosch PJ. Allergic and non-allergic periorbital dermatitis: patch test results of the Information Network of the Departments of Dermatology during a 5-year period. Contact Dermatitis 2004;51:13-19

47 Rastogi SC. Analytical control of preservative labelling on skin creams. Contact Dermatitis 2000;43:339-343

48 Neza E, Centini M. Microbiologically contaminated and over-preserved cosmetic products according Rapex 2008–2014. Cosmetics 2016, 3, 3; doi:10.3390/cosmetics3010003

49 SCCP (Scientific Committee on Consumer Products). Opinion on Methyldibromoglutaronitrile (sensitisation only), 20 June 2006, SCCP/1013/06. Available at: http://ec.europa.eu/health/archive/ph_risk/committees/04_sccp/docs/sccp_o_060.pdf

50 SCCP (Scientific Committee on Consumer Products). Opinion on Methyldibromoglutaronitrile (sensitisation only), 15 March 2005, SCCP/0863/05. Available at: http://ec.europa.eu/health/archive/ph_risk/committees/04_sccp/docs/sccp_o_00f.pdf

51 SCCNFP (Scientific Committee on Cosmetics and Non Food Products). Opinion concerning methyldibromo glutaronitrile, 23 April 2004, SCCNFP/0806/04. Available at: http://ec.europa.eu/health/archive/ph_risk/committees/sccp/documents/out269_en.pdf

52 SCCNFP (Scientific Committee on Cosmetics and Non Food Products). Opinion concerning methyldibromo glutaronitrile, 4 June 2002, SCCNFP/0585/02. Available at: http://ec.europa.eu/health/archive/ph_risk/committees/sccp/documents/out169_en.pdf

53 Laguna C, de la Cuadra J, Martín-González B, Zaragoza V, Martínez-Casimiro L, Alegre V. Allergic contact dermatitis to cosmetics. Actas Dermosifiliogr 2009;100:53-60

54 Bruze M, Gruvberger B, Agrup G. Sensitization studies in the guinea pig with the active ingredients of EuxylR K 400. Contact Dermatitis 1988;18:37-39

55 Warshaw EM, Maibach HI, Taylor JS, Sasseville D, DeKoven JG, Zirwas MJ, et al. North American Contact Dermatitis Group patch test results: 2011-2012. Dermatitis 2015;26:49-59

56 Warshaw EM, Belsito DV, Taylor JS, Sasseville D, DeKoven JG, Zirwas MJ, et al. North American Contact Dermatitis Group patch test results: 2009 to 2010. Dermatitis 2013;24:50-59

57 Fransway AF, Zug KA, Belsito DV, Deleo VA, Fowler JF Jr, Maibach HI, et al. North American Contact Dermatitis Group patch test results for 2007-2008. Dermatitis 2013;24:10-21

58 Zug KA, Warshaw EM, Fowler JF Jr, Maibach HI, Belsito DL, Pratt MD, et al. Patch-test results of the North American Contact Dermatitis Group 2005-2006. Dermatitis 2009;20:149-160

59 Warshaw EM, Belsito DV, DeLeo VA, Fowler JF Jr, Maibach HI, Marks JG, et al. North American Contact Dermatitis Group patch-test results, 2003-2004 study period. Dermatitis 2008;19:129-136

60 Pratt MD, Belsito DV, DeLeo VA, Fowler JF Jr, Fransway AF, Maibach HI, et al. North American Contact Dermatitis Group patch-test results, 2001–2002 study period. Dermatitis 2004;15:176-183

61 De Groot AC, de Cock PAJJM, Coenraads PJ, van Ginkel CJW, Jagtman BA, van Joost, Th, et al. Methyldibromo-glutaronitrile is an important contact allergen in The Netherlands. Contact Dermatitis 1996;34:118-120

62 De Groot AC, Bruynzeel DP, Coenraads PJ, Crijns MB, van Ginkel CJW, van Joost Th, et al. Frequency of allergic reactions to methyldibromoglutaronitrile (1,2-dibromo-2,4-dicyanobutane) in The Netherlands. Contact Dermatitis 1991;25:270-271

63 Mathias CGT. Contact dermatitis to a new biocide (Tektamer 38®) used in a paste glue formulation. Contact Dermatitis 1983;9:418

64 Pigato PD, Bigardi A, Legori A, Altomare GF, Carminati G. Allergic contact dermatitis from Tektamer 38® (dibromocyanobutane). Contact Dermatitis 1991;25:138

65 Torres V, Pinto Soares A. Contact allergy to dibromodicyanobutane in a cosmetic cream. Contact Dermatitis 1992;27:114-115

66 O'Donnell BF, Foulds IS. Contact dermatitis due to dibromodicyanobutane in cucumber eye gel. Contact Dermatitis 1993;29:99-100

67 Fernández E, Navarro JA, del Pozo L, Fernández de Corrès L. Allergic contact dermatitis due to dibromodicyanobutane in cosmetics. Contact Dermatitis 1995;32:109-110

68 Okkerse A, Beursen-Reitsma AM, van Joost Th. Contact allergy to methyldibromoglutaronitrile and certain other preservatives. Contact Dermatitis 1996;34:151

69 Wahlkvist, H, Boman A, Montelius J, Wahlberg JE. Sensitizing potential in mice, guinea pig and man of the preservative Euxyl® K 400 and its ingredient methyldibromo glutaronitrile. Contact Dermatitis 1999;41:330-338

70 Armstrong DKB, Smith HR, Rycroft RJG. Contact allergy to methyldibromo glutaronitrile presenting as severe scalp seborrhoeic eczema. Contact Dermatitis 1999;40:335

71 Tosti A, Vincenzi C, Smith KA. Provocative use testing of methyldibromo glutaronitrile in a cosmetic shampoo. Contact Dermatitis 2000;42:64-67

72 Erdmann SM, Sachs B, Merk HF. Allergic contact dermatitis due to methyldibromo glutaronitrile in Euxyl K 400 in an ultrasonic gel. Contact Dermatitis 2001;44:39-40

73 Leitner B, Hemmer W, Focke M, et al. Kontaktdermatitis auf Ultraschallgel. Dermatosen 1999;47:164-165 (article in German)

74 Wong CSM, Beck MH. Occupational contact allergy to methyldibromo glutaronitrile in abrasive cleansers and work creams. Contact Dermatitis 2001;44:311-312

75 Wilkinson JD, Shaw S, Andersen KE, Brandão FM, Bruynzeel DP, Bruze M, et al. Monitoring levels of preservative sensitivity in Europe. A 10-year overview (1991–2000). Contact Dermatitis 2002;46:207-210

76 Diba VC, Chowdhury MMU, Adisesh A, Statham BN. Occupational allergic contact dermatitis in hospital workers caused by methyldibromo glutaronitrile in a work soap. Contact Dermatitis 2003;48:118-119

77 Zachariae C, Rastogi S, Devantier C, Menné T, Johansen JD. Methyldibromo glutaronitrile: clinical experience and exposure-based risk assessment. Contact Dermatitis 2003;48:150-154

78 Gruvberger B, Bruze M, Tammela M. Preservatives in moisturizers on the Swedish market. Acta Derm Venereol 1998;78:52-56

79 De Groot AC, Weyland JW. Contact allergy to methyldibromoglutaronitrile in the cosmetics preservative Euxyl K 400. Am J Cont Dermat 1991;2:31-32

80 Banerjee P, McFadden JP, Ross JS, Rycroft RJG, White IR. Increased positive patch test reactivity to methyldibromo glutaronitrile. Contact Dermatitis 2003;49:111-113

81 Young HS, Beck MH. Post-coital contact dermatitis from methyldibromo glutaronitrile. Contact Dermatitis 2004;50:48

82 Pedersen LK, Haslund P, Johansen JD, Held E, Vølund A, Agner T. Influence of a detergent on skin response to methyldibromo glutaronitrile in sensitized individuals. Contact Dermatitis 2004;50:1-5

83 Gruvberger B, Bjerkemo M, Bruze M. Stability of patch test preparations of methyldibromo glutaronitrile in petrolatum. Contact Dermatitis 2004;51:315-316

84 Sánchez-Pérez, J, Del Rio MJ, Jiménez YD, García-Diez A. Allergic contact dermatitis due to methyldibromo glutaronitrile in make-up removal wipes. Contact Dermatitis 2005;53:357-358

85 Jensen CD, Johansen JD, Menné T, Andersen KE. Methyldibromo glutaronitrile contact allergy: effect of single versus repeated daily exposure. Contact Dermatitis 2005;52:88-92

86 Bruze M, Goossens A, Gruvberger B. Recommendation to include methyldibromo glutaronitrile in the European standard patch test series. Contact Dermatitis 2005;52:24-28

87 Gruvberger B, Andersen KE, Brandão FM, Bruynzeel DP, Bruze M, Frosch PJ, et al. Patch testing with methyldibromo glutaronitrile, a multicentre study within the EECDRG. Contact Dermatitis 2005;52:14-18

88 Zachariae C, Johansen JD, Rastogi SC, Menné T. Allergic contact dermatitis from methyldibromo glutaronitrile – clinical cases from 2003. Contact Dermatitis 2005;52:6-8

89 Johansen JD, Veien NK, Laurberg G, Kaaber K, Thormann J, Lauritzen M, Avnstorp C, on Behalf Of The Danish Contact Dermatitis Group. Contact allergy to methyldibromo glutaronitrile – data from a 'front line' network. Contact Dermatitis 2005;52:138-141

90 Schnuch A, Kelterer D, Bauer A, Schuster Ch, Aberer W, Mahler V, et al. Quantitative patch and repeated open application testing in methyldibromo glutaronitrile-sensitive patients. Contact Dermatitis 2005;52:197-206

91 Gruvberger B, Andersen KE, Brandão FM, Bruynzeel DP, Bruze M, Frosch PJ, et al. Repeated open application test with methyldibromo glutaronitrile, a multicentre study within the EECDRG. Contact Dermatitis 2005;52:19-23

92 Bruze M, Gruvberger B, Goossens A, Hindsén M, Pontén A. Allergic contact dermatitis from methyldibromo-glutaronitrile. Dermatitis 2005;16:80-86

93 Bruze M, Gruvberger B, Zimerson E. A clinically relevant contact allergy to methyldibromo glutaronitrile at 1% (0.32 mg/cm2) detected by a patch test. Contact Dermatitis 2006;54:14-17

94 Jong CT, Statham BN. Methyldibromoglutaronitrile contact allergy – the beginning of the end? Contact Dermatitis 2006;54:229

95 Zoller L, Bergman R, Weltfriend S. Preservatives sensitivity in Israel: a 10-year overview (1995–2004). Contact Dermatitis 2006;55:227-229

96 Jensen CD, Johansen JD, Menné T, Andersen KE. Increased retest reactivity by both patch and use test with methyldibromoglutaronitrile in sensitized individuals. Acta Derm Venereol 2006;86:8-12

97 Luján-Rodríguez D, Peñate-Santana Y, Hernández-Machín B, Borrego L. Connubial allergic contact dermatitis to Euxyl K 400. Contact Dermatitis 2006;54:122-123

98 Williams JD, Frowen KE, Nixon RL. Allergic contact dermatitis from methyldibromo glutaronitrile in a sanitary pad and review of Australian clinic data. Contact Dermatitis 2007;56:164-167

99 Marcano ME, Heras F, Conde-Salazar L. Occupational allergic contact dermatitis to methyldibromoglutaronitrile in hand degreasing toilet paper. Contact Dermatitis 2007;57:126-127

100 Isaksson M, Gruvberger B, Bruze M. Repeated open application tests with methyldibromoglutaronitrile in dermatitis patients with and without hypersensitivity to methyldibromoglutaronitrile. Dermatitis 2007;18:203-207

101 Thyssen JP, Johansen JD, Menné T. Contact allergy epidemics and their controls. Contact Dermatitis 2007;56:185-195

102 Fischer LA, Johansen JD, Menné T. Methyldibromoglutaronitrile allergy: relationship between patch test and repeated open application test thresholds. Br J Dermatol 2008;159:1138-1143

103 Bordel-Gómez MT, Miranda-Romero A. Contact sensitization to Euxyl K-400. Actas Dermosifiliogr 2009;100:201-204

104 Javvaji S, Belsito DV. Patch testing with methyldibromoglutaronitrile in a localized population in the United States. Dermatitis 2010;21:321-326

105 Pratt MD, Belsito DV, DeLeo VA, Fowler JF Jr, Fransway AF, Maibach HI, et al. North American Contact Dermatitis Group patch-test results, 2001–2002 study period. Dermatitis 2004;15:176-183

106 Marks JG Jr, Belsito DV, DeLeo VA, Fowler JF Jr, Fransway AF, Maibach HI, et al. North American Contact Dermatitis Group patch-test results, 1998–2000. Am J Contact Dermat 2003;14:59-62

107 Kynemund-Pedersen L, Agner T, Held E, Johansen JD. Methyldibromo glutaronitrile in leave-on products elicits contact allergy at low concentration. Br J Dermatol 2004;151:817-822

108 Geier J, Uter W, Lessmann H, Schnuch A. Aktuelle Kontaktallergene. Hautarzt 2011;62:751-756

109 Beliauskiene A, Valiukeviciene S, Uter W, Schnuch A. The European baseline series in Lithuania: results of patch testing in consecutive adult patients. J Eur Acad Dermatol Venereol 2011;25:59-63

110 Uter W, Lessmann H, Geier J, Schnuch A. Contact allergy to hairdressing allergens in female hairdressers and clients – current data from the IVDK, 2003–2006. JDDG 2007;5:993-1001

111 Toholka R, Wang Y-S, Tate B, Tam M, Cahill J, Palmer A, Nixon R. The first Australian Baseline Series: Recommendations for patch testing in suspected contact dermatitis. Australas J Dermatol 2015;56:107-115

112 Zhao J, Li LF. Contact sensitization to cosmetic series of allergens in a general population in Beijing. J Cosmet Dermatol 2014;13:68-71

113 Zaragoza-Ninet V, Blasco Encinas R, Vilata-Corell JJ, Pérez-Ferriols A, Sierra-Talamantes C, Esteve-Martínez A, de la Cuadra-Oyanguren J. Allergic contact dermatitis due to cosmetics: A clinical and epidemiological study in a tertiary hospital. Actas Dermosifiliogr 2016;107:329-336

114 Dinkloh A, Worm M, Geier J, Schnuch A, Wollenberg A. Contact sensitization in patients with suspected cosmetic intolerance: results of the IVDK 2006-2011. J Eur Acad Dermatol Venereol 2015;29:1071-1081

115 Uter W, Rämsch C, Aberer, W, Ayala F, Balato A, Beliauskiene A, et al. The European baseline series in 10 European Countries, 2005/2006 – Results of the European Surveillance System on Contact Allergies (ESSCA). Contact Dermatitis 2009;61:31-38

116 Schwensen JF, Johansen JD, Veien NK, Funding AT, Avnstorp C, Østerballe M, et al. Occupational contact dermatitis in hairdressers: an analysis of patch test data from the Danish Contact Dermatitis Group, 2002–2011. Contact Dermatitis 2014;70:233-237

117 Uter W, Gefeller O, John SM, Schnuch A, Geier J. Contact allergy to ingredients of hair cosmetics – a comparison of female hairdressers and clients based on IVDK 2007–2012 data. Contact Dermatitis 2014;71:13-20

118 Warshaw EM, Wang MZ, Mathias CGT, Maibach HI, Belsito DV, Zug KA, et al. Occupational contact dermatitis in hairdressers/cosmetologists; retrospective analysis of North American Contact Dermatitis Group data, 1994 to 2010. Dermatitis 2012;23:258-268

119 Uter W, Yazar K, Kratz EM, Mildau G, Lidén C. Coupled exposure to ingredients of cosmetic products: II. Preservatives. Contact Dermatitis 2014;70:219-226

120 Giménez-Arnau AM, Deza G, Bauer A, Johnston GA, Mahler V, Schuttelaar ML, et al. Contact allergy to preservatives: ESSCA* results with the baseline series, 2009-2012. J Eur Acad Dermatol Venereol 2017;31:664-671

121 Lubbes S, Rustemeyer T, Sillevis Smitt JH, Schuttelaar ML, Middelkamp-Hup MA. Contact sensitization in Dutch children and adolescents with and without atopic dermatitis - a retrospective analysis. Contact Dermatitis 2017;76:151-159

122 Erfurt-Berge C, Geier J, Mahler V. The current spectrum of contact sensitization in patients with chronic leg ulcers or stasis dermatitis - new data from the Information Network of Departments of Dermatology (IVDK). Contact Dermatitis 2017;77:151-158

123 Chow ET, Avolio AM, Lee A, Nixon R. Frequency of positive patch test reactions to preservatives: The Australian experience. Australas J Dermatol 2013;54:31-35

124 Uter W, Amario-Hita JC, Balato A, Ballmer-Weber B, Bauer A, Belloni Fortina A, et al. European Surveillance System on Contact Allergies (ESSCA): results with the European baseline series, 2013/14. J Eur Acad Dermatol Venereol. 2017 Jun 19. doi: 10.1111/jdv.14423. [Epub ahead of print]

125 Vigan M, Brechat N, Girardin P. Un nouvel allergène: Le dibromodicyuanobutane. Compte rendu d'une étude portant sur 310 malades de Janvier à Décembre 1994. Ann Dermatol Venereol 1996;123:322-324

126 Bauer A, Oehme S, Geier J. Contact sensitization in the anal and genital area. Curr Probl Dermatol 2011;40:133-141

2.294   METHYLDIBROMO GLUTARONITRILE/PHENOXYETHANOL*

Not an INCI name

IDENTIFICATION

Description/definition : Methyldibromo glutaronitrile/phenoxyethanol is a mixture of methyldibromo glutaronitrile and phenoxyethanol in a 1:4 concentration, most commonly encountered trade name: Euxyl® K 400; for identification data see Chapter 2.293 Methyldibromo glutaronitrile and Chapter 2.356 Phenoxyethanol

Other name(s)   : Euxyl® K 400

CAS registry number (s) : 98668-04-3

Function(s) in cosmetics : EU: formerly used as preservative; prohibited; delisted in 2008 (methyldibromo glutaronitrile). USA: preservatives

Patch testing   : 0.1% pet. (SmartPracticeCanada); 1% pet. (SmartPracticeEurope, SmartPracticeCanada); 2% pet. (SmartPracticeCanada). Clinically relevant reactions to Euxyl K 400 1.5-2.5% pet. may sometimes be observed with negative reactions to both methyldibromo glutaronitrile and phenoxyethanol (47,56); irritant reactions to percentages of 2% and higher are not infrequent (67)

Molecular formula   : $C_6H_6Br_2N_2$ (methyldibromo glutaronitrile)
                          $C_8H_{10}O_2$ (phenoxyethanol)

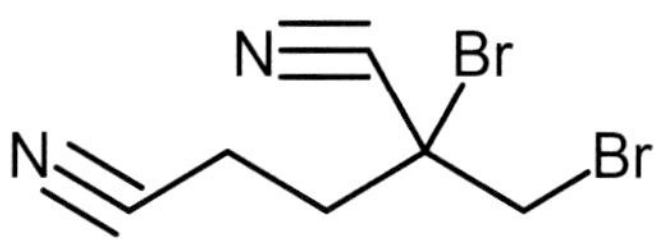

Methyldibromo glutaronitrile 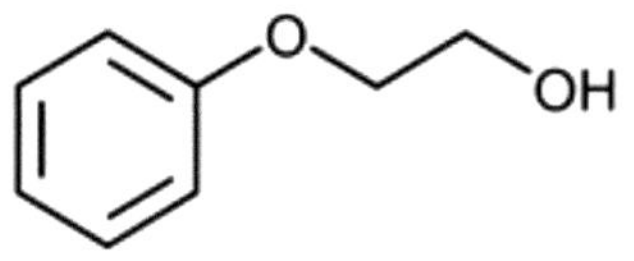   Phenoxyethanol

GENERAL

Methyldibromo glutaronitrile/phenoxyethanol (best known trade name: Euxyl K 4007; Isocide FG; Merguard 1105,1200, MCP; Chemynol K, abbreviated as MDBGN/PE) is a preservative system containing two active ingredients, 2-phenoxyethanol and methyldibromo glutaronitrile (1,2-dibromo-2,4-dicyanobutane) in a ratio of 4:1. Manufacturers began using this preservative system, mostly Euxyl K 400, in cosmetics because guinea pig testing showed no sensitizing potential of the separate ingredients (7) and a substitute for MCI/MI (see Chapter 2.292 Methylchloroisothiazolinone [and] methylisothiazolinone) was urgently needed (45). However, this sensitization study was later challenged and Euxyl K 400 and methyldibromo glutaronitrile *were* found to have allergenic potential (studies summarized in ref. 15). The preservative system was introduced in Europe in 1984 and in the United States approximately 5 years later. It is equally effective against bacteria, yeasts, and fungi at a low concentration of 0.1%. Euxyl K 400 was not only used as a preservative in cosmetics, predominantly in creams and lotions, but also in occupational products such as paint and cleaning agents. It soon became popular because of its effectiveness: in 1995. 25-35% of all cosmetics and 2/3 of all moistened toilet tissues in the Netherlands contained Euxyl K 400 (6).

The first cases of contact allergy to Euxyl K 400 were reported from Germany in 1989 (9). It was soon found that the sensitizer was nearly always methyldibromo glutaronitrile (MDBGN) (43,47,49,52). An increase in the prevalence of Euxyl K 400 and methyldibromo glutaronitrile contact allergy was soon observed in many European countries (6,10,47,49,62) from both stay-on and rinse-off cosmetics (43,47). In The Netherlands, nearly half of all cases were patients with perianal allergic contact dermatitis from Euxyl K 400 in moistened toilet tissues (6,10). Methyldibromo glutaronitrile (and consequently, Euxyl K 400) was banned in the EU from leave-on cosmetic products in 2003 and finally also in rinse-off products in 2007. In the United stated the preservative may still be used in maximum concentrations of 0.125% Euxyl K 400 (0.025% MDBGN) in stay-on and a maximum concentration of 0.3% (containing 0.06% MDBGN) in rinse-off products (15) following the advice of the Cosmetic Ingredient Review Expert Panel (17).

The literature on contact allergy to Euxyl K 400 and methyldibromo glutaronitrile up to 1996 has been reviewed by the author (6). A very useful review article was published in 2011 (15). Euxyl K 400 and other preservatives were also reviewed in 2004 (75). See also Chapter 2.293   Methyldibromo glutaronitrile and Chapter 2.356 Phenoxyethanol.

Although in most publications (especially the early ones) the trade name Euxyl K 400 was used, in this chapter the preservative mixture is termed methyldibromo glutaronitrile/phenoxyethanol, abbreviated as MDBGN/PE.

CONTACT ALLERGY

Contact allergy in the general population and subgroups
Estimates of the 9-year prevalence (1992-2000) of contact allergy to methyldibromo glutaronitrile/phenoxyethanol in the general population of Germany based on the CE-DUR method ranged from 0.2%-0.3% (medium case scenario) to 0.4%-0.7% (worst case scenario) (16,36).

Patch testing in groups of patients
Results of studies testing MDBGN/PE in consecutive patients suspected of contact dermatitis (routine testing) back to 1990 are shown in table 2.294.1. Results of testing in groups of *selected* patients (e.g., patients suspected of cosmetic dermatitis, individuals with eyelid / periorbital dermatitis, hairdressers, patients suspected of occupational dermatitis) back to 1994 are shown in table 2.294.2.

Patch testing in consecutive patients suspected of contact dermatitis: routine testing
There are many data available on routine testing with MDBGN/PE, especially from the USA, where the preservative system has since over 25 years been part of the screening series of the North American Contact Dermatitis Group (NACDG), which publishes its results biannually. There have also been many reports from European countries and from the ESSCA (European Surveillance System on Contact Allergies), with participants from 9-12 countries (5,29,72,73). Unfortunately, many different test concentrations have been used (all in petrolatum): 0.4%, 0.5%, 1%, 1.5%, 2% and 2.5%. Irritant reactions to percentages of MDBGN/PE 2% and higher are not infrequent (47,67), but lower concentrations may result in false-negative reactions (47). In studies where 2 test concentrations were used, the higher test concentration always gave a higher frequency of positive reactions (22,23,24,63), but in most of these (22,23,24), the higher test concentration was 2.5% pet., which is known to induce irritant reactions.

Taken all studies and concentrations together, frequencies of sensitization to MDBGN/PE have ranged from 1.4% to 11.7%; most studies had rates of >3%. The lower frequencies were seen especially before 1995, when MDBGN/PE was still an 'emerging' allergen. In the NACDG studies, relevance rates were low, 'definite' + 'probable' relevance nearly always scoring below 30%. In most other studies, relevance was not mentioned, but in the studies that did address this issue, relevance rates were 33% (43), 42% (64), 67% (47) and 'most' (52). Incriminated products were always cosmetics, both stay-on and rinse-off products.

Table 2.294.1 Patch testing in groups of patients: Routine testing

Years and Country	Test conc. & vehicle	Number of patients tested | positive (%)		Selection of patients (S); Relevance (R); Comments (C)	Ref.
2013-14 USA, Canada	2% pet.	4855	179 (3.7%)	R: definite + probable relevance: 24%	70
2011-12 USA, Canada	2% pet.	4231	157 (3.7%)	R: definite + probable relevance: 26%	18
2009-2012, 12 European countries [b]	1.5% pet.	4590	(2.0%) [a]	R: not stated; C: range per country: one country only	73
2009-10 USA, Canada	2% pet.	4303	164 (3.8%)	R: definite + probable relevance: 26%	19
2006-2010 USA	1.5% pet.	3077	(6.6%)	R: 35%	32
2001-2010 Australia	0.5% pet.	5133	142 (2.8%)	R: 22%	69
1994-2009 USA	various	1753	70 (4.0%)	R: definite + probable relevance: 8% for the + reactions, 38% for the ++ and +++ reactions	67
2007-8 USA, Canada	2.5% pet.	5083	(5.5%)	R: definite + probable relevance 28%	12
2005-6 USA, Canada	2.5% pet.	4437	(5.8%)	R: definite + probable relevance: 31%	11
2005-6 10 European countries [b]	1% pet.	1242	41 (3.3%)	R: not stated; C: prevalences ranged from 0.9 to 4.0%	72
2000-2005 Spain		1092	15 (1.4%)	R: probably not stated; C: 11 of the patients reacted to the methyldibromo glutaronitrile component, 2 to phenoxyethanol and 2 to neither of the constituents	66
2000-2005 USA	1.5% pet.	3839	(6.1%)	R: 46%	2
1998-2004 IVDK	1% pet.	60,936	2593(3.9%) [a]	R: not stated	4
2004, 11 European countries [b]	1% pet.	1658	76 (4.0%) [a]	R: not stated; C: range positives: 1.9%-6.7%	5
2003-4 USA, Canada	2.5% pet.	5140	315 (6.1%)	R: not stated	13
2002-2003, 9 European countries [b]	1% pet.	3525	(4.1%)	R: not stated; C: prevalence range per center (n=17) 0.9%-6.8%	29
2001-2002 USA	2.5% pet.	4897	(5.8%)	R: definite + probable relevance: 18%	22
	4% pet. [c]	4897	(2.7%)	R: definite + probable relevance: 23%	
1998-00 USA, Canada	2.5% pet.	5778	(6.0%)	R: definite + probable relevance: 10%	23
	0.4% pet.	5797	(3.5%)	R: definite + probable relevance: 12%	
1998-1999 Spain	0.5% pet.	528	5 (1.0%)	R: not found	53

Table 2.294.1 Patch testing in groups of patients: Routine testing (*continued*)

Years and Country	Test conc. & vehicle	Number of patients tested	positive (%)		Selection of patients (S); Relevance (R); Comments (C)	Ref.
1996-98 USA, Canada	2.5% pet.	4054		(7.6%)	R: definite + probable + possible relevance: 59%	24
	1% pet.	4053		(2.7%)	R: definite + probable + possible relevance: 74%	24
<1998 USA	2.5% and 1% pet.	163	19	(11.7%)	R: definite relevance in 8 patients, probable in 5; many used one particular brand of moisturizing lotion; there were many Irritant reactions	64
1997-1998 IVDK	1% pet.	4615		(3.5%)	R: not stated; C: the authors stated that testing with 1% identifies more allergic patients than with 0.5%	63
	0.5% pet.	4615		(2.3%)		
1994-1996 USA	1% pet.	3074		(2.0%)	R: definite + probable relevance: 15%	25
1993-5 Netherlands	0.5% pet.	1019	24	(2.4%)	R: most patients had contact with products, notably cosmetics, containing Euxyl K 400; C: all 24 patients also reacted to methyldibromo glutaronitrile, the allergenic component of the preservative mixture	52
1992-1994 USA	1% pet.	3481		(1.5%)	R: present relevance: 23%	26
1991-1994 Italy	2.5% pet.	3455	64	(2.8%)	R: In 2/3 of the cases, patients used cosmetics containing MDBGN/PE, both stay-on and rinse-off cosmetics	47
1990-1994 Germany	0.5% pet.	25,584	444	(1.8%)	R: not stated	27
1988-1990 Italy	2.5% pet. and alc.	2057	24	(1.2%)	R: eight cases were caused by cosmetics containing Euxyl K 400; C: both stay-on and rinse-off products were responsible; increase in frequency of sensitization from 1988 to 1990	43

[a] age-standardized and sex-standardized proportions
[b] study performed by the ESSCA (European Surveillance System on Contact Allergies)
[c] possibly a mistake, should likely be 0.4%
IVDK: Information Network of Departments of Dermatology, Germany, Austria, Switzerland

Patch testing in groups of selected patients

Results of testing MDBGN/PE in groups of *selected* patients (e.g., patients suspected of cosmetic dermatitis, individuals with eyelid / periorbital dermatitis, hairdressers, patients suspected of occupational dermatitis) back to 1994 are shown in table 2.294.2. In 11 investigations, frequencies of sensitization have ranged from 1.4% to 6.9%, generally not higher than in routine testing. The highest frequency was seen in a group of female hairdressers with present or past occupational contact dermatitis, but the relevance of the observed reactions was not mentioned (34).

Table 2.294.2 Patch testing in groups of patients: Selected patient groups

Years and Country	Test conc. & vehicle	Number of patients tested	positive (%)		Selection of patients (S); Relevance (R); Comments (C)	Ref.
2010-2011 Korea	1.5% pet.	584	25	(4.3%)	S: patients suspected of allergic cosmetic dermatitis; R: not stated	31
2006-2011 Singapore	1.5% pet.	345	7	(2.0%)	S: not specified; R: not stated; C: prevalence in men was 3.2%, in women 1.8%	33
2006-2010 USA	1.5% pet.	100	6	(6%)	S: patients with eyelid dermatitis; R: not stated	14
2000-2010 IVDK		1433	39	(2.7%)	S: patients with periorbital dermatitis; R: not stated	20
2000-2007 USA	1.5% pet.	938	53	(5.7%)	S: patients tested with a supplemental cosmetic screening series; R: 98%; C: weak study: a. high rate of macular erythema and weak reactions; b. relevance figures included 'questionable' and 'past' relevance	1
1993-2006 Australia	1.5% pet.	5628		(3.3%)	S: not stated; R: 20%	74
1993-2003 IVDK	1% pet.	1222	32	(2.6%)	S: patients with scalp dermatitis; R: not stated	30
1995-2002 IVDK		884		(6.9%)	S: female hairdressers with present or past occupational contact dermatitis; R: not specified	34
		1217		(2.7%)	S: clients of hairdressers suspected to react to hairdressing cosmetics or hair care products; R: not specified	
1995-1999 IVDK	1% pet.	937		(1.4%)	S: patients with allergic periorbital contact dermatitis; R: not stated	39
1989-1996 Finland	0.5% pet.	736	11	(1.5%)	S: patients suspected of occupational contact dermatitis; R: 3 reactions were relevant, two of which were from occupational contact with soap and a dishwashing detergent	50
1990-1994 Germany	0.5% pet.	11,422	263	(2.3%)	S: patients tested with a preservative series; R: not stated	27

IVDK: Information Network of Departments of Dermatology, Germany, Austria, Switzerland

Case reports and case series

Case series

In the period 2011-2014, 79 patients with a positive patch test reaction to an allergen identified with a wet wipe source were investigated by the members of the NACDG. MDBGN/PE was the (or an) allergen in 5% of the cases (4 patients). Patients with wipe allergy were 15 times more likely to have anal/genital dermatitis compared with those without wipe allergy (77). In the period 1996-2013, in a tertiary referral center in Valencia, Spain, 5419 patients were patch tested. Of these, 628 individuals had allergic contact dermatitis to cosmetics. Methyldibromo glutaronitrile/phenoxyethanol was the responsible allergen in 23 cases (71, overlap with ref. 41). In the period 2000-2007, 202 patients with allergic contact dermatitis caused by cosmetics were seen in Valencia, Spain. In this group, 16 individuals reacted to MDBGN/PE from its presence in moisturizing cream (n=7), in cleansing wipes (n=4), in gel/soap (n=2), in makeup (n=2), and in sunscreen (n=1) (41, overlap with ref. 71). In a group of 2193 patients (1582 women, 611 men) with (presumed) cosmetic allergy, 8.3% of the women and 11.8% of the men had positive patch tests to MDBGN/PE, which were related to a cosmetic source, in a study of the NACDG, 2001-2004 (3).

In a group of 60 patients with allergic contact cheilitis seen by the members of the NACDG between 2001 and 2004, 3 cases (5.0%) were caused by MDBGN/PE in unspecified cosmetics (35). In a group of 83 patients with cheilitis, seen in Bologna, Italy in the period 2001-2005, 3 reacted to MDBGN/PE in (unspecified) cosmetics (38). In a group of 24 patients reacting to MDBGN/PE in Italy, 8 had allergic cosmetic dermatitis. Three patients had facial contact dermatitis from a moisturizing cream, one diffuse dermatitis from multiple products containing the preservative, three had dermatitis from soap (2 hand dermatitis, the 3rd diffuse eczema) and one woman had facial dermatitis from a rinse-off facial cleansing lotion (43).

Case reports

A woman had contact allergy to MDBGN/PE in an anti-ageing day cream (21). One patient had axillary dermatitis from contact allergy to MDBGN/PE in a deodorant, another reacted to the preservative in a moisturizer and developed allergic contact dermatitis of the face (40). Two women had severe eyelid dermatitis from contact allergy to MDBGN/PE in an eye gel (44); a third reacted to both MDBGN/PE and to MDBGN (59). One patient had allergic contact dermatitis of the face from MDBGN in MDBGN/PE in an anti-wrinkle lotion (9). A masseur developed occupational allergic contact dermatitis of the hands from MDBGN in Euxyl K 400 in a massage lotion (9). A woman had allergic contact dermatitis of the face from MDBGN/PE in a sunscreen that she used for polymorphic light eruption (51). One patient had allergic contact dermatitis of the axillae spreading to the trunk and the limbs from MDBGN/PE in a natural cosmetic containing deer fat (54). Another patient had ACD from MDBGN/PE in a self-made skin care product (58).

A woman had contact dermatitis of the forehead from contact allergy to MDBGN/PE present in a cosmetic protecting cream, which was applied before a permanent wave (55). A female patient developed acute ACD of the face and neck from contact allergy to MDBGN in Euxyl K 400 present in a night cleansing cream (60). Another woman had contact allergy to MDBGN in MDBGN/PE in a cleansing milk and make up causing facial dermatitis, whereas a body milk preserved with the preservative system was the cause of hand eczema (61). One patient had chronic perianal eczema from contact allergy to MDBGN/PE in moist toilet paper (37). Four more patients had perianal dermatitis from sensitization to methyldibromo glutaronitrile in MDBGN/PE present in moist toilet tissues (57). A man had active allergic contact dermatitis from MDBGN in a moist toilet paper preserved with MDBGN/PE (45,48).

Contact allergy to MDBGN/PE in non-cosmetic products

One patient developed allergic contact dermatitis on the abdomen after sonography from MDBGN/PE in the ultra-sound gel used (46). One individual had occupational allergic contact dermatitis of the hands from MDBGN/PE in a hand cleanser, another from a liquid dishwashing detergent (50). A female farmer had occupational allergic contact dermatitis of the hands from MDBGN/PE in a 'milking cream' that she used for the udders of her cows after milking (76). A process technician in a 'commercial product manufacturing plant' became sensitized to MDBGN/PE, with which he had contact at work. The nature of the contact material was not mentioned (28).

Cross-reactions, pseudo-cross-reactions and co-reactions

Pseudo-cross-reactions may be observed to methyldibromo glutaronitrile and – to a far lesser degree – to phenoxyethanol, which are the constituents of MDBGN/PE. MDBGN is virtually always the allergenic ingredient (43,47,49,52).

Provocation tests

Five of 11 patients (45%) (43) and 8 of 14 (57%) (47), who were patch test positive to MDBGN/PE 2.5% pet., had a positive ROAT to a lotion preserved with 0.1% MDBGN/PE. A group of 39 patients sensitized to MDBGN/PE performed ROATs with ointments containing various concentrations of this preservative system. There were 15 negative and 24 positive tests. Of the 24 with positive ROATs, 13 patients reacted to an ointment with 50 ppm MDBGN (250 ppm Euxyl K 400), 8 to 100 ppm (500 ppm Euxyl K 400) and 3 to only the highest concentration of 250 ppm MDBGN (1250 ppm Euxyl K 400) (65).

Presence in cosmetic products and chemical analyses
In July 2017, methyldibromo glutaronitrile/phenoxyethanol was present in zero of 64,655 cosmetic products of which the composition is known in EWG's Skin Deep Cosmetics Database, USA (http://www.ewg.org/skindeep/). In the USA, in April 2017, MDBGN/PE was present in zero of 56,714 cosmetic products of which the composition is known in FDA's Voluntary Cosmetic Registration Program (VCRP) (data obtained from FDA, May 2017). It should be realized that methyldibromo glutaronitrile/phenoxyethanol is not an INCI name, used neither in CosIng nor in the Personal Care Products Council Ingredient Database. Hence, products containing MDBGN/PE may either be classified as containing methyldibromo glutaronitrile, as phenoxyethanol or both. Unfortunately, both chemicals are also used as single preservatives. As a consequence, determining the frequency of use of MDBGN/PE in cosmetics in the USA at the moment seems impossible.

In The Netherlands, in 1990, approximately 13% of all cosmetic products were preserved with MDBGN/PE (45). In 1995, the percentage had risen to 25% to 35%, including some of the most widely used brands (6). In that year, two thirds of all moistened toilet tissues in The Netherlands were preserved with Euxyl K 400 (6). In Germany in 1993, MDBGN/PE was said to be present in no more than 20 cosmetic products (8). However, two years later, and estimated 5% of cosmetic products in Germany contained methyldibromo glutaronitrile (personal communication, J. Ellis, October 1995, cited in ref. 6).

OTHER INFORMATION
Sensitization studies (e.g., 7,8,42) are discussed in ref. 15.

LITERATURE
1   Wetter DA, Yiannias JA, Prakash AV, Davis MD, Farmer SA, el-Azhary RA, et al. Results of patch testing to personal care product allergens in a standard series and a supplemental cosmetic series: an analysis of 945 patients from the Mayo Clinic Contact Dermatitis Group, 2000-2007. J Am Acad Dermatol 2010;63:789-798
2   Davis MD, Scalf LA, Yiannias JA, Cheng JF, El-Azhary RA, Rohlinger AL, et al. Changing trends and allergens in the patch test standard series. Arch Dermatol 2008;144:67-72
3   Warshaw EM, Buchholz HJ, Belsito DV et al. Allergic patch test reactions associated with cosmetics: Retrospective analysis of cross-sectional data from the North American Contact Dermatitis Group, 2001-2004. J Am Acad Dermatol 2009;60:23-38
4   Schnuch A, Lessmann H, Geier J, Uter W. Contact allergy to preservatives. Analysis of IVDK data 1996-2009. Br J Dermatol 2011;164:1316-1325
5   ESSCA Writing Group. The European Surveillance System of Contact Allergies (ESSCA): results of patch testing the standard series, 2004. J Eur Acad Dermatol Venereol 2008;22:174-181
6   De Groot AC, van Ginkel CJW, Weijland JW. Methyldibromoglutaronitrile (Euxyl K 400): An important 'new' allergen in cosmetics. J Am Acad Dermatol 1996;35:743-747
7   Bruze M, Gruvberger B, Agrup G. Sensitization studies in the guinea pig with the active ingredients of Euxyl[R] K 400. Contact Dermatitis 1988;18:37-39
8   Hausen BM. The sensitizing potency of Euxyl[R] K 400 and its components 1,2-dibromo-2,4-dicyanobutane and 2-phenoxyethanol. Contact Dermatitis 1993;28:149-153
9   Senff H, Exner M, Gortz J, Goos M. Allergic contact dermatitis from Euxyl K 400. Contact Dermatitis 1989;20:381-382 (also published in Dermatosen 1989;37:45-46)
10   Van Ginkel CJW, Rundervoort GJ. Increasing incidence of contact allergy to the new preservative 1,2-dibromo-2,4-dicyanobutane (methyldibromoglutaronitrile). Br J Dermatol 1995;132:918-920
11   Zug KA, Warshaw EM, Fowler JF Jr, Maibach HI, Belsito DL, Pratt MD, et al. Patch-test results of the North American Contact Dermatitis Group 2005-2006. Dermatitis 2009;20:149-160
12   Fransway AF, Zug KA, Belsito DV, Deleo VA, Fowler JF Jr, Maibach HI, et al. North American Contact Dermatitis Group patch test results for 2007-2008. Dermatitis 2013;24:10-21
13   Warshaw EM, Belsito DV, DeLeo VA, Fowler JF Jr, Maibach HI, Marks JG, et al. North American Contact Dermatitis Group patch-test results, 2003-2004 study period. Dermatitis 2008;19:129-136
14   Wenk KS, Ehrlich AE. Fragrance series testing in eyelid dermatitis. Dermatitis 2012;23:22-26
15   Aakhus AE, Warshaw EM. Allergy to methyldibromoglutaronitrole/phenoxyethanol (Euxyl K 400): Regulatory issues, epidemiology, clinical characteristics, and management. Dermatitis 2011;22:127-140
16   Brasch J, Becker D, Aberer W Bircher A, Kränke B, Denzer-Fürst S, et al. Contact Dermatitis. J Dtsch Dermatol Ges 2007;5:943-951

17 Cosmetic Ingredient Review Expert Panel. Final report on the safety assessment of methyldibromo glutaronitrile. J Am Coll Toxicol 1996;15:140-165

18 Warshaw EM, Maibach HI, Taylor JS, Sasseville D, DeKoven JG, Zirwas MJ, et al. North American Contact Dermatitis Group patch test results: 2011-2012. Dermatitis 2015;26:49-59

19 Warshaw EM, Belsito DV, Taylor JS, Sasseville D, DeKoven JG, Zirwas MJ, et al. North American Contact Dermatitis Group patch test results: 2009 to 2010. Dermatitis 2013;24:50-59

20 Landeck L, John SM, Geier J. Periorbital dermatitis in 4779 patients – patch test results during a 10-year period. Contact Dermatitis 2014;70:205-212

21 Silva R, Almeida LMS, Brandão FM. Photoallergy to oxybenzone in cosmetic creams. Contact Dermatitis 1995;32:176

22 Pratt MD, Belsito DV, DeLeo VA, Fowler JF Jr, Fransway AF, Maibach HI, et al. North American Contact Dermatitis Group patch-test results, 2001–2002 study period. Dermatitis 2004;15:176-183

23 Marks JG Jr, Belsito DV, DeLeo VA, Fowler JF Jr, Fransway AF, Maibach HI, et al. North American Contact Dermatitis Group patch-test results, 1998–2000. Am J Contact Dermat 2003;14:59-62

24 Marks JG Jr, Belsito DV, DeLeo VA, Fowler JF Jr, Fransway AF, Maibach HI, et al. North American Contact Dermatitis Group patch test results, 1996–1998. Arch Dermatol 2000;136:272-273

25 Marks JG Jr, Belsito DV, DeLeo VA, Fowler JF Jr, Fransway AF, Maibach HI, et al. North American Contact Dermatitis Group patch test results for the detection of delayed-type hypersensitivity to topical allergens. J Am Acad Dermatol 1998;38:911-918

26 Marks JG, Belsito DV, DeLeo VA, Fowler JF, Fransway AF, Maibach HI, et al. North American Contact Dermatitis Group standard tray patch test results 1992 through 1994. Am J Contact Dermatitis 1995;6:160-165

27 Schnuch A, Geier J, Uter W, Frosch PJ. Patch testing with preservatives, antimicrobials and industrial biocides. Results from a multicentre study. Br J Dermatol 1998;138:467-476

28 Primka EJ 3rd, Taylor JS. Three cases of contact allergy after chemical burns from methylchloroisothiazolinone/ methylisothiazolinone: one with concomitant allergy to methyldibromoglutaronitrile/phenoxyethanol. Am J Cont Dermat 1997;8:43-46

29 Uter W, Hegewald J, Aberer W, Ayala F, Bircher AJ, Brasch J, et al. The European standard series in 9 European countries, 2002/2003 –First results of the European Surveillance System on Contact Allergies. Contact Dermatitis 2005;53:136-145

30 Hillen U, Grabbe S, Uter W. Patch test results in patients with scalp dermatitis: analysis of data of the Information Network of Departments of Dermatology. Contact Dermatitis 2007;56:87-93

31 Lee SS, Hong DK, Jeong NJ, Lee JH, Choi YS, Lee AY, et al. Multicenter study of preservative sensitivity in patients with suspected cosmetic contact dermatitis in Korea. J Dermatol 2012;39:677-681

32 Wentworth AB, Yiannias JA, Keeling JH, Hall MR, Camilleri MJ, Drage LA, et al. Trends in patch-test results and allergen changes in the standard series: a Mayo Clinic 5-year retrospective review (January 1, 2006, to December 31, 2010). J Am Acad Dermatol 2014;70:269-275

33 Cheng S, Leow YH, Goh CL, Goon A. contact sensitivity to preservatives in Singapore: frequency of sensitization to 11 common preservatives 2006–2011. Dermatitis 2014;25:77-82

34 Uter W, Lessmann H, Geier J, Schnuch A. Contact allergy to ingredients of hair cosmetics in female hairdressers and clients: an 8-year analysis of IVDK data. Contact Dermatitis 2003;49:236-240

35 Zug KA, Kornik R, Belsito DV, DeLeo VA, Fowler JF Jr, Maibach HI, et al. Patch-testing North American lip dermatitis patients: Data from the North American Contact Dermatitis Group, 2001 to 2004. Dermatitis 2008;19:202-208

36 Schnuch A, Uter W, Geier J, Gefeller O (for the IVDK study group). Epidemiology of contact allergy: an estimation of morbidity employing the clinical epidemiology and drug-utilization research (CE-DUR) approach. Contact Dermatitis 2002;47:32-39

37 Blecher P, Korting HC. Tolerance to different toilet paper preparations: Toxicological and allergological aspects. Dermatology 1995;191:299-304

38 Zoli V, Silvani S, Vincenzi C, Tosti A. Allergic contact cheilitis. Contact Dermatitis 2006;54:296-297

39 Herbst RA, Uter W, Pirker C, Geier J, Frosch PJ. Allergic and non-allergic periorbital dermatitis: patch test results of the Information Network of the Departments of Dermatology during a 5-year period. Contact Dermatitis 2004;51:13-19

40 Held E, Johansen JD, Agner T, Menné T. Contact allergy to cosmetics: testing with patients' own products. Contact Dermatitis 1999;40:310-315

41 Laguna C, de la Cuadra J, Martín-González B, Zaragoza V, Martínez-Casimiro L, Alegre V. Allergic contact dermatitis to cosmetics. Actas Dermosifiliogr 2009;100:53-60

42 Wahlkvist H, Boman A, Montelius J, Wahlberg JE. Sensitizing potential in mice, guinea pig and man of the preservative Euxyl® K 400 and its ingredient methyldibromo glutaronitrile. Contact Dermatitis 1999;41:330-338

43 Tosti A, Guerra L, Bardazzi F, Gasparri F. Euxyl K 400: a new sensitizer in cosmetics. Contact Dermatitis 1991;25:89-93

44 Ross JS, Crokin E, White IR, Rycroft RJG. Contact dermatitis from Euxyl K 400 in cucumber eye gel. Contact Dermatitis 1992;26:60

45 De Groot AC, Weyland JW. Contact allergy to methyldibromoglutaronitrile in the cosmetics preservative Euxyl K 400. Am J Cont Derm 1991;2:31-32

46 Gebhart M, Stuhlert A, Knopf B. Allergic contact dermatitis due to Euxyl® K 400 in an ultrasonic gel. Contact Dermatitis 1993;29:272

47 Tosti A, Vincenzi C, Trevisi P, Guerra L. Euxyl K 400: incidence of sensitization, patch test concentration and vehicle. Contact Dermatitis 1995;33:193-195

48 De Groot AC, Baar TJM, Terpstra H, Weyland JW. Contact allergy to most toilet paper. Contact Dermatitis 1991;24:135-136

49 Schnuch A, Geier J. Die häufigsten Kontaktallergene im zweiten Halbjahr 1993. Dermatosen 1994;42:210 -211

50 Aalto-Korte K, Jolanki R, Estlander T, Alanko K, Kanerva L. Occupational allergic contact dermatitis caused by Euxyl K 400. Contact Dermatitis 1996;35:193-194

51 Silvestre JF, Rodrogiez-Serna M, Miquel JF, Gauchía R, Aliaga A. Allergic contact dermatitis from Euxyl K 400 in a sunscreen cream. Contact Dermatitis 1996;35:315

52 Okkerse A, Beursen-Rettsma AM, van Joost Th. Contact allergy to methyldibromoglutaronitrile and certain other preservatives. Contact Dermatitis 1996;34:151

53 Guimaraens D, Hernandez MI, Gonzalez MA, Conde-Salazar L. Contact allergy to Euxyl K 400 in consecutively patch-tested patients. Contact Dermatitis 2000;43:55

54 Hillen U, Franckson T, Goos M. Allergic contact dermatitis due to deer-fat cream (Hirschtalgcreme). Contact Dermatitis 2001;44:51-52

55 Kelterer D, Kaatz M, Bauer HI, Thiele J, Elsner P. Contact allergy to methyldibromo glutaronitrile in Euxyl® K 400 in a cosmetic cream for protection against a permanent wave solution. Contact Dermatitis 2002;46:250

56 Owen JL, del Rosario E, Cruz P. Conundrums of patch testing to Euxyl K 400 and its components. Dermatitis 2014;25:210

57 Hulsmans R-FHJ, Lucker GPH, van der Kley AMJ, et al. Kathon CG and methyldibromoglutaronitrile: important contact allergens in patients with perianal dermatitis. Aktuelle Koloproktologie 1992;9:275-286

58 Keilig W. Kontaktallergie auf einen neuen Konservierungsstof (Euxyl K 400). Parfumerie Kosmetik 1991;72:167-168

59 O'Donnell BF, Foulds IS. Contact dermatitis due to dibromodicyanobutane in cucumber eye gel. Contact Dermatitis 1993;29:99-100

60 Torres V, Pinto Soares A. Contact allergy to dibromodicyanobutane in a cosmetic cream. Contact Dermatitis 1992;27:114-115

61 Fernandez E, Navarro JA, del Pozo L, Fernández de Corrès L. Allergic contact dermatitis due to dibromodicyanobutane in cosmetics. Contact Dermatitis 1995;32:109-110

62 Wilkinson JD, Shaw S, Andersen KE, Brandao FM, Bruynzeel DP, Bruze M, et al. Monitoring levels of preservative sensitivity in Europe. A 10-year overview (1991-2000). Contact Dermatitis 2002;46:207-210

63 Geier J, Schnuch A, Brasch J, Gefeller O. Patch testing with methyldibromoglutaronitrile. Am J Contact Dermatitis 2000;11:207-212

64 Jackson JM, Fowler JF Jr. Methyldibromoglutaronitrile (Euxyl K 400): a new and important sensitizer in the United States? J Am Acad Dermatol 1998;38:934-937

65 Schnuch A, Kelterer D, Bauer A, Schuster Ch, Aberer W, Mahler V, et al. Quantitative patch and repeated open application testing in methyldibromo glutaronitrile-sensitive patients. Contact Dermatitis 2005;52:197-206

66 Bordel-Gómez MT, Miranda-Romero A. Contact sensitization to Euxyl K-400. Actas Dermosifiliogr 2009;100:201-204

67 Javvaji S, Belsito DV. Patch testing with methyldibromoglutaronitrile in a localized population in the United States. Dermatitis 2010;21:321-326

68 Bruze M, Goossens A, Gruvberger B. Recommendation to include methyldibromo glutaronitrile in the European standard patch test series. Contact Dermatitis 2005;52:24-28

69 Toholka R, Wang Y-S, Tate B, Tam M, Cahill J, Palmer A, Nixon R. The first Australian Baseline Series: Recommendations for patch testing in suspected contact dermatitis. Australas J Dermatol 2015;56:107-115

70 DeKoven JG, Warshaw EM, Belsito DV, Sasseville D, Maibach HI, Taylor JS, et al. North American Contact Dermatitis Group Patch Test Results: 2013-2014. Dermatitis. 2016 Oct 21. [Epub ahead of print]

71 Zaragoza-Ninet V, Blasco Encinas R, Vilata-Corell JJ, Pérez-Ferriols A, Sierra-Talamantes C, Esteve-Martínez A, de la Cuadra-Oyanguren J. Allergic contact dermatitis due to cosmetics: A clinical and epidemiological study in a tertiary hospital. Actas Dermosifiliogr 2016;107:329-336

72 Uter W, Rämsch C, Aberer, W, Ayala F, Balato A, Beliauskiene A, et al. The European baseline series in 10 European Countries, 2005/2006 – Results of the European Surveillance System on Contact Allergies (ESSCA). Contact Dermatitis 2009;61:31-38

73 Giménez-Arnau AM, Deza G, Bauer A, Johnston GA, Mahler V, Schuttelaar ML, et al. Contact allergy to preservatives: ESSCA* results with the baseline series, 2009-2012. J Eur Acad Dermatol Venereol 2017;31:664-671

74 Chow ET, Avolio AM, Lee A, Nixon R. Frequency of positive patch test reactions to preservatives: The Australian experience. Australas J Dermatol 2013;54:31-35

75 Sasseville D. Hypersensitivity to preservatives. Dermatol Ther 2004;17:251-263

76 Haapasaari K-M, Niinimäki A. Allergic contact dermatitis from alkylammonium amidobenzoate (Osmaron B®). Contact Dermatitis 2000;42:244-245

77 Warshaw EM, Aschenbeck KA, Zug KA, Belsito DV, Zirwas MJ, Fowler JF Jr, Taylor JS, et al. Wet wipe allergens: Retrospective analysis from the North American Contact Dermatitis Group 2011-2014. Dermatitis 2017;28:64-69

2.295   METHYL DIHYDROXYBENZOATE

IDENTIFICATION

Description/definition	: Methyl dihydroxybenzoate is the organic compound that conforms to the formula shown below
Chemical class(es)	: Esters
Chemical/IUPAC name	: Benzoic acid, 2,5-dihydroxy-, methyl ester
Other names	: Methyl gentisate; methyl 2,5-dihydroxybenzoate
CAS registry number (s)	: 2150-46-1
EC number(s)	: 218-427-8
Function(s) in cosmetics	: EU: chelating. USA: chelating agents
Patch testing	: 0.05% pet. (1); 0.5% alcohol (2); this test preparation is not irritant (2)
Molecular formula	: $C_8H_8O_4$

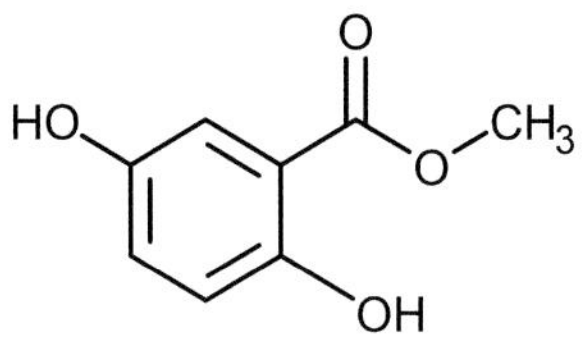

GENERAL

Methyl dihydroxybenzoate is the methyl ester of dihydroxybenzoic acid (gentisic acid). It is a natural product derived from the roots of plants of the genus Gentiana. It is a relatively new skin-lightening agent and is structurally similar to hydroquinone. Methyl gentisate *in vitro* inhibits pigmentation in melanocytes, inhibits tyrosinase selectivity, and has reduced cytotoxicity as compared to hydroquinone (1).

CONTACT ALLERGY

Case reports and case series

A non-atopic woman reported having developed a strong eczematous reaction on the face within a few days of daily applications of a skin-lightening gel. Patch testing with the SIDAPA standard series and the patient's gel as is showed positive reaction to the bleaching gel at D2 and D4. A ROAT performed with the cream in the antecubital fossa was positive within 2 days. Later, the ingredients of the cosmetic product were tested, which yielded a positive response to the active bleaching ingredient, methyl gentisate (methyl dihydroxybenzoate) 0.5% alc. This test preparation was negative in 20 controls (2).

A female patient used a skin lightening face mask containing methyl gentisate because of melasma, which gave cosmetic improvement. Five years later, she used the face mask again, but now she developed severe facial erythema followed by edema affecting both cheeks. After healing, a provocation test was performed, which resulted in the same reaction. Patch tests with the Spanish baseline series, a cosmetic series, and the face mask gave positive reactions to the mask and to methyl gentisate 0.05% in pet.; hydroquinone, which she had also used, was negative (1). In this publication, a similar case was presented of a woman who developed allergic contact dermatitis of the cheeks, spreading to the eyelids and the forehead, caused by methyl gentisate as active ingredient in a skin lightening face mask (1).

Cross-reactions, pseudo-cross-reactions and co-reactions
Not to hydroquinone (1).

Presence in cosmetic products and chemical analyses
In the USA, in April 2017, methyl dihydroxybenzoate was present in 1 of 56,714 cosmetic products of which the composition is known in FDA's Voluntary Cosmetic Registration Program (VCRP) (data obtained from FDA, May 2017). In March 2017, methyl dihydroxybenzoate was present in zero of 65,431 cosmetic products of which the composition is known in EWG's Skin Deep Cosmetics Database, USA (http://www.ewg.org/skindeep/).

LITERATURE
1   Serra-Baldrich E, Rincón C, Guedes A, Tribó MJ, Barco D, Allomar A. Allergic contact dermatitis to methyl gentisate. Contact Dermatitis 2009;60:225-226.
2   Gallo R, Baldary M. Allergic contact dermatitis from methyl gentisate in a bleaching cream. Contact Dermatitis 2006;54:220-221

2.296   METHYLENE BIS-BENZOTRIAZOLYL TETRAMETHYLBUTYLPHENOL

IDENTIFICATION

Description/definition   : Methylene bis-benzotriazolyl tetramethylbutylphenol is the heterocyclic compound that conforms to the formula shown below

Chemical class(es)   : Heterocyclic compounds; phenols

Chemical/IUPAC name   : 2,2'-Methylene-bis[4-(1,1,3,3-tetramethylbutyl)-6-benzotriazol-2-ylphenol]

Other names   : Bisoctrizole; Tinosorb® M (in this commercial sunscreen, methylene bis-benzotriazolyl tetramethylbutylphenol is the active ingredient)

CAS registry number (s)   : 103597-45-1

EC number(s)   : 403-800-1

SCCS opinion(s)   : SCCS/1546/15 (13); SCCS/1460/11 (14); SCCNFP, 17 February 1999 (15)

Function(s) in cosmetics : EU: UV-filter. USA: sunscreen agents

EU cosmetic restrictions : Regulated in Annex VI/23 of the Regulation (EC) No. 1223/2009

Patch testing   : 10.0% pet. (Chemotechnique)

Molecular formula   : $C_{41}H_{50}N_6O_2$

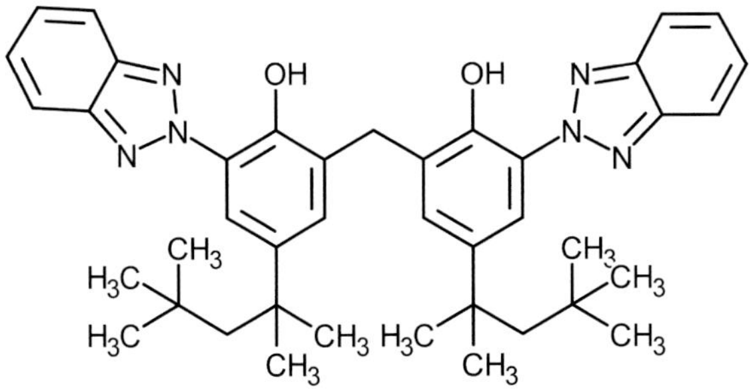

GENERAL

Methylene bis-benzotriazolyl tetramethylbutylphenol is a relatively new UVA/B filter with UV absorbance maxima ($\lambda_{max,1}$, $\lambda_{max,2}$) at 305 and 360 nm (17). It is present as the active ingredient in the commercial sunscreen Tinosorb® M at a concentration of 45-55%. Tinosorb® M (see Chapter 2.461 Tinosorb® M also contains decyl glucoside (6-10%), propylene glycol (0.2-0.6%), xanthan gum (0.1-0.5%) and water (40-42%). It is the first sunscreen of this kind that combines the advantages of organic and physical filters. Its active compound forms small microparticles that are poorly soluble either in water or oil; therefore, they are stabilized by decyl glucoside to achieve dispersion in the aqueous phase of the cosmetic emulsions.

There are several reports of (photo)contact allergy to 'methylene bis-benzotriazolyl tetramethylbutylphenol' (1,2,4,10). It should be appreciated, however, that these were actually reactions to Tinosorb® M, because the commercial patch test preparation was not the sunscreen chemical *per se,* but Tinosorb® M (9). The pure UV-filter first became available on January 1, 2014 from Chemotechnique Diagnostics. Also, materials provided for ingredient patch testing by producers of cosmetics labelled as 'methylene bis-benzotriazolyl tetramethylbutyl phenol' were actually Tinosorb® M (3). In fact, both names were often used as synonyms (10). Decyl glucoside is the usual contact allergen in Tinosorb® M (3,5,6,7; see Chapter 2.134 Decyl glucoside), in one case it was xanthan gum (8). Up to now, there are no proven cases of (photo)contact allergy to methylene bis-benzotriazolyl tetramethylbutylphenol.

Contact allergy to 'methylene bis-benzotriazolyl tetramethylbutylphenol', that was probably Tinosorb® M, is discussed in Chapter 2.461 Tinosorb® M. The literature on adverse reactions to sunscreens has been reviewed in several recent and older publications (19-24). A review of photocontact allergy to sunscreens was published in 2010 (18).

Presence in cosmetic products and chemical analyses

In June 2017, methylene bis-benzotriazolyl tetramethylbutylphenol was present in 10 (Tinosorb M) of 68,866 cosmetic products of which the composition is known in EWG's Skin Deep Cosmetics Database, USA (http://www.ewg.org/skindeep/). It should be realized that sunscreen products containing UV-filters are classified as drugs in the USA, not as cosmetics; the number mentioned here, therefore, is that of cosmetics containing the UV-filter, but it does *not* include their presence in sunscreens. In the USA, in April 2017, methylene bis-benzotriazolyl tetramethylbutylphenol was present in 11 of 56,714 cosmetic products of which the composition is known in FDA's Voluntary Cosmetic Registration Program (VCRP) (data obtained from FDA, May 2017).

In 2012, in Switzerland, 116 cosmetics from seven widely used leave-on product categories (19 lip care products, 8 lipsticks, 29 face creams, 11 liquid makeup foundations, 3 aftershaves, 7 hand creams and 39 sunscreens) were investigated to determine the frequency of occurrence and concentrations of 22 organic UV filters in these products.

Methylene bis-benzotriazolyl tetramethylbutylphenol was found in 9% of the products in a concentration range of 0.24-6.55%, mean 2.84% (16). In a sample of 337 sunscreens marketed in the UK in 2010, methylene bis-benzotriazolyl tetramethylbutylphenol was present in 32% (12). The UV-filter was present in 8% of 329 sunscreen products (incl. 21 lipstick sunscreens) marketed in the UK in 2005 (11).

LITERATURE

1   O'Connell M, Wilkinson M. Allergic contact dermatitis to methylene-*bis*-benzotriazolyl tetramethylbutylphenol. Br J Dermatol 2010;163 (suppl 1):79

2   Travassos AR, Claes L, Boey L, Drieghe J, Goossens A. Non-fragrance allergens in specific cosmetic products. Contact Dermatitis 2011;65:276-285

3   O'Connell M, Kirk S, Wilkinson MS. Allergic contact dermatitis caused by Tinosorb® M. Contact Dermatitis 2011;65:48-49

4   The European Multicentre Photopatch Test Study (EMCPPTS) Taskforce. A European multicentre photopatch test study. Br J Dermatol 2012;166:1002-1009

5   Pereira N, Coutinho I, Andrade P, Gonçalo M. The UV filter Tinosorb M, containing decyl glucoside, is a frequent cause of allergic contact dermatitis. Dermatitis 2013;24:41-43

6   Andrade P, Gonçalo M, Figueiredo A. Allergic contact dermatitis to decyl glucoside in Tinosorb® M. Contact Dermatitis 2010;62:119-120

7   Andersen KE, Goossens A. Decyl glucoside contact allergy from a sunscreen product. Contact Dermatitis 2006;54:349-350

8   Aerts O, Clinck B, Schramme M, Lambert J. Contact allergy caused by Tinosorb® M: let us not forget about xanthan gum. Contact Dermatitis 2015;72:121-123

9   De Groot AC, van Zuuren EJ, Hissink D. Contact allergy to Tinosorb® M: recommendations for diagnostic improvement. Contact Dermatitis 2014;70:251-254

10   González-Pérez R, Trébol I, García-Río I, Arregui MA, Soloeta R. Allergic contact dermatitis from methylene-bisbenzotriazolyl tetramethylbutylphenol (Tinosorb M). Contact Dermatitis 2007;56:121

11   Wahie S, Lloyd JJ, Farr PM. Sunscreen ingredients and labelling: a survey of products available in the U.K. Clin Exp Dermatol 2007;32:359-364

12   Kerr AC. A survey of the availability of sunscreen filters in the U.K. Clin Exp Dermatol 2011;36:541-543

13   SCCS (Scientific Committee on Consumer Safety). Opinion on 2,2'-methylene-bis-(6(2H-benzotriazol-2-yl)-4-(1,1,3,3-tetramethylbutyl)phenol), SCCS/1546/15, 25 March 2015. Available at: http://ec.europa.eu/health/scientific_committees/consumer_safety/docs/sccs_o_168.pdf

14   SCCS (Scientific Committee on Consumer Safety). Opinion on 2,2'-methylene-bis-(6(2H-benzotriazol-2-yl)-4-(1,1,3,3-tetramethylbutyl)phenol), 18 March 2013, revision of 23 July 2013, SCCS/1460/11. Available at: http://ec.europa.eu/health/scientific_committees/consumer_safety/docs/sccs_o_129.pdf

15   SCCNFP (Scientific Committee on Cosmetics and Non Food Products). Opinion concerning 2,2'-Methylene-bis-(6-(2H-benzotriazol-2-yl)-4-(1,1,3,3-tetramethylbutyl)phenol), 17 February 1999. Available at: http://ec.europa.eu/health/scientific_committees/consumer_safety/opinions/sccnfp_opinions_97_04/sccp_out55_en.htm

16   Manová E, von Goetz N, Hauri U, Bogdal C, Hungerbühler K. Organic UV filters in personal care products in Switzerland: A survey of occurrence and concentrations. Int J Hyg Environ Health 2013;216:508-514

17   Shaath NA. Ultraviolet filters. Photochem Photobiol Sci 2010;9:464-469

18   Shaw T, Simpson B, Wilson B, Oostman H, Rainey D, Storrs F. True photoallergy to sunscreens is rare despite popular belief. Dermatitis 2010;21:185-198

19   Heurung AR, Raju SI, Warshaw EM. Adverse reactions to sunscreen agents: epidemiology, responsible irritants and allergens, clinical characteristics, and management. Dermatitis 2014;25:289-326

20   Heurung AR, Raju SI, Warshaw EM. Contact allergen of the year. Benzophenones. Dermatitis 2014;25:3-10 (contains many mistakes; Erratum in Dermatitis 2014;25:92-95)

21   Avenel-Audran M. Sunscreen products: finding the allergen. Eur J Dermatol 2010;20:161-166

22   Scheuer E, Warshaw E. Sunscreen allergy: a review of epidemiology, clinical characteristics, and responsible allergens. Dermatitis 2006;17:3-11

23   Funk JO, Dromgoole SH, Maibach HI. Sunscreen intolerance: contact sensitization, photocontact sensitization, and irritancy of sunscreen agents. Dermatol Clin 1995;13:473-481

24   Dromgoole SH, Maibach HI. Sunscreening agent intolerance: Contact and photocontact sensitization and contact urticaria. J Am Acad Dermatol 1990;22:1068-1078

25   Schauder S. Survey of the literature on adverse reactions to preparations containing UV filters (1947-1989) (Literaturübersicht über Unverträglichkeitsreaktionen auf lichtfilterhaltige Produkte von 1947 bis 1989). Z Hautkr 1990;65:982-998 (article in German)

2.297   METHYL GLUCOSE DIOLEATE

IDENTIFICATION

Description/definition   : Methyl glucose dioleate is the diester of a methyl glucoside and oleic acid, which
        conforms to the formula shown below
Chemical class(es)   : Carbohydrates; esters; polyols
Chemical/IUPAC name   : [(2R,3S,4S,5R)-3,4-Dihydroxy-6-methoxy-5-[(E)-octadec-9-enoyl]oxyoxan-2-yl]methyl
        (E)-octadec-9-enoate
Other names   : D-Glucopyranoside methyl 2,6-dioleate
CAS registry number (s)   : 82933-91-3
EC number(s)   : 280-069-3
CIR review(s)   : Final report, September 2013 (access: www.cir-safety.org/ingredients)
Function(s) in cosmetics   : EU: emollient; humectant; skin conditioning. USA: skin-conditioning agent - emollient
Patch testing   : 5% - 10% pet.
Molecular formula   : $C_{43}H_{78}O_8$

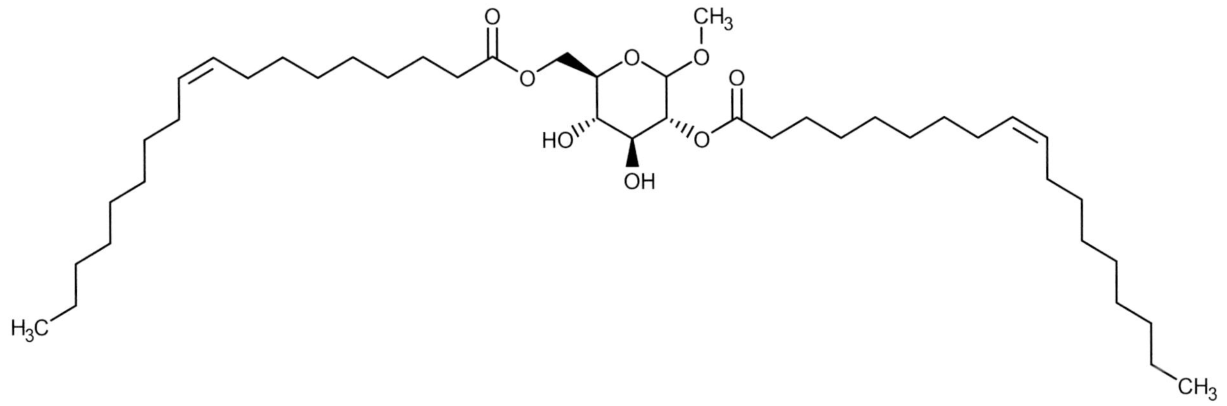

GENERAL

Methyl glucose dioleate is the diester of methyl glucoside and oleic acid. It is used as a water-in-oil emulsifier, emollient, humectant and skin conditioning agent in cosmetics, and may also be present in topical pharmaceutical products and insect repellents (2).

CONTACT ALLERGY

Case reports and case series

A woman was seen with a very itchy erythematous papulovesicular eruption, symmetrically located on the breasts, and spreading to the arms and the upper part of the abdomen. She had been breastfeeding her baby and had applied a 'nursing comfort balm' on the breasts. Patch tests with the European baseline series, a dye and textile-finish series and her personal products gave a strongly positive reaction to the balm. Later, when tested with its ingredients, the patient reacted to methyl glucose dioleate 5% pet.; 5 controls were negative (2). A woman reacted to an antidandruff-shampoo containing methyl glucose dioleate, possibly as a cross-reaction to primary sensitization to decyl glucoside (1). One patient had allergic contact dermatitis from methyl glucose dioleate in a cosmetic cream (7, article not read, data cited in ref.2).

Contact allergy to methyl glucose dioleate in non-cosmetic products

A woman with leg ulcers had used a topical antibiotic pharmaceutical product for 2 weeks. Erythematous and vesicular lesions had developed on both legs, associated with intense itching, which cleared after cessation of the ointment and application of a corticosteroid preparation. Patch tests with the European standard series and the ointment gave a positive reaction to the ointment. Later, when tested with its ingredients, the patient reacted to methyl glucose dioleate 5% pet. A ROAT with methyl glucose dioleate 5% pet. was strongly positive after 4 days. Patch tests in twenty controls and ROATs in 5 controls were negative (4).

Another woman presented with a 4-day history of a pruritic erythematous and vesicular dermatitis of the legs, spreading to the trunk and face, which had begun on her left leg 5 days after she had started applying the same antibiotic ointment as the previous patient. Patch tests were positive to the ointment and, later, to methyl glucose dioleate. Next, the patient was patch tested with the components of methyl glucose dioleate, methyl glucoside and oleic acid, and there was a positive reaction to oleic acid, tested 'as is'. Control tests were performed, but it is not entirely certain that this applied to oleic acid also (5). A female individual developed an itchy erythematous edematous dermatitis of the legs and abdomen after applying a paste to a suspected interdigital mycosis on her left foot, where the dermatitis had started a few days later. The causative ingredient was methyl glucose dioleate, tested 10% pet. (6).

A man presented with a widespread persistent itching erythematous and edematous dermatitis of the arms and legs. The patient stated that he had used an insect repellent the day before the onset of the dermatitis. An open test with the commercial product resulted in an itching erythematous reaction only a few hours after the first application. Patch tests with the constituents of the insect repellent product were positive to methyl glucose dioleate 10% pet. and to the active principle picaridin (9). A similar case of a woman with widespread dermatitis from methyl glucose dioleate in the same repellent product had been described one year earlier (8).

Cross-reactions, pseudo-cross-reactions and co-reactions
Cross-reactivity from primary methyl glucose sesquistearate sensitization (3); reaction to oleic acid, one of the components of methyl glucose dioleate (5). Possible cross-reaction from primary decyl glucoside sensitization (1).

Presence in cosmetic products and chemical analyses
In the USA, in April 2017, methyl glucose dioleate was present in 19 of 56,714 cosmetic products of which the composition is known in FDA's Voluntary Cosmetic Registration Program (VCRP) (data obtained from FDA, May 2017). In May 2017, methyl glucose dioleate was present in 9 of 66,658 cosmetic products of which the composition is known in EWG's Skin Deep Cosmetics Database, USA (http://www.ewg.org/skindeep/).

LITERATURE

1   Blondeel A. Contact allergy to the mild surfactant decylglucoside. Contact Dermatitis 2003;49:304-305
2   Deswysen A-C, Dekeuleneer V, Goossens A, Baeck M. Allergic contact dermatitis caused by a nursing comfort balm: methyl glucose dioleate as the sensitizing ingredient. Contact Dermatitis 2013;68:315-316
3   Dooms-Goossens A, Vandekerckhove M, Verschave H, Degreef H. Cosmetic dermatitis due to methyl glucose sesquistearate. Contact Dermatitis 1984;10:312-313
4   Foti C, Vena GA, Mazzarella F, Angelini G. Contact allergy due to methyl glucose dioleate. Contact Dermatitis 1995;32:303-304
5   Schianchi S, Calista D, Landi G. Widespread contact dermatitis due to methyl glucose dioleate. Contact Dermatitis 1996;35:257-258
6   Corazza M, Levratti A, Virgili A. Allergic contact dermatitis due to methyl glucose dioleate. Contact Dermatitis 2001;45:308
7   Corazza M, Elide C, Levratti A, Virgili A. Methyl glucose dioleate: an often overlooked allergen? Ann Ital Allergol Dermatol 2002;56:63- 64 (in Italian) (data cited in ref. 2)
8   Rossi G, Steffens W. Allergic contact dermatitis from Autan® spray: methyl glucose dioleate as sensitizing ingredient. Contact Dermatitis 2004;50:324
9   Corazza M, Borghi A, Zampino MR, Virgili A. Allergic contact dermatitis due to an insect repellent: double sensitization to picaridin and methyl glucose dioleate. Acta Derm Venereol 2005;85:264-265

2.298   METHYL GLUCOSE SESQUISTEARATE

IDENTIFICATION

Description/definition	: Methyl glucose sesquistearate is a mixture of mono- and diesters of a methyl glucoside and stearic acid
Chemical class(es)	: Carbohydrates; esters; polyols
Chemical/IUPAC name	: (2R,3S,4S,5R)-2-(Hydroxymethyl)-6-methoxyoxane-3,4,5-triol; octadecanoate
Other names	: D-Glucopyranoside, methyl, octadecanoate (2:3); methyl glucoside sesquistearate
CAS registry number (s)	: 68936-95-8
EC number(s)	: 273-049-0
CIR review(s)	: Final report, September 2013 (access: www.cir-safety.org/ingredients)
Function(s) in cosmetics	: EU: emollient; emulsifying; skin conditioning. USA: skin-conditioning agents – emollient
Patch testing	: 5% pet. (1)
Molecular formula	: $C_{68}H_{133}O_{18}$

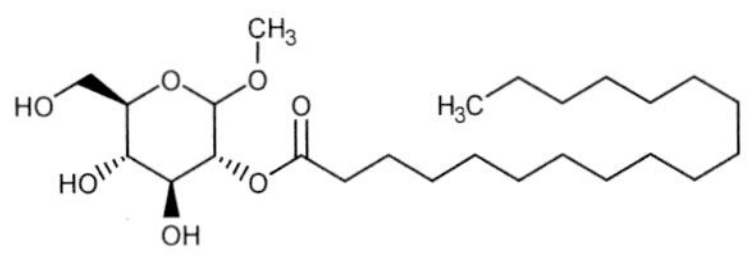

methyl glucose stearate

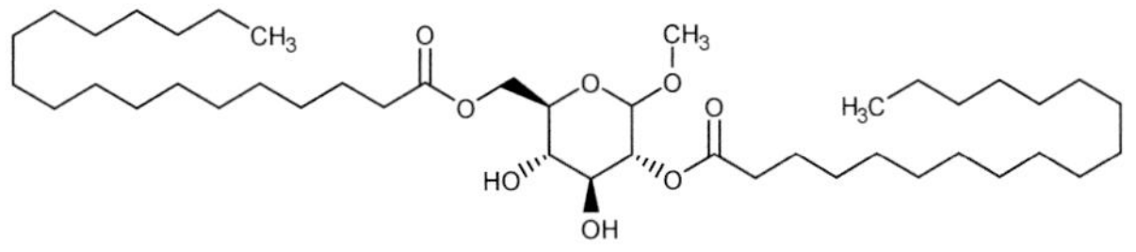

methyl glycose distearate

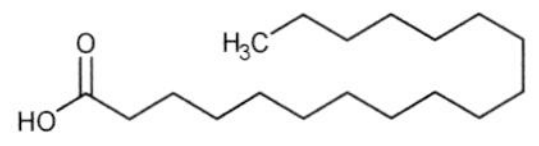

stearic acid

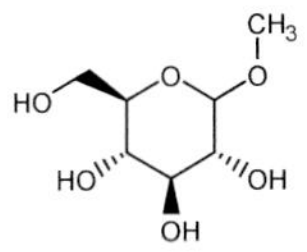

methyl glucoside

CONTACT ALLERGY

Case reports and case series

In a 4-month-period in 1996, 475 patients with contact allergy to 'cosmetic ingredients' were collected in 5 centers in Belgium, UK and Germany. There was 1 reaction to methyl glucose sesquistearate; relevance was not stated (2). A female patient presented with a severe itchy papular and vesicular eruption on her legs. The lesions had begun a week after she had stopped using a tanning lotion, which the patient had applied for 3 weeks. Patch tests with the standard series and the suspected product were negative. However, a ROAT with the lotion was positive after 2 days, at which time the patch test had also become positive. When patch tested with the ingredients, she reacted to methyl glucose sesquistearate 5% pet., which was negative in 20 controls. Half a year later, the patient returned and said that she had developed an itchy red papular eruption on her face and neck two days after having used a facial cream. A ROAT performed by herself was positive. Patch testing with coded ingredients from the manufacturer yielded one positive reaction; the manufacturer confirmed that it was methyl glucose sesquistearate (1).

Cross-reactions, pseudo-cross-reactions and co-reactions

Methyl glucose dioleate (1). Not to sorbitan sesquistearate (1).

Presence in cosmetic products and chemical analyses

In the USA, in April 2017, methyl glucose sesquistearate was present in 200 of 56,714 cosmetic products of which the composition is known in FDA's Voluntary Cosmetic Registration Program (VCRP) (data obtained from FDA, May 2017). In March 2017, methyl glucose sesquistearate was present in 58 of 65,431 cosmetic products of which the composition is known in EWG's Skin Deep Cosmetics Database, USA (http://www.ewg.org/skindeep/).

LITERATURE

1   Dooms-Goossens A, Vandekerckhove M, Verschave H, Degreef H. Cosmetic dermatitis due to methyl glucose sesquisterarate. Contact Dermatitis 1984;10:312-313
2   Goossens A, Beck MH, Haneke E, McFadden JP, Nolting S, Durupt G, Ries G. Adverse cutaneous reactions to cosmetic allergens. Contact Dermatitis 1999;40:112-113

2.299   METHYLISOTHIAZOLINONE

IDENTIFICATION

Description/definition   : Methylisothiazolinone is the heterocyclic organic compound that conforms to the
                           formula shown below
Chemical class(es)   : Heterocyclic compounds
Chemical/IUPAC name   : 2-Methyl-1,2-thiazol-3-one
Other names   : 2-Methyl-4-isothiazolin-3-one; examples of trade names are Euxyl K220, Neolone 950,
                           Microcare MT, Kordek MLX
CAS registry number(s)   : 2682-20-4
EC number(s)   : 220-239-6
CIR review(s)   : J Am Coll Toxicol 1992;11:75-128; Int J Toxicol 2010;29(Suppl.3):187-213 (20); Final
                           report, December 2014 (access: www.cir-safety.org/ingredients)
SCCS opinion(s)   : SCCS/1557/15 (124); SCCS/1521/13, revision of 27 March 2014 (125); SCCNFP/0805/04
                           (18); SCCNFP/0625/02 (19)
Merck Index monograph   : 7433
Function(s) in cosmetics : EU: preservative. USA: preservatives
Patch testing   : 0.05% water (SmartPracticeEurope, SmartPracticeCanada); 0.2% water (Chemotech-
                           nique, SmartPracticeCanada); 0.2% water is included in the European baseline series
                           since November 2013 (69); rationale for choosing this test concentration: ref. 58;
                           methylisothiazolinone was also added to the NACDG screening series in 2013 (101)
EU cosmetic restrictions : Regulated in Annex V/57 of the Regulation (EC) No. 1223/2009
Molecular formula   : C_4H_5NOS

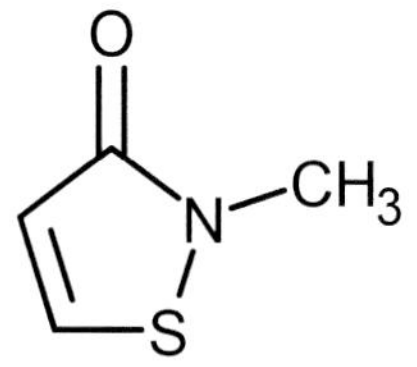

GENERAL

Methylisothiazolinone (MI) has been used since the late 1970s in a 1:3 combination with methylchloroisothiazolinone as a preservative system (MCI/MI, best known trade names: Kathon CG, Euxyl K 100) for cosmetics, household products and a large variety of industrial applications (see the Chapter 2.292 Methylchloroisothiazolinone (and) methyl-isothiazolinone). In the 1980s, this preservative caused an 'epidemic' of allergic contact dermatitis in European countries (90). Although a few patch test reactions were observed to methylisothiazolinone in patients allergic to Kathon CG (89), the chlorinated part (methylchloroisothiazolinone) had the strongest sensitizing capacity and was considered to be the main allergen in MCI/MI (70,89).

Methylisothiazolinone *per se* (single agent, stand-alone) has been used as a preservative in industrial products such as paints, lacquers, varnishes, polishing agents, industrial cleaning/washing agents, toners, printing inks and cutting oils since the early 2000s without concentration limits. Household products containing MI include dishwashing liquid soaps, laundry detergents, laundry stain removers, fabric softeners and all-purpose cleaners. Some years later, manufacturers began using MI in cosmetic products. Reported applications of methylisothiazolinone are shown in table 2.299.1. Trade names include Euxyl K220, Neolone 950, Microcare MT, and Kordek MLX (69).

Table 2.299.1 Reported applications of methylisothiazolinone (examples) [a]

Products	References
Absorbents and adsorbents	55
Adhesives/glues	6,55,127,141,181
Air cleansers and anti-odor agents	55
All-purpose cleaners	
Binding agents	55,181
Biocides (concentrated solutions)	29,46,55
Car care products	29,55,181
Cleaning / washing agents	29,45,55,71,74,127,181
Coloring agents	55,181
Construction materials	127,181

Table 2.299.1 Reported applications of methylisothiazolinone (examples) [a] (*continued*)

Products	References
Contact gel for 'waist reduction belt'	81
Cosmetics, stay-on	6,23,28,29,31,34,48,72,94,110,122,142
Cosmetics, rinse-off	25,72,94,108,109,147,149,151,163
Cutting oils	
Dishwashing liquids	29,52,64,71,94
Fabric softeners	
Filling agents	55,127,181
Floor cleaning detergent	45
Flooring agents	55,127,181
Gel pad	142
Glues	46,127,141
Hand cleaners	29,113
Hand wash	113
Hand wipes	29
Hardeners	127
Impregnating agents / proofing	55,127,181
Industrial cleaning/washing agents	55
Lacquers	55
Latex emulsions	
Laundry detergents/stain removers	175
Leather care products	147
Liquid soaps	29,38
Lubricants	181
Metal surface treatment remedies	181
Metalworking fluids	29,38
Mineral slurries	
Moist toilet paper	6,83,100,109
Paints / lacquers / varnishes	6,10,27,29,39,47,49,51,55,59,65,73,77,78,87,96,104,106, 144,161,162,164,171,181
Pharmaceutical products (topical)	94
Pigment dispersions	29,55
Polishing products	55,127,168
Preservative for recycled water	80
Printing inks	55,127,181
Raw materials and intermediate products	55
Rinsing agents	55,181
Rust inhibitors	55,181
Shoe glue	163
Solvents	55,181
Spectacles	140
Sponge for scrubbing the skin	139
Surface active agents	55,181
Surface treatment for papers, cardboard and other non-metals	181
Tackifiers	
Toners	55,181
Ultrasound gel	53
Varnishes	
Wet wipes for cleaning	30,72
Wet wipes for personal hygiene	6,83,98,100,107,109,118
Wood cleaners	

[a] See also tables 2.299.2 and 2.299.3 for products containing MI causing allergic contact dermatitis

CONTACT ALLERGY

Fairly soon after the introduction of methylisothiazolinone (MI) as single preservative agent, the first cases of allergic contact dermatitis (ACD) caused by MI in industrial products were published (2004 and 2006), after handling of paint and wallpaper glue, respectively (10,46). In 2003, the Scientific Committee on Cosmetic Products and Non-food Products Intended for Consumers (SCCNFP) stated, in their first opinion on MI (SCCNFP/0625/02) in 2003, that no adequate risk assessment of MI could be carried out, as the genotoxicity/mutagenicity studies were inadequate (19). The issue of sensitization to MI was considered to be adequately addressed in this first opinion. It was concluded that 'the number of new sensitizations induced by exposure to MI through the use of cosmetic and toiletry products is expected to be low' (19). However, using the local lymph node assay, it was shown in the same year that MI has strong sensitizing capabilities (17). Unfortunately, this information was not included in the second opinion and no new data regarding sensitization to MI were submitted by industry for inclusion in this second opinion on MI (SCCNFP/0805/04) (18). In this expert document it was concluded that 'the proposed use of methylisothiazolinone as a preservative at a maximum concentration of 0.01% (100 ppm) in the finished cosmetic products does not pose a risk to the health of the consumer' (18). Later, the Cosmetic Ingredient Review in the USA would reach the same conclusion (20).

In 2005, methylisothiazolinone was permitted as a preservative in cosmetic products, both leave-on and rinse-off products, in the EU in a maximum concentration of 100 ppm (0.01%) (Annex V/57 of the Cosmetic Regulation (EC) 1223/2009, Cosmetic Directive 2005/42/EC). Before 2005, the maximum permitted concentration of MI (in the MCI/MI mixture) in cosmetic products in the EU was 3.75 ppm (one quarter of the maximum allowed 15 ppm MCI /MI). The introduction of MI alone thus led to a more than 25-times increase in the permitted concentration of MI in cosmetics. Inevitably, in August 2010, the first cases of cosmetic-related allergic contact dermatitis from MI were published (6). Soon afterwards, Danish dermatologists warned that 'there is a considerable risk that MI will cause an epidemic of contact allergy' and recommended that the permitted concentration of MI be reduced (11). The prevalence of MI sensitization in Denmark between 2006 and 2010 was relatively stable (1.1-2.2%, mean 1.5%) (5) and fairly low, but already somewhat increasing prevalences were noted in Finland (1,4) and Germany (3). However, from 2010 on, the prevalence of MI contact allergy has increased at an alarming rate (7,35,38,40,63,71, 76,79,88,114), and several countries have confirmed the existence of an MI 'epidemic', primarily from its use in cosmetic products, with prevalence rates of 6-12% in consecutively tested patients suspected of contact dermatitis in many European countries (37,40,96,117,130,136,150), Australia (93) and the USA (101). The members of the North American Contact Dermatitis Group started testing MI in 2013 and found a 10.9% frequency of sensitization in their 2013-2014 study period (131). Methylisothiazolinone was named allergen of the year by the American Contact Dermatitis Society in 2013 to raise awareness of this important allergen (99).

At the same time, an increase in the prevalence of MCI/MI sensitization and of co-reactivity to MCI/MI was observed, which was very likely caused by increased primary sensitization to methylisothiazolinone and subsequent (pseudo)-cross-reactivity to MCI/MI (7,40,71,79). Meanwhile, the European Society of Contact Dermatitis raised strong concerns on the use of MI in cosmetics (68). Until 2013, MI was stated and erroneously recognized as possessing weak (70) or moderate (14) sensitizing capabilities, based on a review article of compilations of potency values, that is, reporting modelling studies on a large set of local lymph node assay data (14). However, MI actually has strong sensitizing capabilities (16,17,41,125).

The at that moment well-recognized epidemic of MI contact allergy in several member states of the EU prepared the ground for a revision of the opinion on MI (SCCS/1521/13), published in December 2013 (125). The SCCS concluded that no safe level of MI had been determined for leave-on cosmetic products (e.g. lotions and wet-wipes), and that, for rinse-off cosmetic products (e.g., soaps and shampoos), a maximum concentration of 15 ppm MI was safe from the point of view of sensitization (125). In July 2015, an additional and final re-assessment concerning the risk of sensitization to rinse-off products and leave-on hair care products containing MI in concentrations up to 100 ppm was done. The SCCS again concluded that the concentration of MI in rinse-off cosmetic products and leave-on hair care products should not exceed 15 ppm (124). However, the EU did not act upon the advice of its independent advisory committee, but did act on the request of industry to ask the SCCS to re-evaluate its opinion that MI is not safe for use in rinse-off products and hair care products at 100 ppm (22,42). Meanwhile, in 2013, Cosmetics Europe, following discussions with the European Society of Contact Dermatitis, recommended its members that the use of MI in leave-on skin products including cosmetic wet wipes be discontinued, but did not comment on its use in rinse-off products (67).

In July 2016, the European Commission decided that MI in the EU will be prohibited in stay-on cosmetic products from 12 February 2017 on (26). Yet, it is still allowed in rinse-off products at a maximum concentration of 0.01% (100 ppm). At the same time, a modification was proposed by the European Commission for public consultation, restricting the use of MI to 15 ppm in rinse-off products, with the obligation of a 'contains methylisothiazolinone' labeling and banning the use of MI as a preservative in hair leave-on cosmetic products (9).

Currently, for products other than cosmetics and household cleaning products, there are no legal restrictions or labelling demands for methylisothiazolinone, making it difficult for consumers and workers to consciously avoid exposure to MI. A major concern is that products containing this preservative are now being used extensively in public, domestic, and occupational settings, increasing overall exposure and thereby the risk of developing allergic contact dermatitis (86,95).

Editorials and review articles on allergy to methylisothiazolinone can be found in refs. 8,42,66,68,69,95,99,105, 135 and 138. An overview of non-cosmetic and unusual cosmetic sources of isothiazolinone derivatives (also MCI/MI, benzisothiazolinone, octylisothiazolinone) was published in 2017 (180).

The reader is also referred to Chapter 2.292 Methylchloroisothiazolinone (and) methylisothiazolinone. In some studies, no clear difference is made between results of testing with methylchloroisothiazolinone (and) methylisothia-zolinone (MCI/MI) and with methylisothiazolinone *per se* (MI), combining the results.

Patch testing in groups of patients

Results of routine patch testing (testing in consecutive patients suspected of contact dermatitis) back to 2006 (when MI as single agent was first patch tested) are shown in table 2.299.2. Results of testing MI in groups of *selected* patients (e.g., patients tested with a cosmetic series or preservative series, children with dermatitis, nurses with occupational contact dermatitis) in the same period are shown in table 2.299.3. In most studies, the currently advised test preparation of 2000 ppm in water (0.02%) has been used. Others researchers, however, especially in earlier studies, have utilized lower concentrations of 0.05% or even 0.02%. It is possible that such concentrations, especially the 0.02% concen-tration (63) have resulted in missed cases of sensitization (false-negative reactions). From serial dilution testing, it was shown that nearly all patients reacting to 0.2% also have a positive patch test to 0.05%. However, some of these individuals did *not* react to MI 0.02%, which confirms that this concentration will result in some false-negative results (11,92).

Patch testing in consecutive patients suspected of contact dermatitis: routine testing

Results of routine patch testing with MI are shown in table 2.299.2. Up to 2010, frequencies of sensitization to MI in European countries were generally low, ranging from 0.6% to 2.6% (1,4,5,8). From then on, rates rapidly increased in the years 2011,2012 and 213 in studies from Sweden (88), Denmark (63,71), France (38), UK (40,79), Belgium (35) and Spain (114). Rates in moist studies rose to >5%, and in some studies, over 10% of all routinely tested patients were allergic to methylisothiazolinone (37,150,169). In 2013-2014 the epidemic had spread to North America, where the members of the NACDG documented a 10.9% prevalence of contact allergy to MI (131,176).

Relevance rates have generally been high, ranging from about half to 100%. Causative products were mostly cosmetics (both stay-on cosmetics including wet wipes and rinse-off products such as shampoos), followed by household products (e.g., detergents such as dishwashing liquids) and – to a far lesser degree and mostly in a few countries – occupational products including paint (table 2.299.2).

In the UK, it appeared that the epidemic of contact allergy to MI reached its peak in 2014. In one center, in that year, the prevalence of sensitization was 9.1%, and in the year 2015, 'only' 4.8% positive reactions were observed (173). This decrease is likely the result the 2013 recommendation of Cosmetics Europe, following discussions with the European Society of Contact Dermatitis, that the use of MI in leave-on skin products including cosmetic wet wipes be discontinued. A further decrease is to be expected from the total ban of MI in stay-on cosmetic products in 2017 and – possibly – from future legislation restricting the concentration on MI in rinse-off products to 15 ppm.

Table 2.299.2 Patch testing in groups of patients: Routine testing

Years and Country	Test conc. & vehicle	Number of patients tested | positive (%)		Selection of patients (S); Relevance (R); Comments (C)	Ref.
2015 UK	0.2% water	997	(4.8%)	R: not stated; C: there was a strong decrease in the prevalence of sensitization compared to 2014, when it still was 9.1%	173
2015 eight European countries [c]	0.2% water	3434	205 (6.0%)	R: 73%, mostly (83%) from cosmetics, both from rinse-off (39%) and leave-on products (25%) or from both (20%); 19 reacted to household products, mainly dishwashing detergents; 7% had previously had an allergic reaction from newly painted rooms; C: the frequency per center ranged from 2.6% to 13%	96, 170
2014 9 Countries [d]	0.2% water	3865	284 (7.3%)	R: in 63% the eczema was caused or aggravated by products containing either MI or MCI/MI, mostly cosmetics; C: 67% co-reactivity to MCI/MI; ranger per center: 0.8%-10.9%	177
2014 UK	0.2% water	3897	418 (10.7%)	R: not stated; C: although the frequency was still extremely high, 2014 was the first year in which it was (slightly) lower than the year before	150
2014 Italy	0.2% water	250	18 (7.2%)	R: all relevant; in >50% of the patients the allergens were	117

Table 2.299.2 Patch testing in groups of patients: Routine testing (*continued*)

Years and Country	Test conc. & vehicle	Number of patients tested | positive (%)		Selection of patients (S); Relevance (R); Comments (C)	Ref.
2013-2014 12 European countries, 46 departments [b]	0.02% water 0.05% water 0.2% water	4383 6713 6677	(10.7%) (7.4%) (7.8%)	found in both leave-on and rinse-off cosmetics R: not stated; C: results of 6 occupational dermatology clinics and one pediatric clinic not included in these figures; range of positive reactions: 6.9%-19.6% (test material 0.02%), 0.6%-19.9% (0.05% test material) and 6.4%-20.8% (0.2% test material)	169
2013-14 USA, Canada	0.2% water	4857	527 (10.9%)	R: definite + probable relevance: 53%, mostly from cosmetics, both stay-on an rinse-off products; C: the data from ref 176 are slightly different from those of ref. 131	131, 176
2012-2014 USA	0.02%, later 0.2% water	703	52 (7.4%)	R: 70%, notably from wet wipes, shampoos and detergents; C: the prevalence of MI allergy *alone* (with negative MCI/MI) rose from 2.5% in 2012 to 5.6% in 2013 and to 6.8% in 2014	101
2012-2014 Italy	0.2% water	2028	106 (5.2%)	R: 52% reactions to MI and/or MCI were relevant from stay-on cosmetics (approx. 37%), rinse-off cosmetics (approx. 35%) and household products (approx. 15%); C: unexpected large number of men from a widely used cheap aftershave	143
2011-2014 Canada	0.2% water	322	15 (4.7%)	R: not specified for MI alone	116
2013 Spain	0.05% water	?	? (6.6%)	R: not specified; most were relevant	130
2012-2013 Finland	0.05% water	3682	415 (11.3%)	R: In the majority of patients, the dermatitis was caused by one or more cosmetic products; C: the prevalence rose from 10.3% in 2012 to 13.2% in the first five months of 2013	37
2011-2013 Denmark	0.2% water	1655	? ?	R: not specified for MI alone; C: the prevalence rose from 4.8% in 2011 to 6.5% in 2013	63
	0.02% water	1511	? ?	R: not specified for MI alone; C: the prevalence rose from 3.5% in 2011 to 3.8% in 2013	
2011-2013 Spain	0.05% water	404	21 (5.2%)	R: 100%, all caused by cosmetics, of which one case of occupational contact dermatitis in a beautician	112
2011-2013 Spain	0.2% water	490	22 (4.5%)	R: 21/22 were caused by cosmetics and/or household products; C: the prevalence rose from 1% in 2011 to 3.6% in 2012 and 7.7% in 2013	114
2010-2013 Belgium	0.05% water	5979	324 (5.4%)	R: >60% of the allergen sources were cosmetics; C: the prevalence rose from 3.1% and 3.2% in 2010/2011 to 6.0% in 2012 and 7.2% in 2013; many cases with airborne distribution, notably from water-based paints	35
2010-2013 British Isles	0.02% or 0.05% or 0.2% water	12,592	841 (6.7%)	R: not specified; most cases caused by cosmetics; C: the prevalence rose from 1.7% in 2010 to 2.9% in 2011 to 7.1% in 2012 and to 11.1% in 2013	40
2012 Sweden	0.2% water	1498	106 (7.1%)	R: not stated	136
2011-2012 UK	0.2% water	563	24 (4.3%)	R: not stated C: the prevalence rose from 3.8% in 2011 to 4.6% in 2012	79
2011-2012 Australia	0.02% water	653	43 (6.6%)	R: 53%, mostly caused by cosmetics including baby wipes; 3 occupational cases from hand cleansers; C: 7 patients were parents of young children with hand dermatitis from using baby wipes on their children	93
2010-2012 France	0.02% or 0.05% water	7874	297 (3.8%)	R: 80-90%; 73% caused by cosmetics (notably rinse-off products), 17% household products; 7% wet wipes (both for personal and for occupational use); these percentages are in the group where the causative product was identified!; C: the prevalence rose from 1.5% in 2010 to 3.3% in 2011 and 5.6% in 2012	38
2010-2012 Denmark	0.2% water	2766	82 (3.0%)	R: 63%; 62% of the relevant cases were caused by cosmetics, (of which 55% were rinse-off products), 25% by paints and 5% by cleansing agents; C: the prevalence rose from 1.1-1.7% in 2006-2009 to 2.0% in 2010, 3.0% in 2011 and 3.7% in 2012	71
2009-2012, 12 European countries [b]	0.05% water 0.2% water	4755 3382	(4.9%) [a] (4.5%) [a]	R: not stated; C: range per country 3.1-6.5% R: not stated; C: range per country 2.4-5.1%	155
2003-2010 and 2011-2012, Sweden	from 0.0475 to 0.2% in water	5881	101 (1.7%)	R: not specified; C: in the years 2003-2009, prevalences were 0.5-1.9%; from 2010 the prevalence rose from 2.9% in 2010 to 6.5% in 2012	88
2006-2010 Denmark	0.2% water	2536	37 (1.5%)	R: 2/3 relevant, about half occupational (notably painters) dermatitis and half from exposure to cosmetics (75% rinse-	5

Table 2.299.2 Patch testing in groups of patients: Routine testing (*continued*)

Years and Country	Test conc. & vehicle	Number of patients tested	positive (%)		Selection of patients (S); Relevance (R); Comments (C)	Ref.
					off-products, notably shampoo, conditioner and liquid soap)	
2007-2008 Denmark [b]	0.2% water	1280		(1.4%) [a]	R: not stated	1
2007-2008 Finland [b]	0.03% water	281		(1.1%) [a]	R: not stated	1
	0.1% water	281		(1.7%) [a]	R: not stated	
2007-08 Netherlands [b]	0.05% water	245		(2.6%) [a]	R: not stated	1
2006-2008 Finland	0.1% water	10,821	147	(1.4%)	R: not stated; the frequency of sensitization rose from	4
	0.03% water	10,821	69	(0.6%)	0.9% in 2006 to 1.8% in 2008; C: 30% positive ROAT with a product containing 100 ppm MI for 2 weeks	

[a] age-standardized and sex-standardized proportions
[b] study of the ESSCA (European Surveillance System on Contact Allergy' network)
[c] study of the EECDRG (European Environmental Contact Dermatitis Research Group)
[d] members of the ICDRG (International Contact Dermatitis Research Group); participating countries: Japan, Belgium, Sweden, India, Denmark, Singapore, United Kingdom, Uruguay, Germany

Patch testing in groups of selected patients

Data on patch testing with MI in groups of selected patients (e.g., patients tested with a cosmetic series or preservative series, children with dermatitis, nurses with occupational contact dermatitis) are summarized in table 2.299.3. In 14 investigations, frequencies of sensitization have ranged from 0.5% to 41%. Frequencies of >10% have been observed in a small group of 80 patients with facial dermatitis from Ireland (11.3% [119]) and an extremely high rate of 41% in a small group of 54 patients tested with a cosmetic series in a study from Thailand; however, the relevance of the positive patch test reactions was not mentioned (115).

In a 2007-2012 IVDK study, 8.2% of 496 female hairdressers with current or previous occupational contact dermatitis reacted to MI, which percentage is high considering that the period of investigation included the years 2007-2010, when rates of sensitization to MI were still low. However, in this study also, no relevance data were provided (154). In fact, in 12/14 studies, relevance was either not provided or specified for MI. In two studies that did address the relevancy issue, 69% (76) and 82% (167) of the positive patch tests were considered to be relevant. Causative products were mentioned in 2 studies only and were cosmetics and moist toilet wipes (76,119)

Clinical picture of contact allergy to methylisothiazolinone and causative products

Contact allergy to MI usually presents as eczematous lesions, frequently of the hands and/or of the face (5,39,96, 101,102,170,177), with frequent involvement of the eyelids, and may be accompanied by complaints of burning and severe swelling (35,36,39,96). Generalized dermatitis and perianal dermatitis are not infrequently observed. The causative products are mostly cosmetics, followed by household products such as dishwashing liquids and other cleaning products. Occupational materials as source of sensitization or elicitation of ACD are less often implicated (<20% [170]), though important in some countries such as Denmark (5,71). In most studies, about 2/3 of all patients were women. The implicated cosmetic products are both stay-on cosmetics, including many cases of wet wipes, but also a large percentage (sometimes the majority) of rinse-off products including shampoos and soaps (5,38,71,96, 102). Women aged > 40 years are overrepresented (36,38,39,76). In patients with dermatitis of the hands, household products such as dishwashing liquids and other cleaning products may be involved (96,102).

Anogenital dermatitis, either in children (100,107,109,118) or in adults (6,98,107) may be caused by wet wipes and is quite frequent. These products may also cause hand dermatitis in parents of children for who the wet wipes are used (83). It is estimated that – depending on the country – five to 20% of all sensitizations are from occupational exposure (96,145), causing work-related contact dermatitis, notably of the hands and forearms, e.g., from paints (5,10, 39,71,86,87) (which may also cause airborne contact dermatitis [78,144]), liquid hand soaps and other hand cleansers (29,83), or metalworking fluids (29). Cosmetics may also cause occupational allergic contact dermatitis, for example in beauticians (29,36), masseuses and hairdressers (94,101).

Patch tests with the MI-containing products causing ACD may both be positive (especially stay-on products) (e.g., 139,142,144) or negative.

Atypical manifestations

Many reports of airborne allergic contact dermatitis caused by emission of methylisothiazolinone (MI) from freshly painted walls have been published (6,27,35,47,49,73,86). Such patients have been observed frequently in Denmark (86), where virtually all water-based wall paints appear to contain MI and concentrations of 10-300 ppm have been found, with amounts of >100 ppm in about half of these products (82). Airborne allergic contact dermatitis from paints has also occurred in children (47,65,77). People affected by the emission of MI are often not able to live in their houses/apartments for a long period of time (27,49), as MI in paints can evaporate for at least 6 weeks (97). One patient even developed allergic contact dermatitis from MI in paint used by his neighbor (104).

Table 2.299.3 Patch testing in groups of patients: Selected patient groups

Years and Country	Test conc. & vehicle	Number of patients		Selection of patients (S); Relevance (R); Comments (C)	Ref.
		tested	positive (%)		
2013-2015 USA		818	49 (6.0%)	S: children 0-18 years suspected of contact dermatitis; R: 82%	167
2014 Thailand	0.2% water	54	22 (41%)	S: patients tested with a cosmetics series; R: not stated	115
2012-2014 Ireland	0.2% water	80	9 (11.3%)	S: patients with facial dermatitis; R: not specified for MI alone; in the group of patients who reacted to MI and/or MI/MCI, 86% were relevant, all caused by cosmetics	119
2003-2014 IVDK	0.05% water	<4216	(1.7%)	S: patients with stasis dermatitis / chronic leg ulcers; R: not stated	157
2011-2013 UK	0.2% water	310	2 (0.6%)	S: pediatric patients (16 years or younger); R: not stated	84
2011-2013 IVDK	0.05% water	6176	(6.8%)	S: not specified; R: not specified	91
1996-2013 Netherlands	0.05% water	290	4 (1.4%)	S: children aged 0-17 years with dermatitis; R: not stated	156
2010-2012 UK	0.05% water	1289	52 (4.0%)	S: patients tested with a cosmetic/face series; R: 69% definite relevance, mostly from cosmetics and moist tissue wipes; C: areas most affected were the face (69%), generalized (12%) and groin/perineum/genitals; C: the prevalence rose from 0.5% in 2010 to 3.5% in 2011 and 5.7% in 2012	76
2009-2012 IVDK	0.05% water	28,922	1109 (3.8%)	S: patients tested with a cosmetic preservative series; R: not specified (in %); C: the prevalence increased from 1.9% in 2009 to 6.1% in 2012 and was mainly driven by female patients aged ≥ 40 years, patients with face dermatitis, and the use of cosmetics	36
2007-2012 IVDK	0.05% water	496	29 (8.2%)	S: female hairdressers with current or previous occupational contact dermatitis; R: not stated	154
		1035	26 (2.3%)	S: female patients, clients of hairdressers, in who hair cosmetics were regarded as a cause of dermatitis, and who had never worked as hairdressers; R: not stated	
2003-2012 IVDK		1025	44 (4.3%)	S: nurses with occupational contact dermatitis; R: not stated	120
2011 China	0.2% water	201	1 (0.5%)	S: healthy student volunteers 19-30 years; R: not stated	128
2009-2011 IVDK	0.05% water	21,274	(3.3%)	S: patients tested with a preservative series; R: not stated; C: the frequency of sensitization rose from 1.9% in 2009 to 3.4% in 2010 and to 4.4% in 2011	7
2005-2009 IVDK	0.05% water	13,433	215 (1.5%) [a]	S: not stated; R: not stated; C: increasing prevalence of Sensitization in the study period	3

[a] age-standardized and sex-standardized proportions
IVDK: Information Network of Departments of Dermatology, Germany, Austria, Switzerland

The presenting features of allergic reactions to MI vapor are dermatitis at skin sites not covered by clothes, such as the face and neck, sometimes accompanied by respiratory symptoms (dyspnea, dry cough, wheezing, rhinitis), dizziness, conjunctivitis, headache or malaise (27,49,59,73,86,96,144). Quite remarkably, the affected patients are the inhabitants of the painted apartments/houses in 80% of the cases; occupational contact dermatitis in painters is far less frequently diagnosed (161).

Systemic contact dermatitis from inhalation of MI may present as dermatitis in the popliteal and antecubital fossa and flare-up reactions, such as hand eczema (47,78,96). Usually, the patients were previously sensitized to MI through the use of cosmetic products or moist toilet paper (6,47,65), but primary airborne sensitization could often not be excluded (102).

Skin exposure to high concentrations of MI in commercial MI biocide solutions can cause severe chemical burns, which may be followed by primary sensitization (46). Allergic contact dermatitis from MI may mimic other eczematous reactions, such as seborrheic, asteatotic (35) and atopic dermatitis (47), the latter particularly in widespread reactions such as in cases of airborne exposure (47,35). The lesions may also be lichenified and infiltrated, with follicular accentuation, or present as sharply delineated plaques, and can sometimes be photo-aggravated (35,146,174).

Photo-induced ACD (photoallergic contact dermatitis) has been observed (146,174). MI allergy may also be mistaken for a drug eruption (35). Genital dermatitis causing relapsing episodes of bacterial cellulitis (35), contact dermatitis masquerading as folliculitis decalvans induced by a hair gel (48), contact dermatitis from a facial cream mimicking a photodermatosis (110), airborne-induced lymphomatoid contact dermatitis (45) and lichenoid allergic contact dermatitis (149) have been reported rarely. MI, present in a dishwashing liquid used to clean a dental prosthesis, may have caused primary mucosal sensitization, leading to a flare-up of a long-standing, but inactive, oral lichen planus (52). A boy with atopic dermatitis developed the clinical picture of superinfection with herpes simplex virus (Kaposi's varicelliform eruption, Kaposi-Juliusberg syndrome), which was, in fact airborne allergic contact dermatitis from MI (and MCI/MI) in paint that had been used to paint the ceiling over his bed (171).

Case reports and case series

Case series

Methylisothiazolinone was stated to be the (or an) allergen in 103 patients in a group of 603 individuals suffering from cosmetic dermatitis, seen in the period 2010-2015 in Leuven, Belgium (123). In the period 1996-2013, in a tertiary referral center in Valencia, Spain, 5419 patients were patch tested. Of these, 628 individuals had allergic contact dermatitis to cosmetics. MI was the responsible allergen in 29 cases; it should be realized, that MI was tested only from 2012 on (130). Methylisothiazolinone was responsible for 23 out of 959 cases of non-fragrance cosmetic allergy where the causal allergen was identified, Belgium, 2000-2010 (2). In the period 2011-2014, 79 patients with a positive patch test reaction to an allergen identified with a wet wipe source were identified by the members of the NACDG. Methylisothiazolinone was the (or an) allergen in 59% of the cases. Patients with wipe allergy were 15 times more likely to have anal and/or genital dermatitis compared with those without wipe allergy (160).

Case reports

Stay-on cosmetics

Two women had axillary dermatitis from contact allergy to MI in deodorant (94). A woman had dermatitis of both axillae due to a new deodorant. She reacted to MCI/MI, MI and the deodorant. A ROAT with the product was already positive on D2. Curiously, although the title of the article points at MI as the responsible allergen, it was not mentioned that the deodorant in fact contained this chemical (23). A man had contact allergy from MI in hair gel, causing ACD of the scalp masquerading as folliculitis decalvans (48). In one hospital in Paris, France, in a period of 6 months, four patients were seen who had dermatitis of the scalp and/or the face and/or the neck from contact allergy to MI in hair gel (34). A woman had facial dermatitis caused by contact allergy to MI in an eye cleansing lotion (6). Another female patient developed sensitization to and facial dermatitis from a cream containing MI. Later, she had an extensive dermatitis from a spray tan containing MCI/MI, sprayed over the entire body surface in a cabin. The trunk was unaffected, which could not be explained (31).

One patient had ACD from MI in a cosmetic serum, present in a concentration of 188 ppm (28). A woman had recurrent eczematous lesions around the eyes, on the face, and in the neck caused by MI in her facial cream; previously, she had experienced ACD around the eyes from MI in gel pads used during an eyelash extension procedure (142). Another woman had ACD from MI in a body milk and cleansing oil (72). One patient with hand dermatitis reacted to MI in an emollient (94). The dermatitis of the hands and forearms in one individual was caused by contact allergy to MI in an emollient and a sunscreen (94).

A woman had ACD of the face, neck and proximal arms, mimicking a photodermatosis, from a facial ointment containing MI (110). A man with longstanding atopic dermatitis and photosensitivity reacted to multiple benzophenones and to MI in a sunscreen (122).

Moistened toilet tissues (wet wipes)

Six patients had perianal dermatitis from MI in wet wipes used for hygiene, containing 90-100 ppm MI; one of them later developed airborne ACD from water-based wall paint (6). Four adult patients had severe perianal dermatitis, one of them also of the genital area; all four used moist toilet paper and reacted to MCI/MI. The reactions were ascribed to MCI/MI, and the authors stated that the toilet papers contained the preservative. This is rather curious, as they also provided a list of ingredients, mentioning 'methylisothiazolinone' as component (98). In a Letter to the Editor, their mistake was politely pointed out (24). Six parents had hand dermatitis from contact allergy to MI in wet wipes used for the hygiene of their children (83). Six pediatric patients had chronic dermatitis of the perianal area, and two also around the mouth, from contact allergy to MI in wet wipes (100). An unknown number of patients suffered from MI in wet wipes (107). A 9-year-old boy had chronic perianal dermatitis caused by contact allergy to MI in wet wipes (118). Two children presented with ACD of the buttocks and perianal region from MI present in wet wipes (109).

Rinse-off cosmetic products

A child had vesicular hand dermatitis that may have been aggravated by contact allergy to MI present in liquid soaps (151). One patient had a photodistributed lichenoid contact dermatitis from MI present in a body-wash at a concentration of 95 ppm (149). A child, allergic to MI, had dermatitis of the head, face and buttocks which disappeared after stopping the use of a shampoo containing MI; the product itself also gave a strongly positive patch test reaction (109). A man suffering from atopic dermatitis had superimposed allergic contact dermatitis to MI manifesting as chronic axillary and areolar dermatitis after recurrent full-body cutaneous exposure to an MI-containing body-wash (108). One patient had ACD of the face and V of the neck from MI present in a shampoo and in a hair and body cleanser (25). Contact allergy to MI in a shampoo caused eczema of the hands and wrist in one woman (72). Another woman, allergic to MI, had scalp dermatitis, which disappeared after discontinuation of a shampoo containing MI (163).

Miscellaneous

Data on 8 patients allergic to MI seen in an occupational medicine clinic in Finland with patch test results to MCI/MI, MI, benzisothiazolinone, octylisothiazolinone, occupation, isothiazolinone-related diagnosis, exposures and comments were published in 2017. There were both cases of non-occupational and of occupational allergic contact dermatitis; some were caused by cosmetics, others by non-cosmetic products (165).

Occupational allergic contact dermatitis from methylisothiazolinone in cosmetics

A beautician had occupational ACD from MI in a skin care product (29). A hairdresser had ACD of the hands and wrists from contact with shampoos containing MI (94).

Contact allergy to methylisothiazolinone in non-cosmetic products

Non-occupational ACD from non-cosmetic products

A woman developed ACD from MI in gel pads (surface concentration: 47 ppm) used during an eyelash extension procedure (142). One individual developed ACD on the abdomen from MI in contact gel for 'waist reduction belt'; he had probably previously been sensitized by moist toilet tissues (81). A woman had ACD from MI in a moist household tissue. The tissue was free of MI, according to the manufacturer, but its presence was confirmed by analysis, at a concentration of 26 ppm (72). A woman had airborne allergic contact dermatitis from MI in glass shower screen cleaning spray (74). Contact with personal objects, e.g. a leather sofa (35) or a water bed mattress (103), contaminated with MI present in cleaning products, has caused allergic contact dermatitis in patients sensitized to MI. One individual had dermatitis of the hands and wrist from contact allergy to MI in dishwashing liquid (94). MI, present at 183 ppm in a dishwashing liquid used to clean a dental prosthesis, may have caused primary mucosal sensitization, leading to a flare-up of a long-standing, but inactive, oral lichen planus (52).

A woman had lymphomatoid ACD of the face from MI present in a floor cleaning detergent containing the preservative in a concentration of 181 ppm (45). A woman with chronic dermatitis had worsening of long-standing hand eczema. She proved to be allergic to MI, which was present in a dishwashing liquid. She did protect her hands with natural rubber gloves, but it was demonstrated (by means of patch testing) that MI penetrated the glove (64). Another female patient had facial dermatitis from a scrubbing sponge, produced from the konnyaku plant *Amorphophallus konjac*, which is intended to remove dead cells and cleanse the skin. This product proved to contain approx. 400 ppm MI, to which the patient was allergic (139). A 53-year old man, known to suffer from small plaque parapsoriasis, presented with a recurrent and severe generalized dermatitis, except the face and body folds. He was patch test positive to MI. Methylisothiazolinone was found to be an ingredient of a leather-care product used on a leather seat, relevant for his body lesions; a shampoo preserved with MI accounted for the dermatitis on the scalp and partly on the neck (147).

One individual had ACD of the legs from MI in a NSAID gel (94). A man suffering from recurrent eczema had acute facial dermatitis. He suspected two causes: first, rooms in the home had been newly painted with water-based paint; and second, he had used an old pair of spectacles, which had previously caused itching dermatitis on the temples. Indeed, the acute dermatitis was pronounced in the temple regions where the sidebars of the spectacles touched the skin. The material proved to contain 12 ppm MI, to which the patient was strongly allergic (patch test reaction down to 33 ppm). The function of MI in the solid spectacle material remained a mystery, but it was demonstrated that it was not there as a contaminant from facial cosmetics (140).

A woman had allergic contact dermatitis of the feet from the presence of 10 ppm MI in the shoe glue (163). Contact allergy to methylisothiazolinone in a shoe polish contributed to the hand eczema of a man (168). A 7-year-old girl had dermatitis involving the trunk and proximal extremities, most prominent in the axillae and periaxillary skin, buttocks, and abdomen, which was caused by MI in a laundry detergent (175). In one patient, MI in the leather from a sofa may have contributed to allergic contact dermatitis primarily caused by octylisothiazolinone in the leather (182).

Airborne contact dermatitis from paints

Allergic reactions to MI in newly painted rooms are frequent and were experienced by 13 of 166 (7.8%) patients allergic to MI in a 2015 investigation in 8 European countries. Usually the patients have airborne contact dermatitis, but rhinitis and conjunctivitis were also observed (96,170). One patient developed airborne ACD from using water-based wall paint; she had previously become sensitized to MI in a moist wipe (6). Two patients had airborne CD from MI in wall paint; in one of the products, the concentration of MI was 187 ppm (49). A young woman had facial dermatitis with periorbital edema, which progressed to vesicular dermatitis. When present in the restaurant where she worked and that had just been painted, she felt a burning sensation on the cheeks, malaise, and dizziness. These complaints were caused by contact allergy to MI, present in the paint (73). A woman had airborne ACD from MI in paint used in her new apartment, that was so severe and long-lasting, that she was offered another apartment, which she accepted (27). A 4-year-old girl had allergic contact dermatitis caused by MI as a primary sensitizer in baby wipes, followed by airborne – and partly systemic – dermatitis (presumably by inhalation), the latter mimicking atopic dermatitis, elicited by a wall paint containing 53 ppm MI (47).

A 3-month-old boy became sensitized to MI from its presence in wall paint and later developed airborne ACD in freshly painted rooms and dermatitis from various cosmetic products preserved with MCI/MI and/or MI (77). One patient developed ACD from MI in paint used by his neighbor (contact dermatitis *by proxy*) (104). A woman developed airborne ACD with dyspnea on two occasions when painting her living room with paint containing 100 ppm methylisothiazolinone, to which preservative she had a strongly positive patch test (59). A child, previously sensitized to MI from moist wipes, later developed airborne ACD of the face from MI in paint by moving into a newly painted apartment (65). A woman had suffered from two episodes of acute facial dermatitis following exposure to freshly painted environments. Three days after commencing painting, she developed an intensely pruritic facial rash and periorbital edema that progressed to involve the neck and upper chest with an associated nocturnal cough and wheeze. The subsequent episode occurred 2 months later when her workplace was painted. The cause was contact allergy to MI (and MCI) present in wall paint (106). A young boy developed airborne ACD from MI and MCI/MI in paint; he had probably previously become sensitized from the use of wet wipes, which caused dermatitis in the diaper area (162). A woman had airborne ACD from MI in 4 wall paints containing the preservative at 50-100 ppm (164).

In France and Belgium, 44 patients who had suffered from allergic airborne contact dermatitis caused by isothiazolinones in paints, diagnosed in the period beginning of 2012 to January 2016, were collected (161). Eighty per cent of the reactions took place in a private, non-occupational setting and, in nearly half of the cases, the patients had painted the room themselves. There were only 3 painters with occupational allergic contact dermatitis. Most patients developed reactions within 1-3 days (they were already sensitized); in 3 individuals, there was a delay of 13 to 21 days, potentially indicating active (primary) sensitization (161). Most patients presented with dermatitis limited to non-covered body parts, and ten (23%) also had mucosal symptoms, such as breathing difficulties and/or rhinoconjunctivitis (161). Symptoms were often severe, necessitating repeated consultations (86%), hospitalization (9%), and/or sick leave (20%), and treatment with topical or systemic (27%) corticosteroids. When patch tested, 43 of 44 patients showed positive reactions to MI and 36/44 to MCI/MI. The isothiazolinones octylisothiazolinone (OIT) and benzisothiazolinone (BIT) were patch tested in 21 and 15 patients, respectively, with only OIT showing allergic reactions in 9 of 21 cases. Information on the composition of the incriminated paints could be retrieved in 19 cases, in which BIT, MI, MCI/MI, and OIT were identified in 15, 14, 10 and 2 cases, respectively, Often, different isothiazolinones were used together (161).

Occupational allergic contact dermatitis from non-cosmetic products

In a hospital in Helsinki, Finland, 5 patients with occupational allergic contact dermatitis from MI in non-cosmetic products were seen (purely from MI, not from MCI/MI): a paint factory worker reacted to MI in biocides for paints, two machinists reacted to MI in a metalworking fluid, a café worker to a dishwashing liquid and 2 detergents, and a coating worker to an anti-condensation paint (29). A painter was sensitized to and developed occupational ACD from MI in wallpaper glue; this was the first reported case of sensitization to MI (46). A technician working for a manufacturer of starch for the paper mill industry accidentally spilled a commercial 2.5% MI solution on his shoes, which led to irritant dermatitis of the feet followed by sensitization: one week later, a vesicular dermatitis appeared. One year after the spilling accident, outdoors in wet weather, he again wore the shoes he had worn at the plant and developped a blistering dermatitis on the dorsal surfaces of his feet, despite having laundered the shoes in a washing machine right after the accident (46). Two patients (professions unknown) had ACD of the hands from MI present in hand cleansers (83).

A woman working at a pharmaceutical production facility, operating a machine used for auto-matic labelling of insulin pens, had hand eczema involving the second to fourth fingers on both hands, which was caused by MI in the adhesive of the labels (141). A female laboratory scientist had hand dermatitis from MI in a hand wash she used at work (113). A female nurse developed ACD of the hands from gel she used for making ultrasound scans of pregnant women (53). A nurse had occupational ACD of the hands from MI in wet wipes she used for cleaning at work; the product was mislabeled, the presence of MI was not indicated (30).

Occupational allergic contact dermatitis from paints
Painters are at high risk of developing contact allergy to MI (39,181) and exposure to this preservative (and to MCI/MI) is one of the most common causes of occupational contact dermatitis in this occupational group in Denmark (87,181). In a period of two years (2004-2005), 4 of 14 workers in a paint production facility working with an open system (thereby increasing the risk of contamination) became sensitized to MI after the introduction of a 7%-10% MI-containing additive (10). A woman working in a paint factory became sensitized to MI in paints and developed ACD of the hands, neck and face. Later, she was reallocated at work, where entering rooms containing paint vapors were unavoidable, leading to recurrences of dermatitis and a maculopapular rash. The authors considered this to be systemic contact dermatitis from inhalation of MI (78). A foreman in a construction company specializing in renovation work had dry cough and rhinitis. A few days following these first symptoms, an eczematous eruption appeared, located on the face, eyelids, chest, the nape of his neck, and the folds of the elbows, resembling atopic dermatitis. Both the respiratory and the dermatological symptoms were caused by airborne exposure to MI in water-based paints and to MI and MCI/MI in pulverized indoor facade renders. The patient reacted to both MCI/MI and MI, and also to the paint and to the indoor facade render (144).

Miscellaneous
Data on 8 patients allergic to MI seen in an occupational medicine clinic in Finland with patch test results to MCI/MI, MI, benzisothiazolinone, octylisothiazolinone, occupation, isothiazolinone-related diagnosis, exposures and comments were published in 2017. There were both cases of non-occupational and of occupational allergic contact dermatitis; some were caused by cosmetics, others by non-cosmetic products (165).

Cross-reactions, pseudo-cross-reactions and co-reactions
Cross-reactivity of MI to and (to a lesser degree) from methylchloroisothiazolinone is well known but not obligatory (7,57,62,166). Between 15% (112) and 40-70% of patients with a positive patch test to MI also react to MCI/MI (3,4,5,6,38,39,71,117,170,172,176,177). In Sweden, the percentage was higher (81%), which is explained by the higher test con-centration of MCI/MI (200 ppm) (88) and a percentage of 79 co-reactivity was observed in Australia (93). In a study in Spain, all patients positive to MI 0.2% in water also reacted to MCI/MI 200 ppm water, but only 68% to MCI/MI 100 ppm water (114).

There are strong indications that patients primarily sensitized to MI may cross-react to octylisothiazolinone (35,46,57,129,142,147,161,165,172). This has been corroborated in animal studies (43). Using a modified local lymph node assay in mice, cross-reactivity between methylisothiazolinone and octylisothiazolinone was found, when the potency of the chemical was taken into account in the choice of the challenge concentration (43). Conversely, primary sensitization to octylisothiazolinone may also result in cross-sensitization to methylisothiazolinone (15). Evidence of possible cross-reactivity from MI to benzisothiazolinone is scant (44,129,165). However, in the study mentioned above, using a modified local lymph node assay in mice, cross-reactivity between methylisothiazolinone and benzisothiazolinone was found, but the potency of the chemical had to be taken into account in the choice of the challenge concentration (43).

Patients with MI allergy are often polysensitized, i.e. that they also react to a number of chemically unrelated allergens (113). These are notably fragrances and preservatives (especially formaldehyde and formaldehyde-releasers) (33,170). In fact, contact allergies to MI and/or MCI/MI are significantly associated with reactions to formaldehyde and the two fragrance mixes FM I and FM II (80). These co-reactions are from concomitant or successive sensitization in the same or other (cosmetic) products rather than from cross-reactivity.

Patch test sensitization
There has been one case reported with suspected active sensitization to MI at 1000 ppm (15 μl applied to a Finn Chamber® with a diameter of 8 mm; 30 μg/cm^2) (152).

Provocation tests
Ten of 33 patients (30%) reacting to MI 0.05% and/or 0.1% water had a positive ROAT (twice daily for 2 weeks) with a leave-on lotion containing 100 ppm MI; they all also had positive patch tests to MCI/MI (4). Of 9 MI-allergic patients, 5 (56%) had a positive ROAT (twice daily for two weeks) to a cream containing 100 ppm MI (62). Of 3 patient reacting to MCI/MI, but not to MI, all reacted to the same cream, which is explained by cross-sensitization from methylisothiazolinone to methylchloroisothiazolinone allergy (62). Ten patients allergic to MI performed ROATs with MI in a water/ethanol vehicle containing (recalculated from the amount applied per cm^2) 100, 50 and 5 ppm MI. Eight (90%) reacted positively to 100 and 50 ppm and 2 had a positive ROAT to the 5 ppm MI solution (11).

In a group of 10 patients allergic to MI, all had a positive ROAT (five times daily on the ventral side of the forearm, application to moist skin, the soap was rinsed off after 20-25 seconds) to liquid soap containing 100 ppm MI and 7/9 (78%) reacted to a soap with 50 ppm MI (92). There were no reactions to a control soap without MI in the MI-allergic patients. None of 19 controls reacted to a 21-day ROAT with liquid soap containing 50 ppm, 100 ppm or no MI. This clearly indicates that rinse-off products containing permitted (at that time 100 ppm) concentrations of MI can cause allergic contact dermatitis in patients previously sensitized to MI (92).

Patch test studies with dilution series
In a group of 10 patients allergic to MI tested with a dilution series (2000 ppm down to 0.35 ppm), all 10 (100%) reacted down to 440 ppm, 8 of these (80%) to 220 ppm, and 7 of these (70%) to 147 ppm. The lowest concentration that gave positive reactions was 74 ppm, in six patients (60%) (11). In serial dilution patch testing in nineteen patients allergic to MI, 3 had a lowest threshold of 16 ppm, 13 (68%) of 100 ppm, 1 of 250 ppm and 2 of 500 ppm (92). Some patients have reacted to patch test concentrations of MI as low as 10 and 30 ppm (6).

Presence of methylisothiazolinone in cosmetic products
In the USA, in April 2017, methylisothiazolinone (possibly also in combination with methylchloroisothiazolinone) was present in 5601 of 56,714 cosmetic products of which the composition is known in FDA's Voluntary Cosmetic Registration Program (VCRP) (data obtained from FDA, May 2017). In May 2017, MI was present in 2776 of 66,835 cosmetic products of which the composition is known in EWG's Skin Deep Cosmetics Database, USA (http://www. ewg.org/skindeep/). Methylisothiazolinone was present in 195 of 4737 (4.1%) commonly used cosmetic products of which the full composition was known in 2016 in The Contact Allergen Management Program (CAMP) database of the American Contact Dermatitis Society (158). MI was present in 4 (2.2%) of 178 facial wipes for which ingredient information was obtained online and from retail stores, USA, 2016 (178). MI was present in 3 (5.6%) of 54 personal hygiene wet wipes for which ingredient information was obtained online and from retail stores, USA, 2016 (179).

In 2015-2016, 100 USA-made personal care products from different brands were randomly selected and 15 products (15%) were labeled to contain MI (153). In the USA, in 2015-2016, 63 diaper wipes and 41 topical diaper preparations from a large retailer were screened for the presence of potential sensitizers. MI was found in 4/63 (6%) disposable diaper wipes and in none of 41 topical diaper preparations (159). Of 63 disposable diaper wipes available online from one large USA company in November 2015, 4 (6.3%) contained MI (148). In May and June 2015, the ingredient labels of 1266 cosmetics and 125 baby products marketed in Switzerland were screened for the presence of MI. In addition, product information was collected from online websites and from manufacturers. MI was labelled on 4% of the cosmetics and 6.4% of the baby products (137). Of 152 cosmetic products specifically marketed for babies and children in the USA and surveyed in 2014, 30 (20%) contained MI. Facial or body wipes and hair products were the categories with the greatest percentage of MI-containing products. Cosmetics marketed as 'gentle', 'sensitive', 'organic' or 'hypoallergenic' often contained MI (111).

In 2014, in Thailand, the labels of 1000 cosmetic products (593 leave-on, 407 rinse-off products) were examined for the presence of preservatives. These were partly purchased in shops and on markets and partly brought in by patients. MI was present in 61 products (6%); in the leave-on products, the percentage was 3.7 and in the rinse-off products 9.6 (133). Of 179 emollients available in Poland in 2014, 6 (3.3%) contained MI (126). MI was present in 215 of 7500 cosmetic products (2.9%) registered by the Helsinki Asthma and Allergy Association in Finland in 2013 (37). MI was present in 60 of 1795 (3.3%) cosmetic products bought in supermarkets in 2013 in Denmark. Of the 60 products, 25 (42%) were leave-on, 22 (37%) were rinse-off, six (10%) were hair waxes, four (7%) were wet wipes, and three (5%) were paints for nails (71).

In 2010, in Denmark, 19 of 1272 (1.5%) cosmetic products sold in eight retail stores and a department store were labeled with MI (8); 12 were rinse-off products, three were leave-on and four were wet wipes (8). More than 2400 US cosmetic products on file with FDA (total number of files unknown) were found to be preserved with MI in 2010 (134). The number of cosmetics in the USA containing MI doubled between 2007 and 2010 (no details known) (54,56). In the period 2006-2009, 4680 cosmetics (1500 creams, 459 make-up products, 245 shampoos, 384 shower products, 87 soaps, 454 hair products, 463 sun products) were investigated by a German government office. MI was present, according to the labelling, in 42 products (0.9%). The category with the highest percentage of products containing MI was that of sunscreen products (3.7%), followed by shower products (1.8%) and shampoos (1.6%) (60). Methylisothiazolinone was present in 28/3541 (0.7%) randomly sampled leave-on cosmetic products, Germany, 2006-2009 (21). In 2008, a survey in Sweden on preservatives in 204 cosmetic products (92 shampoos, 61 hair conditioners, 34 liquid soaps, 17 wet tissues) showed that only one product (0.5%) was preserved with MI (12). According to information supplied to the US Food and Drug Administration by industry as part of the Voluntary Cosmetic Ingredient Registration Program, MI was used in a total of 1125 cosmetic products in the United States in 2007; 24% were shampoos, 18% conditioners, and 10% baby soaps and detergents In 2010, three years later, the number of cosmetics containing MI had more than doubled and risen to 2408 (ref. lost during writing). In 2005, 217 of 1142 (19%) toiletries/cosmetics on file in the Danish Product Register Database PROBAS contained MI (127).

Presence of methylisothiazolinone in non-cosmetic products
In May and June 2015, the ingredient labels of 557 detergents marketed in Switzerland were screened for the presence of MI and other isothiazolinones. Product information was also collected from online websites and from

manufacturers. Of the detergents products, 43% were preserved with an isothiazolinone, but the percentage for MI was not specified (137). In the Danish Product Register Database (PROBAS), a database in which the composition of, primarily, hazardous chemical products for occupational use is registered, MI in 2013 was the second most frequently registered isothiazolinone, with 884 different products registered. The top three product types containing MI were paints and varnishes (n=471), cleaning/washing agents (n=87), and polishing agents (n=60). MI was registered in concentrations ranging from 0.01 ppm to 10%, the higher concentrations being the commercial concentrated MI biocide solutions (55). MI was present in 830 of 38,000 active 'substances and materials' registered in 2014 PROBAS as active on the Danish market (181). MI was most frequently registered in paints and varnishes (n=446), cleaning agents (n=88), and polishing agents (n=48) (181). It has been stated that MI was present in nearly all water-based paints in Denmark in 2011 (73).

In 2008, a survey in Sweden on preservatives showed that 16 (16%) out of 97 detergents (multipurpose cleaners and washing-up liquids) were labeled to contain MI (12). In Italy, in 2008, 30 (10%) out of 291 household cleaning products were preserved with MI (13). In Denmark, the total number of products on file in the Danish Product Register Database PROBAS, containing MI, increased from 1872 in 2002 to 3563 in 2005. The categories containing MI were (number provided + percentage of products containing MI in that particular category): paints/lacquers 2145 (16%), printing inks 164 (4.3%), cleaning agents 142 (2.2%), polishes 122 (14%), impregnating agents 39 (7.5%), filling agents 28 (1.5%), hardeners 25 (0.8%), adhesives/glues 23 (1.3%), construction materials 11 (1.1%), flooring agents 8 (2%) and hardeners 25 (0.8%) (127).

Chemical analysis of methylisothiazolinone in cosmetic products

In 2015-2016, 100 USA-made personal care products from different brands were randomly selected. The ingredient labels were examined and the products were analyzed with HPLC for the content of MI. According to labeling, fifteen products (15%) contained MI. Three products not labeled to contain MI or MCI/MI showed positive results on HPLC (not specified for MI and MCI/MI). Of 35 products labeled to contain MCI/MI or MI, five showed negative results upon HPLC analysis (not specified for MI and MCI/MI). Of the 15 products labeled to contain MI, five contained MI > 100 ppm. It was concluded that personal care products are an important source of exposure to MI. Labeling inaccuracies and concentrations above the maximum allowed were identified (153).

In 2015, in the USA, 17 cosmetic products (7 shampoos/conditioners, 10 skin care products), labeled as containing methylisothiazolinone, were analyzed. They all contained MI in concentrations ranging from 0.2 to 12 µg/g in the rinse-off products and 0.3-20 µg/g (ppm) in the 10 skin care products (132). In Switzerland, in 2015, a sample of 19 cosmetics preserved with isothiazolinones (MI, MCI/MI, benzisothiazolinone, octylisothiazolinone) was selected for chemical analysis by liquid chromatography–high-resolution mass spectrometry after ultrasonic extraction. MI was detected in 12 of 19 (63%) investigated cosmetics in concentrations ranging from 1.3-133 ppm (137).

In Belgium, in 2014, of 7 leave-on cosmetics labeled as containing MI, 6 had concentrations of >150 ppm (max. 188); of 6 rinse-off products, 2 had concentrations of >100 ppm (128 and 163 ppm). Some cosmetics labeled as not containing MI did in fact contain the preservative (28). MI was present in 7 of 60 (12%) cosmetics purchased in Israel in 2014, in concentrations ranging from 2.7 to 107 ppm (85). In 2010, in Denmark, 19 cosmetic products sold in eight retail stores and a department store and labeled with MI were analyzed with HPLC-UV-MS. The concentration of MI in the different products ranged from 2 to 100 ppm. Fourteen (74%) of the 19 products contained more than 50 ppm MI and five (26%) more than 95 ppm (8). Use concentrations in cosmetic products in the USA ranged from <1 ppm to 0.01% (100 ppm) (20).

Chemical analysis of methylisothiazolinone in non-cosmetic products

Five types of scrub sponges were investigated for the presence of MI by gas chromatography–mass spectrometry and they all contained MI in concentrations ranging from 320 to 441 ppm (139). In Switzerland, in 2015, a sample of 69 detergents preserved with isothiazolinones (MI, MCI/MI, benzisothiazolinone, octylisothiazolinone) was selected for chemical analysis by liquid chromatography–high-resolution mass spectrometry after ultrasonic extraction. MI was detected in 27 of 69 detergents (39%) in concentrations ranging from 3.5 to 279 ppm (137).

In Belgium, in 2014, 8 detergents and 4 paints were analysed for the presence of MI. Four of 8 detergents (50%) contained MI in a concentration range of 2-181 ppm. All 4 paints had MI as constituent, in concentrations ranging from 8 to 225 ppm (28). In December 2013 and January 2014, 71 wall paints were randomly purchased in retail outlets in five European countries. The paints were quantitatively analyzed for their contents of MI by high-performance liquid chromatography coupled to tandem mass spectrometry. MI was found in 93% (n=66) of the paints, with concentrations ranging from 0.7 to 181 ppm (51). All of 19 wall paints purchased in Denmark in 2011 contained MI in concentrations ranging from 10 to 300 ppm; in half of these, MI concentrations were >100 ppm (82,97)

Other information

Methylisothiazolinone cannot be tested in petrolatum, because it cannot be evenly dispersed (121). Rubber gloves may not protect against skin penetration of MI (64). Some products not labeled as containing MI may sometimes contain the preservative after all (28,30,72).

OTHER SIDE EFFECTS

Irritant contact dermatitis

In one patient, an accidental contact with a solution containing 2.5% MI and 2.5% benzisothiazolinone resulted in irritant contact dermatitis (chemical burn) followed by primary sensitization to methylisothiazolinone (46).

Photosensitivity

Some patients sensitized to MCI/MI and/or MI may show photoaggravated dermatitis and/or persistent photosensitivity for which photopatch tests and phototests are useful diagnostic procedures. The clinical picture in such patients is sometimes difficult to differentiate from airborne allergic contact dermatitis (50). A woman presented with an 18-month history of a photosensitive eruption on exposed sites. She was negative on patch testing to MI, but had a positive reaction to MI on the last reading as part of a photopatch series. The diagnosis was photo-induced ACD (photoallergic contact dermatitis) from MI, but the causative product(s) were not mentioned (146,174). Another 3 patients had dermatitis of the face and (in one) other exposed sites that appeared to be photosensitive. All three had stronger reactions to the photopatch test with MI than to the patch test, which suggests, according to the authors, that these individuals had photoaggravated allergic contact dermatitis. In only one were the incriminated products mentioned (moisturizer and shampoo) (146,174). Not mentioning the causative products is curious, as the authors stated that all reactions were clinically relevant.

Other non-eczematous contact reactions

Rhinitis and airway symptoms have been observed repeatedly, usually in combination with airborne allergic contact dermatitis and mostly from paints (see the sections 'Airborne contact dermatitis from paints' and 'Occupational allergic contact dermatitis from paints' above).

LITERATURE

1   Uter W, Aberer W, Armario-Hita JC, Fernandez-Vozmediano JM, Ayala F, Balato A, et al. Current patch test results with the European baseline series and extensions to it from the 'European Surveillance System on Contact Allergy' network, 2007-2008. Contact Dermatitis 2012;67:9-19

2   Travassos AR, Claes L, Boey L, Drieghe J, Goossens A. Non-fragrance allergens in specific cosmetic products. Contact Dermatitis 2011;65:276-285

3   Schnuch A, Lessmann H, Geier J, Uter W. Contact allergy to preservatives. Analysis of IVDK data 1996-2009. Br J Dermatol 2011;164:1316-1325

4   Ackermann L, Aalto-Korte K, Alanko K, Hasan T, Jolanki R, Lammintausta K, et al. Contact sensitization to methylisothiazolinone in Finland – a multicentre study. Contact Dermatitis 2011;64:49-53

5   Lundov MD, Thyssen JP, Zachariae C, Johansen JD. Prevalence and cause of methylisothiazolinone contact allergy. Contact Dermatitis 2010;63:164-167

6   García-Gavín J, Vansina S, Kerre S, Naert A, Goossens A. Methylisothiazolinone, an emerging allergen in cosmetics? Contact Dermatitis 2010;63:96-101

7   Geier J, Lessmann H, Schnuch A, Uter W. Recent increase in allergic reactions to methylchloroisothiazolinone/methylisothiazolinone: is methylisothiazolinone the culprit? Contact Dermatitis 2012;67:334-341

8   Lundov MD, Krongaard T, Menné TL, Johansen JD. Methylisothiazolinone contact allergy: a review. Br J Dermatol 2011;165:1178-1182+

9   Public consultation on Methylisothiazolinone (MI) in the framework of Regulation (EC) No. 1223/2009 - rinse-off cosmetic products. Available at:
    http://ec.europa.eu/growth/tools-databases/newsroom/cf/itemdetail.cfm?item_id=8740

10 Thyssen JP, Sederberg-Olsen N, Thomsen JF, Menné T. Contact dermatitis from methylisothiazolinone in a paint factory. Contact Dermatitis 2006;54:322-324

11 Lundov MD, Zachariae C, Johansen JD. Methylisothiazolinone contact allergy and dose–response relationship. Contact Dermatitis 2011;64:330-336

12 Yazar K, Johnsson S, Lind M-L, Boman A, Lidén C. Preservatives and fragrances in selected consumer-available cosmetics and detergents. Contact Dermatitis 2011;64:265-272

13 Magnano M, Silvani S, Vincenzi C, Nino M, Tosti A. Contact allergens and irritants in household washing and cleaning products. Contact Dermatitis 2009;61:337-341

14 Gerberick GF, Ryan CA, Kern PS, Schlatter H, Dearman RJ, Kimber I, et al. Compilation of historical local lymph node data for evaluation of skin sensitization alternative methods. Dermatitis 2005;16:157-202

15 Leysen J, Goossens A, Meert H, Apers J, Lambert J, Aerts O. Octylisothiazolinone is a relevant nonoccupational contact allergen in leather goods and may show cross-reactivity to methylisothiazolinone. Contact Dermatitis 2016;75(Suppl.1):65

16 Kimber I, Basketter DA, Butler M, Gamer A, Garrigue JL, Gerberick GF, et al. Classification of contact allergens according to potency: proposals. Food Chem Toxicol 2003;41:1799-1809

17 Basketter DA, Gilmour NJ, Wright Z, Walters T, Boman A, Lidén C. Biocides: characterization of the allergenic hazard of methylisothiazolinone. Cut Ocul Toxicol 2003;22:187-199

18 Scientific Committee on Cosmetic Products and Non-food Products Intended for Consumers (SCCNFP), Opinion on Methylisothiazolinone (P94) – Submission, 23 April 2004, SCCNFP/0805/04, 2004. Available at: http://ec.europa.eu/health/ph_risk/committees/sccp/documents/out270_en.pdf

19 Scientific Committee on Cosmetic Products and Non-food Products Intended for Consumers (SCCNFP), Opinion on Methylisothiazolinone (P94) – Submission, 18 March 2003, SCCNFP/0625/02. 2003. Available at: http://ec.europa.eu/health/ph_risk/committees/sccp/documents/out_201.pdf

20 Burnett CL, Bergfeld WF, Belsito DV, Klaassen CD, Marks JG Jr, Shank RC, et al. Final report of the safety assessment of methylisothiazolinone. Int J Toxicol 2010;29 (Suppl.3):187-213

21 Schnuch A, Mildau G, Kratz E-M, Uter W. Risk of sensitization to preservatives estimated on the basis of patch test data and exposure, according to a sample of 3541 leave-on products. Contact Dermatitis 2011;65:167-174

22 Schwensen JF, White IR, Thyssen JP, Menné T, Johansen JD. Failures in risk assessment and risk management for cosmetic preservatives in Europe and the impact on public health. Contact Dermatitis 2015;73:133-141

23 Amaro C, Santos R, Cardoso J. Contact allergy to methylisothiazolinone in a deodorant. Contact Dermatitis 2011;64:298-299

24 Garcia-Gavin J, Goossens A. Moist toilet paper: allergy to nonhalogenated derivative methylisothiazolinone preservative alone. Arch Dermatol 2010;146:1186

25 Goossens A, Baret I, Swevers A. Allergic contact dermatitis caused by tetrahydroxypropyl ethylenediamine in cosmetic products. Contact Dermatitis 2011;64:161-164

26 Commission Regulation (EU) 2016/1198 of 22 July 2016 amending Annex V to Regulation (EC) No 1223/2009 of the European Parliament and of the Council on cosmetic products. Official Journal of the European Union, 23 July 2016, L 198/10.

27 Lundov MD, Friis UF, Menné T, Johansen JD. Methylisothiazolinone in paint forces a patient out of her apartment. Contact Dermatitis 2013;69:252-253

28 Aerts O, Meert H, Goossens A, Janssens S, Lambert J, Apers S. Methylisothiazolinone in selected consumer products in Belgium: Adding fuel to the fire? Contact Dermatitis 2015;73:142-149

29 Vauhkala A-R, Pesonen M, Suomela S, Kuuliala O, Suuronen K, Aalto-Korte K. Occupational contact allergy to methylchloroisothiazolinone/methylisothiazolinone and methylisothiazolinone. Contact Dermatitis 2015;73:150-156

30 Schwensen JF, Menné T, Friis UF, Johansen JD. Undisclosed methylisothiazolinone in wet wipes for occupational use causing occupational allergic contact dermatitis in a nurse. Contact Dermatitis 2015;73:182-184

31 Madsen JT, Andersen F, Andersen KE. Generalized allergic contact dermatitis caused by methylisothiazolinone in a spray tan. Contact Dermatitis 2015;73:184-185

32 Warburton KL, Wilkinson M. Contact allergy to methylisothiazolinone: Has there been any change? Experience of a UK centre. Contact Dermatitis 2015;72:398-400

33 Martin-Gorgojo A, Curto-Barredo L, Rovira-López R, Pujol RM, Gimenez-Arnau A. Is methylisothiazolinone contact allergy a risk factor for polysensitization? Contact Dermatitis 2015;72:400-402

34 Badaoui A, Bayrou O, Fite C, Frances C, Soria A, Pecquet C. Allergic contact dermatitis caused by methylisothiazolinone in hair gel. Contact Dermatitis 2015;73:364-366

35 Aerts O, Baeck M, Constandt L, Dezfoulian B, Jacobs MC, Kerre S, et al. The dramatic increase in the rate of methylisothiazolinone contact allergy in Belgium: a multicentre study. Contact Dermatitis 2014;71:41-48

36 Uter W, Geier J, Bauer A, Schnuch A. Risk factors associated with methylisothiazolinone contact sensitization. Contact Dermatitis 2013;69:231-238

37 Lammintausta K, Aalto-Korte K, Ackerman L, Alanko K, Berry P, Hasan T, et al. An epidemic of contact allergy to methylisothiazolinone in Finland. Contact Dermatitis 2014;70:184-185

38 Hosteing S, Meyer N, Waton J, Barbaud A, Bourrain J-L, Raison-Peyron N, et al. Outbreak of contact sensitization to methylisothiazolinone: an analysis of French data from the REVIDAL-GERDA network. Contact Dermatitis 2014;70:262-269

39 Schwensen JF, Menné T, Andersen KE, Sommerlund M, Johansen J D. Occupations at risk of developing contact allergy to isothiazolinones in Danish contact dermatitis patients: results from a Danish multicentre study (2009–2012). Contact Dermatitis 2014;71:295-302

40 Johnston GA, Contributing Members of the British Society for Cutaneous Allergy (BSCA). The rise in prevalence of contact allergy to methylisothiazolinone in the British Isles. Contact Dermatitis 2014;70:238-240

41 Roberts DW. Methylisothiazolinone is categorized as a strong sensitizer in the murine local lymph node assay. Contact Dermatitis 2013;69:261-262

42 Bruze M, Uter W, Gonçalo M, Lepoittevin J-P, Diepgen T, Orton D. Incompetence and failure to regulate methylisothiazolinone. Contact Dermatitis 2015;72:353-354

43 Schwensen JF, Menné Bonefeld C, Zachariae C, Agerbeck CH, Petersen T, Geisler C, et al. Cross-reactivity between methylisothiazolinone, octylisothiazolinone and benzisothiazolinone using a modified local lymph node assay. Br J Dermatol. 2017 Jan;176(1):176-183.

44 Geier J, Lessmann H, Schnuch A, Uter W. Concomitant reactivity to methylisothiazolinone, benzisothiazolinone, and octylisothiazolinone. International Network of Departments of Dermatology data, 2009–2013. Contact Dermatitis 2015;72:337-339

45 Van Steenkiste E, Goossens A, Meert H, Apers S, Aerts O. Airborne-induced lymphomatoid contact dermatitis caused by methylisothiazolinone. Contact Dermatitis 2015;72:237-240

46 Isaksson M, Gruvberger B, Bruze M. Occupational contact allergy and dermatitis from methylisothiazolinone after contact with wall covering glue and after a chemical burn from a biocide. Dermatitis 2004;15:201-205

47 Aerts O, Cattaert N, Lambert J, Goossens A. Airborne and systemic dermatitis, mimicking atopic dermatitis, caused by methylisothiazolinone in a young child. Contact Dermatitis 2013;68:250-251

48 Aerts O, Van Dyck F, Dandelooy J, Mellaerts T, Lambert J. Contact dermatitis masquerading as folliculitis decalvans: methylisothiazolinone strikes again! Dermatitis 2014;25:276

49 Lundov MD, Mosbech H, Thyssen JP, Menné T, Zachariae C. Two cases of airborne allergic contact dermatitis caused by methylisothiazolinone in paint. Contact Dermatitis 2011;65:176-179

50 Aerts O, Goossens A, Marguery M-C, Castelain M, Boursault L, Giordano-Labadie F, Lambert J, Milpied B. Photoaggravation and persistent photosensitivity in patients sensitized to methylchloroisothiazolinone/methyl-isothiazolinone and methylisothiazolinone in Belgium and France: a report of nine cases. Contact Dermatitis 2016;75(Suppl.1):66

51 Schwensen JF, Lundov MD, Bossi R, Banerjee P, Gimenez-Arnau E, Lepoittevin J-P, et al. Methylisothiazolinone and benzisothiazolinone are widely used in paint: a multicentre study of paints from five European countries. Contact Dermatitis 2015;72:127-138

52 Aerts O, Meert H, Janssens S, Sprengers M, Chapelle K, Bensch L, et al. A sudden flare-up of a quiescent oral lichen planus: methylisothiazolinone as the prime suspect? Contact Dermatitis 2015;72:186-189

53 Madsen JT, Broesby-Olsen S, Andersen KE. Undisclosed methylisothiazolinone in an ultrasound gel causing occupational allergic contact dermatitis. Contact Dermatitis 2014;71:312-313

54 Food and Drug Administration. Frequency of Use of Cosmetic Ingredients. FDA Database, Submitted by FDA in Response to FOI Request F06-18753: Washington, DC, FDA, 2007.

55 Fischer Friis U, Menné T, Flyvholm M-A, Ellekilde Bonde JP, Lepoittevin J-P, Le Coz CJ, et al. Isothiazolinones in commercial products at Danish workplaces. Contact Dermatitis 2014;71:65-74

56 Steinberg D. Preservatives for Cosmetics, 3rd edition. Carol Stream, IL: Allured Books, 2012.

57 Isaksson M, Gruvberger B, Bruze M. Patch testing with serial dilutions of various isothiazolinones in patients hypersensitive to methylchloroisothiazolinone/methylisothiazolinone. Contact Dermatitis 2014;70:270-275

58 Isaksson M, Andersen KE, Gonçalo M, Goossens A, Gruvberger B, Johansen JD, et al. Multicentre patch testing with methylisothiazolinone by the European Environmental and Contact Dermatitis Research Group. Contact Dermatitis 2014;70:317-320

59 Alwan W, White IR, Banerjee P. Presumed airborne contact allergy to methylisothiazolinone causing acute severe facial dermatitis and respiratory difficulty. Contact Dermatitis 2014;70:320-321

60 Uter W, Yazar K, Kratz E-M, Mildau G, Lidén C. Coupled exposure to ingredients of cosmetic products: II. preservatives. Contact Dermatitis 2014;70:219-226

61 Gameiro A, Coutinho I, Ramos L, Gonçalo M. Methylisothiazolinone: second 'epidemic' of isothiazolinone sensitization. Contact Dermatitis 2014;70:242-243

62 Isaksson M, Gruvberger B, Gonçalo M, Goossens A, Le Coz C-J, Bruze M. Repeated open application test with methylisothiazolinone in individuals sensitive to methylchloroisothiazolinone/methylisothiazolinone. Contact Dermatitis 2014;70:244-246

63 Madsen JT, Andersen KE. Further evidence of the methylisothiazolinone epidemic. Contact Dermatitis 2014;70:246-247

64 Espasandín-Arias M, Goossens A. Natural rubber gloves might not protect against skin penetration of methylisothiazolinone. Contact Dermatitis 2014;70:249-251

65 Madsen JT, Andersen KE. Airborne allergic contact dermatitis caused by methylisothiazolinone in a child sensitized from wet wipes. Contact Dermatitis 2014;70:183-184

66   Editorial. The methylisothiazolinone epidemic: Is the fire out or is Rome still burning? Contact Dermatitis 2014;70:67-68

67   Cosmetics Europe 2013. Cosmetics Europe issues recommendation to discontinue use of MIT in leave-on skin cosmetic products, 13 December 2013. Available at: https://www.cosmeticseurope.eu/news-a-events/news/647-cosmetics-europe-recommendation-on-mit.html

68   Gonçalo M, Goossens A. Whilst Rome Burns: The epidemic of contact allergy to methylisothiazolinone. Contact Dermatitis 2013;68:257-258

69   Bruze M, Engfeldt M, Gonçalo M, Goossens A. Recommendation to include methylisothiazolinone in the European baseline patch test series – on behalf of the European Society of Contact Dermatitis and the European Environmental and Contact Dermatitis Research Group. Contact Dermatitis 2013;69:263-270

70   Bruze M, Fregert S, Gruvberger B, Persson K. Contact allergy to the active ingredients of Kathon CG in the guinea pig. Acta Derm Venereol 1987;67:315-320

71   Lundov MD, Opstrup MS, Johansen JD. Methylisothiazolinone contact allergy – a growing epidemic. Contact Dermatitis 2013;69:271-275

72   Vanneste L, Persson L, Zimerson E, Bruze M, Luyckx R, Goossens A. Allergic contact dermatitis caused by methylisothiazolinone from different sources, including 'mislabelled' household wet wipes. Contact Dermatitis 2013;69:311-312

73   Kaae J, Menné T, Thyssen JP. Presumed primary contact sensitization to methylisothiazolinone from paint: a chemical that became airborne. Contact Dermatitis 2012;66:341-342

74   Pastor-Nieto MA, Gática-Ortega ME, González-Muñoz P, Perna-Monroy C, Gil-Redondo R, Pérez-Mesonero R, Melgar-Molero V, et al. Airborne bullous allergic contact dermatitis from methyl isothiazolinone contained in a glass shower screen cleaning spray. Contact Dermatitis 2016;75(Suppl.1):67

75   Aerts O, Cattaert N, Lambert J, Goossens A. Airborne and systemic dermatitis, mimicking atopic dermatitis, caused by methylisothiazolinone in a young child. Contact Dermatitis 2013;68:250-251

76   McFadden JP, Mann J, White JML, Banerjee P, White IR. Outbreak of methylisothiazolinone allergy targeting those aged ≥40 years. Contact Dermatitis 2013;69:53-55

77   Bregnbak D, Johansen JD. Airborne sensitization to isothiazolinones observed in a 3-month-old boy. Contact Dermatitis 2013;69:55-56

78   Bregnbak D, Lundov MD, Zachariae C, Menné T, Johansen JD. Five cases of severe chronic dermatitis caused by isothiazolinones. Contact Dermatitis 2013;69:57-59

79   Urwin R, Wilkinson M. Methylchloroisothiazolinone and methylisothiazolinone contact allergy: a new 'epidemic'. Contact Dermatitis 2013;68:253-255

80   Pontén A, Bruze M, Engfeldt M, Hauksson I, Isaksson M. Concomitant contact allergies to formaldehyde, methylchloroisothiazolinone/methylisothiazolinone, methylisothiazolinone, and fragrance mixes I and II. Contact Dermatitis 2016;75:285-289

81   Uter W, Uter M, Steen-Schuberth B, Schnuch A. Allergic contact dermatitis caused by methylisothiazolinone from a 'waist reduction belt'. Contact Dermatitis 2012;66:347-348

82   Lundov MD, Bossi R, Kolarik B, Gunnarson L, Johansen JD. Methylisothiazolinone – direct and indirect exposure from paint. Contact Dermatitis 2012;66(suppl.2):30-31

83   Lee A, Boyapati A, Tam M, Tate B, Palmer A, Nixon R. Allergic contact dermatitis to methylisothiazolinone in Australia. Contact Dermatitis 2012;66(suppl.2):57-58

84   Patel AN, Wootton CL, English JS. Methylisothiazolinone allergy in the paediatric population: the epidemic begins? Br J Dermatol 2014;170:1200-1201

85   Horev L, Isaksson M, Engfeldt M, Persson L, Ingber A, Bruze M. Preservatives in cosmetics in the Israeli market conform well to the EU legislation. J Eur Acad Dermatol Venereol 2015;29:761-766

86   Lundov MD, Zachariae C, Menné T, Johansen JD. Airborne exposure to preservative methylisothiazolinone causes severe allergic reactions. BMJ 2012;345:e8221

87   Mose AP, Lundov MD, Zachariae C, Menné T, Veien NK, Laurberg G, et al. Occupational contact dermatitis in painters - an analysis of patch test data from the Danish Contact Dermatitis Group. Contact Dermatitis 2012;67:293-297

88   Isaksson M, Hauksson I, Hindsén M, Pontén A, Svedman C, Bruze M. Methylisothiazolinone contact allergy is rising to alarming heights also in southern Sweden. Acta Derm Venereol 2015;95:31-34

89   Bruze M, Dahlquist I, Fregert S, Gruvberger B, Persson K. Contact allergy to the active ingredients of Kathon®CG. Contact Dermatitis 1987;16:183-188

90   De Groot AC, Herxheimer A. Isothiazolinone preservative: cause of a continuing epidemic of cosmetic dermatitis. The Lancet 1989;i:314-316

91   Mahler V, Geier J, Schnuch A. Current trends in patch testing – new data from the German Contact Dermatitis Research Group (DKG) and the Information Network of Departments of Dermatology (IVDK). J Dtsch Dermatol Ges 2014;12:583-592

92 Yazar K, Lundov MD, Faurschou A, Matura M, Boman A, Johansen JD, et al. Methylisothiazolinone in rinse-off products causes allergic contact dermatitis: a repeated open-application study. Br J Dermatol 2015;173:115-122

93 Boyapati A, Tam M, Tate B, Lee A, Palmer A, Nixon R. Allergic contact dermatitis to methylisothiazolinone: exposure from baby wipes causing hand dermatitis. Australas J Dermatol 2013;54:264-267

94 Macias VC, Fernandes S, Amaro C, Santos R, Cardoso J. Sensitization to methylisothiazolinone in a group of methylchloroisothiazolinone/methylisothiazolinone allergic patients. Cutan Ocul Toxicol 2013;32:99 101

95 Schwensen JF, Bregnbak D, Johansen JD. Recent trends in epidemiology, sensitization and legal requirements of selected relevant contact allergens. Expert Rev Clin Immunol 2016;12:289-300

96 Schwensen JF, Uter W, Bruze M, Svedman C, Goossens A, Wilkinson M, et al. The methylisothiazolinone epidemic: a pan-European prospective study. Contact Dermatitis 2016;75(Suppl.1):68-69

97 Lundov MD, Kolarik B, Bossi R, Gunnarsen L, Johansen JD. Emission of isothiazolinones from water-based paints. Environ Sci Technol 2014;48:6989-6994

98 Gardner KH, Davis MD, Richardson DM, Pittelkow MR. The hazards of moist toilet paper: allergy to the preservative methylchloroisothiazolinone/ methylisothiazolinone. Arch Dermatol 2010;146:886-890

99 Castanedo-Tardana M, Zug K. Methylisothiazolinone. Dermatitis 2013;24:2-6

100 Chang MW, Nakrani R. Six children with allergic contact dermatitis to methylisothiazolinone in wet wipes (baby wipes). Pediatrics 2014;133:e434-e438

101 Yu SH, Sood A, Taylor JS. Patch testing for methylisothiazolinone and methylchloroisothiazolinone-methylisothiazolinone contact allergy. JAMA Dermatol 2016;152:67-72

102 Aerts O, Goossens A, Giordano-Labadie F. Contact allergy caused by methylisothiazolinone: the Belgian-French experience. Eur J Dermatol 2015;25:228-233

103 Vandevenne A, Goossens A, Verreycken E, et al. Dermite de contacto alérgica ao metilcloro- e etilisotiazolinona numa cama de água? Allergic contact dermatitis from methylchloro- and methylisothiazolinone from a waterbed? J Port Soc Derm Venereol 2012;70:223-225 (in Portuguese) (article not read)

104 Horst N, Lambert J, Aerts O. Aërogeen contacteczeem door methylisothiazolinone. Ned Tijdschr Dermatol Venereol 2013;23:329-331 (in Dutch)

105 Latheef F, Wilkinson SM. Methylisothiazolinone outbreak in the European Union. Curr Opin Allergy Clin Immunol 2015;15:461-466

106 Wright AM, Cahill JL. Airborne exposure to methylisothiazolinone in paint causing allergic contact dermatitis: An Australian perspective. Australas J Dermatol 2016;57:294-295

107 Cahill JL, Toholka RW, Nixon RL. Methylisothiazolinone in baby wipes: a rising star among causes of contact dermatitis. Med J Aust 2014;200:208

108 Hamann CR, Brankov N, Hamann D, Hamann C. Chronic areolar dermatitis due to methylisothiazolinone-containing bodywash. Clin Exp Dermatol 2016 Jan;41:114-115

109 Quenan S, Piletta P, Calza AM. Isothiazolinones: sensitizers not to miss in children. Pediatr Dermatol 2015;32:e86-88

110 Gäbelein-Wissing N, Lehmann P, Hofmann SC. Allergic contact eczema to a long-used cosmetic: Methylisothiazolinon, a type IV-allergen. Hautarzt 2015;66:462-464 (Article in German)

111 Schlichte MJ, Katta R. Methylisothiazolinone: an emergent allergen in common pediatric skin care products. Dermatol Res Pract Volume 2014 (2014), Article ID 132564, 4 pages

112 de Unamuno B, Zaragoza Ninet V, Sierra C, de la Cuadra J. Descriptive study of sensitization to methylchloroisothiazolinone and methylisothiazolinone in a skin allergy unit. Actas Dermosifiliogr 2014;105:854-859

113 Palmer MJ, Nixon R. Polysensitisation in a laboratory scientist associated with allergic contact dermatitis from methylisothiazolinone in skin cleansers. Australas J Dermatol 2015;56:56-58

114 Leiva-Salinas M, Frances L, Marin-Cabanas I, Maria Bouret A, Silvestre JF. Methylchloroisothiazolinone/ methylisothiazolinone and methylisothiazolinone allergies can be detected by 200 ppm of methylchloroisothiazolinone/methylisothiazolinone patch test concentration. Dermatitis 2014;25:130-134

115 Puangpet P, Chawarung A, McFadden JP. Methylchloroisothiazolinone/methylisothiazolinone and methylisothiazolinone allergy. Dermatitis 2015;26:99-101

116 Ham K, Posso-De Los Rios CJ, Gooderham M. Methylisothiazolinone testing at 2000 ppm: a prevalent sensitizer for allergic contact dermatitis. Dermatitis 2015;26:166-169

117 Milanesi N, Gola. The utility of patch testing methylisothiazolinone 2000 ppm aqua. Dermatitis 2015;26:242

118 Admani S, Matiz C, Jacob SE. Methylisothiazolinone: a case of perianal dermatitis caused by wet wipes and review of an emerging pediatric allergen. Pediatr Dermatol 2014;31:350-352

119 Murad A, Marren P. Prevalence of methylchloroisothiazolinone and methylisothiazolinone facial dermatitis: a single centre Irish study. JEADV 2016;30:60-62contact allergy in

120 Molin S, Bauer A, Schnuch A, Geier J. Occupational contact allergy in nurses: results from the Information Network of Departments of Dermatology 2003–2012. Contact Dermatitis 2015;72:164-171

121 Isaksson M, Gruvberger B, Bruze M. Can methylisothiazolinone be patch tested in petrolatum? Contact Dermatitis 2014;70:240-242

122 Sasseville D, Nantel-Battista M, Molinari R. Multiple contact allergies to benzophenones. Contact Dermatitis 2011;65:179-180

123 Goossens A. Cosmetic contact allergens. Cosmetics 2016;3. doi: 10.3390/cosmetics3010005

124 SCCS (Scientific Committee on Consumer Safety). Opinion on Methylisothiazolinone (MI) (P94) (sensitisation only), 25 June 2015, SCCS/1557/15, final opinion December 2015. Available at: http://ec.europa.eu/health/scientific_committees/consumer_safety/docs/sccs_o_178.pdf

125 SCCS (Scientific Committee on Consumer Safety). Opinion on Methylisothiazolinone (P94) – Submission II, (sensitization only), 12 December 2013, SCCS/1521/13, revision of 27 March 2014. Available at: http://ec.europa.eu/health/scientific_committees/consumer_safety/docs/sccs_o_145.pdf

126 Osinka K, Karczmarz A, Krauze A, Feleszko W. Contact allergens in cosmetics used in atopic dermatitis: analysis of product composition. Contact Dermatitis 2016;75:241-243

127 Flyvholm M A. Preservatives in registered chemical products. Contact Dermatitis 2005; 53:27-32

128 Zhao J, Li LF. Contact sensitization to cosmetic series of allergens in a general population in Beijing. J Cosmet Dermatol 2014;13:68-71

129 Urwin R, Wilkinson M, Latheef F. Cross-reactivity of isothiazolinones: a clinical perspective. Contact Dermatitis 2016;75(Suppl.1):68-69

130 Zaragoza-Ninet V, Blasco Encinas R, Vilata-Corell JJ, Pérez-Ferriols A, Sierra-Talamantes C, Esteve-Martínez A, de la Cuadra-Oyanguren J. Allergic contact dermatitis due to cosmetics: A clinical and epidemiological study in a tertiary hospital. Actas Dermosifiliogr 2016;107:329-336

131 DeKoven JG, Warshaw EM, Belsito DV, Sasseville D, Maibach HI, Taylor JS, et al. North American Contact Dermatitis Group Patch Test Results: 2013-2014. Dermatitis 2017;28:33-46

132 Wittenberg JB, Canas BJ, Zhou W, Wang PG, Rua D, Krynitsky AJ. Determination of methylisothiazolinone and methylchloroisothiazolinone in cosmetic products by ultra high performance liquid chromatography with tandem mass spectrometry. J Sep Sci 2015;38:2983-2988

133 Bunyavaree M, Kasemsarn P, Boonchai W. Cosmetic preservative labelling on the Thai market. Contact Dermatitis 2016;74:217-221

134 Steinberg DC. Preservatives for Cosmetics, Carol Stream, IL: Allured Books, 2012

135 Yim E, Baquerizo Nole KL, Tosti A. Contact dermatitis caused by preservatives. Dermatitis 2014;25:215-231

136 Engfeldt M, Bråred-Christensson J, Isaksson M, Matura M, Ryberg K, Stenberg B, Svedman C, Bruze M. Swedish experiences from patch testing methylisothiazolinone separately. Acta Derm Venereol 2015;95:717-719

137 Garcia-Hidalgo E, Sottas V, von Goetz N, Hauri U, Bogdal C, Hungerbühler K. Occurrence and concentrations of isothiazolinones in detergents and cosmetics in Switzerland. Contact Dermatitis 2017;76:96-106

138 Editorial. Methylisothiazolinone: Quo vadis? Contact Dermatitis 2016;75:263-264

139 Madsen J, Andersen K, Nielsen D, Hvid L, El-Houri RB, Christensen LP. Undisclosed presence of methylisothiazolinone in "100% natural" Konjac® sponge. Contact Dermatitis 2016;75:308-309

140 El-Houri R, Christensen L. Persson C, et al. Methylisothiazolinone in a designer spectacle frame - a surprising finding. Contact Dermatitis 2016;75:310-312

141 Bennike N, Johansen J, Zachariae C. Please, label the label; a case report of occupational allergic contact dermatitis caused by methylisothiazolinone in adhesive labels. Contact Dermatitis 2016;75:314-315

142 Dahlin J, Hindsén M, Persson C, Isaksson M. What lash stylists and dermatologists should know! Contact Dermatitis 2016;75:317-319

143 Gallo R, Signori A, Gervasio S, Parodi A. Methylisothiazolinone contact allergy – are rinse-off cosmetics and household products relevant sources of exposure? Contact Dermatitis 2016;75:319-321

144 Herry J, Esquirol Y. Giordano-Labadie F. An intriguing occupational atypical dermatitis with respiratory symptoms. Contact Dermatitis 2016;75:322-323

145 Schwensen J, Bregnbak D, Johansen J. Recent trends in epidemiology, sensitization and legal requirements of selected relevant contact allergens. Expert Rev Clin Immunol 2015;30:1-12

146 Trokoudes D, Fityan A, McFadden J, Sarkany R, White I, White J, Banerjee P. Photoinduced and photoaggra-vated allergic contact dermatitis due to methylisothiazolinone. Contact Dermatitis 2016;75:(Suppl.1):41

147 Vandevenne A, Vanden Broecke K, Goossens A. Allergic contact dermatitis from Methylisothiazolinone in a leather-care product. Contact Dermatitis 2014;70(Suppl.1):44

148 Yu J, Treat J, Chaney K, Brod B. Potential allergens in disposable diaper wipes, topical diaper preparations, and disposable diapers: under-recognized etiology of pediatric perineal dermatitis. Dermatitis 2016;27:110-118

149 Raymond J, Konya J, Bakis-Petsoglou S. Lichenoid contact dermatitis secondary to methylisothiazolinone (MI). JAAD Case Rep 2016;2:380-383

150 Venables ZC, Bourke JF, Buckley DA, Campbell F, Chowdhury MM, Abdul-Ghaffar S, et al. Has the epidemic of allergic contact dermatitis due to methylisothiazolinone reached its peak? Br J Dermatol 2017;177:276-278

151 Khanna S, Reeder M. Vesicular hand dermatitis in a child: allergy to methylisothiazolinone. Pediatr Dermatol 2016;33:e272-273

152 Isaksson M, Gruvberger B, Bruze M. Patch testing with isothiazolinones in patients hypersensitive to methylchloroisothiazolinone/methylisothiazolinone (In manuscript). Data cited in ref. 69. The article in manuscript to which is referred here is ref. 57, but in that publication, no mention of patch test sensitization is made (57)

153 Castanedo-Tardan MP, Engfeldt M, Zug KA, Bruze M. Methylchloroisothiazolinone/methylisothiazolinone (MCI/MI) and methylisothiazolinone (MI) in common personal care products in the American market. Dermatitis 2016;27(6):e11

154 Uter W, Gefeller O, John SM, Schnuch A, Geier J. Contact allergy to ingredients of hair cosmetics – a comparison of female hairdressers and clients based on IVDK 2007–2012 data. Contact Dermatitis 2014;71:13-20

155 Giménez-Arnau AM, Deza G, Bauer A, Johnston GA, Mahler V, Schuttelaar ML, et al. Contact allergy to preservatives: ESSCA* results with the baseline series, 2009-2012. J Eur Acad Dermatol Venereol 2017;31:664-671

156 Lubbes S, Rustemeyer T, Sillevis Smitt JH, Schuttelaar ML, Middelkamp-Hup MA. Contact sensitization in Dutch children and adolescents with and without atopic dermatitis - a retrospective analysis. Contact Dermatitis 2017;76:151-159

157 Erfurt-Berge C, Geier J, Mahler V. The current spectrum of contact sensitization in patients with chronic leg ulcers or stasis dermatitis - new data from the Information Network of Departments of Dermatology (IVDK). Contact Dermatitis 2017;77:151-158

158 Beene KM, Scheman A, Severson D, Reeder MJ. Prevalence of preservatives across all product types in the Contact Allergen Management Program. Dermatitis 2017;28:81-87

159 Yu J, Treat J, Chaney K, Brod B. Potential allergens in disposable diaper wipes, topical diaper preparations, and disposable diapers: under-recognized etiology of pediatric perineal dermatitis. Dermatitis 2016;27:110-118

160 Warshaw EM, Aschenbeck KA, Zug KA, Belsito DV, Zirwas MJ, Fowler JF Jr, Taylor JS, et al. Wet wipe allergens: Retrospective analysis from the North American Contact Dermatitis Group 2011-2014. Dermatitis 2017;28:64-69

161 Amsler E, Aerts O, Raison-Peyron N, Debons M, Milpied B, Giordano-Labadie F, et al. and on behalf of the Dermatology Allergy Group (DAG) of the French Society of Dermatology. Airborne allergic contact dermatitis caused by isothiazolinones in water-based paints: a retrospective study of 44 cases. Contact Dermatitis 2017;77:163-170

162 Andersson AM, Opstrup MS, Zachariae C, Friis UF, Thyssen JP, Johansen JD. The importance of a complete declaration of isothiazolinones in products beyond cosmetics. Contact Dermatitis 2017;77:171-172

163 Silva CA, El-Houri RB, Christensen LP, Andersen F. Contact allergy caused by methylisothiazolinone in shoe glue. Contact Dermatitis 2017;77:175-176

164 Goodier MC, Ljungberg L, Persson C, Engfeldt M, Bruze M, Warshaw EM. Allergic contact dermatitis from methylisothiazolinone in residential wall paint. Dermatitis 2017;28:284-287

165 Aalto-Korte K, Suuronen K. Patterns of concomitant allergic reactions in patients suggest cross-sensitization between octylisothiazolinone and methylisothiazolinone. Contact Dermatitis 2017 Jul 28. doi: 10.1111/cod.12855. [Epub ahead of print]

166 Lynch MD, White JM, McFadden JP, Wang Y, White IR, Banerjee P. A dynamic landscape of allergen associations in delayed-type cutaneous hypersensitivity. Br J Dermatol 2017;176:184-196

167 Goldenberg A, Mousdicas N, Silverberg N, Powell D, Pelletier JL, Silverberg JI, et al. Pediatric Contact Dermatitis Registry inaugural case data. Dermatitis 2016;27:293-302

168 Wuyts L, van Hoof T, Lambert J, Aerts O. Allergic contact dermatitis caused by aftershave creams containing *Glycyrrhiza inflata*. Contact Dermatitis 2017;77:49-51

169 Uter W, Amario-Hita JC, Balato A, Ballmer-Weber B, Bauer A, Belloni Fortina A, et al. European Surveillance System on Contact Allergies (ESSCA): results with the European baseline series, 2013/14. J Eur Acad Dermatol Venereol. 2017 Jun 19. doi: 10.1111/jdv.14423. [Epub ahead of print]

170 Schwensen JF, Uter W, Bruze M, Svedman C, Goossens A, Wilkinson M, et al.; European Environmental Contact Dermatitis Research Group. The epidemic of methylisothiazolinone: a European prospective study. Contact Dermatitis 2017;76:272-279

171 Du-Thanh A, Lalande M, Raison-Peyron N, Dereure O. Atypical and severe airborne isothiazolinone contact dermatitis mimicking Kaposi-Juliusberg syndrome. Contact Dermatitis 2017;76:297-298

172 Craig S, Urwin R, Latheef F, Wilkinson M. Patch test clinic experience of potential cross-reactivity of isothiazolinones. Contact Dermatitis 2017;76:299-300

173 Urwin R, Craig S, Latheef F, Wilkinson M. Methylisothiazolinone: the epidemic is declining - but not gone. Contact Dermatitis 2017;76:301-302

174 Trokoudes D, Banerjee P, Fityan A, Sarkany R, White IR, White JM, McFadden JP. Photoaggravated contact dermatitis caused by methylisothiazolinone. Contact Dermatitis 2017;76:303-304

175 Cotton CH, Duah CG, Matiz C. Allergic contact dermatitis due to methylisothiazolinone in a young girl's laundry detergent. Pediatr Dermatol 2017;34:486-487

176 Zirwas MJ, Hamann D, Warshaw EM, Maibach HI, Taylor JS, Sasseville D, et al. Epidemic of isothiazolinone allergy in North America: prevalence data from the North American Contact Dermatitis Group, 2013-2014. Dermatitis 2017;28:204-209

177 Isaksson M, Ale I, Andersen KE, Elsner P, Goh CL, Goossens A, et al. Multicenter patch testing with methylisothiazolinone and methylchloroisothiazolinone/methylisothiazolinone within the International Contact Dermatitis Research Group. Dermatitis 2017;28:210-214

178 Aschenbeck KA, Warshaw EM. Allergenic ingredients in facial wet wipes. Dermatitis 2017 Mar 23. doi: 10.1097/DER.0000000000000268. [Epub ahead of print]

179 Aschenbeck KA, Warshaw EM. Allergenic ingredients in personal hygiene wet wipes. Dermatitis 2017 Mar 23. doi: 10.1097/DER.0000000000000275. [Epub ahead of print]

180 Aerts O, Goossens A, Lambert J, Lepoittevin JP. Contact allergy caused by isothiazolinone derivatives: an overview of non-cosmetic and unusual cosmetic sources. Eur J Dermatol 2017;27:115-122

181 Schwensen JF, Friis UF, Menné T, Flyvholm MA, Johansen JD. Contact allergy to preservatives in patients with occupational contact dermatitis and exposure analysis of preservatives in registered chemical products for occupational use. Int Arch Occup Environ Health 2017;90:319-333.

182 Raison-Peyron N, Amsler E, Pecquet C, Du-Thanh A, Naessens T, Apers S, Aerts O. Severe allergic contact dermatitis caused by octylisothiazolinone in a leather sofa: two new cases. Contact Dermatitis 2017;77:176-178

2.300   METHYL METHACRYLATE

IDENTIFICATION

Description/definition	: Methyl methacrylate is the organic compound that conforms to the formula shown below
Chemical class(es)	: Esters
Chemical/IUPAC name	: Methyl 2-methylprop-2-enoate; 2-propenoic acid, 2-methyl, methyl ester
CAS registry number (s)	: 80-62-6
EC number(s)	: 201-297-1
CIR review(s)	: Report terminated, June 2003 (access: www.cir-safety.org/ingredients)
Function(s) in cosmetics	: EU: anticaking; opacifying. USA: anticaking agents; artificial nail builders; dispersing agents – nonsurfactant; opacifying agents
Patch testing	: 2.0% pet. (Chemotechnique, SmartPracticeEurope, SmartPracticeCanada)
Molecular formula	: $C_5H_8O_2$

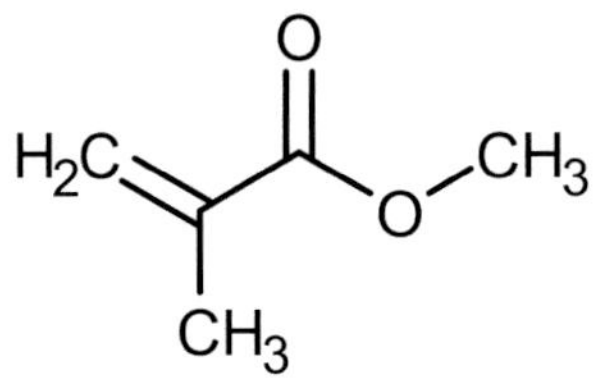

GENERAL

Discussion of contact allergy to (meth)acrylates *from non-cosmetic sources* is considered to fall outside the scope of this book. Therefore, only contact allergy from their presence in cosmetics is presented, which virtually always is from artificial nails. There are many reports of contact allergy to artificial nails, but the specific sensitizers have rarely been identified and – consequently - such publications are not presented in this and other acrylate and methacrylate monographs. Discussion is limited to publications in which the culprit (meth)acrylates have been identified, e.g., from information found in Material Data Safety Sheets, data obtained from the manufacturer or from chemical analyses.

Patients often react to many (meth)acrylates on patch testing. Primary sensitization to methacrylates may result in both methacrylate and acrylate cross-sensitization. Conversely, patients sensitized to acrylates are unlikely to show cross-sensitization to methacrylates (19).

General aspects of acrylates and methacrylates are presented in Chapter 2.219 HEMA (hydroxyethyl methacrylate). A discussion of general aspects of artificial nails, contact allergy to these products, the clinical picture of allergic contact dermatitis and other side effects of sculptured nails can also be found there. A very useful review of contact sensitization to allergens in nail cosmetics, with emphasis on acrylic manicures, was published in 2017 (37).

CONTACT ALLERGY

Contact allergy to methyl methacrylate monomer from its use in cold-cured artificial nails (nail extenders) has been reported for the first time in 1956 (5,17,18). Numerous reports of sensitization to methyl methacrylate eventually led, in 1974, to a Food and Drug Administration ban of this chemical for use in artificial nails (20).

Patch testing in groups of patients

Results of routine patch testing (testing in consecutive patients suspected of contact dermatitis) back to 1994 are shown in table 2.300.1. Results of testing in groups of *selected* patients (e.g., hairdressers and cosmetologists, patients with eyelid dermatitis, patients with a history of acrylate exposure) back to 1994 are shown in table 2.300.2 (example studies, not a full literature review).

Patch testing in consecutive patients suspected of contact dermatitis: routine testing

Methyl methacrylate has been included in the screening tray of the North American Contact Dermatitis Group (NACDG) since 1992. Hence, there are many data on methyl methacrylate contact allergy available, notably from the USA + Canada, where the NACDG publishes their patch test results biannually. In the NACDG studies, frequencies of sensitization between 1992 and 2014 have been fairly constant and have ranged from 0.8% to 1.6%. From other USA centers, similar sensitization rates were reported in the range of 0.9-1.5% (2,25,27). In the first NACDG study, 2/3 of all positive patch test reactions were considered to be of present relevance (24). Thereafter, between 31% and 53% had 'definite + probable' relevance scores.

Table 2.300.1 Patch testing in groups of patients: Routine testing

Years and Country	Test conc. & vehicle	Number of patients tested	positive (%)		Selection of patients (S); Relevance (R); Comments (C)	Ref.
2013-14 USA, Canada	2% pet.	4859	64	(1.3%)	R: definite + probable relevance: 36%	30
2011-12 USA, Canada	2% pet.	4236	37	(0.9%)	R: definite + probable relevance: 40%	13
2009-10 USA, Canada	2% pet.	4305	34	(0.8%)	R: definite + probable relevance: 44%	14
2006-2010 USA	2% pet.	3086		(1.5%)	R: 42%	27
2007-8 USA, Canada	2% pet.	5077		(1.2%)	R: definite + probable relevance: 53%	9
2005-2007 Sweden	2% pet.	1609	2	(0.1%)	R: not specified	34
2005-6 USA, Canada	2% pet.	4427		(1.0%)	R: definite + probable relevance: 44%	8
2000-2005 USA	2% pet.	3848		(1.4%)	R: 54%	2
2003-4 USA, Canada	2% pet.	5143	81	(1.6%)	R: not stated	10
2001-2 USA, Canada	2% pet.	4900		(1.4%)	R: definite + probable relevance: 31%	21
1998–2000 USA	2% pet.	1321		(0.9%)	R: not stated	25
1996-1998 USA	2% pet.	4099		(1.6%)	R: definite + probable + possible relevance: 67%	22
1994-1996 USA	2% pet.	3080		(1.2%)	R: definite + probable relevance: 53%	23
1992-1994 USA	2% pet.	3472		(1.1%)	R: present relevance: 67%	24

Patch testing in groups of selected patients

Data on patch testing with methyl methacrylate in groups of selected patients back to 1994 are summarized in table 2.300.2. Somewhat elevated frequencies of sensitization were observed in 2 studies only, one small study with patients with eyelid dermatitis (11) and an Australian study in which the mode of selecting the patients was not mentioned (29). Relevance, if mentioned, ranged from 60% to 100%. In one non-NACDG USA study, all 16 positive patch test reactions observed between 2000 and 2007were considered to be relevant; however, relevance figures here included 'questionable' and 'past' relevance (1).

Table 2.300.2 Patch testing in groups of patients: Selected patient groups [a]

Years and Country	Test conc. & vehicle	Number of patients tested	positive (%)		Selection of patients (S); Relevance (R); Comments (C)	Ref.
2006-2010 USA	2% pet.	100	4	(4%)	S: patients with eyelid dermatitis; R: not stated	11
2001-2010 Australia	2% pet.	494	201	(4.0%)	S: not stated; R: 60%	29
1994-2010 USA, Canada	2% pet.	432	?	(?)	S: hairdressers/cosmetologists; R: in the group of 187 patients who had at least one relevant occupationally related reaction, 9 (4.8%) reacted to methyl methacrylate	32
2000-2007 USA	2% pet.	943	16	(1.7%)	S: patients tested with a supplemental cosmetic screening series; R: 100%; C: weak study: a. high rate of macular erythema and weak reactions; b. relevance figures included 'questionable' and 'past' relevance	1
2003-2004 USA	2% pet.	268	3	(1.1%)	S: patients with pure eyelid dermatitis; R: this was the number of relevant reactions	28
1998-04 USA, Canada	2% pet.	1253	11	(0.9%)	S: health care workers; R: only occupation-related (=relevant) reactions were recorded; C: the frequency was significantly higher than the rate of occupation-related reactions in non-health care workers (0.2%); the causative products were dentistry materials	35
1991-1994 Finland	2% pet.	124	8	(6.5%)	S: patients with a history of acrylate exposure; R: not stated	36

[a] examples

Case reports and case series

Case series

Methyl methacrylate was stated to be the (or an) allergen in 3 patients in a group of 603 individuals suffering from cosmetic dermatitis, seen in the period 2010-2015 in Leuven, Belgium (26). In the period 1996-2013, in a tertiary referral center in Valencia, Spain, 5419 patients were patch tested. Of these, 628 individuals had allergic contact dermatitis to cosmetics. Methyl methacrylate was the responsible allergen in three cases (31). Methyl methacrylate was responsible for 4 out of 959 cases of non-fragrance cosmetic allergy where the causal allergen was identified, Belgium, 2000-2010 (3). In 1582 female patients with (presumed) cosmetic allergy, 65 reactions (4.1%) were caused by methyl methacrylate in a study of the NACDG, 2001-2004 (4). Four patients had allergic contact dermatitis, paronychia and nail changes from contact allergy to methyl methacrylate used in cold-cured acrylic nails (5).

Case reports
A cosmetician teaching other cosmeticians how to make artificial nails developed occupational contact dermatitis of the hands and face from contact allergy to methyl methacrylate in monomer liquid for sculptured nails. Gas chromatography – mass spectrometry (GC-MS) showed the product to contain 0.5% methyl methacrylate (15). An eyelash extension technician developed occupational allergic contact dermatitis of the hands in an eyelash from methyl methacrylate in the glue (*sensu stricto* not a cosmetic product) (12).

A dentist became sensitized to methyl methacrylate monomer from preparing artificial nails from methyl methacrylate monomer and polymer powder; when she subsequently worked in het practice, dermatitis of the hands relapsed from contact with dental acrylates and she had to wear gloves to prevent allergic reactions to acrylates during work (7). One patient had occupational ACD from (probably) methyl methacrylate while applying artificial nails to her customers (17). One patient was apparently sensitized to methyl methacrylate *polymer* in artificial nail material; patch testing may have been unreliable (18).

Patch test sensitization
In early days, methyl methacrylate was tested in London, UK, at 100%, which caused many cases of patch test sensitization (33).

Presence in cosmetic products and chemical analyses
In the USA, in April 2017, methyl methacrylate was present in an unknown number of 56,714 cosmetic products of which the composition is known in FDA's Voluntary Cosmetic Registration Program (VCRP) (accidentally no data requested from FDA). In August 2017, methyl methacrylate was present in 17 of 70,693 cosmetic products of which the composition is known in EWG's Skin Deep Cosmetics Database, USA (http://www.ewg.org/skindeep/).

Miscellaneous side effects
One patient had permanent loss of the fingernails and persistent paresthesia 6 years after an allergic reaction to methyl methacrylate in cold-cured artificial nails (16).

LITERATURE
1   Wetter DA, Yiannias JA, Prakash AV, Davis MD, Farmer SA, el-Azhary RA, et al. Results of patch testing to personal care product allergens in a standard series and a supplemental cosmetic series: an analysis of 945 patients from the Mayo Clinic Contact Dermatitis Group, 2000-2007. J Am Acad Dermatol 2010;63:789-798
2   Davis MD, Scalf LA, Yiannias JA, Cheng JF, El-Azhary RA, Rohlinger AL, et al. Changing trends and allergens in the patch test standard series. Arch Dermatol 2008;144:67-72
3   Travassos AR, Claes L, Boey L, Drieghe J, Goossens A. Non-fragrance allergens in specific cosmetic products. Contact Dermatitis 2011;65:276-285
4   Warshaw EM, Buchholz HJ, Belsito DV, Maibach HI, Fowler JF Jr, Rietschel RL, et al. Allergic patch test reactions associated with cosmetics: Retrospective analysis of cross-sectional data from the North American Contact Dermatitis Group, 2001-2004. J Am Acad Dermatol 2009;60:23-38
5   Fisher AA, Franks A, Glick H. Allergic sensitization of the skin and nails to acrylic plastic nails. J Allergy 1957;28:84-88
6   Sasseville D. Acrylates in contact dermatitis. Dermatitis 2012;23:6-16
7   Macedo NA, Carmona C, Piñeyro I. Contact dermatitis from acrylic nails. Contact Dermatitis 1995;32:362
8   Zug KA, Warshaw EM, Fowler JF Jr, Maibach HI, Belsito DL, Pratt MD, et al. Patch-test results of the North American Contact Dermatitis Group 2005-2006. Dermatitis 2009;20:149-160
9   Fransway AF, Zug KA, Belsito DV, Deleo VA, Fowler JF Jr, Maibach HI, et al. North American Contact Dermatitis Group patch test results for 2007-2008. Dermatitis 2013;24:10-21
10 Warshaw EM, Belsito DV, DeLeo VA, Fowler JF Jr, Maibach HI, Marks JG, et al. North American Contact Dermatitis Group patch-test results, 2003-2004 study period. Dermatitis 2008;19:129-136
11 Wenk KS, Ehrlich AE. Fragrance series testing in eyelid dermatitis. Dermatitis 2012;23:22-26
12 Pesonen M, Kuuliala O, Henriks-Eckerman M-L, Aalto-Korte K. Occupational allergic contact dermatitis caused by eyelash extension glues. Contact Dermatitis 2012;67:307-308
13 Warshaw EM, Maibach HI, Taylor JS, Sasseville D, DeKoven JG, Zirwas MJ, et al. North American Contact Dermatitis Group patch test results: 2011-2012. Dermatitis 2015;26:49-59
14 Warshaw EM, Belsito DV, Taylor JS, Sasseville D, DeKoven JG, Zirwas MJ, et al. North American Contact Dermatitis Group patch test results: 2009 to 2010. Dermatitis 2013;24:50-59
15 Kanerva L, Lauerma A, Estlander T, Alanko K, Henriks-Eckerman ML, Jolanki R. Occupational allergic contact dermatitis caused by photobonded sculptured nails and a review of (meth)acrylates in nail cosmetics. Am J Cont Derm 1996;7:109-115

16 Fisher AA. Permanent loss of fingernails from sensitization and reaction to acrylic in a preparation designed to make artificial nails. J Dermatol Surg Oncol 1980;6:70 -71

17 Canizares O. Contact dermatitis due to the acrylic materials used in artificial nails. Arch Dermatol 1956;74:141-143

18 Lane CW, Kost LB. Sensitivity to artificial nails. Arch Dermatol 1956;74:671-672

19 Aalto-Korte K, Henriks-Eckerman M-L, Kuuliala O, Jolanki R. Occupational methacrylate and acrylate allergy – cross-reactions and possible screening allergens. Contact Dermatitis 2010;63:301-312

20 Food and Drug Administration seizure actions. FDA Consumer 1974;8:374

21 Pratt MD, Belsito DV, DeLeo VA, Fowler JF Jr, Fransway AF, Maibach HI, et al. North American Contact Dermatitis Group patch-test results, 2001–2002 study period. Dermatitis 2004;15:176-183

22 Marks JG Jr, Belsito DV, DeLeo VA, Fowler JF Jr, Fransway AF, Maibach HI, et al. North American Contact Dermatitis Group patch test results, 1996–1998. Arch Dermatol 2000;136:272-273

23 Marks JG Jr, Belsito DV, DeLeo VA, Fowler JF Jr, Fransway AF, Maibach HI,et al. North American Contact Dermatitis Group patch test results for the detection of delayed-type hypersensitivity to topical allergens. J Am Acad Dermatol 1998;38:911-918

24 Marks JG, Belsito DV, DeLeo VA, Fowler JF, Fransway AF, Maibach HI,et al. North American Contact Dermatitis Group standard tray patch test results 1992 through 1994. Am J Contact Dermatitis 1995;6:160-165

25 Wetter DA, Davis MDP, Yiannias JA, Cheng JF, Connolly SM, el-Azhary RA, et al. Patch test results from the Mayo Contact Dermatitis Group, 1998–2000. J Am Acad Dermatol 2005;53:416-421

26 Goossens A. Cosmetic contact allergens. Cosmetics 2016, 3, 5; doi:10.3390/cosmetics3010005

27 Wentworth AB, Yiannias JA, Keeling JH, Hall MR, Camilleri MJ, Drage LA, et al. Trends in patch-test results and allergen changes in the standard series: a Mayo Clinic 5-year retrospective review (January 1, 2006, to December 31, 2010). J Am Acad Dermatol 2014;70:269-275

28 Rietschel RL, Warshaw EM, Sasseville D, Fowler JF Jr, DeLeo VA. Belsito DV, et al. Common contact allergens associated with eyelid dermatitis: data from the North American Contact Dermatitis Group 2003-2004 study period. Dermatitis 2007;18:78-81

29 Toholka R, Wang Y-S, Tate B, Tam M, Cahill J, Palmer A, Nixon R. The first Australian Baseline Series: Recommendations for patch testing in suspected contact dermatitis. Australas J Dermatol 2015;56:107-115

30 DeKoven JG, Warshaw EM, Belsito DV, Sasseville D, Maibach HI, Taylor JS, et al. North American Contact Dermatitis Group Patch Test Results: 2013-2014. Dermatitis. 2016 Oct 21. [Epub ahead of print]

31 Zaragoza-Ninet V, Blasco Encinas R, Vilata-Corell JJ, Pérez-Ferriols A, Sierra-Talamantes C, Esteve-Martínez A, de la Cuadra-Oyanguren J. Allergic contact dermatitis due to cosmetics: A clinical and epidemiological study in a tertiary hospital. Actas Dermosifiliogr 2016;107:329-336

32 Warshaw EM, Wang MZ, Mathias CGT, Maibach HI, Belsito DV, Zug KA, et al. Occupational contact dermatitis in hairdressers/cosmetologists; retrospective analysis of North American Contact Dermatitis Group data, 1994 to 2010. Dermatitis 2012;23:258-268

33 Calnan CD. Studies in contact dermatitis XX. Active sensitization. Transactions of the St John's Hospital Dermatological Society 1967;53:128-134

34 Goon AT, Bruze M, Zimerson E, Goh CL, Soo-Quee Koh D, Isaksson M. Screening for acrylate/methacrylate allergy in the baseline series: our experience in Sweden and Singapore. Contact Dermatitis 2008;59:307-313

35 Warshaw EM, Schram SE, Maibach HI, Belsito DV, Marks JG Jr, Fowler JF Jr, et al. Occupation-related contact dermatitis in North American health care workers referred for patch testing: cross-sectional data, 1998 to 2004. Dermatitis 2008;19:261-274

36 Kanerva L, Estlander T, Jolanki R, Tarvainen KL. Statistics on allergic patch test reactions caused by acrylate compounds, including data on ethyl methacrylate. Am J Cont Derm 1995;6:75-77

37 Chou M, Dhingra N, Strugar TL. Contact sensitization to allergens in nail cosmetics. Dermatitis 2017;28:231-240

2.301 METHYL NICOTINATE

IDENTIFICATION

Description/definition : Methyl nicotinate is an ester of methyl alcohol and nicotinic acid, which conforms to the formula shown below
Chemical class(es) : Esters; heterocyclic compounds
Chemical/IUPAC name : Methyl pyridine-3-carboxylate
Other names : Nicotinic acid methyl ester
CAS registry number (s) : 93-60-7
EC number(s) : 202-261-8
Merck Index monograph : 7443
Function(s) in cosmetics : EU: soothing; tonic. USA: external analgesics; fragrance ingredients; skin-conditioning agents - miscellaneous
Patch testing : 1% pet. (2)
Molecular formula : $C_7H_7NO_2$

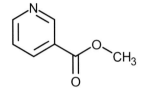

GENERAL

Methyl nicotinate is often used in rubefacients, which are popular topical preparations, often bought without prescription, which by counter-irritation bring comfort in painful lesions of muscles, tendons, and joints and in non-articular rheumatism (7).

CONTACT ALLERGY

Case reports and case series

Methyl nicotinate was stated to be the (or an) allergen in one patient in a group of 603 individuals suffering from cosmetic dermatitis, seen in the period 2010-2015 in Leuven, Belgium (1).

Presence in cosmetic products and chemical analyses

In the USA, in April 2017, methyl nicotinate was present in 32 of 56,714 cosmetic products of which the composition is known in FDA's Voluntary Cosmetic Registration Program (VCRP) (data obtained from FDA, May 2017). In March 2017, methyl nicotinate was present in 7 of 64,431 cosmetic products of which the composition is known in EWG's Skin Deep Cosmetics Database, USA (http://www.ewg.org/skindeep/).

OTHER SIDE EFFECTS

Immediate-type reactions

Methyl nicotinate is a well-known inducer of non-immunological immediate contact reactions (contact urticaria) (3,4,5,6). A young woman twice used a popular proprietary preparation containing methyl nicotinate 1% and capsaicin 0.12% in a cream base. On the first occasion she had rubbed about 2-3 g of the rubefacient on to her back. Ten minutes later she felt a curious burning sensation internally in her abdomen and felt faint but recovered after 10 minutes. About a month later she rubbed a larger quantity, at most 5 gram, on to a painful knee and within five minutes felt nauseated, experienced the internal pain even more unpleasantly, and fainted. When seen some 20 minutes later she was conscious, pale but not shocked, and with a normal pulse and blood pressure. There was intense erythema over the area of application on her knee and lower thigh. Skin patch testing was performed to identify which ingredient might be responsible, and she reacted with erythema to the methyl nicotinate and to the whole preparation, but without any systemic effects, probably as much smaller quantities were used (7).

LITERATURE

1   Goossens A. Cosmetic contact allergens. Cosmetics 2016, 3, 5; doi:10.3390/cosmetics3010005
2   De Groot AC. Patch Testing, 3rd Edition. Wapserveen, The Netherlands: acdegroot publishing, 2008 (ISBN 978-90-813233-1-4)

3   Coverly J, Peters L, Whittle E, Basketter DA. Susceptibility to skin stinging, non-immunologic contact urticaria and acute skin irritation; is there a relationship? Contact Dermatitis 1998;38:90-95

4   Roussaki-Schulze AV, Zafiriou E, Nikoulis D, Klimi E, Rallis E, Zintzaras E. Objective biophysical findings in patients with sensitive skin. Drugs Exp Clin Res 2005;31(Suppl):17-24

5   Larmi E, Lahti A, Hannuksela M. Effects of infra-red and neodymium yttrium aluminium garnet laser irradiation on non-immunologic immediate contact reactions to benzoic acid and methyl nicotinate. Derm Beruf Umwelt 1989;37:210-214

6   Ylipieti S, Lahti A. Effect of the vehicle on non-immunologic immediate contact reactions. Contact Dermatitis 1989;21:105-106

7   Fergusson DA. Systemic symptoms associated with a rubefacient. BMJ 1988;297:1339

2.302   METHYLPARABEN

IDENTIFICATION

Description/definition   : Methylparaben is the ester of methyl alcohol and *p*-hydroxybenzoic acid, which
                              conforms to the formula shown below
Chemical class(es)   . Esters, phenols
Chemical/IUPAC name   : Methyl 4-hydroxybenzoate
Other names   : Methyl parahydroxybenzoate
CAS registry number (s)   : 99-76-3
EC number(s)   : 202-785-7
CIR review(s)   : J Am Coll Toxicol 1984;3:147-209; Int J Toxicol 2008;27(Suppl. 4):1-82 (access:
                              www.cir-safety.org/ingredients)
SCCS opinion(s)   : SCCS/1348/10 (17); SCCP/0874/05 (18)
Merck Index monograph : 7450
Function(s) in cosmetics : EU: preservative. USA: fragrance ingredients; preservatives
EU cosmetic restrictions : Regulated in Annex V/12 of the Regulation (EC) No. 1223/2009
Patch testing   : 3.0% pet. (Chemotechnique; SmartPracticeEurope; SmartPracticeCanada); also present
                              in the paraben mix (see there)
Molecular formula   : $C_8H_8O_3$

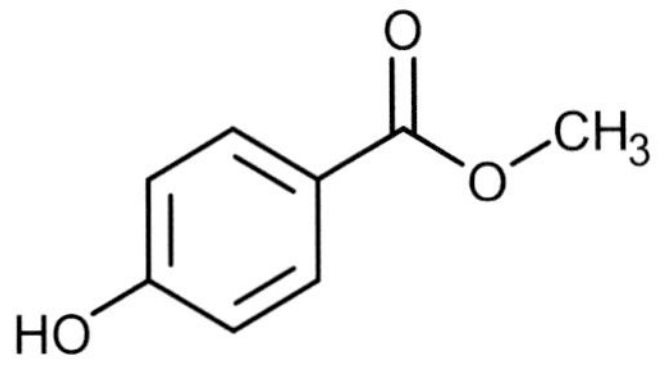

GENERAL

For general information on paraben esters see Chapter 2.333 Paraben mix. The literature on contact allergy to and other information on parabens, in which the ester is not specified ('paraben mix', 'paraben', 'parabens'), is also discussed in that chapter. The literature on contact allergy to methylparaben and other paraben esters from before 1991 has been reviewed in ref. 19. Other, more recent, useful reviews were published in 2005 (parabens) (41), 2004 (42) and 2014 (60) (parabens and other preservatives. A review of the health aspects of methylparaben is provided in ref. 58. The subject of possible endocrine effects of parabens is discussed in the section 'Systemic side effects' of Chapter 2.333 Paraben mix).

CONTACT ALLERGY

Patch testing in groups of patients

Routine testing
In 1985, in The Netherlands, 627 consecutive patients suspected of contact dermatitis were patch tested with methylparaben 5% pet. and 1 patient (0.2%) had a positive reaction. Its relevance was not stated (12).

Testing in groups of selected patients
Between 1971 and 1986, in Denmark, 60 patients previously reacting to the paraben mix (benzyl-, butyl-, ethyl-, methyl- and propylparaben) were tested with all five components at 5% pet. Forty (67%) reacted to one or more of the paraben-esters, most of who reacted to 2 or more. There were 25 reactions (42%) to methylparaben. The relevance of these positive patch test reactions was not mentioned (23). Sixty-three selected patients, with features suggestive of allergic contact dermatitis and histories of prolonged use of numerous topical preparations, or of exacerbation or spread of dermatitis following the use of such preparations, were patch tested in India before 1990 and 5 (8%) reacted to methylparaben 3% pet. The relevance of the positive patch test reactions was not mentioned (54). Also in India, before 1985, 100 patients suspected of ACD from topical medicaments were patch tested with methylparaben and 4 (4%) had a positive reaction; relevance was not mentioned (55).

Case reports and case series
A child, known to be allergic to methyl- and propylparaben, developed vesicular hand dermatitis from a liquid soap containing parabens (7). Four patients had contact allergy to methylparaben present in a moisturizing cream (9).

Another individual had allergic contact dermatitis from methylparaben in a sunscreen (11). Two patients reacted to skin care products from contact allergy to methylparaben used a preservative in these cosmetics (13). A woman had dermatitis of the eyelids from contact allergy to methyl- and propylparaben in a hypoallergenic eye cream (29). One individual suffered from lymphomatoid ACD on the buttocks caused by methylparaben in moist wipes (51).

Contact allergy to methylparaben in non-cosmetic products

Topical pharmaceutical preparations

Three patients reacted to methylparaben in a topical pharmaceutical (2,24,57). In a group of 31 patients allergic to a topical pharmaceutical product, methylparaben was the allergen or one of the allergens in 6 individuals (3). One patient had allergic contact dermatitis from methylparaben in capsicum oleoresin gel (4). A patient with periorbital dermatitis reacted to methylparaben in eye drops (6). One patient had ACD from methylparaben in an antibiotic ointment applied to stasis dermatitis (20). Another individual developed contact dermatitis from allergy to methylparaben and other parabens in multiple topical pharmaceutical preparations (22). (Probably) three patients had ACD from methylparaben (and presumably also from other parabens) in topical pharmaceuticals (28).

Four patients had ACD from topical pharmaceutical preparations. They all reacted to methylparaben and three also to ethyl-, propyl- and butylparaben. It was not mentioned which of the parabens were present in the topical drugs used with the exception of methylparaben, which was present in an antibiotic powder (35). Three patients developed ACD from the application of a corticosteroid cream. They all reacted to the paraben mix. The cream contained methylparaben and butylparaben, but it was not explicitly stated that these paraben-esters were tested separately and whether they gave positive reactions (14). One patient reacted to methylparaben in a corticosteroid cream (63).

Other non-cosmetic products

One individual had ACD from methylparaben in a compress (5). A woman, who had probably been sensitized to methylparaben in topical pharmaceutical products used on a leg ulcer previously, developed generalized dermatitis after an intramuscular injection of ampicillin solution, which was preserved with methyl- and propylparaben (10). A girl had ACD of the hands from play gel. She reacted to the paraben mix. The play gel containing methyl- and propylparaben, also gave a positive patch test. Methyl- and propylparaben were not tested separately (7). A man had ACD from methylparaben and propylparaben in an ultrasonic gel (38). One patient (probably) had widespread dermatitis after oral administration of a preparation containing methylparaben (details unknown) (30). A patient had ACD from methylparaben in Unna boots (25). Another individual developed severe allergic contact dermatitis of the lower legs from contact allergy to methyl- and propylparaben in bandages (43).

Cross-reactions, pseudo-cross-reactions and co-reactions

Co-reactions with other paraben-esters are seen frequently (19,22,23). As most patients are exposed to more than one paraben, it is difficult to determine whether these co-reactions result from cross-sensitivity or from concomitant sensitization (27). Methylparaben is very often combined with propylparaben as preservative system for different products. See also this section in Chapter 2.333 Paraben mix.

Presence in cosmetic products and chemical analyses

In the USA, in April 2017, methylparaben was present in 13753 of 56,714 cosmetic products of which the composition is known in FDA's Voluntary Cosmetic Registration Program (VCRP) (data obtained from FDA, May 2017). In February 2017, methylparaben was present in 4056 of 64,482 cosmetic products of which the composition is known in EWG's Skin Deep Cosmetics Database, USA (http://www.ewg.org/skindeep/). Methylparaben was present in 42(24%) of 178 facial wipes for which ingredient information was obtained online and from retail stores, USA, 2016 (61). Methylparaben was present in 11 (20%) of 54 personal hygiene wet wipes for which ingredient information was obtained online and from retail stores, USA, 2016 (62). Of 179 emollients available in Poland in 2015, 56 (31%) contained methylparaben (37).

In Germany, in 2006-2009, the labels of 4680 cosmetic products were screened for the presence of preservatives. Methylparaben was present in 37% of the products, according to labeling information (52). Methylparaben was present in 41% of 204 cosmetic products (92 shampoos, 61 hair conditioners, 34 liquid soaps, 17 wet tissues) in Sweden, 2008 (1). Methylparaben was present in 390 of 1774 (22%) cosmetics and toiletries in 2002 resp. in 335 of 1170 (29%) such products in 2005, filed in the Danish Product Register Database (PROBAS) (15).

In a group of 67 samples of skin creams, randomly selected from retail outlets in Denmark in 1999, 57 (85%) contained methylparaben in a concentration range of 0.007% to 0.409% (16). In the beginning of the 1990s, 215 cosmetic products, 158 leave-on cosmetics and 57 rinse-off cosmetics, from 79 cosmetic-producing companies, collected in Denmark, were analysed for paraben content with high performance liquid chromatography (HPLC) (36).Of all the products investigated, 93% were found to contain paraben(s). Paraben was detected in 77% of the rinse-off products and in 99% of the leave-on products. Total paraben content in the paraben-positive cosmetics was 0.01%-0.59%, except in one sun-lotion that contained 0.87% parabens. Rinse-off cosmetics contained 0.01-0.50% parabens and the paraben content in leave-on products was 0.01-0.59%. Methylparaben was present in 98% of the paraben-positive products in a concentration range of 0.01% to 0.32% (w/w) (36).

Provocation tests

In 14 patients reacting to the paraben mix, a placebo-controlled oral challenge with a mixture of 100 mg methylparaben and 100 mg propylparaben was performed. Two of the 14 patients had flares of their usual dermatitis (which was recurrent vesicular hand dermatitis) after challenge with the paraben mix but not after the placebo. Subsequently, a diet avoiding items containing parabens did not result in improvement of their dermatitis. It was concluded that oral challenge is not a useful test procedure in patients sensitive to the paraben mix. Although specific reactions were seen in 2 paraben-sensitive patients with recurrent vesicular hand eczema, the significance of this finding remained uncertain (8).

Miscellaneous side effects

One patient had systemic contact dermatitis from methylparaben in a mucolytic drug; oral provocation with 200 mg methylparaben reproduced the eruption, a placebo test was negative (4). A patient had ACD from parabens (unspecified) in a topical pharmaceutical product. Later, he developed widespread dermatitis after local anesthesia with a preparation containing methylparaben; this was considered to be systemic contact dermatitis (26). A patient developed a generalized eczematous eruption after receiving an oral preparation of haloperidol syrup containing methylparaben. Testing by macrophage inhibition factor indicated paraben sensitivity (39).

OTHER SIDE EFFECTS

Immediate-type reactions

A man had contact urticaria from moisturizing preparations and other common skin products containing parabens. He also developed marked swelling, erythema and itching around the injection site of a local anesthetic containing methylparaben. An open test with methylparaben was positive. A Prausnitz-Küstner test was also positive, indicating that this was an immunologic immediate contact reaction and type-I allergy to methylparaben (34). One case of contact urticaria from methylparaben; details unknown (56).

In one individual, local anesthesia with procaine preserved with methylparaben resulted in erythema, hives, itching on the hip, thigh, and lower part of the abdomen and a 'fainting' sensation experienced by the patient. Intracutaneous tests were positive to procaine and various other related anesthetics and to methylparaben; a Prausnitz-Küstner reaction was also positive to methylparaben, indicating immediate-type (type-I) allergy (31).

A hydrocortisone preparation containing methylparaben and propylparaben provoked bronchospasm and generalized pruritus within minutes after being given intravenously to an asthmatic patient. No urticaria, angioedema or hypotension were noted. Another hydrocortisone preparation without paraben preservative did not provoke any allergic symptoms. Intradermal tests and passive transfer (Prausnitz-Küstner) skin tests for immediate hypersensitivity were positive to both parabens (32).

A man had experienced the occurrence of transient skin rashes, itching, and hives following the administration of local anesthetic agents at the dentist on several occasions. An intradermal test with a local anesthetic containing methylparaben was positive, and later methylparaben, tested separately, also gave a positive response (33). A patient had an immediate-type reaction with generalized pruritus from allergy to methylparaben and propylparaben in a heparin solution, injected intravenously (40). One individual had a type-I allergy to methylparaben in anesthetic solutions (clinical data are lacking), as demonstrated by positive intradermal tests (59).

A child developed an anaphylactic shock after receiving a hypertonic rectal enema. The reaction was ascribed to allergy to methylparaben, which was present as preservative in the enema. However, proper diagnostic tests were not performed (44). One individual developed urticaria shortly after air-contrast barium enema studies of the colon. The patient had a positive prick skin test to methylparaben, which was the preservative in the barium mixture used and, therefore, was presumed to be the responsible allergen (45). Similar anaphylactic reactions from barium enemas have been observed, where methylparaben was the suspected causative ingredient of the enema. Tests to substantiate allergy to methylparaben were, however, not performed (46,47). Methylparaben has also been incriminated as causing allergic reactions in local anesthetics without proper diagnostic testing (48,49,50).

OTHER INFORMATION

Methylparaben and other additives in foods and drugs have been held responsible for exacerbations of chronic idiopathic urticaria by some authors. A recent study in 100 such patients, who were challenged wit 11 additives including methylparaben, showed with 95% confidence intervals, that sensitivity to any of the 11 food and drug additives occurs in fewer than 1% of patients with chronic idiopathic urticaria (53).

LITERATURE

1   Yazar K, Johnsson S, Lind M-L, Boman A, Lidén C. Preservatives and fragrances in selected consumer-available cosmetics and detergents. Contact Dermatitis 2011;64:265-272

2   Sagara R, Nakada T, Iijima M. Paraben allergic contact dermatitis in a patient with livedo reticularis. Contact Dermatitis 2008;58:53-54

3   Pecegueiro M, Brandao M, Pinto J, Concalo S. Contact dermatitis to Hirudoid® cream. Contact Dermatitis 1987:17:290-293

4   Sánchez-Pérez J, Ballesteros Diez M, Alonso Pérez A, Delgado Jiménez Y, Diez G. Allergic and systemic contact dermatitis to methylparaben. Contact Dermatitis 2006;54:117-118

5   Oiso N, Fukai K, Ishii M. Allergic contact dermatitis caused by parabens in a compress. Contact Dermatitis 2004;50:317

6   Vilaplana J, Romaguera C. Contact dermatitis from parabens used as preservatives in eyedrops. Contact Dermatitis 2000;43:248

7   Verhaeghe I, Dooms-Goossens A. Multiple sources of allergic contact dermatitis from parabens. Contact Dermatitis 1997;36:269-270

8   Veien NK, Hattel, T, Laurberg G. Oral challenge with parabens in paraben-sensitive patients. Contact Dermatitis 1996;34:433

9   Batten, TL, Wakeel RA, Douglas WS, Evans C, White MI, Moody R, Ormerod AD. Contact dermatitis from the old formula E45 cream. Contact Dermatitis 1994;30:159-161

10   Carradori S, Peluso AM, Faccioli M. Systemic contact dermatitis due to parabens. Contact Dermatitis 1990;22:238-239

11   Edwards EK Jr, Edwards EK. Allergic reaction to triethanolamine stearate in a sunscreen. Cutis 1983:31: 195-196

12   De Groot AC, Weyland JW, Bos JD, Jagtman BA. Contact allergy to preservatives (I). Contact Dermatitis 1986;14:120-122

13   Cronin E. Contact Dermatitis. Edinburgh: Churchill Livingstone, 1980:670-671

14   Fisher AA. Cortaid cream dermatitis and the 'paraben paradox'. J Am Acad Dermatol 1982;6:116-117

15   Flyvholm, MA. Preservatives in registered chemical products. Contact Dermatitis 2005;53:27-32

16   Rastogi SC. Analytical control of preservative labelling on skin creams. Contact Dermatitis 2000;43:339-343

17   SCCS (Scientific Committee on Consumer Safety). Opinion on parabens, 14 December 2010, revision of 22 March 2011, SCCS/1348/10. Available at:
http://ec.europa.eu/health/scientific_committees/consumer_safety/docs/sccs_o_041.pdf

18   SCCP (Scientific Committee on Consumer Products). Extended Opinion on Parabens, underarm cosmetics and breast cancer, 28 January 2005, SCCP/0874/05. Available at:
http://ec.europa.eu/health/archive/ph_risk/committees/04_sccp/docs/sccp_o_00d.pdf

19   Fransway AF. The problem of preservation in the 1990s: III. Agents with preservative function independent of formaldehyde release. Am J Cont Derm 1991;2:145-174

20   Sarkany I. Contact dermatitis from paraben. Br J Dermatol 1960;72:345-347

21   Schorr WP, Mohajerin AH. Paraben sensitivity. Arch Dermatol 1966;93:721-723

22   Hjorth N, Trolle-Lassen C. Skin reactions to ointment bases. Trans St John Hosp Derm Soc 1963;49:127-140

23   Menné T, Hjorth N. Routine patch testing with paraben esters. Contact Dermatitis 1988;19:189-191

24   Schamberg IL. Allergic contact dermatitis to methyl and propyl paraben. Arch Dermatol 1967;95:626-628

25   Praditsuwan P, Taylor JS, Roenigk HH Jr. Allergy to Unna boots in four patients. J Am Acad Dermatol 1995;33(5 Pt. 2):906-908

26   Aeling JL, Nuss DD. Systemic eczematous "contact-type" dermatitis medicamentosa caused by parabens. Arch Dermatol 1974;110:640

27   Hansen J, Møllgaard B, Avnstorp C, Menné T. Paraben contact allergy: Patch testing and in vitro absorption/metabolism. Am J Cont Derm 1993;4:78-86

28   Schorr WF. Paraben allergy. A cause of intractable dermatitis. JAMA 1968;204:859-862

29   Calnan CD. Quinazoline yellow dermatitis (D&C Yellow 11) in an eye cream. Contact Dermatitis 1981;7:271

30   Kaminer Y, Apter A, Tyano S, Livini E, Wijsenbeek H. Delayed hypersensitivity reaction to orally administered methylparaben. Clin Pharm 1982;1:469-470

31   Aldrete JA, Johnson DA. Allergy to local anesthetics. JAMA 1969;207:356-357

32   Nagel JE, Fuscaldo JT, Fireman P. Paraben allergy. JAMA 1977;237:1594-1595

33   Latronica RJ, Goldberg AF, Wightman JR. Local anesthetic sensitivity: Report of a case. Oral Surg 1969;28:439-441

34   Henry JC, Tchen EH, Becker LE. Contact urticaria to parabens. Arch Dermatol 1979;115:1231-1232

35   Wuepper KD. Paraben contact dermatitis. JAMA 1967;202:579-581

36 Rastogi SC, Schouten A, de Kruijf N, Weijland JW. Contents of methyl-, ethyl-, propyl-, butyl- and benzylparaben in cosmetic products. Contact Dermatitis 1995;32:28-30

37 Osinka K, Karczmarz A, Krauze A, Feleszko W. Contact allergens in cosmetics used in atopic dermatitis: analysis of product composition. Contact Dermatitis 2016;75:241-243

38 Eguino P, Sánchez A, Agesta N, Lasa O, Ratón JA, Diaz-Pérez JL. Allergic contact dermatitis due to propylene glycol and parabens in an ultrasonic gel. Contact Dermatitis 2003;48:290

39 Kaminer Y, Apter A, Tyano S, Livni E, Wijsenbeek H. Delayed hypersensitivity reaction to orally administered methylparaben. Clin Pharm 1982;1:469-470

40 Sato K, Kazama JJ, Wada Y, Maruyama H, Narita I, Gejyo F, Sugiyama K, Satoh H. Hypersensitivity to paraoxybenzoic acid esters (parabens) in a dialysis patient. Nephron 2002;92:728-729

41 Cashman AL, Warshaw EM. Parabens: A review of epidemiology, structure, allergenicity, and hormonal properties. Dermatitis 2005;16:57-66

42 Sasseville D. Hypersensitivity to preservatives. Dermatol Ther 2004;17:251-263

43 Lindner K, Cramer HJ, Köhler R. Do Varicosan bandages really rarely cause contact eczema? Case report of allergic contact dermatitis caused by propyl hydroxybenzoate following the use of Varicosan bandages. Dermatol Monatsschr 1989;175:655-657

44 Raulin-Gaignard H, Berlengi N, Gatin A, Loeb O, Borsa-Dorion A, Monin P. Severe allergic reaction due to a rectal enema. Arch Pediatr 2013;20:1329-1332 (article in French)

45 Schwartz EE, Glick SN, Foggs MB, Silverstein GS. Hypersensitivity reactions after barium enema examination. AJR Am J Roentgenol 1984;143:103-104

46 Larsen CF. Allergic side-effects after radioscopic examination of the colon with a barium sulfate suspension. Ugeskr Laeger 1981;143:937-938 (article in Danish)

47 Javors BR, Applebaum Y, Gerard P. Severe allergic reaction: an unusual complication of barium enema. Gastrointest Radiol 1984;9:357-358

48 Lederman DA, Freedman PD, Kerpel SM, Lumerman H. An unusual skin reaction following local anesthetic injection. Review of the literature and report of four cases. Oral Surg Oral Med Oral Pathol. 1980;49(1):28-33.

49 Fine PG, Dingman DL. Hypersensitivity dermatitis following suction-assisted lipectomy: a complication of local anesthetic. Ann Plast Surg 1988;20:573-575

50 Fukuda T, Dohi S. Anaphylactic reaction to fentanyl or preservative. Can Anaesth Soc J 1986;33:826-827

51 Knackstedt TJ, Zug KA. T cell lymphomatoid contact dermatitis: a challenging case and review of the literature. Contact Dermatitis 2015;72:65-74

52 Uter W, Yazar K, Kratz EM, Mildau G, Lidén C. Coupled exposure to ingredients of cosmetic products: II. Preservatives. Contact Dermatitis 2014;70:219-226

53 Rajan JP, Simon RA, Bosso JV. Prevalence of sensitivity to food and drug additives in patients with chronic idiopathic urticaria. J Allergy Clin Immunol Pract 2014;2:168-171

54 George ND, Srinivas CR, Balachandran C, Shenoi SD. Sensitivity to various ingredients of topical preparations following prolonged use. Contact Dermatitis 1990;23:367-368

55 Bajaj AK, Chatterjee AK. Paraben contact hypersensitivity. Ind J Derm Venereol Leprol 1985;51:319-321

56 Kojima M. A case of contact urticaria to methyl paraben. Skin Research 1992;34:578-582

57 Batty KT. Hypersensitivity to methylhydroxybenzoate: a case for additive labeling of pharmaceuticals. Med J Aust 1986;144:107-108

58 Soni MG, Taylor SL, Greenberg NA, Burdock GA. Evaluation of the health aspects of methyl paraben: a review of the published literature. Food Chem Toxicol 2002;40:1335-1373

59 Johnson WT, DeStigter T. Hypersensitivity to procaine, tetracaine, mepivacaine, and methyl paraben: report of a case. J Am Dent Ass 1983;106:53-56

60 Yim E, Baquerizo Nole KL, Tosti A. Contact dermatitis caused by preservatives. Dermatitis 2014;25:215-231

61 Aschenbeck KA, Warshaw EM. Allergenic ingredients in facial wet wipes. Dermatitis 2017 Mar 23. doi: 10.1097/DER.0000000000000268. [Epub ahead of print]

62 Aschenbeck KA, Warshaw EM. Allergenic ingredients in personal hygiene wet wipes. Dermatitis 2017 Mar 23. doi: 10.1097/DER.0000000000000275. [Epub ahead of print]

63 Coskey RJ. Contact dermatitis due to multiple corticosteroid creams. Arch Dermatol 1978;114:115-117

2.303   MISCELLANEOUS COSMETIC INGREDIENTS

2.303.1 ALUMINUM COMPOUNDS (UNSPECIFIED)

Case reports and case series
Two patients, previously sensitized to aluminum by hyposensitization injections, had axillary dermatitis from using antiperspirants containing (unspecified) aluminum salts (1,2). A nurse developed pruritic nodules from hepatitis B vaccinations; she had previously suffered from several episodes of axillary dermatitis caused by antiperspirants containing (unspecified) aluminum salts (3). In three children sensitized to aluminum by vaccinations, itchy vesicular dermatitis appeared on the face or on the back after the use of aluminum-containing sun protection lotions. Lotions free from aluminum caused no reactions. The exact nature of the aluminum compound was not mentioned (4).

Literature
1   Veien NK, Hattel T, Justesen 0, Nerholm A. Aluminium allergy. Contact Dermatitis 1986;15:295-297
2   Clemmensen 0, Knudsen HE. Contact sensitivity to aluminium in a patient hyposensitized with aluminium precipitated grass pollen. Contact Dermatitis 1980;6:305-308
3   Frost L, Johansen P, Pedersen S, Veien N, Aabel 0stergaard P, Nielsen MH. Persistent subcutaneous nodules in children hyposensitized with aluminium-containing allergen extracts. Allergy 1985;40:368-372
4   Bergfors E, Bjorkelund C, Trollfors B. Nineteen cases of persistent pruritic nodules and contact allergy to aluminum after injection of commonly used aluminum-adsorbed vaccines. Eur J Pediatr 2005;164:691-697

2.303.2 BOTANICAL PRODUCTS (MISCELLANEOUS)

Case reports and case series
In a private practice entirely dedicated to contact dermatitis and eczema in Little Rock, AR, USA, 215 patients presenting between April 2001 and October 2003 with an initial complaint of eyelid dermatitis, with or without involvement of other areas, were investigated and patch tested. Many ingredients of personal care products were available. Ingredient lists of products used were reviewed, and patients were tested to available ingredients that were found in products they had used. A total of 54 (25%) individuals reacted to personal care products or ingredients in them. There were 20 who reacted to plant materials other than wood tar, turpentine or colophonium. Twelve of these were allergic to botanicals in personal care products, including 'grapeseed, grapefruit seed, nettles, green tea, ginger, sunflower, wheat, sage, oatmeal, ginseng, anise, cocoa butter and yucca'. Because testing was only done with ingredients in products used by each individual, exposure was documented, and relevance was probable (1).

Literature
1   Guin JD. Eyelid dermatitis: A report of 215 patients. Contact Dermatitis 2004;50:87-90

2.303.3 CI 15880 (D&C RED NO. 34)

Case reports and case series
An unspecified number of patients with eyelid dermatitis had allergic reactions to D&C red no. 34 present in personal care products (1). INCI name EU: CI 15880; INCI name USA: Red 34; CAS number: 6417-83-0; EC number: 229-142-3.

Literature
1   Guin JD. Eyelid dermatitis: A report of 215 patients. Contact Dermatitis 2004;50:87-90

2.303.4 EUPHORBIA EXTRACT (UNSPECIFIED)

Case reports and case series
Euphorbia extract was responsible for 2 out of 959 cases of non-fragrance cosmetic allergy where the causal allergen was identified, Belgium, 2000-2010 (1).

Literature
1   Travassos AR, Claes L, Boey L, Drieghe J, Goossens A. Non-fragrance allergens in specific cosmetic products. Contact Dermatitis 2011;65:276-285

2.303.5 α-GLYCEROL ESTER OF *o*-AMINO-*m*-(2,3-DIHYDROXYPROPOXY)BENZOIC ACID

Case reports and case series
One patient had allergic contact dermatitis of the face from the α-glycerol ester of *o*-amino-*m*-(2,3-dihydroxypropo-xy)benzoic acid (5% and 10% pet.) in a sunscreen. Information on this chemical is lacking. The patient did not react to para-amino compounds (PABA, isobutyl PABA, ethyl aminobenzoate [benzocaine]) (1).

Literature
1   Van Ketel WG. Allergic contact dermatitis from an aminobenzoic acid compound used in sunscreens. Contact Dermatitis 1977;3:283

2.303.6 LABILIN®

Case reports and case series
Labilin® is (or was) a product which contains casein hydrolyzed with papain and 2.5% methylparaben. Labilin® is (or was) added in concentrations of maximum 1% to various preparations of the brand Fissan®, which consists of topical pharmaceuticals and cosmetics, notably for babies and pregnant women (1). Three patients reacted to Fissan products (one to a cosmetic, one to a pharmaceutical, one to both) and to Labilin, in two tested undiluted and in one as a '2% suspension'. Control tests were not performed. Another two patients had strongly positive patch test reactions to Fissan products, but the ingredients were not tested separately.

Five years later, the manufacturer, in a Letter to the Editor, which was co-signed by the author of the first study, reported that in the guinea pig maximization test, Labilin showed no sensitizing potential at all (2). They concluded 'In view of this, the positive patch test results obtained in patients with eczema may be atypical and should be viewed with caution. This judgment of the sensitization potential of Labilin is also supported by the fact that, after those 5 cases, no further patients were seen with even a suspicion of such a contact sensitization (2).

However, it appears that the trademark registration of Labilin was cancelled in 1990 (https://trademarks.justia.com/733/70/labilin-73370616.html).

Literature
1   Ippen H. Labilin®– a little-known contact allergen. Contact Dermatitis 1985;13:200-201
2   Grob W, Ippen H. Labilin. Contact Dermatitis 1990;23:62-63

2.303.7 LIPACIDE-CAS

Case reports and case series
A woman presented with a 2-month history of dermatitis on the face, hands and feet. It had started after using jogging cream to prevent blisters during walking trips. A patch test with the cream as it was positive. When tested with its ingredients, the patient reacted to Lipacide-cas (10% pet.), palmitoyl hydrolyzed milk protein, palmitoyl collagen amino acids and Arnica extract. No data on the nature of Lipacide-cas were provided, nor can anything be found in literature or on the internet (1).

Literature
1   De Leeuw J, den Hollander P. A patient with a contact allergy to jogging cream. Contact Dermatitis 1987;17:260-261

2.303.8 MERCURY

Case reports and case series

A man diagnosed with Addison's disease complained of chronic, severe, generalized pruritus of 20 years duration. Slightly erythematous macules and papules were present, mainly on the face, thorax and dorsa of the hands. Contact dermatitis was suspected as a superimposed phenomenon. Patch tests were positive to mercury 0.5% pet., an eau de cologne and a toilet soap. The soap had been used by the patient for 20 years. Atomic absorption spectrophotometry revealed that it contained 15 ppm of mercury. The use of cosmetics was discontinued. The pruritus stopped completely and in a few days, the cutaneous inflammatory eruption disappeared leaving only the hyperpigmentation of Addison's disease (1). Another patient had allergic contact dermatitis from mercury in a bleaching cream (2).

See also the chapters on other mercurials: Ammoniated mercury and Thimerosal.

Literature

1   Alomar A, Camarasa JG, Barnadas M. Addison's disease and contact dermatitis from mercury in a soap. Contact Dermatitis 1983;9:76
2   Fisher AA. Case presentations from the patch test clinic. American Academy of Dermatology, San Francisco, December 5, 1978. Cutis 1979;23:743,746,753,847,852,855,863,871

2.303.9 MIRANOL® MSA

Case reports and case series

One patient had allergic contact dermatitis from Miranol® MSA in a facial cleansing cream and mousse. The chemical was described as 2-nonyl-2-imidazolinium lauryl sulfate-1(2-hydroxyethyl)-1-carboxymethyl, disodium salt, and it was patch tested at a concentration of 3% in water (1, cited in ref. 2). No identifiers of this chemical have been found.

Literature

1   Verbov JL. Contact dermatitis from miranols. Trans St John's Hosp Derm Soc 1969;55:192-195
2   Dooms-Goossens A, Blockeel I. Allergic contact dermatitis and photoallergic contact dermatitis due to soaps and detergents. Clin Dermatol 1996;14:67-76

2.303.10 POLYESTER RESIN (TRIMELLITIC ANHYDRIDE, ADIPIC ACID, NEOPENTYL GLYCOL AND CYCLOHEXANEDIMETHANOL)

Case reports and case series

A woman from the UK presented with an intermittent rash of 1 year's duration on her neck and upper arms. This often occurred when she was abroad. The rash was erythematous, burning rather than vesicular and itchy, but faded to scaly patches which had the characteristic oval shape of nail varnish sensitivity. This also fitted with the timing of the rash: she painted her nails with a 'hypoallergenic' nail varnish when she went abroad. Patch testing revealed a positive reaction to the polyester resin in the nail varnish on two occasions and to her own nail varnish (open test). The chemical nature of the resin which caused the sensitivity was trimellitic anhydride, adipic acid, neopentyl glycol and cyclohexanedimethanol 70% in butyl acetate. The patient has had no further dermatitis since discontinuing the use of the nail varnish (1).

Literature

1   Shaw S. A case of contact dermatitis from 'hypoallergenic' nail varnish. Contact Dermatitis 1989;20:385

2.303.11 PROCAINE

Case reports and case series

A woman known to be allergic to various para-amino compounds including *p*-phenylenediamine, *p*-aminoazobenzene, *p*-aminobenzoic acid (PABA) and local anesthetics including benzocaine (ethyl-*p*-aminobenzoate and procaine (2-di-ethylamino-ethyl *p*-aminobenzoate hydrochloride, Novocain®) presented with an acute itchy, red, papular dermatitis of both ears, the neck and eyelids. The clinical picture suggested a reaction to a hair-care product. While she herself used no such product except shampoo, her husband used Gerovital®, a Rumanian cosmeceutical lotion for the stimulation of hair growth. A few days later, the patient applied the lotion to the inside of her elbow and obtained a strongly positive reaction. The label on the lotion stated that it should not be used by people sensitive to procaine. Her husband admitted that he had once switched pillows, hers being the softer. When he stopped using the lotion, his wife became symptom-free (1). This is a classic example of 'connubial contact dermatitis' (synonym: 'consort contact dermatitis'). Previously, two patients had been reported with allergic reactions to procaine in the same lotion purchased in Rumania (2).

Another female patient was admitted to hospital with an intense, red, swollen and vesicular eruption on the face. It had appeared after application of a cosmetic product with a Gerovital® base imported from Rumania. The patient had suffered from allergic gingivostomatitis previously following the application of a procaine-based local anesthetic for treatment of a decayed tooth. Patch test were positive to Gerovital® cream, procaine and benzocaine. UV spectrophotometric comparison of the absorption peaks for Gerovital® cream and procaine showed that procaine was present in the cosmetic used by the patient. Analytical weighing and a series of chloroform extractions indicated that Gerovital® cream contained about 1% procaine (3).

Procaine in those days was already prohibited in cosmetics in the EEC (European Economic Community).

Literature
1   Dooms-Goossens A, Swinnen E, VanderMaesen J, Marien K, Dooms M. Connubial dermatitis from a hair lotion. Contact Dermatitis 1987;16:41-42
2   Förström L, Hannuksela M, Idänpään-Heikkilä J, Salo OP. Hypersensitivity reactions to Gerovital. Dermatologica 1977;154:367-369
3   Goitre M, Bedello PG, Cane D, Roncarolo G. Contact dermatitis from novocaine in Gerovital® cream. Contact Dermatitis 1985;12:234-235

2.303.12 SODIUM DIHYDROXYCETYL PHOSPHATE ISOPROPYL HYDROXYCETYL ETHER

Case reports and case series

A man started applying a 12% ammonium lactate lotion twice daily for dry skin on his left leg. Five days later, he developed a very pruritic erythema, which then became eczematous, in the affected area. After discontinuing application of the lotion, and with the administration of topical corticosteroids, the process remitted in a few days. Patch tests with the GEIDC standard series and the lotion, as is, gave a positive reaction to the lotion. Later, the components of this cosmetic product were tested separately, which yielded a positive reaction to the emulsifier Dragophos® S at 1% and 5% in water. Fifteen controls were negative to the lotion and Dragophos S 5% in water. The chemical name given for Dragophos S was sodium dihydroxycetyl phosphate isopropyl hydroxycetyl ether (1).

Literature
1   Goday Bujan JJ, Bayona IY, Güemes MG, Lorentzen RI, Arechavala RS. Allergic contact dermatitis from Dragophos S, a new emulsifier. Contact Dermatitis 1996;34:158

2.303.13 ZIRCONIUM COMPOUNDS

Case reports and case series

In 1956-1958, American dermatologists were confronted with a unique and highly distinctive entity. The dermatosis was invariably found in the axillae, and was characterized by a chronic papular eruption. Pruritus and acute inflammation were occasionally present. Most patients were women, who were in the habit of shaving their axillae. All used deodorants containing zirconium salts, notably sodium zirconium lactate. The eruption was often chronic, persisting for months or years. No therapy was effective, and in most cases there has been gradual spontaneous involution. Histologically, a granulomatous reaction was observed in the dermis (1,3,4,5). Six such cases were presented in ref. 1; the authors also reviewed 64 cases reported previously. It was demonstrated that the 'zirconium deodorant granulomas' were allergic in nature. Patch tests were always negative, but the hypersensitivity was demonstrated by intradermal testing (1). Granulomas from zirconium in deodorants have also been reported from

Germany (2). In the 1950s and 1960s, insoluble zirconium compounds in over-the-counter poison ivy medications were also linked to cases of zirconium granulomas (1,6,8,9,10).

Sodium zirconium lactate and other zirconium salts were eliminated from aerosol-type deodorants in 1978 by a voluntary agreement with the manufacturers (7). Aluminum-zirconium complexes replaced zirconium salts in antiperspirants, and they have rarely caused similar reactions (7,12). One patient was reported with a reaction to an antiperspirant containing aluminum zirconium tetrachlorohydrex glycerin. The patient had used this antiperspirant only for at least 3 years and had a mass in one axilla for approximately 1 year before it became acutely inflamed. Histopathology gave the characteristic histologic features of an epitheloid granulomatous reaction and the aluminum-zirconium complex was demonstrated in the tissue and in the antiperspirant, suggesting both a foreign body reaction and a hypersensitivity reaction (7). A very similar patient with bilateral papular involvement of the axillae was reported some years later. The exact nature of the aluminum-zirconium complex was unknown (11).

Presence in cosmetic products and chemical analyses

In the USA, the use of zirconium-containing complexes in aerosol cosmetic products is prohibited because of their toxic effect on lungs of animals, as well as the formation of granulomas in human skin (FDA, 21 CFR 700.16). Zirconium powder, and some salts and derivatives are mentioned in the Personal Care Products Council Ingredient Database: zirconium chlorohydrate (reported function: cosmetic adstringents), zirconium dioxide (opacifying agents), zirconium powder (antiperspirant agents), zirconium silicate (abrasives; opacifying agents), and diallyloxyneohexyl zirconium tridecanoate (dispersing agents – nonsurfactant). However, for none of these chemicals, reported product categories were mentioned, which probably means that they are not used anymore in the USA. In the EU, zirconium powder and its compounds diallyloxyneohexyl zirconium tridecanoate, zirconium chlorohydrate, zirconium dioxide, zirconium silicate, zirconyl chloride, and zirconyl dioxide are prohibited for use in cosmetic products (Regulation (EC) No. 1223/2009, Annex II/391).

In May 2017, zirconium powder was present in 21 older products of 68,675 cosmetic products of which the composition is known in EWG's Skin Deep Cosmetics Database, USA (http://www.ewg.org/skindeep/). In the USA, in April 2017, zirconium was present in zero of 56,714 cosmetic products of which the composition is known in FDA's Voluntary Cosmetic Registration Program (VCRP) (data obtained from FDA, May 2017).

Literature

1   Shelley WB, Hurley HJ. The allergic origin of zirconium deodorant granulomas. Br J Derm 1958;70:75-101
2   Kleinhans D, Knoth W. Granulomas of axillae (zirconium?). Dermatologica 1976;152:161-167
3   Weber L, Neuhauser I. Tuberculide (?). Rubin L. Case for diagnosis. Discussion. Arch Dermatol 1957;75:597-600
4   Rubin L, Slepyan HH, Weber LF, Neuhauser I. Granulomas of the axilla caused by deodorants. JAMA 1956;162:953-955
5   Saunders TS. Granulomas of the axillas caused by deodorants. Arch Dermatol 1957;76:619-621
6   LePresti P, Hambrick GW. Zirconium granuloma following treatment of Rhus dermatitis. Arch Dermatol 1965;92:188-191
7   Skelton HG 3rd, Smith KJ, Johnson FB, Cooper CR, Tyler WF, Lupton GP. Zirconium granuloma resulting from an aluminum zirconium complex: a previously unrecognized agent in the development of hypersensitivity granulomas. J Am Acad Dermatol 1993;28:874-876
8   Williams RM, Skipworth GB. Zirconium granulomas of the glabrous skin following treatment of the Rhus dermatitis. Arch Dermatol 1959;80:273-276
9   Baler GR. Granulomas from topical zirconium in poison ivy dermatitis. Arch Dermatol 1965;91:145-148
10   Epstein WL, Allen JR. Granulomatous hypersensitivity after use of zirconium-containing poison oak lotions. JAMA 1964;190:940-942
11   Montemarano AD, Sau P, Johnson FB, James WD. Cutaneous granulomas caused by an aluminum-zirconium complex: an ingredient of antiperspirants. J Am Acad Dermatol 1997;37:496-498

2.304 MONOBENZONE[*]

* Not an INCI name

IDENTIFICATION

Description/definition   : Monobenzone is the aromatic ether that conforms to the structural formula shown
                             below
Chemical class(es)   : Aromatic compounds; ethers; alcohols
INCI name USA   : Not in the Personal Care Products Council Ingredient Database
Chemical/IUPAC name   : 4-Phenylmethoxyphenol
Other names   : Monobenzyl ether of hydroquinone; 4-benzyloxyphenol
CAS registry number (s)   : 103-16-2
EC number(s)   : 203-083-3
Merck Index monograph   : 7604
Function(s) in cosmetics   : EU: formerly used for skin bleaching (not an official cosmetic function)
EU cosmetic restrictions   : Regulated in Annex II/178 of the Regulation (EC) No. 1223/2009 (prohibited)
Patch testing   : 1.0% pet. (Chemotechnique, SmartPracticeEurope, SmartPracticeCanada)
Molecular formula   : $C_{13}H_{12}O_2$

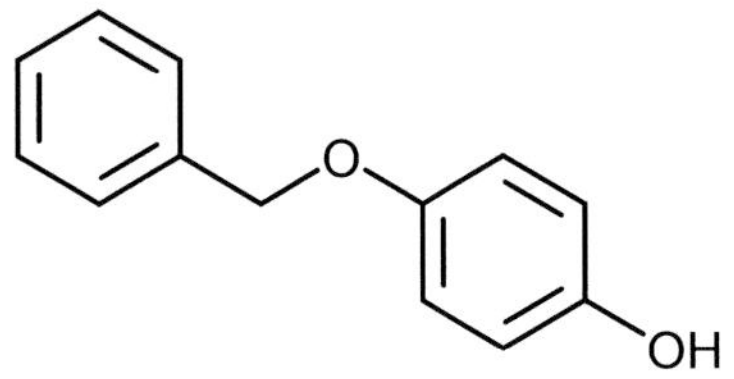

GENERAL

Monobenzone (monobenzyl ether of hydroquinone) has been used since the beginning of the 1950s to treat several forms of hyperpigmentation (11). After some years, cases were being reported of dermatitis, depigmentation (long-lasting and sometimes permanent [7]) and hyperpigmentation. In countries where monobenzone preparations were available without prescription, many such cases were seen (8,12). From the 1970s on, it was, and still is (4,17) used mainly to depigment residual pigmented areas in patients with very extensive therapy-resistant vitiligo (7).

Monobenzone was banned in the USA and in the EU in cosmetic products, but it is approved by the U.S. Food and Drug Administration for use in patients with extensive vitiligo (17).

CONTACT ALLERGY

Case reports and case series

A woman with a 16-year history of extensive vitiligo was given a depigmenting cream containing 20% monobenzone to clear residual areas of normal pigmentation. Over the subsequent 6 weeks, she developed dermatitis at the sites of application. The patient undertook a ROAT with monobenzone 5% cream at an unaffected site and this produced a similar dermatitis. Patch tests were positive to 1% monobenzone in pet. and in two other vehicles; she did not co-react to hydroquinone (1). A man had pigmented areas on the face; no precise diagnosis was made. Treatment with a 2% hydroquinone cream for 3 months did not improve the situation. He was then advised to use a cream containing 5% monobenzone, but 2 days after the first application, an acute dermatitis developed. Patch tests were positive to the cream, to monobenzone 2% pet. and to hydroquinone 2% pet. It was suggested that the patient had previously become sensitized to hydroquinone and now had a reaction from cross-sensitization to monobenzone (3).

It has been suggested that 5% of all patients treated with monobenzone cream become sensitized (16). Indeed, contact dermatitis from a 20% preparation was frequent, up to 13% of those treated (9,11). This was usually termed 'sensitization', but without patch tests being performed or on the basis of a positive patch test with the 20% monobenzone cream without proper controls.

As part of a clinical study to determine the effectiveness of monobenzone as a depigmenting agent, simulated use tests were done on a group of 43 middle-aged and older dark-skinned subjects with normal skin. Monobenzone in a vanishing cream base 1%, 4%, 7% and 10% was applied for 4 months plus the base itself. Inflammatory reactions during the course of treatment were observed in 23. No reactions were observed until after the 4th week of treatment. In general, erythematous reactions were observed on all areas except where the base was applied. In all cases where these reactions were observed, complete subsidence usually took about 2 weeks even though regular applications were continued. Several subjects experienced subsequently 2 or 3 similar episodes of erythema. In every case, with the exception of one, these reactions subsided despite continued applications (which would virtually exclude contact allergy). At the end of 4 months of the simulated use test, 26 of the 42 that completed the study showed depigmentation. This depigmentation was not uniform but was mottled and was more pronounced in those subjects who had experienced the more severe inflammatory reactions. After 2 years, 33 of the subjects were re-examined. Persistent leukoderma was present in 13 of this group. A patch test with the 10% monobenzone cream was applied to 12 who had leukoderma. All of these had a positive patch test which after 2 months revealed an early hypopigmentation at the patch test site. One can argue that the test concentration of 10% is too high (currently advised: 1% pet.), but the same patch test was applied on 16 of the remaining 20 who did *not* show any evidence of leukoderma and all had negative patch tests (13).

Cross-reactions, pseudo-cross-reactions and co-reactions
Not to hydroquinone (1). Cross-reactivity from hydroquinone (3); cross-reactivity from diethylstilbestrol (21).

OTHER SIDE EFFECTS

Irritant contact dermatitis
Contact dermatitis from the use of 20% monobenzone preparations has been observed frequently (9,11), up to 13% of those treated. This was usually termed 'sensitization', but without patch tests being performed or on the basis of a positive patch test with the 20% monobenzone cream without proper controls. As (erythematous) dermatitis during treatment often disappeared despite continued treatment, irritant dermatitis may have been present in a number of these patients (13). Sometimes, in patients with vitiligo, dermatitis (unknown whether irritant or allergic), was limited to pigmented areas (14). In 45% of vitiligo patients treated with monobenzone cream (concentration not stated), it caused concentration-dependent irritation of the skin (17).

Other non-eczematous contact reactions
Monobenzone in rubber gloves was found to cause occupational leukoderma among factory workers in 1939 and 1940. Later reports implicated monobenzone in other rubber products as the cause of leukoderma, including rubber covered wire-disk trays, hat bands, contraceptive diaphragms, rubber finger cots, rubber clothing, rubber aprons, powdered rubber condoms, rubber dolls, neoprene (literature reviewed in ref. 7) and leather wallets (18).

From the late 1950s on, many cases of leukoderma, hyperpigmentation, and combinations of leukoderma and hyperpigmentation (leukomelanoderma), often with bizarre or confetti-like patterns were reported from the use of commercial ointments / creams containing (up to 20%) monobenzone (e.g., 7,8,9,10,12,19). An epidemic of patchy leukomelanoderma in Africans was caused by the use of creams containing monobenzone (8). Creams containing 1.5% monobenzone also caused confetti-like depigmentation (15). Often the depigmentation from monobenzone was permanent and, therefore, monobenzone was later used for this purpose to depigment residual pigmented areas in patients with extensive therapy-resistant vitiligo (1,4,7,17).

Systemic side effects
Percutaneous absorption in patients treated with monobenzone may have caused depigmentation at sites distant from the site of skin application (4,5,17,20). Conversely, the development of pigmentation in the cornea and conjunctival melanosis in patients with vitiligo has also been ascribed to the use of monobenzone (6).

Miscellaneous side effects
A patient was tested with monobenzone 1% pet. in a shoe series and developed hypopigmentation at the test site without contact allergy (2). Positive patch tests to monobenzone creams have frequently resulted in subsequent leukoderma at the patch test sites beginning after 2 months (13).

LITERATURE

1   Lyon CC, Beck MH. Contact hypersensitivity to monobenzyl ether of hydroquinone used to treat vitiligo. Contact Dermatitis 1998;39:132-133
2   Sanzde Galdeano C, Aguirre A, Zabala R, Ratón JA, Diaz-Pérez JL. Achromic patch test from hydroquinone monobenzyl ether. Contact Dermatitis 1993;29:43-44
3   Van Ketel WG. Sensitization to hydroquinone and the monobenzyl ether of hydroquinone. Contact Dermatitis 1984;10:253
4   Harris JE. Chemical-Induced vitiligo. Dermatol Clin 2017;35:151-161
5   Grojean M-F, Thivolet J, Perrot H. leucomélanodermies accidentelles provoquées par les topicuqes depigmentants. Ann Derm Venereol 1982;109:641-644
6   Hedges TR III, Kenyon KR, Hanninen LA, Mosher DB. Corneal and conjunctival effects of monobenzone in patients with vitiligo. Arch Ophthalmol 1983;101-64-67

7   Mosher DB, Parrish JA, Fitzpatrick TB. Monobenzylether of hydroquinone. A retrospective study of treatment of 18 vitiligo patients and a review of the literature. Br J Dermatol 1977;97:669-679

8   Dogliotti M, Caro I, Hartdegen RG, Whiting DA. Leucomelanoderma in blacks. S Afr Med J !974;48:1555

9   Dorsey CS. Dermatitis and pigmentary reactions to monobenzyl ether of hydroquinone: Report of two cases. Arch Dermatol 1960;81:245-248

10 Sidi E, Gourgeois-Spinasse J. Depigmentation resulting from the application of hydroquinone-monobenzyl ether. Semaine Hôp (Paris) 1958;5:34

11 Lerner AB, Fitzpatrick TB. Treatment of melanin hyperpigmentation. JAMA 1953;152:577-582

12 Canizares O, Jaramillo FU, Vegas FK. Leukomelanoderma subsequent to the application of monobenzyl ether of hydroquinone: A vitiligoid reaction observed in Columbia and Venezuela, AMA Arch Dermat 1958;77:220-223

13 Spencer MC. Leukoderma following monobenzyl ether of hydroquinone bleaching. Arch Dermatol 1962;86:615-618

14 Nordlund JJ, Forget B, Kirkwood J, Lerner AB. Dermatitis produced by applications of monobenzone in patients with active vitiligo. Arch Dermatol 1985;121:1141-1143

15 Catona A, Lanzer D. Monobenzone, Superfade, vitiligo and confetti-like depigmentation. Med J Austral 1987;146:320-321

16 Fisher AA. Contact Dermatitis. Philadelphia: Lea and Febiger, 1973: 235

17 Tan ES, Sarkany R. Topical monobenzyl ether of hydroquinone is an effective and safe treatment for depigmentation of extensive vitiligo in the medium term: a retrospective cohort study of 53 cases. Br J Dermatol 2015;172:1662-1664

18 Bajaj AK1, Gupta SC, Chatterjee AK. Contact depigmentation of the breast. Contact Dermatitis 1991;24:58

19 Heilgemeir GP, Balda BR. Irreversible toxic depigmentation. Observations following use of hydroquinonemonobenzylether-containing skin bleaching preparations. MMW Munch Med Wochenschr 1981;123:47-48 (Article in German)

20 Lubowe IL, Morse JL, Gonzales V. Diffuse leukoderma following use of monobenzone. Arch Dermatol 1965;92:211-212

21 De Groot AC, Weyland JW, Nater JP. Unwanted effects of cosmetics and drugs used in dermatology, 3rd Edition. Amsterdam – London – New York – Tokyo: Elsevier, 1994, page 23

2.305　MYRISTIC ACID

IDENTIFICATION

Description/definition　: Myristic acid is the organic acid that conforms to the formula shown below
Chemical class(es)　: Fatty acids
Chemical/IUPAC name　: Tetradecanoic acid
CAS registry number (s)　: 544-63-8
EC number(s)　: 208-875-2
CIR review(s)　: J Am Coll Toxicol 1987;6:321-401; Int J Toxicol 2010;29(Suppl.3):162-186 (access: www.cir-safety.org/ingredients)
Merck Index monograph : 7689
Function(s) in cosmetics　: EU: cleansing; emulsifying; perfuming. USA: fragrance ingredients; opacifying agents; surfactants - cleansing agents
Patch testing　: 2% alc. (1)
Molecular formula　: $C_{14}H_{28}O_2$

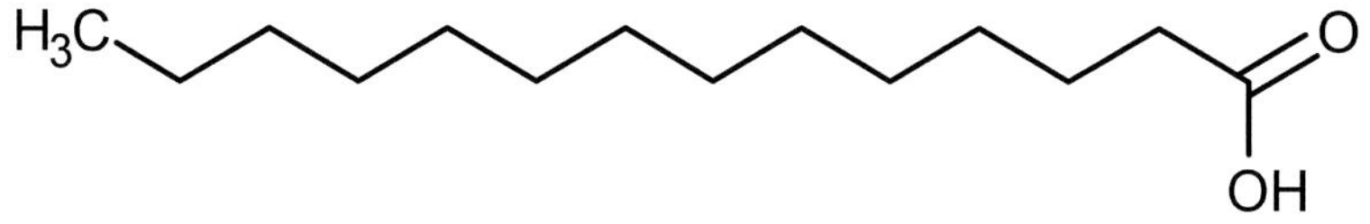

CONTACT ALLERGY

Case reports and case series

A man had suffered from intense outbreaks of seborrheic dermatitis, which improved with topical corticosteroids and ketoconazole but recurred on ceasing medication. For the past 3 months, papular, erythematous, intensely pruriginous lesions had been appearing on sun-exposed areas of the face, neck and hands. Patch tests and photopatch tests with the standard series were negative at 2 and 4 days, as were his cosmetics and toiletries with the single exception of a shaving foam, as is, which gave a strongly positive patch test reaction at both readings. Patch and photopatch tests were then carried out with the ingredients of this product supplied by the manufacturer and he had positive patch test reactions to 6 ingredients including myristic acid 2% in alcohol. There were no positive reactions in 25 controls. The patient was retested 7 months later to all 6 ingredients previously positive and reacted again at 2 and 4 days to myristic acid (1).

Presence in cosmetic products and chemical analyses

In the USA, in April 2017, myristic acid was present in 408 of 56,714 cosmetic products of which the composition is known in FDA's Voluntary Cosmetic Registration Program (VCRP) (data obtained from FDA, May 2017). In March 2017, myristic acid was present in 97 of 65,431 cosmetic products of which the composition is known in EWG's Skin Deep Cosmetics Database, USA (http://www.ewg.org/skindeep/).

LITERATURE

1　Vilaplana J, Lecha M, Romaguera C, Alsina A, Mascaro JM, Castel, T. A polysensitized HIV-positive patient. Contact Dermatitis 1993;29:101-102

2.306   MYRISTYL ALCOHOL

IDENTIFICATION

Description/definition	: Myristyl alcohol is the fatty alcohol that conforms generally to the formula shown below
Chemical class(es)	: Fatty alcohols
Chemical/IUPAC name	: Tetradecan-1-ol
Other names	: Tetradecanol; tetradecyl alcohol
CAS registry number (s)	: 112-72-1
EC number(s)	: 204-000-3
CIR review(s)	: J Am Coll Toxicol 1988;7:359-413 (access: www.cir-safety.org/ingredients)
Merck Index monograph	: 7691
Function(s) in cosmetics	: EU: emollient; emulsion stabilising; foam boosting; skin conditioning; viscosity controlling. USA: emulsion stabilizers; fragrance ingredients; skin-conditioning agents – emollient; surfactants – foam boosters; viscosity increasing agents – aqueous / nonaqueous
Patch testing	: 5% pet (2,7); 10% pet. appears to be (slightly) irritant (2,9)
Molecular formula	: $C_{14}H_{30}O$

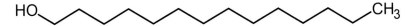

CONTACT ALLERGY

Patch testing in groups of patients
Results of studies patch testing myristyl alcohol in consecutive patients suspected of contact dermatitis (routine testing) and in groups of selected patients are shown in table 2.306.1. In routine testing, a 3.5% rate of sensitization was found in a small Italian study, but relevance was not mentioned (14). In 2 groups of selected patients, frequencies of sensitization were 2.1% and 2.8% (table 2.306.1). In one study, the test concentration of 10% pet. was found to be slightly irritant (9). Relevance was either not mentioned (9) or not specified (6).

Table 2.306.1 Patch testing in groups of patients

Years and Country	Test conc. & vehicle	Number of patients tested	positive (%)	Selection of patients (S); Relevance (R); Comments (C)	Ref.
Routine testing					
2015 Italy	5% pet.	310	11 (3.5%)	R: not stated	14
Testing in groups of selected patients					
2004-2005 Germany, Sweden	10% pet.	144	4 (2.8%)	S: patients tested with a metalworking fluid series; R: not stated; C: test concentration is slightly irritant	9
1992-1995 Italy	5% alc.	146	3 (2.1%)	S: patients suspected of contact allergy to cosmetics or topical pharmaceutical products; R: not specified, but one patient also reacted to a cosmetic containing the alcohol	6

Case reports and case series
In a group of 119 patients with allergic contact dermatitis from cosmetics, investigated in The Netherlands in 1986-1987, two cases were caused by myristyl alcohol in skin care products (11,12, same patients as in ref. 7). In a group of 75 patients allergic to cosmetic products, seen in a private practice in The Netherlands in the period 1981-1986, one case was caused by myristyl alcohol in a skin care product (13). In a 4-month-period in 1996, 475 patients with contact allergy to 'cosmetic ingredients' were collected in 5 centers in Belgium, UK and Germany. There was one reaction to myristyl alcohol; relevance was not stated (10).

A woman had ACD from myristyl alcohol in a deodorant; the patient also reacted to ceteareth-2 and ceteareth-3 in the product, and was also allergic to cetyl alcohol, stearyl alcohol and cetearyl alcohol (1). Three patients had ACD from myristyl alcohol in the same moisturizing cream (7). One patient had a positive patch test to a cosmetic product (unspecified) and its ingredient myristyl alcohol (6).

Contact allergy to myristyl alcohol in non-cosmetic products
Several patients had contact allergy to myristyl alcohol in a topical pharmaceutical product (4). In a group of 31 patients allergic to a topical pharmaceutical product, myristyl alcohol was the / an allergen in seven patients (3). One

or more patients reacted to myristyl alcohol in Eucerin, a lanolin derivative (8). Contact allergy to myristyl alcohol was also demonstrated in two other German publications, but specific data are unknown (15,16).

Cross-reactions, pseudo-cross-reactions and co-reactions
Cetyl alcohol, stearyl alcohol, cetearyl alcohol (1); oleyl alcohol (6). Cetyl alcohol used in cosmetics often contains some 10% myristyl alcohol (5).

Presence in cosmetic products and chemical analyses
In May 2017, myristyl alcohol was present in 131 of 66,669 cosmetic products of which the composition is known in EWG's Skin Deep Cosmetics Database, USA (http://www.ewg.org/skindeep/). In the USA, in April 2017, myristyl alcohol was present in 337 of 56,714 cosmetic products of which the composition is known in FDA's Voluntary Cosmetic Registration Program (VCRP) (data obtained from FDA, May 2017).

LITERATURE
1   Corazza M, Zauli S, Bianchi A, Benetti S, Borghi A, Virgili A. Contact dermatitis caused by fatty alcohols: may polyethoxylation of the fatty alcohols influence their sensitizing potential?. Contact Dermatitis 2013;68:189-190
2   Geier J, Lessmann H, Fuchs T, Andersen KE. Patch testing with myristyl alcohol. Contact Dermatitis 2006;55:366-367
3   Pecegueiro M, Brandao M, Pinto J, Concalo S. Contact dermatitis to Hirudoid® cream. Contact Dermatitis 1987;17:290-293
4   Edman B, Möller H. Medicament contact allergy. Derm Beruf Umwelt 1986;34:139-142
5   Kcomamura H, Dor T, Inui S, Yoshikawa K. A case of contact dermatitis due to impurities of cetyl alcohol. Contact Dermatitis 1997;36:44-46
6   Tosti A, Vincenzi C, Guerra L, Andrisano E. Contact dermatitis from fatty alcohols. Contact Dermatitis 1996;35:287-289
7   De Groot AC, Bruynzeel DP, van Joost T, Weyland JW. Cosmetic allergy from myristyl alcohol. Contact Dermatitis 1988;19:76-77
8   Peter G, Schropl F, Franzwa H. Expenmentelle Untersuchungen über die allergene Wirkung von Wollwachsalkoholen. Hautarzt 1969;20:450-455
9   Geier J, Lessmann H, Becker D, Bruze M, Frosch PJ, Fuchs T, et al. Patch testing with components of water-based metalworking fluids: results of a multicentre study with a second series. Contact Dermatitis 2006;55:322-329
10 Goossens A, Beck MH, Haneke E, McFadden JP, Nolting S, Durupt G, Ries G. Adverse cutaneous reactions to cosmetic allergens. Contact Dermatitis 1999;40:112-113
11 De Groot AC, Bruynzeel DP, Bos JD, van der Meeren HL, van Joost T, Jagtman BA, Weyland JW. The allergens in cosmetics. Arch Dermatol 1988;124:1525-1529
12 De Groot AC. Adverse reactions to cosmetics. PhD Thesis, University of Groningen, The Netherlands: 1988, chapter 3.4, pp.105-113
13 De Groot AC. Contact allergy to cosmetics: Causative ingredients. Contact Dermatitis 1987;17:26-34
14 Corazza M, Virgili A, Ricci M, Bianchi A, Borghi A. Contact sensitization to emulsifying agents: an underrated issue? Dermatitis 2016;27:276-281
15 Maak C, Masuch E, Zesch A. Zur lokalen Überempfindlichkeit von häufig verwendeten Externa-Hilfsstoffen. Allergologie 1983;6:437-449 (data cited in ref. 2)
16 Auth R, Pevny I, Peter G. Ein Beitrag zur Wollwachsallergie. Aktuelle Derm 1984;10:215-220 (data cited in ref. 2)

2.307 MYRISTYL GLUCOSIDE

IDENTIFICATION

Description/definition : Myristyl glucoside is the product obtained by the condensation of myristyl alcohol with glucose

Chemical class(es) : Carbohydrates

Other names : Myristyl D-glucopyranoside; tetradecyl D-glucopyranoside; tetradecyl D-glucoside

CIR review(s) : Int J Toxicol 2013;32(Suppl.3):22-48 (access: www.cir-safety.org/ingredients)

Function(s) in cosmetics : EU: cleansing. USA: surfactants – cleansing agents

Patch testing : No data available; suggested: 3-5% pet.

Molecular formula : $C_{20}H_{40}O_6$

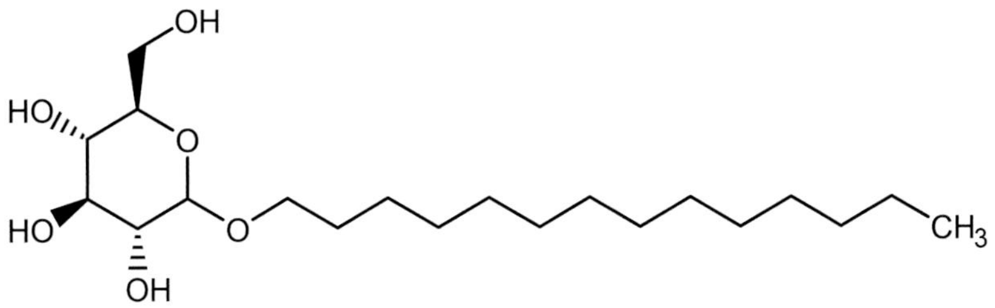

GENERAL

Myristyl glucoside is one of the alkyl glucosides, a family of organic molecules of vegetal origin. They are produced by the condensation of a sugar, usually a cyclic form of glucose (D-glucopyranose), with a fatty alcohol composed of a linear side chain ranging from 2 to 22 carbons. Fatty alcohol is extracted from palm, coconut, or rapeseed oil, and glucose can be obtained from corn, wheat starch, and potato. The average number of carbon atoms composing the alcohol side chain determines the name of the alkyl glucoside. Members of the alkyl glucoside family include butyl, caprylyl, decyl, lauryl, coco-, cetearyl, undecyl, myristyl, hexadecyl, octadecyl, arachidyl, and caprylyl/capryl glucoside, C10-16, C12-18, C12-20, and C20-22 alkyl glucosides, branched isostearyl glucoside, and octyldodecyl glucoside.

Most of the alkyl glucosides are primarily used as mild non-ionic surfactants in cosmetics and cleansing products for human skin, mostly as a mixture of several alkyl glucosides, as it is difficult to obtain individual glucosides at high purity. They can also sometimes function as emulsion stabilizers in sunscreens, skin and hair cleansing agents, and humectants. They can be found in certain baby products such as wipes and cleansers and in antiseptic solutions (4).

Other alkyl glucosides which have caused cosmetic allergy include arachidyl glucoside, cetearyl glucoside, coco-glucoside, decyl glucoside and lauryl glucoside. These are discussed in their respective chapters. A comprehensive review of contact allergy to alkyl glucosides has been published in 2017 (5,6).

CONTACT ALLERGY

Case reports and case series

One patient with eczema of the face from contact allergy to decyl glucoside in Tinosorb® M, present in a facial sunscreen, had positive patch test reactions to an unknown number of his facial cosmetics containing myristyl glucoside (1,2).

Cross-reactions, pseudo-cross-reactions and co-reactions

Often, a mixture of several alkyl glucosides is present in cosmetic products, as it is very difficult to obtain individual glucosides of high purity (3). Because of this and of their chemical similarity, concomitant reactivity or cross-reactions may occur with the various glucosides (2).

Presence in cosmetic products and chemical analyses

In the USA, in April 2017, myristyl glucoside was present in 5 of 56,714 cosmetic products of which the composition is known in FDA's Voluntary Cosmetic Registration Program (VCRP) (data obtained from FDA, May 2017). In February 2017, myristyl glucoside was present in 4 of 64,631 cosmetic products of which the composition is known in EWG's Skin Deep Cosmetics Database, USA (http://www.ewg.org/skindeep/).

LITERATURE

1   Andrade P, Gonçalo M, Figueiredo A. Allergic contact dermatitis to decyl glucoside in Tinosorb® M. Contact Dermatitis 2010;62:119-120

2   Pereira N, Coutinho I, Andrade P, Gonçalo M. The UV filter Tinosorb M, containing decyl glucoside, is a frequent cause of allergic contact dermatitis. Dermatitis 2013;24:41-43

3   Le Coz CJ, Meyer MT. Contact allergy to decyl glucoside in antiseptic after body piercing. Contact Dermatitis 2003;48:279-280

4   Fiume MM, Heldreth B, Bergfeld WF, Belsito DV, Hill RA, Klaassen CD, et al. Safety assessment of decyl glucoside and other alkyl glucosides as used in cosmetics. Int J Toxicol 2013;32(Suppl.5):22S-48S

5   Loranger C, Alfalah M, Ferrier Le Bouedec M-C, Sasseville Denis. Alkyl glucosides in contact dermatitis: a systematic review. Dermatitis Dermatitis 2017;28:5-13

6   Alfalah M, Loranger C, Sasseville D. Contact allergen of the year. Alkyl glucosides. Dermatitis 2017;28:3-4

2.308   2,7-NAPHTHALENEDIOL

IDENTIFICATION

Description/definition   : 2,7-Naphthalenediol is the bicyclic phenol that conforms to the formula shown below
Chemical class(es)   : Color additives hair; phenols
Chemical/IUPAC name   : Naphthalene-2,7-diol
Other names   : CI 76645; 2,7-dihydroxynaphthalene
CAS registry number (s)   : 582-17-2
EC number(s)   : 209-478-7
SCCS opinion(s)   : SCCS/1366/10 (2)
Function(s) in cosmetics   : EU: hair dyeing. USA: hair colorants
EU cosmetic restrictions   : Annex III/216 of the Cosmetics Regulation (EC) No. 1223/2009, amended by
                             (EC) No. 344/2013
Patch testing   : 0.1% water (1)
Molecular formula   : $C_{10}H_8O_2$

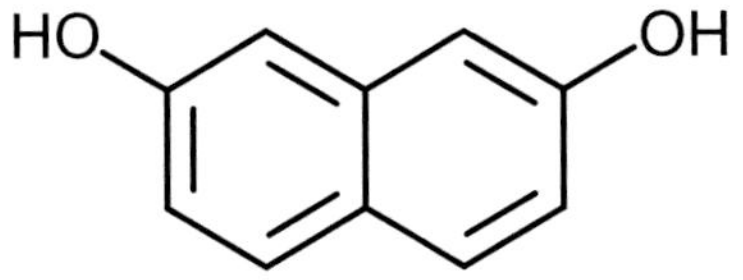

GENERAL

2,7-Naphthalenediol is used as a coupler in oxidative hair dying products. For the chemistry of hair dying see Chapter 2.359 *p*-Phenylenediamine.

CONTACT ALLERGY

Case reports and case series

A woman developed an exceptionally severe skin eruption on her scalp, face, upper chest and upper extremities. She needed oral corticosteroids and had to take a one-month sick leave. The cause remained unknown. Her skin eruption relapsed 2 months later, after her hair had been dyed. Patch testing with the standard series was negative, including *p*-phenylenediamine. The authors then obtained from the manufacturer 22 constituents of the hair dye, and further patch testing was performed. 2,7-Dihydroxynaphthalene 0.1% water elicited a strongly positive reaction, whereas the other constituents were negative. A use test on the lower arm with the hair dye also provoked a reaction. Twenty control persons were patch tested with 2,7-dihydroxynaphthalene 0.1% water: 19 were negative, but one without any history of hair dye dermatitis had a positive reaction (1).

Cross-reactions, pseudo-cross-reactions and co-reactions

Not to *p*-phenylenediamine (1).

Presence in cosmetic products and chemical analyses

In the USA, in April 2017, 2,7-naphthalenediol was present in 1 of 56,714 cosmetic products of which the composition is known in FDA's Voluntary Cosmetic Registration Program (VCRP) (data obtained from FDA, May 2017). In March 2017, 2,7-naphthalenediol was present in zero of 63,983 cosmetic products of which the composition is known in EWG's Skin Deep Cosmetics Database, USA (http://www.ewg.org/skindeep/). In southern Germany, in 2013-2014, the labels of 924 permanent oxidative hair dyes were checked for the presence of hair dye components. There were 334 retail products (of seven different brands) and 590 professional products (of six different brands). The 924 products analyzed revealed a total of 58 different hair dye components, with retail products containing 32 and professional products 52. 2,7-Naphthalenediol was present in 22 (2.4%) of the 924 products (4). In 2011, labels and other information on 365 hair dye products (282 permanent dyes, 79 semi-permanent dyes, 4 direct dyes) available on the Danish market (159 hair dyes for private use, 206 for professional use by hairdressers) were collected to identify the presence of sensitizers. 2,7-Naphthalenediol was present in 8 (2.2%) products (3).

In April 2010, in Spain, 111 consumer-available oxidative hair dye products of 19 brands were purchased to check the labeling for sensitizers. A systematic selection of products to be purchased from each hair dye brand was applied, including the darkest blonde shade available, one 'regular' light brown shade, one 'regular' dark brown shade, one 'regular' black shade, and two further shades with different colours (red, blue, purple, etc.). In this group of 111 hair dyes, 2,7-naphthalenediol was present in two (2%) of the products (6). In August - October 2008, the labels of 122 oxidative hair dye products on the Swedish market were examined for the presence of hair dye substances categorized as potent skin sensitizers. 2,7-Naphthalenediol was present in 5 (4%) of these products (5).

LITERATURE

1   Eskelinen A, Molitor C, Kanerva L. Allergic contact dermatitis from 2,7-dihydroxynaphthalene in hair dye. Contact Dermatitis 1997;36:312-313
2   SCCS (Scientific Committee on Consumer Safety). Opinion on 2,7-naphthalenediol, 21 September 2010, SCCS/1366/10. Available at:
     http://ec.europa.eu/health/scientific_committees/consumer_safety/docs/sccs_o_034.pdf
3   The Danish Environmental Protection Agency. Survey and occurrence of PPD, PTD and other allergenic hair dye substances in hair dyes. Copenhagen, Denmark: The Danish Environmental Protection Agency, 2013 (ISBN 978-87-92903-92-1). Available at: http://www2.mst.dk/Udgiv/publications/2013/02/978-87-92903-92-1.pdf
4   Kirchlecher S, Hübner A, Uter W. Survey of sensitizing constituents of oxidative hair dyes (retail and professional products) in Germany. J Dtsch Dermatol Ges 2016;14:707-715
5   Yazar K, Boman A, Lidén C. Potent skin sensitizers in oxidative hair dye products on the Swedish market. Contact Dermatitis 2009;61:269-275
6   Yazar K, Boman A, Lidén C. p-Phenylenediamine and other hair dye sensitizers in Spain. Contact Dermatitis 2012;66:27-32

2.309 NEOPENTYL GLYCOL DIISOOCTANOATE*
* Not an INCI name

IDENTIFICATION

Description/definition	: Neopentyl glycol diisooctanoate is the organic substance that conforms to the formula shown below
Chemical class(es)	: Esters
INCI name USA	: Neither in Cosing nor in the Personal Care Products Council Ingredient Database
Chemical/IUPAC name	: [2,2-Dimethyl-3-(6-methylheptanoyloxy)propyl] 6-methylheptanoate
Other names	: 2,2-Dimethyl-1,3-propanediyl isooctanoate
CAS registry number (s)	: 129726-86-9
Patch testing	: 20% and 50% pet. (1)
Molecular formula	: $C_{21}H_{40}O_4$

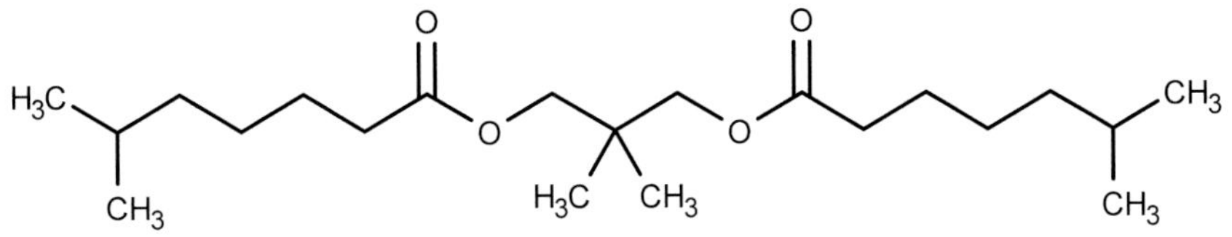

GENERAL
Neopentyl glycol diisooctanoate is a synthetic ester commonly used in cosmetics in Japan in the mid-1990s, especially in milky lotions and face creams. It has weak irritancy as shown by the Draize technique and patch tests (as is) in rabbits (1).

CONTACT ALLERGY

Case reports and case series
A woman developed an itchy reddish eruption on her face. The day before, she had applied a sunscreen product that she used regularly. The patient had a 30-year history of discoid lupus erythematosus (DLE) and a 2-year history of intolerance to fragrances. She was treated with topical corticosteroids and the lesions disappeared. The patient was first patch tested with her cosmetics, sunscreen products and 29 allergens of a cosmetics series. Positive reactions were observed to the sunscreen product that she had used before the onset of the eruption, synthetic sandalwood and benzyl salicylate; there were dubious positive (?+) reactions to jasmine absolute and cananga oil. Subsequently, she was tested with the 9 ingredients of the sunscreen; the component neopentyl glycol diisooctanoate gave a positive response. Later, this chemical was patch tested in a dilution series at 50%, 20%, 10% and 5% in petrolatum. She reacted to all 4 concentrations at D4, but the reactions to 5% and 10% were ?+ at D3. Twenty controls were negative to all concentrations at D3. The incriminated sunscreen contained neopentyl glycol diisooctanoate in a concentration of 57.25% (1).

Presence in cosmetic products and chemical analyses
In the USA, in April 2017, neopentyl glycol diisooctanoate was present in zero of 56,714 cosmetic products of which the composition is known in FDA's Voluntary Cosmetic Registration Program (VCRP) (data obtained from FDA, May 2017). In February 2017, neopentyl glycol diisooctanoate was present in zero of 64,480 cosmetic products of which the composition is known in EWG's Skin Deep Cosmetics Database, USA (http://www.ewg.org/skindeep/).

LITERATURE
1   Nishioka K, Murata M, Ishikawa T. Contact allergy to neopentyl glycol di-iso-octanoate. Contact Dermatitis 1995;33:208-209

2.310   NICKEL*
Not an INCI name

IDENTIFICATION

Description/definition	: Nickel is a metal, which may be present in pigmented make-up products as a contaminant
Chemical class(es)	: Elements, transition metals
INCI name USA	: Neither in CosIng nor in the Personal Care Products Council Ingredient Database
CAS registry number (s)	: 7440-02-0
EC number(s)	: 231-111-4
Merck Index monograph	: 7853
Function(s) in cosmetics	: No function, contaminant
EU cosmetic restrictions	: Regulated in Annex II/1093 of the Regulation (EC) No. 1223/2009 (prohibited)
Patch testing	: Nickel(II)sulfate hexahydrate 5.0% pet. (Chemotechnique, SmartPracticeEurope, SmartPracticeCanada); nickel(II)sulfate hexahydrate 2.5% pet. (Chemotechnique, SmartPracticeCanada)

GENERAL

Discussion of side effects of nickel in this chapter is limited to reactions from its presence in cosmetic products.

CONTACT ALLERGY

The prevalence of metal allergy is high in the general population, and it is estimated that up to 17% of women and 3% of men are allergic to nickel (2). Pigmented make-up products may contain nickel and other metal allergens (3). Nickel is not added as such to make-up and is prohibited in cosmetics in the EU (13), but exists as an impurity among other ingredients, such as in iron oxides. However, an association between eyelid dermatitis and nickel in make-up products remains somewhat controversial. Seventeen patients with a positive patch test reaction to nickel did *not* react to 4 makeup products containing pigments with nickel as impurity nor to 4 individual pigments (2 black iron oxides, titanium dioxide, bismuth oxychloride) 50% in petrolatum, concomitantly patch tested. However, the level of nickel was not analyzed (1). In a cross-sectional general population study, no association between having nickel allergy and reporting cosmetic dermatitis caused by mascara or eye shadow use was found (4). Nevertheless, no guarantee of skin tolerance to pigmented make-up products can be given to extremely sensitive individuals (4).

It has been postulated that low nickel content of an eye pencil (or other eye make-up product) can elicit allergic contact dermatitis by repeated application, leading to accumulation of the allergen. Moreover, the eyelids are particularly prone to the development of allergic contact dermatitis, even at low concentrations of the allergen, or with short exposure times (9). Indeed, eyelid dermatitis has been observed among several nickel-allergic dermatitis patients following exposure to nickel-containing eye pencil, mascara or eye shadow (6,9,10,11,12). Such reactions may also be caused by metal instruments such as an eyelash curler (15,16). In groups of patients with periorbital dermatitis, however, nickel allergy is rarely relevant (17,18,19), so nickel in eye cosmetics is either a rare cause of eyelid dermatitis or may go unrecognized. In a very large group of 4779 patients with periorbital dermatitis, however, nickel was the most frequent allergen. As female sex was overrepresented in this group as compared with controls, the authors suggested that sensitization to nickel may be a coincidence, and does not necessarily reflect problems of the skin around the eyes (21).

Case reports and case series

In the period 1996-2013, in a tertiary referral center in Valencia, Spain, 5419 patients were patch tested. Of these, 628 individuals had allergic contact dermatitis to cosmetics. Nickel was the responsible allergen in one case (5). Nickel sulfate was responsible for 3 out of 959 cases of non-fragrance cosmetic allergy where the causal allergen was identified, Belgium, 2000-2010 (8). One female patient had allergic contact dermatitis to nickel in a green eye pencil containing 0.028µg nickel/g color (ppm) (6). Another woman developed eyelid dermatitis from a blue eye pencil containing 0.015 µg nickel/g (ppm) color (9). A similar case was caused by an eye pencil containing 1.4 ppm nickel (10). In all these cases, there were also positive patch test reactions to the colored pencil material itself.

A female patient with eyelid dermatitis reacted to nickel sulfate and to a brown colored eyeshadow and mascara, which proved to contain 76 and 102 ppm of nickel respectively (11,22). Another patient had eyelid dermatitis and reacted to nickel, but not to her eye cosmetics; one eyeshadow contained 87 ppm nickel, another eyeshadow and mascara both 10 ppm (11,22).

One female patient, known to be allergic to costume jewellery, developed edema and eczema of the eyelids after using a new blue eyeshadow that proved to contain 16.9 µg nickel/g (ppm). The patch test with the product was negative, but the dermatitis cleared after avoidance of this eye cosmetic (12). Five women allergic to nickel had facial dermatitis and reacted to one of their foundations each. Testing with the individual ingredients remained negative. The reactions were ascribed to nickel in iron oxide pigments CI 77492, CI 77489, CI 77499 and/or CI 77491 present in the foundations, but nickel levels were not mentioned (14). Two women, known to be allergic to nickel, had contact cheilitis from lipsticks in metal containers. They both had positive patch tests to lipsticks packed in metal containers, but not to lipsticks in plastic containers (23).

Analysis of allergen in products
A Finnish study on metals in eye shadows performed in 2000 showed that, among 49 eye shadows, the nickel content was up to 44 ppm and that no products contained less than 1 ppm nickel (3). In Denmark, the Information Centre for Environment & Health, after repeatedly receiving complaints from nickel allergic consumers who reported eyelid dermatitis from mascara use, investigated 19 mascaras and found them to contain 16-41 ppm nickel (cited in ref. 4). A thorough review of the literature on studies analysing the amounts of nickel in cosmetic products has been published in 2014 (20).

OTHER INFORMATION

Other information
Several nickel-allergic patients, not having eyelid dermatitis, have shown positive patch test reactions to a nickel-contaminated mascara (7).

LITERATURE
1   Lodén M, Nilsson G, Parvadeh M, Neimert Carne K, Berg M. No skin reactions to mineral powders in nickel-sensitive subjects. Contact Dermatitis 2012;66:210-214
2   Thyssen JP, Menné T. Metal allergy – a review on exposures, penetration, genetics, prevalence, and clinical implications. Chem Res Toxicol 2010;23:309-318
3   Sainio EL, Jolanki R, Hakala E, Kanerva L. Metals and arsenic in eye shadows. Contact Dermatitis 2000;42:5-10
4   Thyssen JP, Linneberg A, Menné T, Nielsen NH, Johansen JD. No association between nickel allergy and reporting cosmetic dermatitis from mascara or eye shadow: a cross-sectional general population study. J Eur Acad Dermatol Venereol 2010;24:722-725
5   Zaragoza-Ninet V, Blasco Encinas R, Vilata-Corell JJ, Pérez-Ferriols A, Sierra-Talamantes C, Esteve-Martínez A, de la Cuadra-Oyanguren J. Allergic contact dermatitis due to cosmetics: A clinical and epidemiological study in a tertiary hospital. Actas Dermosifiliogr 2016;107:329-336
6   Travassos AR, Bruze M, Dahlin J, Goossens A. Allergic contact dermatitis caused by nickel in a green eye pencil. Contact Dermatitis 2011;65:307-308
7   Karlberg A-T, Lidén C, Ehrin E. Colophony in mascara as a cause of eyelid dermatitis. Chemical analyses and patch testing. Acta Derm Venereol 1991;71:445-447
8   Travassos AR, Claes L, Boey L, Drieghe J, Goossens A. Non-fragrance allergens in specific cosmetic products. Contact Dermatitis 2011;65:276-285
9   Verhulst L, Persson L, Zimerson E, Bruze M, Vanden Broecke K, Goossens A. Palpebral eczematous dermatitis caused by nickel in an eye pencil. Contact Dermatitis 2014;70:247-249
10   Zemba C, Ramaguera C, Vilaplana J. Allergic contact dermatitis from nickel in an eye pencil. Contact Dermatitis 1992;27:116
11   Van Ketel WG, Liem DH. Eyelid dermatitis from nickel contaminated cosmetics. Contact Dermatitis 1981;7:217
12   Goh CL, Ng SK, Kwok SF. Allergic contact dermatitis from nickel in eyeshadow. Contact Dermatitis 1989;20:380-381
13   European Commission Regulation no. 1223/2009 of the European Parliament and of the Council of 30 November 2009 on cosmetic products: annex II: 1093
14   Foulds IS. Facial eczema due to colour pigments in foundation makeup in nickel-sensitive patients. Contact Dermatitis 2006;55 (Suppl. 1):11
15   Brandrup F. Nickel eyelid dermatitis from an eyelash curler. Contact Dermatitis 1991;25:77
16   Henke U, Boehncke W. Eyelid dermatitis caused by an eyelash former. Contact Dermatitis 2005;53:237
17   Feser A, Plaza T, Vogelgsang L, Mahler V. Periorbital dermatitis – a recalcitrant disease: causes and differential diagnoses. Br J Dermatol 2008;159:858-863
18   Guin JD. Eyelid dermatitis: a report of 215 patients. Contact Dermatitis 2004;50:87-90
19   Temesvari E, Ponyai G, Nemeth I, Hidvégi B, Sas A, Kárpáti S. Periocular dermatitis: a report of 401 patients. J Eur Acad Dermatol Venereol 2009;23:124-128

20 Bocca B, Pino A, Alimonti A, Forte G. Toxic metals contained in cosmetics. A status report. Regul Toxicol Pharmacol 2014;68:447-462

21 Landeck L, John SM, Geier J. Periorbital dermatitis in 4779 patients – patch test results during a 10-year period. Contact Dermatitis 2014;70:205-212

22 Van Ketel WG, Bruynzeel DP. Allergic contact dermatitis from nickel in eyeshadow. Contact Dermatitis 1989;21:355

23 Hathaway JC. Dermatitis caused by lipsticks in metallic containers. Arch Derm Syph 1941;43:703

2.311 NITROCELLULOSE

IDENTIFICATION

Description/definition   : Nitrocellulose is a variable mixture which consists chiefly of cellulose tetranitrate
Chemical class(es)   : Biological polymers and their derivatives; carbohydrates
Other names   : Pyroxylin; cellulose, nitrate; collodion (flexible)
CAS registry number (s)   : 9004-70-0
Merck Index monograph   : 9395
CIR review(s)   : Final report, June 2013 (access: www.cir-safety.org/ingredients)
Function(s) in cosmetics   : EU: film forming. USA: dispersing agents – non-surfactants; film formers
Patch testing   : 10% in isopropyl alcohol (2)
Molecular formula   : HNO_3.x-unspecified

CONTACT ALLERGY

Case reports and case series

In the period 1996-2013, in a tertiary referral center in Valencia, Spain, 5419 patients were patch tested. Of these, 628 individuals had allergic contact dermatitis to cosmetics. Nitrocellulose was the responsible allergen in five cases (overlap with the cases in ref. 4) (5). In the period 2000-2007, 202 patients with allergic contact dermatitis caused by cosmetics were seen in Valencia, Spain. In this group, three individuals reacted to nitrocellulose from its presence in nail polishes (overlap with the cases in ref. 5) (4). Nitrocellulose was responsible for 1 out of 399 cases of cosmetic allergy where the causal allergen was identified in a study of the NACDG, USA, 1977-1983 (1).

A woman had dermatitis of the neck, recurrent for 15 years and permanent for 3 months. She had used a wide range of cosmetics. Patch tests with her own products showed contact allergy to 2 nail varnishes. Stopping the use of these products resulted in rapid improvement of the dermatitis. Patch tests with the European standard series and a cosmetics series showed a positive reaction to tosylamide/formaldehyde resin, which was present in both nail varnishes, during which the dermatitis flared. The patient was advised to use an experimental nail product which did not contain the resin. However, when applying it to the forearm, she experienced an acute contact dermatitis there with spreading to the neck and face. Patch tests to components of this varnish showed positive reactions to nitrocellulose when tested in two (complex) solvents at the same concentration as used in the varnish, at 50% and at 10% of the concentration. Over 100 controls were negative (2).

Nitrocellulose used in varnishes was already reported in 1944 as a potential allergen. Of 30 patients allergic to nail lacquers, 9 reacted to a 10% nitrocellulose solution; 10 controls were negative (3).

Presence in cosmetic products and chemical analyses

In the USA, in April 2017, nitrocellulose was present in 951 of 56,714 cosmetic products of which the composition is known in FDA's Voluntary Cosmetic Registration Program (VCRP) (data obtained from FDA, May 2017). In April 2017, nitrocellulose was present in 1167 of 66,485 cosmetic products of which the composition is known in EWG's Skin Deep Cosmetics Database, USA (http://www.ewg.org/skindeep/).

LITERATURE

1   Adams RM, Maibach HI, Clendenning WE, Fisher AA, Jordan WJ, Kanof N, et al. A five-year study of cosmetic reactions. J Am Acad Dermatol 1985;13:1062-1069
2   Castelain M, Veyrat S, Laine G, Montastier C. Contact dermatitis from nitrocellulose in a nail varnish. Contact Dermatitis 1997;36:266-267
3   Dobes WL, Nippert Ph. Contact eczema due to nail polish. Arch Derm Syph 1944;49:183-187
4   Laguna C, de la Cuadra J, Martín-González B, Zaragoza V, Martínez-Casimiro L, Alegre V. Allergic contact dermatitis to cosmetics. Actas Dermosifiliogr 2009;100:53-60
5   Zaragoza-Ninet V, Blasco Encinas R, Vilata-Corell JJ, Pérez-Ferriols A, Sierra-Talamantes C, Esteve-Martínez A, de la Cuadra-Oyanguren J. Allergic contact dermatitis due to cosmetics: A clinical and epidemiological study in a tertiary hospital. Actas Dermosifiliogr 2016;107:329-336

2.312   3-NITRO-P-HYDROXYETHYLAMINOPHENOL

IDENTIFICATION

Description/definition   : 3-Nitro-*p*-hydroxyethylaminophenol is the substituted aromatic compound phenol that
                              corresponds to the structure shown below
Chemical class(es)   : Amines; color additives – hair; phenols
Chemical/IUPAC name   : 4-((2-Hydroxyethyl)amino)-3-nitrophenol
Other names   : HC red B54; 4-hydroxyethylamino-3-nitrophenol; *N*-(β-hydroxyethyl)-2-nitro-4-
                              hydroxyaminobenzene (probably incorrect name used in ref. 1); 1-hydroxy-3-nitro-4-β-
                              hydroxyethyl-aminobenzene (probably incorrect name used in ref. 7)
CAS registry number(s)   : 65235-31-6
EC number(s)   : 265-648-0
CIR review(s)   : Int J Toxicol 2009;28(Suppl.3):217-251 (access: www.cir-safety.org/ingredients)
SCCS opinion(s)   : SCCP/1036/06 (2)
Function(s) in cosmetics   : EU: hair dyeing. USA: hair colorants
EU cosmetic restrictions   : Regulated in Annex III/248 of the Regulation (EC) No. 344/2013
Patch testing   : 1% pet.
Molecular formula   : $C_8H_{10}N_2O_4$

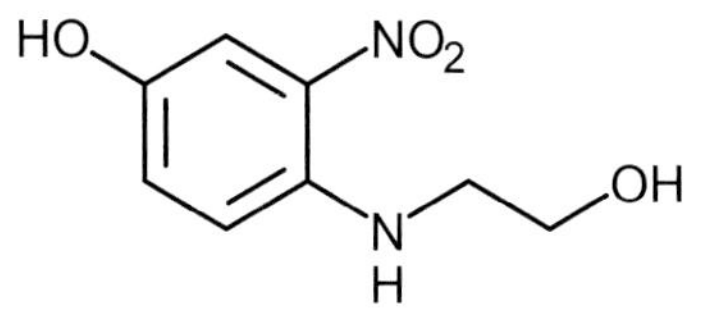

GENERAL

3-Nitro-*p*-hydroxyethylaminophenol belongs to the aminophenol class and is used as a hair colorant, particularly in semi-permanent hair dye preparations (3).

CONTACT ALLERGY

Testing in groups of patients

In 2007-2008, 3-nitro-*p*-hydroxyethylaminophenol 1% pet. was patch tested in 914 consecutive patients seen for suspected contact dermatitis (routine testing) in three European countries. There were 2 (0.2%) positive reactions, but their relevance was not specified (4).

Case reports and case series

One patient had psoriasis-like ACD from 3-nitro-*p*-hydroxyethylaminophenol (termed *N*-(β-hydroxyethyl)-2-nitro-4-hydroxyaminobenzene) in a semi-permanent hair dye (1). A woman developed acute allergic contact dermatitis of the head and neck with severe edema 24 hours after the application of a temporary hair dye. Patch tests with its ingredients were positive to 3-nitro-*p*-hydroxyethylaminophenol tested at 1.35% in ethanol. The hair dye, applied as is on the forearm and rinsed off after 20 minutes, gave a positive reaction after 2 days (3). Two days after applying a coral-red semi-permanent hair dye, a former hairdresser with known allergy to *p*-phenylenediamine and other para-colors developed itchy erythematous-crusted plaques on and behind the ears and in the neck. These lesions subsided in 4 weeks after frequent shampooing and topical corticosteroids. When patch tested with the components of the hair dye, she reacted to 3-nitro-*p*-hydroxyethylaminophenol, which was termed HC Red B54 and 1-hydroxy-3-nitro-4-β-hydroxyethyl-aminobenzene in that report (7).

A woman wanted to dye her hair with a non-permanent hair dye and made the recommended pre-exposure test without any reaction within one day. Then she dyed her hair, following the recommendations carefully with the help of her husband. After one day, she developed a scalp dermatitis with severe itching which spread to her face, neck and upper part of the thorax. As a further complication, the patient developed vesicular hand eczema for the first time in her life. Treatment with systemic and topical steroids was giving for months, leading to gradually clearing of the dermatitis. When patch tested, there were weak positive reactions to *p*-phenylenediamine, to her own hair collected at day 3 after the hair dying, and a positive reaction to 3-nitro-*p*-hydroxyethylaminophenol, an ingredient of the hair dye that had caused the eruption (8). A similar case was reported from France (9,10).

Cross-reactions, pseudo-cross-reactions and co-reactions

3-Nitro-*p*-hydroxyethylaminophenol may cross-react with structurally related chemicals, notably those with a para-structure. Cross-reactivity between para-compounds is discussed in Chapter 2.359 *p*-Phenylenediamine.

Presence in cosmetic products and chemical analyses

In the USA, in April 2017, 3-nitro-*p*-hydroxyethylaminophenol was present in 38 of 56,714 cosmetic products of which the composition is known in FDA's Voluntary Cosmetic Registration Program (VCRP) (data obtained from FDA, May 2017). In March 2017, 3-nitro-*p*-hydroxyethylaminophenol was present in 1 of 64,983 cosmetic products of which the composition is known in EWG's Skin Deep Cosmetics Database, USA (http://www.ewg.org/skindeep/). In southern Germany, in 2013-2014, the labels of 924 permanent oxidative hair dyes were checked for the presence of hair dye components. There were 334 retail products (of seven different brands) and 590 professional products (of six different brands). The 924 products analyzed revealed a total of 58 different hair dye components, with retail products containing 32 and professional products 52. 3-Nitro-*p*-hydroxyethylaminophenol was present in one (0.1%) of the 924 products (6). In 2011, labels and other information on 365 hair dye products (282 permanent dyes, 79 semi-permanent dyes, 4 direct dyes) available on the Danish market (159 hair dyes for private use, 206 for professional use by hairdressers) were collected to identify the presence of sensitizers. 3-Nitro-*p*-hydroxy-ethylaminophenol was present in 2 (0.5%) products (5).

LITERATURE

1   Perno P, Lisi P. Psoriasis-like contact dermatitis from a hair nitro dye. Contact Dermatitis 1990;23:123-124
2   SCCP (Scientific Committee on Consumer Products). Opinion on 3-nitro-*p*-hydroxyethylaminophenol, SCCP/1036/06, 19 December 2006
3   Le Coz, C-J, Kühne S, Engel F. Hair dye allergy due to 3-nitro-*p*-hydroxyethyl-aminophenol. Contact Dermatitis 2003;49:103
4   Søsted H, Rustemeyer T, Gonçalo M, Bruze M, Goossens A, Giménez-Arnau AM, et al. Contact allergy to common ingredients in hair dyes. Contact Dermatitis 2013;69:32-39
5   The Danish Environmental Protection Agency. Survey and occurrence of PPD, PTD and other allergenic hair dye substances in hair dyes. Copenhagen, Denmark: The Danish Environmental Protection Agency, 2013 (ISBN 978-87-92903-92-1). Available at: http://www2.mst.dk/Udgiv/publications/2013/02/978-87-92903-92-1.pdf
6   Kirchlecher S, Hübner A, Uter W. Survey of sensitizing constituents of oxidative hair dyes (retail and professional products) in Germany. J Dtsch Dermatol Ges 2016;14:707-715
7   Sánchez-Pérez J, Río IGD, Ruiz SA, Diez AG. Allergic contact dermatitis from direct dyes for hair colouration in hairdressers' clients. Contact Dermatitis 2004;50:261-262
8   Søsted H, Menné T. Allergy to 3-nitro-*p*-hydroxyethylaminophenol and 4-amino-3-nitrophenol in a hair dye. Contact Dermatitis 2005;52:317-319
9   Dejobert Y, Piette F, Thomas P. Contact dermatitis to 2-hydroxyethylamino-5-nitroanisole and 3-nitro-*p*-hydroxyethyl aminophenol in a hair dye. Contact Dermatitis 2006;54:217-218
10 Dejobert Y, Piette F, Thomas P. Contact dermatitis to 2-hydroxy ethylamino-5-nitroanisole and to 3-nitro-*p*-hydroxyethyl aminophenol in a hair dye, 12th International Contact Dermatitis Symposium, San Francisco, October 14-18, 1999

2.313   2-NITRO-P-PHENYLENEDIAMINE

IDENTIFICATION

Description/definition	: 2-Nitro-*p*-phenylenediamine is the substituted aromatic amine that conforms to the formula shown below
Chemical class(es)	: Amines; color additives - hair
Chemical/IUPAC name	: 2-Nitrobenzene-1,4-diamine
Other names	: CI 76070; *o*-nitro-*p*-phenylenediamine
CAS registry number (s)	: 5307-14-2
EC number(s)	: 226-164-5
CIR review(s)	: J Am Coll Toxicol 1985;4:161-202 (access: www.cir-safety.org/ingredients)
Function(s) in cosmetics	: EU: formerly used for hair dyeing; delisted in 2008. USA: hair colorants
EU cosmetic restrictions	: Regulated in Annex II/1319 of the Regulation (EC) No. 1223/2009 (prohibited)
Patch testing	: 1.0% pet. (Chemotechnique, SmartPracticeEurope, SmartPracticeCanada)
Molecular formula	: $C_6H_7N_3O_2$

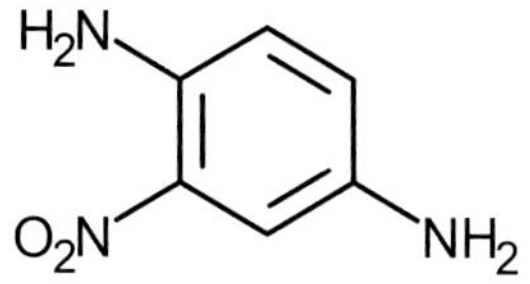

CONTACT ALLERGY

2-Nitro-*p*-phenylenediamine is used in semi-permanent hair dyes; it is also called a 'direct dye' because it does not require mixing with an oxidant. The semi-permanent formulas deposit and adhere to the hair shaft for about 5 to 10 shampoos because dyes are retained by weak, polar and van der Waals forces (4). 2-Nitro-*p*-phenylenediamine was formerly used in the EU and may still be used elsewhere, e.g., in Korea (26).

Patch testing in groups of patients

There are no studies in which 2-nitro-*p*-phenylenediamine was tested in consecutive patients suspected of contact dermatitis (routine testing). However, there are many studies in which the dye has been tested in groups of selected patients, because it is part of most hairdressers series, which is tested in hairdressers and in patients suspected of hair dye allergy. The results of these studies are shown in table 2.313.1. In groups of hairdressers, rates of sensitization ranged from 1.1% in Denmark, 2002-2011 (21) to 23% in Japan (27). In one study, 85% of the 27 positive patch tests were relevant (20); in the other 9 studies in hairdressers, relevance was either not mentioned or not specified. In patients (not hairdressers) suspected of allergy to hair dye or patients tested with a hairdressers series, rates of sensitization ranged from 2.6% (7) to 17.5% (1). Relevance was 100% in two studies (10,23), of which the latter presented only relevant cases. In the other studies, no mention was made of relevance of the positive patch test reactions. The wide range of frequencies of sensitization, both in groups of hairdressers and in non-occupational groups, can likely be explained by different selection criteria.

Case reports and case series

2-Nitro-*p*-phenylenediamine was stated to be the (or an) allergen in 10 patients in a group of 603 individuals suffering from cosmetic dermatitis, seen in the period 2010-2015 in Leuven, Belgium (9). In the period 1996-2013, in a tertiary referral center in Valencia, Spain, 5419 patients were patch tested. Of these, 628 individuals had allergic contact dermatitis to cosmetics. 2-Nitro-*p*-phenylenediamine was the responsible allergen in 18 cases (19, overlap with ref. 16). In the period 2000-2007, 202 patients with allergic contact dermatitis caused by cosmetics were seen in Valencia, Spain. In this group, 7 individuals reacted to 2-nitro-*p*-phenylenediamine from its presence in hair dyes (16, overlap with ref. 19).

In a 4-month-period in 1996, 475 patients with contact allergy to 'cosmetic ingredients' were collected in 5 centers in Belgium, UK and Germany. There were 8 reactions to 2-nitro-*p*-phenylenediamine; relevance was not stated (8). 2-Nitro-*p*-phenylenediamine was responsible for 1 out of 399 cases of cosmetic allergy where the causal allergen was identified in a study of the NACDG, USA, 1977-1983 (2). Two positive patch test reactions to 2-nitro-*p*-phenylenediamine were ascribed to cosmetic allergy (3).

A dental hygienist had allergic contact dermatitis on the inner aspect of her forearm. She reacted to 2-nitro-*p*-phenylenediamine, but not to *p*-phenylenediamine. All her clients were male British soldiers. The author – unconvincingly - ascribed the dermatitis to contact with (still allergenic) dyed hair containing 2-nitro-*p*-phenylenediamine (6). It should be realized that 2-nitro-*p*-phenylenediamine was delisted in 2008 in the EU, which means that recent

European reports of relevant allergy to this dye are virtually impossible, and that the patch test reactions must have been the result of cross-sensitization to other para dyes such as p-phenylenediamine.

Table 2.313.1 Patch testing in groups of patients: Selected patient groups

Years and Country	Test conc. & vehicle	Number of patients tested	positive (%)	Selection of patients (S); Relevance (R); Comments (C)	Ref.
2012-2014 Japan	1% pet.	164	15 (9.1%)	S: patients suspected of allergic contact dermatitis from hair dyes or perming solutions, of who 13% were hairdressers; R: not stated; C: in hairdressers, the frequency of sensitization was 23%, in the non-occupational group 6.5%	27
2002-2011 Denmark		281	3 (1.1%)	S: hairdressers with contact dermatitis; R: not stated	21
2001-2010 Australia	1% pet.	512	96 (15.7%)	S: not stated; R: 33%	17
1993-2010 Australia		164	27 (16.5%)	S: hairdressers and apprentice hairdressers presenting at an occupational dermatology clinic; R: 85%	20
2000-2008 USA	1% pet.	209	(7.2%)	S: patients tested with a hairdresser's series; R: 100%	10
1997-2007 UK	1% pet.	80	14 (17.5%)	S: patients suspected of hair dye allergy; R: not stated	1
1999-2004 UK		428	37 (8.6%)	S: patients tested with the hairdressing series; R: only reactions that were of current or past relevance were collected	23
1994-2003 Spain		300	(7.3%)	S: hairdressers suspected of occupational contact dermatitis; R: not specified	12
2000-2002 Finland		501	(3.2%)	S: patients tested with a hairdressing series; R: not stated	7
<2000 Italy		41	(4.8%)	S: hairdressers with contact dermatitis; R: not specified; C: in the group of 41, sixteen (39%) were diagnosed with occupational allergic contact dermatitis	25
1990-1999 Italy	1% pet.	209	10 (4.7%)	S: hairdressers with contact dermatitis; R: not specified	4
1995-1996 Finland		380	(2.6%)	S: patients tested with a hairdressing series; R: not stated	7
1985-1994 Greece	1% pet.	106	9 (8.4%)	S: hairdressers with contact dermatitis; R: not specified	24
1980-1993 Spain	2% pet.	379	8 (2.1%)	S: hairdressers; R: not specified	14
1988-1991, 8 European countries		798	33 (4.1%)	S: hairdressers with hand dermatitis; R: not stated	13
1985-1990 Italy	1% pet.	261	12 (4.6%)	S: patients with eczema suspected to be caused by hair dying, bleaching or permanent wave solution; R: not stated	11
1985-1990 Italy	1% pet.	302	24 (7.9%)	S: hairdressers with contact dermatitis; R: not specified	15

Cross-reactions, pseudo-cross-reactions and co-reactions

o-Nitro-p-phenylenediamine may cross-react with structurally related chemicals, notably those with a para-structure. Cross-reactivity between para-compounds is discussed in Chapter 2.359 p-Phenylenediamine. No cross-reactions to 11 Food, Drug and Cosmetic (FD&C) dyes were observed in 6 hairdressers allergic to 2-nitro-p-phenylenediamine (5).

Presence in cosmetic products and chemical analyses

In the USA, in April 2017, 2-nitro-p-phenylenediamine was present in of 56,714 cosmetic products of which the composition is known in FDA's Voluntary Cosmetic Registration Program (VCRP) (data obtained from FDA, May 2017). In May 2017, 2-nitro-p-phenylenediamine was present in zero of 66,669 cosmetic products of which the composition is known in EWG's Skin Deep Cosmetics Database, USA (http://www.ewg.org/skindeep/). In 2013-2014, labeled ingredient information from 252 home use and professional hair dye products (210 permanent and 42 non-permanent dyes) from 48 brands sold in Bangkok, Thailand, was collected to identify the type and frequency of potent contact sensitizers. 2-Nitro-p-phenylenediamine was present in 1 (0.4%) products (18). In 2013, in Korea, the labels of 99 oxidative hair dyes produced by Korean domestic manufacturers were examined for potent skin sensitizers. 2-Nitro-p-phenylenediamine was found to be present in 9 (9%) of the hair dyes (26).

In the USA, in 2012, ingredient labels of 107 different consumer oxidative hair dyes from 10 different companies were assessed in stores across the city of Phoenix, Arizona. 2-Nitro-p-phenylenediamine (as free base, sulfate, or HCl) was present in 1 (1%) of the products (22).

LITERATURE

1   Basketter DA, English J. Cross-reactions among hair dye allergens. Cut Ocular Toxicol 2009;28:104-106
2   Adams RM, Maibach HI, Clendenning WE, Fisher AA, Jordan WJ, Kanof N, et al. A five-year study of cosmetic reactions. J Am Acad Dermatol 1985;13:1062-1069
3   Kohl L, Blondeel A, Song M. Allergic contact dermatitis from cosmetics: retrospective analysis of 819 patch-tested patients. Dermatology 2002;204:334-337

4   Iorizzo M, Parente G, Vincenzi C, Pazzaglia M, Tosti A. Allergic contact dermatitis in hairdressers; frequency and source of sensitization. Eur J Dermatol 2002;12:179-182

5   Fautz R, Fuchs A, Van der Walle H, Henny V, Smits L. Hair dye-sensitized hairdressers: the cross-reaction pattern with new generation hair dyes. Contact Dermatitis 2002;46:319-324

6   Hindson C. o-Nitro-paraphenylenediamine in hair dye – an unusual dental hazard. Contact Dermatitis 1975;1:333

7   Hasan T, Rantanen T, Alanko K, Harvima RJ, Jolanki R, Kalimo K, et al. Patch test reactions to cosmetic allergens in 1995–1997 and 2000–2002 in Finland –a multicentre study. Contact Dermatitis 2005;53:40-45

8   Goossens A, Beck MH, Haneke E, McFadden JP, Nolting S, Durupt G, Ries G. Adverse cutaneous reactions to cosmetic allergens. Contact Dermatitis 1999;40:112-113

9   Goossens A. Cosmetic contact allergens. Cosmetics 2016, 3, 5; doi:10.3390/cosmetics3010005

10 Wang MZ, Farmer SA, Richardson DM, Davis MDP. Patch-testing with hairdressing chemicals. Dermatitis 2011;22:16-26

11 Guerra L, Bardazzi F, Tosti A. Contact dermatitis in hairdressers' clients. Contact Dermatitis 1992;26:108-111

12 Valks R, Conde-Salazar L, Malfeito J, Ledo S. Contact dermatitis in hairdressers, 10 years later: patch-test results in 300 hairdressers (1994 to 2003) and comparison with previous study. Dermatitis 2005;16:28-31

13 Frosch PJ, Burrows D, Camarasa JG, Dooms-Goossens A, Ducombs G, Lahti A, et al. Allergic reactions to a hairdressers' series: results from 9 European centres. Contact Dermatitis 1993;28:180-183

14 Conde-Salazar L, Baz M, Guimaraens D, Cannavo A. Contact dermatitis in hairdressers: patch test results in 379 hairdressers (1980-1993). Am J Cont Dermat 1995;6:19-23

15 Guerra L, Tosti A, Bardazzi F, Pigatto P, Lisi P, Santucci B, et al. Contact dermatitis in hairdressers: the Italian experience. Contact Dermatitis 1992;26:101-107

16 Laguna C, de la Cuadra J, Martín-González B, Zaragoza V, Martínez-Casimiro L, Alegre V. Allergic contact dermatitis to cosmetics. Actas Dermosifiliogr 2009;100:53-60

17 Toholka R, Wang Y-S, Tate B, Tam M, Cahill J, Palmer A, Nixon R. The first Australian Baseline Series: Recommendations for patch testing in suspected contact dermatitis. Australas J Dermatol 2015;56:107-115

18 Boonchai W, Bunyavaree M, Winayanuwattikun W, Kasemsarn P. Contact sensitizers in commercial hair dye products sold in Thailand. Contact Dermatitis 2016;74:222-229

19 Zaragoza-Ninet V, Blasco Encinas R, Vilata-Corell JJ, Pérez-Ferriols A, Sierra-Talamantes C, Esteve-Martínez A, de la Cuadra-Oyanguren J. Allergic contact dermatitis due to cosmetics: A clinical and epidemiological study in a tertiary hospital. Actas Dermosifiliogr 2016;107:329-336

20 Lyons G, Roberts H, Palmer A, Matheson M, Nixon R. Hairdressers presenting to an occupational dermatology clinic in Melbourne, Australia. Contact Dermatitis 2013;68:300-306

21 Schwensen JF, Johansen JD, Veien NK, Funding AT, Avnstorp C, Østerballe M, et al. Occupational contact dermatitis in hairdressers: an analysis of patch test data from the Danish Contact Dermatitis Group, 2002–2011. Contact Dermatitis 2014;70:233-237

22 Hamann D, Yazar K, Hamann CR, Thyssen JP, Lidén C. p-Phenylenediamine and other allergens in hair dye products in the United States: a consumer exposure study. Contact Dermatitis 2014;70:213-218

23 Katugampola RP, Statham BN, English JSC, Wilkinson MM, Foulds IS, Green CM, Ormerod AD, et al. A multicentre review of the hairdressing allergens tested in the UK. Contact Dermatitis 2005;53:130-132

24 Katsarou A, Koufou B, Takou K, Kalogeromitros D, Papanayiotou G, Vareltzidis A. Patch test results in hairdressers with contact dermatitis in Greece (1985-1994). Contact Dermatitis 1995;33:347-348

25 Lodi A, Mancini LL, Ambonati M, Coassini A, Ravanelli G, Crosti C. Epidemiology of occupational contact dermatitis in a North Italian population. Eur J Dermatol 2000;10:128-132

26 Kim H, Kim K. Prevalence of potent skin sensitizers in oxidative hair dye products in Korea. Cutan Ocul Toxicol 2016;35:204-207

27 Ito A, Nishioka K, Kanto H, Yagami A, Yamada S, Sugiura M, et al. A multi-institutional joint study of contact dermatitis related to hair colouring and perming agents in Japan. Contact Dermatitis 2017;77:42-48

2.314   NORDIHYDROGUAIARETIC ACID

IDENTIFICATION

Description/definition   : Nordihydroguaiaretic acid is the organic compound that conforms to the formula shown
                            below
Chemical class(es)   : Phenols
Chemical/IUPAC name   : 4-[4-(3,4-Dihydroxyphenyl)-2,3-dimethylbutyl]benzene-1,2-diol
Other names   : 4,4'-(2,3-Dimethyltetramethylene)dipyrocatechol
CAS registry number (s)   : 500-38-9
EC number(s)   : 207-903-0
Merck Index monograph   : 8052
Function(s) in cosmetics : EU: antioxidant. USA: antioxidants
Patch testing   : 2% pet. (1)
Molecular formula   : $C_{18}H_{22}O_4$

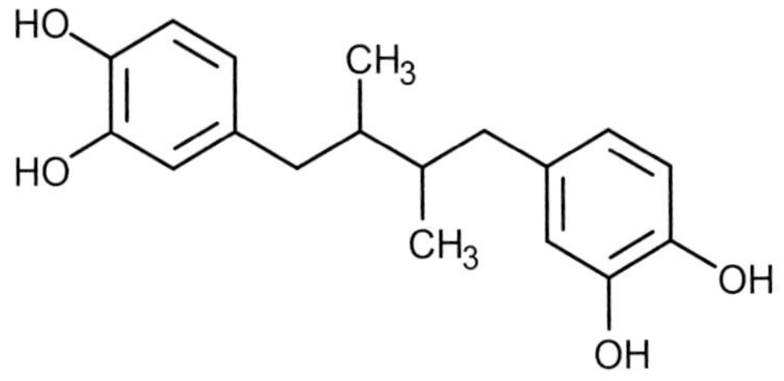

CONTACT ALLERGY

Patch testing in groups of patients

Between 1971 and 1975, 111 selected patients (selection criteria not mentioned) were patch tested with nordihy-droguaiaretic acid 2% pet. and 6 (5.4%) had a positive reaction. Three of them reacted to the antioxidant in lanolin cream, the relevance in the others was unknown (1).

Case reports and case series

Three patients had contact allergy to nordihydroguaiaretic acid in a (lanolin) cream (1). One patient had allergic contact dermatitis from nordihydroguaiaretic acid in the same cream (2). Another individual was allergic to the antioxidant in a cosmetic cream (3).

Contact allergy to nordihydroguaiaretic acid in non-cosmetic products

Preparation of vitamin A-D tablets at a pharmaceutical factory caused occupational dermatitis from nordihydro-guaiaretic acid in one patient (2).

Presence in cosmetic products and chemical analyses

In the USA, in April 2017, nordihydroguaiaretic acid was present in 103 of 56,714 cosmetic products of which the composition is known in FDA's Voluntary Cosmetic Registration Program (VCRP) (data obtained from FDA, May 2017). In March 2017, nordihydroguaiaretic acid was present in 11 of 65,431 cosmetic products of which the composition is known in EWG's Skin Deep Cosmetics Database, USA (http://www.ewg.org/skindeep/).

LITERATURE

1   Roed-Petersen J, Hjorth N. Contact dermatitis from antioxidants. Br J Dermatol 1976;94:233-241
2   Jørgensen G, Hjorth N. Dermatitis from nordihydroguaiaretic acid, an antioxidant in fats. Contact
    Dermatitis Newsletter 1970;7:151
3   Hjorth N. Cited by Fisher AA. Reactions to antioxidants in cosmetics and foods. Cutis 1976;17:21-25

2.315 OCTOCRYLENE

IDENTIFICATION

Description/definition	: Octocrylene is the substituted acrylate that conforms to the formula shown below
Chemical class(es)	: Esters
Chemical/IUPAC name	: 2-Ethylhexyl 2-cyano-3,3-diphenylprop-2-enoate
Other names	: 2-Cyano-3,3-diphenylacrylic acid 2'-ethylhexyl ester; 2'-ethylhexyl 2-cyano-3-phenylcinnamate; 2-ethylhexyl-2-cyano-3,3-diphenylacrylate
CAS registry number (s)	: 6197-30-4
EC number(s)	: 228-250-8
Merck Index monograph	: 8115
Function(s) in cosmetics	: EU: UV-absorber; UV-filter. USA: light stabilizers; sunscreen agents
EU cosmetic restrictions	: Regulated in Annex VI/10 of the Regulation (EC) No. 1223/2009
Patch testing	: 10% pet. (Chemotechnique, SmartPracticeCanada). It appears that photopatch testing with the commercial octocrylene test substance may sometimes be false-negative (48)
Molecular formula	: $C_{24}H_{27}NO_2$

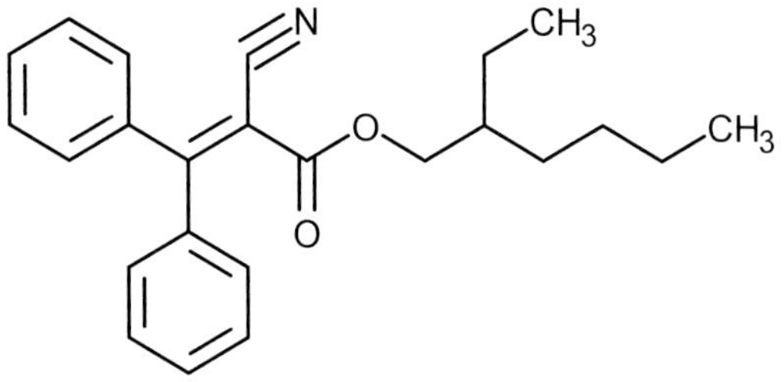

GENERAL

Octocrylene is a relatively new UVB filter with UV absorbance maximum (λ_{max}) at 303 nm (57). It belongs to the cinnamate family, and was introduced in the late 1990s (8). It is not a very effective filter and for this reason, octocrylene is usually combined with other UVB agents to increase the SPF of a sunscreen product, notably other cinnamates (1). However, octocrylene has excellent photostability and is used as stabilizer for other photo-unstable UV-filters (1,5) and to also improve their overall stability and water resistance (3). This applies particularly to the widely used UVA-filter butyl methoxydibenzoylmethane. This UV-absorber is not only used in sunscreen preparations, but also in skin care cosmetics such as day creams and anti-aging creams, to retard photodegradation of the product, extend its shelf-life and protect the consumer from UV-damage (3).

Currently, it appears that, generally speaking, in the USA and European countries, the majority (in some countries >80%) of sunscreens may contain octocrylene; also, this UV-absorber may be present in over 20% of daily skin care cosmetics (4, for details see 'Presence in cosmetic products and chemical analyses' below). A non-cosmetic application of octocrylene is in the protection of plastics, coatings and adhesives from ultraviolet radiation (www.syrgis.com).

Since 2003, several studies have indicated that octocrylene not infrequently causes photocontact allergy / photoallergic contact dermatitis, notably in adult patients previously photosensitized to ketoprofen in topical medications. Allergic contact dermatitis is seen to a lesser degree, usually in children, and is caused by sensitization to octocrylene in sunscreen products (4).

A full review of contact allergy and photocontact allergy to octocrylene up to 2014 is provided in ref. 4. The literature on adverse reactions to (other) sunscreens has been reviewed in several recent and older publications (6,9,16,36,37,47). A review of photocontact allergy to sunscreens was published in 2010 (58).

CONTACT ALLERGY

Patch testing in groups of patients

There is one study in which octocrylene has been patch tested in consecutive patients suspected of contact dermatitis (routine testing), which was performed in 2015-2016 by a subgroup of the IVDK (60). Of 2577 patients tested with octocrylene 10% pet., only 2 (0.1%) had a positive reaction. One of them also reacted to a sunscreen product containing octocrylene (60). Results of testing in groups of *selected* patients (e.g., patients suspected of photosensitivity, patients with dermatitis affecting mainly light-exposed skin or with a history of a skin reaction to a sunscreen or a topical NSAID) are shown in table 2.315.1. In five studies, frequencies of sensitization have ranged from 0.7% to 5%, the latter percentage being the result of 1 positive reaction in a group of 20 patients (18). In two studies, relevance was not mentioned or specified for octocrylene (19,21), in the other relevance was 18% (20) and 100% (17,18).

Table 2.315.1 Patch testing in groups of patients: Selected patient groups

Years and Country	Test conc. & vehicle	Number of patients tested	positive (%)		Selection of patients (S); Relevance (R); Comments (C)	Ref.
2008-2011 12 European countries	10% pet.	1031	7	(0.7%)	S: patients with exposed site dermatitis or history of a reaction to a sunscreen or topical NSAID; R: not specified	21
2001-2010 Canada		160	7	(4.4%)	S: patients with suspected photosensitivity and patients who developed pruritus or a rash after sunscreen application; R: not stated; C: weak study: inadequate reading of test results, erythema only was considered to represent a positive patch test reaction; of the 7 patients, 1 had photo-aggravated allergic contact dermatitis	19
2000-2010 Belgium	10% pet.	172	5	(2.9%)	S: patients with (suspected) adverse reactions to sunscreen products and/or ketoprofen; R: all had sunscreen intolerance and 2/5 had previously used ketoprofen gel; C: 1 of the 5 patients had photo-aggravation from octocrylene and two were photoallergic to ketoprofen (2 others were not tested with ketoprofen) and benzophenone-3 (the two that had used ketoprofen gel); two children (3 and 11), 3 adults	17
2004-2006 Italy	5% pet.	1082	9	(0.8%)	S: patients with histories and clinical features suggestive of photoallergic contact dermatitis; R: 18%; all 9 were cases of photo-aggravated contact allergy	20
2004 Belgium	10% pet.	20	1	(5%)	S: patients suspected of sunscreen allergy; R: 100%	18

IVDK: Information Network of Departments of Dermatology, Germany, Austria, Switzerland

Case reports and case series

Case series

Octocrylene was stated to be the (or an) allergen in 2 patients in a group of 603 individuals suffering from cosmetic dermatitis, seen in the period 2010-2015 in Leuven, Belgium (51). In the period 1996-2013, in a tertiary referral center in Valencia, Spain, 5419 patients were patch tested. Of these, 628 individuals had allergic contact dermatitis to cosmetics. Octocrylene was the responsible allergen in seven cases (54). From 2007 to 2012, 131 positive patch tests and photopatch tests were notified to the French network REVIDAL/GERDA (Réseau de Vigilance en Dermatoallergologie / Groupe d'Etudes et de Recherche en Dermatoallergologie (22) in France. About 20% were young children who mostly suffered from allergic contact dermatitis from octocrylene in sunscreens (80% of the 131 reactions were *photo*allergic). Other clinical data were not provided (23). These data probably include patients from previously published communications (3,24,25,26,27,52). In 2010, 10 children were described who had suffered from allergic contact dermatitis caused by sunscreens containing octocrylene. All had positive patch tests to octocrylene and one or more of the sunscreens (3). In the same study, 6 adults with contact allergy to octocrylene were described (3).

Octocrylene was responsible for 10 out of 959 cases of non-fragrance cosmetic allergy where the causal allergen was identified, Belgium, 2000-2010 (28). Some of these patients have probably been presented in an earlier study (3).

Case reports

Case reports of contact allergy to octocrylene in sunscreen products include one child from Spain (29), two children from Spain (30), a child from Belgium (31), one adult and a child from the UK (32,33), an adult from France (26), a child from Belgium (18), two children from the UK (34), another child from the UK (7), and a young girl suffering from atopic dermatitis and photosensitivity from Denmark (55).

Presence in cosmetic products and chemical analyses

In June 2017, octocrylene was present in 1002 of 68,866 cosmetic products of which the composition is known in EWG's Skin Deep Cosmetics Database, USA (http://www.ewg.org/skindeep/). It should be realized that sunscreen products containing UV-filters are classified as drugs in the USA, not as cosmetics; the number mentioned here, therefore, is that of cosmetics containing the UV-filter, but it does *not* include their presence in sunscreens. In the USA, in April 2017, octocrylene was present in 134 of 56,714 cosmetic products of which the composition is known in FDA's Voluntary Cosmetic Registration Program (VCRP) (data obtained from FDA, May 2017). In The Netherlands, in 2013, >80% of 50 sunscreens randomly collected by The Netherlands Food and Consumer Product Safety Authority proved to contain octocrylene (cited in ref. 4). In Switzerland, in 2011, 33 of 39 sunscreens (85%) contained octocrylene and the UV-filter was present in 17 of 77 (22%) other cosmetic products. Concentrations ranged from 1% to 9.9% with a mean and median of approximately 6%, with similar results in sunscreens and other cosmetics, intended for daily use. This means that the latter widely used product category may be an important source of exposure to octocrylene (15,53). In the UK in 2010, 91% of 337 sunscreens were found to contain octocrylene (13); in a similar UK study performed in 2005, the percentage was only 36 (14).

In the USA, the combination of octocrylene and butyl methoxydibenzoylmethane was not present in any of 48 commercial sunscreens purchased in 1999 in the USA (12). In 2003, it was identified in 12% of 118 sunscreens and in 2009, over half (54%) of 141 commercial sunscreens were found to contain octocrylene + butyl methoxy-dibenzoylmethane. In the same period, the frequency of their combined presence in cosmetic products not specifically intended for protection against UV rose from zero to 23% (12). Also in the USA, sunscreen products were purchased and evaluated in 1997 (n=59), 2003 (n=188) and again in 2009 (n=330) (56). A combination of octocrylene with butyl methoxydibenzoylmethane was found in 0% in 1997, in 12% in 2003 and in 36% of the products in 2009 (56).

In Germany, octocrylene was present in 30.7% of 4447 cosmetic products collected in the period 2006-2009 (2). Of 35 cosmetic products purchased in 2008 in France claiming a SPF between 4 and 30 (6 day creams, 8 anti-aging creams, 10 tinted face creams and foundations, 6 self-tanning lotions, 1 skin lightening cream, 2 anti-redness creams and 2 spot remover creams), ten (29%) contained octocrylene (11). In 2001, in Denmark, 17/75 (23%) sunscreen products, creams and lotions from 30 cosmetic manufacturers contained octocrylene; the concentration range was 1.2-10.4% (10).

OTHER SIDE EFFECTS

Photosensitivity
Photocontact allergy / photoallergic contact dermatitis is the most frequent adverse effect of octocrylene, accounting for some 80% of all reactions and is seen mainly in adults (23). Most such cases are probably secondary to previous photosensitisation to ketoprofen, mostly from topical preparations.

Photopatch testing in groups of patients
There have been several studies in which groups of selected patients (e.g., patients suspected of photosensitivity, patients with dermatitis affecting mainly light-exposed skin or with a history of a skin reaction to a sunscreen or a

Table 2.315.2 Photopatch testing in groups of patients

Years and Country	Test conc. & vehicle	Number of patients tested | positive (%)		Selection of patients (S); Relevance (R); Comments (C)	Ref.
2008-2011 12 European countries	10% pet.	1031	41 (4.0%)	S: patients with exposed site dermatitis or history of a reaction to a sunscreen or topical NSAID; R: 54% current relevance, 34% due to ketoprofen photosensitivity, 15% unknown relevance; C: rates ranged from 0% to 32% in different countries; most frequent photocontact allergen among the UV-filters	21
2000-2010 Belgium	10% pet.	90	18 (20%)	S: patients with (suspected) adverse reactions to sunscreen products and/or ketoprofen; R: 15/18 had sunscreen intolerance, of who 12 previously had used or reacted to ketoprofen gel; 3 had reacted to ketoprofen previously, but had no known sunscreen intolerance; C: 15/18 patients also had a positive photopatch test to ketoprofen (3 were not tested) and 13/18 had a positive photopatch test to benzophenone-3	17
2004-2006 Italy	5% pet.	1082	14 (1.3%)	S: patients with histories and clinical features suggestive of photoallergic contact dermatitis; R: 18%; C: most frequent photocontact allergen among the UV-filters; there were an additional 9 cases of contact allergy with photo-aggravation	20
2004 Belgium	10% pet.	20	1 (5%)	S: patients suspected of sunscreen allergy; R: 100%; the patient was also photoallergic to ketoprofen	18

topical NSAID) have been photopatch tested with octocrylene (table 2.315.2). Rates of photosensitization have ranged from 1.3% to 20%. The latter percentage was found in Belgium and can easily be explained by the fact that topical ketoprofen preparations are widely used in that country and by the fact that the clinic reporting these data is highly specialized in cosmetic allergy (17). In general, high frequencies of reactions to octocrylene were accompanied by high numbers of photosensitization to ketoprofen (17,21). Relevance rates varied from 18% to 100%.

Case series and case reports

Case series

From 2007 to 2012, 131 positive patch tests and photopatch tests were notified to the French network REVIDAL /GERDA (Réseau de Vigilance en Dermatoallergologie / Groupe d'Etudes et de Recherche en Dermatoallergologie (22) in France. About 80% were adult patients with a history of photoallergic contact dermatitis from ketoprofen who mostly suffered from photoallergic contact dermatitis from octocrylene (20% of the 131 were young children who mostly had allergic contact dermatitis from octocrylene in sunscreens). Other clinical data were not provided (abstract) (23). These data probably include patients from previously published communications (3,24,25,26,27).

In 2010, 22 adult patients were described aged 18-69 (mean 40) years, of who nearly all had a history of ketoprofen photoallergic contact dermatitis (3). All had positive photopatch tests to octocrylene and 12 (55%) to one or more of the sunscreens containing octocrylene used by them (3). The other 10 had a history of sunscreen intolerance, so all 22 photopatch test reactions were considered to be relevant (3).

Octocrylene photocontact allergy was responsible for 28 out of 959 cases of (non-fragrance) contact dermatitis, where the causal allergen was identified, Belgium, 2000-2010 (28). Some of these patients have probably been presented in an earlier study (3). Four patients with positive photopatch test reactions to octocrylene and benzophenone-3, of which 3 also photo-reacted to ketoprofen, were reported from Spain. Only one reaction to octocrylene was clinically relevant (35). Other studies in which positive photopatch tests to octocrylene have been reported in relation to ketoprofen photosensitization include refs. 3,21,40,41,43,44 and 45.

Case reports

Case reports of photocontact allergy to octocrylene in sunscreens include a child (29) and two adults (38) from Spain, one (26) and two (39) adult patients from France, an 48-year-old man from Belgium (18) and an adult from Italy (50). Most had a history of photoallergic reactions to ketoprofen gel.

Photocross-reactions, pseudo-cross-reactions and co-reactions

Some patients in early reports on photoallergic contact dermatitis from octocrylene-containing sunscreens (18,39) reported a history of reactions to ketoprofen gel (a non-steroidal anti-inflammatory drug) and the possible relationship was first discussed in 2008 (40) and was later confirmed (3). Topical ketoprofen products have caused many cases of photoallergic contact dermatitis, notably in France, Spain, Italy and Belgium (20,21,40,41,42), countries where these products are widely used. From the data of various studies (3,21,40,41,43,44,45) it has been concluded (4) that ketoprofen photosensitivity in a considerable number of the patients leads to octocrylene (27-80%) and to benzophenone-3 (17-64%) photocontact allergy. Conversely, octocrylene photocontact allergy is in the great majority (probably >80%) of cases the result of ketoprofen photosensitization (3,4,17,21). The co-reactions to benzophenone-3 can be explained as photocross-sensitization to primary ketoprofen photosensitization (46,4), but for octocrylene the pathomechanism of co-reactivity is less clear (4).

Miscellaneous side effects

Erythema multiforme of the oral mucosa was – highly unconvincingly – ascribed to octocrylene in a facial cream (49).

LITERATURE

1   Palm MD, O'Donoghue MN. Update on photoprotection. Dermatol Ther 2007;20:360-376
2   Uter W, Gonçalo M, Yazar K, Kratz E-M, Mildau G, Lidén C. Coupled exposure to ingredients of cosmetic products: III. Ultraviolet filters. Contact Dermatitis 2014;71:162-169
3   Avenel-Audran M, Dutartre H, Goossens A, Jeanmougin M, Comte C, Bernier C, et al. Octocrylene, an emerging photoallergen. Arch Dermatol 2010;146:753-757
4   De Groot AC, Roberts DW. Contact and photocontact allergy to octocrylene: a review. Contact Dermatitis 2014;70:193-204
5   Herzog B, Wehrle M, Quass K. Photostability of UV absorber systems in sunscreens. Photochem Photobiol 2009;85:869-878
6   Heurung AR, Raju SI, Warshaw EM. Adverse reactions to sunscreen agents: epidemiology, responsible irritants and allergens, clinical characteristics, and management. Dermatitis 2014;25:289-326
7   Haylett AK, Chiang YZ, Nie Z, Ling TC, Rhodes LE. Sunscreen photopatch testing: a series of 157 children. Br J Dermatol 2014;171:370-375
8   Kerr A, Ferguson J. Photoallergic contact dermatitis. Photodermatol Photoimmunol Photomed 2010;26:56-65

9   Heurung AR, Raju SI, Warshaw EM. Contact allergen of the year. Benzophenones. Dermatitis 2014;25:3-10
     (contains many mistakes; Erratum in Dermatitis 2014;25:92-95)

10   Rastogi SC. UV filters in sunscreen products - a survey. Contact Dermatitis 2002;46:348-351

11   Séhédic D, Hardy-Boismartel A, Couteau C, Coiffard LJ. Are cosmetic products which include an SPF appropriate
     for daily use? Arch Dermatol Res 2009;301:603-608

12   Wang SQ, Tanner PR, Lim HW, Nash JF. The evolution of sunscreen products in the United States – a 12-year
     cross sectional study. Photochem Photobiol Sci 2013;12:197-202

13   Kerr AC. A survey of the availability of sunscreen filters in the UK. Clin Exp Dermatol 2011;36:541-543

14   Wahie S, Lloyd JJ, Farr PM. Sunscreen ingredients and labelling: a survey of products available in the UK. Clin Exp
     Dermatol 2007;32:359-364

15   Manová E, von Goetz N, Hauri U, Bogdal C, Hungerbühler K. Organic UV filters in personal care products in
     Switzerland: A survey of occurrence and concentrations. Int J Hyg Environ Health 2013;216:508-514

16   Avenel-Audran M. Sunscreen products: finding the allergen. Eur J Dermatol 2010;20:161-166

17   Karlsson I, VandenBroecke K, Martensson J, Goossens A, Börje A. Clinical and experimental studies of
     octocrylene's allergenic potency. Contact Dermatitis 2011;64:343-352

18   Delplace D, Blondeel A. Octocrylene: really non-allergenic? Contact Dermatitis 2006;54:295

19   Greenspoon J, Ahluwalia R, Juma N, Rosen CF. Allergic and photoallergic contact dermatitis: A 10-year
     experience. Dermatitis 2013;24:29-32

20   Pigatto PD, Guzzi G, Schena D, Guarrera M, Foti C, Francalanci S, et al. Photopatch tests: an Italian multicentre
     study from 2004 to 2006. Contact Dermatitis 2008;59:103-108

21   The European Multicentre Photopatch Test Study (EMCPPTS) Taskforce. A European multicentre photopatch test
     study. Br J Dermatol 2012;166:1002-1009

22   Vigan M. REVIDAL-GERDA: Organisation et collaboration avec la pharmaco vigilance. Therapie 2002;57:263-264

23   Avenel-Audran M and the members of the REVIDAL/GERDA. Update on octocrylene (photo)allergy (Abstract).
     Photoderm Photoimmunol Photomed 2012;28:283

24   Avenel-Audran M, Comte C, Dutartre H, Ferrier-Lebouëdec M-C, Benkalfate L, Outtas A, et al. Attention à
     l'octocrylène ! Les cas de photo-allergie se multiplient. La Lettre du GERDA (Numéro spécial) 2008;20:2

25   Du-Thanh A, Comte C, Guillot B, et al. L'octocrylène, un photoallergène rarement incriminé ? Communication
     affichée GERDA Paris 09/2007 (Poster presentation)

26   Avenel-Audran M. L'octocrylène : un photoallergène emergent (Abstract)? Ann Dermatol Venereol
     2007;134:7S273

27   Avenel-Audran M. Vigilance activée sur l'octocrylène, il continue à sévir! (Abstract). Nouv Dermatol
     2008;27(Suppl. 5):65

28   Travassos AR, Claes L, Boey L, Drieghe J, Goossens A. Non-fragrance allergens in specific cosmetic products.
     Contact Dermatitis 2011;65:276-285

29   Agustí-Mejias A, Messeguer F, de la Cuadra J, Martorell-Aragonés A. Contact allergy to octocrylene in children: A
     report of 2 cases. Actas Dermosifiliogr 2014;105:92-93

30   Macías E, González AM, De Lamas C, Ponce V, Muñoz-Bellido F, Moreno E. Allergic contact dermatitis due to
     sensitisation to sunscreen in two infants. Allergol Immunopathol. (Madr) 2013;41:419-420

31   Dumon D, Dekeuleneer V, Tennstedt D, Goossens A, Baeck M. Allergic contact dermatitis caused by octocrylene
     in a young child. Contact Dermatitis 2012;67:240-242

32   Alexandroff AB, Gawkrodger DJ. Update on contact dermatitis 2007: Medical pearls from the annual meeting of
     the British Contact Dermatitis Society at the annual meeting of the British Association of Dermatologists.
     J Derm Sci 2008;51:220-223

33   Kaushal G, Orton D. Contact dermatitis to octocrylene (Abstract). Br J Dermatol 2007;57(Suppl. 1):81

34   Madan V, Beck MH. Contact allergy to octocrylene in sunscreen with recurrence from passive transfer of a
     cosmetic. Contact Dermatitis 2005;53:241-242

35   Curto-Barredo L, Lopez-Aventin D, Pujol RM, et al. Relevance assessment of ultraviolet sunscreen photoallergy as
     an evolving concept (Abstract). Contact Dermatitis 2012;66(Suppl. 2):83

36   Scheuer E, Warshaw E. Sunscreen allergy: a review of epidemiology, clinical characteristics, and responsible
     allergens. Dermatitis 2006;17:3-11

37   Funk JO, Dromgoole SH, Maibach HI. Sunscreen intolerance: contact sensitization, photocontact sensitization,
     and irritancy of sunscreen agents. Dermatol Clin 1995;13:473-481

38   Bennàssar A, Grimalt R, Romaguera C, Vilaplana J. Two cases of photocontact allergy to the new sun filter
     octocrylene. Dermatol Online J 2009;15:14

39   Carrotte-Lefebvre I, Bonnevalle A, Segard M, Delaporte E, Thomas P. Contact allergy to octocrylene – first 2
     cases. Contact Dermatitis 2003;48:46-47

40   Devleeschouwer V, Roelandts R, Garmyn M, Goossens A. Allergic and photoallergic contact dermatitis from
     ketoprofen: results of (photo)patch testing and follow-up of 42 patients. Contact Dermatitis 2008;58:159-166

41 Durbize E, Vigan M, Puzenat E, Girardin P, Adessi B, Desprez PH, et al. Spectrum of cross-photosensitisation in 18 consecutive patients with contact photoallergy to ketoprofen: associated photoallergies to non-benzophenone-containing molecules. Contact Dermatitis 2003;48:144-149

42 Foti C, Bonamonte D, Conserva A, Stingeni L, Lisi P, Lionetti N, et al. Allergic and photoallergic contact dermatitis from ketoprofen: evaluation of cross-reactivities by a combination of photopatch testing and computerized conformational analysis. Curr Pharm Des 2008;14:2833-2839

43 Veyrac G, Leroux A, Ruellan AL, Bernier C, Jolliet P. Kétoprofène gel et octocrylène : étude des réactions photoallergiques associées à partir des cas nantais de la base nationale de pharmacovigilance (Abstract). Rev Franç d'Allergol 2012;52:277

44 Bonnevalle A, Thomas P. Cross-reactions between ketoprofen and octocrylene (abstract). Nouvelles Dermatologiques 2008;27(Suppl. 5):64

45 Le Coz CJ, Bottlaender A, Scrivener JN, Santinelli F, Cribier BJ, Heid E, et al. Photocontact dermatitis from ketoprofen and tiaprofenic acid: cross-reactivity study in 12 consecutive patients. Contact Dermatitis 1998;38:245-252

46 Sugiura M, Hayakawa R, Xie Z, Sugiura K, Hiramoto K, Shamoto M. Experimental study on phototoxicity and the photosensitisation potential of ketoprofen, suprofen, tiaprofenic acid and benzophenone and the photocross-reactivity in guinea pigs. Photodermatol Photoimmunol Photomed 2002;18:82-89

47 Dromgoole SH, Maibach HI. Sunscreening agent intolerance: Contact and photocontact sensitization and contact urticaria. J Am Acad Dermatol 1990;22:1068-1078

48 Aerts O, Goossens A, Bervoets A, Lambert J. Almost missed it! Photo-contact allergy to octocrylene in a ketoprofen-sensitized subject. Dermatitis 2016;27:33-34

49 Farquharson AA, Stoopler ET, Houston AM, Brown RS. Erythema multiforme major secondary to a cosmetic facial cream: first case report. Oral Surg Oral Med Oral Pathol Oral Radiol 2016;121:e10-15

50 Martina E, Rosa L, Postacchini V, Simonetti O, Cataldi I, Offidani A. Photoprotection and photodermatitis: a case. Contact Dermatitis.2017;76:54-55

51 Goossens A. Cosmetic contact allergens. Cosmetics 2016, 3, 5; doi:10.3390/cosmetics3010005

52 Avenel-Audran M, Comte C, Dutartre H, et al. Vigilance activée sur l'octocrylène! Il continue a` sévir.... Nouv Dermatol 2008;27 Suppl.5:65

53 Manová E, von Goetz N, Hungerbühler K. Ultraviolet filter contact and photocontact allergy: consumer exposure and risk assessment for octocrylene from personal care products and sunscreens. Br J Dermatol 2014;171:1368-1374

54 Zaragoza-Ninet V, Blasco Encinas R, Vilata-Corell JJ, Pérez-Ferriols A, Sierra-Talamantes C, Esteve-Martínez A, de la Cuadra-Oyanguren J. Allergic contact dermatitis due to cosmetics: A clinical and epidemiological study in a tertiary hospital. Actas Dermosifiliogr 2016;107:329-336

55 Simonsen AB, Koppelhus, U, Sommerlund M, Deleuran M. Photosensitivity in atopic dermatitis complicated by contact allergy to common sunscreen ingredients. Contact Dermatitis 2016;74:56-58

56 Wang SQ, Tanner PR, Lim HW, Nash JF. The evolution of sunscreen products in the United States- a 12-year cross sectional study. Photochem Photobiol Sci 2013;12:197-202

57 Shaath NA. Ultraviolet filters. Photochem Photobiol Sci 2010;9:464-469

58 Shaw T, Simpson B, Wilson B, Oostman H, Rainey D, Storrs F. True photoallergy to sunscreens is rare despite popular belief. Dermatitis 2010;21:185-198

59 Schauder S. Survey of the literature on adverse reactions to preparations containing UV filters (1947-1989) (Literaturübersicht über Unverträglichkeitsreaktionen auf lichtfilterhaltige Produkte von 1947 bis 1989). Z Hautkr 1990;65:982-998 (article in German)

60 Uter W, Lessmann H, Geier J, for the IVDK. Is octocrylene a frequent contact allergen?. Contact Dermatitis 2017;77:127-128

2.316   OCTYLDODECANOL

IDENTIFICATION

Description/definition   : Octyldodecanol is an aliphatic alcohol that conforms to the formula shown below
Chemical class(es)   : Alcohols
Chemical/IUPAC name   : 2-Octyldodecan-1-ol
CAS registry number (s) : 5333-42-6
EC number(s)   : 226-242-9
CIR review(s)   : J Am Coll Toxicol 1985;4:1-29 (access: www.cir-safety.org/ingredients)
Merck Index monograph   : 8126
Function(s) in cosmetics : EU: emollient; masking; perfuming. USA: fragrance ingredients; skin-conditioning agents
                           - emollient
Patch testing   : 3% pet. (1); 1% water (1);13.5% in liquid paraffin (2) or water (4); 13.5%, 1.35% and
                           0.675% in liquid paraffin (3); 13.5% in water is not irritant (4)
Molecular formula   : $C_{20}H_{42}O$

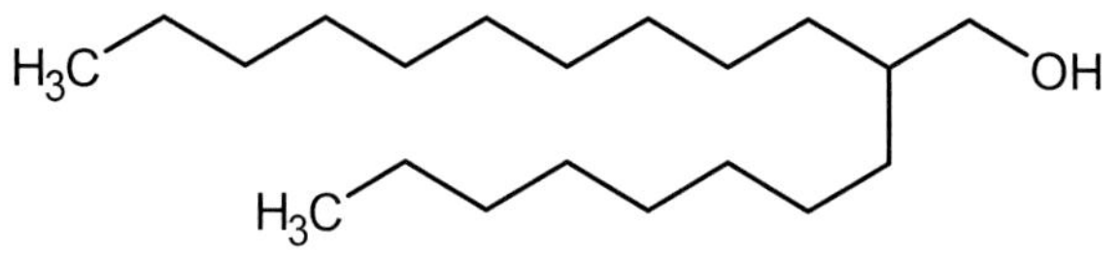

CONTACT ALLERGY

Case reports and case series

Two patients had dermatitis from contact allergy to octyldodecanol in a cosmetic anti-itch cream. One of them, a woman, presented with a 2-year history of perianal irritation, which had recently worsened and spread to the vulval area after applying the anti-itch cream. The second patient, a man, presented with a 5-year history of psoriasis. In the previous 12 months, he had developed a more widespread eczematous eruption confirmed on histology. He had been treated with topical corticosteroids, emollients, and the anti-itch relief cream, which he had bought over the counter 1 year previously. In both patients, patch tests were positive to the cream and its component octyldodecanol (1).

A woman reacted to octyldodecanol in a moisturizing lotion and an antimycotic pharmaceutical product (4). Another female patient had allergic contact cheilitis from octyldodecanol and candelilla wax in a lip balm (6).

Contact allergy to octyldodecanol in non-cosmetic products

Three patient were allergic to octyldodecanol in antimycotic pharmaceutical creams (2,3,4).

Presence in cosmetic products and chemical analyses

In the USA, in April 2017, octyldodecanol was present in 2265 of 56,714 cosmetic products of which the composition is known in FDA's Voluntary Cosmetic Registration Program (VCRP) (data obtained from FDA, May 2017). In April 2017, octyldodecanol was present in 867 of 66,485 cosmetic products of which the composition is known in EWG's Skin Deep Cosmetics Database, USA (http://www.ewg.org/skindeep/).

OTHER SIDE EFFECTS

Other non-eczematous contact reactions

In (somewhat) older literature, octyldodecanol has been suspected of being comedogenic, based on the rabbit ear assay (5).

LITERATURE

1   Singh M, Winhoven SM, Beck MH. Contact sensitivity to octyldodecanol and trometamol in an anti-itch cream. Contact Dermatitis 2007;56:289-290
2   Dawn G, Forsyth A. Genital swelling caused by octyldodecanol contact dermatitis. Clin Exp Dermatol. 2003;28:228-229

3   Dharmagunawardena B, Chrales-Holmes R. Contact dermatitis due to octyldodecanol in clotrimazole cream. Contact Dermatitis 1997;36:231

4   Tucker WFG. Contact dermatitis to Eutanol G. Contact Dermatitis 1983;9:88-89

5   Lanzet M. Comedogenic effects of cosmetic raw materials. Cosmetics & Toiletries 1986;101:63-72

6   Barrientos N, Abajo P, Moreno de Vega M, Domínguez J. Contact cheilitis caused by candelilla wax contained in lipstick. Contact Dermatitis 2013;69:126-127

2.317   OCTYLDODECYL XYLOSIDE

IDENTIFICATION

Description/definition   : Octyldodecyl xyloside is the ether formed by the reaction of xylose and octyldodecanol
Chemical class(es)   : Carbohydrates; ethers; polyols
CAS registry number (s)   : 423772-95-6
Function(s) in cosmetics   : EU: emulsifying; surfactant. USA: surfactants - emulsifying agents
Patch testing   : Mixture with octyldodecanol, 40% pet. (1)

GENERAL

Octyldodecyl xyloside is an alkyl polyglycoside, which structurally belongs to the glycoside group, a family of small organic molecules in which a sugar component (glycone) is bound to a non-carbohydrate component (aglycone) by a glycosidic bond. Other alkyl (poly)glycosides include decyl glucoside, lauryl glucoside, coco-glucoside and cetearyl glucoside. These are all discussed in separate chapters.

CONTACT ALLERGY

Case reports and case series

A woman developed an extensive urticated rash following the use of a cosmetic skin serum applied to her arms, legs and trunk. The reaction developed within 2 hours of application, and persisted for 2 days after removal. The patient had previously experienced similar reactions after using certain brands of soap and laundry detergent. Patch testing with a baseline, photo-patch, facial and fragrance series together with her own products gave a positive reaction only to the serum on two occasions. Twenty controls gave negative results. Patch testing with individual constituents of the serum produced a reaction to octyldodecyl xyloside 6% pet., which was negative in controls. The octyldodecyl xyloside supplied by the manufacturer was a mixture of octyldodecanol 60%, octyldodecyl xyloside 20%, and PEG-30 dipolyhydroxystearate 20%. Octyldodecanol and PEG-30 dipolyhydroxystearate were available as pure materials and contact allergy to them was excluded. Octyldodecyl xyloside was only available as part of a blend with Octyldodeca-nol. Positive reactions were noted to the octyldodecyl xyloside and octyldodecanol mixture at 40%, 20% and 4% in pet. Tests in 20 controls to the 40% concentration gave negative results. By exclusion, it was concluded that octyldodecyl xyloside was the causative contact allergen (1).

Presence in cosmetic products and chemical analyses

In the USA, in April 2017, octyldodecyl xyloside was present in 13 of 56,714 cosmetic products of which the composition is known in FDA's Voluntary Cosmetic Registration Program (VCRP) (data obtained from FDA, May 2017). In March 2017, octyldodecyl xyloside was present in 13 of 65,431 cosmetic products of which the composition is known in EWG's Skin Deep Cosmetics Database, USA (http://www.ewg.org/skindeep/).

LITERATURE

1   Wilkinson M, Powis RA. Octyldodecyl xyloside: a novel contact allergen. Contact Dermatitis 2011;65:302-304

2.318 OLAFLUR

IDENTIFICATION

Description/definition : Olaflur is the substituted amine salt that conforms to the formula shown below
Chemical class(es) : Alkoxylated amines, Amines
Chemical/IUPAC name : 2-[3-[bis(2-Hydroxyethyl)amino]propyl-octadecylamino]ethanol
Other names : *N*'-Octadecyltrimethylendiamine-*N,N,N*'-tris(2-ethanol)-dihydrofluoride; stearyl
trihydroxyethyl propylenediamine dihydrofluoride; ethanol, 2,2'-[[3-[(2-
hydroxyethyl)octadecylamino]propyl]imino] bis-, dihydrofluoride
CAS registry number (s) : 6818-37-7
EC number(s) : 229-891-6
Merck Index monograph : 8182
Function(s) in cosmetics : EU: antiplaque; hair fixing; oral care. USA: oral care agents
Patch testing : 0.9% water (2)
Molecular formula : $C_{27}H_{60}F_2N_2O_3$

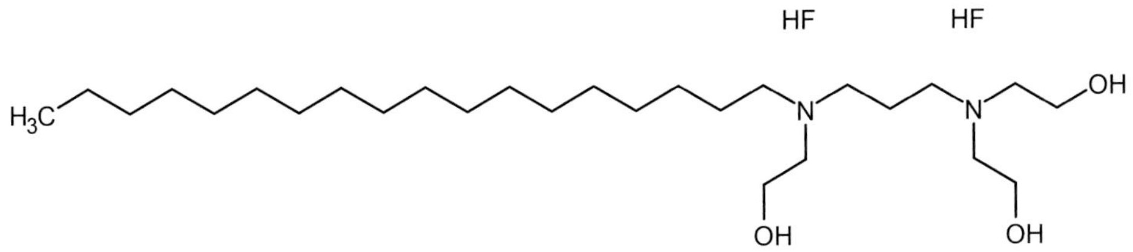

GENERAL

Amine fluorides, used in toothpastes to deliver fluoride to the teeth and combat caries, were developed at the end of the 1950's. The most widely used amine fluorides are olaflur (though only in one brand) and octadecenylammonium fluoride (synonym: dectaflur). In some articles, the exact nature of the 'amine fluoride' was not ascertained (1,3).

CONTACT ALLERGY

Case reports and case series

A woman had suffered from itchy, red and dry lips with painful angular cheilitis for 9 months. She only applied Vaseline®, and did not use nail varnish. The patient was patch tested with the European baseline series and the toothpaste and had a positive reaction to the toothpaste, tested 1% water. Nineteen coded constituents were obtained from the manufacturer in the same concentrations as in the finished product. On patch testing, there was again a positive reaction to the toothpaste Itself (tested 'as is' this time) and also one of the constituents reacted, which was, according to the manufacturer, olaflur. Requests for more material for serial dilution and control testing were denied by the manufacturer. After the patient had changed to another brand of toothpaste, the symptoms disappeared (2).

Previously, in Italy, a patient was described with allergic contact cheilitis caused by 'amine fluoride' in a toothpaste (1). She had a positive patch test reaction to the toothpaste 3% pet., and a positive repeated open application test result with the toothpaste 'as is', and reacted later to the ingredient 'amine fluoride' 5% water. Ten controls showed negative results with the toothpaste 3% pet. and with amine fluoride 5% water. Neither the brand of the toothpaste nor the exact nature of the amine fluoride was mentioned (1). However, the first author of this article was contacted, and she confirmed that the toothpaste in this report was the same as used by the patient described above, which means that the 'amine fluoride' very likely was olaflur. In both cases, the reported concentration of amine fluoride in the test substance was 5% water. However, the 5% concentration proved to be 5% of a stock solution used by the manufacturer, and the actual test concentration of olaflur was 0.9%, containing 700 ppm fluoride, according to personal communication with the manufacturer after further inquiry (2).

A young boy had cheilitis, papules and plaques around the mouth and vesicles in the oral mucosa, which were ascribed to the use of an anti-caries gel (same brand as the toothpastes in the cases described above), He had positive patch test reactions to the gel, diluted with 0.9% NaCl solution and tested at 50% 10%, 1% and 0.1% and to 'amine fluoride' 3.7% water, which was the concentration in the gel. Five control patients were negative. The amine fluoride was a mixture of olaflur and dectaflur; these chemicals could not be tested separately (3).

Cross-reactions, pseudo-cross-reactions and co-reactions
Not to fluoride (2).

Presence in cosmetic products and chemical analyses

In the USA, in April 2017, olaflur was present in zero of 56,714 cosmetic products of which the composition is known in FDA's Voluntary Cosmetic Registration Program (VCRP) (data obtained from FDA, May 2017). In March 2017, olaflur was present in zero of 65,431 cosmetic products of which the composition is known in EWG's Skin Deep Cosmetics Database, USA (http://www.ewg.org/skindeep/).

LITERATURE

1   Foti C, Romita Paolo, Ficco D, Bonamonte D, Angelini G. Allergic contact cheilitis to amine fluoride in a toothpaste. Dermatitis 2014;25:209
2   De Groot A, Tupker R, Hissink D, Woutersen M. Allergic contact cheilitis caused by olaflur in toothpaste. Contact Dermatitis 2017;76:61-62
3   Ganter G, Disch R, Borelli S, Simon D. Contact dermatitis and stomatitis due to amine fluoride. Contact Dermatitis 1997;37:248

2.319   OLEAMIDE DEA

IDENTIFICATION

Description/definition	: Oleamide DEA is a mixture of ethanolamides of oleic acid, which conforms generally to the formula shown below
Chemical class(es)	: Alkanolamines
Chemical/IUPAC name	: N,N-bis(2-Hydroxyethyl)-(Z)-9-octadecenamide
Other names	: Oleic acid diethanolamide; diethanololeamide
CAS registry number (s)	: 93-83-4; 5299-69-4
EC number(s)	: 202-281-7
CIR review(s)	: J Am Coll Toxicol 1986;5:415-454; Int J Toxicol 2013;32(Suppl.1):36-58 (access: www.cir-safety.org/ingredients)
Function(s) in cosmetics	: EU: antistatic; foam boosting; viscosity controlling. USA: surfactants – foam boosters; viscosity increasing agents - aqueous
EU cosmetic restrictions	: Regulated in Annex III/60 of the Regulation (EC) No. 1223/2009
Patch testing	: No data available; suggested: 0.5% pet.
Molecular formula	: $C_{22}H_{43}NO_3$

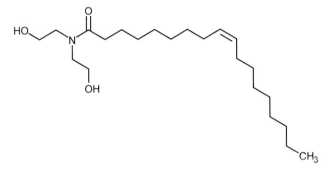

CONTACT ALLERGY

Case reports and case series

Oleamide DEA was responsible for 1 out of 399 cases of cosmetic allergy where the causal allergen was identified in a study of the NACDG, USA, 1977-1983 (1).

Cross-reactions, pseudo-cross-reactions and co-reactions

Possibly pseudo-cross-reactivity to cocamide DEA, as coconut oil contains oleic acid and, as a consequence, oleamide DEA may is present in cocamide DEA (2).

Presence in cosmetic products and chemical analyses

In the USA, in April 2017, oleamide DEA was present in 16 of 56,714 cosmetic products of which the composition is known in FDA's Voluntary Cosmetic Registration Program (VCRP) (data obtained from FDA, May 2017). In March 2017, oleamide DEA was present in 2 older products of 65,431 cosmetic products of which the composition is known in EWG's Skin Deep Cosmetics Database, USA (http://www.ewg.org/skindeep/).

Contact allergy from non-cosmetic products

One patient possibly had occupational allergic contact dermatitis from oleamide DEA in an industrial hand cleanser. Oleamide DEA itself was not patch tested, but the patient reacted to cocamide DEA, which contains oleamide DEA (2).

LITERATURE

1   Adams RM, Maibach HI, Clendenning WE, Fisher AA, Jordan WJ, Kanof N, et al. A five-year study of cosmetic reactions. J Am Acad Dermatol 1985;13:1062-1069
2   Aalto-Korte K, Pesonen M, Kuuliala O, Suuronen K. Occupational allergic contact dermatitis caused by coconut fatty acids diethanolamide. Contact Dermatitis 2014;70:169-174

2.320 OLEAMIDOPROPYL DIMETHYLAMINE

IDENTIFICATION

Description/definition	: Oleamidopropyl dimethylamine is the amidoamine that conforms generally to the formula shown below
Chemical class(es)	: Amines
Chemical/IUPAC name	: (Z)-N-[3-(Dimethylamino)propyl]octadec-9-enamide
Other name(s)	: Dimethylaminopropyl oleamide
CAS registry number (s)	: 109-28-4
EC number(s)	: 203-661-5
CIR review(s)	: Final report, June 2014 (access: www.cir-safety.org/ingredients)
Function(s) in cosmetics	: EU: antistatic. USA: antistatic agents
Patch testing (conc/veh)	: 0.1% water (Chemotechnique); 0.1% alc. (SmartPracticeCanada); this test concentration may induce irritant reactions (1,7)
Molecular formula	: $C_{23}H_{46}N_2O$

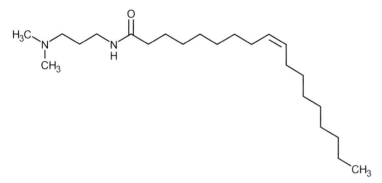

CONTACT ALLERGY

Patch testing in groups of patients

Results of routine patch testing with oleamidopropyl dimethylamine (testing in consecutive patients suspected of contact dermatitis) back to 1992 are shown in table 2.320.1. Results of testing in groups of *selected* patients (e.g., patients with eyelid dermatitis, patients previously reacting to surfactants, hairdressers/cosmetologists) back to 2004 are shown in table 2.320.2.

Patch testing in consecutive patients suspected of contact dermatitis: routine testing

Oleamidopropyl dimethylamine has been added to the NACDG screening series in 2009 and results of patch testing with it have been reported biannually (with the exception of 2011-2012, where a mistake in nomenclature made interpretation impossible [23]). In routine testing, frequencies of sensitization have ranged from 1.8% to 4.5% (table 2.320.1). Rates of sensitization in the NACDG studies ranged from 1.8% to 3.5%, but 'definite + probable' relevance was only 27% as maximum (5,10,17). In Italy, in the first half of the 1990s, despite rare use of oleamidopropyl dimethyla-mine in cosmetics, relatively high rates of sensitization ranging from 2.4% to 4.5% (6,19,20) were observed. In these studies, higher concentrations were used for patch testing, pointing at irritancy as explanation for a number of positive 'allergic' reactions. Some authors suggested that these patients were actually sensitized to dimethylamino-propylamine (DMAPA) by the use of shampoos containing cocamidopropyl betaine (in which DMAPA is an impurity) and now reacted positively to DMAPA, which is also present as a contaminant in oleamidopropyl dimethylamine (6).

Table 2.320.1 Patch testing in groups of patients: Routine testing

Years and Country	Test conc. & vehicle	Number of patients tested | positive (%)		Selection of patients (S); Relevance (R); Comments (C)	Ref.
2013-14 USA, Canada	0.1% water	4859	172 (3.5%)	R: definite + probable relevance: 18%	17
2009-14 USA, Canada	0.1% water	10,877	248 (2.3%)	R: not stated	10
2009-10 USA, Canada	0.1% water	4300	77 (1.8%)	R: definite + probable relevance: 27%	5
<1995 Italy	0.5% water	285	14 (2.9%)	R: not specified; C: 12% irritant reactions; co-reactivity with cocamidopropyl betaine and 3-dimethylaminopropylamine	6
<1994 Italy		?	? (2.4%)	R: unknown; C: data cited in ref. 6	20
1992 Italy		155	7 (4.5%)	R: not stated	19

Patch testing in groups of selected patients

Data on patch testing with oleamidopropyl dimethylamine in groups of selected patients back to 2004 are summarized in table 2.320.2. Frequencies of sensitization ranged from 0.6% (patients suspected of occupational contact dermatitis and tested with a 'coconut series' [1]) to 34% in patients previously reacting to one or more surfactants present in the NACDG screening series (16). Most (1) or all (11) reactions were considered to be relevant and were caused by liquid soap and shampoo in one study (1). Whether the reactions to oleamidopropyl dimethylamine in the 16 patients previously reacting to other surfactants were relevant was not mentioned by the authors (16).

A very high frequency of sensitization to oleamidopropyl dimethylamine of 7.9% was seen in another US study, which had, however, certain flaws (2). As oleamidopropyl dimethylamine is rarely used in cosmetics in the USA, it may be assumed that many reactions have been false-positive (irritant). Indeed, other authors have shown that the test concentration of 0.1%, which was used in these studies, may induce irritant reactions (1,7). A 99% relevance in the US study is also unlikely and may be caused by inclusion of questionable' and 'past' relevance (2).

Table 2.320.2 Patch testing in groups of patients: Selected patient groups

Years and Country	Test conc. & vehicle	Number of patients tested	positive (%)	Selection of patients (S); Relevance (R); Comments (C)	Ref.
2015-2016 USA	0.1% water	47	16 (34%)	S: patients previously reacting to one or more surfactants present in the NACDG screening series; R: not stated; C: there were also 11 doubtful reactions	16
1994-2010 USA, Canada	0.1% water	?	? (?)	S: hairdressers/cosmetologists; R: in the group of 24 patients who had at least one relevant occupationally related reaction, one (4.2%) reacted to oleamidopropyl dimethylamine	18
2002-2009 Finland	0.1% water	1092	7 (0.6%)	S: patients suspected of occupational contact dermatitis and tested with a 'coconut series'; R: most reactions were relevant and caused by liquid soap and shampoo; C: there were 104 (10%) irritant patch test reactions	1
2000-2007 USA	0.1% water	941	73 (7.9%)	S: patients tested with a supplemental cosmetic screening series; R: 99%; C: weak study: a. high rate of macular erythema and weak reactions; b. relevance figures included 'questionable' and 'past' relevance; obviously many irritant reactions	2
1994-2004 USA		46	5 (10.9%)	S: patients with allergic contact dermatitis of the eyelids; R: all were relevant, but the source products were not mentioned	11

Case reports and case series

In a group of 119 patients with allergic contact dermatitis from cosmetics, investigated in The Netherlands in 1986-1987, thirteen cases (10.9%) were caused by oleamidopropyl dimethylamine in skin care products for babies (but used by their mothers to remove eyeshadow) (12,13). In a group of 75 patients allergic to cosmetic products, seen in a private practice in The Netherlands in the period 1981-1986, eight cases were caused by oleamidopropyl dimethylamine in skin care products (intended for babies, but used by their mothers to remove eye makeup (14, overlap with ref. 9). Three patient had ACD from oleamidopropyl dimethylamine in a baby body lotion (9). One patient had relevant positive patch test reactions to a moisturizer, another to a sun protection lotion and a third individual to a make-up remover and to their ingredient oleamidopropyl dimethylamine (15). The Dutch experience with oleamidopropyl dimethylamine has been summarized in ref. 22.

Cross-reactions, pseudo-cross-reactions and co-reactions

In The Netherlands, 13 patients who had previously shown positive patch tests to oleamidopropyl dimethylamine 0.4% water, were tested with 10 structurally related amide-type surfactants; the results are shown in table 2.320.3. It has been suggested that the co-reactions may have been due to the presence of the impurity 3-dimethylaminopropylamine (which is used the synthesis of these surfactants) in both oleamidopropyl dimethylamine and the co-reacting test substances (6).

Co- or cross-reactions have also been observed to cocamidopropyl betaine (6,10,16), dimethylaminopropylamine (6), cocamidopropyl dimethylamine (1,16), stearamidopropyl dimethylamine ('amidoamine') (10), sodium lauroyl sarcosinate (16), isostearamidopropyl morpholine lactate (16), disodium lauroamphodiacetate (16) and possibly to myristamidopropyl dimethylamine (24). In some cases, dimethylaminopropylamine, present as contaminant, may have been the actual sensitizer in oleamidopropyl dimethylamine and (some) co-reacting substances (6,21).

There is an unexplained high positivity rate to oleamidopropyl dimethylamine (13%) and cocamidopropyl betaine (27%) in patients reacting to ascaridole, an allergen in Melaleuca alternifolia (tea tree) oil (3).

Table 2.320.3 Cross-reaction pattern of oleamidopropyl dimethylamine in 13 patients (8)

Surfactant	Test conc. and vehicle	Nr. and (%) of positive reactions	
Ricinoleamidopropyl dimethylamine lactate	0.5% w/v water	11	(85%)
Tallowamidopropyl dimethylamine	0.3% w/v water	11	(85%)
Lauramidopropyl dimethylamine	0.2% w/v water	9	(75%) [a]
Myristamidopropyl dimethylamine	0.05% w/v water	6	(46%)
Cocamidopropyl dimethylamine	0.1% w/v water	5	(42%) [a]
Isostearamidopropyl dimethylamine	0.3% w/v water	5	(38%)
Minkamidopropyl dimethylamine	0.1% w/v water	5	(38%)
Behenamidopropyl dimethylamine	0.5% w/v water	2	(15%)
Stearamidopropyl dimethylamine lactate	0.5% w/v water	2	(15%)
Palmitamidopropyl dimethylamine	0.025% w/v water	1	(8%)

[a] tested in 12 patients

Presence in cosmetic products and chemical analyses

In the USA, in April 2017, oleamidopropyl dimethylamine was present in 2 of 56,714 cosmetic products of which the composition is known in FDA's Voluntary Cosmetic Registration Program (VCRP) (data obtained from FDA, May 2017). In February 2017, oleamidopropyl dimethylamine was present in one of 64,613 cosmetic products of which the composition is known in EWG's Skin Deep Cosmetics Database, USA (http://www.ewg.org/skindeep/). In 1986, oleamidopropyl dimethylamine was contained in 23 of approximately 19,000 cosmetic formulations on file with the US Food and Drug Administration (FDA) (8). Oleamidopropyl dimethylamine may contain dimethylamino-propylamine (DMAPA) (1,6) and cocamidopropyl dimethylamine (1). The levels of DMAPA and cocamidopropyl dimethylamine are reported to be between 0.0002% (the detection limit) and <0.5% (4).

LITERATURE

1   Suuronen K, Pesonen M, Aalto-Korte K. Occupational contact allergy to cocamidopropyl betaine. Contact Dermatitis 2012;66:286-292
2   Wetter DA, Yiannias JA, Prakash AV, Davis MD, Farmer SA, el-Azhary RA, et al. Results of patch testing to personal care product allergens in a standard series and a supplemental cosmetic series: an analysis of 945 patients from the Mayo Clinic Contact Dermatitis Group, 2000-2007. J Am Acad Dermatol 2010;63:789-798
3   Bakker C, Blömeke B, Coenraads PJ, Schuttelaar M-L. Ascaridole, a sensitizing component of tea tree oil, patch tested at 1% and 5% in two series of patients. Contact Dermatitis 2012;65:240-241
4   Burnett CL, Bergfeld WF, Belsito DV, Hill RA, Klaassen CD, Liebler D, et al. Final report of the Cosmetic Ingredient Review Expert Panel on the safety assessment of cocamidopropyl betaine (CAPB). Int J Toxicol 2012;31(suppl. 1): 77S-111S
5   Warshaw EM, Belsito DV, Taylor JS, Sasseville D, DeKoven JG, Zirwas MJ, et al. North American Contact Dermatitis Group patch test results: 2009 to 2010. Dermatitis 2013;24:50-59
6   Foti C, Rigano L, Vena GA, Grandolfo M, Liguoril G, Angelini G. Contact allergy to oleamidopropyl dimethylamine and related substances. Contact Dermatitis 1995;33:132-133
7   Bruynzeel DP, Niklasson B. The patch test dilution of oleamidopropyl dimethylamine. Contact Dermatitis 1992;27:190-191
8   De Groot AC, Jagtman BA, van der Meeren HLM, Bruynzeel DP, Bos JD, den Hengst CW, Weyland JW. Cross-reaction pattern of the cationic emulsifier oleamidopropyl dimethylamine. Contact Dermatitis 1988;19:284-289
9   De Groot AC, Liem DH. Contact allergy to oleamidopropyl dimethylamine. Contact Dermatitis 1984;11:298-301
10   Fowler JF Jr, Shaughnessy CN, Belsito DV, DeKoven JG, Deleo VA, Fransway AF, et al. Cutaneous delayed-type hypersensitivity to surfactants. Dermatitis 2015;26:268-270
11   Amin KA, Belsito DV. The aetiology of eyelid dermatitis: a 10-year retrospective analysis. Contact Dermatitis 2006;55:280-285
12   De Groot AC, Bruynzeel DP, Bos JD, van der Meeren HL, van Joost T, Jagtman BA, Weyland JW. The allergens in cosmetics. Arch Dermatol 1988;124:1525-1529
13   De Groot AC. Adverse reactions to cosmetics. PhD Thesis, University of Groningen, The Netherlands: 1988, chapter 3.4, pp.105-113
14   De Groot AC. Contact allergy to cosmetics: Causative ingredients. Contact Dermatitis 1987;17:26-34
15   Held E, Johansen JD, Agner T, Menné T. Contact allergy to cosmetics: testing with patients' own products. Contact Dermatitis 1999;40:310-315
16   Grey KR, Hanson J, Hagen SL, Hylwa SA, Warshaw EM. Epidemiology and co-reactivity of novel surfactant allergens: a double-blind randomized controlled study. Dermatitis 2016;27:348-354

17 DeKoven JG, Warshaw EM, Belsito DV, Sasseville D, Maibach HI, Taylor JS, et al. North American Contact Dermatitis Group Patch Test Results: 2013-2014. Dermatitis 2017;28:33-46

18 Warshaw EM, Wang MZ, Mathias CGT, Maibach HI, Belsito DV, Zug KA, et al. Occupational contact dermatitis in hairdressers/cosmetologists; retrospective analysis of North American Contact Dermatitis Group data, 1994 to 2010. Dermatitis 2012;23:258-268

19 Motolese A, Seidenari S. Patch test reading: a comparison between 2 application methods. Contact Dermatitis 1994;30:49-50

20 Brusi C, Giorgini S, Francalanci F, Acciai M C, Sertoli A. Evaluation of oleamidopropyl dimethylamine patch test reactions by means of evaporimetry and colorimetry. In: Abstract Book of 2nd Congress of the European Society of Contact Dermatitis. Barcelona, Spain, 6-8 October 1994 (data cited in ref. 2)

21 Moreau L, Sasseville D. Allergic contact dermatitis from cocamidopropyl betaine, cocamidoamine, 3-(dimethylamino)propylamine, and oleamidopropyl dimethylamine: co-reactions or cross-reactions? Dermatitis. 2004;15:146-149

22 De Groot AC. Oleamidopropyl dimethylamine. Derm Beruf Umwelt 1989;37:101-105

23 Warshaw EM, Maibach HI, Taylor JS, Sasseville D, DeKoven JG, Zirwas MJ, et al. North American Contact Dermatitis Group patch test results: 2011-2012. Dermatitis 2015;26:49-59

24 Cressey BD, Scheinman PL. Systemic allergic dermatitis of the lips resulting from allergy to an antimicrobial agent in a contact lens disinfecting solution. Contact Dermatitis 2012;67:239-240

2.321   C30-38 OLEFIN/ISOPROPYL MALEATE/MA COPOLYMER

IDENTIFICATION

Description/definition   : C30-38 Olefin /isopropyl maleate/MA copolymer is the copolymer of maleic anhydride,
                               isopropyl maleate and C30-38 olefin monomers
Chemical class(es)   : Synthetic polymers
CAS registry number (s)   : 75535-27-2
EC number(s)   : 278-251-2
Function(s) in cosmetics   : EU: emulsifying; surfactant; viscosity controlling. USA: surfactants – emulsifying agents;
                               viscosity increasing agents - nonaqueous
Patch testing   : 5% or 10% pet. (1,2); the 10% test material is non-irritant (2)
Molecular formula   : $C_7H_{10}O_4.C_4H_2O_3$.unspecified

GENERAL

Copolymers are important ingredients in cosmetics, added because of their antistatic, film-forming, binding, suspending, viscosity-increasing, skin-conditioning, and emulsion-stabilizing properties. Copolymers have been underestimated for a long time as to their sensitizing capacities because of their large structures and high molecular weights. Allergic contact dermatitis to copolymers in cosmetics, however, does occur, but the exact nature of the hapten is unknown. The copolymers are not likely to be haptens themselves in view of their large molecular weights. The sensitizer could be an additive, an impurity, a product that forms during polymerization, a residual monomer, or a degradation product (5).

CONTACT ALLERGY

Case reports and case series

C30-38 Olefin/isopropyl maleate/MA copolymer was stated to be the (or an) allergen in 3 patients in a group of 603 individuals suffering from cosmetic dermatitis, seen in the period 2010-2015 in Leuven, Belgium (6). Four patients were investigated in the UK who all had extensive allergic contact dermatitis from the use of one particular sunscreen product. When patch tested, they reacted to the product's ingredient C30-38 olefin/isopropyl maleate/MA copolymer, tested at 10% pet. It was not stated, but highly likely, that the sunscreen itself also gave positive patch test reactions. Thirty controls were negative to C30-38 olefin/isopropyl maleate/MA copolymer 10% pet. (2,4). Shortly thereafter, two more patients were reported, one from Belgium and the other from The Netherlands, who reacted to the same sunscreen and its ingredient C30-38 olefin/isopropyl maleate/MA copolymer. In one of them, the copolymer was also found to be present in a SPF30 face cream (1). One patient with allergic contact dermatitis from C30-38 olefin/isopropyl maleate/MA copolymer in a sunscreen was identified in a cosmetovigilance survey in The Netherlands. Possibly, this was the same individual as the Dutch patient reported in ref. 1 (3).

Presence in cosmetic products and chemical analyses

In the USA, in April 2017, C30-38 olefin/isopropyl maleate/MA copolymer was present in zero of 56,714 cosmetic products of which the composition is known in FDA's Voluntary Cosmetic Registration Program (VCRP) (data obtained from FDA, May 2017). In March 2017, C30-38 olefin /isopropyl maleate/MA copolymer was present in 26 of 64,983 cosmetic products of which the composition is known in EWG's Skin Deep Cosmetics Database, USA (http://www.ewg.org/skindeep/).

LITERATURE

1   Swinnen I, Goossens A, Rustemeyer Th. Allergic contact dermatitis caused by C30-38 olefin/isopropyl
    maleate/MA copolymer in cosmetics. Contact Dermatitis 2012;67:318-320
2   Kai AC, White JML, White IR, Johnston G, McFadden JP. Contact dermatitis caused by C30-38 olefin/isopropyl
    maleate/MA copolymer in a sunscreen. Contact Dermatitis 2011;64:353-354
3   Salverda JGW, Bragt PJC, de Wit-Bos L, Rustemeyer T, Coenraads PJ, Tupker R, et al. Results of a
    cosmetovigilance survey in The Netherlands. Contact Dermatitis 2013;68:139-148
4   Kai A, Khorshid M, McFadden J. Allergic contact dermatitis to copolymers. Br J Dermatol 2010;163 (Suppl. 1):87
5   Quartier S, Garmyn M, Becart S, Goossens A. Allergic contact dermatitis to copolymers in cosmetics – case report
    and review of the literature. Contact Dermatitis 2006;55:257-267
6   Goossens A. Cosmetic contact allergens. Cosmetics 2016, 3, 5; doi:10.3390/cosmetics3010005

2.322   OLETH-3 PHOSPHATE

IDENTIFICATION

Description/definition : Oleth-3 phosphate is a complex mixture of esters of phosphoric acid and oleth-3
Chemical class(es) : Phosphorus compounds
Chemical/IUPAC name : Poly(oxy-1,2-ethanediyl),α-9-octadecenyl-ω-hydroxy- (Z)-, phosphate (3 mol EU average molar ratio)
Other names : PEG-3 oleyl ether phosphate; polyoxyethylene (3) oleyl ether phosphate
CAS registry number (s) : 39464-69-2 (generic)
Function(s) in cosmetics : EU: surfactant. USA: surfactants – emulsifying agents
Patch testing : 1% pet. (1)
Molecular formula : $(C_{18}H_{36}O).(C_2H_4O)_n.x(H_3.PO_4)$

CONTACT ALLERGY

Case reports and case series

A man with a long-standing history of chronic stable plaque psoriasis presented with a 1-week history of a pruritic red rash on his hands, scalp and face soon after he was started on cyclosporin. Despite discontinuation of this drug, his rash intermittently worsened over the subsequent weeks and was very itchy. Examination revealed an urticarial papular eruption on the hands, scalp and face. Patch tests with the European standard series, preservatives, balsam and perfumes series were all negative. The patient habitually used a finishing hair wax during the working week, and told that his rash was less prominent over the weekends when he temporarily stopped using this hair product. Next, patch testing was performed with this cosmetic product (which was probably positive) and later with its ingredients, obtained from the manufacturer. The ingredients oleth-3-phosphate and oleth-5 were tested at 1% pet and both gave strongly positive vesicular and bullous patch test reactions at D2 and D4. Both chemicals were patch tested on 20 control patients and no positive reactions were observed. After avoiding products containing oleth-3 phosphate and oleth-5, the patient has remained free of dermatitis (1).

Cross-reactions, pseudo-cross-reactions and co-reactions

Possibly to oleth-5 (1).

Presence in cosmetic products and chemical analyses

In the USA, in April 2017, oleth-3- phosphate was present in 17 of 56,714 cosmetic products of which the composition is known in FDA's Voluntary Cosmetic Registration Program (VCRP) (data obtained from FDA, May 2017). In March 2017, oleth-3 phosphate was present in 70 of 65,431 cosmetic products of which the composition is known in EWG's Skin Deep Cosmetics Database, USA (http://www.ewg.org/skindeep/).

LITERATURE

1   Abdullah A, Walker S, Tan CY, Foulds IS. Sensitization to oleth-3-phosphate and oleth-5 in a hair wax. Contact Dermatitis 1997;37:188

2.323   OLETH-5

IDENTIFICATION

Description/definition	: Oleth-5 is the polyethylene glycol ether of oleyl alcohol, which conforms generally to the formula shown below, where n has an average value of 5
Chemical class(es)	: Alkoxylated alcohols
Chemical/IUPAC name	: Poly(oxy-1,2-ethanediyl),α-9-(Z)-octadecenyl-ω-hydroxy (5 mol EO average molar ratio)
Other names	: PEG-5 oleyl ether; polyoxyethylene (5) oleyl ether
CAS registry number (s)	: 5353-27-5; 9004-98-2 (generic)
CIR review(s)	: Int J Toxicol 1999;18(Suppl.2):17-24; Int J Toxicol 2012;31(Suppl.2):169-244 (access: www.cir-safety.org/ingredients)
Function(s) in cosmetics	: EU: emulsifying. USA: fragrance ingredients; surfactants - emulsifying agents
Patch testing	: 1% pet. (1)
Structural formula	: $CH_3(CH_2)_7CH=CH(CH_2)_7CH_2(OCH_2CH_2)_nOH$

CONTACT ALLERGY

Case reports and case series

A man with a long-standing history of chronic stable plaque psoriasis presented with a 1-week history of a pruritic red rash on his hands, scalp and face soon after he was started on cyclosporin. Despite discontinuation of this drug, his rash intermittently worsened over the subsequent weeks and was very itchy. Examination revealed an urticarial papular eruption on the hands, scalp and face. Patch tests with the European standard series, preservatives, balsam and perfumes series were all negative. The patient habitually used a finishing hair wax during the working week, and told that his rash was less prominent over the weekends when he temporarily stopped using this hair product. Next, patch testing was performed with this cosmetic product (which was probably positive) and later with its ingredients, obtained from the manufacturer. The ingredients oleth-5 and oleth-3-phosphate were tested at 1% pet and both gave strongly positive vesicular and bullous patch test reactions at D2 and D4. Both chemicals were patch tested on 20 control patients and no positive reactions were observed. After avoiding products containing oleth-5 and oleth-3 phosphate, the patient has remained free of dermatitis (1).

Cross-reactions, pseudo-cross-reactions and co-reactions

Possibly to oleth-3 phosphate (1).

Presence in cosmetic products and chemical analyses

In the USA, in April 2017, oleth-5 was present in 203 of 56,714 cosmetic products of which the composition is known in FDA's Voluntary Cosmetic Registration Program (VCRP) (data obtained from FDA, May 2017). In March 2017, oleth-5 was present in 69 of 65,431 cosmetic products of which the composition is known in EWG's Skin Deep Cosmetics Database, USA (http://www.ewg.org/skindeep/).

LITERATURE

1   Abdullah A, Walker S, Tan CY, Foulds IS. Sensitization to oleth-3-phosphate and oleth-5 in a hair wax. Contact Dermatitis 1997;37:188

2.324   OLEYL ALCOHOL

IDENTIFICATION

Description/definition	: Oleyl alcohol is the unsaturated fatty alcohol that conforms generally to the formula shown below
Chemical class(es)	: Fatty alcohols
Chemical/IUPAC name	: (Z)-octadec-9-enol
Other names	: Hydroxyoctadec-9-ene
CAS registry number (s)	: 143-28-2; 593-47-5
EC number(s)	: 205-597-3; 209-791-9
CIR review(s)	: J Am Coll Toxicol 1985;4:1-29 (access: www.cir-safety.org/ingredients)
Merck Index monograph	: 8194
Function(s) in cosmetics	: EU: emollient; emulsifying; opacifying; viscosity controlling. USA: fragrance ingredients; skin-conditioning agents - emollient; solvents; viscosity increasing agents - nonaqueous
Patch testing	: 10% pet. (3,6)
Molecular formula	: $C_{18}H_{36}O$

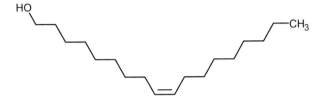

GENERAL

Oleyl alcohol is a long-chain fatty alcohol often used as an emulsifier in the production of lubricants, papers, printing inks, cutting fluids, cosmetics and topical drugs (3). Oleyl alcohol is said to be frequently present as an impurity in commercial cetyl and stearyl alcohols (10) and it has been suggested that the impurity may be the actual sensitizer in these products (11).

CONTACT ALLERGY

Patch testing in groups of patients

Results of patch testing oleyl alcohol in consecutive patients suspected of contact dermatitis (routine testing) and of testing groups of *selected* patients (patients tested with a metalworking fluid series, patients suspected of contact allergy to cosmetics or topical pharmaceutical products) are shown in table 2.324.1. In one small Italian study performing routine testing, there was only one reaction among 310 patients tested (0.3%); relevance was not mentioned (13). In two studies testing groups of selected patients, a low frequency of sensitization of 0.7% was observed in 144 patients tested with a metalworking fluid series (12).

An unlikely high rate of 22.6% sensitization was found in a 1992-1995 Italian study in a group pf 146 patients suspected of contact allergy to cosmetics or topical pharmaceutical products (7). 25/33 reactions (76%) were relevant, mostly from cosmetics (n=18) and from topical pharmaceutical preparations (n=5) (7). It seems likely that that many of these reactions to oleyl alcohol 30% in alcohol have been irritant in nature.

Table 2.324.1 Patch testing in groups of patients

Years and Country	Test conc. & vehicle	Number of patients tested | positive (%)		Selection of patients (S); Relevance (R); Comments (C)	Ref.
Routine testing					
2015 Italy	30% pet.	310	1 (0.3%)	R: not stated	13
Testing in groups of selected patients					
2004-2005 Germany, Sweden	10% pet.	144	1 (0.7%)	S: patients tested with a metalworking fluid series; R: not stated	12
1992-1995 Italy	30% alc.	146	33 (22.6%)	S: patients suspected of contact allergy to cosmetics or topical pharmaceutical products; R: 25 (or 24) were relevant, of which 18 from cosmetics and 5 from topical pharmaceutical preparations; C: the purity of oleyl alcohol was >99%	7

Case reports and case series

Oleyl alcohol was responsible for 1 out of 399 cases of cosmetic allergy where the causal allergen was identified in a study of the NACDG, USA, 1977-1983 (1). One patient had allergic contact cheilitis from oleyl alcohol in lipsticks (2). Three patients reacted to (purified) oleyl alcohol in lipstick(s) (4). Another one also had contact allergy to oleyl alcohol in lipstick (6). Ten individuals reacted to oleyl alcohol in cosmetic products (7). Three patients had contact allergy to oleyl alcohol in respectively a sun lotion, hair lotion and cleansing milk; a 4th possibly reacted to oleyl alcohol in a liquid soap (10).

Contact allergy to oleyl alcohol in non-cosmetic products

One patient had allergic contact dermatitis from oleyl alcohol in a topical pharmaceutical product (3). A man had occupational allergic contact dermatitis from oleyl alcohol in a cutting fluid (8). A female patient reacted to stearyl alcohol, ethyl alcohol and cetyl alcohol present in topical pharmaceutical preparations (11); she did not react to pure cetyl alcohol and stearyl alcohol, but had positive patch test reactions to oleyl alcohol and n-decyl alcohol, which may be present as impurities in stearyl and cetyl alcohol (11).

Cross-reactions, pseudo-cross-reactions and co-reactions

Lanolin alcohol (6); *not* to oleic acid (6); possibly to ricinoleic acid (6) (?); myristyl alcohol (7); stearyl alcohol (7,9). Oleyl alcohol is said to be frequently present as an impurity in cetyl and stearyl alcohols (10) and may, according to some authors, be the actual sensitizer in these products (11).

Presence in cosmetic products and chemical analyses

In July 2017, oleyl alcohol was present in 249 of 69,543 cosmetic products of which the composition is known in EWG's Skin Deep Cosmetics Database, USA (http://www.ewg.org/skindeep/). In the USA, in April 2017, oleyl alcohol was present in 723 of 56,714 cosmetic products of which the composition is known in FDA's Voluntary Cosmetic Registration Program (VCRP) (data obtained from FDA, May 2017).

OTHER SIDE EFFECTS

Other non-eczematous contact reactions

In (somewhat) older literature, oleyl alcohol has been suspected of being comedogenic in 'people with more sensitive complexions or acne-prone problems', based on rabbit ear assays (5,14).

LITERATURE

1   Adams RM, Maibach HI, Clendenning WE, Fisher AA, Jordan WJ, Kanof N, et al. A five-year study of cosmetic reactions. J Am Acad Dermatol 1985;13:1062-1069

2   Inui S, Azukizawa H, Katayama I. Recurrent contact cheilitis because of glyceryl isostearate, diisostearyl maleate, oleyl alcohol, and Lithol Rubine BCA in lipsticks. Contact Dermatitis 2009;60:231-232

3   Andersen KE, Broesby-Olsen S. Allergic contact dermatitis from oleyl alcohol in Elidel® cream. Contact Dermatitis 2006;55:354-356

4   Calnan CD, Sarkany I. Studies in contact dermatitis (XII). Sensitivity to oleyl alcohol. Trans St Johns Hosp Dermatol Soc 1960;44:47-50

5   Lanzet M. Comedogenic effects of cosmetic raw materials. Cosmetics & Toiletries 1986;101:63-72

6   Tan BB, Noble AL, Roberts ME, Lear JT, English JSC. Allergic contact dermatitis from oleyl alcohol in lipstick cross-reacting with ricinoleic acid in castor oil and lanolin. Contact Dermatitis 1997;37:41-42

7   Tosti A, Vincenzi C, Guerra L, Andrisano E. Contact dermatitis from fatty alcohols. Contact Dermatitis 1996;35:287-289

8   Koch P. Occupational allergic contact dermatitis from oleyl alcohol and monoethanolamine in a metalworking fluid. Contact Dermatitis 1995;33:273

9   Fisher AA. Contact dermatitis from stearyl alcohol and propylene glycol. Arch Dermatol 1974;110:636

10 Guidetti, MS, Vincenzi C, Guerra L, Tosti A. Contact dermatitis due to oleyl alcohol. Contact Dermatitis 1994;31:260-261

11 Ishiguro N, Kawashima M. Contact dermatitis from impurities in alcohol. Contact Dermatitis 1991;25:257

12 Geier J, Lessmann H, Becker D, Bruze M, Frosch PJ, Fuchs T, et al. Patch testing with components of water-based metalworking fluids: results of a multicentre study with a second series. Contact Dermatitis 2006;55:322-329

13 Corazza M, Virgili A, Ricci M, Bianchi A, Borghi A. Contact sensitization to emulsifying agents: an underrated issue? Dermatitis 2016;27:276-281

14 Fulton JE Jr, Pay SR, Fulton JE 3rd. Comedogenicity of current therapeutic products, cosmetics, and ingredients in the rabbit ear. J Am Acad Dermatol 1984;10:96-105

2.325 OSMARON® B*
* Not an INCI name, but name according to ChemIDPlus, Chemicalbook and Merck Index

IDENTIFICATION

Description/definition : Osmaron B is a complex chemical mixture composed of benzoates of primary aliphatic fatty amines obtained from palm kernel oil and corn oil as starting materials, preponderantly dodecylammonium benzoate and tetradecylammonium benzoate

Chemical class(es) : Quaternary ammonium compounds; benzoates

INCI name EU/USA : Neither in CosIng nor in the Personal Care Products Council Ingredient Database

Chemical/IUPAC name : Alkylammonium amidobenzoate

CAS registry number (s) : 8031-66-1

Merck Index monograph : 8257

Patch testing : 0.1% pet. (1,13); 0.5% paraff. liq. (4); 0.3% pet. (3); test concentrations of 1% and higher in petrolatum induce irritant reactions (1,5)

GENERAL

Osmaron B is a disinfectant, which is used especially in udder creams and ointments and milking fats. It is an oily yellow-brown liquid, added as an antiseptic, disinfecting and preserving agent of milking fats since 1934 (4). Osmaron B is composed of benzoates of primary aliphatic fatty amines obtained from palm kernel oil and corn oil as starting materials, preponderantly dodecylammonium benzoate and tetradecylammonium benzoate. Its total nitrogen is 4.15% and average benzoic acid content 27.6% by analysis (www.druglead.com/cds/osmaron-b.html).

In the 1950s and 1960s, in Germany, many cases of occupational allergic contact dermatitis in farmers and milkers from Osmaron B have been reported (7-11). Such cases became less frequent as machine milking super-seded hand milking (1,2,4,5,6), although case series of 3 (5) and 9 patients (6) were still being reported in the beginning of the 1990s. However, udder creams containing Osmaron B are very popular in household medicine (2) and have produced allergic contact dermatitis when used for skin care repeatedly.

It can be doubted that udder fat products containing Osmaron B can be considered as cosmetics. The cases are presented here, though, because these products (which are still called udderfat or udder ointment or milk fat) are widely used as cosmetic products for skin care and are in fact marketed by the manufacturers as skin care products rather than as products to use on cow's udders, but are also advised for the treatment of atopic dermatitis, neurodermatitis and psoriasis (13).

CONTACT ALLERGY

Patch testing in groups of patients

In the period 1990-1994, in Germany, Austria and Switzerland (IVDK) 3135 patients were selected to be tested with a preservative series including Osmaron B 0.3% pet. Sixty-three patients (2.0%) had a positive patch test reaction; their relevance was not mentioned (3). The high frequency of sensitization was ascribed to 'natural cosmetics' (2). In the subgroups of younger women (age <40 years), Osmaron B was even the leading allergen of the preservatives series (2).

In the period 1992-1995, an unknown number of nurses was patch tested with Osmaron B (probably 0.3% pet.) by the members of the IVDK and 5.1% had a positive reaction. The relevance was not specified, but it was stated that Osmaron B is contained in udder ointments which are used more and more often as an 'alternative' cream (12). There is without doubt overlap in these two studies (3,12).

Case reports and case series

A farmer had occupational ACD from Osmaron B in udder ointment (1). A woman had subacute contact dermatitis of the hands and the face. She had used melkfett for skin care for more than 2 years. Patch tests were positive to the product and its ingredient Osmaron B, tested 0.5% and 1% in paraffinum liquidum (to which 10 controls were nega-tive) (4). Nine patients had allergic reactions to Osmaron B in milking fat; one of them, a masseur, had occupational allergic contact dermatitis (6). Three patients became sensitized from Osmaron B in udderfat used for skin care (5). They all had positive patch tests to the product itself, tested 'as is' and to its ingredient Osmaron B 1% and 0.1% pet. (5). A ship technician developed occupational allergic contact dermatitis from Osmaron B in an udder ointment, which was used as hand ointment at his work (13).

Presence in cosmetic products and chemical analyses

In May 2017, Osmaron B was present in zero of 66,975 cosmetic products of which the composition is known in EWG's Skin Deep Cosmetics Database, USA (http://www.ewg.org/skindeep/). In the USA, in April 2017, Osmaron B was present in zero of 56,714 cosmetic products of which the composition is known in FDA's Voluntary Cosmetic Registration Program (VCRP) (data obtained from FDA, May 2017).

LITERATURE

1   Haapasaari K-M, Niinimäki A. Allergic contact dermatitis from alkylammonium amidobenzoate (Osmaron B®). Contact Dermatitis 2000;42:244-245
2   Schnuch A. Osmaron B® is a rare occupational, but a frequent cosmetic, allergen. Contact Dermatitis 2001;44:134
3   Schnuch A, Geier J, Uter W, Frosch P J. Patch testing with preservatives, antimicrobials and industrial biocides. Results from a multicenter study (IVDK). Br J Dermatol 1998;138:467-476
4   Schubert HJ. Contact allergy to Osmaron B® in milking fat. Contact Dermatitis 1993;28:245-246
5   Goldermann R, Scharffetter-Kochanek K, Brunner M, Merk H, Goerz G. 3 cases of contact dermatitis from alkylammonium amidobenzoate (Osmaron BA). Contact Dermatitis 1992;27:337-339
6   Hausen BM, Post B. Allergische Reaktionen auf Osmaron B in Melkfett. Akt Dermatol 1992;18:108-111
7   Pettker K, Schultheiss E. Uberempfindlichkeit gegenüber amidosulfosauren Salzen höhermolekularer aliphatischer Amide. Z Hautkr 1957;22:310-312
8   Von Preyss JA. Melkfettekzeme. Berufsdermatosen 1958;6:287-290
9   Reinhard M. Derzeitige Häufigkeit beruflicher Schadstoffe. Berufsdermatosen 1973;21:62-68
10   Schroeder KH. Zur Analyse des Melkerekzems. Berufsdermatosen 1956;4:157-166
11   Wagner G, Wezel G. Art und Häufigkeit hautschädigender Berufsnoxen in Schleswig-Holstein. Berufsdermatosen 1966;14:1-40
12   Schnuch A, Uter W, Geier J, Frosch PJ, Rustemeyer Th. Contact allergies in healthcare workers. Results from the IVDK. Acta Dermato-venereologica 1998;78:358-363
13   Kanerva L, Estlander T, Jolanki R. Occupational allergic contact dermatitis from alkylammonium amidobenzoate. Eur J Dermatol 2001;11:240-243

2.326 OXYQUINOLINE

IDENTIFICATION

Description/definition : Oxyquinoline is the heterocyclic compound that conforms to the formula shown below
Chemical class(es)   : Heterocyclic compounds; phenols
Chemical/IUPAC name   : Quinolin-8-ol
Other names   : 8-Hydroxyquinoline; 8-quinolinol; phenopyridine
CAS registry number (s) : 148-24-3
EC number(s)   : 205-711-1
CIR review(s)   : J Am Coll Toxicol 1992;11:497-507; Int J Toxicol 2006;25(Suppl.1):1-9 (access:
                          www.cir-safety.org/ingredients)
Merck Index monograph   : 6151
Function(s) in cosmetics : EU: stabilizing. USA: chelating agents; cosmetic biocides
EU cosmetic restrictions : Regulated in Annexes II/395 and III/51 of the Regulation (EC) No. 1223/2009
Patch testing   : No data available; suggested: 5% pet.
Molecular formula   : C_9H_7NO

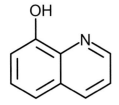

GENERAL
Discussion of oxyquinoline in this its effects in cosmetics.

CONTACT ALLERGY

Case reports and case series
Oxyquinoline was responsible for out 1of 399 cases of cosmetic allergy where the causal allergen was identified in a study of the NACDG, USA, 1977-1983 (1).

Presence in cosmetic products and chemical analyses
In the USA, in April 2017, oxyquinoline was present in 4 of 56,714 cosmetic products of which the composition is known in FDA's Voluntary Cosmetic Registration Program (VCRP) (data obtained from FDA, May 2017). In March 2017, oxyquinoline was present in one of 65,431 cosmetic products of which the composition is known in EWG's Skin Deep Cosmetics Database, USA (http://www.ewg.org/skindeep/).

LITERATURE
1   Adams RM, Maibach HI, Clendenning WE, Fisher AA, Jordan WJ, Kanof N, et al. A five-year study of cosmetic reactions. J Am Acad Dermatol 1985;13:1062-1069

2.327 PABA

IDENTIFICATION

Description/definition   : PABA is the aromatic acid that conforms to the formula shown below; member of the
vitamin B complex
Chemical class(es)   : Amines; amino acids; PABA derivatives
Chemical/IUPAC name   : 4-Aminobenzoic acid
Other names   : p-Aminobenzoic acid
CAS registry number (s)   : 150-13-0
EC number(s)   : 205-753-0
SCCS opinion(s)   : SCCP/1008/06 (54)
Merck Index monograph   : 1688
Function(s) in cosmetics   : Formerly used as UV-absorber and UV-filter; delisted in 2009. USA: light stabilizers;
sunscreen agents
EU cosmetic restrictions   : Regulated in Annex II/167 of the Regulation (EC) No. 1223/2009 (prohibited)
Patch testing   : 5% pet. (Chemotechnique, SmartPracticeEurope); 5% alc. (Chemotechnique); 10% pet.
(Chemotechnique, SmartPracticeCanada); photopatch tests may sometimes be false-
negative when PABA is tested in petrolatum (18)
Molecular formula   : $C_7H_7NO_2$

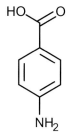

GENERAL

In its naturally occurring form, PABA is synthesized by intestinal bacteria as an intermediate during the synthesis of folic acid. Small amounts of the substance naturally occur in cereal, eggs, milk and meat. As a consequence, detectable levels are normally present in human body fluids. PABA is also promoted as a dietary supplement under the name of vitamin Bx, allegedly contributing to healthy hair and to the formation of red blood cells (62).

PABA is also a UVB filter with UV absorbance maximum (λ_{max}) at 283 nm, which has been used in Europe since 1948 (25,44,57). PABA was formerly a widely used sunscreen ingredient and a leading cause of sunscreen photoallergy (17). In recent years, it has almost disappeared from sunscreens due to concerns over its allergic and photoallergic potential (2,24,45,46) and it is prohibited in the EU. Many patients may have become allergic to PABA from prior sensitization to benzocaine, p-phenylenediamine or other para-substituted compounds (cross-reactivity) (34).

The literature on adverse reactions to sunscreens has been reviewed in several recent and older publications (17,47-51,68). A review of photocontact allergy to sunscreens was published in 2010 (58).

CONTACT ALLERGY

Patch testing in groups of patients

Results of routine patch testing (testing in consecutive patients suspected of contact dermatitis) with PABA and results of testing in groups of *selected* patients (e.g., patients suspected of photosensitivity, patients with dermatitis affecting mainly light-exposed skin or with a history of a sunscreen skin reaction) back to 1990 are shown in table 2.327.1. Test concentrations used have been 1% pet., 2% pet., 2% water 5% pet., 10% pet. and 5% alc.; the higher test con-centrations have not clearly resulted in more positive reactions, the mode of selection probably being the more important determinant. PABA has been routinely tested in one early (1980) study only, yielding a rate of sensitization of 0.6%; the reaction was not relevant (33).

In 14 studies testing groups of selected patients, frequencies of sensitization have ranged from 0.2% to 11.9%. In 9 of the 14 studies, rates were 1.1% or lower. The high frequency of 11.9% was seen in a study from Canada, which had certain weaknesses (23). When tested with PABA 5% alc., 19 of 160 (11.9%) patients had a positive patch test, whereas 3.1% in the same group reacted to PABA 5% pet. This points at many irritant reactions to the 5% alc. test material rather than false-negative reactions to the 5% pet. test material, also considering the fact that this 3.1% is already one of the highest percentages of positive reactions in all 14 studies.

In a 2005-2014 Chinese study, a stunning 9.6% positive reactions to PABA was observed in a large group of patients suspected of photodermatoses (56). However, in a subgroup of this population (nearly 75%) previously reported (55), the percentage of reactions to PABA was given as 0.4%, so there is no doubt that a serious mistake has been made in one (or both?) investigations (55,56). In all but three investigations, the relevance of the positive patch test reactions to PABA was either not stated or specified for the UV-filter. In the three where relevance was mentioned, its rate ranged from 0% to 100%, but the number of positive patients were very small (n=1-3) (2,20,41). Causative products were never mentioned.

Table 2.327.1 Patch testing in groups of patients

Years and Country	Test conc. & vehicle	Number of patients tested	positive (%)	Selection of patients (S); Relevance (R); Comments (C)	Ref.
Routine testing					
1980 Denmark	5% alc.	161	1 (0.6%)	R: none; C: all consecutive patients suspected of contact dermatitis were photopatch tested with PABA; one individual may have become sensitized (plain contact allergy) from the test procedure	33
Testing in groups of selected patients					
2005-2014 China	2% water	5032	481 (9.6%)	S: patients suspected of photodermatoses; R: not stated; C: same center as in ref. 55	56
2006-2012 China	2% water	3718	14 (0.4%)	S: patients with suspected photodermatoses; R: not stated; C: same center as in ref. 56	55
2001-2010 Canada	5% alc.	160	19 (11.9%)	S: patients with suspected photosensitivity and patients who developed pruritus or a rash after sunscreen applica- tion; R: not stated; C: very weak study: inadequate reading of test results, erythema only was considered to represent a positive patch test reaction	23
	5% pet.	160	5 (3.1%)		
2000-2007 USA	10% pet.	835	3 (0.4%)	S: patients tested with a supplemental cosmetic screening series; R: 100% (for both 5% and 10% pet.); C: weak study: a. high rate of macular erythema and weak reactions; b. relevance figures included 'questionable' and 'past' relevance	20
	5% pet.	107	3 (2.8%)		
2000-2005 USA	10% pet.	141	1 (0.7%)	S: patients photopatch tested for suspected photoderma- titis; R: not relevant	41
	5% alc.	178	2 (1.1%)	S: patients photopatch tested for suspected photoderma- titis; R: 1 reaction was relevant	
2000-2002 UK, I, NL	10% pet.	1155	3 (0.3%)	S: patients suspected of photosensitivity or reaction to a sunscreen; R: current relevance 1, exposed but no dermatitis 1, past relevance 1	2
1995-1999 Germany	10% pet.	638	1 (0.2%)	S: patients tested with a 'para-amino series'; R: not stated	1
1996-1998 UK	10% pet.	167	1 (0.6%)	S: patients with suspected photosensitivity; R: 'most cases' in the total study group were considered relevant	13
1983-1998 UK	2% or 10% pet.	2715	7 (0.3%)	S: patients suspected of photosensitivity or with (a history of) dermatitis at exposed sites; R: not stated	4
1990-1996 Sweden	5% alc.	355	1 (0.3%)	S: patients suspected of photosensitivity; R: not stated	38
1981-1996 Germany	5% or 10% pet.	355	3 (0.8%)	S: patients suspected of clinical photosensitivity; R: not stated	9
1990-1994 France	5% or 10% pet.	370	1 (0.3%)	S: patients with suspected photodermatitis; R: not specified, 72% of all reactions in the study were considered relevant	15
1989-1991 UK	2% pet.	99	2 (2%)	S: 45 patients with photosensitivity dermatitis/actinic reticuloid syndrome and 54 with polymorphic light eruption; R: not specified	10
1985-1990 USA	1% pet.	187	3 (1.6%)	S: patients with a history of photosensitivity; R: not stated	12

I: Ireland; NL: Netherlands; UK: United Kingdom

Case reports and case series
One positive patch test reaction to PABA was ascribed to cosmetic allergy (21). In the period 1978-1991, there were 6 relevant patch test reactions to PABA in one center in Leuven, Belgium (34). PABA was responsible for 3 out of 399 cases of cosmetic allergy where the causal allergen was identified in a study of the NACDG, USA, 1977-1983 (16). Six patients had allergic contact dermatitis from PABA in sunscreens (5). Two individuals had photoaggravated allergic contact dermatitis from PABA in sunscreens (42). One patient with xeroderma pigmentosum (3) and another one (30) had combined contact allergy and photocontact allergy to PABA in sunscreens. Several authors described single case reports of patients with allergic contact dermatitis from PABA in sunscreens (27,28,52).

Reports of positive patch tests to PABA with unspecified relevance
In a group of 73 patients referred to a contact dermatitis clinic in Melbourne, Australia, 1990-1991, who reported a history of reactions to sunscreens, there were 4 positive patch tests to PABA; the relevance of these reactions was not specified, but at that time, no sunscreens containing PABA were available in Australia (43). In the period 1978-1991, there were 54 non-relevant positive patch test reactions to PABA and/or isobutyl PABA (not specified) in Leuven, Belgium. Forty sensitizations represented cross-reactions to chemically-related para-substituted compounds, particularly p-phenylenediamine, benzocaine, diaminodiphenylmethane and sulfanilamide (34).

Contact allergy from PABA in non-cosmetic products
One patient developed DRESS syndrome (Drug Rash with Eosinophilia and Systemic Symptoms) while taking potassium p-aminobenzoate for induratio penis plastica. A patch test with the ground drug was positive. Unfortunately, the patient was not subsequently tested with PABA or potassium p-aminobenzoate to exclude a reaction to an excipient of the drug, and no controls were performed to exclude irritancy of the test preparation (63).

Cross-reactions, pseudo-cross-reactions and co-reactions (including photoreactions)
PABA may cross-react with structurally related chemicals, notably those with a para-structure. Cross-reactivity between para-compounds is discussed in Chapter 2.359 p-Phenylenediamine. Octyl dimethyl PABA (27,32); pentyl dimethyl PABA (11,30); glyceryl PABA (11,18,33); sulfonamides (34,60), p-phenylenediamine (34,60,61), benzocaine (11, 17,18,30,34), diaminodiphenylmethane (34). *Not* to glyceryl, pentyl or ethylhexyl dimethyl PABA (29).

Patch test sensitization
One patient may have become sensitized from a patch and photopatch with PABA 5% alcohol (33).

Presence in cosmetic products and chemical analyses
In June 2017, PABA was present in 2 of 68,985 cosmetic products of which the composition is known in EWG's Skin Deep Cosmetics Database, USA (http://www.ewg.org/skindeep/). It should be realized that sunscreen products containing UV-filters are classified as drugs in the USA, not as cosmetics; the number mentioned here, therefore, is that of cosmetics containing the UV-filter, but it does *not* include their presence in sunscreens. In the USA, in April 2017, PABA was present in 18 of 56,714 cosmetic products of which the composition is known in FDA's Voluntary Cosmetic Registration Program (VCRP) (data obtained from FDA, May 2017).

In 2009, in the USA, the ingredient lists of 796 hair products from one company were screened for the presence of PABA. PABA was present in 0% of 279 shampoos, in 1% of 231 conditioners, and in 1% of 286 styling products (53). PABA was present in 0.4% of 4447 cosmetic products collected in Germany, 2006-2009 (24). PABA was present in 0.6% of 329 sunscreen products (incl. 21 lipstick sunscreens) marketed in the UK in 2005 (45). PABA was found by HPLC to be present in two of 97 sunscreens and 15 after-sun products in Sweden, 1989 (64).

OTHER SIDE EFFECTS

Photosensitivity

Photopatch testing in groups of patients
Results of photopatch testing PABA in groups of selected patients (e.g., patients suspected of photosensitivity, patients with dermatitis affecting mainly light-exposed skin or with a history of a sunscreen skin reaction) back to 1981 are shown in table 2.327.2. Test concentrations used have been 1% pet., 2% pet., 2% water, 5% pet., 5% alc. and 10% pet.; the higher test concentrations have not clearly resulted in more positive reactions, the mode of selection probably being the more important determinant. In 21 studies photopatch testing groups of selected patients, frequencies of sensitization have ranged from 0.1% to 14.7%. In 15 of the 21 studies, rates were 2.6% or lower.

High frequencies of 11.9% and 14.7% were seen in two studies from the same center in China, where 5032 and 3718 patients with suspected photodermatoses were photopatch tested with PABA 2% (55,56). There is an overlap between these two investigations, as the entire patient group in ref. 55 (2006-2012) must also have been presented in ref. 56 (2005-2014), explaining the high percentage *in both* studies. Why these percentages are so high, is unknown. The authors themselves provide no other explanation than 'p-Aminobenzoic acid is a widely used sunscreen ingredient and a leading cause of photodermatitis (56).

In all but four investigations, the relevance of the positive photopatch test reactions to PABA was either not stated or specified for the UV-filter. In the four where relevance was mentioned, its rate ranged from 25% to 100%, but the number of positive patients were very small (n=1-4) (22,36,37,41). Causative products were mentioned in one study only: sunscreen product (37).

Table 2.327.2 Photopatch testing in groups of patients

Years and Country	Test conc. & vehicle	Number of patients tested	positive (%)	Selection of patients (S); Relevance (R); Comments (C)	Ref.
2005-2014 China	2% water	5032	601 (11.9%)	S: patients suspected of photodermatoses; R: not stated; C: same center as in ref. 55	56
2006-2012 China	2% water	3718	546 (14.7%)	S: patients with suspected photodermatoses; R: not stated; C: same center as in ref. 56	55
2000-2011 UK	10% pet.	157	1 (0.6%)	S: children <18 years suspected of photosensitivity; R: the reaction was caused by a sunscreen product	37
2001-2010 Canada	5% alc.	160	6 (3.8%)	S: patients with suspected photosensitivity and patients who developed pruritus or a rash after sunscreen applica-	23
	5% pet.	160	3 (1.9%)	tion; R: not stated; C: very weak study: inadequate reading of test results, erythema only was considered to represent a positive photopatch test reaction	
2003-2007 Portugal	10% pet.	83	1 (1.2%)	S: patients with suspected photoaggravated facial dermati-tis or systemic photosensitivity; R: all sunscreen photopatch tests were of current or past relevance	36
2004-2006 Italy	5% pet.	1082	2 (0.2%)	S: patients with histories and clinical features suggestive of photoallergic contact dermatitis; R: 100%	22
1993-2006 USA	5% alc.	76	4 (5.3%)	S: not stated; R: 56% of all reactions to sunscreens were considered 'probably relevant'	19
2000-2005 USA	10% pet.	141	4 (2.8%)	S: patients photopatch tested for suspected photoderma-titis; R: 1 reaction was relevant	41
	5% alc.	178	2 (1.1%)	S: patients photopatch tested for suspected photoderma-titis; R: 1 reaction was relevant	
2000-2002 UK, I, NL	10% pet.	1155	1 (0.1%)	S: patients suspected of photosensitivity or reaction to a sunscreen; R: past relevance	2
1993-2000 Australia	5% pet.	172	3 (2.0%)	S: patients suspected of photosensitivity; R: of 17 patient who had contact or photocontact reactions to a panel of 10 sunscreens, 10 were considered to have relevant reactions	35
1983-1998 UK	2% or 10% pet.	2715	5 (0.2%)	S: patients suspected of photosensitivity or with (a history of) dermatitis at exposed sites; R: 37% for all photoallergens together	4
1991-97 Ger, Au, Swi	10% pet.	1261	3 (0.2%)	S: patients suspected of photosensitivity; R: not stated	6
1990-1996 Sweden	5% alc.	355	2 (0.6%)	S: patients suspected of photosensitivity; R: not stated	38
1981-1996 Germany	5% or 10% pet.	355	2 (0.6%)	S: patients suspected of clinical photosensitivity; R: not stated	9
1990-1994 France	5% or 10% pet.	370	1 (0.3%)	S: patients with suspected photodermatitis; R: not specified, 72% of all reactions in the study were considered relevant	15
1986-1993 USA	5% pet. or 5% alc.	138	3 (2.2%)	S: patients suspected of photosensitivity; R: not stated	14
1985-1993 Italy		1050	7 (0.7%)	S: patients suspected of photoallergic contact dermatitis; R: not specified (97% for all sunscreens together)	7
1991-1993 Singapore	2% pet.	62	1 (2%)	S: patients with clinical features suggestive of photosensiti-vity; R: not stated	59
1985-1990 USA	1% pet.	187	5 (2.7%)	S: patients with a history of photosensitivity; R: all relevant	12
1980-85 Ger, Au, Swi	5% pet.	1129	1 (0.1%)	S: patients suspected of photoallergy, polymorphic light eruption, phototoxicity and skin problems with photo-distribution; R: not stated	8
1980-1981 4 Scandi-navian countries	5% alc.	745	19 (2.6%)	S: patients suspected of sun-related skin disease; R: not stated	40

Au: Austria; Ger: Germany; I: Ireland; NL: Netherlands; UK: United Kingdom; Swi: Switzerland

Case reports and series

Five patients had photoallergic contact dermatitis from PABA in sunscreens (5). One patient, who previously was diagnosed with contact allergy to benzocaine, developed photocontact allergy to PABA (26). Another individual had combined contact and photocontact allergy to PABA in a sunscreen (30). One patient photoreacted to PABA in a sunscreen (18). Of 280 patients tested with sunscreens in London, 1985-1987, one had photoallergic contact dermatitis from PABA in a sunscreen (39). In a group of 73 patients referred to a contact dermatitis clinic in Melbourne, Australia, 1990-1991, who reported a history of reactions to sunscreens, there were 2 positive photopatch tests to PABA; the relevance of these reactions was not specified, but at that time, no sunscreens containing PABA were available in Australia (43).

In a center in France, between 1982 and 1992, 283 patients with suspected photodermatitis were patch and photopatch tested and there were 17 cases of photocontact allergy to PABA and its derivatives. Details are unknown (66, article not read). An unknown number of patients had photoallergic contact dermatitis from PABA in sunscreens (67).

Photosensitization from non-cosmetic sources

A man suffered from an acute eczematous rash confined to the air- and light-exposed areas of the skin. There had been intensive holiday-associated sun exposure, but the patient did not use any sunscreen agents. However, several weeks before the onset of skin eruptions, conservative treatment of Peyronie's disease with oral potassium para-aminobenzoate had been started. Photopatch testing revealed photoallergy to PABA. Thus, this patient had photoallergic dermatitis from PABA acting as a systemic photosensitizer (62).

Other non-eczematous contact reactions

One patient developed milia on the extensor and flexor aspects of the forearms after resolution of allergic contact dermatitis from PABA in a sunscreen (65).

Miscellaneous side effects

PABA has a tendency to discolor white clothing or fabrics if these are wetted and then exposed to sunlight. It has been suggested that contact allergy to PABA, notably when combined with oral intake of related drugs such as sulfonamides, may lead to autoimmune responses, especially systemic lupus erythematosus and dermatomyositis (60).

LITERATURE

1   Uter W, Lessmann H, Geier J, Becker D, Fuchs T, Richter G. The spectrum of allergic (cross-)sensitivity in clinical patch testing with 'para amino' compounds. Allergy (Eur J All Clin Immmunol) 2002;57:319-322

2   Bryden A, Moseley H, Ibbotson S, Chowdhury MM, Beck MH, Bourke J, et al. Photopatch testing of 1155 patients: results of the U.K. multicenter photopatch test study group. Brit J Dermatol 2006;155:737-747

3   Horio T, Hituchi T. Photocontact dermatitis from p-aminobenzoic acid. Dermatologica (Basel) 1978;156:124-128

4   Darvay A, White I, Rycroft R, Jones AB, Hawk JL, McFadden JP. Photoallergic contact dermatitis is uncommon. Br J Dermatol 2001;145:597-601

5   Thune P. Contact and photocontact allergy to sunscreens. Photodermatol 1984;1:5-9

6   Neumann NJ, Hölzle E, Plewig G, Schwarz T, Panizzon RG, Breit R, et al. Photopatch testing: The 12-year experience of the German, Austrian and Swiss Photopatch Test Group. J Am Acad Dermatol 2000;42:183-192

7   Pigatto PD, Legori A, Bigardi AS, Guarrera M, Tosti A, Santucci B, et al. Gruppo Italiano recerca dermatiti da contatto ed ambientali Italian multicenter study of allergic contact photodermatitis: epidemiological aspects. Am J Contact Dermatitis 1996;17:158-163

8   Hölzle E, Neumann N, Hausen B, Przybilla B, Schauder S, Hönigsmann H, et al. Photopatch testing: the 5-year experience of the German, Austrian and Swiss Photopatch Test Group. J Am Acad Dermatol 1991;25:59-68

9   Schauder S, Ippen H. Contact and photocontact sensitivity. Review of a 15-year experience and of the literature to suncreens. Contact Dermatitis 1997;37:221-232

10   Bilsland D, Ferguson J. Contact allergy to sunscreen chemicals in photosensitivity dermatitis/actinic reticuloid syndrome (PD/AR) and polymorphic light eruption. Contact Dermatitis 1993;29:70-73

11   Marmelzat J, Rapaport MJ. Photodermatitis with PABA. Contact Dermatitis 1980;6:230-231

12   DeLeo VA, Suarez SM, Maso MJ. Photoallergic contact dermatitis. Results of photopatch testing in New York, 1985 to 1990. Arch Dermatol 1992;128:1513-1518

13   Bell HK, Rhodes LE. Photopatch testing in photosensitive patients. Br J Dermatol 2000;142:589-590

14   Fotiades J, Soter NA, Lim HW. Results of evaluation of 203 patients for photosensitivity in a 7.3 year period. J Am Acad Dermatol 1995;33:597-602

15   Journe F, Marguery M-C, Rakotondrazafy J, El Sayed F, Bazex J. Sunscreen sensitization: a 5-year study. Acta Derm Venereol (Stockh) 1999;79:211-213

16   Adams RM, Maibach HI, Clendenning WE, Fisher AA, Jordan WJ, Kanof N, et al. A five-year study of cosmetic reactions. J Am Acad Dermatol 1985;13:1062-1069

17   Dromgoole SH, Maibach HI. Sunscreening agent intolerance: Contact and photocontact sensitization and contact urticaria. J Am Acad Dermatol 1990;22:1068-1078

18   Mathias CGT, Maibach HI, Epstein J. Allergic contact photodermatitis to para-aminobenzoic acid. Arch Derm 1978; 114:1665-1666

19 Victor FC, Cohen DE, Soter NA. A 20-year analysis of previous and emerging allergens that elicit photoallergic contact dermatitis. J Am Acad Dermatol 2010;62:605-610

20 Wetter DA, Yiannias JA, Prakash AV, Davis MD, Farmer SA, el-Azhary RA, et al. Results of patch testing to personal care product allergens in a standard series and a supplemental cosmetic series: an analysis of 945 patients from the Mayo Clinic Contact Dermatitis Group, 2000-2007. J Am Acad Dermatol 2010;63:789-798

21 Kohl L, Blondeel A, Song M. Allergic contact dermatitis from cosmetics: retrospective analysis of 819 patch-tested patients. Dermatology 2002;204:334-337

22 Pigatto PD, Guzzi G, Schena D, Guarrera M, Foti C, Francalanci S, et al. Photopatch tests: an Italian multicenter study from 2004 to 2006. Contact Dermatitis 2008;59:103-108

23 Greenspoon J, Ahluwalia R, Juma N, Rosen CF. Allergic and photoallergic contact dermatitis: A 10-year experience. Dermatitis 2013;24:29-32

24 Uter W, Gonçalo M, Yazar K, Kratz E-M, Mildau G, Lidén C. Coupled exposure to ingredients of cosmetic products: III. Ultraviolet filters. Contact Dermatitis 2014;71:162-169

25 Shaath NA. Evolution of modern sunscreen chemicals. In: Lowe NJ, Shaath NA, Pathak MA, eds. Sunscreens: Development, evaluation, and regulatory aspects, 2nd edition. New York: Marcel Dekker Inc., 1997: 3-33.

26 Waters AJ, Sandhu DR, Lowe G, Ferguson J. Photocontact allergy to PABA in sunscreens: the need for continued vigilance. Contact Dermatitis 2009;60:172-173

27 Camarasa JG, Serra-Baldrich E. Allergic contact dermatitis to sunscreens. Contact Dermatitis 1986;15:253-254

28 Romaguera C, Grimalt F. Dermatitis from PABA and hydroquinone. Contact Dermatitis 1983;9:226

29 Thune P. Photosensitivlty and allergy to cosmetics. Contact Dermatitis 1981;7:54-55

30 Marmelzat J, Rapaport MJ. Photodermatitis with PABA. Contact Dermatitis 1980;6:230-231

31 Trevisi P, Vincenzi C, Chieregato C, Guerra L, Tosti A. Sunscreen sensitization: a three-year study. Dermatology 1994;189:55-57

32 Crowe MJ, Banks SL, Guin JD. Photoallergic and allergic contact dermatitis to butyl-methoxydibenzoylmethane. Am J Cont Derm 1992;3:33-34

33 Kroon S. Standard photopatch testing with Waxtar®, para-aminobenzoic acid, potassium dichromate and balsam of Peru. Contact Dermatitis 1983;9:5-9

34 Theeuwes M, Degreef H, Dooms-Goossens A. Para-aminobenzoic acid (PABA) and sunscreen allergy. Am J Cont Derm 1992;3:206-207

35 Crouch RB, Foley PA, Baker CS. The results of photopatch testing 172 patients to sunscreening agents at the photobiology clinic, St Vincent's Hospital, Melbourne. Australas J Dermatol 2002;43:74

36 Cardoso J, Canelas MM, Gonçalo M, Figueiredo A. Photopatch testing with an extended series of photoallergens: a 5-year study. Contact Dermatitis 2009;60:325-329

37 Haylett AK, Chiang YZ, Nie Z, Ling TC, Rhodes LE. Sunscreen photopatch testing: a series of 157 children. Br J Dermatol 2014;171:370-375

38 Berne B, Ross AM. 7 years experience of photopatch testing with sunscreen allergens in Sweden. Contact Dermatitis 1998;38:61-64

39 English JSC, White IR, Cronin K. Sensitivity to sunscreens. Contact Dermatitis 1987;17:159-162

40 Wennersten G, Thune P, Brodthagen H, Jansen C, Rystedt I, Crames M, et al. The Scandinavian multicenter photopatch study. Contact Dermatitis 1984;10:305-309

41 Scalf LA, Davis MDP, Rohlinger AL, Connolly SM. Photopatch testing of 182 patients: A 6-year experience at the Mayo Clinic. Dermatitis 2009;20:44-52

42 Freeman S, Frederiksen P. Sunscreen allergy. Am J Cont Derm 1990;1:240-243

43 Nixon RL, Frowen KE, Lewis AE. Skin reactions to sunscreens. Australas J Dermatol 1997;38:S83-S85.

44 Kerr A, Ferguson J. Photoallergic contact dermatitis. Photodermatol Photoimmunol Photomed 2010;26:56-65

45 Wahie S, Lloyd JJ, Farr PM. Sunscreen ingredients and labelling: a survey of products available in the U.K. Clin Exp Dermatol 2007;32:359-364

46 Scheuer E, Warshaw E. Sunscreen allergy: a review of epidemiology, clinical characteristics, and responsible allergens. Dermatitis 2006;17:3-11

47 Heurung AR, Raju SI, Warshaw EM. Adverse reactions to sunscreen agents: epidemiology, responsible irritants and allergens, clinical characteristics, and management. Dermatitis 2014;25:289-326

48 Heurung AR, Raju SI, Warshaw EM. Contact allergen of the year. Benzophenones. Dermatitis 2014;25:3-10 (contains many mistakes; Erratum in Dermatitis 2014;25:92-95)

49 Avenel-Audran M. Sunscreen products: finding the allergen. Eur J Dermatol 2010;20:161-166

50 Scheuer E, Warshaw E. Sunscreen allergy: a review of epidemiology, clinical characteristics, and responsible allergens. Dermatitis 2006;17:3-11

51 Funk JO, Dromgoole SH, Maibach HI. Sunscreen intolerance: contact sensitization, photocontact sensitization, and irritancy of sunscreen agents. Dermatol Clin 1995;13:473-481

52 Held E, Johansen JD, Agner T, Menné T. Contact allergy to cosmetics: testing with patients' own products. Contact Dermatitis 1999;40:310-315

53 Scheman A, Jacob S, Katta R, Nedorost S, Warshaw E, Zirwas M, et al. Part 2 of a 4 part series. Hair cosmetics: trends and alternatives. Data from the American Contact Alternative Group. J Clin Aesthet Dermatol 2011;4:42-46

54 SCCP (Scientific Committee on Consumer Products). Opinion on 4-Aminobenzoic acid (PABA), 20 June 2006, SCCP/1008/06. Available at:
http://ec.europa.eu/health/archive/ph_risk/committees/04_sccp/docs/sccp_o_058.pdf

55 Gao L, Hu Y, Ni C, Xu Y, Ma L, Yan S, Dou X. Retrospective study of photopatch testing in a Chinese population during a 7-year period. Dermatitis 2014;25:22-26

56 Hu Y, Wang D, Shen Y, Tang H. Photopatch testing in Chinese patients over 10 years. Dermatitis 2016;27:137-142

57 Shaath NA. Ultraviolet filters. Photochem Photobiol Sci 2010;9:464-469

58 Shaw T, Simpson B, Wilson B, Oostman H, Rainey D, Storrs F. True photoallergy to sunscreens is rare despite popular belief. Dermatitis 2010;21:185-198

59 Leow YH, Wong WK, Ng SK, Goh CL. 2 years experience of photopatch testing in Singapore. Contact Dermatitis 1994;31:181-182

60 Mackie B, Mackie L. The PABA story. Australas J Dermatol 1999;40:51-53

61 Mackie BS, Mackie LE. Cross-sensitization in dermatitis due to hair dyes. Australas J Dermatol 1964;4:189-201

62 Stoevesandt J, Kürzinger N, Bröcker EB, Trautmann A. Uro-dermatological problems of a construction worker: paraaminobenzoic acid as a systemic photosensitizer. Eur J Dermatol 2010;20:217-219

63 Viehweg A, Stein A, Bauer A, Spornraft-Ragaller P. Potassium-paraaminobenzoic acid (Potaba®)-associated DRESS syndrome. Dermatitis 2013;24:257-258

64 Bruze M, Gruvberger B, Thulin I. PABA, benzocaine, and other PABA esters in sunscreens and after-sun products. Photodermatol Photoimmunol Photomed 1990;7:106-108

65 Ibbotson SH, Taylor WD, Farr PM. Milia as unusual sequelae to allergic contact dermatitis. Contact Dermatitis 1996;35:49-50

66 Szczurko C, Dompmartin A, Michel M, Moreau A, Leroy D. Photocontact allergy to oxybenzone: ten years of experience. Photodermatol Photoimmunol Photomed 1994;10:144-147

67 Kaminester LH. Allergic reaction to sunscreen products. Arch Dermatol 1981;117:66

68 Schauder S. Survey of the literature on adverse reactions to preparations containing UV filters (1947-1989) (Literaturübersicht über Unverträglichkeitsreaktionen auf lichtfilterhaltige Produkte von 1947 bis 1989). Z Hautkr 1990;65:982-998 (article in German)

2.328   PALMITOYL COLLAGEN AMINO ACIDS

IDENTIFICATION

Description/definition   : Palmitoyl collagen amino acids is the condensation product of palmitic acid chloride and collagen amino acids

Chemical class(es)   : Amino acids

Other names   : Amino acids, collagen, 1-oxohexadecyl derivatives; palmitoyl animal collagen amino acids

CIR review(s)   : Final report, January 2014 (access: www.cir-safety.org/ingredients)

Function(s) in cosmetics : EU: antistatic; cleansing. USA: hair conditioning agents; skin-conditioning agents – miscellaneous; surfactants - cleansing agents

Patch testing   : 5% pet. (1)

GENERAL

Palmitoyl collagen amino acids is obtained from a condensation reaction between palmitic acid and a collagen hydrolysate, which is rarely used in cosmetics. It is supposed to have anti-inflammatory, anti-pruriginous and wound-healing properties, and is therefore used in the treatment of insect bites, napkin dermatitis, sunburn, and contact dermatitis (2).

CONTACT ALLERGY

Case reports and case series

A female teacher presented with a 2-month history of dermatitis on the face, hands and feet. It had started after using 'jogging cream' to prevent blisters during walking trips. Her only known allergy was to penicillin, which she had not taken recently. Neither the patient nor her blood relatives had symptoms of atopy or psoriasis. A patch test with the jogging cream was positive at D2 and D3. Patch tests with the ICDRG standard series were negative. After discontinuing the use of the jogging cream, no relapse occurred. Next, the ingredients of the cream were patch tested, which yielded positive results to palmitoyl collagen amino acids 5% pet. and some other components (1).

Contact allergy to palmitoyl collagen amino acids in non-cosmetic products

An atopic woman presented with chronic radiodermatitis on the left side of her neck due to radiotherapy performed in childhood to treat scrofuloderma. After electrocauterisation, a cream was applied to prevent the formation of keloids. Three days later, the patient noticed erythema and an itchy vesicular eczema at the site of application. She was patch tested with the Portuguese Group standard series, a series of 25 cosmetic allergens and with her own cosmetics. Only the anti-keloid cream was positive. This cream was composed of 23 constituents, which were all tested individually. There were positive reactions to 'palmitoyl collagenic acid', tested at 1% and 10% pet. only. There were no reactions to other collagen-derivatives. A control group of 80 subjects suspected of cosmetic dermatitis was patch tested with palmitoyl collagenic acid, but there were no positive reactions (2).

Cross-reactions and pseudo-cross-reactions

Co-reaction to palmitoyl hydrolyzed milk protein (1).

Presence in cosmetic products and chemical analyses

In the USA, in April 2017, palmitoyl collagen amino acids was present in 1 of 56,714 cosmetic products of which the composition is known in FDA's Voluntary Cosmetic Registration Program (VCRP) (data obtained from FDA, May 2017). In March 2017, palmitoyl collagen amino acids was present in one of 65,431 cosmetic products of which the composition is known in EWG's Skin Deep Cosmetics Database, USA (http://www.ewg.org/skindeep/).

LITERATURE

1   De Leeuw J, den Hollander P. A patient with a contact allergy to jogging cream. Contact Dermatitis 1987;17:260-261

2   Bordalo O, Brandao FM. Contact allergy to palmitoyl collagenic acid in an anti-keloid cream. Contact Dermatitis 1991;24:316

2.329   PALMITOYL HYDROLYZED MILK PROTEIN

IDENTIFICATION

Description/definition   : Palmitoyl hydrolyzed milk protein is the condensation product of palmitic acid chloride
                              and hydrolyzed milk protein
Chemical class(es)   : Protein derivatives
Other names   : Protein hydrolyzates, milk, 1-oxohexadecyl derivatives
Function(s) in cosmetics   : EU: antistatic; cleansing. USA: hair conditioning agents; skin-conditioning agents –
                              miscellaneous; surfactants - cleansing agents
Patch testing   : 10% pet. (1)

CONTACT ALLERGY

Case reports and case series
A female teacher presented with a 2-month history of dermatitis on the face, hands and feet. It had started after using 'jogging cream' to prevent blisters during walking trips. Her only known allergy was to penicillin, which she had not taken recently. Neither the patient nor her blood relatives had symptoms of atopy or psoriasis. A patch test with the jogging cream was positive at D2 and D3. Patch tests with the ICDRG standard series were negative. After discontinuing the use of the jogging cream, no relapse occurred. Next, the ingredients of the cream were patch tested, which yielded positive results to palmitoyl hydrolyzed milk protein 10% pet. and some other components (1).

Cross-reactions, pseudo-cross-reactions and co-reactions
Co-reaction to palmitoyl collagen amino acids (1)

Presence in cosmetic products and chemical analyses
In the USA, in April 2017, palmitoyl hydrolyzed milk protein was present in 2 of 56,714 cosmetic products of which the composition is known in FDA's Voluntary Cosmetic Registration Program (VCRP) (data obtained from FDA, May 2017). In March 2017, palmitoyl hydrolyzed milk protein was present in zero of 65,431 cosmetic products of which the composition is known in EWG's Skin Deep Cosmetics Database, USA (http://www.ewg.org/skindeep/).

LITERATURE
1   De Leeuw J, den Hollander P. A patient with a contact allergy to jogging cream. Contact Dermatitis 1987;17:260-
     261

2.330 PALMITOYL HYDROLYZED WHEAT PROTEIN

IDENTIFICATION

Description/definition	: Palmitoyl hydrolyzed wheat protein is the condensation product of palmitic acid chloride and hydrolyzed wheat protein
Chemical class(es)	: Protein derivatives
Other names	: Protein hydrolyzates, wheat (*Triticum vulgare*), 1-oxohexadecyl derivatives
Function(s) in cosmetics	: EU: cleansing; surfactant. USA: hair conditioning agents; skin-conditioning agents – miscellaneous; surfactants – cleansing agents
Patch testing	: 50% water (1)

GENERAL

Animal and/or plant-derived hydrolyzed proteins are added to skin cosmetics because of their moisturizing and cleansing properties. Such proteins are also added to foods, presumably for their binding properties. Among these proteins, hydrolyzed wheat protein is often used in both the cosmetic and food industries. Hydrolyzed wheat proteins can be associated with manifestations of immediate hypersensitivity ranging from urticaria to anaphylaxis, and less frequently with allergic contact dermatitis (2).

CONTACT ALLERGY

Case reports and case series

A 3-year-old girl with a history of moderate atopic dermatitis presented with an intolerance to a common emollient containing hydrolyzed wheat protein. Scaly erythematous dermatitis-like skin lesions were observed at sites atypical for atopic dermatitis including the knees. There was no evidence of associated contact urticaria. Patch tests with the European standard series and the emollient gave a positive reaction to the cosmetic product. Additional patch tests with individual components of the emollient were positive only for palmitoyl hydrolyzed wheat protein at D2 and D3 (patch test concentration and vehicle not mentioned). A prick test, open test and open patch test with this material were negative. Prick- and RAST tests for wheat were also negative (2). The hydrolysis of wheat proteins is associated with the formation of new epitopes, which are not present in unmodified wheat proteins. This explains hypersensitivity to palmitoyl hydrolyzed wheat protein in the absence of allergy to wheat (2).

An atopic child had allergic contact dermatitis from palmitoyl hydrolyzed wheat protein present in a moisturizer. The child had a positive patch test reaction to the material 50% water (1).

Presence in cosmetic products and chemical analyses

In the USA, in April 2017, palmitoyl hydrolyzed wheat protein was present in 13 of 56,714 cosmetic products of which the composition is known in FDA's Voluntary Cosmetic Registration Program (VCRP) (data obtained from FDA, May 2017). In March 2017, palmitoyl hydrolyzed wheat protein was present in one of 65,431 cosmetic products of which the composition is known in EWG's Skin Deep Cosmetics Database, USA (http://www.ewg.org/skindeep/).

LITERATURE

1   Mailhol C, Lauwers-Cances V, Rancé F, Paul C, Giordano-Labadie F. Prevalence and risk factors for allergic contact dermatitis to topical treatment in atopic dermatitis: a study in 641 children. Allergy 2009;64:801-806
2   Livideanu C, Giordano-Labadie F, Paul C. Contact dermatitis to hydrolyzed wheat protein. Contact Dermatitis 2007;57:283-284

2.331 PANTHENOL

Description/definition   : Panthenol is the alcohol that conforms to the formula shown below
Chemical class(es)   : Alcohols; amides
Chemical/IUPAC name   : (2R)-2,4-Dihydroxy-N-(3-hydroxypropyl)-3,3-dimethylbutanamide
Other names   : Dexpanthenol; pantothenol; provitamin B5
CAS registry number (s)   : 81-13-0; 16485-10-2
EC number(s)   : 201-327-3; 240-540-6
CIR review(s)   : J Am Coll Toxicol 1987;6:139-162 (access: www.cir-safety.org/ingredients)
Merck Index monograph   : 4219
Function(s) in cosmetics   : EU: antistatic; hair conditioning; skin conditioning. USA: hair conditioning agents
Patch testing   : 5% pet. (SmartPracticeEurope, SmartPracticeCanada)
Molecular formula   : $C_9H_{19}NO_4$

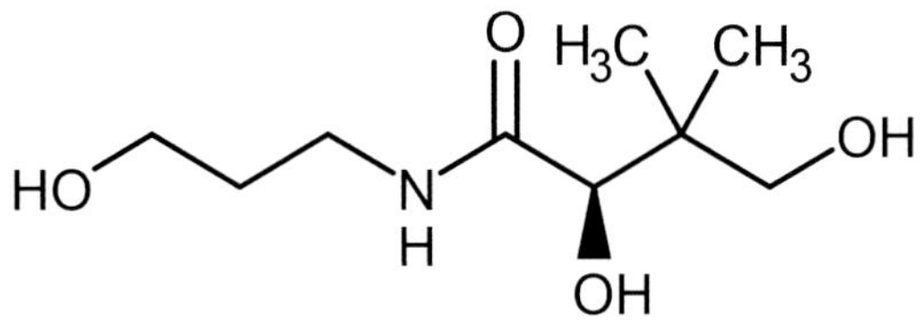

GENERAL

Panthenol is the stable alcoholic analogue of pantothenic acid, a water-soluble vitamin (B5) that is essential for the biosynthesis of coenzyme A (1). Panthenol is commonly used in the pharmaceutical and cosmetic industries, because of its moisturizing and conditioning properties. It is said to maintain skin softness and elasticity, to reduce transepidermal water loss, improve hydration of the stratum corneum, stabilize the epidermal barrier function, and accelerate skin re-epithelialization and activation of fibroblast proliferation (12). It is a frequent component of shampoos and hair conditioners as it coats and seals the hair surface, making hair appear more shiny (11). Panthenol is also added to other products, including wipes, cosmetic makeup, cleansers, and nail polish (6). It is also found in topical treatments for rhinitis, conjunctivitis, sunburn and for wound healing (ulcers, burns, bed sores, and excoriations) (10,12). It is present as 'active ingredient' in a concentration of 5% in the widely used Bepanthen® / Bepanthol® / Bepanthenol® creams and ointments.

The literature on contact allergy to panthenol has been reviewed in 1995 (15). Up to then, 40 cases had been reported. Most patients also reacted to several other allergens, mostly ingredients of cosmetic or pharmaceutical products (15).

CONTACT ALLERGY

Patch testing in groups of patients

Results of studies patch testing panthenol in consecutive patients suspected of contact dermatitis (routine testing) and in groups of selected patients are shown in table 2.331.1. In one study performing routine testing, the frequency of sensitization was 0.3%; 4 out of 5 positive reactions were considered to be relevant, of which three were caused by cosmetic products (14). In 7 studies patch testing panthenol in groups of selected patients (e.g., patients tested with a pharmaceutical and/or cosmetic series, patients with leg ulcers), rates of sensitization ranged from 0.3% to 7%; 5 had a score of 0.7% or lower. The 7% frequency was seen in a small study of 75 patients with venous leg ulcers and dermatitis of the surrounding skin, of who 5 had a positive reaction. However, their relevance was not mentioned and the patch test concentration was 30% pet., which is unusually high (27) (panthenol 30% in water was negative in 12 controls, though [6]).

In most studies, no relevance data were provided, but in a large group of 23 patients with contact allergy to panthenol, all were relevant. Four reactions were caused by a cosmeceutical cream or ointment with panthenol as active ingredient, the other 19 were related to the use of cosmetic products (28).

Case reports and case series

In the period 1990-2017, in Belgium, 23 patients with allergic contact dermatitis from panthenol were seen. Four subjects were sensitized through Bepanthen or Bepanthol cream or ointment, in which panthenol is the main active ingredient, and 19 through various (other) cosmetic products, particularly moisturizing facial and body-care products (n=12), but also shampoos and sunscreen products (n=3 each), hand creams, hair care products, 'repairing balms', deodorants, and eye make-up removers (n=2 each), and a tanning product, a shower gel, and a lipstick (n=1 each) (28, overlap with refs. 4 and 22). Panthenol was stated to be the (or an) allergen in 3 patients in a group of 603 individuals suffering from cosmetic dermatitis, seen in the period 2010-2015 in Leuven, Belgium (22, overlap with ref. 28). Panthenol was responsible for 8 out of 959 cases of non-fragrance cosmetic allergy where the causal allergen was identified, Belgium, 2000-2010 (4, overlap with ref. 28). Five positive patch test reactions to panthenol were ascribed to cosmetic allergy (5). In a 4-month-period in 1996, 475 patients with contact allergy to 'cosmetic ingredients' were collected in 5 centers in Belgium, UK and Germany. There were 3 reactions to panthenol; their relevance was not mentioned (21).

Table 2.331.1 Patch testing in groups of patients

Years and Country	Test conc. & vehicle	Number of patients tested | positive (%)		Selection of patients (S); Relevance (R); Comments (C)	Ref.
Routine testing					
1996/1997 Austria	5% pet.	1474	5 (0.3%)	R: 4 (80%) were considered relevant, of which three were from cosmetic products	14
Testing in groups of selected patients					
1990-2017 Belgium	5% pet.	3301	23 (0.7%)	S: patients tested with a pharmaceutical series, a cosmetic series, and individuals in who aimed patch testing was done; R: all were relevant, 4 were due to a cream or ointment with panthenol as active ingredient, 19 patients had ACD from various cosmetic products, notably moisturizing facial and body-care products	28
2010-2015 Denmark	5% pet.	431	1 (0.2%)	S: not stated; the reaction was relevant and published as a case report (23)	23
1990-2004 IVDK	5% pet.	450	7 (1.6%)	S: housewives from a group of 2633, tested with a pharmaceutical series; R: not stated	18
2000-2002 Finland		5102	(0.5%)	S: patients tested with a cosmetic series; R: not stated	20
2000-2002 Serbia	30% pet.	75	5 (7%)	S: patients with venous leg ulcers and dermatitis of the surrounding skin; R: not stated	27
1995-1996 Finland		286	(0.7%)	S: patients tested with a cosmetic series; R: not stated	20
1990-1993 Austria		273	2 (0.7%)	S: unknown; R: both reactions were probably caused by topical pharmaceutical products	15

IVDK: Information Network of Departments of Dermatology, Germany, Austria, Switzerland

A woman with post-thrombotic syndrome had extensive leg ulcers and stasis dermatitis on both legs. Skin grafting was performed; the autologous grafts were well accepted, but the skin around the ulcers and the donor site at the thigh showed persistent erythema, vesicles and oozing. The contact dermatitis proved to be caused by allergy to panthenol in Bepanthen ointment (7). Two patients from Portugal also reacted to panthenol in Bepanthen cream used for the treatment of stasis dermatitis on the legs in one patient and for local application after radiotherapy for basal cell carcinoma of the face in the other. The patient with stasis dermatitis subsequently developed generalized dermatitis (1). Another patient allergic to panthenol in Bepanthen cream had both a positive patch test to the cream and to panthenol and a positive lymphocyte transformation test; clinical details were not provided (17). Five patients had allergic contact dermatitis from panthenol-containing ointments applied to the face (2). An 11-year-old girl presented with a history of two episodes of facial eczema, which developed one day after the application of make-up that was removed with 'hypoallergenic' facial wipes. She was patch test positive to the wipe and its ingredient panthenol, tested 30% in water, to which 12 controls were negative (6).

A young man suffered for 2 years from an edematous erythema of the face which only appeared during winter sports and which was caused by contact allergy to panthenol in 2 sunscreen products (8). A woman had dermatitis of the face from panthenol in a moisturizing lotion (10); in another female individual, allergic contact dermatitis of the face was caused by a hydrating lotion (11). One patient had dermatitis from a baby cream. After avoidance, some eczema remained, notably on the hands. Oral challenge with calcium panthotenate resulted in worsening of the dermatitis on two occasions and dietary avoidance of vitamin B5 in improvement; change-over to B5-rich nutrition provoked worsening of facial and hand eczema within one week (14). During the testing for skin irritation of a sun protective and baby care lotion in epicutaneous tests over 24 hours, an eczematous test reaction appeared in one subject, which was caused in both products by panthenol (9). A 3-year-old girl with severe recalcitrant atopic dermatitis had superimposed allergic contact dermatitis from panthenol (and bisabolol) in a moisturizing ointment (19).

A woman developed allergic contact dermatitis caused by panthenol in a cream used as aftercare for a tattoo (23). Another female individual had ACD from panthenol in an 'intolerance repairing cream and soothing moisturizer' and a body lotion (24). Seven cases of contact allergy to panthenol were reported from Austria; details are unknown, but the causative products were most likely cosmetics and topical pharmaceutical preparations (15). A woman had perioral dermatitis from contact allergy to panthenol in two lip balms. Previously, she had suffered from facial dermatitis from a cream also containing panthenol (31).

Contact allergy to panthenol in non-cosmetic products
Pharmaceutical products for the treatment of leg ulcers / stasis dermatitis caused allergic contact dermatitis from their ingredient panthenol (2,16). An unknown number of patients reacted to panthenol in unknown products (25,26). Seven cases of contact allergy to panthenol were reported from Austria; details are unknown, but the causative products were most likely topical pharmaceutical preparations and cosmetics (15).

Provocation tests
One patient had dermatitis from a baby cream. After avoidance, some eczema remained, notably on the hands. Oral challenge with calcium panthotenate resulted in worsening of the dermatitis on two occasions and dietary avoidance of vitamin B5 in improvement; change-over to B5-rich nutrition provoked worsening of facial and hand eczema within one week (14).

Presence in cosmetic products and chemical analyses
In May 2017, panthenol was present in 4369 of 66,669 cosmetic products of which the composition is known in EWG's Skin Deep Cosmetics Database, USA (http://www.ewg.org/skindeep/). In the USA, in April 2017, panthenol was present in 586 of 56,714 cosmetic products of which the composition is known in FDA's Voluntary Cosmetic Registration Program (VCRP) (data obtained from FDA, May 2017). Panthenol derivatives were present in 36 (20%) of 178 facial wipes for which ingredient information was obtained online and from retail stores, USA, 2016 (30).

OTHER SIDE EFFECTS

Irritant contact dermatitis
An 8-year-old girl presented with pruriginous pustular lesions, pustule remnants and thin scales over erythematous and eczematous areas on the face and neck. These lesions had appeared 2 days after application of a moisturizing cream containing panthenol. A skin biopsy showed subcorneal pustules, spongiosis and an inflammatory infiltrate composed mainly of lymphocytes and some eosinophils and neutrophils. A patch test with the European baseline series and panthenol was negative. The authors diagnosed this child with 'pustular irritant contact dermatitis caused by dexpanthenol' (29). This may be incorrect, as the reaction was caused by *the cream containing panthenol*, and it cannot be concluded that panthenol was the causative ingredient. Also, the product itself has apparently not been patch tested, so contact allergy to another ingredient of the cream cannot be ruled out.

Immediate-type reactions
A woman was admitted to the emergency department with edema of the face including the eyelids and tongue, and dyspnea, dizziness and faintness. The symptoms had started 20 minutes after breakfast. She took multivitamin tablets more or less regularly after breakfast with orange juice. Scratch tests with the patient's three tablets were all positive. Fifteen minutes after scratch testing, the patient felt a tightness in her throat and she developed a facial edema and breathlessness. Under emergency conditions, a further skin scratch test was performed to identify the causative ingredient; they were negative to vitamin B1, B2, B6, B12 and folic acid. Testing of panthenol by a friction test (panthenol 5% in purified petrolatum) led to pruritus and erythema in the tested skin area and to pruritus on the lips and a coated tongue. Discussing the skin test results, the patient remembered that panthenol-containing sun cream had caused pruritus and local urticaria previously (3).

Another female patient presented with a history of facial edema, erythema and pruritus within a minute after application of a new hair conditioner with panthenol. She had no shortness of breath but did have diffuse pruritus on her trunk. There was gradual improvement of her symptoms over an hour, after washing off the conditioner. The patient had previously used panthenol-containing hair coloring products at her hairdresser, with pruritus occurring at the hairline. Open tests with panthenol 30% pet. and her conditioner 1:5 diluted with water were negative, but prick tests were positive to both substances. Later, the patient had one more episode of pruritus and swelling at the hairline after her hairdresser again used panthenol-containing hair coloring (13).

LITERATURE
1   Fernandes S, Macias V, Cravo M, Amaro C, Santos R, Cardoso J. Allergic contact dermatitis caused by dexpanthenol: report of two cases. Contact Dermatitis 2012;66:160-161
2   Schulze-Dirks A, Frosch PJ. Contact allergy to dexpanthenol. Hautarzt 1988;39:375-377
3   Röckmann H, Goerdt S, Bayerl C. Anaphylaxis after dexpanthenol exposure by multivitamin tablets. Clin Exp Dermatol 2005;30:714-716

4   Travassos AR, Claes L, Boey L, Drieghe J, Goossens A. Non-fragrance allergens in specific cosmetic products. Contact Dermatitis 2011;65:276-285

5   Kohl L, Blondeel A, Song M. Allergic contact dermatitis from cosmetics: retrospective analysis of 819 patch-tested patients. Dermatology 2002;204:334-337

6   Chin MF, Hughes TM, Stone NM. Allergic contact dermatitis caused by panthenol in a child. Contact Dermatitis 2013;69:321-322

7   Gollhausen R, Przybilla B, Ring J. Contact allergy to dexpanthenol. Contact Dermatitis 1985;13:38

8   Jeanmougin M, Manchet J R, Moulin J P, Blanc F, Pons A, Civatte J. Contact allergy to dexpanthenol in unscreens. Contact Dermatitis 1988;18:240

9   Ippen H. Kontaktallergie auf Dexpanthenol. Dermatosen 1981;29:45

10   Stables GI, Wilkinson SM. Allergic contact dermatitis due to panthenol. Contact Dermatitis 1998;38:236-237

11   Roberts H, Williams J, Tate B. Allergic contact dermatitis to panthenol and cocamidopropyl PG dimonium chloride phosphate in a facial hydrating lotion. Contact Dermatitis 2006;55:369-370

12   Ebner F, Heller A, Rippke F, Tausch I. Topical use of dexpanthenol in skin disorders. Am J Clin Dermatol 2002;3:427-433

13   Schalock PC, Storrs FJ, Morrison L. Contact urticaria from panthenol in hair conditioner. Contact Dermatitis 2000;43:223

14   Hemmer W, Bracun R, Wolf-Abdolvahab S, Focke M, Götz M, Jarisch R. Maintenance of hand eczema by oral pantothenic acid in a patient sensitized to dexpanthenol. Contact Dermatitis 1997;37:51

15   Schmid-Grendelmeier P, Wyss M, Elsner P. Contact allergy to dexpanthenol – a report of seven cases and review of the literature. Dermatosen 1995;43:175-178.

16   Keilig W. Kontaktallergie auf Dexpanthenol. Dermatosen 1987;35:206-208

17   Hahn C, Röseler S, Fritzsche R, Schneider R, Merk HF. Allergic contact reaction to dexpanthenol: lymphocyte transformation test and evidence for microsomal-dependent metabolism of the allergen. Contact Dermatitis 1993;28:81-83

18   Ockenfels hm, Seemann u, Goos M. Kontaktekzeme bei Hausfrauen. Update nach 1986 unter Berücksichtigung der Epikutantestergebnisse von 2633 Patienten. Hautarzt 1998;49:280-290

19   Jacob SE, Matiz C, Herro EM. Compositae-associated allergic contact dermatitis from bisabolol. Dermatitis 2011;22:102-105

20   Hasan T, Rantanen T, Alanko K, Harvima RJ, Jolanki R, Kalimo K, et al. Patch test reactions to cosmetic allergens in 1995–1997 and 2000–2002 in Finland –a multicentre study. Contact Dermatitis 2005;53:40-45

21   Goossens A, Beck MH, Haneke E, McFadden JP, Nolting S, Durupt G, Ries G. Adverse cutaneous reactions to cosmetic allergens. Contact Dermatitis 1999;40:112-113

22   Goossens A. Cosmetic contact allergens. Cosmetics 2016, 3, 5; doi:10.3390/cosmetics3010005

23   Bregnbak D, Johansen JD, Zachariae C. Contact dermatitis caused by panthenol used for aftercare treatment of a new tattoo. Contact Dermatitis 2016;75:50-52

24   Van Steenkiste E, Goossens A, Meert H, Apers S, Aerts O. Airborne-induced lymphomatoid contact dermatitis caused by methylisothiazolinone. Contact Dermatitis 2015;72:237-240

25   Lampe P. Kontaktallergie gegen Dexpanthenol. Allergologie 1984;7:153

26   Schulz KH. Kontaktallergie durch Dexpanthenol. Dermatosen 1981;29:80

27   Jankićević J, Vesić S, Vukićević J, Gajić M, Adamic M, Pavlović MD. Contact sensitivity in patients with venous leg ulcers in Serbia: comparison with contact dermatitis patients and relationship to ulcer duration. Contact Dermatitis 2008;58:32-36

28   Clerens I, Goossens A. Allergic contact dermatitis caused by panthenol: a rare but relevant sensitizer. Contact Dermatitis 2017;76:122-123

29   Gulec AI, Albayrak H, Uslu E, Başkan E, Aliagaoglu C. Pustular irritant contact dermatitis caused by dexpanthenol in a child. Cutan Ocul Toxicol 2015;34:75-76

30   Aschenbeck KA, Warshaw EM. Allergenic ingredients in facial wet wipes. Dermatitis 2017 Mar 23. doi: 10.1097/DER.0000000000000268. [Epub ahead of print]

31   Verheyden M, Rombouts S, Lambert J, Aerts O. Contact allergy to castor oil, but not to castor wax. Cosmetics 2017, 4, 5; doi:10.3390/cosmetics4010005

2.332   PANTHENYL ETHYL ETHER

IDENTIFICATION

Description/definition : Panthenyl ethyl ether is the ethyl ether of panthenol, which conforms to the formula shown below
Chemical class(es) : Alcohols; amides; ethers
Chemical/IUPAC name : (2R)-N-(3-Ethoxypropyl)-2,4-dihydroxy-3,3-dimethylbutanamide
Other names : Pantothenyl ethyl ether
CAS registry number (s) : 667-83-4
EC number(s) : 211-569-1
Function(s) in cosmetics : EU: antistatic; hair conditioning. USA: hair conditioning agents
Patch testing : 30% pet. (1,2)
Molecular formula : $C_{11}H_{23}NO_4$

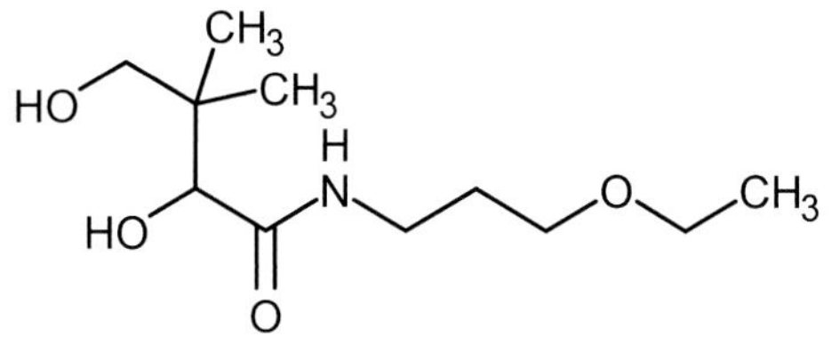

GENERAL

Panthenyl ethyl ether is a yellowish to colorless, slightly viscous liquid that is used for its emollient and conditioning properties in several skin and hair products; it is also a source of vitamin B5 (2).

CONTACT ALLERGY

Case reports and case series

A woman had a relapsing dermatitis of the face, especially on the temples and the ears, as well as on the neck. She had applied two cosmetic hair lotions recommended to people with greasy hair. Patch tests with the two lotions were positive, but there were no reactions to the ICDRG standard series. One of the lotions contained alcohol, Ricinus communis (castor) seed oil, lactic acid, panthenyl ethyl ether, two dyes, a UV-absorber and 14 fragrance ingredients. There was a strong positive patch test reaction to panthenyl ethyl ether 30% pet., which gave negative results in 10 controls (1).

A woman suffering from palmoplantar psoriasis was referred with intense itching eczematous dermatitis on her feet. Her psoriasis was treated with oral acitretin and daily topical application of an emollient stick used to improve the re-epithelization of fissured heels. During the treatment, her hands healed quickly, but she experienced worsening of the skin lesions on the feet during the last month of therapy. Patch testing with the baseline series and the emollient stick gave a positive reaction to the stick only at D2 and D4. When tested with its ingredients, the patient reacted to panthenyl ethyl ether 30% pet. There was no reaction to panthenol 5% and 10% pet. A repeated open application test with panthenyl ethyl ether 30% pet. was positive after 4 applications already. Twenty controls were negative. After discontinuing the use of the emollient stick and with topical corticosteroid ointment, the dermatitis quickly healed (2).

Cross-reactions, pseudo-cross-reactions and co-reactions

Not to panthenol (2).

Presence in cosmetic products and chemical analyses

In the USA, in April 2017, panthenyl ethyl ether was present in 395 of 56,714 cosmetic products of which the composition is known in FDA's Voluntary Cosmetic Registration Program (VCRP) (data obtained from FDA, May 2017). In March 2017, panthenyl ethyl ether was present in 396 of 65,431 cosmetic products of which the composition is known in EWG's Skin Deep Cosmetics Database, USA (http://www.ewg.org/skindeep/).

LITERATURE

1   Van Ketel WG. Hair lotion dermatitis with sensitization to d-panthenyl ethyl ether. Contact Dermatitis 1984;10:48
2   Foti C, Romita P, Bufano T, Antelmi A. Allergic contact dermatitis caused by panthenyl ethyl ether in a patient with psoriasis. Contact Dermatitis 2017;76:181-182

2.333 PARABEN MIX AND UNSPECIFIED PARABENS

Description/definition : The paraben mix is a mixture of paraben esters for patch testing. It contains four parabens, each in a concentration of 3% or 4%: butylparaben, ethylparaben, methylparaben and propylparaben. See the individual chapters of these chemicals for their specific data

Patch testing : 12.0% pet. (Chemotechnique); 16.0% pet. (Chemotechnique, SmartPracticeEurope, SmartPracticeCanada); 15.0% pet. (SmartPracticeCanada); the 15.0% test substance contains butyl-, ethyl-, methyl- and propylparaben *plus* benzylparaben (3% each)

GENERAL

The family of alkyl esters of *p*-hydroxybenzoic acid includes methyl-, ethyl-, propyl-, and butylparaben. They are present in many natural products, such as some fruits and vegetables, strawberries, grape juice, yeast extracts, barley, vinegar, cheeses, royal jelly and propolis (74). These compounds were introduced in the 1930s in cosmetics and foods, as well as in topical and systemic medicaments and various industrial products. The parabens have the particularity of being odorless and tasteless, of having no bleaching power, and very low acute and chronic toxicity. They are easily hydrolyzed by non-specific enzymes; studies have shown that they are degraded once applied on the skin, which accounts for the low systemic exposure for consumers (74). Because of their different solubility and spectrum of activity, they are commonly combined, and methyl- and ethylparabens are most frequently used. Parabens are more effective against fungi than bacteria, and antibacterial activity is greatest against gram-positive organisms. For extended coverage against gram-negative bacteria, especially *Pseudomonas aeruginosa*, parabens are used synergistically with other biocides such as formaldehyde-releasers, isothiazolinones, or phenoxyethanol. Parabens are the most commonly used preservatives in cosmetics, but they became less popular in topical medicaments once contact hypersensitivity was described. In both types of products, the usual concentrations range between 0.1% and 0.8% (66).

The parabens are – contrary to what is thought by the public and many physicians – infrequent sensitizers and belong to the least allergenic of all preservatives (115). Patients mostly become sensitized from topical medicaments; individuals with stasis dermatitis and leg ulcers are at particular risk (47,96,116). In Denmark, creams, ointments, and powders containing ethyl paraben 5% were popular remedies for athlete's foot since 1935, explaining for at least half of the 340 cases of paraben sensitivity diagnosed at the Finsen Institute in that country and reported at the beginning of the 1960s (87). In cosmetics, the parabens are considered to be generally safe. In the general population, recent investigations have shown frequencies of sensitization of 0 - 0.1% in various European countries (54, table 2.333.1). Many people who have become allergic to parabens from topical medicaments (used on diseased skin) can safely use paraben-containing cosmetic products on normal, healthy, intact skin. This has been termed the 'paraben-paradox' (28,29,91,92,93).

This chapter discusses both literature on the paraben mix and reactions to *unspecified* parabens. See also the chapters on butylparaben, ethylparaben, methylparaben and propylparaben. The literature on contact allergy to paraben esters from before 1991 has been reviewed in ref. 86. Other, more recent, useful reviews were published in 2005 (parabens) (111), 2004 (66) and in 2014 (parabens and other preservatives) (113).

CONTACT ALLERGY

Contact allergy in the general population and subgroups
There have been investigations in several European countries, in which random samples of the population of certain age groups have been patch tested with paraben mix (table 2.333.1). Frequencies of sensitization were consistently low, ranging from 0% to 0.4% (54,55,56,57). In two Danish studies, the patch tests were read only at day 2, which may have resulted in underestimation of the actual rate of sensitization (55,56).

In subgroups of the general population, slightly higher rates of sensitization to the paraben mix have been observed in male soldiers without skin disease (0.7% [61]) and in adults aged 28-78 years, comprising a large percentage (>50%) of atopic individuals (0.6% [59,62]). In the latter study, the use of moisturizers applied to atopic dermatitis or otherwise mildly damaged atopic skin, may have resulted in a slightly increased rate of sensitization (59,62).

Estimates of the 9-year prevalence (1992-2000) of contact allergy to parabens in the general population of Germany based on the CE-DUR method ranged from 0.2% (medium case scenario) to 0.5% (worst case scenario) (11,53).

Patch testing in groups of patients
Results of routine patch testing (testing in consecutive patients suspected of contact dermatitis) with the paraben mix back to 2000 are shown in table 2.333.2. Results of testing in groups of *selected* patients (e.g., patients with leg

ulcers, patients suspected of cosmetic dermatitis, individuals with periorbital eczema) back to 1989 are shown in table 2.333.3.

Table 2.333.1 Contact allergy in the general population and subgroups

Year and country	Selection and number tested	Prevalence of contact allergy			Comments	Ref.
		Total	Women	Men		
General population						
2008-11 five European countries	general population, random sample, 18-74 years, n=3119	0.1%	0.2%	0%		54
2006 Denmark	general population, random sample, 18-69 years, n=3460	0%	0%	0%	patch tests were read on day 2 only	55
2005 Norway	general population, random sample, 18-69 years, n=1236	0.1%	0%	0.2%		57
1990 Denmark	general population, random sample, 18-69 years, n=543	0.4%	0.4%	0.4%	patch tests were read on day 2 only; data from 15-17 years old are excluded in the data presented here	56
Subgroups						
1997-1998 Germany	adults 28-78 years, with a large percentage (>50%) of atopic individuals, n=1141	0.6%	0.5%	0.7%		59, 62
1995-1996 Denmark	8th grade school children, 12-16 years, n=1146	0.1%	0.2%	0%		58, 60
1989 Italy	male soldiers without skin disease, 18-28 years, n=593	0.7%				61

Patch testing in consecutive patients suspected of contact dermatitis: routine testing

As the paraben mix is included in the European Baseline Series, the screening tray of the North American Contact Dermatitis Group (NACDG) and most other national series routinely tested in consecutive patients suspected of contact dermatitis, there are many data on paraben contact allergy available, notably from European countries and from the USA + Canada, where the NACDG publishes their patch test results biannually. The results of these and other studies are shown in table 2.333.2. Rates of sensitization have been fairly low and constant, ranging mostly between 0.6% and 1.4%. The highest frequency of sensitization has been 2.6% in Singapore, which was ascribed to the widespread use of cosmetics from Japan in Singapore, many of which are preserved with parabens (50). In most European studies, relevance percentages were not provided. In a 2000 multicenter UK study, however, 90% of 34 positive patch tests to paraben mix were considered to be relevant (38). In the NACDG studies, rates of 'definite' + 'probable' relevance have ranged from 28% to 73%.

Table 2.333.2 Patch testing in groups of patients: Routine testing

Years and Country	Test conc. & vehicle	Number of patients tested | positive (%)			Selection of patients (S); Relevance (R); Comments (C)	Ref.
2013-2014[b] 12 European countries, 46 departments	16% pet.	28596		(0.5%)	R: not stated; C: results of 6 occupational dermatology clinics and one pediatric clinic not included in these figures; range of positive reactions: 0%-2.4%	124
2013-14 USA, Canada	12% pet.	4859	30	(0.6%)	R: definite + probable relevance: 40%	79
2011-12 USA, Canada	12% pet.	4231	59	(1.4%)	R: definite + probable relevance: 73%	15
2009-2012, 12 European countries [b]	16% pet.	52,586		(0.7%) [a]	R: not stated; C: range per country 0.5-1.9%	118
2006-2011 Singapore	16% pet.	3177	82	(2.6%)	R: not stated; C: prevalence was 2.4% in men, 2.7% in women; the high prevalence may be related to the use of cosmetics from Japan, of which many are preserved with parabens	50
2002-2011 France		3374	55	(1.6%)	R: not stated; C: the prevalence decreased from 3.1% in 2002-2004 to 1.5% in 2005-2009 to 0.2% in 2010-2011	74
2009-10 USA, Canada	12% pet.	4304	34	(0.8%)	R: definite + probable relevance: 53%	16
2006-2010 USA	16% pet.	3090		(1.7%)	R: 45%	49
2001-2010 Australia	12% pet.	5138	45	(0.9%)	R: 27%	77
2009 Sweden	16% pet.	3112		(0.3%)	R: not stated	45
1996-2009 IVDK	16% pet.	121,247		(1.3%) [a]	R: not stated; C: test preparation slightly irritant, may result in false-positive patch test reactions; C: 1752 positive reactions	7
2007-2008, 11 Euro-	16% pet.	23,008	192	(0.8%) [a]	R: not stated; C: prevalences ranged from 0.1% (Denmark)	1

Table 2.333.2 Patch testing in groups of patients: Routine testing (*continued*)

Years and Country	Test conc. & vehicle	Number of patients tested | positive (%)		Selection of patients (S); Relevance (R); Comments (C)	Ref.
pean countries [b]				to 3.4% (Lithuania)	
2007-8 USA, Canada	12% pet.	5082	(1.1%)	R: definite + probable relevance: 57%	12
2005-6 USA, Canada	12% pet.	4439	(1.2%)	R: definite + probable relevance: 60%	10
2005-6 10 European countries [b]	16% pet.	17,197	186 (1.1%)	R: not stated; C: prevalences in the four regions (Central, West, Northeast and South Europe) ranged from 0.7 to 2.3%	83
1993-2006 Australia	16% pet.	6845	(1.1%)	R: 21%	90
2004-2005 UK	16% pet.	6958	(1.9%)	R: not stated	36
2000-2005 USA	16% pet.	3841	(1.7%)	R: 56%	5
2004, 11 European countries [b]	16% pet.	9166	92 (1.0%) [a]	R: not stated; range positives per center was 0%-7.6%	8
2003-4 USA, Canada	12% pet.	5142	58 (1.1%)	R: not stated	13
1998-2004 Israel	16% pet.	2156	12 (0.6%)	R: not stated	39
1992-2004 Turkey	16% pet.	1038	3 (0.2%)	R: not stated; C: prevalence in women 0.1%, in men 0.6%	40
2002-2003, 9 European countries [b]	12% or 16% pet.	8857	(1.2%)	R: not stated; C: prevalence range per center (n=17) 0%-3.7%	41
2001-2 USA, Canada	12% pet.	4898	(0.6%)	R: definite + probable relevance: 28%	34
1999-2001 Sweden	12% pet.	3790	(0.4%)	R: not stated; C: prevalence in women 0.4%, in men 0.5% (standardized prevalences)	37
1997-2001 Czech Rep.	16% pet.	12,058	158 (1.3%)	R: not stated; C: prevalence in men 1.2%, in women 1.4%	42
2000 United Kingdom	16% pet.	3063	(1.1%)	R: 90% (current and past relevance in one center)	38
1998-2000 USA	12% pet.	5803	(1.0%)	R: definite + probable relevance: 24%	35
1996-2000 Europe	16% pet.	26,210	(0.6%)	R: not stated; C: prevalence in women 0.6%, in men 0.6%; C: ten centers, seven countries, EECDRG study	43

[a] age-standardized and sex-standardized proportions
[b] study of the ESSCA (European Surveillance System on Contact Allergies)
EECDRG: European Environmental and Contact Dermatitis Research Group
IVDK: Information Network of Departments of Dermatology, Germany, Austria, Switzerland

Patch testing in groups of selected patients

Data on patch testing with the paraben mix in groups of selected patients back to 1989 (examples) are summarized in table 2.333.3. As expected, high frequencies of sensitization of 12% and 14% were seen only in patients with leg ulcers with or without surrounding dermatitis (47,116). In a recent IVDK study, the prevalence was far lower, 2.6%, but this was still significantly higher than in a control group (120). Slightly elevated rates of sensitization compared with routine testing of 3.1% were seen in one group of patients suspected of cosmetic dermatitis (46) and in another group of patients with leg ulcers (44). Relevance rates were provided in one study only, a 2000-2007 study in patients tested with a cosmetics series. All 9 positive patch test reactions were scored as relevant, but this included 'questionable' and 'past' relevance (3).

Case reports and case series

Case series

'Parabens' were stated to be the (or an) allergen in one patient in a group of 603 individuals suffering from cosmetic dermatitis, seen in the period 2010-2015 in Leuven, Belgium (48). In the period 1996-2013, in a tertiary referral center in Valencia, Spain, 5419 patients were patch tested. Of these, 628 individuals had allergic contact dermatitis to cosmetics. Parabens were the responsible allergens in eleven cases (80, overlap with ref. 73). Parabens were responsible for 25 out of 959 cases of non-fragrance cosmetic allergy where the causal allergen was identified, Belgium, 2000-2010 (2). In the period 2000-2007, 202 patients with allergic contact dermatitis caused by cosmetics were seen in Valencia, Spain. In this group, one individual reacted to parabens in a moisturizing cream (73, overlap with ref. 80). In a group of 2193 patients (1582 women, 611 men) with (presumed) cosmetic allergy, 23 reactions were caused by parabens in a study of the NACDG, 2001-2004 (6).

In a group of 75 patients allergic to cosmetic products, seen in a private practice in The Netherlands in the period 1981-1986, one case was caused by parabens in a skin care product (64). In 3 clinics in Belgium, in the period 1978-1985, 279 patients with allergic contact dermatitis exclusively caused by cosmetics were seen. In this group, there were 6 reactions to parabens. It was implied that parabens were the cause of the allergic reactions (76). 'Paraben, unspecified' was responsible for 19 out of 399 cases of cosmetic allergy where the causal allergen was identified in a study of the NACDG, USA, 1977-1983 (4).

Table 2.333.3 Patch testing in groups of patients: Selected patient groups

Years and Country	Test conc. & vehicle	Number of patients tested	positive (%)		Selection of patients (S); Relevance (R); Comments (C)	Ref.
2005-2014 China	15% pet.	6013	87	(1.4%)	S: patients suspected of photodermatoses; R: not stated	82
2003-2014 IVDK	16% pet.	5202		(2.6%)	S: patients with stasis dermatitis / chronic leg ulcers; R: not stated; C: percentage of reactions significantly higher than in a control group of routine testing	120
1996-2013 Netherlands	16% pet.	1001	9	(0.9%)	S: children aged 0-17 years; R: not stated	119
2011 China	16% pet.	201	1	(0.5%)	S: healthy student volunteers 19-30 years; R: not stated	78
2010-2011 Korea	16% pet.	584	18	(3.1%)	S: patients suspected of allergic cosmetic dermatitis; R: not stated	46
2006-2011 IVDK	16% pet.	10,124	103	(1.1%)	S: patients suspected of cosmetic intolerance; R: not stated	81
2004-2008 France	16% pet.	423	13	(3.1%)	S: patients with leg ulcers; R: not stated	44
2000-2007 USA	16% pet.	941	9	(1.0%)	S: patients tested with a supplemental cosmetic screening series; R: 100%; C: weak study: a. high rate of macular erythema and weak reactions; b. relevance figures included 'questionable' and 'past' relevance	3
2000-2002 Serbia	16% pet.	75	9	(12%)	S: patients with venous leg ulcers and dermatitis of the surrounding skin; R: not stated	116
1982-2001 UK		146	1	(0.7%)	S: patients with cheilitis; R: only relevant reactions were reported in this study	33
1990-1994 IVDK		589	13	(2.2%)	S: patients with periorbital eczema; R: not stated	84
1988-1989 UK		81	11	(14%)	S: patients with leg ulcers; R: not specified	47

IVDK: Information Network of Departments of Dermatology, Germany, Austria, Switzerland

Case reports

One patient reacted to parabens in moisturizing cream (17). A baby had contact dermatitis from allergy to parabens in various skin care products (18). One individual had ACD from parabens in a moisturizing cream (23). A child, known to be allergic to methyl- and propylparaben, developed vesicular hand dermatitis from a liquid soap containing parabens (103). One individual reacted to paraben esters (unspecified) in a shampoo (27). Another patient had ACD of the face from parabens which were present in 6 different makeup products (30). Three individuals reacted to parabens in skin care products and one also to the preservative in a sunscreen (65). A woman had ACD of the face and neck from parabens in various cosmetics (85).

Another woman had irritant contact dermatitis of the hands from frequent hand washing in the hospital where she worked. Later, she developed superimposed ACD from parabens in a moisturizer (85). One woman became allergic to parabens in a tar shampoo; she reacted to butyl-, ethyl- and propylparaben. It was not mentioned which paraben(s) the shampoo (which can also be regarded as topical pharmaceutical product) contained (20).

Contact allergy to parabens in non-cosmetic products

Topical pharmaceutical products

One patient (19), two individuals (99) and a girl (103) had ACD from unspecified paraben(s) in topical pharmaceutical preparations. One individual reacted to parabens present in a corticosteroid ointment and in pharmaceuticals to treat leg ulcers (31). Two patient were allergic to parabens in corticosteroid creams (32). A man had ACD from parabens in a topical pharmaceutical product. Later, he developed widespread dermatitis after local anesthesia with a preparation containing methylparaben; this was considered to be systemic contact dermatitis (94). Two patients had allergic contact dermatitis from parabens; details unknown (97). Four patients had ACD from topical pharmaceuticals. They all reacted to methylparaben and three to ethyl-, propyl- and butylparaben. It was not mentioned which of the parabens were present in the topical pharmaceuticals used with the exception of methylparaben, which was present in an antibiotic powder (102).

Three patients developed ACD from the application of a corticosteroid cream. They all reacted to the paraben mix. The cream contained methylparaben and butylparaben, but it was not explicitly stated that these paraben-esters were tested separately and that they were both positive (112).

Other non-cosmetic products

A young boy had acute vesicular dermatitis of the palms and fingers from contact allergy to parabens in gelatinous play material (21). One individual reacted to parabens in an ECG electrode gel (26). A patient had allergic contact dermatitis of the legs from a medicated bandage containing parabens (28), another one from parabens in paste bandages (17). Two patients had ACD from Unna boots (paste bandages). Both had positive patch tests to the paraben mix. The paste bandages contained methyl- and propylparaben, but these esters were not tested separately (88).

A girl had ACD of the hands from play gel. She reacted to the paraben mix. The play gel, containing methyl- and propylparaben, also gave a positive patch test. Methyl- and propylparaben were not tested separately (103). A man developed a severe eczematous reaction in the genital area after using a condom containing a retarding cream formulated with benzocaine and parabens. There were positive patch tests to the cream, to benzocaine and to the paraben mix (110). There have been reports of hand dermatitis in cooks and food handlers from contact allergy to parabens used for preserving foods (105).

Cross-reactions, pseudo-cross-reactions and co-reactions

Co-reactions of various paraben-esters are seen frequently (24,86,87). As most patients are exposed to more than one paraben, it is difficult to determine whether these co-reactions result from cross-sensitivity or from concomitant sensitization (96). There are (weak) indications that some patients sensitized to p-phenylenediamine may cross-react to parabens (95). Some authors have reported cross-reactivity between parabens and other para-compounds such as benzocaine (ethyl p-aminobenzoate) and sulfonamides (100,101), other investigators have not been able to confirm such cross-sensitivity (95).

Presence in cosmetic products and chemical analyses

Parabens were present in 42 (24%) of 178 facial wipes for which ingredient information was obtained online and from retail stores, USA, 2016 (121). Parabens were present in 983 of 4737 (20.8%) commonly used cosmetic products of which the full composition was known in 2016 in The Contact Allergen Management Program (CAMP) database of the American Contact Dermatitis Society (123). Parabens were present in 11 (20%) of 54 personal hygiene wet wipes for which ingredient information was obtained online and from retail stores, USA, 2016 (122). In the USA, in 2015-2016, 63 diaper wipes and 41 topical diaper preparations from a large retailer were screened for the presence of potential sensitizers. Parabens were found in 6/63 (10%) disposable diaper wipes and in 10/41 (24%) topical diaper preparations (22).

In 2014, in Thailand, the labels of 1000 cosmetic products (593 leave-on, 407 rinse-off products) were examined for the presence of preservatives. These were partly purchased in shops and on markets and partly brought in by patients. Parabens were present in 432 products (43%); in the leave-on products, the percentage was 54 and in the rinse-off products 27 (104). In 2013, 60 cosmetic products manufactured and purchased in Israel (40 stay-on and 20 rinse-off products) were investigated for preservatives. According to the labeling, 21 (35%) cosmetics contained parabens (esters not specified). In the stay-on products (hand and body creams), the percentage was 43, whereas four of the 20 shampoos and soaps (20%) were preserved with parabens (89).

In 2009, in the USA, the ingredient lists of 1591 facial cosmetics from one company were screened for the presence of parabens. One or more parabens were present in 87% of 132 blushers and 38 bronzers, in 77% of 90 concealers, in 0% of 174 eyeliners, in 82% of 304 eyeshadows, in 85% of 457 foundations, in 66% of 140 loose and pressed powders, and in 90% of 256 mascaras (69). In 2009, in the USA, the ingredient lists of 796 hair products from one company were screened for the presence of parabens. One or more parabens were present in 30% of 279 shampoos, in 0% of 231 conditioners, and in 0% of 286 styling products (70). In 2009, in the USA, the ingredient lists of 730 lip cosmetics and dental care products from one company were screened for the presence of parabens. One or more parabens were present in 77% of 31 lip liners, in 82% of 429 lipsticks, in 27% of 92 lip moisturizers, in 0% of 153 toothpastes, and in 0% of 25 mouth washes (71). In 2009, in the USA, the ingredient lists of 657 miscellaneous cosmetics from one company were screened for the presence of parabens. One or more parabens were present in 0% of 195 antiperspirants/deodorants, in 0% of 41 powders, in 0% of 167 shaving products, in 30% of 201 sun blocks, and in 23% of 53 wipes (72).

In Germany, in 2006-2009, the labels of 4680 cosmetic products were screened for the presence of preservatives. Parabens were present in 39% of the products, according to labeling information (114). Parabens were present in 1474/3541 (39%) randomly sampled leave-on cosmetic products, Germany, 2006-2009 (9). Of 276 moisturizers sold in the USA in 2007, 170 (62%) contained parabens (14). Parabens were present in 19 out of 166 (11%) corticosteroid preparations collected in 2007 in the USA (51). Of 38 cosmetic products marketed for babies in the UK in 2007, 22 (58%) contained parabens (63).

In the beginning of the 1990s, 215 cosmetic products, 158 leave-on cosmetics and 57 rinse-off cosmetics, from 79 cosmetic-producing companies, collected in Denmark, were analysed for paraben content with high performance liquid chromatography (HPLC) (98). Of all the products investigated, 93% were found to contain paraben(s). Paraben was detected in 77% of the rinse-off products and in 99% of the leave-on products. Total paraben content in the paraben-positive cosmetics was 0.01%-0.59%, except in one sun-lotion that contained 0.87% parabens. Rinse-off cosmetics contained 0.01-0.50% parabens and the paraben content in leave-on products was 0.01-0.59% (98). The results for the individual paraben-esters (butylparaben, ethylparaben, methylparaben and propylparaben) are shown in their respective chapters.

Other information

The ester linkage of the parabens is hydrolyzed in the skin, generating the corresponding alcohol (butyl, ethyl, methyl or propyl alcohol) and *p*-hydroxybenzoic acid. The alcohols are not suspected sensitizers. Neither is *p*-hydroxybenzoic acid, as a common metabolite, the sensitizer in patients reacting to one or more paraben-esters (96). Ingestion of foods preserved with parabens does not seem to cause contact dermatitis or exacerbation of pre-existing contact dermatitis in paraben-allergic individuals (106,107).

OTHER SIDE EFFECTS

Photosensitivity

In the period of 2005-2014, in China, 6017 patients with suspected photodermatoses were photopatch tested with the paraben mix 15%. Seventy-one (1.2%) reacted positively, but the relevance of the positive photopatch tests was not mentioned (82).

Immediate-type reactions

Of 50 individuals who had open tests with paraben mix 15% pet. on the forearm, seven showed local macular erythema after 45 minutes, which was termed 'contact urticaria' by the authors (67). In a group of 664 patch tested patients, there were 30 (4.5%) immediate contact reactions to paraben mix as shown by 'well distinguished erythema' after 30 minutes. However, the clinical relevance of these reactions was not addressed (68).

Systemic side effects

Parabens have been accused of having disruptive endocrine effects. However, a recent review of the literature concluded that, even if parabens exert very weak estrogenic activity *in vitro* and *in vivo*, evidence of paraben-induced developmental and reproductive toxicity lacks consistency and coherence (75). Suggestions that parabens in antiperspirants may increase the risk of breast cancer have been refuted (74). The literature has been reviewed recently and the authors concluded that 'Any effect caused by the doses of parabens received from topical consumer products is likely to be insignificant compared with natural estrogens' (108). Indeed, the American Cancer Society has concluded that studies have not shown any direct link between parabens and any health problems, including breast cancer (109).

LITERATURE

1   Uter W, Aberer W, Armario-Hita JC, Fernandez-Vozmediano JM, Ayala F, Balato A, et al. Current patch test results with the European baseline series and extensions to it from the 'European Surveillance System on Contact Allergy' network, 2007-2008. Contact Dermatitis 2012;67:9-19

2   Travassos AR, Claes L, Boey L, Drieghe J, Goossens A. Non-fragrance allergens in specific cosmetic products. Contact Dermatitis 2011;65:276-285

3   Wetter DA, Yiannias JA, Prakash AV, Davis MD, Farmer SA, el-Azhary RA, et al. Results of patch testing to personal care product allergens in a standard series and a supplemental cosmetic series: an analysis of 945 patients from the Mayo Clinic Contact Dermatitis Group, 2000-2007. J Am Acad Dermatol 2010;63:789-798

4   Adams RM, Maibach HI, Clendenning WE, Fisher AA, Jordan WJ, Kanof N, et al. A five-year study of cosmetic reactions. J Am Acad Dermatol 1985;13:1062-1069

5   Davis MD, Scalf LA, Yiannias JA, Cheng JF, El-Azhary RA, Rohlinger AL, et al. Changing trends and allergens in the patch test standard series. Arch Dermatol 2008;144:67-72

6   Warshaw EM, Buchholz HJ, Belsito DV et al. Allergic patch test reactions associated with cosmetics: Retrospective analysis of cross-sectional data from the North American Contact Dermatitis Group, 2001-2004. J Am Acad Dermatol 2009;60:23-38

7   Schnuch A, Lessmann H, Geier J, Uter W. Contact allergy to preservatives. Analysis of IVDK data 1996-2009. Br J Dermatol 2011;164:1316-1325

8   ESSCA Writing Group. The European Surveillance System of Contact Allergies (ESSCA): results of patch testing the standard series, 2004. J Eur Acad Dermatol Venereol 2008;22:174-181

9   Schnuch A, Mildau G, Kratz E-M, Uter W. Risk of sensitization to preservatives estimated on the basis of patch test data and exposure, according to a sample of 3541 leave-on products. Contact Dermatitis 2011;65:167-174

10   Zug KA, Warshaw EM, Fowler JF Jr, Maibach HI, Belsito DL, Pratt MD, et al. Patch-test results of the North American Contact Dermatitis Group 2005-2006. Dermatitis 2009;20:149-160

11   Brasch J, Becker D, Aberer W Bircher A, Kränke B, Denzer-Fürst S, et al. Contact Dermatitis. J Dtsch Dermatol Ges 2007;5:943-951

12   Fransway AF, Zug KA, Belsito DV, Deleo VA, Fowler JF Jr, Maibach HI, et al. North American Contact Dermatitis Group patch test results for 2007-2008. Dermatitis 2013;24:10-21

13 Warshaw EM, Belsito DV, DeLeo VA, Fowler JF Jr, Maibach HI, Marks JG, et al. North American Contact Dermatitis Group patch-test results, 2003-2004 study period. Dermatitis 2008;19:129-136

14 Zirwas MJ, Stechschulte SA. Moisturizer allergy. Diagnosis and management. J Clin Aesthetic Dermatol 2008;1:38-44

15 Warshaw EM, Maibach HI, Taylor JS, Sasseville D, DeKoven JG, Zirwas MJ, et al. North American Contact Dermatitis Group patch test results: 2011-2012. Dermatitis 2015,26.49-59

16 Warshaw EM, Belsito DV, Taylor JS, Sasseville D, DeKoven JG, Zirwas MJ, et al. North American Contact Dermatitis Group patch test results: 2009 to 2010. Dermatitis 2013;24:50-59

17 Kulozik M, Powell SM, Cherry G, Ryan TJ. Contact sensitivity in community-based leg ulcer patients. Clin Exp Dermatol 1988;13:82-84

18 Nardelli A, Morren MA, Goossens A. Contact allergy to fragrances and parabens in an atopic baby. Contact Dermatitis 2009;60:107-109

19 Dejobert Y, Delaporte E, Piette F, Thomas P. Vesicular eczema and systemic contact dermatitis from sorbic acid. Contact Dermatitis 2001;45:291

20 Cooper SM, Shaw S. Allergic contact dermatitis from parabens in a tar shampoo. Contact Dermatitis 1998;39:140

21 Downs AMR, Sansom JE, Simmons I. Let Rip! Fun Pot® dermatitis. Contact Dermatitis 1998;38:234

22 Yu J, Treat J, Chaney K, Brod B. Potential allergens in disposable diaper wipes, topical diaper preparations, and disposable diapers: under-recognized etiology of pediatric perineal dermatitis. Dermatitis 2016;27:110-118

23 Reynolds NJ, Harman RRM. Allergic contact dermatitis from chlorhexidine diacetate in a skin swab. Contact Dermatitis 1990;22:103-104

24 Menné T, Hjorth N. Routine patch testing with paraben esters. Contact Dermatitis 1988;19:189-191

25 Tomb RR, Rivara G, Foussereau J. Contact dermatitis after ultrasonography and electrocardiography. Contact Dermatitis 1987;17:149-152

26 Fisher AA. Dermatologic hazards of electrocardiography. Cutis 1977;20:686 (further pages unknown, data cited in ref. 25)

27 Van Haute N, Dooms-Goossens A. Shampoo dermatitis due to cocobetaine and sodium lauryl ether sulphate. Contact Dermatitis 1983;9:169

28 Fisher AA. Paraben dermatitis due to a new medicated bandage: The "paraben paradox". Contact Dermatitis 1979; 5:273-274

29 Fisher AA. The paraben paradox. Cutis 1973;12:830-832

30 Simpson JR. Dermatitis due to parabens in cosmetic creams. Contact Dermatitis 1978;4:311-312

31 Malten KE. Sensitization to solcoseryl and methylanisate (fragrance ingredient). Contact Dermatitis 1977;3:219

32 Fisher AA. Allergic paraben and benzyl alcohol hypersensitivity relationship of the "delayed" and "immediate" varieties. Contact Dermatitis 1975;1:281-284

33 Strauss RM, Orton DI. Allergic contact cheilitis in the United Kingdom: a retrospective study. Am J Contact Dermat 2003;14:75-77

34 Pratt MD, Belsito DV, DeLeo VA, Fowler JF Jr, Fransway AF, Maibach HI, et al. North American Contact Dermatitis Group patch-test results, 2001–2002 study period. Dermatitis 2004;15:176-183

35 Marks JG Jr, Belsito DV, DeLeo VA, Fowler JF Jr, Fransway AF, Maibach HI, et al. North American Contact Dermatitis Group patch-test results, 1998–2000. Am J Contact Dermat 2003;14:59-62

36 Jong CT, Statham BN, Green CM, King CM, Gawkrodger DJ, Sansom JE, et al. Contact sensitivity to preservatives in the UK 2004–2005: results of a multicenter study. Contact Dermatitis 2007;57:165-168

37 Lindberg M, Edman B, Fischer T, Stenberg B. Time trends in Swedish patch test data from 1992 to 2000. A multi-centre study based on age- and sex-adjusted results of the Swedish standard series. Contact Dermatitis 2007;56:205-210

38 Britton JE, Wilkinson SM, English JSC, Gawkrodger DJ, Ormerod AD, Sansom JE, et al. The British standard series of contact dermatitis allergens: validation in clinical practice and value for clinical governance. Br J Dermatol 2003;148:259-264

39 Lazarov A. European Standard Series patch test results from a contact dermatitis clinic in Israel during the 7-year period from 1998 to 2004. Contact Dermatitis 2006;55:73-76

40 Akyol A, Boyvat A, Peksari Y, Gurgey E. Contact sensitivity to standard series allergens in 1038 patients with contact dermatitis in Turkey. Contact Dermatitis 2005;52:333-337

41 Uter W, Hegewald J, Aberer W, Ayala F, Bircher AJ, Brasch J, et al. The European standard series in 9 European countries, 2002/2003 –First results of the European Surveillance System on Contact Allergies. Contact Dermatitis 2005;53:136-145

42 Machovcova A, Dastychova E, Kostalova D, et al. Common contact sensitizers in the Czech Republic. Patch test results in 12,058 patients with suspected contact dermatitis. Contact Dermatitis 2005;53:162-166

43 Bruynzeel DP, Diepgen TL, Andersen KE, Brandão FM, Bruze M, Frosch PJ, et al (EECDRG). Monitoring the European Standard Series in 10 centres 1996–2000. Contact Dermatitis 2005;53:146-152

44 Barbaud A, Collet E, Le Coz CJ, Meaume S, Gillois P. Contact allergy in chronic leg ulcers: results of a multicentre study carried out in 423 patients and proposal for an updated series of patch tests. Contact Dermatitis 2009;60:279-287

45 Fall S, Bruze M, Isaksson M, Lidén C, Matura M, Stenberg B, Lindberg M. Contact allergy trends in Sweden – a retrospective comparison of patch test data from 1992, 2000, and 2009. Contact Dermatitis 2015;72:297-304

46 Lee SS, Hong DK, Jeong NJ, Lee JH, Choi YS, Lee AY, et al. Multicenter study of preservative sensitivity in patients with suspected cosmetic contact dermatitis in Korea. J Dermatol 2012;39:677-681

47 Wilson CC, Cameron J, Powell SM, Cherry G, Ryan TJ. High incidence of contact dermatitis in leg ulcer patients – implications for management. Clin Exp Dermatol 1991;16:250-253

48 Goossens A. Cosmetic contact allergens. Cosmetics 2016, 3, 5; doi:10.3390/cosmetics3010005

49 Wentworth AB, Yiannias JA, Keeling JH, Hall MR, Camilleri MJ, Drage LA, et al. Trends in patch-test results and allergen changes in the standard series: a Mayo Clinic 5-year retrospective review (January 1, 2006, to December 31, 2010). J Am Acad Dermatol 2014;70:269-275

50 Cheng S, Leow YH, Goh CL, Goon A. contact sensitivity to preservatives in Singapore: frequency of sensitization to 11 common preservatives 2006–2011. Dermatitis 2014;25:77-82

51 Coloe J, Zirwas MJ. Allergens in corticosteroid vehicles. Dermatitis 2008;19:38-42

52 Thyssen JP, Uter W, Schnuch A, Linneberg A, Johansen JD. 10-year prevalence of contact allergy in the general population in Denmark estimated through the CE-DUR method. Contact Dermatitis 2007;57:265-272

53 Schnuch A, Uter W, Geier J, Gefeller O (for the IVDK study group). Epidemiology of contact allergy: an estimation of morbidity employing the clinical epidemiology and drug-utilization research (CE-DUR) approach. Contact Dermatitis 2002;47:32-39

54 Diepgen TL, Ofenloch RF, Bruze M, Bertuccio P, Cazzaniga S, Coenraads P-J, et al. Prevalence of contact allergy in the general population in different European regions. Br J Dermatol 2016;174:319-329

55 Thyssen JP, Linneberg A, Menné T, Nielsen NH, Johansen JD. Contact allergy to allergens of the TRUE-test (panels 1 and 2) has decreased modestly in the general population. Br J Dermatol 2009;161:1124-1129

56 Nielsen SH, Menné T. Allergic contact sensitization in an unselected Danish population. The Glostrup Allergy Study, Denmark. Acta Derm Venereol 1992;72:456-460

57 Dotterud LK, Smith-Sivertsen T. Allergic contact sensitization in the general adult population: a population-based study from Northern Norway. Contact Dermatitis 2007;56:10-15

58 Mortz CG, Lauritsen JM, Bindslev-Jensen C, Andersen KE. Contact allergy and allergic contact dermatitis in adolescents: prevalence measures and associations. Acta Derm Venereol 2002;82:352-358

59 Schäfer T, Böhler E, Ruhdorfer S, Weigl L, Wessner D, Filipiak B, et al. Epidemiology of contact allergy in adults. Allergy 2001;56:1192-1196

60 Mortz CG, Lauritsen JM, Bindslev-Jensen C, Andersen KE. Prevalence of atopic dermatitis, asthma, allergic rhinitis, and hand and contact dermatitis in adolescents. The Odense Adolescence Cohort Study on Atopic Diseases and Dermatitis. Br J Dermatol 2001;144:523-532

61 Seidenari S, Manzini BM, Danese P, Motolese A. Patch and prick test study of 593 healthy subjects. Contact Dermatitis 1990; 23:162-167

62 Uter W, Ludwig A, Balda BR, Schnuch A, Pfahlberg A, Schäfer T, Wichmann HE, Ring J. The prevalence of contact allergy differed between population-based data and clinic–based data. J Clin Epidemiol 2004;57:627-632

63 White JML, McFadden JP. Exposure to haptens/contact allergens in baby cosmetic products. Contact Dermatitis 2008;59:176-177

64 De Groot AC. Contact allergy to cosmetics: Causative ingredients. Contact Dermatitis 1987;17:26-34

65 Cronin E. Contact Dermatitis. Edinburgh: Churchill Livingstone, 1980:670-671

66 Sasseville D. Hypersensitivity to preservatives. Dermatol Ther 2004;17:251-263

67 Emmons WW, Marks JG. Immediate and delayed reactions to cosmetic ingredients. Contact Dermatitis 1985;13:258-265

68 Katsarou A, Armenaka M, Ale I, Koufou V, Kalogeromitros, D. Frequency of immediate reactions to the European standard series. Contact Dermatitis 1999;41:276-279

69 Scheman A, Jacob S, Katta R, Nedorost S, Warshaw E, Zirwas M, et al. Part 1 of a 4 part series. Facial cosmetics: trends and alternatives. Data from the American Contact Alternative Group. J Clin Aesthet Dermatol 2011;4:25-30

70 Scheman A, Jacob S, Katta R, Nedorost S, Warshaw E, Zirwas M, et al. Part 2 of a 4 part series. Hair cosmetics: trends and alternatives. Data from the American Contact Alternative Group. J Clin Aesthet Dermatol 2011;4:42-46

71 Scheman A, Jacob S, Katta R, Nedorost S, Warshaw E, Zirwas M, et al. Part 3 of a 4 part series. Lips and common Dental Care products: trends and alternatives. Data from the American Contact Alternative Group. J Clin Aesthet Dermatol 2011;4:50-53

72 Scheman A, Jacob S, Katta R, Nedorost S, Warshaw E, Zirwas M, et al. Part 4 of a 4 part series. Miscellaneous products: trends and alternatives in deodorants, antiperspirants, sunblocks, shaving products, powder, and wipes. Data from the American Contact Alternative Group. J Clin Aesthet Dermatol 2011;4:35-39

73 Laguna C, de la Cuadra J, Martín-González B, Zaragoza V, Martínez-Casimiro L, Alegre V. Allergic contact dermatitis to cosmetics. Actas Dermosifiliogr 2009;100:53-60

74 Castelain F, Castelain M. Parabens: a real hazard or a scare story? Eur J Dermatol 2012;22:723-727

75 Witorsch RJ, Thomas JA. Personal care products and endocrine disruption: A critical review of the literature. Crit Rev Toxicol 2010;40(Suppl. 3):1-30

76 Dooms-Goossens A, de Boulle K, Dooms M, Degreef H. Imidazolidinyl urea dermatitis. Contact Dermatitis 1986;14:322-324

77 Toholka R, Wang Y-S, Tate B, Tam M, Cahill J, Palmer A, Nixon R. The first Australian Baseline Series: Recommendations for patch testing in suspected contact dermatitis. Australas J Dermatol 2015;56:107-115

78 Zhao J, Li LF. Contact sensitization to cosmetic series of allergens in a general population in Beijing. J Cosmet Dermatol 2014;13:68-71

79 DeKoven JG, Warshaw EM, Belsito DV, Sasseville D, Maibach HI, Taylor JS, et al. North American Contact Dermatitis Group Patch Test Results: 2013-2014. Dermatitis 2017;28:33-46

80 Zaragoza-Ninet V, Blasco Encinas R, Vilata-Corell JJ, Pérez-Ferriols A, Sierra-Talamantes C, Esteve-Martínez A, de la Cuadra-Oyanguren J. Allergic contact dermatitis due to cosmetics: A clinical and epidemiological study in a tertiary hospital. Actas Dermosifiliogr 2016;107:329-336

81 Dinkloh A, Worm M, Geier J, Schnuch A, Wollenberg A. Contact sensitization in patients with suspected cosmetic intolerance: results of the IVDK 2006-2011. J Eur Acad Dermatol Venereol 2015;29:1071-1081

82 Hu Y, Wang D, Shen Y, Tang H. Photopatch testing in Chinese patients over 10 years. Dermatitis 2016;27:137-142

83 Uter W, Rämsch C, Aberer, W, Ayala F, Balato A, Beliauskiene A, et al. The European baseline series in 10 European Countries, 2005/2006 – Results of the European Surveillance System on Contact Allergies (ESSCA). Contact Dermatitis 2009;61:31-38

84 Ockenfels H, Seemann U, Goos M. Contact allergy in patients with periorbital eczema: an analysis of allergens. Dermatology 1997;195:119-124

85 Mowad CM. Allergic contact dermatitis caused by parabens: 2 case reports and a review. Am J Contact Derm 2000;11:53-56

86 Fransway AF. The problem of preservation in the 1990s: III. Agents with preservative function independent of formaldehyde release. Am J Cont Derm 1991;2:145-174

87 Hjorth N, Trolle-Lassen C. Skin reactions to ointment bases. Trans St John Hosp Derm Soc 1963;49:127-140

88 Praditsuwan P, Taylor JS, Roenigk HH Jr. Allergy to Unna boots in four patients. J Am Acad Dermatol 1995;33(5 Pt. 2):906-908

89 Horev L, Isaksson M, Engfeldt M, Persson L, Ingber A, Bruze M. Preservatives in cosmetics in the Israeli market conform well to the EU legislation. J Eur Acad Dermatol Venereol 2015;29:761-766

90 Chow ET, Avolio AM, Lee A, Nixon R. Frequency of positive patch test reactions to preservatives: The Australian experience. Australas J Dermatol 2013;54:31-35

91 Fisher AA. Esoteric contact dermatitis. Part I: the paraben paradox. Cutis 1996;57:65-66

92 Fisher AA. Esoteric contact dermatitis. Part II: the paraben paradox. Cutis. 1996;57:135-138

93 Fisher AA: The parabens: Paradoxical preservatives. Cutis 1993;51:405-406

94 Aeling JL, Nuss DD. Systemic eczematous "contact-type" dermatitis medicamentosa caused by parabens. Arch Dermatol 1974;110:640

95 Turchin I, Moreau L, Warshaw E, Sasseville D. Cross-reactions among parabens, para-phenylenediamine, and benzocaine: a retrospective analysis of patch testing. Dermatitis 2006;17:192-195

96 Hansen J, Møllgaard B, Avnstorp C, Menné T. Paraben contact allergy: Patch testing and in vitro absorption/metabolism. Am J Cont Derm 1993;4:78-86

97 Fisher AA. Management of selected types of allergic contact dermatitis through the proper substitutes. Cutis 1967;3:498-504 (data cited in ref. 98)

98 Rastogi SC, Schouten A, de Kruijf N, Weijland JW. Contents of methyl-, ethyl-, propyl-, butyl- and benzylparaben in cosmetic products. Contact Dermatitis 1995;32:28-30

99 Fisher AA. Allergic paraben and benzyl alcohol hypersensitivity relationship of the 'delayed' and 'immediate' varieties. Contact Dermatitis 1975;1:281-284

100 Maucher OM. Beitrag zur Kreuz- oder Kopplingsallergie zur Parahydroxybenzoesäure-ester. Berufsdermatosen 1974;22:183-187

101 Rietschel RL, Fowler JF Jr. Allergy to preservatives and vehicles in cosmetics and toiletries. In: Rietschel RL, Fowler JF Jr, editors. Fisher's contact dermatitis, 5th ed. Philadelphia: Lippincott Williams & Wilkins, 2001:211-259

102 Wuepper KD. Paraben contact dermatitis. JAMA 1967;202:579-581

103 Verhaeghe I, Dooms-Goossens A. Multiple sources of allergic contact dermatitis from parabens. Contact Dermatitis 1997;36:269

104 Bunyavaree M, Kasemsarn P, Boonchai W. Cosmetic preservative labelling on the Thai market. Contact Dermatitis 2016;74:217-221

105 Fisher AA. Contact dermatitis due to food additives. Cutis 1982;30:304,308,312,318,414

106 Schorr WF. The skin and chemical additives to foods. Arch Dermatol 1972;105:131

107 Veien NK, Hattel T. Laurberg G: Oral challenge with parabens in paraben-sensitive patients. Contact Dermatitis 1996;34:433

108 Sasseville D, Alfalah M, Lacroix J-P. 'Parabenoia' debunked, or 'who's afraid of parabens'? Dermatitis 2015;26:254-259

109 American Cancer Society. Antiperspirants and breast cancer risk. Available at: https://www.cancer.org/cancer/cancer-causes/antiperspirants-and-breast-cancer-risk.html Immunopharmacol Immunotoxicol. 2004 Aug;26(3):481-5.

110 Foti C, Bonamonte D, Antelmi A, Conserva A, Angelini G. Allergic contact dermatitis to condoms: description of a clinical case and analytical review of current literature. Immunopharmacol Immunotoxicol 2004;26:481-485

111 Cashman AL, Warshaw EM. Parabens: A review of epidemiology, structure, allergenicity, and hormonal properties. Dermatitis 2005;16:57-66

112 Fisher AA. Cortaid cream dermatitis and the 'paraben paradox'. J Am Acad Dermatol 1982;6:116-117

113 Yim E, Baquerizo Nole KL, Tosti A. Contact dermatitis caused by preservatives. Dermatitis 2014;25:215-231

114 Uter W, Yazar K, Kratz EM, Mildau G, Lidén C. Coupled exposure to ingredients of cosmetic products: II. Preservatives. Contact Dermatitis 2014;70:219-226

115 Hafeez F, Maibach H. An overview of parabens and allergic contact dermatitis. Skin Therapy Lett 2013;18:5-7

116 Jankićević J, Vesić S, Vukićević J, Gajić M, Adamic M, Pavlović MD. Contact sensitivity in patients with venous leg ulcers in Serbia: comparison with contact dermatitis patients and relationship to ulcer duration. Contact Dermatitis 2008;58:32-36

117 Rytter M, Walther T, Süss E, Haustein UF. Allergic reactions of the immediate and delayed type following prednisolone medication (article in German). Dermatol Monatsschr 1989;175:44-48

118 Giménez-Arnau AM, Deza G, Bauer A, Johnston GA, Mahler V, Schuttelaar ML, et al. Contact allergy to preservatives: ESSCA* results with the baseline series, 2009-2012. J Eur Acad Dermatol Venereol 2017;31:664-67

119 Lubbes S, Rustemeyer T, Sillevis Smitt JH, Schuttelaar ML, Middelkamp-Hup MA. Contact sensitization in Dutch children and adolescents with and without atopic dermatitis - a retrospective analysis. Contact Dermatitis 2017;76:151-159

120 Erfurt-Berge C, Geier J, Mahler V. The current spectrum of contact sensitization in patients with chronic leg ulcers or stasis dermatitis - new data from the Information Network of Departments of Dermatology (IVDK). Contact Dermatitis 2017;77:151-158

121 Aschenbeck KA, Warshaw EM. Allergenic ingredients in facial wet wipes. Dermatitis 2017 Mar 23. doi: 10.1097/DER.0000000000000268. [Epub ahead of print]

122 Aschenbeck KA, Warshaw EM. Allergenic ingredients in personal hygiene wet wipes. Dermatitis 2017 Mar 23. doi: 10.1097/DER.0000000000000275. [Epub ahead of print]

123 Beene KM, Scheman A, Severson D, Reeder MJ. Prevalence of preservatives across all product types in the Contact Allergen Management Program. Dermatitis 2017;28:81-87

124 Uter W, Amario-Hita JC, Balato A, Ballmer-Weber B, Bauer A, Belloni Fortina A, et al. European Surveillance System on Contact Allergies (ESSCA): results with the European baseline series, 2013/14. J Eur Acad Dermatol Venereol. 2017 Jun 19. doi: 10.1111/jdv.14423. [Epub ahead of print]

2.334 PARAFFINUM LIQUIDUM

IDENTIFICATION

Description/definition : Paraffinum liquidum is a highly refined petroleum mineral oil consisting of a complex combination of hydrocarbons obtained from the intensive treatment of a petroleum fraction with sulfuric acid and oleum, or by hydrogenation, or by a combination of hydrogenation and acid treatment. Additional washing and treating steps may be included in the processing operation. Paraffinum liquidum consists of saturated hydrocarbons having carbon numbers predominantly in the range of C15 through C50

Chemical class(es) : Hydrocarbons

INCI name USA : Mineral oil

Chemical / IUPAC name : Paraffin oils; liquid hydrocarbons from petroleum

Other names : Mineral oil; white mineral oil; liquid paraffin; paraffinum perliquidum; hydrocarbon oils; liquid petrolatum; petrolatum, liquid

CAS registry number (s) : 8012-95-1; 8042-47-5; 8020-83-5

EC number(s) : 232-384-2; 232-455-8

Merck Index monograph : 8571

Function(s) in cosmetics : EU: antistatic; emollient; skin protecting; solvent. USA: fragrance ingredients; hair conditioning agents; skin protectants; skin-conditioning agents – emollient; skin-conditioning agents – occlusive; solvents

Patch testing : pure, 20% in olive oil (10)

CONTACT ALLERGY

Case reports and case series

Mineral oil was responsible for 1 out of 399 cases of cosmetic allergy where the causal allergen was identified in a study of the NACDG, USA, 1977-1983 (1). In a group of 119 patients with allergic contact dermatitis from cosmetics, investigated in The Netherlands in 1986-1987, one case was caused by mineral oil in an eyeshadow (3,4). A man had hand dermatitis from contact allergy to liquid petrolatum in a hair tonic; quite curiously, the scalp was not affected (5). Three patients reacted to paraffinum liquidum used as emollient in skin care products (6). The first patient had atopic dermatitis and had recently developed eczema of the face. A patch test and an open test with her 'complexion cream' were positive, and of its constituents she reacted only to the mineral oil, but did so on two occasions. The oil did not contain any additives according to the manufacturer (6).

The second patient was a woman who recently had developed dermatitis of the eyelids. A patch test with her foundation cream was strongly positive, and of its components only the mineral oil elicited a definitely positive response; however, she attended only for the first reading at D2 (6). The third patient had an acute exudative dermatitis on her face. On patch testing she had several positive reactions, one of which was to a baby lotion. She was tested to the ingredients and had irritant reactions to propylene glycol and sodium dioctyl sulfosuccinate, both tested undiluted, but she was also positive to the mineral oil which had been applied well away from the irritant patch tests (6). The author stated that it seems improbable to her that white mineral oil could act as a sensitizer and that the more reasonable interpretation of these results is that they were mild irritant reactions. Control series with the mineral oils were not done, and the patch test concentration was not mentioned, though likely it had been applied undiluted (6).

Presence in cosmetic products and chemical analyses

In the USA, in April 2017, paraffin (probably, but not certain, liquid) was present in 1401 of 56,714 cosmetic products of which the composition is known in FDA's Voluntary Cosmetic Registration Program (VCRP) (data obtained from FDA, May 2017). In April 2017, mineral oil was present in 1752 of 66,485 cosmetic products of which the composition is known in EWG's Skin Deep Cosmetics Database, USA (http://www.ewg.org/skindeep/).

OTHER SIDE EFFECTS

Photosensitivity

A metal polishing mechanic had had an acute-on-chronic eczematous eruption on sun-exposed skin for 2 years. It improved in winter. At work, he had been using an insoluble oil as a cutting oil for 20 years. The cutting oil itself and mineral oil, which was one of its ingredients, showed positive reactions on photopatch testing (2).

Other non-eczematous contact reactions

In older literature, paraffinum liquidum has been suspected of being comedogenic and causing 'pomade acne' (7,8). In more recent investigations, however, paraffin was found to be non-comedogenic in the rabbit ear assay (9).

Other side effects

Apparently, skin diseases have developed in cable workers exposed to mineral oils. No details are known (article not read, in Norwegian) (11).

LITERATURE

1   Adams RM, Maibach HI, Clendenning WE, Fisher AA, Jordan WJ, Kanof N, et al. A five-year study of cosmetic reactions. J Am Acad Dermatol 1985;13:1062-1069
2   Sakakibara S, Kawabe Y, Mizuno N. Photoallergic contact dermatitis due to mineral oil. Contact Dermatitis 1989;20:291-294
3   De Groot AC, Bruynzeel DP, Bos JD, van der Meeren HL, van Joost T, Jagtman BA, Weyland JW. The allergens in cosmetics. Arch Dermatol 1988;124:1525-1529
4   De Groot AC. Adverse reactions to cosmetics. PhD Thesis, University of Groningen, The Netherlands: 1988, chapter 3.4, pp.105-113
5   Niles HD. Dermatitis of hands caused by liquid petrolatum in a proprietary hair tonic. Arch Derm Syph 1941;43:689-691
6   Cronin E. Contact Dermatitis. Edinburgh: Churchill Livingstone, 1980:102-103
7   Plewig G, Fulton JE, Kligman AM. Pomade acne. Arch Dermatol 1970;101:580-584
8   Berlin C. Acne comedo in children due to paraffin oil applied on the head. Arch Dermatol 1954;69:683-687
9   Nguyen SH, Dang TP, Maibach HI. Comedogenicity in rabbit: some cosmetic ingredients/vehicles. Cutan Ocul Toxicol 2007;26:287-292
10   De Groot AC. Patch Testing, 3rd Edition. Wapserveen, The Netherlands: acdegroot publishing, 2008 (ISBN 978-90-813233-1-4)
11   Skyberg K, Rønneberg A. Skin diseases in cable workers exposed to mineral oils. Tidsskr Nor Laegeforen 1986;106:657-659 (Article in Norwegian)

2.335 PARAFORMALDEHYDE

IDENTIFICATION

Description/definition   : Paraformaldehyde is a linear polymer of formaldehyde which has the formula shown
                            below; the number of formaldehyde units averages about 30 but may range from 8 to
                            100
Chemical class(es)   : Polymers; aldehydes
INCI name USA   : Not in the Personal Care Council Database
Chemical/IUPAC name   : Polyoxymethylene
Other names   : Formaldehyde resin; paraform; polyacetal; polyacetal resin
CAS registry number (s)   : 30525-89-4
EC number(s)   : 200-001-8
Merck Index monograph   : 8399
SCCS opinion(s)   : SCCNFP/587/02 (2)
Function(s) in cosmetics   : EU: preservative
Patch testing   : 5% pet. (1); 10% pet. (3)

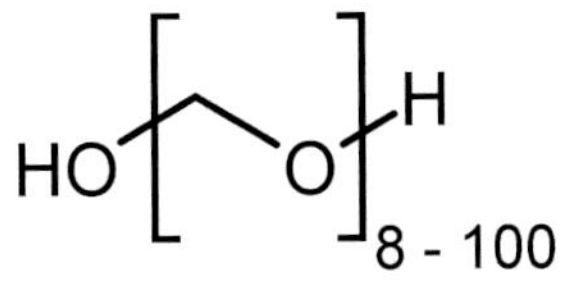

GENERAL

Paraformaldehyde is a linear solid-phase polymer of formaldehyde. It is a white, crystalline powder and is used as a fumigant, disinfectant, and fungicide, in root-canal therapy and as a curing agent for phenol-formaldehyde resins. Higher molecule homopolymer is a hard engineering plastic (polyoxymethylene plastic), which is strong, rigid, and has good moisture, heat, and solvent resistance. As paraformaldehyde is essentially a solid form of formaldehyde, it therefore has the same uses as formaldehyde (4). In aqueous environment, paraformaldehyde releases formaldehyde, possibly most of all formaldehyde-releasers used in cosmetics such as diazolidinyl urea, DMDM hydantoin, quaternium-15 , imidazolidinyl urea, methenamine and 2-bromo-2-nitropropane-1,3-diol (5).

CONTACT ALLERGY

Case reports and case series

A man had suffered from intense outbreaks of seborrheic dermatitis, which improved with topical corticosteroids and ketoconazole but recurred on ceasing medication. For the past 3 months, papular, erythematous, intensely pruriginous lesions had been appearing on sun-exposed areas of the face, neck and hands. Patch tests and photopatch tests with the standard series were negative at 2 and 4 days, as were his cosmetics and toiletries with the single exception of a shaving foam, tested as is, which gave a strongly positive patch test reaction at both readings. Patch and photopatch tests were then carried out with the ingredients of this product supplied by the manufacturer and he had positive patch test reactions to 6 ingredients including paraformaldehyde 5% pet. There were no positive reactions in 25 controls. The patient was retested 7 months later to all 6 allergens previously positive and reacted again at 2 and 4 days to paraformaldehyde 5% pet. (1).

Contact allergy to paraformaldehyde in non-cosmetic products

A woman was seen because of pruritic erythema and swelling on her left side of the oral mucosa and cheek. She had received a root canal filling in the upper jaw on the morning of the day before and noticed her symptoms 12 hours later. She had previously received two such treatments. The dental filling contained four components: paraform-aldehyde, copal, silicic anhydride and isoamyl acetate. Prick tests were negative. Patch tests with the ingredients gave positive reactions to copal and to paraformaldehyde 10% pet., but reactions to paraformaldehyde 1% pet. and 0.1% pet. were negative. Five controls were negative (3). It appears that a standard series with formaldehyde in it was not tested, which is unfortunate, as formaldehyde itself may well have been responsible. Allergic reactions to formaldehyde and paraformaldehyde from tooth root treatments have been reported earlier from Switzerland (6).

Cross-reactions, pseudo-cross-reactions and co-reactions

Not to formaldehyde (1). Co-reaction to formaldehyde (7).

Presence in cosmetic products and chemical analyses

In the USA, in April 2017, paraformaldehyde was present in zero of 56,714 cosmetic products of which the composition is known in FDA's Voluntary Cosmetic Registration Program (VCRP) (data obtained from FDA, May 2017). In April 2017, paraformaldehyde was present in zero of 66,485 cosmetic products of which the composition is known in EWG's Skin Deep Cosmetics Database, USA (http://www.ewg.org/skindeep/).

OTHER SIDE EFFECTS

Immediate-type reactions

A woman who had experienced urticaria following dental treatment several times for the past 3 years, was treated for acute odontitis with a paraformaldehyde-containing root canal disinfectant. Three hours later, she noticed itchy urticarial erythema on her arms, legs and trunk. On the following day, she was again treated, this time with another paraformaldehyde-containing disinfectant and 8 hours later, she developed a wheal and flare reaction on her entire body accompanied by systemic symptoms, including wheezing, cough, dyspnea, and dysphagia. IgE radioallergo-sorbent tests showed a high titre of specific IgE against formaldehyde. Prick testing showed positive reactions to paraformaldehyde 1% water and formaldehyde 1% water at 20 minutes. Delayed-type responses to formaldehyde and paraformaldehyde were noted at the prick test sites at D3. Patch tests with these chemicals were also positive. The case was diagnosed as anaphylaxis due to type-I allergy to formaldehyde contained in dental root-canal fillings. It was speculated that the delay in the manifestation of her symptoms was due to gradual formaldehyde release from paraformaldehyde and time lag of penetrating and diffusing of formaldehyde outside the dentin, gradually increase-ing in the circulating blood after root-canal treatment, finally reaching the threshold to trigger allergic symptoms after 2-12 hours (7). A similar case, where the patient developed generalized urticaria, was reported from Poland (8).

A man had recurrent generalized urticaria several hours after endodontic treatment where paraformaldehyde was used. Prick tests to latex, lidocaine, and formaldehyde showed negative reactions. However, swelling and redness at the formaldehyde prick site continued for several days. The level of formaldehyde-specific IgE was high (class 4). Thus, the patient was deemed to have experienced an IgE-mediated hypersensitivity reaction caused by the paraformaldehyde used in the root canal disinfectant (9).

LITERATURE

1   Vilaplana J, Lecha M, Romaguera C, Alsina A, Mascaro JM, Castel, T. A polysensitized HIV-positive patient. Contact Dermatitis 1993;29:101-102
2   SCCNFP (Scientific Committee on Cosmetics and Non Food Products). Opinion concerning a clarification on the formaldehyde and para-formaldehyde entry in Directive 76/768/EEC on cosmetic products, 17 December 2002, SCCNFP/587/02. Available at:
    http://ec.europa.eu/health/archive/ph_risk/committees/sccp/documents/out187_en.pdf
3   Kimura M, Miura S, Ozawa S, Kawada A. Allergic contact stomatitis from paraformaldehyde and copal in a dental root canal filling. Contact Dermatitis 2003;49:164
4   De Groot AC, Geier J, Flyvholm MA, Lensen G, Coenraads PJ. Formaldehyde-releasers: relationship to formaldehyde contact allergy. Part 2: Metalworking fluids and remainder. Contact Dermatitis 2010;63:129-139
5   Lv C, Hou J, Xie W, Cheng H. Investigation on formaldehyde release from preservatives in cosmetics. Int J Cosm Sci 2015;37:474-478
6   Fehr B, Huwyler T, Wüthrich B. Formaldehyde and paraformaldehyde allergy. Allergic reactions to formaldehyde and paraformaldehyde after tooth root treatments. Schweiz Monatsschr Zahnmed 1992;102:94-97
7   Kunisada M, Adachi A, Asano H, Horikawa T. Anaphylaxis due to formaldehyde released from root-canal disinfectant. Contact Dermatitis 2002;47:215-218
8   Adamowicz Z, Doboszyńska A, Tomaszewska I, Siemieniuk A. Allergy to formaldehyde. Pol Merkur Lekarski 2004;99:271-272 (Article in Polish)
9   Jang JH, Park SH, Jang HJ, Lee SG, Park JH, Jeong JW, Park CS. A case of recurrent urticaria due to formaldehyde release from root-canal disinfectant. Yonsei Med J 2017;58:252-254

2.336   PEG-4 DILAURATE

IDENTIFICATION

Description/definition	: PEG-4 dilaurate is the polyethylene glycol diester of lauric acid that conforms to the formula shown below, where n has an average value of 4
Chemical class(es)	: Alkoxylated carboxylic acids
Chemical/IUPAC name	: Poly(oxy-1,2-ethanediyl),α-(1-oxododecyl)-ω-[(1-oxododecyl)oxy]- (4 mol EO average molar ratio)
Other names	: Polyethylene glycol 200 dilaurate; polyoxyethylene (4) dilaurate
CAS registry number (s)	: 9005-02-1
CIR review(s)	: Int J Toxicol 2000;19(Suppl.2):29-41; Final report, March 2015 (access: www.cir-safety.org/ingredients)
Function(s) in cosmetics	: EU: emulsifying. USA: surfactants - emulsifying agents
Patch testing	: No data available; suggested: 10% pet.
Molecular formula	: $C_{32}H_{62}O_7$

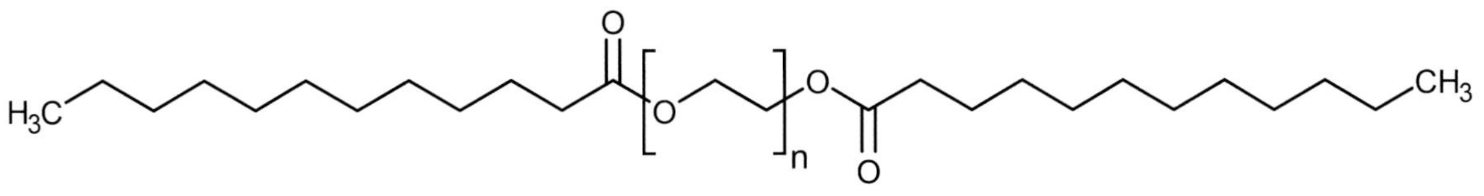

CONTACT ALLERGY

Case reports and case series
PEG-4 dilaurate was responsible for 1 out of 399 cases of cosmetic allergy where the causal allergen was identified in a study of the NACDG, USA, 1977-1983 (1).

Presence in cosmetic products and chemical analyses
In the USA, in April 2017, PEG-4 dilaurate was present in 34 of 56,714 cosmetic products of which the composition is known in FDA's Voluntary Cosmetic Registration Program (VCRP) (data obtained from FDA, May 2017). In March 2017, PEG-4 dilaurate was present in 27 of 65,431 cosmetic products of which the composition is known in EWG's Skin Deep Cosmetics Database, USA (http://www.ewg.org/skindeep/).

LITERATURE
1   Adams RM, Maibach HI, Clendenning WE, Fisher AA, Jordan WJ, Kanof N, et al. A five-year study of cosmetic reactions. J Am Acad Dermatol 1985;13:1062-1069

2.337   PEG-4 DIMETHACRYLATE

IDENTIFICATION

Description/definition	: PEG-4 dimethacrylate is the organic compound that conforms to the formula shown below
Chemical class(es)	: Alkoxylated carboxylic acids
Chemical/IUPAC name	: 2-[2-[2-[2-(2-Methylprop-2-enoyloxy)ethoxy]ethoxy]ethoxy]ethyl 2-methylprop-2-enoate
Other names	: Tetraethylene glycol dimethacrylate; polyethylene glycol (4) dimethacrylate; polyoxyethylene (4) dimethacrylate
CAS registry number (s)	: 109-17-1
EC number(s)	: 203-653-1
CIR review(s)	: Int J Toxicol 2005;24(Suppl.5):53-100 (access: www.cir-safety.org/ingredients)
Function(s) in cosmetics	: EU: binding; film forming. USA: artificial nail builders
Patch test allergens	: 2% pet.
Molecular formula	: $C_{16}H_{26}O_7$

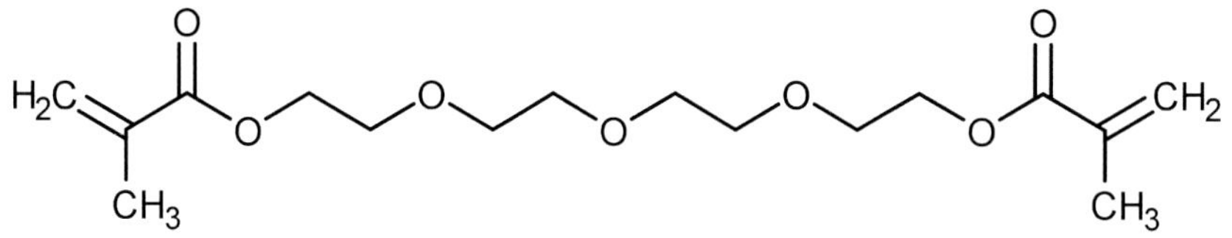

GENERAL

Discussion of contact allergy to (meth)acrylates *from non-cosmetic sources* is considered to fall outside the scope of this book. Therefore, only contact allergy from their presence in cosmetics is presented, which virtually always is from artificial nails. There are many reports of contact allergy to artificial nails, but the specific sensitizers have rarely been identified and – consequently - such publications are not presented in this and other acrylate and methacrylate monographs. Discussion is limited to publications in which the culprit (meth)acrylates have been identified, e.g., from information found in Material Data Safety Sheets, data obtained from the manufacturer or from chemical analyses.

Patients often react to many (meth)acrylates on patch testing. Primary sensitization to methacrylates may result in both methacrylate and acrylate cross-sensitization. Conversely, patients sensitized to acrylates are unlikely to show cross-sensitization to methacrylates (2).

General aspects of acrylates and methacrylates are presented in Chapter 2.219 HEMA (hydroxyethyl methacrylate). A discussion of general aspects of artificial nails, contact allergy to these products, the clinical picture of allergic contact dermatitis and other side effects of sculptured nails can also be found there. A very useful review of contact sensitization to allergens in nail cosmetics, with emphasis on acrylic manicures, was published in 2017 (4).

CONTACT ALLERGY

Patch testing in groups of patients
Studies in which consecutive patients suspected of contact dermatitis have been tested with PEG-4 dimethacrylate (routine testing) and studies testing groups of selected patients are planned to be discussed in a future publication.

Case reports and case series
In the period 1996-2013, in a tertiary referral center in Valencia, Spain, 5419 patients were patch tested. Of these, 628 individuals had allergic contact dermatitis to cosmetics. PEG-4 dimethacrylate (tetraethylene glycol dimethacrylate) was the responsible allergen in three cases (3).

In the period 2000-2007, 202 patients with allergic contact dermatitis caused by cosmetics were seen in the same clinic in Valencia, Spain (overlap with ref. 3). In this group, there were 10 beauticians with occupational allergic contact dermatitis of the hands, who reacted to multiple (meth)acrylates from their presence in artificial nail materials. Of these ten individuals, one reacted to PEG-4 dimethacrylate, which reaction was apparently relevant (although it can be doubted that the presence of these specific chemicals in the products could always be verified) (1).

Presence in cosmetic products and chemical analyses

In the USA, in April 2017, PEG-4 dimethacrylate was present in 4 of 56,714 cosmetic products of which the composition is known in FDA's Voluntary Cosmetic Registration Program (VCRP) (data obtained from FDA, May 2017). In February 2017, PEG-4 dimethacrylate was present in zero of 64,480 cosmetic products of which the composition is known in EWG's Skin Deep Cosmetics Database, USA (http://www.ewg.org/skindeep/).

LITERATURE

1   Laguna C, de la Cuadra J, Martín-González B, Zaragoza V, Martínez-Casimiro L, Alegre V. Allergic contact dermatitis to cosmetics. Actas Dermosifiliogr 2009;100:53-60
2   Aalto-Korte K, Henriks-Eckerman M-L, Kuuliala O, Jolanki R. Occupational methacrylate and acrylate allergy – cross-reactions and possible screening allergens. Contact Dermatitis 2010;63:301-312
3   Zaragoza-Ninet V, Blasco Encinas R, Vilata-Corell JJ, Pérez-Ferriols A, Sierra-Talamantes C, Esteve-Martínez A, de la Cuadra-Oyanguren J. Allergic contact dermatitis due to cosmetics: A clinical and epidemiological study in a tertiary hospital. Actas Dermosifiliogr 2016;107:329-336
4   Chou M, Dhingra N, Strugar TL. Contact sensitization to allergens in nail cosmetics. Dermatitis 2017;28:231-240

2.338 PEG-4 RAPESEEDAMIDE

IDENTIFICATION

Description/definition	: PEG-4 rapeseedamide is the polyethylene glycol amide of the fatty acids derived from rapeseed oil with an average of 4 moles of ethylene oxide
Chemical class(es)	: Alkoxylated amides
Chemical/IUPAC name	: Polyoxyethylene rapeseedamide
Other names	: Polyethylene glycol 200 rapeseedamide; polyoxyethylene (4) rapeseedamide
CAS registry number (s)	: 85536-23-8
Function(s) in cosmetics	: EU: viscosity controlling. USA: surfactants - emulsifying agents; viscosity increasing agents - aqueous
Patch testing	: 0.03%-3% pet. (1)

CONTACT ALLERGY

Case reports and case series

A woman had suffered from dermatitis on the flexor wrists and forearms for 4 months. She had had mild atopic dermatitis as a child, but as an adult had been free of eczema until she started working as a masseuse. After one month, dermatitis had appeared on skin exposed to massage oils. When patch tested, she reacted to two massage oils. Later, she was tested with their components, and there were reactions to PEG-4 rapeseedamide in a concentration range of 3.0% down to 0.003% in water and in pet. This chemical was present in both oils in a concentration of 3%. 28 controls tested with PEG-4 rapeseedamide 0.3% pet. were negative. The patient stopped her work as masseuse and her dermatitis cleared. Several months later, however, an itchy, papular dermatitis appeared behind the ears and around the hair margin, the scalp turning red and itchy, a few hours after she had colored her hair with a brown permanent hair dye. The label stated that PEG-4 rapeseedamide was an ingredient of the dye. She was tested with the PEG-rapeseedamide and again had multiple positive reactions to a dilution series. The patient also reacted to the intermediate product rapeseedamide 0.5% pet., but not to its parent compounds rapeseed oil and monoethanolamine (1).

Cross-reactions, pseudo-cross-reactions and co-reactions

Rapeseedamide (1). Not to the two raw materials to produce the chemical, rapeseed oil and monoethanolamine (1).

Presence in cosmetic products and chemical analyses

In the USA, in April 2017, PEG-4 rapeseedamide was present in 281 of 56,714 cosmetic products of which the composition is known in FDA's Voluntary Cosmetic Registration Program (VCRP) (data obtained from FDA, May 2017). In March 2017, PEG-4 rapeseedamide was present in 42 of 65,431 cosmetic products of which the composition is known in EWG's Skin Deep Cosmetics Database, USA (http://www.ewg.org/skindeep/).

LITERATURE

1   Isaksson, M. Occupational allergic contact dermatitis from PEG-4 rapeseed amide in a massage oil. Contact Dermatitis 2002;47:175-176

2.339 PEG-5 LANOLATE

IDENTIFICATION

Description/definition : PEG-5 lanolate is the polyethylene glycol ester of lanolin acid that conforms generally to the formula shown below, where RCO- represents the fatty acids derived from lanolin and n has an average value of 5

Chemical class(es) : Alkoxylated carboxylic acids; lanolin and lanolin derivatives

Chemical/IUPAC name : Fatty acids, lanolin, ethoxylated (5 mol EO average molar ratio)

Other names : Polyethylene glycol (5) lanolate; polyoxyethylene (5) lanolate; Lanpol® 5

CAS registry number (s) : 68459-50-7 (generic)

Function(s) in cosmetics : EU: emulsifying. USA: surfactants - emulsifying agents

Patch testing : 5% pet. (1)

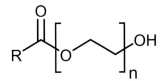

CONTACT ALLERGY

Case reports and case series

A young woman presented with a 6-month history of cracking and swelling of both upper and lower lips (cheilitis). She had a past history of atopic dermatitis. The patient knew she was allergic to adhesive tape and had previously suffered from dermatitis of the eyelids after using a lanolin-based eye make-up. Patch tests with the standard series of contact allergens produced a positive reaction to colophonium, but there was no reaction to several 'lanolins': wool alcohols, hydrogenated lanolin, Eucerit or Amerchol® L 101. On testing with her various cosmetics, she reacted to a lipstick and a lipstick sealant. Further patch testing to the individual ingredients of these 2 cosmetic lip preparations gave positive reactions to PEG-5 lanolate (Lanpol® 5) 5% pet., an ingredient of the lipstick, and to shellac in the lip sealant (1).

Cross-reactions, pseudo-cross-reactions and co-reactions

Not to lanolin (-derivatives) (1).

Presence in cosmetic products and chemical analyses

In the USA, in April 2017, PEG-5 lanolate was present in zero of 56,714 cosmetic products of which the composition is known in FDA's Voluntary Cosmetic Registration Program (VCRP) (data obtained from FDA, May 2017). In March 2017, PEG-5 lanolate was present in zero of 65,431 cosmetic products of which the composition is known in EWG's Skin Deep Cosmetics Database, USA (http://www.ewg.org/skindeep/).

LITERATURE

1   Rademaker M, Kirby JD, White IR. Contact cheilitis to shellac, Lanpol 5 and colophony. Contact Dermatitis 1986;15:307-308

2.340   PEG-5 SOY STEROL

IDENTIFICATION

Description/definition	: PEG-5 soy sterol is a polyethylene glycol derivative of sterols found in Glycine soja (soybean) oil with an average of 5 moles of ethylene oxide
Chemical class(es)	: Alkoxylated alcohols; sterols
Other names	: Sterols, soya (*Glycine soja*), ethoxylated (5 mol EO average molar ratio); polyethylene glycol (5) soy sterol; polyoxyethylene (5) soy sterol
CIR review(s)	: Int J Toxicol 2004;23(Suppl.2):23-47; Int J Toxicol 2000;19(Suppl.1):29-46 (access: www.cir-safety.org/ingredients)
Function(s) in cosmetics	: EU: emulsifying. USA: skin-conditioning agents - miscellaneous; surfactants – emulsifying agents
Patch testing	: No data available

CONTACT ALLERGY

Case reports and case series
In the period 1996-2013, in a tertiary referral center in Valencia, Spain, 5419 patients were patch tested. Of these, 628 individuals had allergic contact dermatitis to cosmetics. PEG-5 soy sterol was the responsible allergen in one case (1).

Presence in cosmetic products and chemical analyses
In the USA, in April 2017, PEG-5 soya sterol was present in 28 of 56,714 cosmetic products of which the composition is known in FDA's Voluntary Cosmetic Registration Program (VCRP) (data obtained from FDA, May 2017). In March 2017, PEG-5 soy sterol was present in 3 of 65,431 cosmetic products of which the composition is known in EWG's Skin Deep Cosmetics Database, USA (http://www.ewg.org/skindeep/).

LITERATURE
1   Zaragoza-Ninet V, Blasco Encinas R, Vilata-Corell JJ, Pérez-Ferriols A, Sierra-Talamantes C, Esteve-Martínez A, de la Cuadra-Oyanguren J. Allergic contact dermatitis due to cosmetics: A clinical and epidemiological study in a tertiary hospital. Actas Dermosifiliogr 2016;107:329-336

2.341   PEG-6

IDENTIFICATION

Description/definition	: PEG-6 is the polymer of ethylene oxide that conforms generally to the formula shown below
Chemical class(es)	: Alkoxylated alcohols; polymeric ethers
Chemical/IUPAC name	: 2-[2-[2-[2-[2-(2-Hydroxyethoxy)ethoxy]ethoxy]ethoxy]ethoxy]ethanol
Other names	: Hexaethylene glycol; polyoxyethylene (6); polyethylene glycol 300; PEG-300
CAS registry number (s)	: 25322-68-3 (polyethylene glycol); 2615-15-8
EC number(s)	: 220-045-1
CIR review(s)	: J Am Coll Toxicol 1993;12:429-457; Final report, June 2010 (access: www.cir-safety.org/ingredients)
Merck Index monograph	: 8958 (Polyethylene glycol)
Function(s) in cosmetics	: EU: humectant; solvent. USA: humectants; solvents
Patch testing	: Polyethylene glycol ointment pure (SmartPracticeCanada, MW unknown); PEG-400 (SmartPracticeEurope, SmartPracticeCanada); PEG-6 4% pet. (8)
Molecular formula	: $C_{12}H_{26}O_7$

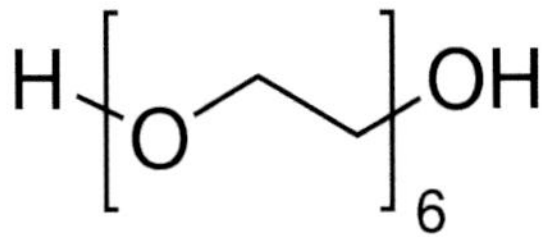

GENERAL

Polyethylene glycol (PEG) is a polyether compound with many applications from industrial manufacturing to medicine. PEG is also known as polyethylene oxide (PEO) or polyoxyethylene (POE), depending on its molecular weight. The structure of PEG is commonly expressed as $H(OCH_2CH_2)_nOH$, in which n = 3-200; its molecular weight varies from 200-7500. The abbreviations PEG, PEO, or POE refer to an oligomer or polymer of ethylene oxide. The three names are chemically synonymous, but historically polyethylene glycols (PEG) is preferred in the biomedical field, whereas PEO is more prevalent in the field of polymer chemistry (Wikipedia). The low molecular weight (MW) polyethylene glycols are liquids, whereas MWs 1000 to 6000 are solid. They are used extensively as vehicles in topical medicaments, suppositories, shampoos, detergents, hair dressings, insect repellents, cosmetics, toothpastes, contraceptives and many other products (2).

CONTACT ALLERGY

Patch testing in groups of patients
In the period 2004 to 2008, in France, 423 patients with leg ulcers were patch tested with a combination of PEG-6 and PEG-32, tested pure, and 3 individuals (0.7%) had positive reactions. The relevance of these reactions was not mentioned (6). In Germany, in the 1960s, routine tests in 92 dermatological patients with contact allergies gave 4% positive reactions to PEG-6 (polyethylene glycol 300). Their relevance and causative products are unknown (1).

Case reports and case series
One patient was allergic to PEG-6 in a soap; possibly, the patient had been sensitized from experimental contact sensitization studies (7).

Contact allergy to PEG-6 in non-cosmetic products
Three patients had contact allergy to PEG-6 (polyethylene glycol 300) in topical pharmaceutical preparations (1). One patient reacted to polyethylene glycol 300 (PEG-6) in a pharmaceutical dressing, another one caused allergic contact dermatitis from its presence in an antibiotic solution (4); the same patients were probably also reported in ref. 9. Another patient reacted to both nitrofurazone and polyethylene glycol 300 (PEG-6) in nitrofurazone topical pharmaceutical ointment (8).

Cross-reactions, pseudo-cross-reactions and co-reactions
In 12 subjects allergic to PEG-6 (polyethylene glycol 300), 5 also reacted to PEG-400 and 1 to polyethylene glycol 1500 (PEG-32) and to PEG 6000 (1). Cross-reaction from and/or to PEG-400 (3,8,9). Cross-reactivity to polyethylene glycols (PEG) 600, 1000, 4000 and 6000 (5).

Presence in cosmetic products and chemical analyses

In the USA, in April 2017, PEG-6 was present in 175 of 56,714 cosmetic products of which the composition is known in FDA's Voluntary Cosmetic Registration Program (VCRP) (data obtained from FDA, May 2017). In April 2017, PEG-6 was present in 22 of 66,485 cosmetic products of which the composition is known in EWG's Skin Deep Cosmetics Database, USA (http://www.ewg.org/skindeep/).

OTHER SIDE EFFECTS

Immediate-type reactions

A patient had immediate contact reactions from polyethylene glycol 300 (PEG-6) in an ear medication (4); probably, the patient was also presented in ref. 9.

LITERATURE

1   Braun W. Contact allergies to polyethylene glycols. Z Haut und Geschl Krankh 1969;44:385-388.
2   Bajaj AK, Gupta SC, Chatterjee AK,Singh KG. Contact sensitivity to polyethylene glycols. Contact Dermatitis 1990; 22:291-292
3   Stenveld HJ, Langendijk PNJ, Bruynzeel DP. Contact sensitivity to polyethylene glycols. Contact Dermatitis 1994;30:184-185
4   Fisher AA. Contact urticaria due to polyethylene glycol. Cutis 1977;19:409-412
5   Maibach HI. Polyethyleneglycol: allergic contact dermatitis potential. Contact Dermatitis 1975;1:247
6   Barbaud A, Collet E, Le Coz CJ, Meaume S, Gillois P. Contact allergy in chronic leg ulcers: results of a multicentre study carried out in 423 patients and proposal for an updated series of patch tests. Contact Dermatitis 2009;60:279-287
7   Marzulli F, Maibach HI. Use of graded concentration in studying skin sensitizers. Experimental contact sensitization in man. Food Chem Toxicol 1974;12:219-228
8   Guijarro SC, Sánchez-Pérez J, García-Díez A. Allergic contact dermatitis to polyethylene glycol and nitrofurazone. Am J Contact Dermat 1999;10:226-227
9   Fisher AA. Immediate and delayed allergic contact reactions to polyethylene glycol. Contact Dermatitis 1978;4:135-138

2.342   PEG-7 HYDROGENATED CASTOR OIL

IDENTIFICATION

Description/definition	: PEG-7 hydrogenated castor oil is a polyethylene glycol derivative of hydrogenated castor oil with an average of 7 moles of ethylene oxide
Chemical class(es)	: Alkoxylated alcohols
Other names	: Castor oil (*Ricinus communis*), hydrogenated, ethoxylated (7 mol EO average molar ratio); polyoxyethylene (7) hydrogenated castor oil
CAS registry number (s)	: 61788-85-0 (generic)
CIR review(s)	: Int J Toxicol 2014;33(Suppl.4):13-39 (access: www.cir-safety.org/ingredients)
Function(s) in cosmetics	: EU: emulsifying; surfactant. USA: fragrance ingredients; skin-conditioning agents – emollient; surfactants - emulsifying agents
Patch testing	: 10% pet. (1)

CONTACT ALLERGY

Case reports and case series

A non-atopic male patient presented with an eczematous eruption on the face and neck after application of a sunscreen lotion. Patch testing with an extended British Contact Dermatitis Society standard series, medicament series, facial series, photoallergic series and patient's own sunscreen was performed. Photopatch testing with the photoallergic series and patient's own sunscreen was also performed. The only positive reaction was to the sunscreen lotion on non-irradiated and irradiated skin, indicating a non-photosensitive allergic contact dermatitis. Further patch testing with the individual ingredients of the sunscreen lotion, obtained from the manufacturers, showed a positive reaction to PEG-7 hydrogenated castor oil 10% in petrolatum. There were negative reactions to all the other ingredients including PEG-8 (1).

Cross-reactions, pseudo-cross-reactions and co-reactions

Not to PEG-8 (1).

Presence in cosmetic products and chemical analyses

In the USA, in April 2017, PEG-7 hydrogenated castor oil was present in 15 of 56,714 cosmetic products of which the composition is known in FDA's Voluntary Cosmetic Registration Program (VCRP) (data obtained from FDA, May 2017). In March 2017, PEG-7 hydrogenated castor oil was present in 20 of 65,431 cosmetic products of which the composition is known in EWG's Skin Deep Cosmetics Database, USA (http://www.ewg.org/skindeep/).

LITERATURE

1   Kalavala M, Hughes TM, Stone NM. Allergic contact dermatitis to polyethylene glycol-7 hydrogenated castor oil. Contact Dermatitis 2007;56:287-288

2.343   PEG-7 OLEATE

IDENTIFICATION

Description/definition   : PEG-7 oleate is the polyethylene glycol ester of oleic acid that conforms to the formula
                             shown below, where n has an average value of 7
Chemical class(es)   : Alkoxylated carboxylic acids
Other names   : Polyethylene glycol (7) monooleate; polyoxyethylene (7) monooleate
CAS registry number (s)   : 9004-96-0
Function(s) in cosmetics   : EU: emulsifying; surfactant. USA: surfactants – emulsifying agents
Patch testing   : pure (1)
Molecular formula   : $C_{32}H_{62}O_9$

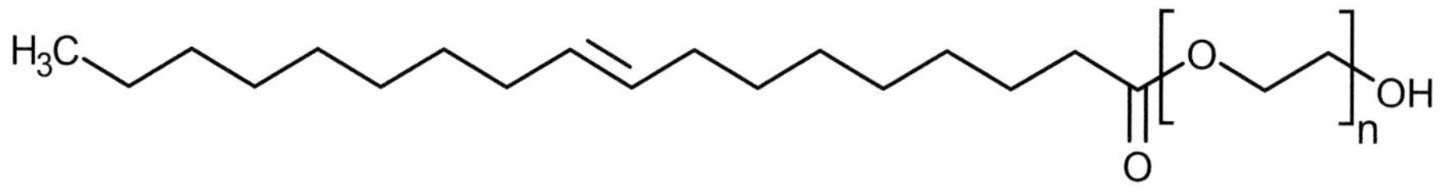

CONTACT ALLERGY

Case reports and case series

A female atopic physiotherapist had suffered for 6 months from dermatitis on the palmar and lateral aspects of both hands and wrists. The eruption improved with the use of topical corticosteroids. She suspected two products that she used at work to massage her clients. The patient was patch tested with the baseline, cosmetic and fragrance series and her own products. There was a strongly positive patch test reaction to one massage oil, tested undiluted. The ingredients of this product were obtained from the manufacturer and patch tested on the patient, which yielded a positive reaction at D2 and D4 to PEG-7 oleate (termed polyethylene glycol (PEG)-7 monooleate), tested 'as is'. Eight controls were negative to this material. Subsequently, the patient was tested with oleic acid and several PEG derivatives, but there were no positive reactions to any of them (1).

Cross-reactions, pseudo-cross-reactions and co-reactions

Not to oleic acid and several 'PEG derivatives' (1).

Presence in cosmetic products and chemical analyses

In the USA, in April 2017, PEG-7 oleate was present in zero of 56,714 cosmetic products of which the composition is known in FDA's Voluntary Cosmetic Registration Program (VCRP) (data obtained from FDA, May 2017). In March 2017, PEG-7 oleate was present in zero of 65,431 cosmetic products of which the composition is known in EWG's Skin Deep Cosmetics Database, USA (http://www.ewg.org/skindeep/).

LITERATURE

1   Conejero C, Loidi L, Hervella M. Contact dermatitis caused by polyethylene glycol-7 monooleate. Contact
      Dermatitis 2015;72:185-186

2.344 PEG-22/DODECYL GLYCOL COPOLYMER

IDENTIFICATION

Description/definition	: PEG-22/dodecyl glycol copolymer is the polyoxyethylene, polydodecyl glycol block polymer that conforms generally to the formula shown below, in which the average value of x, y, and z are 4.5, 22 and 4.5 respectively
Chemical class(es)	: Alkoxylated alcohols; synthetic polymers
Chemical/IUPAC name	: Poly(oxy-1,2-ethanediyl), α-(12-hydroxydodecyl)-θ-[(12-hydroxydodecyl)oxy]-s;
Other names	: Poly(oxy-1,2-ethanediyl), α-hydro-ω-hydroxy-, diethers with 1,2-dodecanediol homopolymer (22 mol EO, 9 mol dodecanediol average molar ratio)
CAS registry number (s)	: 78336-31-9
Function(s) in cosmetics	: EU: emulsifying; stabilising. USA: emulsion stabilizers; skin-conditioning agents – emollient
Patch testing	: 20% pet.

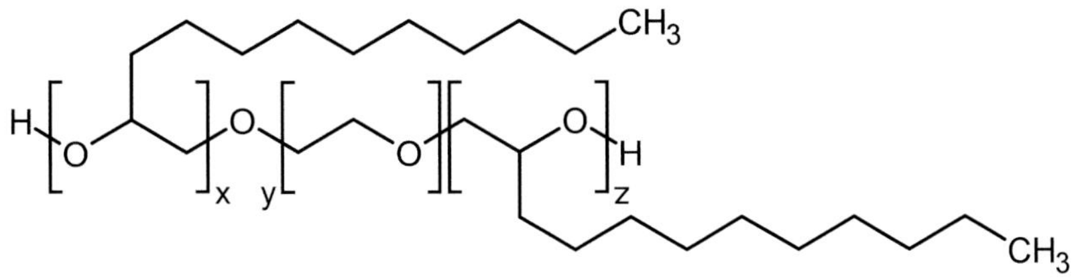

CONTACT ALLERGY

Case reports and case series

A woman developed acute dermatitis around the surgical scar of her thyroidectomy 20 days after the operation. She had applied a cosmetic 'skin-repair' cream twice daily for 2 days when the cutaneous lesions occurred. The symptoms subsided within 2 weeks with application of topical corticosteroids and ceasing the use of this product. A ROAT with the cream was positive after 4 days. Patch test with the European baseline series, a cosmetics series and with all ingredients of the product obtained from the manufacturer gave a positive reaction to PEG-22/dodecyl glycol copolymer 20% pet. (1). Controls tests were not performed.

Presence in cosmetic products and chemical analyses

In July 2017, PEG-22/dodecyl glycol copolymer was present in one of 69,548 cosmetic products of which the composition is known in EWG's Skin Deep Cosmetics Database, USA (http://www.ewg.org/skindeep/).

LITERATURE

1 Amsler E, Al-Raddadi R, Frances C. Allergic contact dermatitis caused by PEG-22/dodecyl glycol copolymer in a skin-repairing cream. Contact Dermatitis 2017;77:54-55

2.345   PEG-32 STEARATE

IDENTIFICATION

Description/definition	: PEG-32 stearate is the polyethylene glycol ester of stearic acid that conforms to the formula shown below, where n has an average value of 32
Chemical class(es)	: Alkoxylated carboxylic acids
Chemical/IUPAC name	: Poly(oxy-1,2-ethanediyl),α-(1-oxooctadecyl)-ω-hydroxy- (32 mol EO average molar ratio)
Other names	: Polyethylene glycol 1540 monostearate; polyoxyethylene (32) monostearate
CAS registry number (s)	: 9004-99-3 (generic)
CIR review(s)	: J Am Coll Toxicol 1983;2:17-34 (access: www.cir-safety.org/ingredients)
Function(s) in cosmetics	: EU: emulsifying; surfactant. USA: surfactants – cleansing agents; surfactants – solubilizing agents
Patch testing	: 20% pet. (3)

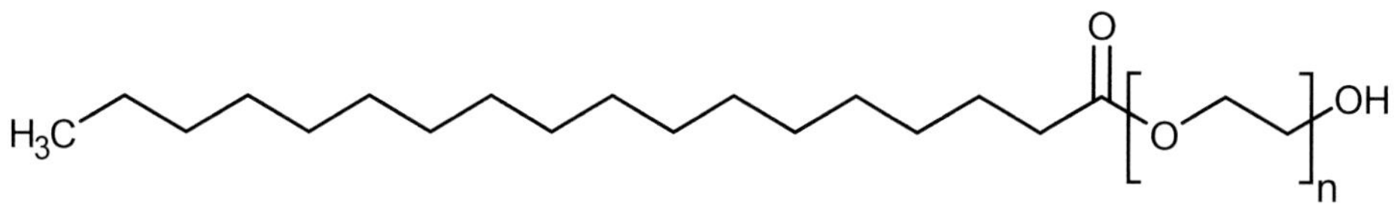

CONTACT ALLERGY

Case reports and case series

In a group of 119 patients with allergic contact dermatitis from cosmetics, investigated in The Netherlands in 1986-1987, one case was caused by PEG-32 stearate in a skin care product (1,2).

Presence in cosmetic products and chemical analyses

In the USA, in April 2017, PEG-32 stearate was present in 50 of 56,714 cosmetic products of which the composition is known in FDA's Voluntary Cosmetic Registration Program (VCRP) (data obtained from FDA, May 2017). In March 2017, PEG-32 stearate was present in 8 older products of 65,431 cosmetic products of which the composition is known in EWG's Skin Deep Cosmetics Database, USA (http://www.ewg.org/skindeep/).

LITERATURE

1   De Groot AC, Bruynzeel DP, Bos JD, van der Meeren HL, van Joost T, Jagtman BA, Weyland JW. The allergens in c cosmetics. Arch Dermatol 1988;124:1525-1529
2   De Groot AC. Adverse reactions to cosmetics. PhD Thesis, University of Groningen, The Netherlands: 1988, chapter 3.4, pp.105-113
3   De Groot AC. Patch Testing, 3rd Edition. Wapserveen, The Netherlands: acdegroot publishing, 2008 (ISBN 978-90-813233-1-4)

2.346 PEG-40 SORBITAN LANOLATE

IDENTIFICATION

Description/definition	: PEG-40 sorbitan lanolate is an ethoxylated sorbitan derivative of lanolin acid with an average of 40 moles of ethylene oxide
Chemical class(es)	: Lanolin and lanolin derivatives; sorbitan derivatives
Chemical/IUPAC name	: Sorbitan, ethoxylated, esters with lanolin fatty acids (40 mol EO average molar ratio)
Other names	: Polyethylene glycol 2000 sorbitan lanolate; polyoxyethylene (40) sorbitol lanolate; Atlas® G 1441
CAS registry number (s)	: 8036-77-9
CIR review(s)	: Int J Toxicol 2000;19(Suppl.2):43-89; Final report, June 2015 (access: www.cir-safety.org/ingredients)
Function(s) in cosmetics	: EU: emulsifying. USA: surfactants - cleansing agents; surfactants – solubilising agents
Patch testing	: 20% pet.

CONTACT ALLERGY

Patch testing in groups of patients

Routine testing

In Finland, in 1975, 1132 consecutive patients suspected of contact dermatitis were patch tested with PEG-40 sorbitan lanolate (routine testing) and 5 (0.4%) had a positive patch test. The relevance of these reactions was not mentioned (2).

Testing in groups of selected patients

In the period 1972 to 1974, in Finland, a group of 412 selected patients was patch tested with PEG-40 sorbitan lanolate 20% pet. and 2 (0.5%) had a positive patch test reaction. The mode of selecting the patients was not mentioned and neither was the relevance of the two positive reactions (3). In Switzerland, before 1994, 47 patients with chronic or recurrent (> 1 year) inflammatory skin diseases, using or having used topical preparations, were tested with a battery of emulsifiers; PEG-40 sorbitan lanolate 20% pet. was tested in 31 of these patients. Among the 47 patients, 23 had chronic leg ulcers, 15 had contact dermatitis, 1 had nummular eczema, 6 had psoriasis and 2 had atopic dermatitis. There were two positive reactions to PEG-40 sorbitan lanolate. Relevance for these reactions was not found (4).

Case reports and case series

A man had a 4-month history of dermatitis of the forehead after using a styling gel for 1 month. Patch tests with the GIRDCA standard series, a rubber series, the lining of his crash helmet and his own cosmetics were positive to the hair gel, tested as is, at D2 and D3. Additional patch testing with textile, preservative and emulsifier series was positive to Atlas G 1441 (PEG-40 sorbitan lanolate) 20% pet. at D2 and D3. Ceasing the use of the styling gel rapidly improved the dermatitis. Enquiry of the manufacturer of the styling gel revealed that it indeed contained PEG-40 sorbitan lanolate. Patch tests with PEG-40 sorbitan lanolate 20% pet. in 50 healthy volunteers were negative (1).

Presence in cosmetic products and chemical analyses

In the USA, in April 2017, PEG-40 sorbitan lanolate was present in zero of 56,714 cosmetic products of which the composition is known in FDA's Voluntary Cosmetic Registration Program (VCRP) (data obtained from FDA, May 2017). In April 2017, PEG-40 sorbitan lanolate was present in zero of 64,485 cosmetic products of which the composition is known in EWG's Skin Deep Cosmetics Database, USA (http://www.ewg.org/skindeep/).

LITERATURE

1   Pazzagelia M, Vincenzi C, Spiller M, Tosti A. Contact sensitivity to Atlas G-1441. Contact Dermatitis 1995;33:208
2   Hannuksela M, Kousa M, Pirilä V. Contact sensitivity to emulsifiers. Contact Dermatitis 1976;2:201-204
3   Hannuksela M, Kousa M, Pirilä V. Allergy to ingredients of vehicles. Contact Dermatitis 1976;2:105-110
4   Pasche-Koo F, Piletta P-A, Hunziker N, Hauser C. High sensitization rate to emulsifiers in patients with chronic leg ulcers. Contact Dermatitis 1994;31:226-228

2.347 PENTAERYTHRITYL ROSINATE

IDENTIFICATION

Description/definition	: Pentaerythrityl rosinate is the ester of rosin acids derived from rosin (colophonium), with the polyol, pentaerythritol
Chemical class(es)	: Esters
Other names	: Resin acids and rosin acids, esters with pentaerythritol; pentaerythritol rosinate
CAS registry number (s)	: 8050-26-8
EC number(s)	: 232-479-9
CIR review(s)	: J Am Coll Toxicol 1994;13:395-399; Int J Toxicol 1998;17(Suppl.4):83-94 (access: www.cir-safety.org/ingredients)
Function(s) in cosmetics	: EU: film forming. USA: skin-conditioning agents – emollient; viscosity increasing agents – nonaqueous
Patch testing	: 5% pet. (2)

CONTACT ALLERGY

Case reports and case series
A woman developed erythema, papules and swelling on her lips two days after she started to use a new lipstick. Patch tests with the standard series of the Japanese Society for Contact Dermatitis and the lipstick, tested 'as is', gave a positive reaction to the lipstick only at D2 and D3. Later the patient was patch tested with the ingredients and she now reacted to pentaerythrityl rosinate 0.1% pet, 0.5% pet, 1% pet. and 5% pet. The cheilitis healed quickly under treatment with corticosteroid ointment. She has remained free of symptoms since using lipsticks without pentaerythrityl rosinate. The patient was also tested with 'related chemicals', but there were no reactions to abietic acid, colophonium or glyceryl rosinate (2). A Japanese woman also had allergic contact cheilitis from pentaerythrityl rosinate (and isopalmityl diglyceryl sebacate) in lipsticks. Details are unknown (article not read, in Japanese) (1).

Cross-reactions, pseudo-cross-reactions and co-reactions
Patients may (3) or may not (2) cross-react to unmodified colophonium in the European baseline series. Glyceryl rosinate (3).

Presence in cosmetic products and chemical analyses
In the USA, in April 2017, pentaerythrityl rosinate was present in 2 of 56,714 cosmetic products of which the composition is known in FDA's Voluntary Cosmetic Registration Program (VCRP) (data obtained from FDA, May 2017). In April 2017, pentaerythrityl rosinate was present in 10 of 66,485 cosmetic products of which the composition is known in EWG's Skin Deep Cosmetics Database, USA (http://www.ewg.org/skindeep/).

LITERATURE
1 Adachi A, Yamada Y. Allergic contact cheilitis due to isopalmityl diglyceryl sebacate and pentaerythritol rosinate in the lipsticks. Environ Dermatol 2003;10:70-74 (in Japanese)
2 Ichihashi K, Soga F, Katoh N, Kishimoto S. Allergic contact cheilitis from pentaerythritol rosinate in a lipstick. Contact Dermatitis 2003;49:213
3 Inoue A, Shoji A, Aso S. Allergic lipstick cheilitis due to ester gum and ricinoleic acid. Contact Dermatitis 1998;39:39

2.348 PENTAERYTHRITYL TETRACAPRYLATE/TETRACAPRATE

IDENTIFICATION

Description/definition	: Pentaerythrityl tetracaprylate/tetracaprate is the tetraester of pentaerythritol and a blend of caprylic and capric acids
Chemical class(es)	: Esters
Chemical/IUPAC name	: 2,2-Bis(hydroxymethyl)propane-1,3-diol;decanoic acid;octanoic acid
Other names	: Decanoic acid, mixed esters with octanoic acid and pentaerythritol; pentaerythrityl tetracaprylate/caprate
CAS registry number (s)	: 68441-68-9
EC number(s)	: 270-472-2
Function(s) in cosmetics	: EU: emollient. USA: skin-conditioning agents - occlusive; viscosity increasing agents – nonaqueous
Patch testing	: 5% pet.
Molecular formula	: $C_{23}H_{48}O_8$

CONTACT ALLERGY

Case reports and case series

A woman developed dermatitis of the face after she had started using a new cosmetic night cream. After one overnight application, she developed a pruritic and erythematous papular eruption with marked edema. Later, the patient was patch tested with the North American Contact Dermatitis Group baseline series and her suspected personal product 'as is'. There was a dubiously positive reaction to the cream only. When patch tested with the 19 separate ingredients, she showed a positive reaction to pentaerythrityl tetracaprylate/tetracaprate 5% pet. Patch testing in 5 control subjects was negative (1). .

Presence in cosmetic products and chemical analyses

In July 2017, pentaerythrityl tetracaprylate/tetracaprate was present in 55 of 69,548 cosmetic products of which the composition is known in EWG's Skin Deep Cosmetics Database, USA (http://www.ewg.org/skindeep/).

LITERATURE

1   Al Ali A, Mireault J, Tremblay C, Sasseville D. Allergic contact dermatitis caused by pentaerythrityl tetracaprylate/tetracaprate. Contact Dermatitis 2017;77:58-59

2.349   PENTAERYTHRITYL TRIACRYLATE

IDENTIFICATION

Description/definition	: Pentaerythrityl triacrylate is the triester of pentaerythritol and acrylic acid
Chemical class(es)	: Esters
Chemical/IUPAC name	: [2-(Hydroxymethyl)-3-prop-2-enoyloxy-2-(prop-2-enoyloxymethyl)propyl] prop-2-enoate
Other names	: Pentaerythritol triacrylate
CAS registry number (s)	: 3524-68-3; 1245638-61-2
EC number(s)	: 222-540-8; 629-850-6
Function(s) in cosmetics	: EU: binding; film forming. USA: binders; film formers
Patch testing	: 0.1% pet. (SmartPracticeEurope, SmartPracticeCanada)
Molecular formula	: $C_{14}H_{18}O_7$

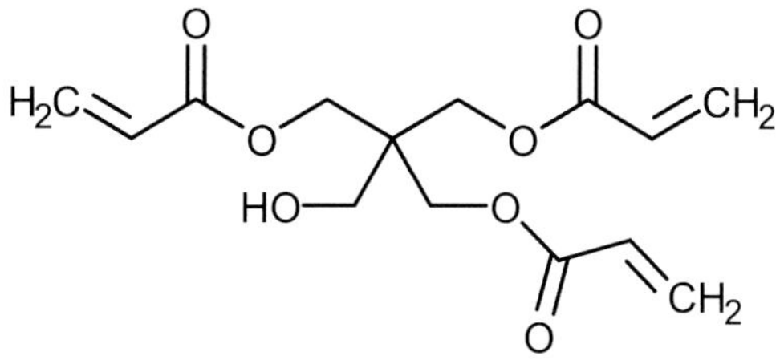

GENERAL

Discussion of contact allergy to (meth)acrylates *from non-cosmetic sources* is considered to fall outside the scope of this book. Therefore, only contact allergy from their presence in cosmetics is presented, which virtually always is from artificial nails. There are many reports of contact allergy to artificial nails, but the specific sensitizers have rarely been identified and – consequently - such publications are not presented in this and other acrylate and methacrylate monographs. Discussion is limited to publications in which the culprit (meth)acrylates have been identified, e.g., from information found in Material Data Safety Sheets, data obtained from the manufacturer or from chemical analyses.

Patients often react to many (meth)acrylates on patch testing. Primary sensitization to methacrylates may result in both methacrylate and acrylate cross-sensitization. Conversely, patients sensitized to acrylates are unlikely to show cross-sensitization to methacrylates (2).

General aspects of acrylates and methacrylates are presented in Chapter 2.219 HEMA (hydroxyethyl methacrylate). A discussion of general aspects of artificial nails, contact allergy to these products, the clinical picture of allergic contact dermatitis and other side effects of sculptured nails can also be found there. A very useful review of contact sensitization to allergens in nail cosmetics, with emphasis on acrylic manicures, was published in 2017 (3).

Case reports and case series

Pentaerythrityl triacrylate was stated to be the (or an) allergen in one patient in a group of 603 individuals suffering from cosmetic dermatitis, seen in the period 2010-2015 in Leuven, Belgium (1).

Presence in cosmetic products and chemical analyses

In the USA, in April 2017, pentaerythrityl triacrylate was present in zero of 56,714 cosmetic products of which the composition is known in FDA's Voluntary Cosmetic Registration Program (VCRP) (data obtained from FDA, May 2017). In March 2017, pentaerythrityl triacrylate was present in zero of 65,431 cosmetic products of which the composition is known in EWG's Skin Deep Cosmetics Database, USA (http://www.ewg.org/skindeep/).

LITERATURE

1   Goossens A. Cosmetic contact allergens. Cosmetics 2016, 3, 5; doi:10.3390/cosmetics3010005
2   Aalto-Korte K, Henriks-Eckerman M-L, Kuuliala O, Jolanki R. Occupational methacrylate and acrylate allergy – cross-reactions and possible screening allergens. Contact Dermatitis 2010;63:301-312
3   Chou M, Dhingra N, Strugar TL. Contact sensitization to allergens in nail cosmetics. Dermatitis 2017;28:231-240

2.350   PENTYL DIMETHYL PABA

IDENTIFICATION

Description/definition   : Pentyl dimethyl PABA is the ester of pentyl alcohol and dimethyl *p*-aminobenzoic acid,
                                          which conforms to the formula shown below
Chemical class(es)   : PABA derivatives
Chemical/IUPAC name   : Pentyl 4-(dimethylamino)benzoate
Other names   : Amyl dimethyl PABA; padimate A
CAS registry number (s)   : 14779-78-3
EC number(s)   : 238-849-6
Function(s) in cosmetics : EU: formerly used as UV-absorber; delisted in 1990. USA: light stabilizers
EU cosmetic restrictions : Regulated in Annex II/381 of the Regulation (EC) No. 1223/2009 (prohibited)
Patch testing   : 5% or 10% pet.
Molecular formula   : $C_{14}H_{21}NO_2$

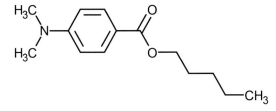

GENERAL

Pentyl dimethyl PABA is a UVB filter with UV absorbance maximum (λ_{max}) at 310 nm (22). The literature on adverse reactions to sunscreens has been reviewed in several recent and older publications (10,15-19,24). A review of photocontact allergy to sunscreens was published in 2010 (23). Because of phototoxicity issues (3), it is safe to assume that pentyl dimethyl PABA is hardly, if at all, used anymore in cosmetic products, and certainly not in the EU (prohibited) and the USA.

CONTACT ALLERGY

Patch testing in groups of patients

There have been no studies in which pentyl dimethyl PABA was tested in consecutive patients suspected of contact dermatitis (routine testing). Results of patch testing pentyl dimethyl PABA in groups of *selected* patients (e.g., patients suspected of photosensitivity, patients with dermatitis affecting mainly light-exposed skin) back to 1990 are shown in table 2.350.1. In 3 investigations, frequencies of sensitization were 0.1% (2), 1.4% (6) and 27% (5). The high percentage of 27 was seen in a very small group of 11 patients with a history of photosensitivity, of who 3 had a positive patch test. One of the 3 reactions (a combined contact/photocontact allergy) was considered to be relevant (5).

Table 2.350.1 Patch testing in groups of patients: Selected patient groups

Years and Country	Test conc. & vehicle	Number of patients tested	positive (%)	Selection of patients (S); Relevance (R); Comments (C)	Ref.
1983-1998 UK	2% or 10% pet.	2715	4 (0.1%)	S: patients suspected of photosensitivity or with (a history of) dermatitis at exposed sites; R: not stated	2
1986-1993 USA	5% pet. or 5% alc.	138	2 (1.4%)	S: patients suspected of photosensitivity; R: one reaction was described as 'clinically irrelevant irritant response'	6
1985-1990 USA	5% pet.	11	3 (27%)	S: patients with a history of photosensitivity; R: one with a combined contact/photocontact allergy was relevant	5

Case reports and case series

Pentyl dimethyl PABA was responsible for 2 out of 399 cases of cosmetic allergy where the causal allergen was identified in a study of the NACDG, USA, 1977-1983 (9). A young girl had allergic contact dermatitis of the face and conjunctivitis from allergy to pentyl dimethyl PABA in lip gloss cosmetic (12). A woman with polymorphic light eruption had aggravation of her skin eruption from contact allergy to pentyl dimethyl PABA in a sunscreen (20).

One more individual had contact allergy to pentyl dimethyl PABA in a sunscreen (21). One patient was presented as having allergic contact dermatitis from pentyl dimethyl PABA in a sunscreen; however, it was only *assumed* that pentyl dimethyl PABA was the culprit, it was not tested separately (13).

Cross-reactions, pseudo-cross-reactions and co-reactions
PABA (10); *not* to PABA (6).

Presence in cosmetic products and chemical analyses
In June 2017, pentyl dimethyl PABA was present in zero of 68,866 cosmetic products of which the composition is known in EWG's Skin Deep Cosmetics Database, USA (http://www.ewg.org/skindeep/). In the USA, in April 2017, pentyl dimethyl PABA was present in zero of 56,714 cosmetic products of which the composition is known in FDA's Voluntary Cosmetic Registration Program (VCRP) (data obtained from FDA, May 2017).

Minimal amounts of PABA and benzocaine were found as contaminants in most batches of pentyl dimethyl PABA (4).

OTHER SIDE EFFECTS

Photosensitivity

Photopatch testing in groups of patients
Results of photopatch testing pentyl dimethyl PABA in groups of selected patients (e.g., patients suspected of photosensitivity, patients with dermatitis affecting mainly light-exposed skin) back to 1985 are shown in table 2.350.2. In 4 investigations, the frequencies of photosensitization were <0.1% (2), 2.9% (1), 3.6% (6) and 18% (5). The high percentage of 18 was seen in a very small group of 11 patients with a history of photosensitivity, in which 2 patients had a positive photopatch test. One of these was considered to be relevant (5).

Table 2.350.2 Photopatch testing in groups of patients

Years and Country	Test conc. & vehicle	Number of patients tested | positive (%)		Selection of patients (S); Relevance (R); Comments (C)	Ref.
1983-1998 UK	2% or 10% pet.	2715	2 (<0.1%)	S: patients suspected of photosensitivity or with (a history of) dermatitis at exposed sites; R: 37% for all photoallergens together	2
1986-1993 USA	5% pet. or 5% alc.	138	5 (3.6%)	S: patients suspected of photosensitivity; R: 3 of 5 reactions were described as 'clinically irrelevant irritant responses'	6
1985-1990 USA	5% pet.	11	2 (18%)	S: patients with a history of photosensitivity; R: both reactions were relevant	5
1980-1985 USA	5% pet.	70	2 (2.9%)	S: not stated; R: not stated	1

Case reports and case series
One patient had photoallergic contact dermatitis from pentyl dimethyl PABA in a sunscreen (21).

Phototoxicity
Twelve of 17 (70%) normal individuals showed phototoxic reactions to pentyl dimethyl PABA 5% in alcohol and an equal percentage to a sunscreen containing pentyl dimethyl PABA (3). Three of nine healthy subjects complained of a burning sensation and developed an immediate bright erythema 30 minutes after application of Blockout, a sunscreen containing 2.5% pentyl dimethyl PABA and 65% alcohol, and exposure to the sun (7). However, testing with a different batch of the sunscreen could not reproduce the symptoms in two of the test subjects (11).

Phototoxicity in four workers manufacturing UV-cured inks was caused by a mixture of pentyl dimethyl PABA (amyl dimethyl *p*-aminobenzoate) and amyl dimethyl *o*-aminobenzoate (14).

Irritant contact dermatitis
Test preparations with 2.5% and 5% pentyl dimethyl PABA have induced burning and irritation of the face in warm weather (8).

LITERATURE

1   Menz J, Muller SA, Connnolly SM. Photopatch testing: A six year experience. J Am Acad Dermatol 1988;18:1044-1047
2   Darvay A, White I, Rycroft R, Jones AB, Hawk JL, McFadden JP. Photoallergic contact dermatitis is uncommon. Br J Dermatol 2001;145:597-601
3   Kaidbey KH, Kligman AM. Phototoxicity to a sunscreen ingredient. Padimate A. Arch Dermatol 1978;114:547-549
4   Bruze M, Fregert S, Gruvberger B. Occurrence of *para*-aminobenzoic acid and benzocaine as contaminants in sunscreen agents of *para*-aminobenzoic acid type. Photodermatology 1984;1:277-285

5 DeLeo VA, Suarez SM, Maso MJ. Photoallergic contact dermatitis. Results of photopatch testing in New York, 1985 to 1990. Arch Dermatol 1992;128:1513-1518

6 Fotiades J, Soter NA, Lim HW. Results of evaluation of 203 patients for photosensitivity in a 7.3 year period. J Am Acad Dermatol 1995;33:597-602

7 Katz SI. Relative effectiveness of selected sunscreens. Arch Derm 1970;101:466-468

8 Willis I, Kligman AM. Aminobenzoic acid and its esters. The quest for more effective sunscreens. Arch Derm 1970;102:405-417

9 Adams RM, Maibach HI, Clendenning WE, Fisher AA, Jordan WJ, Kanof N, et al. A five-year study of cosmetic reactions. J Am Acad Dermatol 1985;13:1062-1069

10 Dromgoole SH, Maibach HI. Sunscreening agent intolerance: Contact and photocontact sensitization and contact urticaria. J Am Acad Dermatol 1990;22:1068-1078

11 Blank H. Immediate cutaneous reactions to sunscreens. Arch Dermatol 1971;103:461

12 Calnan CD. Amyldimethylamino benzoic acid causing lipstick dermatitis. Contact Dermatitis 1980;6:233

13 Thompson G, Maibach H, Epstein J. Allergic contact dermatitis from sunscreen preparations complicating photodermatitis. Arch Dermatol 1977;113:1252-1253

14 Emmett EA, Taphorn BR, Kaminsky JR. Phototoxicity occurring during the manufacture of ultraviolet-cured ink. Arch Dermatol 1977;113:770-775

15 Heurung AR, Raju SI, Warshaw EM. Adverse reactions to sunscreen agents: epidemiology, responsible irritants and allergens, clinical characteristics, and management. Dermatitis 2014;25:289-326

16 Heurung AR, Raju SI, Warshaw EM. Contact allergen of the year. Benzophenones. Dermatitis 2014;25:3-10 (contains many mistakes; Erratum in Dermatitis 2014;25:92-95)

17 Avenel-Audran M. Sunscreen products: finding the allergen. Eur J Dermatol 2010;20:161-166

18 Scheuer E, Warshaw E. Sunscreen allergy: a review of epidemiology, clinical characteristics, and responsible allergens. Dermatitis 2006;17:3-11

19 Funk JO, Dromgoole SH, Maibach HI. Sunscreen intolerance: contact sensitization, photocontact sensitization, and irritancy of sunscreen agents. Dermatol Clin 1995;13:473-481

20 Cronin E. Contact Dermatitis. Edinburgh: Churchill Livingstone, 1980: 452

21 Thune P. Contact and photocontact allergy to sunscreens. Photodermatol 1984;1:5-9

22 Shaath NA. Ultraviolet filters. Photochem Photobiol Sci 2010;9:464-469

23 Shaw T, Simpson B, Wilson B, Oostman H, Rainey D, Storrs F. True photoallergy to sunscreens is rare despite popular belief. Dermatitis 2010;21:185-198

24 Schauder S. Survey of the literature on adverse reactions to preparations containing UV filters (1947-1989) (Literaturübersicht über Unverträglichkeitsreaktionen auf lichtfilterhaltige Produkte von 1947 bis 1989). Z Hautkr 1990;65:982-998 (article in German)

2.351   PENTYLENE GLYCOL

IDENTIFICATION

Description/definition	: Pentylene glycol is the organic compound that conforms to the formula shown below
Chemical class(es)	: Alcohols
Chemical/IUPAC name	: Pentane-1,5-diol
Other names	: 1,2-Dihydroxypentane
CAS registry number (s)	: 5343-92-0
EC number(s)	: 226-285-3
CIR review(s)	: Int J Toxicol 2012;31(Suppl.2):147-168 (access: www.cir-safety.org/ingredients)
Function(s) in cosmetics	: EU: skin conditioning; solvent. USA: preservatives; skin-conditioning agents – miscellaneous; solvents
Patch testing	: 0.5% and 5% water (1); 0.5%-5% and 10% water (2); 5% and 10% pet. (3, 10 controls were negative); 2% pet (4); 2% and 5% pet., 5% water (7)
Molecular formula	: $C_5H_{12}O_2$

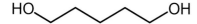

GENERAL

Pentylene glycol is a skin-conditioning agent, solvent and excellent humectant; it also has antimicrobial effects (1). In industry, it serves as a plasticizer, emulsifying agent, solvent, preservative, and initial product for chemicals (4).

CONTACT ALLERGY

Case reports and case series

Pentylene glycol was stated to be the (or an) allergen in 2 patients in a group of 603 individuals suffering from cosmetic dermatitis, seen in the period 2010-2015 in Leuven, Belgium (6). Single case reports have described allergic contact dermatitis from hexylene glycol present in a moisturizing cream (2), a facial cream (1), a prescription moisturizer (3), a hypoallergenic cream (4) and a facial cream and body lotion (5).

Contact allergy to pentylene glycol in non-cosmetic products

A man had ACD from pentylene glycol in a cream containing piroctone olamine and various anti-inflammatory agents to treat seborrheic dermatitis (7).

Cross-reactions, pseudo-cross-reactions and co-reactions

Not to propylene glycol (1,2,3). Not to 1,3-butylene glycol, 1,2-propylene glycol, and 1,5-hexylene glycol (4). Co-reactivity to propylene glycol (5,7). Not to butylene glycol (7).

Presence in cosmetic products and chemical analyses

In the USA, in April 2017, pentylene glycol was present in 1641 of 56,714 cosmetic products of which the composition is known in FDA's Voluntary Cosmetic Registration Program (VCRP) (data obtained from FDA, May 2017). In April 2017, pentylene glycol was present in 473 of 66,485 cosmetic products of which the composition is known in EWG's Skin Deep Cosmetics Database, USA (http://www.ewg.org/skindeep/).

LITERATURE

1   Mortz CG, Otkjær A, Andersen KE. Allergic contact dermatitis to ethylhexylglycerin and pentylene glycol. Contact Dermatitis 2009;61:180
2   Gallo R, Viglizzo G, Vecchio F, Parodi A. Allergic contact dermatitis from pentylene glycol in an emollient cream, with possible co-sensitization to resveratrol. Contact Dermatitis 2003;48:176-177
3   Amado A, Taylor JS, Murray DA, Reynolds JS. Contact dermatitis to pentylene glycol in a prescription cream for atopic dermatitis: case report. Arch Dermatol 2008;144:810-812
4   Hausen BM. Contact allergy to pentylene glycol. Dermatitis 2007;18:99-100
5   Kerre S. Allergic contact dermatitis to pentylene glycol in a cosmetic cream Contact Dermatitis 2008;58:122-123
6   Goossens A. Cosmetic contact allergens. Cosmetics 2016, 3, 5; doi:10.3390/cosmetics3010005
7   Foti C, Bonamonte D, Cassano N, Conserva A, Vena GA. Allergic contact dermatitis to propyl gallate and pentylene glycol in an emollient cream. Australas J Dermatol 2010;51:147-148

2.352 PENTYL RHAMNOSIDE

IDENTIFICATION

Description/definition : Pentyl rhamnoside is the product obtained by the reaction of pentanol with rhamnose that conforms generally to the formula shown below
Chemical class(es) : Carbohydrates; ethers
Chemical/IUPAC name : L-Mannopyranoside, pentyl 6-deoxy-
Other names : Alkyl rhamnoside-C5
CAS registry number (s) : 494844-53-0
Function(s) in cosmetics : EU: skin conditioner. USA: skin-conditioning agents - miscellaneous
Patch testing : 1% water (1); this concentration may be too low
Molecular formula : $C_{11}H_{22}O_5$

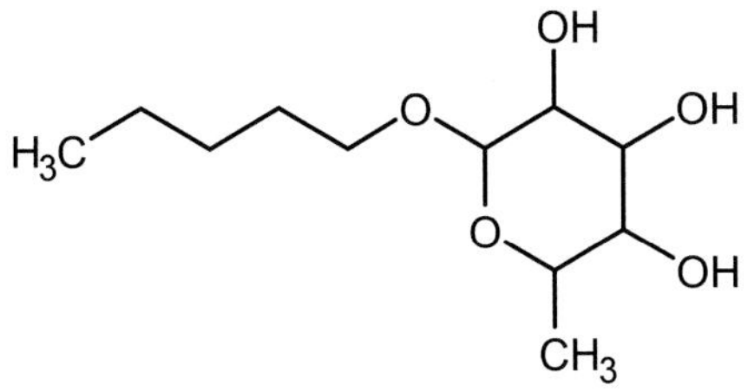

GENERAL

Pentyl rhamnoside belongs to the group of alkyl polysaccharides and is synthesized from l-rhamnose, an important natural sugar. Pentyl rhamnoside is water soluble and used as a co-surfactant for micro-emulsions. Compositions of liquid soaps and moisturizers with pentyl rhamnoside have been well tolerated in use tests (2).

CONTACT ALLERGY

Case reports and case series

A woman had suffered from atopic dermatitis for 6 years. In the previous 2 months she had noticed progressive worsening of the dermatitis on her face, neck, and chest, for which she was hospitalized and treated with systemic and topical corticosteroids. Patch tests with the baseline series of the German Contact Dermatitis Group, additional preservatives and cosmetic allergens, corticosteroids and her own topical preparations gave a strong positive patch test reaction to a moisturizing cream, tested as is. A repeated open application test (ROAT) performed twice daily on the forearm with the cosmetic product was strongly positive on the 7th day showing pruritic papules and vesicles. Later, the 19 ingredients of the product, provided by the manufacturer, were tested and the patient reacted to alkyl rhamnoside-C5 (pentyl rhamnoside) 1% in water. Five controls were negative to this material. At a follow-up visit after 4 weeks the dermatitis on the face, neck, and chest had nearly cleared with intermittent use of a topical corticosteroid and an emollient preparation (1).

Presence in cosmetic products and chemical analyses

In the USA, in April 2017, pentyl rhamnoside was present in zero of 56,714 cosmetic products of which the composition is known in FDA's Voluntary Cosmetic Registration Program (VCRP) (data obtained from FDA, May 2017). In March 2017, pentyl rhamnoside was present in zero of 65,431 cosmetic products of which the composition is known in EWG's Skin Deep Cosmetics Database, USA (http://www.ewg.org/skindeep/).

LITERATURE

1 Kügler K, Mydlach B, Frosch PJ. Contact allergy from alkyl rhamnoside-C5. Contact Dermatitis 2009;61:352-353
2 Houlmont J P, Vercruysse K, Perez E, Rico-Lattes I, Bordat P, Treilhou M. Cosmetic use formulations containing pentyl rhamnoside and cetyl rhamnoside. Intern J Cosmet Sci 2001;23:363-368

2.353 PERSEA GRATISSIMA (AVOCADO) OIL

IDENTIFICATION

Description/definition   : Persea gratissima oil is the fixed oil obtained by pressing the dehydrated sliced flesh of the avocado pear, *Persea gratissima*, Lauraceae. It consists principally of the glycerides of fatty acids

Chemical class(es)   : Fats and oils

INCI name USA   : Persea gratissima (avocado) fruit oil

Other names   : Avocado oil

CAS registry number (s)   : 8024-32-6

EC number(s)   : 232-428-0

CIR review(s)   : J Environ Pathol Toxicol 1980;4:93-103; Int J Toxicol 2003;22(Suppl.1):1-35; Final report, March 2011 (access: www.cir-safety.org/ingredients)

Function(s) in cosmetics : EU: skin conditioning. USA: skin-conditioning agents - occlusive

Patch testing   : pure (1); 30% pet. (6)

CONTACT ALLERGY

Case reports and case series

In a group of 119 patients with allergic contact dermatitis from cosmetics, investigated in The Netherlands in 1986-1987, one case was caused by avocado oil in a sunscreen cream (3,4). One patient had allergic contact dermatitis from avocado oil in a sunscreen product (1, the same patient as in refs. 3 and 4).

Contact allergy to avocado oil in non-cosmetic products

One patient developed a maculopapular rash from to amoxicillin. She had leg ulcers and had taken capsules containing avocado oil for many years. The patient had a positive reaction to a patch test with avocado oil 30% pet. She denied food allergy to avocado. A prick test with avocado was negative. The capsules were orally well tolerated, indicating that the positive patch test had no present relevance to the maculopapular rash. However, the patient had polysensitization to topical drugs used to treat her leg ulcers and she had previously developed contact allergy to and allergic contact dermatitis from an ointment containing avocado oil (2).

Presence in cosmetic products and chemical analyses

In February 2017, Persea gratissima oil was present in 1422 (avocado oil) and 133 (avocado fruit oil) products of 64,631 cosmetic products of which the composition is known in EWG's Skin Deep Cosmetics Database, USA (http://www.ewg.org/skindeep/).

Other information

Twenty-two patients known to be allergic to German chamomile were patch tested with a number of topical herbal pharmaceuticals and cosmetics containing chamomile; in addition, seven individuals, who were known to be allergic to Arnica, were tested with Arnica-containing products . Some who had one or more positive reactions were subsequently tested with the ingredients of the incriminated product(s). One chamomile-allergic patient reacted to Melissa day cream and its ingredient 'avocado oil' and one Arnica-sensitive patient to Melissa day cream and (amongst others) to its ingredient 'avocado oil'; probably, they had never used this product (5).

LITERATURE

1   De Groot AC, van der Meeren HLM, Weyland JW. Contact allergy to avocado oil in a sunscreen. Contact Dermatitis 1987;16:108-109

2   Barbaud A, Trechot P, Reichert-Penetrat S, Commun N, Schmutz JL. Relevance of skin tests with drugs in investigating cutaneous adverse drug reactions. Contact Dermatitis 2001;45:265-268

3   De Groot AC, Bruynzeel DP, Bos JD, van der Meeren HL, van Joost T, Jagtman BA, Weyland JW. The allergens in cosmetics. Arch Dermatol 1988;124:1525-1529

4   De Groot AC. Adverse reactions to cosmetics. PhD Thesis, University of Groningen, The Netherlands: 1988, chapter 3.4, pp.105-113

5   Paulsen E, Christensen LP, Andersen KA. Cosmetics and herbal remedies with Compositae plant extracts – are they tolerated by Compositae-allergic patients? Contact Dermatitis 2008;58:15-23

2.354 PETROLATUM

IDENTIFICATION

Description/definition : Petrolatum is a complex combination of hydrocarbons obtained as a semi-solid from dewaxing paraffinic residual oil. It consists predominantly of saturated crystalline and liquid hydrocarbons having carbon numbers predominantly greater than C25

Chemical class(es) : Hydrocarbons

Other names : Mineral wax; mineral fat; Vaseline®; petroleum jelly; paraffin jelly; white petrolatum; yellow petrolatum

CAS registry number (s) : 8009-03-8

EC number(s) : 232-373-2

Merck Index monograph : 8570

Function(s) in cosmetics : EU: antistatic; emollient. USA: hair conditioning agents; skin protectants; skin-conditioning agents - occlusive

EU cosmetic restrictions : Regulated in Annex II/903 of the Regulation (EC) No. 1223/2009 (prohibited, except if the full refining history is known and it can be shown that the substance from which it is produced is not a carcinogen)

Patch testing : 100% (Chemotechnique, SmartPracticeEurope, SmartPracticeCanada)

GENERAL

Four types of petrolatum can be distinguished: natural, artificial, Gatsch and synthetic, the first three being based on natural petroleum. 'Natural' petrolatum is obtained from petroleum distillation residues or from storage tank sediments containing crude petroleum. 'Artificial' petrolatum is a blend of natural hydrocarbon wax (paraffin wax or other solid hydrocarbons) with paraffin oil. 'Gatsch' or 'slack wax' petrolatum is obtained from the by-products of petroleum distillates used for the production of lubricating oil, and is blended with paraffin oil to obtain the desired consistency, melting point, viscosity, etc. Synthetic petrolatum is made from synthetic hydrocarbons obtained by co-hydrogenation or by catalytic polymerization of ethylene (6). All naturally derived petrolatums are purified by one or a combination of several processes such as treatment with sulfuric acid followed by neutralization with sodium hydroxide; filtration through bleaching earth, charcoal, silica gel, or aluminum silicate; selective solvent extraction or catalytic hydrogenation (6; cited data are 35 years old; not verified if they are currently still accurate). Natural petrolatum is a biological product, the chemical composition of which may vary greatly.

The INCI name petrolatum indicates both yellow and white petrolatum. The only difference is that, in the case of white petrolatum, the purification process is extended until practically all of the yellow color has been removed (9). In view of the differences in sensitizing properties and other toxicological properties between yellow and white petrolatum, only highly purified petrolatum, with the (carcinogenic) aromatic fraction eliminated, should be used, as regulated by national and international pharmacopoeias (22). White petrolatum is used as ointment base in pharmaceuticals and cosmetics and as vehicle for most patch test allergens. Yellow petrolatum may still be used in lubricating machinery, leather grease, shoe polish, rust preventives and modelling clays (22).

Contact allergy to petrolatum occurs very infrequently and is sometimes discovered by positive patch tests to all or most chemicals tested in petrolatum (9,20,23,28,30). Cosmetic allergic contact dermatitis from petrolatum is extremely rare. Most cases of petrolatum allergy are caused by application of the material to damaged skin in topical pharmaceuticals, notably for the treatment of leg ulcers and stasis dermatitis (6,8,9,13,27). The more highly purified white petrolatum appears to be less allergenic than the yellow variety, although some patients both react to yellow and to white petrolatum (8,10,20,35).

CONTACT ALLERGY

Patch testing in groups of patients

Results of patch testing petrolatum in consecutive patients suspected of contact dermatitis (routine testing) and in groups of *selected* patients (e.g., patients suspected of photosensitivity and individuals tested with a topical medicament series) are shown in table 2.354.1. In two studies in which petrolatum was used in routine testing, frequencies of sensitization were extremely low: 0% in a group of 1730 patients tested (6) and 0.03% in a population of 79,365 consecutive patients suspected of contact dermatitis (22). In 3 studies testing selected patient groups, rates were 0.6% (17), 1.2% (1) and 1.3% (37), but the few positive reactions (n=1-3) were either not relevant or their relevance was not mentioned. In addition, in the case of contact allergy to petrolatum, one might have expected many more positive reactions to other haptens patch tested in petrolatum, which was not mentioned as such and therefore most likely did not occur (1,17,37). Therefore, it may be doubted whether these reactions really indicated contact sensitization to petrolatum.

Table 2.354.1 Patch testing in groups of patients

Years and Country	Test conc. & vehicle	Number of patients tested | positive (%)		Selection of patients (S); Relevance (R); Comments (C)	Ref.
Routine testing					
1992-2004 IVDK	pure	79,365	29 (0.03%)	R: none; most + reactions were considered to be irritant; C: of the two +++ reactions, one was negative on retesting (excited skin syndrome) and the other did not react to many other test materials containing exactly the same white petrolatum	22
1979-1981 Belgium	probably pure	1730	0	R: not applicable	6
Testing in groups of selected patients					
2001-2010 Canada	not stated	160	2 (1.2%)	S: patients with suspected photosensitivity and patients who developed pruritus or a rash after sunscreen application; R: not stated; C: weak study: inadequate reading of test results, erythema only was considered to represent a positive patch test reaction	1
2000-2005 USA	pure	178	1 (0.6%)	S: patients photopatch tested for suspected photodermatitis; R: the reaction was not relevant	17
<1955 USA	pure	240	3 (1.3%)	S: patients tested with a topical medicaments series; R: not stated; C: it can be doubted whether these reactions were really allergic, since no mention was made of concurrent reactions to other haptens in petrolatum	37

Case reports and case series

One patient had contact allergy to white soft petrolatum present in a moisturizing cream (3). In a 4-month-period in 1996, 475 patients with contact allergy to 'cosmetic ingredients' were collected in 5 centers in Belgium, UK and Germany. There was one reaction to petrolatum; relevance was not stated (12).

Contact allergy to petrolatum in non-cosmetic products

Causative products known

One patient had an allergic reaction to petrolatum which he used to groom his hair (7). A woman reacted to white and yellow petrolatum from their presence in topical pharmaceuticals used to treat venous ulcers (8). A patient was sensitized to yellow petrolatum used to treat his psoriasis; he also proved allergic to white petrolatum (10). Six patients had allergic contact dermatitis from vaselinum album (white petrolatum) in a topical pharmaceutical product for leg ulcers and thrombophlebitis; however, they did not react to vaselinum flavum (yellow petrolatum, which is less purified). It was suggested that the allergy was caused by chemicals used to bleach the petrolatum (13). A woman was patch tested because of stasis dermatitis with expansion to the arms and trunk. She reacted to all test substances in white petrolatum. Later, she was tested with both white and yellow petrolatum and reacted to both. She had previously used pure petrolatum on her skin, but did not do so anymore because of itching (20). Another female patient had allergic contact dermatitis of the left upper eyelid from white petrolatum in a corticosteroid ointment and other topical pharmaceuticals used to treat seborrheic dermatitis (27).

Causative products unknown

A woman with eczema reacted upon patch testing to all haptens in white petrolatum, but not to those in water or propylene glycol. Later, patch testing with 8 brands of white petrolatum gave positive reactions to 4 of these (30). A patient reacted to both white and yellow petrolatum (35, detail unknown, article not read). A woman suffering from long-standing atopic dermatitis reacted to 69 of 70 petrolatum-based patch test materials, but not to haptens in water. Later patch tests with white petrolatum were positive (28). Another female individual was patch tested with a number of commercial drugs in petrolatum, made by the hospital pharmacy, for the investigation of cutaneous adverse drug reactions. She had positive patch test reactions to 9 of 11 test materials. Later, she reacted to the petrolatum used and some other brands of petrolatum, but not to those used by the suppliers of patch test materials. The primary source of sensitization was not mentioned (23).

One patient had contact allergy to yellow, but not to white petrolatum (details unknown, article not read [18]). Three leg ulcer patients had ACD from the application of yellow petrolatum, but not of white petrolatum (6). When tested later with a large number of white and yellow petrolatums, one reacted to a few white petrolatums and extracts and another to a number of extracts of white petrolatums (one patient was not tested with the extracts) (6). A patient who developed dermatitis of the leg after orthopedic treatment had a positive patch test on 2 occasions to white petrolatum; the relevance of this reaction was not mentioned, probably not found (4). Two patients tested with a leg ulcer series reacted to yellow petrolatum used as vehicle for patch test materials; they did not react to white petrolatum (9).

Cross-reactions, pseudo-cross-reactions and co-reactions
Two patients allergic to yellow petrolatum were further patch tested with white soft paraffins and related products such as liquid paraffin, ozokerite, ceresin, and hard paraffin, with negative results (9). Patients (tested with both types of petrolatum) may be allergic to only white petrolatum (13), to only yellow petrolatum (6,9,18) or to both (8,10,20,35).

Presence in cosmetic products and chemical analyses
In July 2017, petrolatum was present in 1059 (petrolatum) and 34 (white petrolatum) of 69,751 cosmetic products of which the composition is known in EWG's Skin Deep Cosmetics Database, USA (http://www.ewg.org/skindeep/). In the USA, in April 2017, petrolatum was present in 3579 of 56,714 cosmetic products of which the composition is known in FDA's Voluntary Cosmetic Registration Program (VCRP) (data obtained from FDA, May 2017).

Other information
In South Africa, 'vaselien-dermatitis' has long been recognized and is very common among dark-skinned people who use petrolatum as a cosmetic, which reflects a cultural bias not observed in the white population (24,25). Some authors considered this to be a form of photosensitivity, but this has not been proven (25) (details unknown, articles 24 and 25 not read).

In an early study from Poland, white and yellow petrolatums were found to be among the most frequent offenders in a study of 355 patients suffering from leg eczema, occupational dermatoses, or prurigo (26; data cited in ref. 6, details unknown, article not read).

OTHER SIDE EFFECTS

Photosensitivity
Results of photopatch testing with petrolatum are shown in table 2.354.2. In three studies, frequencies of positive photo-patch tests were 0.2% (2), 0.6% (1) and 1.1% (17). In two, their relevance was not mentioned or specified, in the third study, one of 2 reactions was considered to be relevant, but the culprit product was not mentioned (17). It may be doubted whether these patients really had photocontact allergy to petrolatum. In such cases, one might have expected many more photocontact reactions to other haptens patch tested in petrolatum, which was not mentioned as such and therefore most likely did not occur (1,17,37).

Table 2.354.2 Photopatch testing in groups of patients

Years and Country	Test conc. & vehicle	Number of patients tested	positive (%)	Selection of patients (S); Relevance (R); Comments (C)	Ref.
2008-2011 12 European countries	10% pet.	1031	2 (0.2%)	S: patients with exposed site dermatitis or history of a reaction to a sunscreen or topical NSAID; R: 44% current and 11% past relevance for all photoallergens together	2
2001-2010 Canada	not stated	160	1 (0.6%)	S: patients with suspected photosensitivity and patients who developed pruritus or a rash after sunscreen application; R: not stated; C: weak study: inadequate reading of test results, erythema only was considered to represent a positive patch test reaction	1
2000-2005 USA	pure	178	2 (1.1%)	S: patients photopatch tested for suspected photodermatitis; R: one reaction was relevant	17

Immediate-type reactions
A woman with hand eczema had positive patch tests at D2 and D4 to many but not all petrolatum-based materials. The clinical picture was a mixture of urticaria and dermatitis. Repeat patch testing gave the same result. An open test with 'petrolatum' gave an urticarial reaction after 15-30 minutes on 2 occasions. It was suggested that the urticaria remained for 2 and 4 days, but the mechanism was unexplained. It was not mentioned what clinical relevance the reaction had (29).

Other non-eczematous contact reactions
In older literature, petrolatum has been suspected of being comedogenic and causing 'pomade acne' (16). Pomade acne occurred characteristically in adult dark-skinned individuals who apply various grooming substances including petrolatum as part of their daily toilet. These are usually rubbed into the scalp; however, some also lubricate the face. The eruption occurs mainly on the forehead and temples. The pomade may be applied to these areas directly or usually it may drain down from the scalp. The distribution exactly corresponds to the areas of contact. The lesions are closely set, rather uniform, closed comedones with a strictly follicular localization. Expression of the contents with an acne extractor yields the firm, cheesy material so typical of comedones. Ordinarily, inflammation is not conspicuous; a scattering of pustules may be present (16). Previously, it had been reported that pomade acne, or 'vaselinoderma', as the authors called it, was so common in Kenya (East Africa) that they saw 41 cases in two years. This was invariably due to a widespread practice of treating the face of African children frequently, up to twice daily, with petroleum jelly (Vaseline) (33). Such cases represented 1% to 2% of dermatologic outpatients. In the great majority, lesions consisted only of open comedones, with minute inflammation. Almost all the patients were children between the ages of 1 and 12 years (34).

Acne-like eruptions from application of petrolatum and petrolatum-containing products have been described (14,15). The application of white petrolatum may have induced unilateral acne with comedones, papules and pustules in a young acne-prone woman attempting to relieve the effects of Bell's palsy by massaging the affected part of her face nightly for 15 minutes with the white petrolatum (31). However, subsequently, it was argued by others that an increased sebum excretion rate from nerve paresis in Bell's palsy rather than local application of petrolatum probably was the most important factor in the development of unilateral acne, as there is proof of acne developing unilaterally in patients with paraplegia and Bell's paralysis without application of petrolatum (32).

Miscellaneous side effects
Chronic dermatitis and hyperpigmentation of the face in a darkly pigmented man was caused by the use of petrolatum. After petrolatum was stopped and replaced with rose water, the dermatosis cleared completely. Patch and photopatch tests were negative. The mechanism of this side effect remained unclear, but when petrolatum was restarted, a recurrence of the dermatosis was noted within a week (11).

OTHER INFORMATION
The allergens in petrolatum in an earlier study were presumed to be polycyclic aromatic hydrocarbons, most probably phenanthrene derivatives with molecular weights of 230 and 244 (5,6). In a 2007 study, petrolatum was not found to be comedogenic in the rabbit ear assay (19).

LITERATURE
1   Greenspoon J, Ahluwalia R, Juma N, Rosen CF. Allergic and photoallergic contact dermatitis: A 10-year experience. Dermatitis 2013;24:29-32
2   The European Multicentre Photopatch Test Study (EMCPPTS) Taskforce. A European multicentre photopatch test study. Br J Dermatol 2012;166:1002-1009
3   Batten TL, Wakeel RA, Douglas WS, Evans C, White MI, Moody R, Ormerod AD. Contact dermatitis from the old formula E45 cream. Contact Dermatitis 1994;30:159-161
4   Ayadi M, Martin P. Contact allergy to petrolatum. Contact Dermatitis 1987;16:51
5   Dooms-Goossens A, Degreef H. Contact allergy to petrolatums. (II). Attempts to identify the nature of the allergens. Contact Dermatitis 1983;9:247-256
6   Dooms-Goossens A, Degreef H. Contact allergy to petrolatums. (I). Sensitizing capacity of different brands of yellow and white petrolatums. Contact Dermatitis 1983;9:175-185
7   Hollander L. Dermatitis produced by petrolatum. Arch Derm Syphilol 1938;38:49-51
8   Lawrence CM, Smith AG. Ampliative medicament allergy: concomitant sensitivity to multiple medicaments including yellow soft paraffin, white soft paraffin, gentian violet and Span 20. Contact Dermatitis 1982;8:240-245
9   Dooms-Goossens A, Degreef H. Sensitization to yellow petrolatum used as a vehicle for patch testing. Contact Dermatitis 1980;6:146-147
10   Grimalt F, Romaguera C. Sensitivity to petrolatum. Contact Dermatitis 1978;4:377
11   Maibach H. Chronic dermatitis and hyperpigmentation from petrolatum. Contact Dermatitis 1978;4:62
12   Goossens A, Beck MH, Haneke E, McFadden JP, Nolting S, Durupt G, Ries G. Adverse cutaneous reactions to cosmetic allergens. Contact Dermatitis 1999;40:112-113
13   Prins FJ, Smeenk G. Contacteczeem door Hirudoid zalf. Ned T Geneeskd 1971;115:1935-1938
14   Shelly WB, Shelley ED. Chap stick® acne. Cutis 1986;37:459-460
15   Fisher AA. Acne venenata in black skin. Cutis 1986;37:24-26
16   Plewig G, Fulton JE, Kligman AM. Pomade acne. Arch Dermatol 1970;101:580-584

17   Scalf LA, Davis MDP, Rohlinger AL, Connolly SM. Photopatch testing of 182 patients: A 6-year experience at the Mayo Clinic. Dermatitis 2009;20:44-52

18   Malten KE. A case of contact eczema to yellow soft paraffin. Contact Dermatitis Newsletter 1969;5:106

19   Nguyen SH, Dang TP, Maibach HI. Comedogenicity in rabbit: some cosmetic ingredients/vehicles. Cutan Ocul Toxicol 2007;26:287-292

20   Rios Scherrer MA. Allergic contact dermatitis to petrolatum. Contact Dermatitis 2006;54:300 301

21   Tam CC, Elston DM. Allergic contact dermatitis caused by white petrolatum on damaged skin. Dermatitis 2006;17:201-203

22   Schnuch A, Lessmann H, Geier J, Uter W. White petrolatum (Ph. Eur.) is virtually non-sensitizing. Analysis of IVDK data on 80 000 patients tested between 1992 and 2004 and short discussion of identification and designation of allergens. Contact Dermatitis 2006;54:338-343

23   Ulrich G, Schmutz J L, Trechot Ph, Commun N, Barbaud A. Sensitization to petrolatum: an unusual cause of false-positive drug patch-tests. Allergy 2004;59:1006-1009

24   Rubin MG, Pirozzi DJ. Contact dermatitis from carbolated vaseline. Cutis 1973;12:52-55 (data cited in ref. 6)

25   Scott FP, Holland A. Huidreaksies bij die bantoe as gevolg van die gebruik van kosmetiese middels. Geneeskunde 1974;16:39-41 (article in Afrikaans) (data cited in ref. 6).

26   Szarmach H, Pawlik H, Dratwinski Z. Experimental studies on contact allergy to ointment bases. Przeglad Dermatologiczny 1969;56:171-177 (article in Polish) (data cited in ref. 6)

27   Kang H, Choi J, Lee AY. Allergic contact dermatitis to white petrolatum. J Dermatol 2004;31:428-430

28   Kundu RV, Scheman AJ, Gutmanovich A, Hernandez C. Contact dermatitis to white petrolatum. Skinmed 2004;3:295-296

29   Grin R, Maibach HI. Long-lasting contact urticaria from petrolatum mimicking dermatitis. Contact Dermatitis 1999;40:110

30   Conti A, Manzini BM, Schiavi ME, Motolese A. Sensitization to white petrolatum used as a vehicle for patch testing. Contact Dermatitis 1995;33:201-202

31   Frankel EB. Acne secondary to white petrolatum use. Arch Dermatol 1985;121:589-590

32   English JS, Murphy G. Acne secondary to white petrolatum use. Arch Dermatol 1985;121:1240

33   Verhagen AR, Koten JW, Chaddah VK, Patel RI. Skin diseases in Kenya. A clinical and histopathological study of 3,168 patients. Arch Dermatol 1968;98:577-586

34   Verhagen AR. Pomade acne in black skin. Arch Dermatol 1974;110:465

35   Fisher AA. Cutaneous reactions to petrolatum. Cutis 1981;28:23-24,31,57,93

36   Baer RL, Serri F, Weissenbach-Vial C. Studies on allergic sensitization to certain topical therapeutic agents. Arch Derm Syph 1955;71:19-23

2.355   PHENYLETHYL RESORCINOL

IDENTIFICATION

Description/definition : Phenylethyl resorcinol is the organic compound that conforms to the formula shown below
Chemical class(es) : Phenols
Chemical/IUPAC name : 4-(1-Phenylethyl)benzene-1,3-diol
Other names : Phenethyl resorcinol; 1,3-benzenediol, 4-(1-phenylethyl)-
CAS registry number (s) : 85-27-8
Function(s) in cosmetics : EU: antioxidant. USA: antioxidants; skin-conditioning agents - miscellaneous
Patch testing : 0.1% and 1% pet. (1); 2% pet. (2)
Molecular formula : $C_{14}H_{14}O_2$

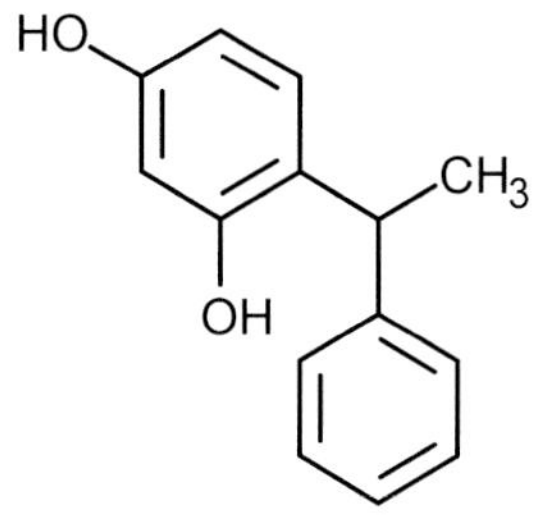

GENERAL

Phenylethyl resorcinol is a potent inhibitor of tyrosinase and a relatively new and apparently highly effective skin lightening agent. The chemical has been used as a skin-lightening agent in cosmetics in Japan since 2000. It is a synthetic compound, and is one of the natural lightening compounds found in *Pinus sylvestris* (1).

CONTACT ALLERGY

Case reports and case series

A female patient presented with a 3-year history of an itchy erythematous rash and hyperpigmented areas on both cheeks. She had been using several steroid ointments and antifungal creams with temporary result. The patient reported that the facial erythema had appeared after application of a skin-lightening essence for hyperpigmentation on the face. Patch tests with her cosmetics and 17 cosmetic allergens gave a positive reaction to the skin-lightening essence. Later, when patch tested with its ingredients, obtained from the cosmetics supplier, there were positive reactions to phenylethyl resorcinol 0.1% and 1% pet. The 1% test material was negative in two control subjects (1). Two other women had facial allergic contact dermatitis from phenylethyl resorcinol present in a sunscreen cream intended to be used in patients with melasma or hyperpigmentation, containing <0.5% phenylethyl resorcinol (2).

Presence in cosmetic products and chemical analyses

In the USA, in April 2017, phenylethyl resorcinol was present in 19 of 56,714 cosmetic products of which the composition is known in FDA's Voluntary Cosmetic Registration Program (VCRP) (data obtained from FDA, May 2017). In March 2017, phenylethyl resorcinol was present in 25 of 65,431 cosmetic products of which the composition is known in EWG's Skin Deep Cosmetics Database, USA (http://www.ewg.org/skindeep/). In 2015, 338 sunscreen, 'anti-ageing' and skin-lightening cosmetic products of 15 brands available in Spain were assessed in order to determine the presence of resorcinol derivatives with skin-lightening properties (phenylethyl resorcinol, hexyl resorcinol, and butyl resorcinol). Phenylethyl resorcinol was present in 6 (1.8%) of these products (2).

LITERATURE

1   Gohara M, Yagami A, Suzuki K, Morita Y, Sano A, Iwata Y, et al. Allergic contact dermatitis caused by phenylethyl resorcinol [4-(1-phenylethyl)-1,3-benzenediol], a skin-lightening agent in cosmetics. Contact Dermatitis 2013;69:319-320
2   Pastor-Nieto M-A, Sánchez-Pedreño P, Martínez-Menchón T, Melgar-Molero V, Alcántara-Nicolás F, de la Cruz-Murie P. Allergic contact dermatitis caused by phenylethyl resorcinol, a skin-lightening agent contained in a sunscreen. Contact Dermatitis 2016;75:250-253

2.356 PHENOXYETHANOL

IDENTIFICATION

Description/definition : Phenoxyethanol is the aromatic ether alcohol that conforms to the formula shown below
Chemical class(es) : Alcohols; ethers
Chemical/IUPAC name : 2-Phenoxyethanol
Other names : Ethylene glycol monophenyl ether; in Euxyl® K 400 with methyldibromo glutaronitrile
CAS registry number (s) : 122-99-6
EC number(s) : 204-589-7
CIR review(s) : J Am Coll Toxicol 1990;9:259-277 (access: www.cir-safety.org/ingredients)
SCCS opinion(s) : SCCS/1575/16 (34)
Merck Index monograph : 7275
Function(s) in cosmetics : EU: preservative. USA: fragrance ingredients; preservatives
EU cosmetic restrictions : Regulated in Annex V/29 of the Regulation (EC) No. 1223/2009
Patch testing : 1% pet. (Chemotechnique, SmartPracticeEurope, SmartPracticeCanada)
Molecular formula : $C_8H_{10}O_2$

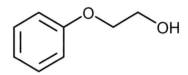

GENERAL

Phenoxyethanol is used as a preservative in cosmetic formulations at a maximum concentration of 1.0%. It is a broad-spectrum preservative which has excellent activity against a wide range of gram-negative and gram-positive bacteria, yeast and mould. It is also used as a solvent and, because of its properties as a solvent, may be present in many blends and mixtures with other preservatives (34). Phenoxyethanol can also be used as a fragrance ingredient (39). In the past, the combination of phenoxyethanol and methyldibromo glutaronitrile (best known trade name: Euxyl® K400) caused an epidemic of allergic contact dermatitis from its component methyldibromo glutaronitrile (see Chapter 2.294 Methyldibromo glutaronitrile/phenoxyethanol [Euxyl® K400] and Chapter 2.293 Methyldibromo glutaronitrile).

CONTACT ALLERGY

In accord with its lack of sensitizing potential in animal studies (5,6), contact allergy to phenoxyethanol is, despite its widespread use for 40 years, rare. In routine testing of more than 6500 patients suspected of having contact dermatitis, for example, only four cases were diagnosed (7-9), two of which were caused by its presence in Euxyl® K400 (9). In 159 patients allergic to this preservative mixture, only four (2.7%) reacted to phenoxyethanol (9-11) and in 39 patients who became sensitized to moisturizers from a preservative system consisting of phenoxyethanol, caprylhydroxamic acid and methylpropanediol, not one allergic reaction was caused by phenoxyethanol (43).

Patch testing in groups of patients

Results of studies patch testing phenoxyethanol in consecutive patients suspected of contact dermatitis (routine testing) and in groups of selected patients are shown in table 2.356.1. In routine testing, frequencies of sensitization have ranged from 0% to 0.2%. In four studies in which phenoxyethanol was tested in groups of selected patients (e.g., patients suspected of allergic cosmetic dermatitis, patients tested with a preservative series), rates of sensitization ranged from 0.1% to 1.7%. The latter frequency was found in a Korean study in a group of 584 patients suspected of cosmetic allergic contact dermatitis. The relevance of the 10 positive patch tests was not mentioned (23).

Case reports and case series

In the period 1996-2013, in a tertiary referral center in Valencia, Spain, 5419 patients were patch tested. Of these, 628 individuals had allergic contact dermatitis to cosmetics. Phenoxyethanol was the responsible allergen in one case (35). Phenoxyethanol was responsible for 13 out of 959 cases of non-fragrance cosmetic allergy where the causal allergen was identified, Belgium, 2000-2010 (1). Two positive patch test reactions to phenoxyethanol were ascribed to cosmetic allergy (3). In a 4-month-period in 1996, 475 patients with contact allergy to 'cosmetic ingredients' were collected in 5 centers in Belgium, UK and Germany. There were 3 reactions to phenoxyethanol; relevance was not stated (24). Of 11 patients allergic to Euxyl® K400, who were tested with its ingredients, one reacted to phenoxyethanol 5% pet. This patient had a positive ROAT with a skin care lotion containing 0.1% Euxyl® K400 (not used by the patient). However, contact allergy to methyldibromo glutaronitrile was not excluded (11). A man became sensitized to phenoxyethanol present in aqueous cream BP, used as a soap substitute (7).

Table 2.356.1 Patch testing in groups of patients

Years and Country	Test conc. & vehicle	Number of patients tested | positive (%)		Selection of patients (S); Relevance (R); Comments (C)	Ref.
Routine testing					
2000-2005 USA	1% pet.	2700	(0.1%)	R: 50%	2
2001-2 USA, Canada	1% pet.	4887	(0.2%)	R: definite + probable relevance: 9%	20
1994-6 USA, Canada	1% pet.	3080	- -		10
1992-4 USA, Canada	1% pet.	3492	(0.2%)	R: present relevance: 38%	21
1991-1994 Italy	5% pet.	3455	2 (0.1%)	R: not stated	9
1985 The Netherlands	5% pet.	501	1 (0.2%)	R: not stated	8
1985 The Netherlands	5% pet.	501	1 (0.2%)	R: not stated	25
<1984 UK	1% pet.	2736	0 -		7
Tested in groups of selected patients					
2010-2011 Korea	1% pet.	584	10 (1.7%)	S: patients suspected of allergic cosmetic dermatitis; R: not stated	23
2006-2011 Singapore	1.5% pet.	300	1 (0.3%)	S: not specified; R: not stated; C: prevalence in men was 0%, In women 0.4%	26
1996-2009 IVDK	1% pet.	6932	20 (0.2%)[a]	S: not specified; R: not specified	4
1990-1994 Germany	1% pet.	11,120	14 (0.1%)	S: patients tested with a preservative series; R: not stated	22

IVDK: Information Network of Departments of Dermatology, Germany, Austria, Switzerland
[a] standardized for sex and age

Contact allergy to phenoxyethanol in non-cosmetic products

One patient had allergic contact dermatitis from phenoxyethanol in a gauze for leg ulcers (18). An 18-month-old boy developed generalized eczema due to phenoxyethanol in DPT vaccine (19). A man had purpuric allergic contact dermatitis from phenoxyethanol in an ultrasound gel. A semi-open test with the ultrasound gel and patch test with phenoxyethanol were positive and also had the purpuric component (47). One individual had allergic contact dermatitis from phenoxyethanol in an antiseptic used for wound care (48).

Cross-reactions, pseudo-cross-reactions and co-reactions

Pseudo-cross-reactions to methyldibromoglutaronitrile/phenoxyethanol (Euxyl® K400) may occur.

Provocation tests

One patient known to be allergic to German Chamomile reacted to a cream containing chamomile extract when patch tested with it (provocation test, the cream had not been used by this individual). The patient was allergic to several of its ingredients including phenoxyethanol (40).

Presence in cosmetic products and chemical analyses

In May 2017, phenoxyethanol was present in 6924 of 66,669 cosmetic products of which the composition is known in EWG's Skin Deep Cosmetics Database, USA (http://www.ewg.org/skindeep/). In the USA, in April 2017, phenoxyethanol was present in 15655 of 56,714 cosmetic products of which the composition is known in FDA's Voluntary Cosmetic Registration Program (VCRP) (data obtained from FDA, May 2017). Phenoxyethanol was present in 96 (54%) of 178 facial wipes for which ingredient information was obtained online and from retail stores, 2016, USA (44). Phenoxyethanol was present in 30 (56%) of 54 personal hygiene wet wipes for which ingredient information was obtained online and from retail stores, 2016, USA (45).

Phenoxyethanol was present in 1132 of 4737 (23.9%) commonly used cosmetic products of which the full composition was known in 2016 in The Contact Allergen Management Program (CAMP) database of the American Contact Dermatitis Society (46). Of 60 different Israeli brand cosmetics, including shampoos, liquid soaps, body creams and hand creams, randomly selected in 2015, thirteen (22%) contained phenoxyethanol; the percentage in rinse-off products was 15, whereas 25% of the stay-on products contained phenoxyethanol (42).

In 2009, in the USA, the ingredient lists of 1591 facial cosmetics from one company were screened for the presence of phenoxyethanol. Phenoxyethanol was present in 25% of 132 blushers and 38 bronzers, in 0% of 90 concealers, in 13% of 174 eyeliners, in 38% of 304 eyeshadows, in 44% of 457 foundations, in 10% of 140 loose and pressed powders, and in 66% of 256 mascaras (30). In 2009, in the USA, the ingredient lists of 796 hair products from one company were screened for the presence of phenoxyethanol. Phenoxyethanol was present in 12% of 279 shampoos, in 0% of 231 conditioners, and in 0% of 286 styling products (31). In 2009, in the USA, the ingredient lists of 730 lip cosmetics and dental care products from one company were screened for the presence of phenoxyethanol. Phenoxyethanol was present in 0% of 31 lip liners, in 0% of 429 lipsticks, in 9% of 92 lip moisturizers, in 0% of 153 toothpastes, and in 0% of 25 mouth washes (32). In 2009, in the USA, the ingredient lists of 657 miscellaneous cosmetics from one company were screened for the presence of phenoxyethanol. Phenoxyethanol was present in 3% of 195 antiperspirants/deodorants, in 0% of 41 powders, in 0% of 167 shaving products, in 13% of 201 sunblocks, and in 19% of 53 wipes (33).

Phenoxyethanol was present in 1111/3541 (29.6%) randomly sampled leave-on cosmetic products, Germany, 2006-2009 (12). In Germany, in 2006-2009, the labels of 4680 cosmetic products were screened for the presence of preservatives. Phenoxyethanol was present in 30.1% of the products, according to labelling information (36). Phenoxyethanol was present in 39% of 204 cosmetic products (92 shampoos, 61 hair conditioners, 34 liquid soaps, 17 wet tissues) in Sweden, 2008 (14). Of 38 cosmetic products marketed for babies in the UK in 2007, 11 (29%) contained phenoxyethanol (27). Phenoxyethanol was the third most commonly used preservative in the USA, 2007 (13). Of 23 brands of moist toilet paper marketed in 2006 in Italy, 14 (61%) contained phenoxyethanol (28). In a group of 67 samples of skin creams, randomly selected from retail outlets in Denmark in 1999, 33 (49%) contained phenoxyethanol in a concentration range of 0.023-0.957%. In 5 products it was present, but not declared (29).

OTHER SIDE EFFECTS

Immediate-type reactions

One patient had an immediate contact reaction from phenoxyethanol in her mother's moisturizer (15). Another reacted to phenoxyethanol and 17 cosmetics products containing the preservative with contact urticarial responses (16). Another case of contact urticaria from phenoxyethanol, present in a body lotion, has been described (17). A man had contact urticaria from phenoxyethanol in an aftershave (38, article cannot be traced).

A woman presented with a 6-month history of hives developing on skin to which any of a large number of products had been applied including moisturizers, sun care products, skin cleansing solutions, shampoos and toothpaste. At one time, on applying a moisturizer, the patient immediately developed hives in the contact zone, followed by rhinorrhea, dyspnea, and dizziness without loss of consciousness. After using a blue ink pen to mark the skin prick tests, hives developed at the ink contact sites. An open test with the moisturizer resulted in immediate whealing. Phenoxyethanol was present in all suspected cosmetic products. An open test with Euxyl® K400 0.1% pet. (containing 20% phenoxyethanol) was strongly positive. A skin prick test with a vaccine containing phenoxyethanol 5mg/mL was positive in the patient and negative in 5 controls (37).

A review of contact urticaria caused by ingredients of cosmetics has been provided in ref. 41.

LITERATURE

1   Travassos AR, Claes L, Boey L, Drieghe J, Goossens A. Non-fragrance allergens in specific cosmetic products. Contact Dermatitis 2011;65:276-285

2   Davis MD, Scalf LA, Yiannias JA, Cheng JF, El-Azhary RA, Rohlinger AL, et al. Changing trends and allergens in the patch test standard series. Arch Dermatol 2008;144:67-72

3   Kohl L, Blondeel A, Song M. Allergic contact dermatitis from cosmetics: retrospective analysis of 819 patch-tested patients. Dermatology 2002;204:334-337

4   Schnuch A, Lessmann H, Geier J, Uter W. Contact allergy to preservatives. Analysis of IVDK data 1996-2009. Br J Dermatol 2011;164:1316-1325

5   Bruze M, Gruvberger B, Agrup G. Sensitization studies in the guinea pig with the active ingredients of Euxyl ® K 400. Contact Dermatitis 1988;18:37-39

6   Hausen BM. The sensitizing potency of Euxyl ® K 400 and its components 1,2-dibromo-2,4-dicyanobutane and 2-phenoxyethanol. Contact Dermatitis 1993;28:149-153

7   Lovell CR, White IR, Boyle J. Contact dermatitis from phenoxyethanol in aqueous cream BP. Contact Dermatitis 1984;11:187

8   De Groot AC, Bos JD, Jagtman BA, Bruynzeel DP, van Joost T, Weyland JW. Contact allergy to preservatives- II. Contact Dermatitis 1986;15:218-222

9   Tosti A, Vincenzi C, Trevisi P, e Guerra L. Euxyl K 400: incidence of sensitization, patch test concentration and vehicle. Contact Dermatitis 1995;33:193-195

10 Marks JG Jr, Belsito DV, DeLeo VA, Fowler JF Jr, Fransway AF, Maibach HI,et al. North American Contact Dermatitis Group patch test results for the detection of delayed-type hypersensitivity to topical allergens. J Am Acad Dermatol 1998;38:911-918

11 Tosti A, Guerra L, Bardazzi F, Gasparri F. Euxyl K 400: a new sensitizer in cosmetics. Contact Dermatitis 1991;25:89-93

12 Schnuch A, Mildau G, Kratz E-M, Uter W. Risk of sensitization to preservatives estimated on the basis of patch test data and exposure, according to a sample of 3541 leave-on products. Contact Dermatitis 2011;65:167-174

13 Steinberg DC. Voluntary registration of cosmetics and 2007 frequency of preservatives use. Cosmetics Toiletries Magazine 2008;123:47-52

14 Yazar K, Johnsson S, Lind M-L, Boman A, Lidén C. Preservatives and fragrances in selected consumer-available cosmetics and detergents. Contact Dermatitis 2011;64:265-272

15 Birnie AJ, English JS. 2-phenoxyethanol-induced contact urticaria. Contact Dermatitis 2006;54:349

16 Hernandez B, Ortiz-Frutos FJ, Garcia M, Palencia S, Garcia MC, Iglesias L. Contact urticaria from 2-phenoxyethanol. Contact Dermatitis 2002;47:54

17 Bohn S, Bircher AJ. Phenoxyethanol-induced urticaria. Allergy 2001;56:922-923

18 Gallo R, Marro I, Sorbara S. Contact allergy from phenoxyethanol in Fitostimoline® gauzes. Contact Dermatitis 2005;53:241

19 Vogt T, Landthaler M, Stolz W. Generalized eczema in an 18-month-old boy due to phenoxyethanol in DPT vaccine. Contact Dermatitis 1998;38:50-51

20 Pratt MD, Belsito DV, DeLeo VA, Fowler JF Jr, Fransway AF, Maibach HI, et al. North American Contact Dermatitis Group patch-test results, 2001–2002 study period. Dermatitis 2004;15:176-183

21 Marks JG, Belsito DV, DeLeo VA, Fowler JF, Fransway AF, Maibach HI,et al. North American Contact Dermatitis Group standard tray patch test results 1992 through 1994. Am J Contact Dermatitis 1995;6:160-165

22 Schnuch A, Geier J, Uter W, Frosch PJ. Patch testing with preservatives, antimicrobials and industrial biocides. Results from a multicentre study. Br J Dermatol 1998;138:467-476

23 Lee SS, Hong DK, Jeong NJ, Lee JH, Choi YS, Lee AY, et al. Multicenter study of preservative sensitivity in patients with suspected cosmetic contact dermatitis in Korea. J Dermatol 2012;39:677-681

24 Goossens A, Beck MH, Haneke E, McFadden JP, Nolting S, Durupt G, Ries G. Adverse cutaneous reactions to cosmetic allergens. Contact Dermatitis 1999;40:112-113

25 De Groot AC, Bos JD, Jagtman BA, Bruynzeel DP, van Joost T, Weyland JW. Contact allergy to preservatives – II. Contact Dermatitis 1986;15:218-222

26 Cheng S, Leow YH, Goh CL, Goon A. contact sensitivity to preservatives in Singapore: frequency of sensitization to 11 common preservatives 2006–2011. Dermatitis 2014;25:77-82

27 White JML, McFadden JP. Exposure to haptens/contact allergens in baby cosmetic products. Contact Dermatitis 2008;59:176-177

28 Zoli V, Tosti A, Silvani S, Vincenzi C. Moist toilet papers as possible sensitizers: review of the literature and evaluation of commercial products in Italy. Contact Dermatitis 2006;55:252-254

29 Rastogi SC. Analytical control of preservative labelling on skin creams. Contact Dermatitis 2000;43:339-343

30 Scheman A, Jacob S, Katta R, Nedorost S, Warshaw E, Zirwas M, et al. Part 1 of a 4 part series. Facial cosmetics: trends and alternatives. Data from the American Contact Alternative Group. J Clin Aesthet Dermatol 2011;4:25-30

31 Scheman A, Jacob S, Katta R, Nedorost S, Warshaw E, Zirwas M, et al. Part 2 of a 4 part series. Hair cosmetics: trends and alternatives. Data from the American Contact Alternative Group. J Clin Aesthet Dermatol 2011;4:42-46

32 Scheman A, Jacob S, Katta R, Nedorost S, Warshaw E, Zirwas M, et al. Part 3 of a 4 part series. Lips and common Dental Care products: trends and alternatives. Data from the American Contact Alternative Group. J Clin Aesthet Dermatol 2011;4:50-53

33 Scheman A, Jacob S, Katta R, Nedorost S, Warshaw E, Zirwas M, et al. Part 4 of a 4 part series. Miscellaneous products: trends and alternatives in deodorants, antiperspirants, sunblocks, shaving products, powder, and wipes. Data from the American Contact Alternative Group. J Clin Aesthet Dermatol 2011;4:35-39

34 SCCS (Scientific Committee on Consumer Safety). Opinion on Phenoxyethanol, 16 March 2016, SCCS/1575/16. Available at: http://ec.europa.eu/health/scientific_committees/consumer_safety/docs/sccs_o_195.pdf

35 Zaragoza-Ninet V, Blasco Encinas R, Vilata-Corell JJ, Pérez-Ferriols A, Sierra-Talamantes C, Esteve-Martínez A, de la Cuadra-Oyanguren J. Allergic contact dermatitis due to cosmetics: A clinical and epidemiological study in a tertiary hospital. Actas Dermosifiliogr 2016;107:329-336

36 Uter W, Yazar K, Kratz EM, Mildau G, Lidén C. Coupled exposure to ingredients of cosmetic products: II. Preservatives. Contact Dermatitis 2014;70:219-226

37 Núñez Orjales R, Carballas Vázquez C, Carballada González F, Boquete París M. 2-Phenoxyethanol-induced contact urticaria and anaphylaxis. J Investig Allergol Clin Immunol 2010;20:354-355

38 Lujan D, Hernandez-Machin B, Peñate Y, Borrego L. Contact urticaria due to phenoxyethanol in an aftershave. Dermatitis 2009;20:E10

39 Scognamiglio J, Jones L, Letizia CS, Api AM. Fragrance material review on 2-phenoxyethanol. Food Chem Toxicol 2012;50(Suppl.2):S244-255

40   Paulsen E, Christensen LP, Andersen KA. Cosmetics and herbal remedies with Compositae plant extracts – are they tolerated by Compositae-allergic patients? Contact Dermatitis 2008;58:15-23

41   Verhulst L, Goossens A. Cosmetic components causing contact urticaria: a review and update. Contact Dermatitis 2016;75:333-344

42   Horev L, Isaksson M, Engfeldt M, Persson L, Ingber A, Bruze M. Preservatives in cosmetics in the Israeli market conform well to the EU legislation. J Eur Acad Dermatol Venereol 2015;29:761 766

43   Ackermann L, Virtanen H, Korhonen L, Laukkanen A, Huilaja L, Riekki R, Hasan T. An epidemic of allergic contact dermatitis caused by a new allergen, caprylhydroxamic acid, in moisturizers. Contact Dermatitis 2017 Apr 19. doi: 10.1111/cod.12787. [Epub ahead of print]

44   Aschenbeck KA, Warshaw EM. Allergenic ingredients in facial wet wipes. Dermatitis 2017 Mar 23. doi: 10.1097/DER.0000000000000268. [Epub ahead of print]

45   Aschenbeck KA, Warshaw EM. Allergenic ingredients in personal hygiene wet wipes. Dermatitis 2017 Mar 23. doi: 10.1097/DER.0000000000000275. [Epub ahead of print]

46   Beene KM, Scheman A, Severson D, Reeder MJ. Prevalence of preservatives across all product types in the Contact Allergen Management Program. Dermatitis 2017;28:81-87

47   Chasset F, Soria A, Moguelet P, Mathian A, Auger Y, Francès C, Barete S. Contact dermatitis due to ultrasound gel: A case report and published work review. J Dermatol 2016;43:318-320

48   Calow T, Oberle K, Bruckner-Tuderman L, Jakob T, Schumann H. Contact dermatitis due to use of Octenisept in wound care. J Dtsch Dermatol Ges 2009;7:759-765 (article in German)

2.357   PHENYLBENZIMIDAZOLE SULFONIC ACID

IDENTIFICATION

Description/definition   : Phenylbenzimidazole sulfonic acid is the aromatic organic compound that conforms to
                             the formula shown below
Chemical class(es)   : Heterocyclic compounds; sulfonic acids
Chemical/IUPAC name   : 2-Phenyl-3H-benzimidazole-5-sulfonic acid
Other names   : Ensulizole; Eusolex® 232
CAS registry number (s)   : 27503-81-7
EC number(s)   : 248-502-0
SCCS opinion(s)   : SCCP/1056/06 (23)
Merck Index monograph   : 4917
Function(s) in cosmetics   : EU: UV-absorber; UV-filter. USA: light stabilizers; sunscreen agents
EU cosmetic restrictions   : Regulated in Annex VI/6 of the Regulation (EC) No. 1223/2009
Patch testing   : 10% pet. (Chemotechnique, SmartPracticeCanada)
Molecular formula   : $C_{13}H_{10}N_2O_3S$

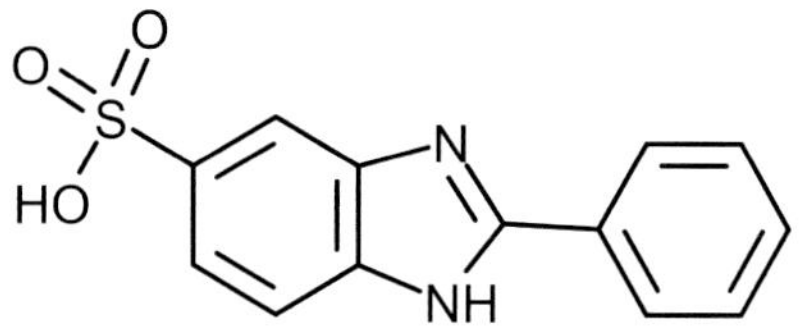

GENERAL

Phenylbenzimidazole sulfonic acid is a UVB filter with UV absorbance maximum (λ_{max}) at 302 nm (25), which has been used in Europe since 1933 (14). The literature on adverse reactions to sunscreens has been reviewed in several recent and older publications (17-22,29). A review of photocontact allergy to sunscreens was published in 2010 (26).

CONTACT ALLERGY

Patch testing in groups of patients

Between 1981 and 1996, in one center in Germany, 378 patients suspected of clinical photosensitivity were patch tested with phenylbenzimidazole 1% water or 10% pet. and 1 (0.3%) positive reaction was observed; its relevance was not mentioned (2).

Case reports and case series

Two patients had allergic contact dermatitis from phenylbenzimidazole sulfonic acid in sunscreens (3); the authors mentioned two more cases (3, note added in proof). Two individuals had photoaggravated allergic contact dermatitis from the sunscreen in moisturizers (8). Two patients suffered from allergic contact dermatitis caused by phenylben-zimidazole sulfonic acid in sunscreens (4,9). In the period 1981-1989, 56 patients (43 women, 13 men) were diagnosed with contact allergy or photocontact allergy to UV-filters in one center in Germany. There was one photo-aggravated contact allergic reaction to phenylbenzimidazole sulfonic acid. All reactions were relevant and all 46 patients who could be (photo)patch tested with their own sunscreens (and a few of them with other cosmetics) had one or more positive (photo)patch tests to these products (28, overlap with refs. 2,3 and 4).

Presence in cosmetic products and chemical analyses

In June 2017, phenylbenzimidazole sulfonic acid was present in 56 of 69,003 cosmetic products of which the composition is known in EWG's Skin Deep Cosmetics Database, USA (http://www.ewg.org/skindeep/). It should be realized that sunscreen products containing UV-filters are classified as drugs in the USA, not as cosmetics; the number mentioned here, therefore, is that of cosmetics containing the UV-filter, but it does *not* include their presence in sunscreens. In the USA, in April 2017, phenylbenzimidazole sulfonic acid was present in 41 of 56,714 cosmetic products of which the composition is known in FDA's Voluntary Cosmetic Registration Program (VCRP) (data obtained from FDA, May 2017). In 2012, in Switzerland, 116 cosmetics from seven widely used leave-on product categories (19 lip care products, 8 lipsticks, 29 face creams, 11 liquid makeup foundations, 3 aftershaves, 7 hand creams and 39 sunscreens) were investigated to determine the frequency of occurrence and concentrations of 22 organic UV filters in these products. Phenylbenzimidazole sulfonic acid and its salts were found in 11% of the products in a concentration range of 0.95-2.29%, mean 1.56% (24).

In a sample of 337 sunscreens marketed in the UK in 2010, phenylbenzimidazole sulfonic acid was present in 6% (16). Phenylbenzimidazole sulfonic acid was present in 11.6% of 4447 cosmetic products collected in Germany, 2006-2009 (7). Phenylbenzimidazole sulfonic acid was present in 4% of 329 sunscreen products (incl. 21 lipstick sunscreens) marketed in the UK in 2005 (15). Phenylbenzimidazole sulfonic acid and its potassium, sodium and triethanolamine salts were present in 2 of 75 (3%) sunscreen creams and lotions from 30 European and US producers purchased in Denmark in 2001 in a concentration range of 1.4-2.5% (11). In The Netherlands, in 1978, 197 sunscreen products of 48 brands were investigated for the presence of UV-filters. Phenylbenzimidazole sulfonic acid was present in 11 brands (number of products not mentioned) in a concentration range of 1.0-6.2%. This chemical was at that time the most prevalent UV-absorber in sunscreen products after ethylhexyl methoxycinnamate (19 brands) (27).

OTHER SIDE EFFECTS

Photosensitivity

Photopatch testing in groups of patients

Results of photopatch testing phenylbenzimidazole sulfonic acid in groups of selected patients (e.g., patients suspected of photosensitivity, patients with dermatitis affecting mainly light-exposed skin) back to 1996 are shown in table 2.357.1. In 6 studies photopatch testing groups of selected patients, frequencies of sensitization have ranged from 0.1% to 1.9%, being 1.2% or lower in all but one investigation. In four of the 6 studies, the relevance of the positive photopatch test reactions to phenylbenzimidazole sulfonic acid was either not stated or specified for the UV-filter. In the two other studies, both positive reactions observed were relevant, but causative products were not mentioned (10,13).

Table 2.357.1 Photopatch testing in groups of patients

Years and Country	Test conc. & vehicle	Number of patients tested | positive (%)		Selection of patients (S); Relevance (R); Comments (C)	Ref.
2003-2007 Portugal	10% pet.	83	1 (1.2%)	S: patients with suspected photoaggravated facial dermatitis or systemic photosensitivity; R: all sunscreen photopatch tests were of current or past relevance	10
2000-2005 USA	10% pet.	177	1 (0.6%)	S: patients photopatch tested for suspected photodermatitis; R: the reaction was relevant	13
2001-2003 Colombia	10% pet.	82	1 (1.2%)	S: patients with a clinical diagnosis of photoallergic contact dermatitis; R: 65% of all reactions in the study were relevant	6
1983-1998 UK	10% pet.	2715	1 (<0.1%)	S: patients suspected of photosensitivity or with (a history of) dermatitis at exposed sites; R: 37% for all photoallergens together	1
1990-1996 Sweden	2% pet.	355	2 (0.6%)	S: patients suspected of photosensitivity; R: not stated	12
1981-1996 Germany	1% water or 10 % pet.	378	7 (1.9%)	S: patients suspected of clinical photosensitivity; R: not stated	2

Case reports and series

In the period 1981-1989, 56 patients (43 women, 13 men) were diagnosed with contact allergy or photocontact allergy to UV-filters in one center in Germany. There was one photoaggravated contact allergic and 4 photoallergic reactions to phenylbenzimidazole sulfonic acid. All reactions were relevant and all 46 patients who could be (photo)patch tested with their own sunscreens (and a few of them with other cosmetics) had one or more positive (photo)patch tests to these products (28, overlap with refs. 2,3 and 4). One patient had photoallergic contact dermatitis from phenylbenzimidazole sulfonic acid in a sunscreen (5). Two individuals had photoaggravated allergic contact dermatitis from the UV-absorber in moisturizers (8).

LITERATURE

1   Darvay A, White I, Rycroft R, Jones AB, Hawk JL, McFadden JP. Photoallergic contact dermatitis is uncommon. Br J Dermatol 2001;145:597-601

2   Schauder S, Ippen H. Contact and photocontact sensitivity. Review of a 15-year experience and of the literature to suncreens. Contact Dermatitis 1997;37:221-232

3   Schauder S, Ippen H. Photoallergic and allergic contact eczema caused by dibenzoylmethane compounds and other sunscreening agents. Hautarzt 1988;39:435-440

4   Schauder S, Ippen H. Photoallergic and allergic contact dermatitis from dibenzoylmethanes. Photodermatology 1986;3:140-147

5   Fagerlund VL, Kalimo K, Jansen CH. Valonsurjaaineet fotokontaktallergien aiheuttajin. Duodecim 1983;99:146-150

6   Rodriguez E, Valbuena M, Rey M, Porras de Quintana L. Causal agents of photoallergic contact dermatitis diagnosed in the national institute of dermatology of Columbia. Photoderm Photoimmunol Photomed 2006;22:189-192

7   Uter W, Gonçalo M, Yazar K, Kratz E-M, Mildau G, Lidén C. Coupled exposure to ingredients of cosmetic products: III. Ultraviolet filters. Contact Dermatitis 2014;71:162-169

8   Nedorost S. Ensulizole (phenylbenzimidazole-5-sulfonic acid) as a cause of facial dermatitis: two cases. Dermatitis 2005;16:148

9   Gonçalo M, Ruas E, Figueiredo A, Gonçalo S. Contact and photocontact sensitivity to sunscreens. Contact Dermatitis 1995;33:278-280

10   Cardoso J, Canelas MM, Gonçalo M, Figueiredo A. Photopatch testing with an extended series of photoallergens: a 5-year study. Contact Dermatitis 2009;60:325-329

11   Rastogi SC. UV filters in sunscreen products – a survey. Contact Dermatitis 2002;46:348-351

12   Berne B, Ross AM. 7 years experience of photopatch testing with sunscreen allergens in Sweden. Contact Dermatitis 1998;38:61-64

13   Scalf LA, Davis MDP, Rohlinger AL, Connolly SM. Photopatch testing of 182 patients: A 6-year experience at the Mayo Clinic. Dermatitis 2009;20:44-52

14   Kerr A, Ferguson J. Photoallergic contact dermatitis. Photodermatol Photoimmunol Photomed 2010;26:56-65

15   Wahie S, Lloyd JJ, Farr PM. Sunscreen ingredients and labelling: a survey of products available in the U.K. Clin Exp Dermatol 2007;32:359-364

16   Kerr AC. A survey of the availability of sunscreen filters in the U.K. Clin Exp Dermatol 2011;36:541-543

17   Heurung AR, Raju SI, Warshaw EM. Adverse reactions to sunscreen agents: epidemiology, responsible irritants and allergens, clinical characteristics, and management. Dermatitis 2014;25:289-326

18   Heurung AR, Raju SI, Warshaw EM. Contact allergen of the year. Benzophenones. Dermatitis 2014;25:3-10 (contains many mistakes; Erratum in Dermatitis 2014;25:92-95)

19   Avenel-Audran M. Sunscreen products: finding the allergen. Eur J Dermatol 2010;20:161-166

20   Scheuer E, Warshaw E. Sunscreen allergy: a review of epidemiology, clinical characteristics, and responsible allergens. Dermatitis 2006;17:3-11

21   Funk JO, Dromgoole SH, Maibach HI. Sunscreen intolerance: contact sensitization, photocontact sensitization, and irritancy of sunscreen agents. Dermatol Clin 1995;13:473-481

22   Dromgoole SH, Maibach HI. Sunscreening agent intolerance: Contact and photocontact sensitization and contact urticaria. J Am Acad Dermatol 1990;22:1068-1078

23   SCCP (Scientific Committee on Consumer Products). Opinion on phenylbenzimidazole sufonic acid and its salts, 19 December 2006, SCCP/1056/06. Available at: http://ec.europa.eu/health/archive/ph_risk/committees/04_sccp/docs/sccp_o_079.pdf

24   Manová E, von Goetz N, Hauri U, Bogdal C, Hungerbühler K. Organic UV filters in personal care products in Switzerland: A survey of occurrence and concentrations. Int J Hyg Environ Health 2013;216:508-514

25   Shaath NA. Ultraviolet filters. Photochem Photobiol Sci 2010;9:464-469

26   Shaw T, Simpson B, Wilson B, Oostman H, Rainey D, Storrs F. True photoallergy to sunscreens is rare despite popular belief. Dermatitis 2010;21:185-198

27   Liem DH, Hilderink LT. UV absorbers in sun cosmetics 1978. Int J Cosmet Sci 1979;1:341-361

28   Schauder S. Adverse reactions to sunscreening agents in 58 patients (part 3). Z Hautkr 1991;66:294-318 (article in German)

29   Schauder S. Survey of the literature on adverse reactions to preparations containing UV filters (1947-1989) (Literaturübersicht über Unverträglichkeitsreaktionen auf lichtfilterhaltige Produkte von 1947 bis 1989). Z Hautkr 1990;65:982-998 (article in German)

lymphoid dermal infiltration chiefly comprising B-cells. Histological examination of a waist lesion revealed chronic eczema. Patch testing was positive for PPD. The cause was hair dye used by the patient's spouse and withdrawal of the allergenic product resulted in complete remission of both types of lesions (311).

A woman presented with violaceous tumors on the right temple and left post-auricular area in close proximity to the hairline. Due to the location of the lesions, history of exposure and pathology, the diagnosis of B-cell pseudo-lymphoma secondary to hair cosmetic allergy was suspected. Patch testing confirmed allergy to PPD which was present in the patient's hair dye. All lesions resolved within 2 months after discontinuation of the dye (219). A man had an itchy facial rash, that later became generalized over the trunk and upper limbs. He had widespread erythematous, tumid plaques, and papules over the cheeks, upper limbs, and trunk. Patch tests were positive to PPD. It transpired that his partner regularly dyed her hair and applications were associated with flares in his rash. Six months later he was seen again, as his skin had flared despite his wife using a different hair dye. He had the same tumid plaques over the face, upper back, hands, and legs. A repeat biopsy showed a lymphomatoid dermatitis picture. The new hair dye contained toluene-2,5-diamine sulfate, and on discontinuing this product his skin cleared. This case was remarkable because the patient reacted to a product used by his partner (consort dermatitis), because of the lymphomatoid dermatitis and because of the atypical clinical picture with tumid plaques (219).

An Indian man had pseudolymphoma (lymphomatoid contact dermatitis) from contact allergy to PPD in moustache dye (305). Another male patient had recurrent dermatitis affecting the left arm. He had noticed that each time his rash flared up, his partner had dyed her hair black. The PPD patch test was positive, as was the dye, his partner's hair was negative (202). A man had ACD from PPD presenting as nummular eczema. He reacted to PPD and to his wife's dyed hair. She was accustomed to reading a book in bed with her head nestled on his armpit (204). A woman had worsening of rosacea from ACD due to PPD in hair dye (197). Two women had extensive erythema multiforme-like ACD from PPD in hair dye (163,168). Unknown number of patients with 'erythema multiforme' from contact allergy to PPD (321). A young girl had erythema multiforme-like ACD from PPD in hair dye (316). Another patient with EM-like lesions from contact allergy to PPD in hair dye was seen in Italy (231).

A woman with alopecia totalis developed acute ACD of the scalp, ears, and limbs with EM-like lesions, target-like appearance at the periphery of the sharply delineated lesions. She had her wig dyed with normal hair dye one day before the onset of the eruption and was allergic to PPD. In the eczematous lesions on the scalp, there later was some hair growth visible (232). Three patients had lichenoid ACD from PPD in hair dyes (177). A woman suffering from vitiligo developed allergic contact dermatitis with hypertrophic features from PPD in a hair dye which had been applied to the skin for ornamental purposes, followed by persistent leukoderma. The positive PPD patch test mimicked the clinical picture with hypertrophic lesions followed by depigmentation (169). A female patient had been using the same hair dye for many years. After another dying session, she developed scalp dermatitis and widespread skin lesions as well as lymphadenopathy and quite possibly dyspnea resembling asthma. The histopathologic findings were atypical and consisted of neutrophilic cellulitis and a marked neutrophilic infiltrate with variable spongiosis. This unique finding was confirmed by histologic analysis of a patch test lesion specimen (253).

A woman developed severe and persistent blepharoconjunctivitis accompanied by centrofacial edema from contact allergy to PPD present in eyelash dye (265). A man dying his moustache with a dye containing PPD and other para-dyes developed pruritic erythematous lesions on the face, lips, penis and scrotum, and psoriasis-like hyperkeratotic lesions on the elbows, knees, and knuckles. The skin beneath the moustache, however, was normal. The patch test with PPD was positive and after discontinuing the moustache dye, all symptoms gradually disappeared (228).

Case reports of allergic hair dye reactions after sensitization to PPD in temporary black henna tattoos

Temporary black henna tattoos have become a potent and considerable source of skin sensitization to PPD in the last 15 years (26,38,67,124). Later, these patients may develop very strong allergic reactions to hair dyes, sometimes necessitating admission to hospital (53,54,59,60,61,62,63,138,139,140,141). There have been many single case reports (53,54,62,66,138,139,140,141,262,300,310,316) and small case series of two (63,230), five (59) and six individuals (60,61), mostly children and adolescents, who had been sensitized to PPD from a temporary black henna tattoo, who later had classic allergic contact dermatitis of the scalp, ears and face from hair dyes. Some patients had fierce reactions of the eyelids from using PPD-containing dye on the eyebrows and/or eyelashes (59,137). All aspects of contact allergy to PPD in temporary black henna tattoos are discussed in Chapter 2.220 Henna, black and have been reviewed in 2013 by the author (124).

Contact allergy to p-phenylenediamine in non-cosmetic products

A patient reacted to PPD in the ink of a copying machine (25). A purpuric eruption was attributed to PPD in black felt hats. The PPD patch test was positive and purpuric, but whether the hats were actually dyed with PPD was unknown (159). Dermatitis on the dorsal aspect of the toes in a young girl was unconvincingly ascribed to allergy to PPD in socks (165). A professional violinist had contact dermatitis in the left side of the neck attributed to contact allergy to PPD in a chin rest made of ebony, which was presumed to have been dyed with PPD (166). A female laboratory worker after 11 years developed occupational ACD of the hand from a 2% PPD solution that she worked with for testing milk samples to check adequate pasteurization (171). A patient had lichenoid ACD of the beard area, which was ascribed to contact allergy to PPD in a net and wooden stick that he used to tie and set his beard; however, its presence in those products was not ascertained (177).

A schoolgirl playing the cello had ACD of her right thumb, index and middle finger from PPD used to stain the bowstring (183). One patient had lymphomatoid contact dermatitis in the axillary folds, inner thighs, on the scrotum and inguinal region. A patch test with PPD was positive, histopathology showed the same lymphomatoid picture as a biopsy of the dermatitis. The reaction was thought to be caused by PPD or substances cross-reacting with PPD in oil products (antioxidants) and in clothing (azo dyes) (192). A man developed erythematous xerotic lesions on the auricle and peri-auricular area from contact allergy to PPD present in the sponge rubber portion of the headphones the patient used to listen to the television (241).

A furrier had erythematous, desquamative, pruriginous lesions on the cheeks, nasolabial folds, neck and eyelids. The skin lesions were worst at work. His job was cutting out dyed fur of animals. Patch tests showed positive reactions to PPD, dyed rabbit hair and dyed lamb hair. Oxidative hair dyes based on PPD were used to dye the furs, according to the manufacturer (314). A woman developed dermatitis of the feet. Orthopedic shoes were suspected to be the cause. She reacted to PPD and to pieces of the outer and inner surface material of the shoes. The manufacturer confirmed that the leather of the shoes was colored with PPD (322). A man had an itchy, red and crusted eruption affecting the sides of the bridge of the nose for 2 years. Patch tests with PPD and scrapings of his black spectacle frame were positive. The manufacturer confirmed that the spectacles had been dyed in a bath of PPD (323).

Cross-reactions, pseudo-cross-reactions and co-reactions
Patients allergic to PPD often cross-react to (and/or from) related chemicals of the 'para'-group in textile dyes, other hair dyes, dyes for other products, drugs (sulfonamides, benzocaine), and PPD-related rubber chemicals used as antioxidants. Examples are provided in table 2.359.7; these are primarily adapted from ref. 124 (cross-reactions in patients sensitized from PPD in black henna tattoos), and expanded with other literature references.

In a group of 134 PPD-sensitized patients, the most frequent co-reactions were to toluene-2,5-diamine sulfate (31%), o-nitro-p-phenylenediamine (25%), p-aminophenol (20%), m-aminophenol (19%), disperse orange 3 (14%), disperse red 1 (7.5%), benzocaine (7.5%), disperse red 17 (6.7%), sulfonamides (6%), and disperse yellow 3 (4.5%) (50). In Germany, in 1995-1999, individuals in a group of 74 patients allergic to PPD most frequently co-reacted to p-aminoazobenzene (66%), toluene-2,5-diamine (46%), disperse orange 3 (39%), 4,4'-diaminodiphenylmethane (32%), and p-aminophenol (14%) (18). In the Netherlands, in a group of 59 patients reacting to PPD, the most frequent co-reactivities were to disperse orange 3 (n=21; 36%), p-aminoazobenzene (n=20; 34%), toluene-2,5-diamine sulfate (n=14; 24%), disperse orange 1 (n=5; 8%), and p-aminophenol and o-nitro-PPD (both n=4; 7%) (195). In 133 PPD-positive patients investigated in 9 European countries, 2007-2008, 67 (50%) co-reacted to toluene-2,5-diamine, 46 (35%) to p-aminophenol, 24 (18.0%) to m-aminophenol and only 2 (1.5%) to resorcinol (256). No cross-reactions were observed to 11 Food, Drug and Cosmetic (FD&C) dyes in 39 hairdressers allergic to PPD (193).

Individuals with strong reactions to PPD may have an increased likelihood of co-reactions to (certain) structurally related chemicals than patients who have weaker sensitivity to PPD (7,268,269,336). Up to 2/3 of patients allergic to PPD or toluene-2,5-diamine were shown to tolerate dying their hair with a dye containing 2-methoxymethyl-p-phenylenediamine (278,283).

Table 2.359.7 Chemicals that may (be able to) cross-react with p-phenylenediamine [a]

Co- or cross-reacting compound	Synonyms	CAS	References
Acid yellow 36	metanil yellow; CI 13065	587-98-4	53
p-Aminoazobenzene	aniline yellow; CI 11000	60-09-3	2,18,25,50,57,175
4-Amino-m-cresol	4-hydroxy-o-toluidine	2835-99-6	61,256
4-Amino-2-hydroxytoluene	5-Amino-o-cresol	2835-95-2	256,326
m-Aminophenol	1-amino-3-hydroxybenzene; 3-aminophenol; CI 76545	591-27-5	2,19,50,53,59,61,63,256,296
p-Aminophenol	1-amino-4-hydroxybenzene; 4-aminophenol; CI 76550	123-30-8	2,18,19,50,53,57,58,59,60,63,256, 296
p-Aminosalicylic acid		65-49-6	217
Aniline	aminobenzene; CI 76000	62-53-3	51,223
Aniline dyes			259
Anthraquinone		84-65-1	259
Basic red 46		12221-69-1	50
Benzocaine	ethyl p-aminobenzoate	**94-09-7**	2,50,53,59,61,216,223
p-Benzoquinone [b]	1,4-cyclohexadienedione	106-51-4	164
N',N'-Bis-(4-aminophenyl)-2,5-diamino-	Bandrowski's base	20048-27-5	164

Table 2.359.7 Chemicals that may (be able to) cross-react with *p*-phenylenediamine [a] (*continued*)

Co- or cross-reacting compound	Synonyms	CAS	References
1,4-quinonediimine [b]			
N,N'-Bis(2-hydroxyethyl)-*p*-phenylene-diamine sulfate		54381-16-7	256
Bismarck brown R	basic brown 4; CI 21010	8005-78-5	53
Black rubber mix			54,58
Butacaine	3-dibutylaminopropyl PABA	149-16-6	58
Butanilicaine	2-butylamino-6'-chloro-*o*-ace-totoluidine	3785-21-5	58
Butyl PABA	butamben; butoform	94-25-7	58
Celecoxib (?)		169590-42-5	217
2-Chloro-*p*-phenylenediamine	2-chlorobenzene-1,4-diamine; CI 76065	615-66-7	182
2,4-Diaminoazobenzene	solvent orange 3; CI 11270:1	495-54-5	54
4,4'-Diaminodiphenylmethane	4,4'-methylenedianiline	101-77-9	2,18,58,261
2,4-Diaminophenoxyethanol HCl		66422-95-5	256
N,N-Diethyl-*p*-phenylenediamine	4-amino-*N,N'*-diethylaniline	93-05-0	173
p-Dimethylaminoazobenzene	solvent yellow 2; CI 11020	60-11-7	175
N,N'-Diphenyl-*p*-phenylenediamine	1-*N*,4-*N*-diphenylbenzene-1,4-diamine	74-31-7	2
Direct orange 34	CI 40215	1325-54-8	18,56
Disperse blue 106	CI 111935	68516-81-4	50,58,62,174,229
Disperse blue 124		15141-18-1	50,58,62,174,175,229
Disperse blue 106/124 mix			53,56
Disperse blue 135	unknown chemical		58
Disperse brown 1	CI 11152	23355-64-8	50,174
Disperse orange 1	CI 11080	2581-69-3	54,56,58,59
Disperse orange 3 [c]	CI 11005	730-40-5	53,54,57,58,59,61,62,174,175,229, 269
Disperse red 1	CI 11110; CI solvent red 14	2872-52-8	54,55,56,58,62,174,175,229
Disperse red 17	CI 11210	3179-89-3	54,59,174
Disperse yellow 3	CI 11855	2832-40-8	50,53,54,55,56,58,59,62,175,229
Disperse yellow 9	CI 10375	6373-73-5	59
Hydroquinone	1,4-dihydroxybenzene	123-31-9	19,53,59,61,296
Hydroxyethyl-*p*-phenylenediamine sulfate		93841-25-9	33
4-Isopropylaminodiphenylamine		101-72-4	259
N-Isopropyl-*N'*-phenyl-*p*-phenylene-diamine	4-(isopropylamino)diphenyl-amine	101-72-4	50,53,56,58,60,61,158,223,258
Mesalazine (?)	5-aminosalicylic acid	89-57-6	212,273
2-Methoxymethyl-*p*-phenylenediamine	1,4-benzenediamine, 2-(me-thoxymethyl)-	337906-36-2	277,282,283
p-Methylaminophenol		150-75-4	256
p-Methylaminophenol sulfate		55-55-0	304
o-Nitro-*p*-phenylenediamine	4-amino-2-nitroaniline; CI 76070	5307-14-2	19,32,50,57,60,193
Octyl dimethyl PABA	ethylhexyl dimethyl PABA	21245-02-3	217
PABA	*p*-aminobenzoic acid	150-13-0	50
Parabens			216
p-Phenylenediamine dihydrochloride	CI 76061	624-18-0	160
N-Phenyl-*p*-phenylenediamine	*p*-aminodiphenylamine	101-54-2	32,52
N-Phenyl-*p*-phenylenediamine HCl	*p*-aminodiphenylamine HCl	2198-59-6	163
Procainamide	*p*-aminobenzoic diethylamino-ethylamide	51-06-09	58
Procaine	2-diethylaminoethyl *p*-amino-benzoate	59-46-1	58,259
Pyrogallol	1,2,3-benzenetriol; CI 76515	87-66-1	2,18,19,53,61,296
Resorcinol	benzene-1,3-diol; CI 76505	108-46-3	19,256
Sesquiterpene lactones (?)			230
Sodium sulfadimidine	sodium sulfamethazine	1981-58-4	58
Sodium sulfamerazine		127-58-2	58
Solvent orange 3	CI 11270:1; chrysoidine Y	495-45-5	54
Sulfaguanidine		57-67-0	58
Sulfanilamide	*p*-aminobenzenesulfonamide	63-74-1	58

Table 2.359.7 Chemicals that may (be able to) cross-react with *p*-phenylenediamine [a] (*continued*)

Co- or cross-reacting compound	Synonyms	CAS	References
Sulfanilic acid	4-aminobenzenesulfonic acid	121-57-3	260
Sulfonamides			217
Sulfonylurea antidiabetic drugs			217
Thiazide diuretics			217,227
Toluene-2,5-diamine	*p*-toluenediamine; CI 76042	95-70-5	2,18,19,52,53,57,58,59,60,61,256
Toluene-2,5-diamine sulfate	*p*-toluenediamine sulfate; CI 76043	615-50-9	32,50,56,193

[a] More relevant literature references can be found in ref. 124; [b] Oxidation product of PPD; [c] Disperse orange 3 and possibly other simple azo dyes can be degraded to PPD within the skin (238), so the co-reactivity may be explained by pseudo-cross-reactivity

Patch test sensitization

p-Phenylenediamine is an extreme sensitizer and patch test sensitization to PPD 1% pet. (and also to PPD 0.4% and 0.5% [130]) has been observed repeatedly (10,11,13,126,127,131). The risk of sensitization was shown to be enhanced by concurrently testing the chemically related and often cross-reacting *p*-aminoazobenzene (128).

Frequencies (estimations) of (possible) active sensitization in patch test populations in various studies were 0.3% in the UK in 1990-1999 (10), 0.2-0.3% in The Netherlands in 1992-1999 (25), 0.01% in Denmark in 1991-2005 (131), and 0.1% in the UK in 2000-2005 (11). In a general population patch tested with the PPD TRUE test twice with an interval of 8 years, none of 365 individuals reacted to the PPD patch test (albeit read at D2 only) in the second session (14). Because of the risk of patch test sensitization, it was first suggested in 2001to delete PPD 1% from the routine series and test this dye on indication only (although in this study from The Netherlands, possible active sensitization / late reactions after 7 days with no clinical relevance, was observed in 0.2-0.3% of all patch tested patients only) (25).

Following this, possible active sensitization, as shown by a >7-day patch test reaction without clinical relevance, occurred in 1.5% of patients patch tested with *p*-phenylenediamine base 1% pet. in Germany, 2003-2004 (13). Seven patients with a late patch test were retested and in five, the reaction was now positive after 3 days, which is highly suggestive of previous patch test sensitization (13). Additional (weak) evidence for possible patch test sensitization was found in a study showing that patients who were tested twice with PPD and had a negative reaction at the first session and a positive in the second, had not been exposed to PPD in 'henna tattoos', dark hair dyes, dark textiles or by working as hairdresser significantly more frequent than individuals who did *not* have a positive second test, suggesting that active sensitization from the first test may have occurred in a number of them (15). Because of these findings, the German Contact Dermatitis Research Group decided in 2005 to delete PPD 1% pet. from the German standard series (13).

It should be realized that not all late reactions are indicative of active sensitization, but may equally be delayed immune responses (11). Indeed, a patient who reacted at day 11 was later retested and again reacted at that time, the response at D2-D4 being entirely negative (12). The same observation was made in the abovementioned German study, where two patients with late reactions to PPD again had late reactions when retested (13). And in one study, of 24 reactions to PPD which were positive after 7 days only, 20 (83%) were nevertheless relevant (195).

In spite of this, it is very likely that not every patient who has a late reaction to PPD will notice this and some who do may not report back to the dermatologist. This means that frequencies reported in literature are all probably an underestimation. On the bright side, it has been postulated, that subsequent allergic contact dermatitis following an alleged patch test sensitization is very rare (131).

Presence in cosmetic products and chemical analyses

General

It is often stated that PPD is present in more than 60% of all oxidative hair dyes (221,224,238). This is an incorrect generalization. Indeed, in several countries >50% of oxidative hair dyes investigated contained PPD: Sweden (50%, small sample, subgroup [117]), Spain (50% [250]; 85%, small sample [312]), Thailand (56% [115]), and USA (78% [297]). In Denmark however, in two studies, low percentages were found of 11 (even in products that had caused allergic contact dermatitis, small sample [257]) and of 22 (281) and in Sweden, in 2008, PPD was present in only 15% of oxidative hair dyes (237). Very recently, in Germany, it was found, that in a very large sample of 924 permanent oxidative hair dyes, only 3 (0.3%) contained PPD (293). Thus, it appears that the percentage of permanent hair dyes containing PPD may differ considerably between countries!

Specific studies

In May 2017, PPD was present in 142 of 66,835 cosmetic products of which the composition is known in EWG's Skin Deep Cosmetics Database, USA (http://www.ewg.org/skindeep/). In the USA, in April 2017, *p*-phenylene-diamine was present in 1350 of 56,714 cosmetic products of which the composition is known in FDA's Voluntary Cosmetic Registration Program (VCRP) (data obtained from FDA, May 2017).

In 2016, in Sweden, the labels of 26 oxidative hair dye products advertised with the signal words organic, natural or similar, or sold/used at a hair dressing salon advertised with the same terminology, were screened for the presence of known contact allergens. p-Phenylenediamine was present in 13 (50%) products (117). In 2013-2014, labeled ingredient information from 252 home use and professional hair dye products (210 permanent and 42 non-permanent dyes) from 48 brands sold in Bangkok, Thailand, was collected to identify the type and frequency of potent contact sensitizers. p-Phenylenediamine was present in 141 (56%) products (115).

Of 15 hair dyes advertised as 'hypoallergenic', 'para-phenylenediamine-free', or 'non-allergenic', purchased in South Korea in 2015, 4 (27%) proved to contain PPD (337). In Germany, in 2013-2014, the labels of 924 permanent oxidative hair dyes were checked for the presence of hair dye components. There were 334 retail products (of seven different brands) and 590 professional products (of six different brands). The 924 products analyzed revealed a total of 58 different hair dye components, with retail products containing 32 and professional products 52 dye ingredients. p-Phenylenediamine was present in only 0.3% of the 924 products (293).

In the USA, in 2012, ingredient labels of 107 different consumer oxidative hair dyes from 10 different companies were assessed in stores across the city of Phoenix, Arizona. PPD (as free base, sulfate, or HCl) was present in 78% of the products (297). In 2011, labels and other information on 365 hair dye products (282 permanent dyes, 79 semi-permanent dyes, 4 direct dyes) available on the Danish market (159 hair dyes for private use, 206 for professional use by hairdressers) were collected to identify the presence of sensitizers. PPD was present in 81 (22%) products (281).

Fifty-two permanent hair dye products from 11 countries in five continents (Arab Emirates, Australia, Brazil, Germany, Greece, Israel, Italy, Kenya, Singapore, Sweden, and USA) were collected during one year from the autumn of 2011 to the autumn of 2012. Twenty-three products were purchased in and 29 outside of Europe. Thirty-five all products (67%) were labelled to contain PPD, of which three had the labelling 'may contain'. Of European products (n=23), 43% contained PPD versus 86% (25/29) of the non-European hair dyes (335).

In Spain, in 2010, 15 brown and 12 blonde dyes were analyzed. PPD was identified in all of the brown dyes, irrespective of whether it was indicated (n = 12) or not (n = 3) on the label. PPD was found in 6 of the 9 blonde dyes that indicated it in the composition and 2 of the 3 in which it was not shown on the label. Semi-quantitative analysis by thin-layer chromatography revealed that the concentration of PPD in brown hair dyes (mean 3%) was higher than in blonde dyes (mean 0.1-0.3%). It was concluded that the presence of PPD in hair dyes is related to the color of the dye. It is consistently present in darker dyes and at low levels in blonde dyes (312).

In April 2010, in Spain, 111 consumer-available oxidative hair dye products of 19 brands were purchased to check the labeling for sensitizers. A systematic selection of products to be purchased from each hair dye brand was applied, including the darkest blonde shade available, one 'regular' light brown shade, one 'regular' dark brown shade, one 'regular' black shade, and two further shades with different colors (red, blue, purple, etc.). In this group of 111 hair dyes, PPD was present in 50% of the products (250). In Sweden, in 2008, PPD was present in 19 of 122 (15%) oxidative hair dyes of 20 brands (237).

Chemical analyses

Of twenty-three hair-coloring products purchased in 2011-2012 in Europe, 9 (39%) were found to contain PPD at a calculated on-head concentration (based on the recommended ratio with which the hair dye should be mixed with developer) range of 0.025%-0.98% on the basis of HPLC analysis. Of twenty-nine products purchased outside Europe, 19 (66%) contained PPD at a calculated on-head concentration in the range of 0.20%-0.96%); one had a calculated on-head concentration of 7.9%, and four products, which lacked information on how to mix the hair dye with the oxidation product had concentrations in the range of 2.2%-14.2%. The PPD concentration was on average higher in hair dyes purchased outside Europe, but the difference was not statistically significant. The hair dyes with black/brown shade contained higher concentrations of PPD compared to the hair dyes with red/blonder shades (335).

In Denmark, in 2001-2002, nine hair coloring products that had caused classic ACD with face, scalp and neck dermatitis developing within 1-2 days (sometimes hours) after hair coloring in nine patients were subjected to chemical analysis. Eight hair dye products contained toluene-2,5-diamine (0.18 to 0.98%). PPD (0.27%) was found in one product, and m-aminophenol (0.015 to 0.38%) and p-aminophenol (0.16 to 2.1%) were found in 3 products. The concentration levels were similar in the patients' products compared to a random control sample of 16 hair dye products (257).

Analyses of PPD in black henna temporary tattoo preparations (inks) have been reviewed in ref. 124.

Provocation and serial dilution tests

An open test was performed in 30 dermatitis patients with diagnosed PPD allergy and in 30 sex-matched and age-matched controls without PPD allergy (132). The test material was a marketed hair dye product containing 1.8% PPD and six other hair dye substances. It was applied without mixing with a developer. The test material was applied to the retro-auricular area on one side, the other side was used as a negative control, and the hair dye was left open for 48 hr without washing. On day 2, all 30 PPD-allergic individuals had erythema and infiltration, and 25 had vesicles. In the control group, 29 reactions were negative and one doubtful. On day 4, reactivity had decreased in most PPD-allergic individuals (132).

A follow-up study included 34 PPD-allergic individuals and 49 sex-matched and age-matched controls (23). The open test was performed in the same manner as in the first study, but this time hair dyes with increasing concentrations of PPD (A = 0.1%, B = 0.5%, C = 1.0%, and D = 1.5%) were tested consecutively, and a negative control substance (0% PPD) was included. The experiment showed that 27 of 34 PPD-allergic individuals reacted to product A (0.1% PPD), 3 of the 7 remaining PPD-allergic individuals reacted to further testing with product B (0.5% PPD), 3 of the 4 remaining reacted to further testing with product C (1.0% PPD), and the last individual, without reactions to products A–C, reacted to product D (1.5% PPD). No controls had positive reactions. In this study also, reactivity was generally stronger on day 2 after application than on to day 4 (23).

Danish investigators have performed occluded serial dilution patch testing in 15 PPD-allergic patients on the back, outer aspects of the arms, and behind the ears (133). One patient reacted to 50 ppm on the back, arm, and behind the ear, 2 patients reacted to 100 ppm on the back and outer aspects of the arm and 3 patients to 100 ppm behind the ears. The threshold values that elicited allergic contact dermatitis in 10% (ED10) of the patients were 38 ppm on the back, 56 ppm on the upper arm, and 75 ppm on the retro-auricular region (133).

In the UK, 16 PPD-allergic patients were patch tested to investigate the elicitation response over time (134). Seven patients were patch-tested with 1% PPD for 15, 30 and 120 minutes. The remaining 9 patients were patch tested with 1%, 0.3%, 0.1% and 0.01% (100 ppm) PPD for 15, 30 and 120 minutes each. With exposure time of 120 minutes, 11 of 16 subjects reacted to 1% PPD and 2 of 9 reacted to 0.01%. With exposure for 15 minutes, 6 of 16 reacted to 1% PPD and 0 of 9 reacted to 0.01% PPD. The study concluded that prolonged exposure and high exposure concentrations increase the risk of elicitation (134).

When PPD-allergic subjects were patch tested with a permanent hair dye product containing 0.5% PPD for, respectively, 30 minutes, 1 hour, and 24 hours, positive reactions were only observed in the 30 minutes group in subjects who had 2+ or 3+ patch test reactions to PPD prior to the study (135). Investigators in the UK performed a ROAT in 18 PPD-allergic patients. Application of 0.2 ml of 1% PPD in petrolatum to the antecubital fossa was performed daily for up to 8 days; each application was rubbed onto the skin for 1 minute, and then left for a further 4 minutes; excess material was then wiped away. After 8 days, 39% of the patients had reacted to the ROAT (136).

It has been shown in experimental studies that pretreatment of the skin with the antioxidant ascorbic acid has an attenuating effect on the elicitation reaction to PPD in patch tests materials and in hair dye formulations in PPD-sensitized individuals (263,264). Elicitation responses after application of a typical hair dye product containing 2% PPD for 30 minutes followed by rinsing (simulating exposure in actual hair dying) were analysed in 38 PPD-allergic individuals with a documented history of hair dye-related allergy. A positive reaction was elicited in 32 patients (84%). Of 20 patients with grades ++ to +++ patch test reactions to PPD, 20 (100%) had a positive reaction versus 12 of 18 (67%) with grade + PPD patch test reactions (284). In weakly sensitized individuals, the PPD exposure becoming available from a 2% PPD-containing hair-dye formulation within 30 minutes is too low to elicit a positive allergic reaction (285).

Miscellaneous side effects

Xanthelasmata palpebrarum

A normolipemic woman, who had been previously sensitized to PPD from a black henna tattoo, developed severe facial ACD from a black eyelash-tinting product (presumably containing PPD) and, thereafter, developed lesions of xanthelasmata palpebrarum. As xanthelasma has been reported previously following erythroderma and inflammatory skin disorders in the presence of normal lipid profiles, the development of xanthelasma in this patient was considered to be causally associated with the preceding allergic contact dermatitis to PPD in hair dye. The authors stated that the mechanism that initiates macrophage accumulation, cholesterol uptake and foam-cell formation in a normolipemic patient following an inflammatory skin disorder is not clearly understood, but that it may be related to increased plasma lipid peroxidation, derived from oxidized low-density lipoprotein (194).

Hair loss

Extensive irreversible follicular damage after repeated use of hair dyes in allergic subjects has been reported; it is unknown whether PPD was the allergenic culprit (208). A mild to moderate telogen effluvium was documented in 4 of 7 patients with allergic scalp contact dermatitis who completed a 6 month follow-up. In all these patients, the hair loss persisted for more than 3 months and was still present at 6 months. The diagnosis of telogen effluvium was confirmed by the pathological findings in the scalp, which showed a normal terminal-vellus ratio and a reduced anagen-telogen ratio in the absence of inflammatory infiltration (190).

Other information

To determine whether gloves are sufficiently protective when hairdressers are exposed to permanent dyes, six gloves from Sweden, Italy and Germany were studied: two vinyl, one natural rubber latex, two nitrile, and one polyethylene glove. The hair dye used for the provocation was a dark shade permanent dye containing PPD. The dye was mixed with hydrogen peroxide, and 8 PPD-sensitized volunteers were tested with the gloves as a membrane between the hair dye and the skin in a cylindrical open chamber system. Three exposure times (15, 30 and 60 minutes) were used. Eczematous reactions were found when natural rubber latex, polyethylene and vinyl gloves were tested with the dye. The nitrile gloves gave good protection, even after 60 minutes of exposure to the hair dye (274). Permeation of PPD through gloves has also been investigated in ref. 333.

Hypertrichosis, hypertrophic and keloidal scarring, hypopigmentation, hyperpigmentation and persistent leukoderma have been observed in patients with allergic reactions to PPD in black henna tattoos (124).

Is hair dyed with PPD allergenic?

In an early investigation, twenty patients with proven contact allergy to PPD were tested on two occasions with hair that had been dyed with PPD 24 hours previously, and none reacted (156,157). It was concluded that dyed hair is not allergenic and that sensitized individuals can have contact with it without risking an allergic reaction. However, there have been several case reports of individuals allergic to PPD who developed ACD – sometimes repeatedly – from contact with the dyed hair of their partners (202,271) or mother (201) or from wearing a wig dyed with PPD (232). Also, in some cases, there were positive patch tests to dyed hair (198,204). Indeed, it has been shown that, when the formation of the final coloring molecules is completed, up to 1.1% of unconsumed (unpolymerized) PPD is still present, which can be auto-oxidized to allergenic oxidation products (239).

OTHER SIDE EFFECTS

Photosensitivity

Two patients had photocontact allergy to PPD, one of who photo-cross-reacted to PABA and benzocaine (21). In China, between 2005 and 2014, 6017 patients suspected of photodermatoses were photopatch tested with PPD 1% pet. and 80 (1.4%) had a positive reaction. Unfortunately, the relevance of the positive photopatch tests was not mentioned (118). Positive photopatch tests to PPD with unknown relevance have also been reported a few times in other investigations (161,162).

Immediate-type reactions

There have been several case reports of immediate contact reactions with symptoms including contact urticaria, respiratory symptoms, anaphylaxis, anaphylactic shock and even one fatal anaphylactic reaction (5). The first case of contact urticaria from PPD in hair dye was reported in 1967; a scratch test with PPD 0.5% pet. provoked an immediate wheal (151). Two patients presented with urticaria localized on the scalp which developed while dying their hair; later, the wheals would spread all over the body. A 20 minute patch test with 1% PPD was positive in both individuals (147). A female doll-maker for some months had experienced painful palms with erythema and edema, which was worse while working with black cotton thread. She then developed urticaria all over the body. A patch test with PPD provoked an urticarial reaction after 20-30 minutes, as did the black cotton thread. The authors postulated that 'it is evident that this patient had occupational contact urticaria from para-phenylenediamine', but the presence of PPD in the thread was not ascertained (147).

Two individuals had combined type IV and type I allergy to PPD with both contact urticaria and allergic contact dermatitis (6,149). One patient had allergic reactions to hair dyes on four occasions. With each of these reactions, the patient's symptoms became progressively worse. These exposures culminated in an anaphylactic reaction, manifested by angioedema, dyspnea, hypotension, tachycardia, and loss of consciousness. Skin testing with the dye and its individual components demonstrated a wheal and flare response to an oxidation product of PPD. This product was N',N'-bis-(4-aminophenyl)-2,5-diamino-1,4-quinonediimine, also known as Bandrowski's base (CAS 20048-27-5). Passive transfer of this sensitivity by the patient's serum to a normal control implicated an IgE-mediated reaction (3).

Three patients from Japan had immediate-type reactions to PPD in hair dyes, of who one with anaphylactic shock; details are unknown (152,153, data cited in ref. 4). A woman had fainted within minutes of using a hair dye. Previously, she experienced wheals on her head and hands 10-30 minutes after applying the dye, which contained PPD. Another time, the itchy bumps had spread over her entire body and she had developed nausea, vomiting, and difficulty in breathing, accompanied by a cold sweat. All these symptoms disappeared spontaneously within 3 hours. Patch tests with the hair dye and its components disclosed an immediate-type allergy to PPD. A passive transfer test to her daughter was positive (4).

A woman had a history of anaphylactic reaction to hair dye 2 years before her death. After using a different hair dye preparation, the patient experienced shortness of breath, collapsed, and died. Autopsy findings were consistent with anaphylaxis (5). A woman who had used the same hair dye without problems for approximately 10 years, became giddy and flushed a few minutes after the application of the dye by the hairdresser. She felt generally ill and her eyesight became blurred, but there was no rash or difficulty in breathing. She went outside for some fresh air and then returned to have her hair finished off. In a next dying session, she became breathless with some chest pain, her speech became slurred and she had two bouts of diarrhea. Later, a challenge test was performed in the hospital. Twenty minutes after applying the dye to the entire scalp, the patient reported palpitations and chest tightness. She then became faint and flushed. The dye was washed off. Shortly afterwards her diastolic pressure began to drop and she developed a generalized urticarial rash. Skin tests to identify the culprit were not performed (145).

A man developed swelling of both eyelids 8 hours after using a hair dye. Subsequently, the whole face and both lips became swollen. He also developed itchy, exudative lesions on the scalp almost simultaneously. On examination, there was extensive periorbital and facial edema, and multiple eczematous lesions on the scalp. He was unable to open his eyes. No respiratory distress was evident. Patch tests showed sensitivity to the dye (10% aq.) and PPD. Prick testing revealed sensitivity to the hair dye (no controls performed). This case was presented as the first report of immediate-type reaction to PPD-containing hair dye from India (148). However, the late start of the reaction only after 8 hours, the eczematous lesions on the scalp and the positive patch tests point at a very strong contact allergic reaction rather than immediate-type hypersensitivity.

A female trainee hairdresser reported that her hands became red when coming into contact with certain hair dyes. Since commencing her training 5 months earlier, her normally very mild asthma had worsened such that while at work, she often found herself with both wheeze and chest tightness. She was scratch tested to 3 hair dyes that she had brought with her. Within 10 minutes, a strong urticarial reaction was seen from 2 of the dyes. Both the products contained PPD, and as the third did not, she was tested to PPD 1% in pet. which showed a positive urticarial reaction. The patient was subsequently examined by a respiratory physician who confirmed that she had occupational asthma to PPD (150).

A hairdresser with contact urticaria and anaphylaxis had a positive skin prick test to PPD (146). For this patient, reference was made to ref. 203, but in that report, the patient reacted to a skin prick test with toluene-2,5-diamine. The patient also had a positive patch test to PPD and a weak ?+ reaction to toluene-2,5-diamine (203). In a group of 664 patch tested patients, there were 2 (0.3%) immediate contact reactions to PPD as shown by 'well distinguished erythema' after 30 minutes (108).

A review of contact urticaria caused by ingredients of cosmetics has been provided in 2016 (123).

Other non-eczematous contact reactions

Depigmentation (leukoderma)

Chemical leukoderma is an acquired depigmentation dermatosis induced by repeated exposure to specific chemical compounds, including PPD. The depigmentation can occur secondarily to a preceding allergic contact dermatitis (especially in patients with vitiligo, Köbner phenomenon) or via direct toxic effects. The chemical structure of *p*-phenylenediamine is similar to tyrosine, which may be converted by tyrosine-related protein 1 into compounds toxic to the melanocyte. This leads to loss of melanocytes within the skin and hair follicle, resulting in skin depigmentation and greying of the hair (46).

Allergic depigmentation

An Indian woman became sensitized to PPD in a hair dye containing the color at 16%, which she left on for 3 hours. An exudative dermatitis of the scalp was followed 3-4 weeks later by depigmentation of the hair and the skin of the scalp and neck. It was concluded that the mechanism was a Köbner phenomenon in an individual susceptible to chemical leukoderma (48). Four cases of a contact leukoderma associated with the use of hair dye were reported in 1993 from the USA (35). Specific allergens were identified in 3 of the 4 patients, including benzyl alcohol and PPD. Three of the patients were not treated, and in only one of them did the pigment gradually return to all the affected areas, except the scalp. The 4th patient was treated with topical psoralen and UVA phototherapy for 18 months, which led to partial perifollicular repigmentation of the skin of the forehead and above the ears (35).

A woman suffering from vitiligo developed allergic contact dermatitis with hypertrophic features from PPD in a hair dye which had been applied to the skin for ornamental purposes, followed by persistent leukoderma. The positive PPD patch test mimicked the clinical picture with hypertrophic lesions followed by depigmentation (169). Contact leukoderma from hair colors was described in 4 patients. Depigmentation was limited to the site of application of the hair dyes. Two of 3 patients patch tested to PPD were positive. The 4th had a positive use test to the hair-coloring product itself. In two patients, the positive PPD patch test depigmented (170). An African-American man developed leukoderma of 30% of the scalp following allergic contact dermatitis to hair dye (235).

A man of Yemenite origin had contact leukoderma ('contact vitiligo') of the beard and temporal region, which was related to contact allergy to PPD in hair dye. The patient was treated using narrow-band UVB light, which led to a complete regression of all vitiliginous lesions after one year (236).

Non-allergic depigmentation

Between 2002 and 2007, in Kolkota, India, 864 patients were diagnosed with 'chemical leukoderma', characterized by sharply demarcated vitiligo-like macules (47). In 237 of these cases (27%), hair dyes were causative or co-causative to the depigmentation. PPD was a 'contributory chemical' in hair dyes, but also in black socks and shoes. Chemical leukoderma from PPD was not preceded by contact dermatitis. Hair dye (PPD)-induced chemical leukoderma was noticed in many cases at the hair margin rather than on the scalp itself. 'Confetti macules' represented an important diagnostic clue, but the differential diagnosis with vitiligo may, according to the authors, be difficult (47).

A woman developed an asymptomatic, depigmented area on her scalp with increased number of grey hair roots 2 days after application of hair dye containing PPD. She had been using the same hair dye for several years. Medical history and family history were non-contributory for vitiligo or autoimmune disease. A patch test with PPD was negative and the diagnosis was chemical leukoderma from PPD in hair dye (46). A man had non-allergic contact leukoderma of the upper lip caused by a moustache-coloring solution with four satellite lesions on the face and neck. He had no history nor physical signs of vitiligo (172).

Hyperpigmentation

A man had pigmented contact cheilitis from PPD in moustache dye (313).

Asthma

PPD is listed as a cause of occupational asthma in 'Asthma in the Workplace' (330), and in the United Kingdom Health and Safety Executive's publication 'Asthmagen? ', it was on the 'Watch List' for being a respiratory sensitizer (331). Based on these data and additional literature studying, PPD in a review article was labeled as a 'potential' cause of occupational asthma (332).

Several hairdressers developed occupational asthma or rhinitis from PPD; the pathogenesis was not mentioned (319). See also the section 'Immediate-type reactions' above.

Systemic side effects

PPD is very toxic when ingested. Patients with PPD poisoning have characteristic angioedema of the face and neck on initial presentation. Symptoms may start after 4-6 hours. There is marked orofacial swelling with swollen hard protruding tongue and edematous bull neck. The patient may have difficulty in breathing secondary to upper respiratory tract edema. The urine has a characteristic chocolate brown color. Other consistent features are rigidity and tenderness of the limbs secondary to rhabdomyolysis and acute renal failure. Toxic features include methemoglobinemia (308), gastritis, hoarseness of the voice, cardiac toxicity, hepatitis, convulsions, coma and sudden cardiac death. Hypotensive shock is recognized and is associated with poor prognosis. Death may occur from acute airway obstruction, acute renal failure and sudden cardiac arrest (154,155,167,287,288,289, 295,307). In Africa, the Middle East, and some Asian countries, PPD is easily accessible and a common poisoning agent (154). PPD has resulted in deaths from accidental, suicidal (299,301,302,309,343), and homicidal (309) ingestions (155). Most suicidal patients appear to be young women (344).

The topical use of henna mixed with p-phenylenediamine to dye the hair in Sudan and other countries has also caused many cases of intoxication, of which some have been fatal (105,106).

The literature on PPD toxicity in children, both from topical application and from ingestion, has been reviewed in 2010 (295).

Exposure to hair dye substances was in some epidemiological studies associated with the development of bladder cancer and non-Hodgkin's lymphoma (315). This controversial subject is considered to fall outside the scope of this book and is not discussed here.

LITERATURE

1   Uter W, Aberer W, Armario-Hita JC, Fernandez-Vozmediano JM, Ayala F, Balato A, et al. Current patch test results with the European baseline series and extensions to it from the 'European Surveillance System on Contact Allergy' network, 2007-2008. Contact Dermatitis 2012;67:9-19

2   Schnuch A, Lessmann H, Frosch PJ, Uter W. para-Phenylenediamine: the profile of an important allergen. Results of the IVDK. Br J Dermatol 2008;159:379-386 and [erratum] Br J Dermatol 2008;159:772

3   Goldberg BJ, Herman FF, Hirata I. Systemic anaphylaxis due to an oxidation product of p-phenylenediamine in a hair dye. Ann Allergy 1987;58:205-208

4   Fukunaga T, Kawagoe R, Hozumi H, Kanzani T. Contact anaphylaxis due to para-phenylenediamine. Contact Dermatitis 1996;35:185-186

5   Belton AL, Chira T. Fatal anaphylactic reaction to hair dye. Am J Forens Med Pathol 1997;18:290-292

6   Edwards EK Jr, Edwards EK. Contact urticaria and allergic contact dermatitis caused by paraphenylenediamine. Cutis 1984;34:877

7   Ho SC, Basketter D, Jefferies D, Rycroft RJ, White IR, McFadden JP. Analysis of para-phenylenediamine allergic patients in relation to strength of patch test reaction. Br J Dermatol 2005;153:364-367

8   Hussain I, Rani Z, Rashid T, Haroon TS. Suitability of the European standard series of patch test allergens in Pakistani patients. Contact Dermatitis 2002;46: 50-51

9   Brancaccio RR, Brown LH, Chang YT, Fogelman JP, Mafong EA, Cohen DE. Identification and quantification of para-phenylenediamine in a temporary black henna tattoo. Am J Contact Dermatitis 2002;13:15-18

10   Dawe SA, White IR, Rycroft RJ, Basketter DA, McFadden JP. Active sensitization to para-phenylenediamine and its relevance: a 10-year review. Contact Dermatitis 2004;51:96-97

11   Gawkrodger DJ, Paul L. Late patch test reactions: delayed immune response appears to be more common than active sensitization. Contact Dermatitis 2008;59:185-187

12   Hellinckx K, Goossens A. Late reactions to para-phenylenediamine are not always an indication of active sensitization: an example. Contact Dermatitis 2008;58:110

13   Hillen U, Jappe U, Frosch PJ, Becker D, Brasch J, Lilie M, et al. Late reactions to the patch-test preparations para-phenylenediamine and epoxy resin: a prospective multicentre investigation of the German Contact Dermatitis Research Group. Br J Dermatol 2006;154:665-670

14   Thyssen JP, Menné T, Nielsen NH, Linneberg A. Is there a risk of active sensitization to PPD by patch testing the general population? Contact Dermatitis 2007;57:133-134

15   Uter W, Hillen U, Geier J. Is incident sensitization to p-phenylenediamine related to particular exposure patterns? Results of a questionnaire study. Contact Dermatitis 2007;56:266-270

16   Thyssen JP, Menné T, Johansen JD. The increase in p-phenylenediamine allergy in Denmark is not explained by an increase in contact allergy to para group chemicals. Contact Dermatitis 2011;64:176-179

17   Wahlberg JE, Tammela M, Anderson C, Björkner B, Bruze M, FischerT, et al. Contact allergy to p-phenylenediamine in Sweden. Follow-up after reversed intervention. Derm Beruf Umwelt 2002;50:51-54

18   Uter W, Lessmann H, Geier J, Becker D, Fuchs T, Richter G. The spectrum of allergic (cross-)sensitivity in clinical patch testing with 'para amino' compounds. Allergy (Eur J All Clin Immmunol) 2002;57:319-322

19   Basketter DA, English J. Cross-reactions among hair dye allergens. Cut Ocular Toxicol 2009;28:104-106

20   Travassos AR, Claes L, Boey L, Drieghe J, Goossens A. Non-fragrance allergens in specific cosmetic products. Contact Dermatitis 2011;65:276-285

21   Wasserman GA, Haberman HF. Photosensitivity: results of investigation in 250 patients. Can Med Assoc J 1975;113:1055-1060

22   Aeby P, Sieber T, Beck H, Gerberick GF, Goebel C. Skin sensitization to p-phenylenediamine: the diverging roles of oxidation and N-acetylation for dendritic cell activation and the immune response. J Invest Dermatol 2009;129:99-109

23   Krasteva M, Cottin M, Cristaudo A, Lainé G, Nohynek G, Orton D, et al. Sensitivity and specificity of the consumer open skin allergy test as a method of prediction of contact dermatitis to hair dyes. Eur J Dermatol 2005;15:18-25

24   Thyssen JP, Giménez-Arnau E, Lepoittevin J-P, Menné T, Boman A, Schnuch A. The critical review of methodologies and approaches to assess the inherent skin sensitizing potential (skin allergies) of chemicals. Part II. Contact Dermatitis 2012;66 (Suppl.1):25-52

25   Devos SA, Van der Valk PGM. The risk of active sensitization to PPD. Contact Dermatitis 2001;44:273-275

26   Kazandjieva J, Grozdev I, Tsankov N. Temporary henna tattoos. Clin Dermatol 2007;25:383-387

27   Wetter DA, Yiannias JA, Prakash AV, Davis MD, Farmer SA, el-Azhary RA, et al. Results of patch testing to personal care product allergens in a standard series and a supplemental cosmetic series: an analysis of 945 patients from the Mayo Clinic Contact Dermatitis Group, 2000-2007. J Am Acad Dermatol 2010;63:789-798

28   Adams RM, Maibach HI, Clendenning WE, Fisher AA, Jordan WJ, Kanof N, et al. A five-year study of cosmetic reactions. J Am Acad Dermatol 1985;13:1062-1069

29   Davis MD, Scalf LA, Yiannias JA, Cheng JF, El-Azhary RA, Rohlinger AL, et al. Changing trends and allergens in the patch test standard series. Arch Dermatol 2008;144:67-72

30   Warshaw EM, Buchholz HJ, Belsito DV et al. Allergic patch test reactions associated with cosmetics: Retrospective analysis of cross-sectional data from the North American Contact Dermatitis Group, 2001-2004. J Am Acad Dermatol 2009;60:23-38

31   ESSCA Writing Group. The European Surveillance System of Contact Allergies (ESSCA): results of patch testing the standard series, 2004. J Eur Acad Dermatol Venereol 2008;22:174-181

32   Iorizzo M, Parente G, Vincenzi C, Pazzaglia M, Tosti A. Allergic contact dermatitis in hairdressers; frequency and source of sensitization. Eur J Dermatol 2002;12:179-182

33   Frosch PJ, Kügler K, Geier J. Patch testing with hydroxyethyl-p-phenylenediamine sulfate – cross-reactivity with p-phenylenediamine. Contact Dermatitis 2011;65:96-100

34   Zug KA, Warshaw EM, Fowler JF Jr, Maibach HI, Belsito DL, Pratt MD, et al. Patch-test results of the North American Contact Dermatitis Group 2005-2006. Dermatitis 2009;20:149-160

35 Taylor JS, Maibach HI, Fisher AA, Bergfeld WF. Contact leukoderma associated with the use of hair colors. Cutis 1993;52:273-280

36 Fransway AF, Zug KA, Belsito DV, Deleo VA, Fowler JF Jr, Maibach HI, et al. North American Contact Dermatitis Group patch test results for 2007-2008. Dermatitis 2013;24:10-21

37 Warshaw EM, Belsito DV, DeLeo VA, Fowler JF Jr, Maibach HI, Marks JG, et al. North American Contact Dermatitis Group patch-test results, 2003-2004 study period. Dermatitis 2008;19:129-136

38 Almeida PJ, Borrego L, Limiñana JM. Age-related sensitization to p-phenylenediamine. Contact Dermatitis 2011;64:172-174

39 Brasch J, Becker D, Aberer W Bircher A, Kränke B, Denzer-Fürst S, et al. Contact Dermatitis. J Dtsch Dermatol Ges 2007;5:943-951

40 Thyssen JP, Carlsen BC, Søsted H, Menné T, Johansen JD. Frequency of p-phenylenediamine (PPD) sensitization among Danish eczema patients tested between 1985 and 2007. Contact Dermatitis 2008;59:184-185

41 Hoeller Obrigkeit D, Vens N, Merk HF, Schroeder CM. Contact allergens in the standard patch test series from 1980–2004 at the University Clinic Aachen. Hautarzt 2005;56:1125-1132

42 Lindberg M, Edman B, Fischer T, Stenberg B. Time trends in Swedish patch test data from 1992 to 2000. A multi-centre study based on age- and sex-adjusted results of the Swedish standard series. Contact Dermatitis 2007;56:205-210

43 Patel S, Basketter DA, Jefferies D, White IR, Rycroft RJ, McFadden JP, et al. Patch test frequency to p-phenylenediamine: follow up over the last 6 years. Contact Dermatitis 2007;56:35-37

44 Malvestio A, Bovenzi M, Hoteit M, Belloni Fortina A, Peserico A, Corradin MT, et al. p-Phenylenediamine sensitization and occupation. Contact Dermatitis 2011;64:37-42

45 Warshaw EM, Wang MZ, Mathias CGT, Maibach HI, Belsito DV, Zug KA, et al. Occupational contact dermatitis in hairdressers/cosmetologists; retrospective analysis of North American Contact Dermatitis Group data, 1994 to 2010. Dermatitis 2012;23:258-268

46 Farsani TT, Jalian HR, Young CL. Chemical leukoderma from hair dye containing para-phenylenediamine. Dermatitis 2012;23:181-182

47 Ghosh S, Mukhopadhyay S. Chemical leucoderma: a clinico-aetiological study of 864 cases in the perspective of a developing country. Br J Dermatol 2009;160:40-47

48 Bajaj AK, Gupta SC, Chatterjee AK, Singh KG, Basu S, Kant A. Hair dye depigmentation. Contact Dermatitis 1996;35:56-57

49 Wenk KS, Ehrlich AE. Fragrance series testing in eyelid dermatitis. Dermatitis 2012;23:22-26

50 Laberge L, Pratt M, Fong B, Gavigan G. A 10-year review of p-phenylenediamine allergy and related para-amino compounds at the Ottawa patch test clinic. Dermatitis 2011;22:332-334

51 Sidbury R, Storrs FJ. Pruritic eruption at the site of a temporary tattoo. Am J Contact Dermat 2000;11:182-183

52 Wakelin SH, Creamer D, Rycroft RJG, White IR, McFadden JP. Contact dermatitis from para-phenylenediamine used as skin paint. Contact Dermatitis 1998;39:92-93

53 Spornraft-Ragaller P, Kämmerer E, Gillitzer C, Schmitt J. Severe allergic reactions to para-phenylenediamine in children and adolescents: should the patch test concentration of PPD be changed? J Dtsch Dermatol Ges 2012;10:258-263

54 Gonzalo-Garijo MA, Fernandéz-Duràn DA, Pérez-Calderòn R, Sánchez-Carvajal J. Allergic contact dermatitis due to a temporary henna tattoo, a hair dye and a marker pen. J Investig Allergol Clin Immunol 2008;18:226-227

55 Di Prisco MC, Puig L, Alomar A. Contact dermatitis due to paraphenylenediamine (PPD) on a temporal tattoo with henna. Cross reaction to azoic dyes. Invest Clin 2006;47:295-299

56 Matulich J, Sullivan J. A temporary henna tattoo causing hair and clothing dye allergy. Contact Dermatitis 2005;53:33-36

57 Le Coz CJ, Lefebvre C, Keller F, Grosshans E. Allergic contact dermatitis caused by skin painting (pseudotattooing) with black henna, a mixture of henna and p-phenylenediamine and its derivatives. Arch Dermatol 2000;136:1515-1517

58 Van den Keybus C, Morren MA, Goossens A. Walking difficulties due to an allergic reaction to a temporary tattoo. Contact Dermatitis 2005;53:180-181

59 Kind F, Scherer K, Bircher AJ. Contact dermatitis to para-phenylenediamine in hair dye following sensitization to black henna tattoos – an ongoing problem. J Dtsch Dermatol Ges 2012;10:572-577

60 Redlick F, DeKoven J. Allergic contact dermatitis to paraphenylenediamine in hair dye after sensitization from black henna tattoos: a report of 6 cases. CMAJ 2007;176:445-446

61 Søsted H, Johansen JD, Andersen KE, Menné T. Severe allergic hair dye reactions in 8 children. Contact Dermatitis 2006;54:87-91

62 Martin JA, Hughes TM, Stone NM. 'Black henna' tattoos: an occult source of natural rubber latex allergy? Contact Dermatitis 2005;52:145-146

63 Jasim ZF, Darling JR, Handley JM. Severe allergic contact dermatitis to paraphenylene diamine in hair dye following sensitization to black henna tattoos. Contact Dermatitis 2005;52:116-117

64 Kluger N, Raison-Peyron N, Guillot B. Tatouages temporaires au henné: des effets indésirables parfois graves. Presse Med 2008;37:1138-1142

65 Ho, White IR, Rycroft RJ, McFadden JP. A new approach to patch testing patients with para-phenylenediamine allergy secondary to temporary black henna tattoos. Contact Dermatitis 2004;51:213-214

66 Jung P, Sesztak-Greinecker G, Wantke F, Götz M, Jarisch R, Hemmer W. The extent of black henna tattoo's complications are not restricted to PPD-sensitization. Contact Dermatitis 2006;55:57

67 Vogel TA, Coenraads P-J, Bijkersma LM, Vermeulen KM, Schuttelaar M-LA and on behalf of the EDEN Fragrance Study Group. p-Phenylenediamine exposure in real life – a case–control study on sensitization rate, mode and elicitation reactions in the northern Netherlands. Contact Dermatitis 2015;72:355-361

68 Warshaw EM, Maibach HI, Taylor JS, Sasseville D, DeKoven JG, Zirwas MJ, et al. North American Contact Dermatitis Group patch test results: 2011-2012. Dermatitis 2015;26:49-59

69 Warshaw EM, Belsito DV, Taylor JS, Sasseville D, DeKoven JG, Zirwas MJ, et al. North American Contact Dermatitis Group patch test results: 2009 to 2010. Dermatitis 2013;24:50-59

70 Janach, M, Kühne A, Seifert B, French LE, Ballmer-Weber B, Hofbauer GFL. Changing delayed-type sensitizations to the baseline series allergens over a decade at the Zurich University Hospital. Contact Dermatitis 2010;63:42-48

71 Landeck L, John SM, Geier J. Periorbital dermatitis in 4779 patients – patch test results during a 10-year period. Contact Dermatitis 2014;70:205-212

72 Goossens A. Cosmetic contact allergens. Cosmetics 2016;3. doi: 10.3390/cosmetics3010005

73 Pratt MD, Belsito DV, DeLeo VA, Fowler JF Jr, Fransway AF, Maibach HI, et al. North American Contact Dermatitis Group patch-test results, 2001–2002 study period. Dermatitis 2004;15:176-183

74 Marks JG Jr, Belsito DV, DeLeo VA, Fowler JF Jr, Fransway AF, Maibach HI, et al. North American Contact Dermatitis Group patch-test results, 1998–2000. Am J Contact Dermat 2003;14:59-62

75 Wetter DA, Davis MDP, Yiannias JA, Cheng JF, Connolly SM, el-Azhary RA, et al. Patch test results from the Mayo Contact Dermatitis Group, 1998–2000. J Am Acad Dermatol 2005;53:416-421

76 Britton JE, Wilkinson SM, English JSC, Gawkrodger DJ, Ormerod AD, Sansom JE, et al. The British standard series of contact dermatitis allergens: validation in clinical practice and value for clinical governance. Br J Dermatol 2003;148:259-264

77 Hasan T, Rantanen T, Alanko K, Harvima RJ, Jolanki R, Kalimo K, et al. Patch test reactions to cosmetic allergens in 1995–1997 and 2000–2002 in Finland –a multicentre study. Contact Dermatitis 2005;53:40-45

78 Lazarov A. European Standard Series patch test results from a contact dermatitis clinic in Israel during the 7-year period from 1998 to 2004. Contact Dermatitis 2006;55:73-76

79 Akyol A, Boyvat A, Peksari Y, Gurgey E. Contact sensitivity to standard series allergens in 1038 patients with contact dermatitis in Turkey. Contact Dermatitis 2005;52:333-337

80 Uter W, Hegewald J, Aberer W, Ayala F, Bircher AJ, Brasch J, et al. The European standard series in 9 European countries, 2002/2003 –First results of the European Surveillance System on Contact Allergies. Contact Dermatitis 2005;53:136-145

81 Machovcova A, Dastychova E, Kostalova D, et al. Common contact sensitizers in the Czech Republic. Patch test results in 12,058 patients with suspected contact dermatitis. Contact Dermatitis 2005;53:162-166

82 Bruynzeel DP, Diepgen TL, Andersen KE, Brandão FM, Bruze M, Frosch PJ, et al (EECDRG). Monitoring the European Standard Series in 10 centres 1996–2000. Contact Dermatitis 2005;53:146-152

83 Fall S, Bruze M, Isaksson M, Lidén C, Matura M, Stenberg B, Lindberg M. Contact allergy trends in Sweden – a retrospective comparison of patch test data from 1992, 2000, and 2009. Contact Dermatitis 2015;72:297-304

84 Amin KA, Belsito DV. The aetiology of eyelid dermatitis: a 10-year retrospective analysis. Contact Dermatitis 2006;55:280-285

85 Wentworth AB, Yiannias JA, Keeling JH, Hall MR, Camilleri MJ, Drage LA, et al. Trends in patch-test results and allergen changes in the standard series: a Mayo Clinic 5-year retrospective review (January 1, 2006, to December 31, 2010). J Am Acad Dermatol 2014;70:269-275

86 Valks R, Conde-Salazar L, Malfeito J, Ledo S. Contact dermatitis in hairdressers, 10 years later: patch-test results in 300 hairdressers (1994 to 2003) and comparison with previous study. Dermatitis 2005;16:28-31

87 Uter W, Lessmann H, Geier J, Schnuch A. Contact allergy to ingredients of hair cosmetics in female hairdressers and clients: an 8-year analysis of IVDK data. Contact Dermatitis 2003;49:236-240

88 Katsarou A, Koufou B, Takou K, Kalogeromitros D, Papanayiotou G, Vareltzidis A. Patch test results in hairdressers with contact dermatitis in Greece (1985-1994). Contact Dermatitis 1995;33:347-348

89 Conde-Salazar L, Baz M, Guimaraens D, Cannavo A. Contact dermatitis in hairdressers: patch test results in 379 hairdressers (1980-1993). Am J Cont Dermat 1995;6:19-23

90 Thyssen JP, Uter W, Schnuch A, Linneberg A, Johansen JD. 10-year prevalence of contact allergy in the general
    population in Denmark estimated through the CE-DUR method. Contact Dermatitis 2007;57:265-272

91 Schnuch A, Uter W, Geier J, Gefeller O (for the IVDK study group). Epidemiology of contact allergy: an estimation
    of morbidity employing the clinical epidemiology and drug-utilization research (CE-DUR) approach. Contact
    Dermatitis 2002;47:32-39

92 Diepgen TL, Ofenloch RF, Bruze M, Bertuccio P, Cazzaniga S, Coenraads P-J, et al. Prevalence of contact allergy in
    the general population in different European regions. Br J Dermatol 2016;174:319-329

93 Mortz CG, Bindslev-Jensen C, Andersen KE. Prevalence, incidence rates and persistence of contact allergy and
    allergic contact dermatitis in The Odense Adolescence Cohort Study: a 15-year follow-up. Brit J Dermatol
    2013;168:318-325

94 Thyssen JP, Linneberg A, Menné T, Nielsen NH, Johansen JD. Contact allergy to allergens of the TRUE-test (panels
    1 and 2) has decreased modestly in the general population. Br J Dermatol 2009;161:1124-1129

95 Nielsen SH, Menné T. Allergic contact sensitization in an unselected Danish population. The Glostrup Allergy
    Study, Denmark. Acta Derm Venereol 1992;72:456-460

96 Dotterud LK, Smith-Sivertsen T. Allergic contact sensitization in the general adult population: a population-based
    study from Northern Norway. Contact Dermatitis 2007;56:10-15

97 Nielsen NH, Linneberg A, Menné T, Madsen F, Frølund L, Dirksen A, et al. Allergic contact sensitization in an
    adult Danish population: two cross-sectional surveys eight years apart (the Copenhagen Allergy Study). Acta
    Derm Venereol 2001;81:31-34

98 White JML, Gilmour NJ, Jeffries D, Duangdeeden I, Kullavanijaya P, Basketter DA, et al. A general population from
    Thailand: incidence of common allergens with emphasis on para-phenylenediamine. Clin Exp Allergy
    2007;37:1848-1853

99 Mortz CG, Lauritsen JM, Bindslev-Jensen C, Andersen KE. Contact allergy and allergic contact dermatitis in
    adolescents: prevalence measures and associations. Acta Derm Venereol 2002;82:352-358

100 Schäfer T, Böhler E, Ruhdorfer S, Weigl L, Wessner D, Filipiak B, et al. Epidemiology of contact allergy in adults.
    Allergy 2001;56:1192-1196

101 Mortz CG, Lauritsen JM, Bindslev-Jensen C, Andersen KE. Prevalence of atopic dermatitis, asthma, allergic
    rhinitis, and hand and contact dermatitis in adolescents. The Odense Adolescence Cohort Study on Atopic
    Diseases and Dermatitis. Br J Dermatol 2001;144:523-532

102 Seidenari S, Manzini BM, Danese P, Motolese A. Patch and prick test study of 593 healthy subjects. Contact
    Dermatitis 1990; 23:162-167

103 Uter W, Ludwig A, Balda BR, Schnuch A, Pfahlberg A, Schäfer T, Wichmann HE, Ring J. The prevalence of contact
    allergy differed between population-based data and clinic–based data. J Clin Epidemiol 2004;57:627-632

104 De Groot AC. Contact allergy to cosmetics: Causative ingredients. Contact Dermatitis 1987;17:26-34

105 D'Arcy PF. Fatalities with the use of a henna dye. Pharmacy Int 1982;3:217

106 El-Ansary EH, Ahmed MEK, Clague HW. Systemic toxicity of para-phenylenediamine. Lancet 1983;1:1341-1343

107 Herbst RA, Uter W, Pirker C, Geier J, Frosch PJ. Allergic and non-allergic periorbital dermatitis: patch test results
    of the Information Network of the Departments of Dermatology during a 5-year period. Contact Dermatitis
    2004;51:13-19

108 Katsarou A, Armenaka M, Ale I, Koufou V, Kalogeromitros, D. Frequency of immediate reactions to the European
    standard series. Contact Dermatitis 1999;41:276-279

109 SCCS (Scientific Committee on Consumer Safety). Opinion on p-phenylenediamine, SCCS/1443/11, 26-27 June
    2012. Available at: http://ec.europa.eu/health/scientific_committees/consumer_safety/docs/sccs_o_094.pdf

110 SCCP (Scientific Committee on Consumer Products). Opinion on p-Phenylenediamine, 10 October 2006, SCCP/
    0989/06. Available at: http://ec.europa.eu/health/archive/ph_risk/committees/04_sccp/docs/sccp_o_069.pdf

111 SCCNFP (Scientific Committee on Cosmetics and Non Food Products). Opinion concerning p-phenylenediami-ne,
    27 February 2002, SCCNFP/0129/99. Available at:
    http://ec.europa.eu/health/archive/ph_risk/committees/sccp/documents/out156_en.pdf

112 Laguna C, de la Cuadra J, Martín-González B, Zaragoza V, Martínez-Casimiro L, Alegre V. Allergic contact
    dermatitis to cosmetics. Actas Dermosifiliogr 2009;100:53-60

113 Toholka R, Wang Y-S, Tate B, Tam M, Cahill J, Palmer A, Nixon R. The first Australian Baseline Series:
    Recommendations for patch testing in suspected contact dermatitis. Australas J Dermatol 2015;56:107-115

114 DeKoven JG, Warshaw EM, Belsito DV, Sasseville D, Maibach HI, Taylor JS, et al. North American Contact
    Dermatitis Group Patch Test Results: 2013-2014. Dermatitis 2017;28:33-46

115 Boonchai W, Bunyavaree M, Winayanuwattikun W, Kasemsarn P. Contact sensitizers in commercial hair dye
    products sold in Thailand. Contact Dermatitis 2016;74:222-229

116 Zaragoza-Ninet V, Blasco Encinas R, Vilata-Corell JJ, Pérez-Ferriols A, Sierra-Talamantes C, Esteve-Martínez A, de
    la Cuadra-Oyanguren J. Allergic contact dermatitis due to cosmetics: A clinical and epidemiological study in a
    tertiary hospital. Actas Dermosifiliogr 2016;107:329-336

117 Thorén S, Yazar K. Contact allergens in 'natural' hair dyes. Contact Dermatitis 2016;74:302-304

118 Hu Y, Wang D, Shen Y, Tang H. Photopatch testing in Chinese patients over 10 years. Dermatitis 2016;27:137-142

119 Uter W, Rämsch C, Aberer, W, Ayala F, Balato A, Beliauskiene A, et al. The European baseline series in 10 European Countries, 2005/2006 – Results of the European Surveillance System on Contact Allergies (ESSCA). Contact Dermatitis 2009;61:31-38

120 Dooms-Goossens A, de Boulle K, Dooms M, Degreef H. Imidazolidinyl urea dermatitis. Contact Dermatitis 1986;14:322-324

121 Raber L. What's that stuff? Chem Eng News 2000;78:52

122 Cathelineau H. Note sur 18 cases d'accidents provoqués par teinture pour cheveux à base de chlorhydrate de PPD. Bull Soc Fr Dermatol Syphil 1898;9:28-35

123 Verhulst L, Goossens A. Cosmetic components causing contact urticaria: a review and update. Contact Dermatitis 2016;75:333-344

124 De Groot AC. Side-effects of henna and semi-permanent 'black henna' tattoos: a full review. Contact Dermatitis 2013;69:1-25

125 Hillen U, Grabbe S, Uter W. Patch test results in patients with scalp dermatitis: analysis of data of the Information Network of Departments of Dermatology. Contact Dermatitis 2007;56:87-93

126 Aalto-Korte K, Alanko K, Kuuliala O, Jolanki R. Late reactions in patch tests: a 4-year review from a clinic of occupational dermatology. Contact Dermatitis 2007;56:81-86

127 Le Coz CJ, El Bakali A, Untereiner F, Grosshans E. Active sensitization to budesonide and para-phenylenediamine from patch testing. Contact Dermatitis 1998;39:153-155

128 Arnold WP, van Joost T, van der Valk PGM. Adding p-aminoazobenzene may increase the sensitivity of the European standard series in detecting contact allergy to dyes, but carries the risk of active sensitization. Contact Dermatitis 1995;33:444

129 Calnan CD. Active sensitization to para and balsam of Peru. Contact Dermatitis 1975;1:126-127

130 Hillen U, Dickel H, Löffler H, Pfützner W, Mahler V, Becker D, et al. Late reactions to patch test preparations with reduced concentrations of p-phenylenediamine: a multicentre investigation of the German Contact Dermatitis Research Group. Contact Dermatitis 2011;64:196-202

131 Jensen, CD, Paulsen E, Andersen KE. Retrospective evaluation of the consequence of alleged patch test sensitization. Contact Dermatitis 2006;55:30-35

132 Krasteva M, Cristaudo A, Hall B, Orton D, Rudzki E, Santucci B, Toutain H, Wilkinson J. Contact sensitivity to hair dyes can be detected by the consumer open test. Eur J Dermatol 2002;12:322-326

133 Søsted H, Menné T, Johansen JD. Patch test dose–response study of p-phenylenediamine: thresholds and anatomical regional differences. Contact Dermatitis 2006;54:145-149

134 McFadden JP, Wakelin SH, Holloway DB, Basketter DA. The effect of patch duration on the elicitation of para-phenylenediamine contact allergy. Contact Dermatitis 1998;39:79-81

135 Jowsey IR, Basketter DA, McFadden JP, Kullavanijaya P, Duangdeeden I. Elicitation response characteristics to permanent hair dye in paraphenylenediamine-allergic volunteers. Contact Dermatitis 2006;55:330-334

136 Hextall JM, Alagaratnam NJ, Glendinning AK, Holloway DB, Blaikie L, Basketter DA, McFadden JP. Dose–time relationships for elicitation of contact allergy to para-phenylenediamine. Contact Dermatitis 2002;47:96-99

137 Schultz E, Mahler V. Prolonged lichenoid reaction and cross-sensitivity to para-substituted amino-compounds due to temporary henna tattoo. Int J Dermatol 2002;41:301-303

138 Marcoux D, Couture-Trudel PM, Riboulet-Delmas G, Sasseville D. Sensitization to para-phenylenediamine from a streetside temporary tattoo. Pediatr Dermatol 2002;19:498-502

139 Hink E, de Winter JP. Hair-dye allergy: a coloured case. Eur J Pediatr 2006;165:195-196

140 Onder M. Temporary holiday 'tattoos' may cause lifelong allergic contact dermatitis when henna is mixed with PPD. J Cosmet Dermatol 2003;2:126-130

141 Castelain M. Allergie a la PPD: une cause inhabitualle de sensibilisation. Lettre du GERDA 1999;16:57-58

142 Clayton TH, Wilkinson SM, Rawcliffe C, Pollock B, Clark SM. Allergic contact dermatitis in children: should pattern of dermatitis determine referral? A retrospective study of 500 children tested between 1995 and 2004 in one U.K. centre. Br J Dermatol 2006;154:114-117

143 Park J, Ro Y. Occupational skin disease in hairdressers: Results of patch test. Korean J Dermatol 2006;44:669-674

144 Uter W, Lessmann H, Geier J, et al. Contact allergy to hairdressing allergens in female hairdressers and clients. Current data from the IVDK, 2003-2006. J Dtsch Dermatol Ges 2007;5:993-1001.

145 Mavroleon G, Begishvili B, Frew A J. Anaphylaxis to hair dye: a case report. Clin Exp Dermatol 1998;28:121-122

146 Helaskoski E, Suolajehto H, Kuuliala O, Aalto-Korte K. Prick testing with chemicals in the diagnosis of occupational contact urticaria and respiratory diseases. Contact Dermatitis 2014;72:20-32

147 Temesvari E. Contact urticaria from paraphenylenediamine. Contact Dermatitis 1984;11:125

148 Sahoo B, Handa S, Penchallaiah K, Kumar B. Contact anaphylaxis due to hair dye. Contact Dermatitis 2000;43:244

149 Wong GA, King CM. Immediate-type hypersensitivity and allergic contact dermatitis due to para-phenylenediamine in hair dye. Contact Dermatitis 2003;48:166

150 Birnie AJ, English JS. Immediate hypersensitivity to paraphenylenediamine. Contact Dermatitis 2007;56:240

151 Calnan CD. Hair dye reaction. Contact Dermatitis Newsletter 1967;1:16

152 Kantoh H, Noike N, Tuyuki S. Summary of hair coloring contact dermatitis for the past 2 years. Hifubyou Sinryou 1990;12:1141-1144 (in Japanese, data cited in ref. 4)

153 Kawai K, Yasuno Y. Anaphylatic shock due to hair dye. Rinsyou Hifuka 1990;44:803-807 (in Japanese, data cited in ref. 4)

154 Ashraf W, Dawling S, Farrow LJ. Systemic paraphenylenediamine (PPD) poisoning: a case report and review. Hum Exp Toxicol 1994;13:167-170

155 Hashim M, Hamza YO, Yahia B, Khogali FM, Suileman GI. Poisoning from henna dye and para-phenylene- diamine mixtures in children in Kartoum. Ann Trop Paediatr 1992;12:3-6

156 Fisher AA. Is hair dyed with para-phenylenediamine allergenic?. Contact Dermatitis 1975;1:266

157 Reiss F, Fisher AA. Is hair dyed with para-phenylenediamine allergenic? Arch Dermatol 1974;109:221-222

158 Schonning L, Hjorth N. Cross-sensitization between hair dyes and rubber chemicals. Berufsdermatosen 1969;17:100-106

159 Shmunes E. Purpuric allergic contact dermatitis to paraphenylenediamine . Contact Dermatitis 1978;4:225-229

160 Storrs FJ, Taylor J, Jordan WP, Maibach HI. Paraphenylenediamine dihydrochloride. Contact Dermatitis 1979;5:126

161 LeVine MJ. Idiopathic photodermatitis with a positive paraphenylenediamine photopatch test. Arch Dermatol 1984;120:1488-1490

162 Wasserman GA, Haberman HF. Photosensitivity results of investigation of 250 patients. Can Med Assoc J 1975;113:1055-1059

163 Tosti A, Bardazzi F, Valeri F, Toni F. Erythema multiforme with contact dermatitis to hair dyes. Contact Dermatitis 1987;17:321-322

164 Möllgaard B, Hansen J, Kreilgård B, Wildfang IL. Cross-sensitization in guinea pigs between p-phenylene diamine and oxidation products thereof. Contact Dermatitis 1990;23:274

165 Saha M, Srinivas CR. Footwear dermatitis possibly due to para-phenylenediamine in socks. Contact Dermatitis 1993;28:295

166 Bork K. Allergic contact dermatitis on a violinist's neck from para-phenylenediamine in a chin rest stain. Contact Dermatitis 1993;28:250-251

167 Averbukh Z, Modai D, Leonov Y, Weissgarten J, Lewinsohn G, Fucs L, et al. Rhabdomyolysis and acute renal failure induced by paraphenylenediamine. Hum Toxicol 1989;8:345-348

168 Vincenzi C, Stinchi C, Guerra L, Piraccini BM, Bardazzi F, Tosti A. Erythema multiformlike contact dermatitis: Report of four cases. Am J Cont Derm 1994;5:90-93

169 Santucci B, Cristaudo A, Cannistraci C, Amantea A, Picardo M. Hypertrophic allergic contact dermatitis from hair dye. Contact Dermatitis 1994;31:169-171

170 Taylor JS, Maibach HI, Fisher AA, Bergfeld WF. Contact ;eikoderma associated with the use of hair colors. Cutis 1993;52:273-280

171 Rebandel P, Rudzki E. Occupational allergy to p-phenylendiamine in milk testers. Contact Dermatitis 1995;33:138

172 Brancaccio R, Cohen DE. Contact leukoderma secondary to para-phenylenediamine. Contact Dermatitis 1995;32:313

173 Weller R, Ormerod A. Water tester's dermatitis due to a para-phenylenediamine derivative. Contact Dermatitis 1996;34:138

174 Nakagawa M, Kawai K, Kawai K. Multiple azo disperse dye sensitization mainly due to group sensitizations to azo dyes. Contact Dermatitis 1996;34:6-11

175 Seidenari S, Mantovani L, Manzini BM, Pignatti M. Cross-sensitizations between azo dyes and para-amino compound. Contact Dermatitis 1997;36:91-96

176 Armstrong DKB, Jones AB, Smith HR, Ross JS, White IR, Rycroft RJG, McFadden JP. Occupational sensitization to p-phenylenediamine: a 17-year review. Contact Dermatitis 1999;41:348-349

177 Sharma VK, Mandal SK, Sethuraman G, Bakshi NA. Para-phenylenediamine-induced lichenoid eruptions. Contact Dermatitis 1999;41:40-41

178 Gallo R, Ghigliotti G, Cozzani E, Balestrero S. Contact dermatitis from para-phenylenediamine used as a skin paint: a further case. Contact Dermatitis 1999;40:57

179 Lodi A, Mancini LL, Ambonati M, Coassini A, Ravanelli G, Crosti C. Epidemiology of occupational contact dermatitis in a North Italian population. Eur J Dermatol 2000;10:128-132

180 Brocq L. Les éruptions eczématiformes provoqués par une teinture pour cheveaux à base de chlorohydrate de paraphénylenediamine. Bull Med 1898;12:237-241

181 Shapiro M, Mowad C, James WD. Contact dermatitis due to printer's ink in a milk industry employee: Case report and review of the allergen paraphenylenediamine. Am J Cont Derm 2001;12:109-112

182 Hansson C, Thorneby-Andersson K. Allergic contact dermatitis from 2-chloro-*p*-phenylenediamine in a cream dye for eyelashes and eyebrows. Contact Dermatitis 2001;45:235-236

183 O'Hagan AH, Bingham EA. Cellist's finger dermatitis. Contact Dermatitis 2001;45:319

184 Han Y-C, Ng S-K, Goh C-L. Positive patch-test reactions to para-phenylenediamine, their clinical relevance and the concept of clinical tolerance. Contact Dermatitis 2001;45:217-220

185 Søsted H, Agner T, Andersen KE, Menné T. 55 cases of allergic reactions to hair dye: a descriptive, consumer complaint-based study. Contact Dermatitis 2002;47:299-303

186 Gerberick F, Robinson MK, Ryan CA, Dearman RJ, Kimber I, Basketter DA, et al. Contact allergenic potency: Correlation of human and local lymph node assay data. Am J Contact Dermatitis 2001;3:156-161

187 Marzulli FN, Maibach HI. The use of graded concentrations in studying skin sensitizers: experimental contact sensitization in man. Fd Cosmet Toxicol 1974;12:219-227

188 Benezra CB, Sigman CC, Bagheri D, Tucker Helmes T, Maibach HI. A systemic Search for structure-activity relationships of skin sensitizers. II. Para-phenylenediamines. Semin Dermatol 1989;8:88-93

189 Wahlberg J, Tammela M, Anderson C, et al. Contact allergy to PPD in Sweden. Dermatol Beruf Umwelt 2002;50:51-54

190 Tosti A, Piraccini BM, van Neste DJJ. Telogen effluvium after allergic contact dermatitis of the scalp. Arch Dermatol 2001;137:187-190

191 Shah M, Lewis FM, Gawkrodger D J. Occupational dermatitis in hairdressers. Contact Dermatitis 1996;35:364-365

192 Calzavara-Pinton P, Capezzera R, Zane C, Brezzi A, Pasolini G, Ubiali A, Facchetti F. Lymphomatoid allergic contact dermatitis from para-phenylenediamine. Contact Dermatitis 2002;47:173-174

193 Fautz R, Fuchs A, Van der Walle H, Henny V, Smits L. Hair dye-sensitized hairdressers: the cross-reaction pattern with new generation hair dyes. Contact Dermatitis 2002;46:319-324

194 Bhat J, Smith AG. Xanthelasma palpebrarum following allergic contact dermatitis from para-phenylenediamine in a black eyelash-tinting product. Contact Dermatitis 2003;49:311

195 Koopmans AK, Bruynzeel DP. Is PPD a useful screening agent? Contact Dermatitis 2003;48:89-92

196 Søsted H, Basketter DA, Estrada E, Johansen JD, Patlewicz GY. Ranking of hair dye substances according to predicted sensitization potency: quantitative structure–activity relationships. Contact Dermatitis 2004;51:241-254

197 Bardazzi F, Manuzzi P, Riguzzi G, Veronesi S. Contact dermatitis with rosacea. Contact Dermatitis 1987;16:298

198 Foussereau J, Reuter G, Petitjean J. Is hair dyed with PPD-like dyes allergenic? Contact Dermatitis 1980;6:143

199 Ibsen Hh, Andersen K E. Picture of the month: contact allergy. Ugeskr Laeger 2000;162:6858 (article in Danish, data cited in ref. 196)

200 Viraben R, Aquilina C, Cambon L, Bazex J. Allergic contact dermatitis in HIV-positive patients. Contact Dermatitis 1994;31:326-327

201 Seidenari S, Manzini BM, Motolese A. Contact sensitization in infants: report of 3 cases. Contact Dermatitis 1992;27:319-320

202 Warin AP. Contact dermatitis to partner's hair dye. Clin Exp Dermatol 1976;1:283-284

203 Helaskoski E, Suojalehto H. Hairdressers' occupational asthma, rhinitis and contact urticaria caused by oxidative hair dyes. Ann Allergy Asthma Immunol 2014;112:46-52

204 Mitchell JC. Allergic dermatitis from paraphenylene diamine presenting as nummular eczema. Contact Dermatitis Newsletter 1972;11:270

205 Cronin E. Dermatitis from wife's dyed hair. Contact Dermatitis Newsletter 1973;13:363

206 Gottlober P, Gall H, Bezold G, Peter RU. Allergic contact dermatitis in beauty parlor clients. Hautarzt 2001;52:401-404 (article in German)

207 Hsu TS, Davis MD, el Azhary R, Corbett JF, Gibson LE. Beard dermatitis due to para-phenylenediamine use in Arabic men. J Am Acad Dermatol 2001;44:867-869

208 Brown AC, Broyles JA. Accumulative scarring of the scalp due to hair dye. In: Brown AC, Crounse RG, eds. Hair, trace elements and human illness. New York, NY: Praeger Publishers, 1980:348-360 (data cited in ref. 190)

209 Matsunaga K, Hosokawa K, Suzuki M, Arima Y, Hayakawa R. Occupational allergic contact dermatitis in beauticians. Contact Dermatitis 1988;18:94-96

210 Li LF, Wang J. A clinical and patch test study of adult widespread eczema. Contact Dermatitis 2002;47:341-344

211 Zhao B, Fan WX. Facial contact dermatitis. Pathogenetic factors in China. Int J Dermatol 1991;30:485-486

212 Charles J, Bourrain JL, Tessier A, Lepoittevin JP, Beani JC. Mesalazine and para-phenylenediamine allergy. Contact Dermatitis 2004;51:313-314

213 Ho SGY, White IR, Rycroft RJG, McFadden JP. Allergic contact dermatitis from para-phenylenediamine in Bigen® powder hair dye. Contact Dermatitis 2004;51:93-94

214 Chey WY, Kim KL, Yoo T-Y, Lee A-Y. Allergic contact dermatitis from hair dye and development of lichen simplex chronicus. Contact Dermatitis 2004;51:5-8

215 Søsted H, Hesse U, Menné T, Andersen KE, Johanson JD. Contact dermatitis to hair dyes in an adult Danish population – an interview based study. Br J Dermatol 2005;153:132-135

216 Turchin I, Moreau L, Warshaw E, Sasseville D. Cross-reactions among parabens, para-phenylenediamine, and benzocaine: a retrospective analysis of patch testing. Dermatitis 2006;17:192-195

217 DeLeo VA. Contact Allergen of the Year. p-Phenylenediamine. Dermatitis 2006;17:53-55

218 Teixeira M, De Wachter L, Ronsyn E, Goossens A. Contact allergy to para-phenylenediamine in a permanent eyelash dye. Contact Dermatitis 2006;55:92-94

219 Veysey EC, Burge S, Cooper S. Consort contact dermatitis to paraphenylenediamine, with an unusual clinical presentation of tumid plaques. Contact Dermatitis 2007;56:366-367

220 McFadden JP, White IR, Frosch PJ, Søsted H, Johansen JD, Menné T. Allergy to hair dye. BMJ 2007;334:220-221

221 Warbrick EV, Dearman RJ, Lea L. Local lymph node assay responses to para-phenylenediamine: intra- and inter-laboratory evaluations. J Appl Toxicol 1999;19:255-260

222 Gorriz-Torres MC, Linares T, Fernández de Rojas, Hernández D. para-Phenylenediamine allergic contact dermatitis in twins. Dermatitis 2007;18:56-57

223 Rudzki E, Rebandel P. Sensitivity to paraphenylenediamine in Warsaw (Poland). Contact Dermatitis 2007;57:347-348

224 Thyssen JP, White JM L. Epidemiological data on consumer allergy to p-phenylenediamine. Contact Dermatitis 2008;59:327-343

225 Thyssen JP, Johansen JD, Menné T. Contact allergy epidemics and their controls. Contact Dermatitis 2007;56:185-195

226 Fregert S. Chemical demonstration of paraphenylenediamine in hair dyes. Hautarzt 1972;23:393-394 (article in German)

227 Jacob S, Zapolanski T, Chayavichitsilp P. Sensitivity to para-phenylenediamine and intolerance to hydrochlorothiazide. Dermatitis 2008;19:E44-E45

228 Chan HP, Maibach HI. Moustache p-phenylenediamine dye allergic contact dermatitis with distant site involvement – an atypical presentation. Contact Dermatitis 2008;58:179-180

229 Winhoven SM, Rutter KJ, Beck MH. Multiple positive allergic reactions from patch testing to p-phenylenediamine and azo dyes. Is this a frequent risk and can it be reduced? Contact Dermatitis 2008;58:182-183

230 Paulsen E, Christensen LP, Andersen KE. Possible cross-reactivity between para-phenylenediamine and sesquiterpene lactones. Contact Dermatitis 2008;58:120-122

231 Seidenari S, Di Nardo, Motolese A, Pincelli C. Eritema polimorfo associate a sensibilizzazione per contatto. G Ital Dermatol Venereol 1990;125:35-40

232 Balato A, Patruno C, Balato N, Gallo L, Ayala F. Erythema multiforme-like eruption because of para-phenylenediamine. Contact Dermatitis 2008;58:65-66

233 Thyssen JP, Andersen KE, , Diepgen T, Giménez-Arnau AM, Gonçalo M, et al. p-Phenylenediamine sensitization is more prevalent in central and southern European patch test centres than in Scandinavian: results from a multicentre study. Contact Dermatitis 2009;60:314-319

234 Krasteva M, Bons B, Ryan C, Gerberick FG. Consumer allergy to oxidative hair coloring products: epidemiologic data in the literature. Dermatitis 2009;20:123-141

235 Saitta P, Cohen D, Brancaccio R. Contact leukoderma from para-phenylenediamine. Dermatitis 2009;20:56-57

236 Trattner A, David M. Hair-dye-induced contact vitiligo treated by phototherapy. Contact Dermatitis 2007;56:115-116

237 Yazar K, Boman A, Lidén C. Potent skin sensitizers in oxidative hair dye products on the Swedish market. Contact Dermatitis 2009;61:269-275

238 McFadden JP, Yeo L, White JL. Clinical and experimental aspects of allergic contact dermatitis to para-phenylenediamine. Clin Dermatol 2011;29:316-324

239 Rastogi SC1, Søsted H, Johansen JD, Menné T, Bossi R. Unconsumed precursors and couplers after formation of oxidative hair dyes. Contact Dermatitis 2006;55:95-100

240 Wang MZ, Farmer SA, Richardson DM, Davis MDP. Patch-testing with hairdressing chemicals. Dermatitis 2011;22:16-26

241 Bassi A, Massimiliano A, D'Erme M, Ricci GL, Francalanci S. Unusual localization of allergic contact dermatitis from p-phenylenediamine. Dermatitis 2011;22:358

242 Spornraft-Ragaller P, Schnuch A, Uter W. Extreme patch test reactivity to p-phenylenediamine but not to other allergens in children. Contact Dermatitis 2011;65:220-226

243 Nosbaum A, Dupin C, Nicolas J-F, Bérard F. Severe immediate hypersensitivity and allergic contact dermatitis caused by hair dyes. Contact Dermatitis 2012;67:52-53

244 Goossens A. Self-testing for contact sensitization to hair dyes. Contact Dermatitis 2012;66:299

245 Thyssen JP, Søsted H, Uter W, Schnuch A, Giménez-Arnau AM, Vigan M, et al. Self-testing for contact sensitization to hair dyes – scientific considerations and clinical concerns of an industry-led screening programme. Contact Dermatitis 2012;66:300-311

246 Krasteva M, Cottin M, Cristaudo A, Lainé G, Nohynek G, Orton D, et al. Sensitivity and specificity of the consumer open skin allergy test as a method of prediction of contact dermatitis to hair dyes. Eur J Dermatol 2006;15:18-25

247 Orton DI. A clinical assessment of a patch test kit marketed to UK hairdressers for detecting hair dye allergy. Br J Dermatol 2007;157:1017-1020

248 Basketter DA, English J. Pre-testing in hair dye users: an assessment of the Colourstart system. Eur J Dermatol 2009;19:232-237

249 Orton D, Basketter D. Hair dye sensitivity testing: a critical commentary. Contact Dermatitis 2012;66:312-316

250 Yazar K, Boman A, Lidén C. p-Phenylenediamine and other hair dye sensitizers in Spain. Contact Dermatitis 2012;66:27-32

251 Lyons G, Roberts H, Palmer A, Matheson M, Nixon R. Hairdressers presenting to an occupational dermatology clinic in Melbourne, Australia. Contact Dermatitis 2013;68:300-306

252 Uchida S, Oiso N, Matsunaga K, Kawada A. Patch test reaction to p-phenylenediamine can persist for more than 1 month. Contact Dermatitis 2013;69:382-383

253 Lönngren V, Young E, Simanaitis M, Svedman C. Neutrophilic and eosinophilic dermatitis caused by contact allergic reaction to paraphenylenediamine in hair dye. Arch Dermatol 2012;148:1299-1301

254 White JLM, Kullavanijaya P, Duangdeeden I, Zazzeroni R, Gilmour NJ, Basketter DA, McFadden JP. p-Phenylenediamine allergy: the role of Bandrowski's base. Clin Exp Allergy 2006;36:1289-1293

255 Geier J, Ballmer-Weber BK, Dickel H, Frosch PJ, Bircher A, Weisshaar E, Hillen U. Monitoring contact sensitization to p-phenylenediamine (PPD) by patch testing with PPD 0.3% in petrolatum. Contact Dermatitis 2013;69:26-31

256 Søsted H, Rustemeyer T, Gonçalo M, Bruze M, Goossens A, Giménez-Arnau AM, et al. Contact allergy to common ingredients in hair dyes. Contact Dermatitis 2013;69:32-39

257 Søsted H, Rastogi SC, Andersen KE, Johansen JD, Menné T. Hair dye contact allergy: quantitative exposure assessment of selected products and clinical cases. Contact Dermatitis 2004;50:344-348

258 Hald M, Menné T, Johansen JD, Zachariae C. Severe occupational contact dermatitis caused by black rubber as a consequence of p-phenylenediamine allergy resulting from a temporary henna tattoo. Contact Dermatitis 2013;68:377-379

259 Andersen KE, White IR, Goossens A. Allergens from the European baseline series. In: Johansen JD, Frosch PJ, Lepoittevin JP, Eds. Contact Dermatitis, 5th edition. Berlin, Heidelberg: Springer-Verlag, 2011: 545-590

260 Sornin de Leysat C, Boone M, Blondeel A, Song M. Two cases of cross-sensitivity in subjects allergic to paraphenylenediamine following ingestion of Polaronil. Dermatology 2003;206:379-380

261 Engfeldt M, Goossens A, Isaksson M, Zimerson E, Bruze M. The outcome of 9 years of consecutive patch testing with 4,4'-diaminodiphenylmethane and 4,4'-diphenylmethane diisocyanate. Contact Dermatitis 2013;68:98-102

262 Haluk Akar H, Adatepe S, Tahan F, Solmaz I. Hair dyes and temporary tattoos are a real hazard for adolescents? Eur Ann Allergy Clin Immunol 2014;46:35-37

263 Basketter DA, White IR, Kullavanijaya P, Tresukosol P, Wichaidit M, McFadden JP. Influence of vitamin C on the elicitation of allergic contact dermatitis to p-phenylenediamine. Contact Dermatitis 2016;74:368-372

264 Coenraads P-J, Vogel TA, Blömeke B, Goebel C, Roggeband R, Schuttelaar MLA. The role of the antioxidant ascorbic acid in the elicitation of contact allergic reactions to p-phenylenediamine. Contact Dermatitis 2016;74:267-272

265 Vogel TA, Coenraads P-J, Schuttelaar M-LA. Allergic contact dermatitis presenting as severe and persistent blepharoconjunctivitis and centrofacial oedema after dyeing of eyelashes. Contact Dermatitis 2014;71:304-306

266 Schuttelaar M-LA, Vogel TA, Rui F, Kręcisz B, Chomiczewska-Skora D, Kieć-Świerczyńska M, et al. ESSCA results with the baseline series, 2002–2012: p-phenylenediamine. Contact Dermatitis 2016;75:165-172

267 Verma P, Yadav P. Paraphenylenediamine dye allergic contact dermatitis of mustache region manifesting as prurigo nodularis–like lesions. Dermatitis 2014;25:91-92

268 Thomas BR, White IR, McFadden JP, Banerjee P. Positive relationship – intensity of response to p-phenylenediamine on patch testing and cross-reactions with related allergens. Contact Dermatitis 2014;71:98-101

269 Goon ATJ, Gilmour NJ, Basketter DA, White IR, Rycroft RJG, McFadden JP. High frequency of simultaneous sensitivity to Disperse Orange 3 in patients with positive patch tests to para-phenylenediamine. Contact Dermatitis 2003; 48:248-250

270 Hamann CR, Love J, Hamann C, Hamann D, Jacob SE. Paraphenyenediamine allergy and mustache dermatitis. Dermatitis 2016;27:e8

271 Lopez I, Turrentine JE., Cruz PD jr. Clues to diagnosis of connubial contact dermatitis to paraphenylenediamine. Dermatitis 2014;25:32-33

272 Gass JK, Todd PM. PPD: is this a connubial dermatitis? Contact Dermatitis 2006;55:309

273 Audran-Avenel MJ, Lepoittevin J-P, Pajot Caroline, Martin L. Are paraphenylenediamine and benzocaine relevant markers of sulfasalazine allergy? Dermatitis 2014;25:40-41

274 Antelmi A, Young E, Svedman C, Zimerson E, Engfeldt M, Foti C, Bruze M. Are gloves sufficiently protective when hairdressers are exposed to permanent hair dyes? An in vivo study. Contact Dermatitis 2015;72:229-236

275 Pónyai G, Diczig BM, Németh I, Temesvári E. para-Phenylenediamine hypersensitivity: a report from Budapest, Hungary, 2007–2014. Dermatitis 2016;27:303-307

276 Jenkins D, Chow ET. Allergic contact dermatitis to para-phenylenediamine. Australas J Dermatol 2015;56:40-43

277 Zahir A, Kindred C, Blömeke B, Goebel C, Gaspari AA. Tolerance to a hair dye product containing 2-methoxymethyl-*p*-phenylenediamine in an ethnically diverse population of *p*-phenylenediamine-allergic individuals. Dermatitis 2016;27:355-361

278 Schuttelaar M-LA, Vogel TA. Contact allergy to hair dyes. Cosmetics 2016,3,21; doi:10.3390/cosmetics3030021

279 Diepgen TL, Naldi L, Bruze M, Cazzaniga S, Schuttelaar ML, Elsner P, et al. Prevalence of contact allergy to *p*-phenylenediamine in the European general population. J Investig Dermatol 2016;136:409-415

280 Da França SA, Dario MF, Esteves VB, Baby AR, Velasco MV. Types of hair dye and their mechanisms of action. Cosmetics 2015, 2, 110-126; doi:10.3390/cosmetics2020110

281 The Danish Environmental Protection Agency. Survey and occurence of PPD, PTD and other allergenic hair dye substances in hair dyes; Copenhagen, Denmark: The Danish Environmental Protection Agency, 2013 (ISBN 978-87-92903-92-1). Available at: http://www2.mst.dk/Udgiv/publications/2013/02/978-87-92903-92-1.pdf

282 Blömeke B, Pot LM, Coenraads PJ, Hennen J, Kock M, Goebel C. Cross-elicitation responses to 2-methoxymethyl-*p*-phenylenediamine under hair dye use conditions in *p*-phenylenediamine-allergic individuals. Br J Dermatol 2015; 172:976-980

283 Kock M, Coenraads PJ, Blömeke B, et al. Continuous usage of a hair dye product containing 2-methoxymethyl-para-phenylenediamine by hairdye-allergic individuals. Br J Dermatol 2016;174:1042-1050

284 Goebel C, Coenraads PJ, Rothe H, Kunze G, Kock M, Schlatter H, et al. Elicitation of the immune response to *p*-phenylenediamine in allergic patients: the role of dose and exposure time. Br J Dermatol 2010;163:1205-1211

285 Pot LM, Coenraads PJ, Goebel C, Blomeke B. Assessment of the elicitation response in subjects weakly sensitized to *p*-phenylenediamine. Br J Dermatol 2014;172:138-144

286 Van Aerde E, Kerre S, Goossens A. Discoid lupus triggered by allergic contact dermatitis caused by a hair dye. Contact Dermatitis 2016;74:61-64

287 Ashar A. Acute angioedema in paraphenylenediamine poisoning. J Pak Med Assoc 2003;53:120-122

288 Bourquia A, Jubrane AJ. Ramdani B, et al. Systemic toxicity of paraphenylenediamine: 4 cases. Presse Med 1988;17:798-800

289 Yagi H, El Hind AM, Khalil SI. Acute poisoning from hair dye. East Afr Med J 1991;68:404-411

290 Young E, Zimerson E, Bruze M, Svedman C. Two sensitizing oxidation products of *p*-phenylenediamine patch tested in patients allergic to *p*-phenylenediamine. Contact Dermatitis 2016;74:76-82

291 Pot LM, Scheitza SM, Coenraads PJ, Blömeke B. Penetration and haptenation of *p*-phenylenediamine. Contact Dermatitis 2013;68:193-207

292 Morel OJX, Christie RM. Current trends in the chemistry of permanent hair dyeing. Chem Rev 2011;111:2537-2561

293 Kirchlecher S, Hübner A, Uter W. Survey of sensitizing constituents of oxidative hair dyes (retail and professional products) in Germany. J Dtsch Dermatol Ges 2016;14:707-715

294 Schwensen JF, Johansen JD, Veien NK, Funding AT, Avnstorp C, Østerballe M, et al. Occupational contact dermatitis in hairdressers: an analysis of patch test data from the Danish Contact Dermatitis Group, 2002–2011. Contact Dermatitis 2014;70:233-237

295 Abdelraheem MB, Hamdouk M, Zijlstra EE. Paraphenylenediamine (hair dye) poisoning in children. Arab J Nephrol Transpl 2010;3:39-43. Available at: http://www.ajol.info/index.php/ajnt/article/viewFile/57599/45978

296 Uter W, Gefeller O, John SM, Schnuch A, Geier J. Contact allergy to ingredients of hair cosmetics – a comparison of female hairdressers and clients based on IVDK 2007–2012 data. Contact Dermatitis 2014;71:13-20

297 Hamann D, Yazar K, Hamann CR, Thyssen JP, Lidén C. *p*-Phenylenediamine and other allergens in hair dye products in the United States: a consumer exposure study. Contact Dermatitis 2014;70:213-218

298 O'Connell RL, White IR, McFadden JP, White JML. Hairdressers with dermatitis should always be patch tested regardless of atopy status. Contact Dermatitis 2010;62:177-181

299 Beshir L, Kaballo B, Young D. Attempted suicide by ingestion of hair dye containing *p*-phenylenediamine: A case report. Ann Clin Biochem 2016 Dec 5. pii: 0004563216685117. [Epub ahead of print]

300 Nacaroglu HT, Yavuz S, Basman E, Bahceci S, Tasdemir M, Yigit Ö, Can D. The clinical spectrum of reactions developed based on paraphenylenediamine hypersensitivity two pediatric cases. Postepy Dermatol Alergol 2015;32:393-395

301 Mendonca S, Barki S, Mishra M, Kumar RS, Gupta D, Gupta P. Acute kidney injury: A rare cause. Saudi J Kidney Dis Transpl 2015;26:980-982

302 Patra AP, Shaha KK, Rayamane AP, Dash SK, Mohanty MK, Mohanty S. Paraphenylenediamine containing hair dye: an emerging household poisoning. Am J Forensic Med Pathol 2015;36:167-171

303 Lee JY, Kim CW, Kim SS. Analysis of the results from the patch test to para-phenylenediamine in the true test in patients with a hair dye contact allergy. Ann Dermatol 2015;27:171-177

304 Chen T, Pratt MD. Photo developer allergic contact dermatitis in a photographer following paraphenylenediamine sensitization from a temporary henna tattoo J Cutan Med Surg 2015,19):73-76

305 Sequeira FF, Jayaseelan E, Stephen J. Paraphenylenediamine-induced cutaneous pseudolymphoma. Indian J Dermatol 2014;59:424

306 van Genderen ME, Carels G, Lonnee ER, Dees A. Severe facial swelling in a pregnant woman after using hair dye. BMJ Case Rep 2014 Mar 31;2014. pii: bcr2013202562. doi: 10.1136/bcr-2013-202562.

307 Elevli M, Civilibal M, Ersoy O, Demirkol D, Gedik AH. Paraphenylene diamine hair dye poisoning: an uncommon cause of rhabdomyolysis. Indian J Pediatr 2014;81:709-711

308 Ryoo SM, Sohn CH, Oh BJ, Kim WY, Lim KS. A case of severe methemoglobinemia caused by hair dye poisoning. Hum Exp Toxicol 2014;33:103-105

309 Abdelraheem MB, Elbushra M, Ali el-T, Ellidir RA, Bushara AI, Abdelraheem WB, Zijlstra EE. Filicide and suicide in a family by paraphenylene diamine poisoning: a mother who committed suicide and poisoned her four children of which one died. Toxicol Ind Health 2014;30:679-682

310 Tukenmez Demirci G, Kivanc Altunay I, Atis G, Kucukunal A. Allergic contact dermatitis mimicking angioedema due to paraphenylendiamine hypersensitivity: a case report. Cutan Ocul Toxicol 2012;31:250-252

311 Hospital V, Amarger S, Franck F, Ferrier Le Bouëdec MC, Souteyrand P, D'Incan M. Dermite de contact lymphomatoïde par procuration (Proxy lymphomatoid contact dermatitis). Ann Dermatol Venereol 2011;138:315-318 (Article in French)

312 Fernández-Vozmediano JM, Padilla-Moreno M, Armario-Hita JC, Carranza-Romero C. Pattern of contact sensitization to paraphenylenediamine and its detection in hair dyes. Actas Dermosifiliogr 2011;102:206-211 (Article in Spanish)

313 Mehta V, Nayak S, Balachandran C. Pigmented contact cheilitis to paraphenylenediamine. Indian J Dermatol 2010;55:119-120

314 Cordoba S, Sanz-Sanchez T, Hernandez-Nuñez A, Borbujo JM. Occupational contact dermatitis from *p*-phenylenediamine in a furrier. J Eur Acad Dermatol Venereol 2008;22:773

315 Kelsh MA, Alexander DD, Kalmes RM, Buffler PA. Personal use of hair dyes and risk of bladder cancer: a meta-analysis of epidemiologic data. Cancer Causes Control 2008;19:549-558

316 Wiedemeyer K, Enk A, Jappe U. Erythema multiforme following allergic contact dermatitis: case report and literature review. Acta Derm Venereol 2007;87:559-561

317 Paley K, Geskin LJ, Zirwas MJ. Cutaneous B-cell pseudolymphoma due to paraphenylenediamine. Am J Dermatopathol 2006;28:438-441

318 Khumalo NP, Jessop S, Ehrlich R. Prevalence of cutaneous adverse effects of hairdressing: a systematic review. Arch Dermatol 2006;142:377-383

319 Moscato G, Pignatti P, Yacoub MR, Romano C, Spezia S, Perfetti L. Occupational asthma and occupational rhinitis in hairdressers. Chest 2005;128:3590-3598

320 Lisi P, Hansel K. Is benzoquinone the prohapten in cross-sensitivity among aminobenzene compounds? Contact Dermatitis 1998;39:304-306

321 Seidenari S, Di Nardo A, Motolese A, Pincelli C. Erythema multiforme associated with contact sensitization. Description of 6 clinical cases. G Ital Dermatol Venereol 1990;125:35-40 (Article in Italian)

322 Romaguera C, Grimalt F, Vilaplana J. Shoe contact dermatitis. Contact Dermatitis 1988;18:178

323 Doherty E, Freeman S. Spectacle frame dermatitis due to paraphenylenediamine. Australas J Dermatol 1988;29:113-115

324 Silberman DE, Sorrell AH. Allergy in fur workers with special reference to paraphenylenediamine. J Allergy 1959;30:11-18

325 Ockenfels H, Seemann U, Goos M. Contact allergy in patients with periorbital eczema: an analysis of allergens. Dermatology 1997;195:119-124

326 Ellis RA, Wilkinson SM. Contact dermatitis to 4-amino-2-hydroxytoluene in hair dye. Contact Dermatitis 2009;60:118-119

327 Ali L, Foulds JS, Abdul Ghaffar S. Severe eyelid allergic contact dermatitis secondary to eyelash tint: two case reports. Contact Dermatitis 2017;77:59-60

328 Ito A, Nishioka K, Kanto H, Yagami A, Yamada S, Sugiura M, et al. A multi-institutional joint study of contact dermatitis related to hair colouring and perming agents in Japan. Contact Dermatitis 2017;77:42-48

329 Gottlöber P, Gall H, Bezold G, Peter RU. Allergic contact dermatitis in beauty parlor clients. Hautarzt 2001;52:401-404 (Article in German)

330 Bernstein IL, Chan-Yeung M, Malo JL, Bernstein DI, Eds. Asthma in the Workplace, 3rd Edn. New York: Taylor & Francis, 2006

331 UK Health and Safety Executive. 2001. Asthmagen? critical assessment of the evidence for agents implicated in occupational asthma. Available at: http://www.hse.gov.uk/asthma/asthmagen.pdf

332 Arrandale VH, Liss GM, Tarlo SM, Pratt MD, Sasseville D, Kudla I, Holness DL. Occupational contact allergens: are they also associated with occupational asthma? Am J Ind Med 2012;55:353-360

333 Lee HS, Lin YW. Permeation of hair dye ingredients, p-phenylenediamine and aminophenol isomers, through protective gloves. Ann Occup Hyg 2009;53:289-296

334 Lubbes S, Rustemeyer T, Sillevis Smitt JH, Schuttelaar ML, Middelkamp-Hup MA. Contact sensitization in Dutch children and adolescents with and without atopic dermatitis - a retrospective analysis. Contact Dermatitis 2017;76:151-159

335 Antelmi A, Bruze M, Zimerson E, Engfeldt M, Young E, Persson L, Foti C, Sörensen Ö, Svedman C. Evaluation of concordance between labelling and content of 52 hair dye products: overview of the market of oxidative hair dye. Eur J Dermatol 2017;27:123-131

336 Vogel TA, Heijnen RW, Coenraads PJ, Schuttelaar MA. Two decades of p-phenylenediamine and toluene-2,5-diamine patch testing - focus on co-sensitizations in the European baseline series and cross-reactions with chemically related substances. Contact Dermatitis 2017;76:81-88

337 Lee HJ, Kim WJ, Kim JY, Kim HS, Kim BS, Kim MB, Ko HC. Patch tests with commercial hair dye products in patients with allergic contact dermatitis to para-phenylenediamine. Indian J Dermatol Venereol Leprol 2016;82:645-650

338 Ortiz Salvador JM, Esteve Martínez A, Subiabre Ferrer D, Victoria Martínez AM, de la Cuadra Oyanguren J, Zaragoza Ninet V. Pediatric allergic contact dermatitis: Clinical and epidemiological study in a tertiary hospital. Actas Dermosifiliogr 2017;108:571-578

339 Vogel TA, Prins TM, Dijkstra A, Coenraads PJ, Schuttelaar MLA. The attitude of patients with p-phenylenediamine or 2,5-toluenediamine contact allergy to hair dyeing. Contact Dermatitis 2017;76:358-361

340 Uter W, Amario-Hita JC, Balato A, Ballmer-Weber B, Bauer A, Belloni Fortina A, et al. European Surveillance System on Contact Allergies (ESSCA): results with the European baseline series, 2013/14. J Eur Acad Dermatol Venereol 2017 Jun 19. doi: 10.1111/jdv.14423. [Epub ahead of print]

341 Belloni Fortina A, Fontana E, Peserico A. Contact sensitization in children: A retrospective study of 2,614 children from a single center. Pediatr Dermatol 2016;33:399-404

342 Goldenberg A, Mousdicas N, Silverberg N, Powell D, Pelletier JL, Silverberg JI, et al. Pediatric Contact Dermatitis Registry inaugural case data. Dermatitis 2016;27:293-302

343 Beshir L, Kaballo B, Young D. Attempted suicide by ingestion of hair dye containing p-phenylenediamine: a case report. Ann Clin Biochem 2017;54:507-510

344 Sanchez L, Handyal H, Kannan S; Siddalingeshwara, Alvarez-Uria G, Gavalda L, Corbella X. Hair dye poisoning: Retrospective analyses of patients admitted to ICU at a rural hospital in India. Indian J Med Res 2016;144:134-137

2.360　O-PHENYLPHENOL

IDENTIFICATION

Description/definition	: *o*-Phenylphenol is the substituted aromatic compound that conforms to the formula shown below
Chemical class(es)	: Phenols
Chemical/IUPAC name	: Biphenyl-2-ol
Other names	: 2-Hydroxydiphenyl; 2-phenylphenol
CAS registry number (s)	: 90-43-7
EC number(s)	: 201-993-5
SCCS opinion(s)	: SCCS/1555/15 (5)
Merck Index monograph	: 8685
Function(s) in cosmetics	: EU: preservative. USA: cosmetic biocides; fragrance ingredients; pesticides; preservatives
EU cosmetic restrictions	: Regulated in Annex V/7 of the Regulation (EC) No. 1223/2009
Patch testing	: 1% pet. (Chemotechnique)
Molecular formula	: $C_{12}H_{10}O$

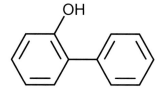

CONTACT ALLERGY

Patch testing in groups of patients

The results of patch testing *o*-phenylphenol in consecutive patients suspected of contact dermatitis (routine testing) and of testing groups of *selected* patients (patients with a cosmetic, preservative or industrial biocide series) are shown in table 2.360.1. *o*-Phenylphenol has routinely tested in one small and early study only, yielding a 1.2% frequency of sensitization. Causative products were not mentioned. In testing in selected patients, low rates of 0.2% to 0.4% sensitization were found. In two studies, relevance was not mentioned (4). In a study from the USA, both positive patch test reactions were scored as relevant, but this included 'questionable' and 'past' relevance (1).

Table 2.360.1 Patch testing in groups of patients

Years and Country	Test conc. & vehicle	Number of patients tested	positive (%)	Selection of patients (S); Relevance (R); Comments (C)	Ref.
Routine testing					
1979-1980 USA	1% pet.	588	7 (1.2%)	R: not stated	2
Testing in groups of selected patients					
2000-2007 USA	1% pet.	871	2 (0.2%)	S: patients tested with a supplemental cosmetic screening series; R: 100%; C: weak study: a. high rate of macular erythema and weak reactions; b. relevance figures included 'questionable' and 'past' relevance	1
1990-1994 Germany	1% pet.	11,418	33 (0.3%)	S: patients tested with a preservative series; R: not stated	4
1990-1994 Germany	1% pet.	1785	7 (0.4%)	S: patients tested with an industrial biocide series; R: not stated	4

Case reports and case series

Two patients had facial allergic contact dermatitis from *o*-phenylphenol in foundation creams. Both reacted to the creams and, when tested with their ingredients, to the preservative *o*-phenylphenol (3). A medical laboratory assistant applied a medicated hand cream to various parts of his body for dry skin. A severe, highly pruritic vesicular eruption developed. Patch testing with the cream and *o*-phenylphenol in 0.5% and 1% concentrations showed strong positive reactions at D3. In the hospital laboratory where he worked, a germicidal cleaning agent containing *o*-phenylphenol was used, but he was careful to avoid contact with it and experienced no further dermatitis (2).

Contact allergy to *o*-phenylphenol in non-cosmetic products
A male machinist had experienced a recurring dermatitis on the hands, arms, trunk, thighs and feet for 25 years. A coolant was suspected as the cause. When patch tested, he reacted to *o*-phenylphenol 1% pet. A 'provocative use test' with the suspected coolant which contained this preservative was positive. When a new coolant with double the concentration of *o*-phenylphenol was introduced into the plant, the patient became so severely affected that he had to leave work entirely (2).

Presence in cosmetic products and chemical analyses
In the USA, in April 2017, *o*-phenylphenol was present in 2 of 56,714 cosmetic products of which the composition is known in FDA's Voluntary Cosmetic Registration Program (VCRP) (data obtained from FDA, May 2017). In April 2017, *o*-phenylphenol was present in one of 66,485 cosmetic products of which the composition is known in EWG's Skin Deep Cosmetics Database, USA (http://www.ewg.org/skindeep/).

OTHER SIDE EFFECTS

Immediate-type reactions
One individual had an immediate contact reactions to *o*-phenylphenol present in plaster cast material (6).

LITERATURE

1 Wetter DA, Yiannias JA, Prakash AV, Davis MD, Farmer SA, el-Azhary RA, et al. Results of patch testing to personal care product allergens in a standard series and a supplemental cosmetic series: an analysis of 945 patients from the Mayo Clinic Contact Dermatitis Group, 2000-2007. J Am Acad Dermatol 2010;63:789-798
2 Adams RM. Allergic contact dermatitis due to o-phenylphenol. Contact Dermatitis 1981;7:332
3 Cronin E. Contact Dermatitis. Edinburgh: Churchill Livingstone, 1980:681
4 Schnuch A, Geier J, Uter W, Frosch PJ. Patch testing with preservatives, antimicrobials and industrial biocides. Results from a multicentre study. Br J Dermatol 1998;138:467-476
5 SCCS (Scientific Committee on Consumer Safety). Opinion on o-Phenylphenol, Sodium o-phenylphenate and Potassium o-phenylphenate, 25 June 2015, SCCS/1555/15, revision of 15 December 2015. Available at: http://ec.europa.eu/health/scientific_committees/consumer_safety/docs/sccs_o_177.pdf
6 Tuer WF, James WD, Summers RJ. Contact urticaria to o-phenylphenate. Ann Allergy 1986;56:19-21

2.361 N-PHENYL-P-PHENYLENEDIAMINE

IDENTIFICATION

Description/definition	: *N*-Phenyl-*p*-phenylenediamine is the aromatic amine salt that conforms to the formula shown below
Chemical class(es)	: Amines; color additives - hair
Chemical/IUPAC name	: 4-*N*-Phenylbenzene-1,4-diamine
Other names	: 4-Aminodiphenylamine; *N*-(4-aminophenyl)aniline; CI 76085
CAS registry number (s)	: 101-54-2
EC number(s)	: 202-951-9
CIR review(s)	: J Am Coll Toxicol 1994;13:374-394 (access: www.cir-safety.org/ingredients)
SCCS opinion(s)	: SCCP/0991/06 (11)
Function(s) in cosmetics	: EU: hair dyeing. USA: hair colorants
EU cosmetic restrictions	: Regulated in Annex III/8 of the Regulation (EC) No. 1223/2009
Patch testing	: 0.25% pet. (SmartPracticeCanada)
Molecular formula	: $C_{12}H_{12}N_2$

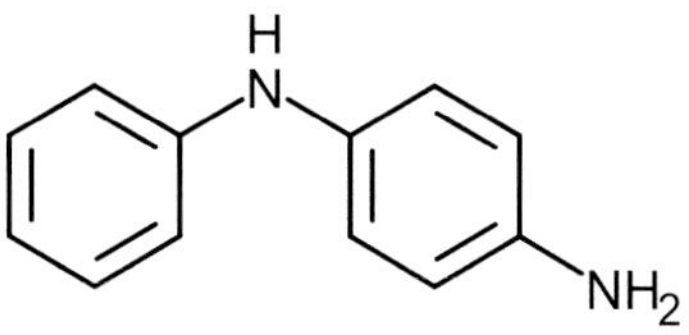

GENERAL

N-Phenyl-*p*-phenylenediamine is used in oxidative hair dying products. The chemistry of oxidative hair dying is discussed in Chapter 2.359 *p*-Phenylenediamine. It has been shown that possibly *N*-phenyl-*p*-phenylenediamine, a metabolite of disperse orange 1 and disperse yellow 3, is a major sensitizer in these colors (14).

CONTACT ALLERGY

Patch testing in groups of patients

There are no studies in which *N*-phenyl-*p*-phenylenediamine has been patch tested in consecutive patients suspected of contact dermatitis (routine testing). Results of testing in groups of *selected* patients (hairdressers with [suspected] contact dermatitis, patients with eczema suspected to be caused by hair dying, bleaching or permanent wave solution) are shown in table 2.361.1. In 7 investigations, frequencies of sensitization to *N*-phenyl-*p*-phenylenediamine have ranged from 2.9% to 10.6%. In none of the studies was the relevance of the positive patch tests stated or specified for *N*-phenyl-*p*-phenylenediamine; culprit products were not mentioned in any investigation (2,3,6,7,8,9, 10).

Table 2.361.1 Patch testing in groups of patients: Selected patient groups

Years and Country	Test conc. & vehicle	Number of patients tested	positive (%)	Selection of patients (S); Relevance (R); Comments (C)	Ref.
1994-2003 Spain		300	(7.7%)	S: hairdressers suspected of occupational contact dermatitis; R: not specified	7
1990-1999 Italy	0.25% pet.	209	8 (3.8%)	S: hairdressers with contact dermatitis; R: not specified	2
1985-1994 Greece	0.25% pet.	106	3 (4.3%)	S: hairdressers with contact dermatitis; R: not specified	3
1980-1993 Spain	0.25% pet.	379	11 (2.9%)	S: hairdressers; R: not specified	9
1988-1991, 8 European countries		365	13 (3.6%)	S: hairdressers with hand dermatitis; R: not stated	8
1985-1990 Italy	0.25% pet.	302	32 (10.6%)	S: hairdressers with contact dermatitis; R: not specified	10
1985-1990 Italy	0.25% pet.	261	11 (4.2%)	S: patients with eczema suspected to be caused by hair dying, bleaching or permanent wave solution; R: not stated	6

Case reports and case series

In the period 1996-2013, in a tertiary referral center in Valencia, Spain, 5419 patients were patch tested. Of these, 628 individuals had allergic contact dermatitis to cosmetics. *N*-Phenyl-*p*-phenylenediamine was the responsible allergen in 2 cases (12). In a 4-month-period in 1996, 475 patients with contact allergy to 'cosmetic ingredients' were collected in 5 centers in Belgium, UK and Germany. There were 2 reactions to *N*-phenyl-*p*-phenylenediamine; relevance was not stated (5).

Contact allergy to *N*-phenyl-*p*-phenylenediamine in non-cosmetic products

Numerous cases of work-related airborne contact dermatitis of the face were encountered in a waste collection facility. Potential allergens contained in the dust at the facility could be identified. In 5 of 7 symptomatic workers contact allergy to *p*-aminodiphenylamine was established. A change in the work routine led to a reduction of dust emissions and afterwards no cases of airborne contact dermatitis of the face recurred (15,16).

Cross-reactions, pseudo-cross-reactions and co-reactions

N-Phenyl-*p*-phenylenediamine may cross-react with structurally related chemicals, notably those with a para-structure. Cross-reactivity between para-compounds is discussed in Chapter 2.359 *p*-Phenylenediamine.

Patch test sensitization

One patient became sensitized by a patch test with *N*-phenyl-*p*-phenylenediamine 0.5% pet. (1).

Presence in cosmetic products and chemical analyses

In July 2017, *N*-phenyl-*p*-phenylenediamine was present in one product of 69,545 cosmetic products of which the composition is known in EWG's Skin Deep Cosmetics Database, USA (http://www.ewg.org/skindeep/). In the USA, in April 2017, *N*-phenyl-*p*-phenylenediamine was present in 20 of 56,714 cosmetic products of which the composition is known in FDA's Voluntary Cosmetic Registration Program (VCRP) (data obtained from FDA, May 2017). In 2016, in Sweden, the labels of 26 oxidative hair dye products advertised with the signal words organic, natural or similar, or sold/used at a hair dressing salon advertised with the same terminology, were screened for the presence of known contact allergens. *N*-Phenyl-*p*-phenylenediamine *sulfate* was present in 10 (38%) products (13).

In 2011, labels and other information on 365 hair dye products (282 permanent dyes, 79 semi-permanent dyes, 4 direct dyes) available on the Danish market (159 hair dyes for private use, 206 for professional use by hairdressers) were collected to identify the presence of sensitizers. *N*-Phenyl-*p*-phenylenediamine was present in 6 (1.6%) products (4).

LITERATURE

1   Kanerva L, Estlander T. Simultaneous active sensitization to multiple chemicals. Contact Dermatitis 1998;38:174-175
2   Iorizzo M, Parente G, Vincenzi C, Pazzaglia M, Tosti A. Allergic contact dermatitis in hairdressers; frequency and source of sensitization. Eur J Dermatol 2002;12:179-182
3   Katsarou A, Koufou B, Takou K, Kalogeromitros D, Papanayiotou G, Vareltzidis A. Patch test results in hairdressers with contact dermatitis in Greece (1985-1994). Contact Dermatitis 1995;33:347-348
4   The Danish Environmental Protection Agency. Survey and occurrence of PPD, PTD and other allergenic hair dye substances in hair dyes. Copenhagen, Denmark: The Danish Environmental Protection Agency, 2013 (ISBN 978-87-92903-92-1). Available at: http://www2.mst.dk/Udgiv/publications/2013/02/978-87-92903-92-1.pdf
5   Goossens A, Beck MH, Haneke E, McFadden JP, Nolting S, Durupt G, Ries G. Adverse cutaneous reactions to cosmetic allergens. Contact Dermatitis 1999;40:112-113
6   Guerra L, Bardazzi F, Tosti A. Contact dermatitis in hairdressers' clients. Contact Dermatitis 1992;26:108-111
7   Valks R, Conde-Salazar L, Malfeito J, Ledo S. Contact dermatitis in hairdressers, 10 years later: patch-test results in 300 hairdressers (1994 to 2003) and comparison with previous study. Dermatitis 2005;16:28-31
8   Frosch PJ, Burrows D, Camarasa JG, Dooms-Goossens A, Ducombs G, Lahti A, et al. Allergic reactions to a hairdressers' series: results from 9 European centres. Contact Dermatitis 1993;28:180-183
9   Conde-Salazar L, Baz M, Guimaraens D, Cannavo A. Contact dermatitis in hairdressers: patch test results in 379 hairdressers (1980-1993). Am J Cont Dermat 1995;6:19-23
10 Guerra L, Tosti A, Bardazzi F, Pigatto P, Lisi P, Santucci B, et al. Contact dermatitis in hairdressers: the Italian experience. Contact Dermatitis 1992;26:101-107
11 Scientific Committee on Consumer Products (SCCP). Opinion on *N*-Phenyl-*p*-phenylenediamine, 19 December 2006, SCCP/0991/06. Available at:
    http://ec.europa.eu/health/archive/ph_risk/committees/04_sccp/docs/sccp_o_089.pdf
12 Zaragoza-Ninet V, Blasco Encinas R, Vilata-Corell JJ, Pérez-Ferriols A, Sierra-Talamantes C, Esteve-Martínez A, de la Cuadra-Oyanguren J. Allergic contact dermatitis due to cosmetics: A clinical and epidemiological study in a tertiary hospital. Actas Dermosifiliogr 2016;107:329-336
13 Thorén S, Yazar K. Contact allergens in 'natural' hair dyes. Contact Dermatitis 2016;74:302-304

14   Malinauskiene L, Zimerson E, Bruze M, Ryberg K, Isaksson M. Patch testing with the textile dyes Disperse Orange 1 and Disperse Yellow 3 and some of their potential metabolites, and simultaneous reactions to para-amino compounds. Contact Dermatitis 2012;67:130-140

15   Skudlik C, Meyer E, Allmers H, Domagalski E, John SM. Endemic air-borne contact dermatitis? Frequent occurrence of a rare contact allergy in a waste collection facility (article in German). Hautarzt 2011;62:765-769

16   Domagalski E, Baratli J, Skudlik C, John SM. *p*-Aminodiphenylenamin – ein bisher kaum bekanntes berufliches Kontaktallergen. Diaklinik – interessante Fälle aus der Welt der DDG (Abstract). J Dtsch Dermatol Ges 2011;9(Suppl.1):255

2.362 PHENYL SALICYLATE

IDENTIFICATION

Description/definition	: Phenyl salicylate is the organic compound that conforms to the formula shown below
Chemical class(es)	: Esters; phenols
Chemical/IUPAC name	: 2-Hydroxybenzoic acid, phenyl ester
Other names	: Phenyl 2-hydroxybenzoate; Salol®; salol
CAS registry number (s)	: 118-55-8
EC number(s)	: 204-259-2
Merck Index monograph	: 8690
Function(s) in cosmetics	: EU: antimicrobial; denaturant; perfuming. USA: cosmetic biocides; denaturants; fragrance ingredients
Patch testing	: 1% pet. (Chemotechnique, SmartPracticeEurope, SmartPracticeCanada)
Molecular formula	: $C_{13}H_{10}O_3$

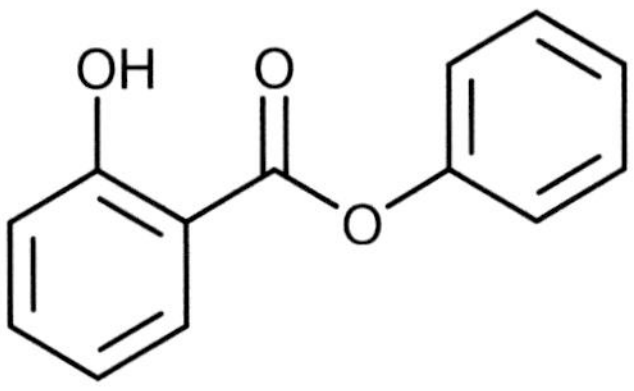

CONTACT ALLERGY

Patch testing in groups of patients

Results of studies patch testing phenyl salicylate in consecutive patients suspected of contact dermatitis (routine testing) and in groups of selected patients are shown in table 2.362.1. In routine testing, the frequency of sensitization in one available study was 2.2%, but the relevance of the 13 reactions was not mentioned. Three studies testing groups of *selected* patients (healthy student volunteers, patients tested with a cosmetic screening series, patients suspected of oral or lip contact allergy) showed rates of 0.5% (17), 1.0% (1) and 2.4% (18) sensitization. In one study from the USA, all 9 positive patch test reactions were scored as relevant, but this included 'questionable' and 'past' relevance (1).

Table 2.362.1 Patch testing in groups of patients

Years and Country	Test conc. & vehicle	Number of patients tested	positive (%)	Selection of patients (S); Relevance (R); Comments (C)	Ref.
Routine testing					
2003-2005 China		599	13 (2.2%)	R: not stated	9
Testing in groups of selected patients					
2014-2016 USA		126	3 (2.4%)	S: patients with suspected oral or lip contact allergy; R: not stated	18
2011 China	1% pet.	201	1 (0.5%)	S: healthy student volunteers 19-30 years; R: not stated	17
2000-2007 USA	1% pet.	866	9 (1.0%)	S: patients tested with a supplemental cosmetic screening series; R: 100%; C: weak study: a. high rate of macular erythema and weak reactions; b. relevance figures included 'questionable' and 'past' relevance	1

Case reports and case series

In 3 clinics in Belgium, in the period 1978-1985, 279 patients with allergic contact dermatitis exclusively caused by cosmetics were seen. In this group, there were 6 reactions to phenyl salicylate. It was implied that this was the cause of the allergic reaction (16). In a 4-month-period in 1996, 475 patients with contact allergy to 'cosmetic ingredients' were collected in 5 centers in Belgium, UK and Germany. There were 2 reactions to phenyl salicylate; relevance was not stated (10). Three positive patch test reactions to phenyl salicylate were ascribed to cosmetic allergy (2).

Five patients had allergic contact cheilitis and perioral dermatitis from phenyl salicylate in a lip salve (6). Phenyl salicylate was incorporated into the formulation of this particular brand as a sunscreen over a period of two years, before it was removed. During this time the company was notified of 15 complaints by dermatologists; in 14 cases, phenyl salicylate had caused contact allergy to the product (6). One patient had cheilitis from phenyl salicylate in a lip salve (7). Three patients reacted to phenyl salicylate in a lipstick causing allergic contact cheilitis (8). Eleven patients were allergic to phenyl salicylate in Dermophil Indien lipstick (13).

Phenyl salicylate (salol) in a toothpaste was already incriminated in lip contact dermatitis in 1900 (12, data cited in ref. 13). In France, in 1936, phenyl salicylate in toothpastes was considered as one of the most frequent causes of lip dermatitis (14, data cited in refs. 11 and 13). One patient reacted to phenyl salicylate in a mouthwash (15).

Contact allergy to phenyl salicylate in non-cosmetic products
One individual had allergic contact dermatitis from a galenic cream containing 10% phenyl salicylate (4). A tool grinder and a worker in a metal foundry had occupational ACD from phenyl salicylate in safety spectacles (5).

Cross-reactions, pseudo-cross-reactions and co-reactions
Resorcinol monobenzoate (3); not to methyl salicylate (7); *p*-nitrophenyl salicylate, *p*-tert-butylphenyl salicylate, *p*-methylphenyl salicylate (13); methyl salicylate (18); benzyl salicylate (18).

Presence in cosmetic products and chemical analyses
In May 2017, phenyl salicylate was present in one of 66,720 cosmetic products of which the composition is known in EWG's Skin Deep Cosmetics Database, USA (http://www.ewg.org/skindeep/). In the USA, in April 2017, phenyl salicylate was present in zero of 56,714 cosmetic products of which the composition is known in FDA's Voluntary Cosmetic Registration Program (VCRP) (data obtained from FDA, May 2017).

LITERATURE

1   Wetter DA, Yiannias JA, Prakash AV, Davis MD, Farmer SA, el-Azhary RA, et al. Results of patch testing to personal care product allergens in a standard series and a supplemental cosmetic series: an analysis of 945 patients from the Mayo Clinic Contact Dermatitis Group, 2000-2007. J Am Acad Dermatol 2010;63:789-798
2   Kohl L, Blondeel A, Song M. Allergic contact dermatitis from cosmetics: retrospective analysis of 819 patch-tested patients. Dermatology 2002;204:334-337
3   Nakagawa M, Kawai K, Kawai K. Cross-sensitivity between resorcinol, resorcinol monobenzoate and phenyl salicylate. Contact Dermatitis 1992;27:199
4   Fimiani M, Casini L, Bocci S. Contact dermatitis from phenyl salicylate in a galenic cream. Contact Dermatitis 1990;22:239
5   Sonnex TS, Rycroft RJG. Dermatitis from phenyl salicylate in safety spectacle frames. Contact Dermatitis 1986;14:268-270
6   Calnan CD, Cronin E, Rycroft RJG. Allergy to phenyl salicylate. Contact Dermatitis 1981;7:208-211
7   Hindson C. Phenyl salicylate (salol) in a lip salve. Contact Dermatitis 1980;6:216
8   Foussereau J. Allergy to Dermophil Indien. Contact Dermatitis 1975;1:257
9   Li L-F, Liu G, Wang J. Patch test in Chinese patients with cosmetic allergic contact dermatitis to common cosmetic allergens from a European cosmetic series. Contact Dermatitis 2007;57:50-54
10 Goossens A, Beck MH, Haneke E, McFadden JP, Nolting S, Durupt G, Ries G. Adverse cutaneous reactions to cosmetic allergens. Contact Dermatitis 1999;40:112-113
11 Sainio E-L, Kanerva L. Contact allergens in toothpastes and a review of their hypersensitivity. Contact Dermatitis 1995;33:100-105
12 Axmann H. Salol Exzem. Arch für Dermatol 1900;52:298-299 (data cited in ref. 13) (article in German).
13 Marchand B, Barbier P, Ducombs G, Foussereau J, Martin P, Benezra C. Allergic contact dermatitis to various salols (phenyl salicylates). Arch Derm Res 1982;272:61-66.
14 Fernet P. Dermites artificielles par les dentifrices. In: Darier J, Sabourad R, Gougerot H, Milian G, et al, eds. Nouvelles pratiques dermatologiques (VIII). Paris: Masson; 1936: 107 (data cited in refs. 11 and 13) (in French)
15 Neisser A (1898) quoted by Bonnevie. In: Aetiologie und Pathogenese der Ekzemkrankheiten. Copenhagen: A. Burck, 1939:250
16 Dooms-Goossens A, de Boulle K, Dooms M, Degreef H. Imidazolidinyl urea dermatitis. Contact Dermatitis 1986;14:322-324
17 Zhao J, Li LF. Contact sensitization to cosmetic series of allergens in a general population in Beijing. J Cosmet Dermatol 2014;13:68-71
18 Scheman A, Te R. Contact allergy to salicylates and cross-reactions. Dermatitis 2017;28:291

2.363 PHTHALIC ANHYDRIDE/TRIMELLITIC ANHYDRIDE/GLYCOLS COPOLYMER

IDENTIFICATION

Description/definition : Phthalic anhydride/trimellitic anhydride/glycols copolymer is a copolymer of phthalic anhydride, trimellitic anhydride, ethylene glycol, and neopentyl glycol monomers

Chemical class(es) : Synthetic polymers

Chemical/IUPAC name : 1,3-Isobenzofurandione, polymer with 5-carboxy-1,3-isobenzofurandione, 1,2-ethanediol and 2,2-dimethyl-1,3-propanediol

Function(s) in cosmetics : EU: film forming; viscosity controlling. USA: film formers; viscosity increasing agents - nonaqueous

CIR review(s) : Final report, September 2016 (access: www.cir-safety.org/ingredients)

Patch testing : 1-5% pet. (1)

GENERAL

Copolymers are important ingredients in cosmetics, added because of their antistatic, film-forming, binding, suspending, viscosity-increasing, skin-conditioning, and emulsion-stabilizing properties. Copolymers have been underestimated for a long time as to their sensitizing capacities because of their large structures and high molecular weights. Allergic contact dermatitis to copolymers in cosmetics, however, does occur, but the exact nature of the hapten is still unknown. The copolymers are not likely to be haptens themselves in view of their large molecular weights. The sensitizer could be an additive, an impurity, a product that forms during polymerization, a residual monomer, or a degradation product (5).

The synthetic polymer phthalic anhydride/trimellitic anhydride/glycols copolymer is a non-aqueous agent, which increases viscosity and is responsible for forming a film when used in nail polish and enamel. It is also used in the manufacture of dyes, pharmaceuticals, insecticides and as a hardener for resins (3).

CONTACT ALLERGY

Case reports and case series

Three patients were sensitized to phthalic anhydride/trimellitic anhydride/glycols copolymer in nail varnish. There were no reactions to the monomers phthalic anhydride, trimellitic anhydride and glycols, performed in 2 patients (1,4). One patient reacted to the copolymer in nail varnish (2). Four patients had ACD from phthalic anhydride/trimellitic anhydride/glycols copolymer in nail varnishes (3).

Presence in cosmetic products and chemical analyses

In May 2017, phthalic anhydride/trimellitic anhydride/glycols copolymer was present in 83 of 68,675 cosmetic products of which the composition is known in EWG's Skin Deep Cosmetics Database, USA (http://www.ewg.org/skindeep/). In the USA, in April 2017, phthalic anhydride/trimellitic anhydride/glycols copolymer was present in 110 of 56,714 cosmetic products of which the composition is known in FDA's Voluntary Cosmetic Registration Program (VCRP) (data obtained from FDA, May 2017). Phthalic anhydride/trimellitic anhydride/glycols copolymer was found in 32 different nail polishes and 10 other nail treatment products in a cosmetics database in Leuven, Belgium (5).

LITERATURE

1 Nassif AS, Le Coz CJ, Collet É. A rare nail polish allergen: phthalic anhydride, trimellitic anhydride and glycols copolymer. Contact Dermatitis 2007;56:172-173

2 Moffitt DL, Sansom JE. Allergic contact dermatitis from phthalic anhydride/trimellitic anhydride/glycol copolymers in nail varnish. Contact Dermatitis 2002;46:236

3 Gach JE, Stone NM, Finch TM. A series of four cases of allergic contact dermatitis to phthalic anhydride/trimellitic anhydride/glycols copolymer in nail varnish. Contact Dermatitis 2005;53:63-64

4 Le Coz CJ, Nassif A, Collet E. Allergy to phthalic anhydride/trimellitic anhydride/glycols copolymer in nail varnishes. Contact Dermatitis 2004;50:169 [abstract FC04.3]

5 Quartier S, Garmyn M, Becart S, Goossens A. Allergic contact dermatitis to copolymers in cosmetics – case report and review of the literature. Contact Dermatitis 2006;55:257-267

2.364   PHYTANTRIOL

IDENTIFICATION

Description/definition   : Phytantriol is the aliphatic alcohol that conforms to the formula shown below
Chemical class(es)   : Polyols
Chemical/IUPAC name   : 3,7,11,15-Tetramethylhexadecane-1,2,3-triol
Other names   : Tetramethyl trihydroxyhexadecane
CAS registry number (s)   : 74563-64-7
EC number(s)   : 277-923-2
CIR review(s)   : Int J Toxicol 2007;26(Suppl.1):107-114 (access: www.cir-safety.org/ingredients)
Merck Index monograph : 8768
Function(s) in cosmetics   : EU: humectant. USA: anticaking agents; hair conditioning agents; skin-conditioning
                             agents - miscellaneous
Patch testing   : 0.02%, 0.2% and 0.5% pet.(1)
Molecular formula   : $C_{20}H_{42}O_3$

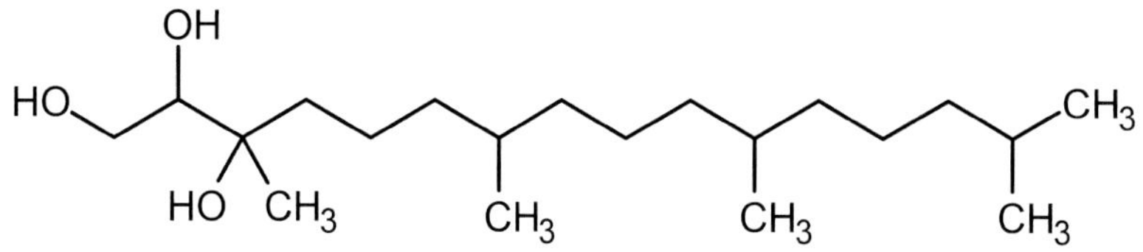

GENERAL

Phytantriol is a viscous light yellow fatty alcohol with a sweetish odor. As an ingredient in cosmetics, phytantriol can enhance the binding of dexpanthenol and amino acids to hair. According to the Cosmetic Ingredient Review (CIR) safety assessment, the chemical can be formulated at concentrations up to 3% without relevant irritation or sensitization (2).

CONTACT ALLERGY

Case reports and case series

A woman developed an acute eruption on her face a few days after starting to use a new face cream and had applied pure almond oil. Previously, she had suffered from reactions to hair dye and other cosmetics. Examination revealed marked erythema of her whole face with marked periorbital swelling and moderate scaling. Avoidance of the face cream and almond oil and treatment with a topical steroid resulted in prompt healing. Later, patch tests with the German Contact Dermatitis Group standard series and the patient's own cosmetic products. were performed showing positive reactions to the face cream and various allergens in the baseline series including fragrance mixes. All her other cosmetic products, including the almond oil, were negative. The manufacturer of the face cream supplied the 27 individual ingredients of the product. When patch tested, there were positive reactions to phytantriol 0.02%, 0.2%, and 0.5% in pet. The concentration of phytantriol in the cosmetic cream was 0.5%. A repeated open application test (ROAT) was then performed on the patient's forearm with 0.5% phytantriol in pet. After four applications on two consecutive days, the ROAT had to be stopped because an acute spreading dermatitis had developed in the test field (1).

Presence in cosmetic products and chemical analyses

In the USA, in April 2017, phytantriol was present in 22 of 56,714 cosmetic products of which the composition is known in FDA's Voluntary Cosmetic Registration Program (VCRP) (data obtained from FDA, May 2017). In March 2017, phytantriol was present in 130 of 65,431 cosmetic products of which the composition is known in EWG's Skin Deep Cosmetics Database, USA (http://www.ewg.org/skindeep/).

LITERATURE

1   Brasch J, Lipowsky F, Kreiselmaier I. Allergic contact dermatitis to phytantriol. Contact Dermatitis 2008;59:251-252
2   Cosmetic Ingredient Review. Final report on the safety assessment of phytantriol. Int J Toxicol 2007;26(Suppl.1):107-114

2.365 PHYTONADIONE

IDENTIFICATION

Description/definition   : Phytonadione is the organic compound that conforms to the formula shown below
Chemical class(es)   : Ketones
Chemical/IUPAC name   : 2-Methyl-3-(3,7,11,15-tetramethylhexadec-2-enyl)-1,4-naphthoquinone
Other names   : Vitamin K1; phylloquinone; phytomenadione
CAS registry number (s)   : 84-80-0; 81818-54-4; 11104-38-4
EC number(s)   : 234-330-3; 279-833-9; 201-564-2
SCCS opinion(s)   : SCCS/1313/10 (11); SCCP/1187/08 (12); SCCP/1105/07 (13)
Merck Index monograph   : 8762
Function(s) in cosmetics : EU: banned in November 2009 (1); USA: skin-conditioning agents - miscellaneous
EU cosmetic restrictions : Regulated in Annex II/1371 of the Regulation (EC) No. 1223/2009 (prohibited)
Patch testing   : 2% pet. (2,16); 1% and 10% pet. (3); 10% pet. was negative in control groups (3,7,15)
Molecular formula   : $C_{31}H_{46}O_2$

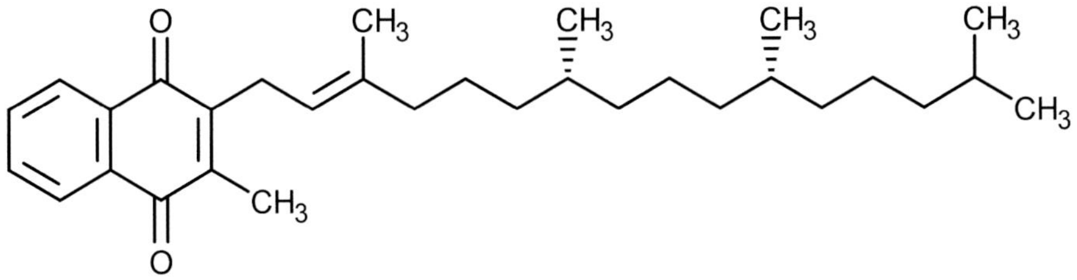

GENERAL

Vitamin K denotes a group of molecules that are needed for the synthesis of certain proteins, mostly required for blood coagulation. Vitamin K exists in 5 forms: vitamin K_1 (phytonadione), the natural form; vitamin K_2 (menaquinone) from intestinal bacterial synthesis; and the synthetic analogues vitamin K_3 (menadione), K_4 (menadiol) and vitamin K_5 (1,2). A deficiency of vitamin K results in symptoms of abnormal bleeding, including epistaxis, hematuria, ecchymoses, and bleeding from the gastrointestinal tract. Vitamin K, commonly in the form of phytonadione (vitamin K_1), is frequently used in the treatment and prevention of both hypoprothrombinemia and hemorrhagic disease of the newborn. In addition, it serves as an antidote to anticoagulants (4,17). Although phytonadione is rather nontoxic, severe adverse reactions can infrequently occur. Phytonadione is available for oral, intramuscular, subcutaneous, or intravenous routes. Especially with repeated injections, cutaneous reactions to vitamin K_1 may arise (17).

In 2004, phytonadione was marketed for topical use in cosmetics (16). Claimed uses for vitamin K_1 in cosmetics included skin lightening, improving periorbital pigmentation, and treatment of actinic and traumatic purpura. For these reasons, these cosmetics were also advised to help clear and prevent bruising associated with cosmetic surgery or laser therapy. Phytonadione-containing skin creams were recommended by some physicians and beauticians as a remedy for dark eye circles, bruising, spider veins, and varicose veins. They were available in prescription strength to over-the-counter products sold in the local drugstore, cosmetics shop, natural food store, or any number of online retailers. These products could be purchased in a range of formulations, containing differing concentrations of phytonadione (2%-5%). In 2009, however, as a result of its sensitizing potential, the substance was prohibited in the EU as an ingredient of cosmetics (1,16).

Adverse reactions

There are 4 types of adverse reactions to phytonadione relevant to the dermatologist / allergist:
1. contact allergy and allergic contact dermatitis from topical products, notably cosmetics;
2. an eczematous form appearing at parenteral (intramuscular, subcutaneous) injection sites with erythematous indurated plaques;
3. a late-appearing local scleroderma/morphea-like reaction at the injection site (intramuscular, subcutaneous) and
4. anaphylactic/anaphylactoid reactions to parenteral phytonadione (notably intravenous)

CONTACT ALLERGY

Case reports and case series

Between December 2003 and February 2006, the French Group REVIDAL-GERDA reported 12 cases of cosmetic allergy from phytonadione, 6 of who had such serious dermatitis that they required hospitalization (5). A woman developed allergic contact dermatitis of the face, particularly around the eyes, from a cream to depigment periorbital hyperpigmentation, containing phytonadione and retinol. Patch tests with the ingredients of this product were positive to vitamin K_1 2% pet. and *trans*-vitamin K 2% pet. All symptoms and signs cleared after she stopped this cosmetic treatment (2). Another female patient developed allergic contact dermatitis of the face with intense edema on the entire application zone from phytonadione in a cosmetic cream prescribed by her dermatologist to treat rosacea (3). On her own account, the patient tested the application repeatedly on the forearm, confirming reactivity. When tested with its ingredients, she reacted only to phytonadione 1% and 10% pet. (3).

Two patients developed allergic contact dermatitis of the eyelids and periorbital areas from a cream intended to decrease hyperpigmentation (4). Contact allergy to vitamin K_1 in 'glycoline lotion 15%' that had been applied to the face of a female patient following a peeling procedure caused a 'major erythematosquamous reaction' (14). Two women had dermatitis of the face from phytonadione in cosmetic creams (15). Another female individual developed dermatitis of the eyelids from phytonadione present in an anti-wrinkle eye cream (16).

Cross-reactions, pseudo-cross-reactions and co-reactions
Vitamin K_3 (1,18); vitamin K_4 (6).

Presence in cosmetic products and chemical analyses
In July 2017, phytonadione was present in 20 recent and 7 older products of 69,545 cosmetic products of which the composition is known in EWG's Skin Deep Cosmetics Database, USA (http://www.ewg.org/skindeep/). In the USA, in April 2017, phytonadione was present in 36 of 56,714 cosmetic products of which the composition is known in FDA's Voluntary Cosmetic Registration Program (VCRP) (data obtained from FDA, May 2017).

OTHER SIDE EFFECTS

Immediate-type reactions
In a patient with eczematous plaques from vitamin K_1-injections with a positive patch test to vitamin K_1, a prick test was positive after 15 min. From this area, a skin eruption reproducing exactly the same clinical characteristics of the adverse skin reaction (erythematous plaques) developed subsequently. An intradermal test with the commercial vitamin K_1 preparation gave a positive reaction after 30 minutes. Ten healthy controls that were also tested with prick and intradermal tests showed negative results (7).

Adverse reactions to parenteral administration of phytonadione

Cutaneous reactions
There are two main types of cutaneous reactions, occurring mainly after repeated intramuscular or subcutaneous administration of phytonadione: 1. erythematous and eczematous plaques and 2. scleroderma-like (morphea-like) reactions.

Erythematous and eczematous plaques
These lesions appear around the injection site 5 days to 4 weeks after one or more injections, either intramuscular or subcutaneous, rarely intravenous (35). Clinical presentations and morphology vary, with reactions consisting of erythematous, indurated plaques, sometimes with vesicles (19) or localized eczematous eruptions at the injection sites, which may sometimes spread (18) or be accompanied by a maculopapular eruption (21,29). The lesions may be tender or (intensely) pruritic (18). Localized urticaria after 3 days has been observed once (8). The plaques can grow to be 30 cm in diameter or more and heal spontaneously after some 4 weeks, sometimes with hyperpigmentation (17), but spontaneous healing can take up to 4 months or longer (10,19,23). Residual erythema in one case lasted for up to 6 months (18). Rarely, patients experience a prolonged course with development of sclerotic plaques 2-4 months after treatment, lasting for years. Hypersensitivity reactions to vitamin K_1 treatment were first described in patients with liver disease secondary to cirrhosis and/or hepatitis. However, this adverse effect is not restricted to those with liver dysfunction and appears to be dose-independent (17,20,33).

Several features of the erythematous and eczematous reaction to vitamin K_1 suggest that the reaction is a manifestation of delayed type hypersensitivity (18,19,21):
a. in most cases, there was an approximate 10-14 day lag between the first dose and appearance of the rash;
b. subsequent patch and/or prick/intradermal testing produces a reaction in 2-3 days (7,10,18,19,21,24,31,34 ,35);
c. a recall phenomenon has been described in several patients, in which patch or intradermal testing at a distant location precipitated an eczematous flare at the original reaction sites (19,21,29,34); and
d. lesional biopsies consistently showed spongiosis of the epidermis, dermal edema, and a perivascular mononuclear and eosinophilic cellular infiltrate, consistent with a delayed-type hypersensitivity reaction (7,10,18,19,21,22,28,29, 34).

Although prophylaxis against hemolytic disease of the newborn with intramuscular vitamin K_1 has been practiced routinely in many countries, there appear to be no reports in the English language literature of cutaneous eruptions due to this medication in neonates. This may be a consequence of the immaturity of the neonatal immune system. However, in some cases, this injection may represent the sensitizing event, as some adults reacted after a single injection (19,21,22,23). Some pediatric cases have been observed (31,32).

Patients with delayed type cutaneous reactions to injections with vitamin K_1 have been presented in refs. 7,10 and 17-35. These reactions seem to be far from rare, considering the many case reports, case series of 6 (21,32) and 4 patients (22,33) and 94 patients reported from Japan (probably not all local hypersensitivity reactions, but also skin rashes from intravenous administration) (27). The relevant literature up to 1994 has been reviewed in ref. 19.

Scleroderma-like reactions

Scleroderma-like reactions are late reactions to vitamin K_1 injections, that resemble localized scleroderma or morphea. The phenomenon is sometimes called Texier's disease, after the first author of the first publication on this rare side effect of phytonadione. The French authors described 9 patients with liver cirrhosis, 7 men and 2 women, who first had erythematous plaques at the sites of intramuscular vitamin K_1 injections, but subsequently developed a scleroderma-like picture that appeared up to 2 years later. The distribution of these sclerotic plaques was described as a 'ceinturon de cowboy avec ses revolvers' ('Cowboy's belt with revolvers'; 'Cowboy gun belt and holsters'), because of its extension around the waist and onto the lateral aspect of the thighs. Intracutaneous tests with vitamin K_1 were performed in 4 patients and they all had positive delayed reactions (37).

This side effect, that has been described in nearly 20 publications (10,37,38-53), many from France, occurs from weeks to 2 years after previous vitamin K_1 injections (38) with an average of about 9 months (9). It may appear with (47,53) or without (38,39,44,46,50,51) a previous *early* erythematous plaque - eczematous reaction (18). Generally, late erythematous plaques develop around the sites of injections and progressively extend from the upper part of the buttock to the lateral aspects of both thighs and around the waist, forming the 'cowboy gun belt and holsters' picture. These erythematous plaques progress in a few months to white dense sclerosis surrounded by a lilac border. After 12 to 18 months of evolution, the lilac border and then the cutaneous sclerosis progressively resolve. Lesions may, however, persist for over 10 years or be permanent (38). Most patients are adults, but a 2-year-old child (40) and 6 other children (46) developed scleroderma-like reactions from the vitamin K_1 injections they had received immediately after his birth.

No systemic or immunologic features of systemic sclerosis are found in these patients (52). Some authors have proposed 4 clinical and histopathological stages of vitamin K_1-induced skin sclerosis: erythematous, erythemato-pigmented, established scleroderma and regression of scleroderma (53). Histopathology of the scleroderma-like reactions shows a picture which is usually indistinguishable from deep morphea or scleroderma: sclerosis involving the reticular dermis and extending to the subcutaneous fat. Collagen bundles are homogenized and thickened. A mild to moderately dense lymphocytic infiltrate is seen among collagen bundles and around blood vessels and the epidermis is normal (19,38). Intradermal tests with vitamin K_1 (usually the commercial product) have consistently been positive when performed (10,38,41,50), but the pathogenesis is unknown.

Anaphylactic / anaphylactoid reactions

Intravenous (and to a far lesser degree intramuscular or subcutaneous) injection of vitamin K_1 (commercial preparations) may result in severe reactions with hypotension, bradycardia or tachycardia, dyspnea, bronchospasm, cardiac arrest, and death. The symptoms occur during or within 20 minutes after administration. The estimated incidence is low, 3 per 10,000 doses, but such reactions from *intravenous* administration may result in death in nearly 1 in every 5 cases (36). These reactions are most consistent with a nonimmune-mediated anaphylactoid mechanism. The majority of reactions have occurred in patients receiving vitamin K_1 solubilized with PEO-CO (polyoxyethylated castor oil), suggesting that the solubilizer may contribute in many of these reactions.

However, some reactions have been reported in patients receiving formulations free of PEO-CO, indicating that vitamin K_1 itself may also be responsible in some reactions. These reactions may be more likely to occur when vitamin K_1 is administered at higher doses, inadequately diluted, or quickly administered, but reactions have been reported despite all precautions being properly followed (36). A full literature review on this subject was published in 2016 (36).

LITERATURE

1   García-Gavín J, Goossens A, Tennstedt D. Allergic contact dermatitis due to cosmetics containing vitamin K1 oxide. Contact Dermatitis 2010;62:248-250
2   Veneziano L, Silvani S, Voudouris S, Tosti A. Contact dermatitis due to topical cosmetic use of vitamin K. Contact Dermatitis 2005;52:113-114

3   Serra-Baldrich E, Dalmau J, Pla C, Muntañola AA. Contact dermatitis due to clarifying cream. Contact Dermatitis 2005;53:174-175

4   Ruiz-Hornillos FJ, Prieto A, De Castro FJ, Martín E, De Barrio M, Tornero P, Sotés MR. Allergic contact dermatitis due to vitamin K1 contained in a cosmetic cream. Contact Dermatitis 2006;55:246-247

5   Vigan M. L'allergie au bufexamac: naissance d'un réseau de vigilance en dermato-allergologie. Rev Fr Allergol Immunol Clin 1999;39:299-300. (cited in ref. 1, but probably wrong reference) (article in French)

6   Sommer S, Wilkinson SM, Peckham D, Wilson C. Type IV hypersensitivity to vitamin K. Contact Dermatitis 2002;46:94-96

7   Giménez–Arnau AM, Toll A, Pujol RM. Immediate cutaneous hypersensitivity response to phytomenadione induced by vitamin K1 in skin diagnostic procedure. Contact Dermatitis 2005;52:284-285

8   Carton FX. Réaction allergique au cours d'un traitement: vitamine K1 +extrait de foie. Bull Soc Fr Dermat 1965;72:228 (article in French)

9   Wilkins K, De Koven J, Assaad D. Cutaneous reactions associated with vitamin K1. J Cutan Med Surg 2000;4:164-168

10   Balato N, Cuccurullo FM, Patruno C, Ayala F. Adverse skin reactions to vitamin K1: report of 2 cases. Contact Dermatitis 1998;38:341-342

11   SCCS (Scientific Committee on Consumer Safety). Opinion on vitamin K1 (phytonadione), 23 March 2010, SCCS/1313/10. Available at: http://ec.europa.eu/health/scientific_committees/consumer_safety/docs/sccs_o_014.pdf

12   SCCP (Scientific Committee on Consumer Products). Opinion on vitamin K1 (Phytonadione), 24 June 2008, SCCP/ 1187/08. Available at:
http://ec.europa.eu/health/archive/ph_risk/committees/04_sccp/docs/sccp_o_140.pdf

13   SCCP (Scientific Committee on Consumer Products). Opinion on Vitamin K1 (phytonadione), 28 September 2007, SCCP/1105/07. Available at:
http://ec.europa.eu/health/archive/ph_risk/committees/04_sccp/docs/sccp_o_107.pdf

14   Mestach L, Goossens A. Allergic contact dermatitis and nail damage mimicking psoriasis caused by nail hardeners. Contact Dermatitis 2016;74:112-114

15   Ramírez Santos A, Fernández-Redondo V, Pérez Pérez L, Concheiro Cao J, Toribio J. Contact allergy from vitamins in cosmetic products. Dermatitis 2008;19:154-156

16   Lopez-Lerma I, Vilaplana J. Contact dermatitis to vitamin K1 in an eye cream. Ann Allergy Asthma Immunol 2013;111:227-228

17   Sousa T, Hunter L, Petitt M, Wilkerson MG. Localized cutaneous reaction to intramuscular vitamin K in a patient with acute fatty liver of pregnancy. Dermatol Online J 2010;16(12):16

18   Wong DA, Freeman S. Cutaneous allergic reaction to intramuscular vitamin K1. Australas J Dermatol 1999;40:147-152

19   Bruynzeel I, Hebeda CL, Folkers E, Bruynzeel DP. Cutaneous hypersensitivity reactions to vitamin K: 2 case reports and a review of the literature. Contact Dermatitis 1995;32:78-82

20   Moreau-Cabarrot A, Giordano-Labadie F, Bazex J. Cutaneous hypersensitivity at the site of injection of vitamin K1. Ann Dermatol Venereol 1996;123:177-179 (article in French)

21   Finkelstein H, Champion MC, Adam JE. Cutaneous hypersensitivity to vitamin K1 injection. J Am Acad Dermatol 1987;16:540-545

22   Lemlich G, Green M, Phelps R, Lebwohl M, Don P, Gordon M. Cutaneous reactions to vitamin K1 injections. J Am Acad Dermatol 1993;28:345-347

23   Joyce JP, Hood AF, Weiss MM. Persistent cutaneous reaction to intramuscular vitamin K injection. Arch Dermatol 1988;124:27-28

24   Piguet B, Bertheuil F. Accidents cutanés allergiques provoqués par une préparation injectable de vitamine K1 synthétique. Bull Soc Fr Dermatol Syph 1964;71:486-491 (article in French)

25   Gettler SL, Fung MA. Off-center fold: indurated plaques on the arms of a 52-year-old man. Diagnosis: Cutaneous reaction to phytonadione injection. Arch Dermatol 2001;137:957-962

26   Lee MM, Gellis S, Dover JS. Eczematous plaques in a patient with liver failure. Fat-soluble vitamin K hypersensitivity. Arch Dermatol 1992;128:260-261

27   Tsuboi R, Ogawa H. Skin eruption caused by fat-soluble vitamin K injection. J Am Acad Dermatol 1988;18:386

28   Tuppal R, Tremaine R. Cutaneous eruption from vitamin K1 injection. J Am Acad Dermatol 1992;27:105-106

29   Barnes HM, Sarkany I. Adverse skin reaction from vitamin K1. Br J Dermatol 1976;95:653-656

30   Keough GC, English JC 3rd, Meffert JJ. Eczematous hypersensitivity from aqueous vitamin K injection. Cutis 1998;61:81-83

31   Pigatto PD, Bigardi A, Fumagalli M, Altomare GF, Riboldi A. Allergic dermatitis from parenteral vitamin K. Contact Dermatitis 1990;22:307-308

32   Bullen AW, Miller JP, Cunliffe WJ, Losowsky MS. Skin reactions caused by vitamin K in patients with liver disease. Br J Dermatol 1978;98:561-565

33 Sanders MN, Winkelmann RK, Rochester PD. Cutaneous reactions to vitamin K. J Am Acad Dermatol 1988;19:699-704

34 Robison JW, Odom RB. Delayed cutaneous reaction to phytonadione. Arch Dermatol 1978;114:1790-1792

35 Heydenreich G. A further case of adverse skin reaction from vitamin K1. Br J Dermatol 1977;97:697

36 Britt RB, Brown JN. Characterizing the severe reactions of parenteral Vitamin K1. Clin Appl Thromb Hemost 2016 Jan. DOI: 10.1177/1076029616674825

37 Texier L, Gendre PH, Gauthier O, Gauthier Y, Surlèvé-Bazeille JE, Boineau D. Hypodermites sclérodermiformes lombo-fessières induites par des injections médicamenteuses intramusculaires associées à la vitamine K1. Ann Derm Syph 1972;99:363-372 (article in French)

38 Pang BK, Munro V, Kossard S. Pseudoscleroderma secondary to phytomenadione (vitamin K1) injections: Texier's disease. Australas J Dermatol 1996;37:44-47

39 Pujol RM, Puig L, Moreno A, Perez M, de Moragas JM. Pseudoscleroderma secondary to phytonadione (vitamin K1) injections. Cutis 1989;43:365-368

40 Rommel A, Saurat JH. Hypodermite fessière sclérodermiforme et injections de vitamine K1 à la naissance. Ann Pediat 1982;29: 64-66 (article in French)

41 Larrègue M, Gallet Ph, Giacomoni P de, Rat JP. Sclérodermie lombofessière consecutive à des injections de vitamin K1. Bull Soc Fr Dermat 1975;82:447-448 (article in French)

42 Duntze F, Durand JR, Vignes P. Sclérodermie en bande secondaire à des injections de vitamine K1. Bull Soc Fr Dermat 1975;82:78-79 (article in French)

43 Misson R, Guenard C, Garrel J, Millet P. Placards sclérodermiformes des régions ilio-trochanteriennes paraissant consécutifs à des injections I.M. contenant de la vitamin K1. Bull Soc Fr Dermat 1972;79:581-582 (article in French)

44 Lembo S, Megna M, Balato A, Balato N. "Cowboy's belt with revolver" scleroderma caused by vitamin K1 injections. G Ital Dermatol Venereol 2012;147:203-205 (article in Italian)

45 Alonso-Llamazares J, Ahmed I. Vitamin K1-induced localized scleroderma (morphea) with linear deposition of IgA in the basement membrane zone. J Am Acad Dermatol 1998;38:322-324

46 Bourrat E, Moraillon I, Vignon-Pennamen MD, Fraitag S, Cavelier-Balloy B, Cordoliani F, et al. Scleroderma-like patch on the thigh in infants after vitamin K injection at birth: six observations. Ann Dermatol Venereol 1996;123:634-648 (article in French)

47 Morel A, Betlloch I. Morphea-like reaction from vitamin K1. Int J Dermatol 1995;34:201-202

48 Bazex A, Dupré A, Christol B, Serres D. Lumbo-buttocks sclerodermiformic reactions after injection of vitamin K1: Presentation of 2 cases. Histological verification. Bull Soc Fr Derm Syph 1972;79:578-581 (article in French).

49 Jean-Pastor MJ, Jean P, Gamby T. Accidents cutanés consecutifs à l'administration parenterale de vitamine K1. Therapie 1981;36:369-374 (article in French)

50 Guidetti MS, Vincenzi C, Papi M, Tosti A. Sclerodermatous skin reaction after vitamin K1 injections. Contact Dermatitis 1994;31:45-46

51 Brunskill NJ, Berth-Jones J, Graham-Brown R AC. Pseudosclerodermatous reaction to phytomenadione injection (Texier's syndrome). Clin Exp Dermatol 1988;13:276-278

52 Janin-Mercier A, Mosser C, Souteyrand P, Bourgees M. Subcutaneous sclerosis with fasciitis and eosinophilia after phytonadione injections. Arch Dermatol 1985;121:1421-1423

53 Mosser C, Janin-Mercier A, Souteyrand P. Les réactions cutanées après administration parenterale de vitamine K1. Ann Dermatol Venereol 1987;114:243-251 (article in French)

2.366 PHYTONADIONE EPOXIDE

IDENTIFICATION

Description/definition : Phytonadione epoxide is the organic compound that conforms to the formula shown below
Chemical class(es) : Ethers; ketones
Chemical/IUPAC name : 1a,7a-Dihydro-1a-methyl-7a-(3,7,11,15-tetramethyl-2-hexadecen-1-yl)-naphth[2,3-b]oxirene-2,7-dione
Other names : Vitamin K1 oxide; phylloquinone oxide; (2,3-epoxyphytyl)menaquinone
CAS registry number (s) : 25486-55-9
EC number(s) : 247-022-9
Merck Index monograph : 8762 (Phylloquinone)
Function(s) in cosmetics : EU: adstringent. USA: drug astringents - skin protectant drugs
Patch testing : 1% pet. (1)
Molecular formula : $C_{31}H_{46}O_3$

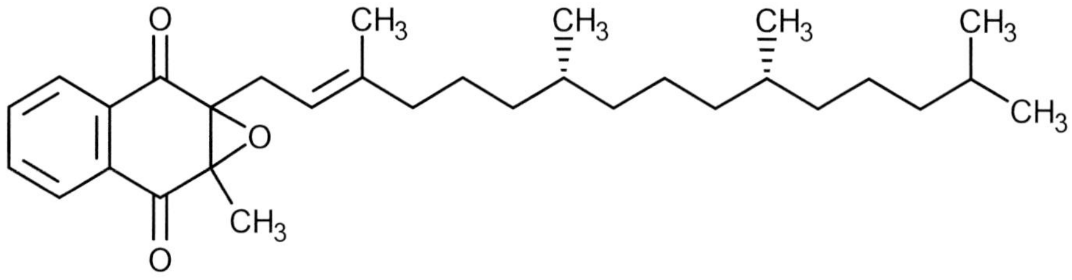

GENERAL

Vitamin K1 oxide, the oxidized isoform of vitamin K1, is claimed to be as effective as the non-oxidized form (vitamin K1, phytonadione) to treat post-procedural purpura after laser therapies. For this reason, cosmetics containing vitamin K1 oxide have replaced those containing the non-oxidized form after this was banned because it caused many cases of sensitization (1).

CONTACT ALLERGY

Case reports and case series

Phytonadione epoxide was stated to be the (or an) allergen in one patient in a group of 603 individuals suffering from cosmetic dermatitis, seen in the period 2010-2015 in Leuven, Belgium (2).

A woman developed eczematous lesions on her legs after the use of a cosmetic gel prescribed to prevent hyperpigmentation after the treatment of varicose veins with pulsed laser therapy. Examination showed slightly rounded perifollicular papules distributed over the anterior surface of both legs. A second woman, with history of breast cancer treated with surgery and radiotherapy, presented with pruritic lesions on the right breast, which she ascribed to the use of the same cosmetic gel, prescribed to treat post-radiotherapy telangiectasia. When she stopped using this product, her dermatitis settled. A third female individual presented with pruritic lesions of 4-month duration on her legs. This patient had applied the same product for a month after surgical treatment of varicose veins. When she stopped using the gel, only slight improvement was noted. Examination revealed erythematous perifollicular papules distributed all over her legs. Topical corticosteroids were prescribed and the lesions cleared completely after 1 month. All three patients were patch tested with the European baseline series, the cosmetic product 'as is', and - later -the vehicle components, provided by the manufacturer. The active component vitamin K1 oxide (phytonadione epoxide) 1% pet. was tested in 2 patients only because of insufficient material. All three patients reacted to the product as is and the 2 that were tested with it also to vitamin K1 oxide. There were no reactions to other ingredients of the gel (1).

Presence in cosmetic products and chemical analyses

In the USA, in April 2017, phytonadione epoxide was present in 12 of 56,714 cosmetic products of which the composition is known in FDA's Voluntary Cosmetic Registration Program (VCRP) (data obtained from FDA, May 2017). In March 2017, phytonadione epoxide was present in 4 of 65,431 cosmetic products of which the composition is known in EWG's Skin Deep Cosmetics Database, USA (http://www.ewg.org/skindeep/).

LITERATURE

1 García-Gavín J, Goossens A, Tennstedt D. Allergic contact dermatitis due to cosmetics containing vitamin K1 oxide. Contact Dermatitis 2010;62:248-250

2 Goossens A. Cosmetic contact allergens. Cosmetics 2016, 3, 5; doi:10.3390/cosmetics3010005

2.367   PIGMENT ORANGE 5

IDENTIFICATION

Description/definition   : Pigment orange 5 is a monoazo color, which conforms to the formula shown below
Chemical class(es)   : Color additives - miscellaneous
Chemical/IUPAC name   : 1-[(2,4-Dinitrophenyl)azo]-2-naphthol
Other names   : CI 12075; D&C orange no. 17; permanent orange
CAS registry number (s)   : 3468-63-1
EC number(s)   : 222-429-4
Function(s) in cosmetics   : EU: prohibited in the EU; delisted in 1992. USA: colorants
EU cosmetic restrictions   : Regulated in Annex II/397 of the Regulation (EC) No. 1223/2009 (prohibited)
Patch testing   : No data available; suggested: 1% pet.
Molecular formula   : $C_{16}H_{10}N_4O_5$

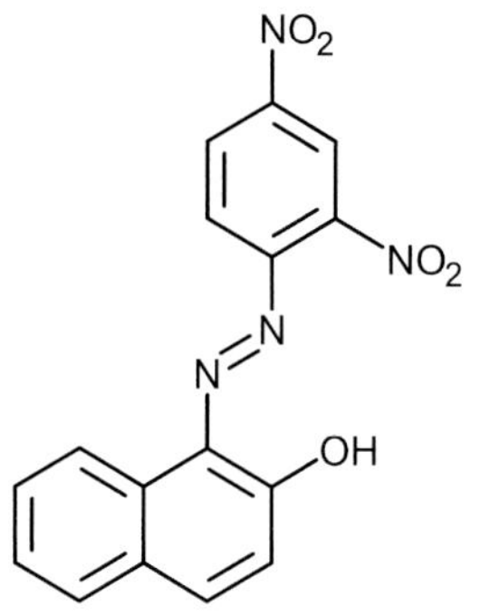

CONTACT ALLERGY

Patch testing in groups of patients

Of 38 Japanese patients with pigmented cosmetic dermatitis, patch tested and photopatch tested with coal tar dyes in 1975-1976, 4 had positive patch tests to pigment orange 5. It was not mentioned (and probably unknown) whether this color was present in the cosmetics used by the patients (1).

Case reports and case series

A woman had allergic contact cheilitis from D&C orange no.17 (pigment orange 5) in a lipstick (2).

Cross-reactions, pseudo-cross-reactions and co-reactions

Other coal tar dyes (1).

Presence in cosmetic products and chemical analyses

In the USA, in April 2017, pigment orange 5 was present in zero of 56,714 cosmetic products of which the composition is known in FDA's Voluntary Cosmetic Registration Program (VCRP) (data obtained from FDA, May 2017). In April 2017, pigment orange 5 was present in zero of 65,434 cosmetic products of which the composition is known in EWG's Skin Deep Cosmetics Database, USA (http://www.ewg.org/skindeep/).

OTHER SIDE EFFECTS

Photosensitivity

Of 38 Japanese patients with pigmented cosmetic dermatitis, patch tested and photopatch tested with coal tar dyes in 1975-1976, 3 had positive photopatch tests to pigment orange 5. It was not mentioned (and probably unknown) whether this color was present in the cosmetics used by the patients (1).

LITERATURE

1   Sugai T, Takahashi Y, Tagaki T. Pigmented cosmetic dermatitis and coal tar dyes. Contact Dermatitis 1977;3:249-256
2   Calnan CD. Reactions to artificial colouring materials. J Soc Cosm Chem 1967;18:215-223

2.368   PIGMENT RED 57:1

IDENTIFICATION

Description/definition   : Pigment red 57:1 is a monoazo color, which conforms to the formula shown below
Chemical class(es)   : Color additives - miscellaneous
INCI name USA   : Pigment red 57:1; red 7 (certified batches)
Chemical/IUPAC name   : Calcium 3-hydroxy-4-[(4-methyl-2-sulphonatophenyl)azo]-2-naphthoate;
Other names   : 4-(o-Sulfo-p-tolylazo)-3-hydroxy-2-naphthoic acid; CI 15850; D&C red 7 calcium lake;
                             Lithol rubin BCA®
CAS registry number (s)   : 5281-04-9
EINECS number(s)   : 226-109-5
Function(s) in cosmetics   : EU: cosmetic colorant. USA: colorants
EU cosmetic restrictions   : Regulated in Annex IV/27 of the Regulation (EC) No. 1223/2009 (
Patch testing   : 20% water (3); 1% pet. (4)
Molecular formula   : $C_{18}H_{14}CaN_2O_6S$

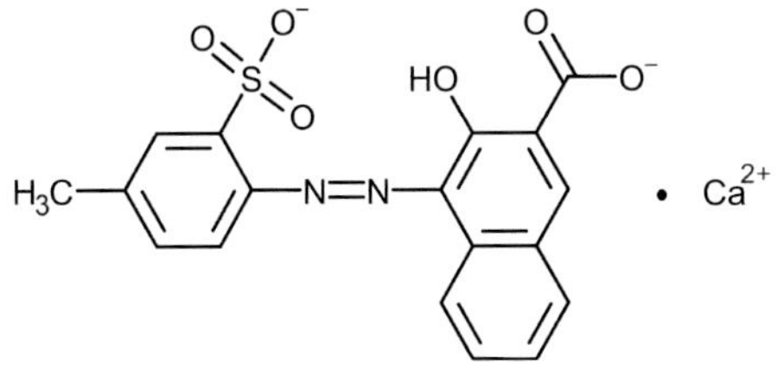

GENERAL
Commercial Lithol rubin BCA® contains calcium rosinate (to adjust color tone) and several subsidiary dyes (4).

CONTACT ALLERGY

Case reports and case series
Three patients had allergic contact cheilitis from pigment red 57:1 in lipsticks (1,2,3). An unknown number of Japanese patients had allergic contact cheilitis from the color in lipsticks (5,6,7, articles in Japanese, data cited in ref. 4). One patient developed pigmented cosmetic dermatitis from pigment red 57:1 in a lipstick; the allergy was shown to be caused by the free acid 4-(o-sulfo-p-tolylazo)-3-hydroxy-2-naphthoic acid (4).

Cross-reactions, pseudo-cross-reactions and co-reactions
4-(m-sulfo-p-tolylazo)-3-hydroxy-2-naphthoic acid (4).

Presence in cosmetic products and chemical analyses
In April 2017, D&C red 7 calcium lake was present in 103 of 66,485 cosmetic products of which the composition is known in EWG's Skin Deep Cosmetics Database, USA (http://www.ewg.org/skindeep/). In the USA, in April 2017, pigment red 57:1 was present in an unknown number of 56,714 cosmetic products of which the composition is known in FDA's Voluntary Cosmetic Registration Program (VCRP) (accidentally no data requested from FDA).

LITERATURE
1   Inui S, Azukizawa H, Katayama I. Recurrent contact cheilitis because of glyceryl isostearate, diisostearyl maleate, oleyl alcohol, and Lithol Rubine BCA in lipsticks. Contact Dermatitis 2009;60:231-232
2   Ando Y, Komanura H, Yoshikawa K. Contact cheilitis due to Lithol Rubine BCA. Environ Dermatol 1998;5:223-227 (in Japanese)
3   Ha JH, Kim HO, Lee JY, Kim CW. Allergic contact cheilitis from D&C Red no. 7 in lipstick. Contact Dermatitis 2003;48:231
4   Hayakawa R, Fujimoto Y, Kaniwa M-A. Allergic pigmented lip dermatitis from lithol rubine BCA. Am J Cont Derm 1994;5:34-37
5   Matsunaga K, Hayakawa R, Arima Y, et al. Contact dermatitis on vermilion border from lipstick. Hifubyoh-Shiryoh 1990;12:223-226 (in Japanese, data cited in ref. 4)
6   Utsumi M, Sugai T, Syouji A, et al. Lipstick dermatitis due to Lithol Rubine BCA. Skin Res 1991;11(suppl.33):238-244 (in Japanese, data cited in ref. 4)
7   Shono M, Kaniwa M, Japan Cosmetic Industry Association. Allergic contact cheilitis from Lithol Rubine BCA in lipstick. Skin Res 1992;14 (Suppl.34):208-213 (in Japanese, data cited in ref. 4)

2.369   PIGMENT RED 172 ALUMINUM LAKE

IDENTIFICATION

Description/definition   : Pigment red 172 aluminum lake is an insoluble pigment composed of the aluminum salt of CI Acid red 51 extended on an appropriate substrate. It conforms to the formula shown below

Chemical class(es)   : Color additives - miscellaneous; halogen compounds

Chemical/IUPAC name   : Dialuminum;2',4',5',7'-tetraiodo-3-oxospiro[2-benzofuran-1,9'-xanthene]-3',6'-diolate

Other names   : CI 45430 (Al); 2',4',5',7'-tetraiodofluorescein, aluminium salt; CI 45430:1; CI acid red 51:1; CI food red 14:1; FD&C red no. 3 - aluminum lake

CAS registry number (s)   : 12227-78-0

EC number(s)   : 235-440-4

Function(s) in cosmetics   : EU: formerly used for hair dyeing. USA: colorants

EU cosmetic restrictions   : Regulated in Annex II/1337 of the Regulation (EC) No. 1223/2009 (prohibited)

Patch testing   : 5% in polyethylene glycol (1)

Molecular formula   : $C_{60}H_{18}Al_2I_{12}O_{15}$

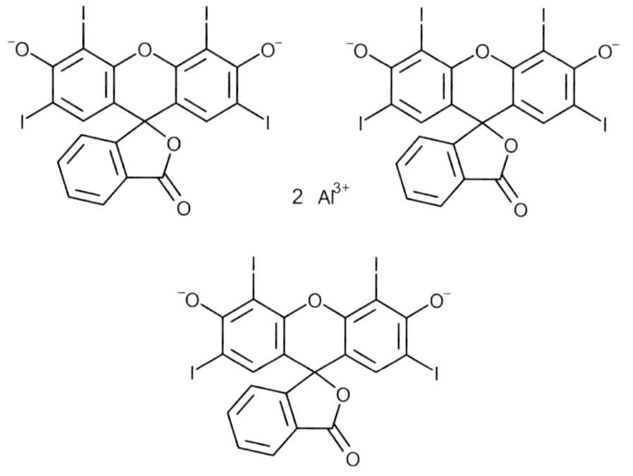

CONTACT ALLERGY

Patch testing in groups of patients

Of 28 Japanese patients with pigmented cosmetic dermatitis, patch tested and photopatch tested with coal tar dyes in 1975-1976, one had a positive patch test to pigment red 172 aluminum lake. It was not mentioned (and probably unknown) whether this color was present in the cosmetics used by the patient (1).

Cross-reactions, pseudo-cross-reactions and co-reactions

Other coal tar dyes (1)

Presence in cosmetic products and chemical analyses

In the USA, in April 2017, pigment red 172 aluminium lake was present in zero of 56,714 cosmetic products of which the composition is known in FDA's Voluntary Cosmetic Registration Program (VCRP) (data obtained from FDA, May 2017). In April 2017, pigment red 172 aluminum lake was present in zero of 65,434 cosmetic products of which the composition is known in EWG's Skin Deep Cosmetics Database, USA (http://www.ewg.org/skindeep/).

OTHER SIDE EFFECTS

Photosensitivity

Of 28 Japanese patients with pigmented cosmetic dermatitis, patch tested and photopatch tested with coal tar dyes in 1975-1976, one had a positive photopatch test to pigment red 172 aluminum lake. It was not mentioned (and probably unknown) whether this color was present in the cosmetics used by the patient (1).

LITERATURE

1   Sugai T, Takahashi Y, Tagaki T. Pigmented cosmetic dermatitis and coal tar dyes. Contact Dermatitis 1977;3:249-256

2.370   PIGMENT YELLOW 12

IDENTIFICATION

Description/definition	: Pigment yellow 12 is the diazo color that conforms to the structural formula shown below
Chemical class(es)	: Color additives - miscellaneous; halogen compounds
Chemical/IUPAC name	: 2-[[4-[4-[(1-anilino-1,3-dioxobutan-2-yl)diazenyl]-3-chlorophenyl]-2-chlorophenyl]diazenyl]-3-oxo-*N*-phenylbutanamide
Other names	: CI 21090; 2,2'-[(3,3'-dichloro[1,1'-biphenyl]-4,4'-diyl)bis(azo)]bis[3-oxo-*N*-phenylbutyramide]; benzidine yellow G
CAS registry number (s)	: 6358-85-6
EC number(s)	: 228-787-8
Function(s) in cosmetics	: EU: formerly used for hair dyeing; prohibited, delisted in 2008. USA: colorants
EU cosmetic restrictions	: Regulated in Annex II/1263 of the Regulation (EC) No. 1223/2009
Patch testing	: 5% in polyethylene glycol (1)
Molecular formula	: $C_{32}H_{26}Cl_2N_6O_4$

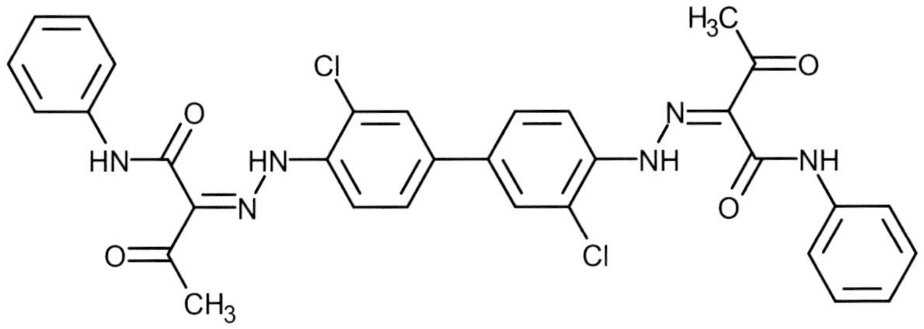

CONTACT ALLERGY

Patch testing in groups of patients

Of 38 Japanese patients with pigmented cosmetic dermatitis, patch tested and photopatch tested with coal tar dyes in 1975-1976, two had positive patch tests to pigment yellow 12. It was not mentioned (and probably unknown) whether this color was present in the cosmetics used by the patients (1).

Cross-reactions, pseudo-cross-reactions and co-reactions

Other coal tar dyes (1).

Presence in cosmetic products and chemical analyses

In the USA, in April 2017, pigment yellow 12 was present in zero of 56,714 cosmetic products of which the composition is known in FDA's Voluntary Cosmetic Registration Program (VCRP) (data obtained from FDA, May 2017). In April 2017, pigment yellow 12 was present in of zero of 65,434 cosmetic products of which the composition is known in EWG's Skin Deep Cosmetics Database, USA (http://www.ewg.org/skindeep/).

OTHER SIDE EFFECTS

Photosensitivity

Of 38 Japanese patients with pigmented cosmetic dermatitis, patch tested and photopatch tested with coal tar dyes in 1975-1976, one had a positive photopatch test to pigment yellow 12. It was not mentioned (and probably unknown) whether this color was present in the cosmetics used by the patient (1).

LITERATURE

1   Sugai T, Takahashi Y, Tagaki T. Pigmented cosmetic dermatitis and coal tar dyes. Contact Dermatitis 1977;3:249-256

2.371 POLYAMINOPROPYL BIGUANIDE

IDENTIFICATION

Description/definition : Polyaminopropyl biguanide is the organic compound that conforms to the formula shown below

Chemical class(es) : Synthetic polymers

Chemical/IUPAC name : 1-(Diaminomethylidene)-2-hexylguanidine

Other names : Polyhexamethylene biguanide hydrochloride; polyhexanide; PHMB; homopolymer of N-(3-aminopropyl)-imidodicarbonimidic diamide

CAS registry number (s) : 32289-58-0; 70170-61-5; 133029-32-0; 28757-47-3

SCCS opinion(s) : SCCS/1535/14, revision of 16 December 2014, 2nd revision of 13 July 2015 (13); SCCS, final opinion, 5 May 2017 (18)

Function(s) in cosmetics : EU: preservative. USA: preservatives

EU cosmetic restrictions : Regulated in Annex V/28- CMR2 from 1st Jan 2015 of the Regulation (EC) No. 1223/2009

Patch testing : 2.5% in water is probably too low; 5% is more appropriate, but may (rarely [16]) be irritant (9); higher concentrations (10-20%) may be necessary in selected cases (11,19)

Molecular formula : $(C_8H_{17}N_5)$mult. (HCl)

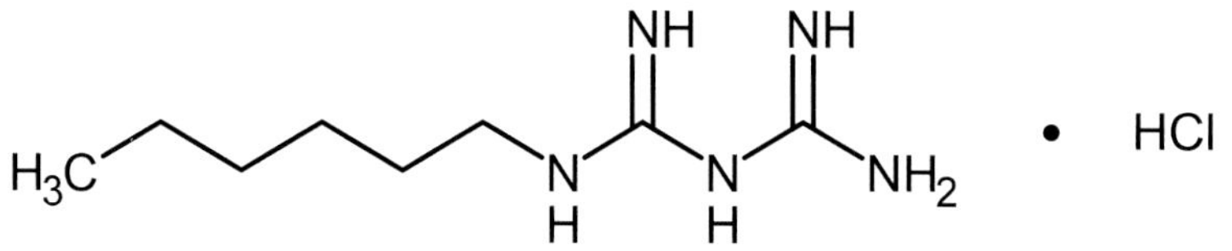

GENERAL

Polyaminopropyl biguanide (frequently used synonym: polyhexamethylene biguanide hydrochloride) is a broad-spectrum, fast-acting bactericide that is now widely used as a preservative for cosmetics, such as make-up removers, toners, facial cleansers, deodorants and (baby) wet wipes. In recent years, there has been increasing use of polyaminopropyl biguanide as wound care antiseptic solutions, gels, and dressings, especially in traumatic and orthopedic surgery, owing to its tissue compatibility. It is also used in non-alcoholic disinfectants and hand rub lotions, which are widely used in hospitals, and in contact lens solutions. Another application is its use as a water disinfectant in the treatment of swimming pools (2,9,15).

The identification of polyaminopropyl biguanide is somewhat confusing. In CosIng, polyaminopropyl biguanide is described as polyhexamethylene biguanide hydrochloride (which is correct). Two of the 4 CAS numbers (32289-58-0, 70170-61-5) indeed refer to polyhexamethylene biguanide hydrochloride, the others (133029-32-0, 28757-47-3) to polyhexamethylene biguanide. In many publications, this name is used and in some chemical databases, the parent compound and its hydrochloride salt are presented as synonyms (www.chemicalbook.com).

CONTACT ALLERGY

Patch testing in groups of patients

Results of studies patch testing polyaminopropyl biguanide in consecutive patients suspected of contact dermatitis (routine testing) and in groups of selected patients are shown in table 2.371.1. In routine testing, frequencies of sensitiza-tion have ranged from 0.5% to 0.9%; the highest frequencies were found with the 5% test material, but 40% of the 'positive' reactions were considered to be irritant (9). Relevance was either not found (9) or not mentioned (1,7). In a group of selected patients (those tested with a cosmetic and medicament series), the sensitization rate was only 0.4%, but the patients were tested with polyaminopropyl biguanide 2.5% in water, which may result in false-negative reactions (10).

Case reports and case series

A woman had therapy-resistant dermatitis of both upper and lower eyelids. Patch tests with the European baseline series, a cosmetic series and her own personal care products, including an eye make-up remover, was negative. However, a ROAT with the remover produced a positive reaction with a marked follicular accentuation. Further patch tests with some of the available ingredients of the make-up remover, among which polyaminopropyl biguanide 5% in water, were negative at D2, but the preservative was positive at D4. After stopping the use of the incriminated cosmetic product, the patient's symptoms healed completely and did not recur (17). A man had chronic and recurrent anogenital dermatitis from polyaminopropyl biguanide in wet wipes (11).

Table 2.371.1 Patch testing in groups of patients

Years and Country	Test conc. & vehicle	Number of patients tested	positive (%)		Selection of patients (S); Relevance (R); Comments (C)	Ref.
Routine testing						
2005 IVDK	2.5% water	1975	10	(0.5%)	R: none found; C: at least 4 of the 10 positive reactions	9
	5% water	1975	16	(0.8%)	were considered to be irritant, as no reactions were seen	
					to the 2.5% test preparation; However, 2.5% is too low to	
					detect all cases of sensitization	
1998 & 2005 IVDK	5% water	3207	30	(0.9%)	R: not stated	1
	2.5% water.	8848	60	(0.6%)	R: not stated	
1998 UK	2.5% water	274	2	(0.5%)	C: no further details present; data cited in refs. 2 and 9	7
Testing in selected groups of patients						
1998 IVDK	2.5% water	1554	6	(0.4%)	S: patients tested with a cosmetics and medicaments	10
					series; R: 1/6, a hospital cleaner working with a polyamino-	
					propyl biguanide-containing disinfectant	

IVDK: Information Network of Departments of Dermatology, Germany, Austria, Switzerland

Contact allergy to polyaminopropyl biguanide in non-cosmetic products

A nurse had occupational allergic contact dermatitis from polyaminopropyl biguanide present in a non-alcoholic hand rub at a concentration of 0.3% (8). A hospital cleaner had dermatitis from contact allergy to polyaminopropyl biguanide present in a disinfectant (10). A woman had allergic contact dermatitis of the legs and hand from polyaminopropyl biguanide in a wound gel applied to leg ulcers (16).

A woman had an itchy reaction involving her left (non-dominant) hand that had been present for 2 years, which she attributed to a particular rinse-off contact lens cleaning solution. Patch tests with the baseline series, a cosmetic series, a fragrance series, a corticosteroid series, and the patient's personal care products gave a doubtful reaction to the contact lens cleaning solution tested 'as is' on day 4. A dilution test and a semi-open test were both positive. Testing with the ingredients of the products revealed positive reactions to polyaminopropyl biguanide 10% and 20% in water. A test with a 2% solution was negative and with 5% weakly positive. Patch tests with polyaminopropyl biguanide 20% water in 10 controls were negative. The patient replaced the solution with another product not containing polyaminopropyl biguanide, but the lesions did not clear. This product proved to labeled with the term 'polyhexanide' (a synonym), which was not recognized by the patient (19).

Cross-reactions, pseudo-cross-reactions and co-reactions

Possibly limited cross-reactivity concerning type-I allergy (IgE-mediated) to the related biguanide derivative chlorhexidine (5).

Presence in cosmetic products and chemical analyses

In the USA, in April 2017, polyaminopropyl biguanide was present in 151 of 56,714 cosmetic products of which the composition is known in FDA's Voluntary Cosmetic Registration Program (VCRP) (data obtained from FDA, May 2017). In January 2017, polyaminopropyl biguanide was present in 138 of 64,655 cosmetic products of which the composition is known in EWG's Skin Deep Cosmetics Database, USA (http://www.ewg.org/skindeep/).

In Spain, in 2016-2017, the ingredients of 2237 products (cosmetics, topical medicines, and household cleaning products) available in Spain were analysed in order to determine the presence of polyaminopropyl biguanide. This preservative was found in eight leave-on cosmetics (0.4%) only: four brands of wet wipes, one eye make-up remover, two micellar solutions, and one moisturizer (19). Polyaminopropyl biguanide was also found to be present in 16 of 35 (46%) contact lens care solutions from five brands at concentrations ranging from 0.00005% to 0.001% (19).

Other information

On the basis of both animal and human studies, polyaminopropyl biguanide is considered to be a sensitizer (6).

OTHER SIDE EFFECTS

Immediate-type reactions

A male patient developed anal pruritus, angioedema and general malaise after the use of a wipe for intimate hygiene. There were positive prick test after 15 minutes to the wipe and to its ingredient polyaminopropyl biguanide

10% in water. A basophil activation test was positive. There was no reaction to chlorhexidine, which is also a biguanide derivative (2). An 18-year-old woman and a 15-year-old boy both had severe immediate reactions when a disinfectant containing polyaminopropyl biguanide was used to clean surgical wounds during orthopedic surgery. Immediate-type hypersensitivity to polyaminopropyl biguanide was shown by positive prick test results. Both patients had previously been exposed to chlorhexidine, but prick testing with this gave negative results (3). A case of anaphylaxis during orthopedic surgery in a young boy following the perioperative use of a solution containing polyaminopropyl biguanide to the wound was observed. Immediate-type hypersensitivity to polyaminopropyl biguanide was assumed but not proven, as no prick or other tests to confirm the diagnosis were performed (4).

A woman developed anaphylaxis with palmar pruritus, flush, swelling of the lips, swallowing difficulties, hypotension and loss of consciousness (stage 3 contact urticaria syndrome) following the use of a new brand of moist toilet tissue containing polyaminopropyl biguanide (5). She had previously experienced three episodes of minor symptoms caused by the same antimicrobial agent in a wound dressing and two episodes following the use of two different wound cleansing products. Prick tests with polyaminopropyl biguanide and with chlorhexidine gave positive results, and ImmunoCAPs revealed specific IgE to both antimicrobials. Limited *in vitro* cross-reactivity was demonstrated, with higher avidity of the patient's IgE antibodies for polyaminopropyl biguanide than for chlorhexidine, which is a very well known cause of immediate-type reactions (see Chapter 2.91 Chlorhexidine digluconate) (5). One patient allergic to a cosmetic had a positive prick test to polyaminopropyl biguanide; clinical details were not provided (12).

A review of contact urticaria caused by ingredients of cosmetics has been provided in ref. 14.

LITERATURE

1   Schnuch A, Lessmann H, Geier J, Uter W. Contact allergy to preservatives. Analysis of IVDK data 1996-2009. Br J Dermatol 2011;164:1316-1325

2   Creytens K, Goossens A, Faber M, Ebo D, Aerts O. Contact urticaria syndrome caused by polyaminopropyl biguanide in wipes for intimate hygiene. Contact Dermatitis 2014;71:307-309

3   Olivieri J, Eigenmann PA, Hauser C. Severe anaphylaxis to a new disinfectant: polyhexanide, a chlorhexidine polymer. Schweiz Med Wochenschr 1998;128:1508-1511

4   Ferrarini A, Baggi M, Flückiger R, Bianchetti MG. Intraoperative anaphylaxis to a chlorhexidine polymer in childhood. Paediatr Anaesth 2006;16:705

5   Kautz O, Schumann H, Degerbeck F, Venemalm L, Jakob T. Severe anaphylaxis to the antiseptic polyhexanide. Allergy 2012;65:1068-1070

6   Committee for Risk Assessment RAC Annex 1. Background Document to the Opinion proposing harmonised classification and labelling at Community level of Polyhexamethylene biguanide or Poly(hexamethylene) biguanide hydrochloride or PHMB, 9 September 2011. Available at: http://echa.europa.eu/documents/10162/2125cf0b-8320-48fc-b213-2f4fe29e3d38

7   McFadden JP, Wakelin S, Holloway DB, Rycroft RJG, White IR, Basketter DA. Positive patch test reactions to polyhexamethylene biguanide. In: Abstract 5th Congress of the European Society of Contact Dermatitis, Helsinki, 1998 (data cited in ref. 2)

8   Pummi K, Kemppi E, Lammintausta K. Occupational sensitization to polyhexamethylene guanidine hydrochloride in a non-alcoholic hand rub. Contact Dermatitis 2012;66:348-349

9   Schnuch A, Geier J, Uter W, Basketter DA, Jowsey IR. The biocide polyhexamethylene biguanide remains an uncommon contact allergen. Contact Dermatitis 2007;56:235-239

10   Schnuch A, Geier J, Brasch J, Fuchs Th, Pirker C, Schulze-Dirks A, Basketter DA. Polyhexamethylene biguanide: a relevant contact allergen? Contact Dermatitis 2000;42:302-303

11   Leysen J, Goossens A, Lambert J, Aerts O. Polyhexamethylene biguanide is a relevant sensitizer in wet wipes. Contact Dermatitis 2014: 70: 323-325

12   Goossens A. Cosmetic contact allergens. Cosmetics 2016, 3, 5; doi:10.3390/cosmetics3010005

13   SCCS (Scientific Committee on Consumer Safety). Opinion on the safety of poly(hexamethylene) biguanide hydrochloride or polyaminopropyl biguanide (PHMB) in cosmetic products, 18 June 2014, SCCS/1535/14, revision of 16 December 2014, 2nd revision of 13 July 2015. Available at: http://ec.europa.eu/health/scientific_committees/consumer_safety/docs/sccs_o_157.pdf

14   Verhulst L, Goossens A. Cosmetic components causing contact urticaria: a review and update. Contact Dermatitis 2016;75:333-344

15 Kaehn K. Polyhexanide: a safe and highly effective biocide. Skin Pharmacol Physiol 2010;23(Suppl): 7-16

16 Bervoets A, Aerts O. Polyhexamethylene biguanide in wound care products: a non-negligible cause of peri-ulcer dermatitis. Contact Dermatitis 2016;74:53-55

17 Aerts O, Smeets J, Adriaenssens K, Lambert J, Goossens A. Contact allergy to biguanides might explain cases of unresolved eyelid dermatitis. J Eur Acad Dermatol Venereol 2015;29:2064-2065

18 Opinion of the scientific committee on consumer safety (SCCS) – Final opinion on Polyaminopropyl Biguanide (PHMB) - Submission III- in cosmetic products, Regulatory Toxicology and Pharmacology 2017, doi: 10.1016/j.yrtph.2017.04.013

19 Pastor-Nieto MA, González-Muñoz P, Pérez-Mesonero R, Melgar-Molero V, Pastor-Nieto MB, Zarallo-Gallardo J, Martín-Alcalde E, De Eusebio-Murillo E. Allergic contact dermatitis caused by poly(hexamethylene) biguanide hydrochloride in contact lens care solutions. Contact Dermatitis 2017;76:373-376

2.372   POLYESTER-8

IDENTIFICATION

Description/definition   : Polyester-8 is a copolymer of adipic acid and neopentyl glycol end-capped with either octyldodecanol or a cyanodiphenylpropenoyl group. It conforms generally to the formula shown below

Chemical class(es)   : Synthetic polymers
Other names   : Polycrylene®
CAS registry number (s)   : 862993-96-2
Function(s) in cosmetics : EU: film forming; skin conditioning. USA: film formers; skin-conditioning agents – miscellaneous
Patch testing   : 3% pet. (1)

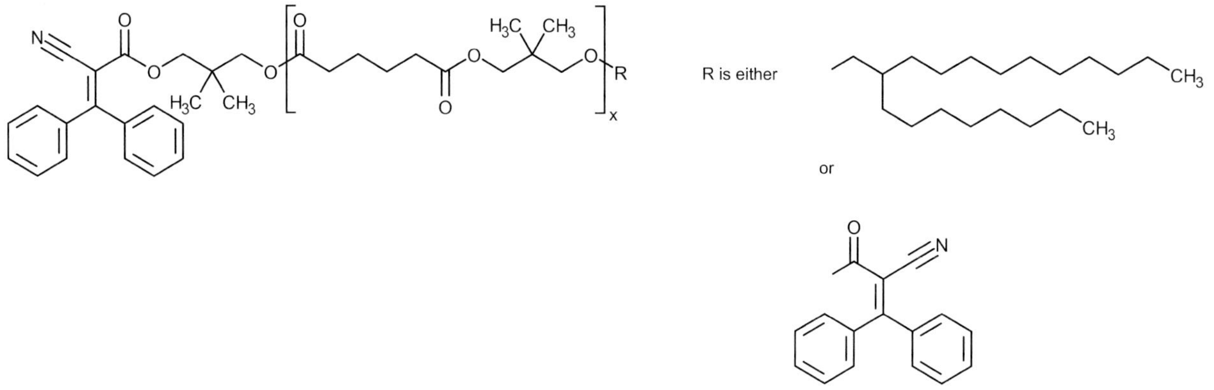

GENERAL

Polyester-8 is a novel photostabilizer used in sunscreens. It is a copolymer, with part of the molecule having structural similarities to octocrylene. The cyanodiphenyl propenoate moiety has the ability to absorb in the UVB range. Like octocrylene, polyester-8 photostabilizes the UVA absorber butyl methoxydibenzoylmethane to provide SPF enhancement. It also improves the waterproofing of sunscreen formulations as measured by their resistance to water. The hapten in one reported case of contact allergy to polyester-8 is unknown (1).

CONTACT ALLERGY

Case reports and case series

A woman developed severe dermatitis from a SPF25 moisturizer during the summer. She had used the product for a number of days prior to developing the reaction on her cheeks and upper neck, which resolved after a week. Patch tests with the British Society of Cutaneous Allergy baseline series, cosmetic series, fragrance and sunscreen series, and the suspected product (the product and the sunscreen series were also photopatch tested) gave positive reactions to the SPF25 moisturizer on both covered and uncovered sites. The sunscreen series, including octocrylene, was entirely negative. The patient was patch-tested in a second session with the 50 ingredients of the cream, and retested with the cream 'as is'. A positive reaction was observed to polyester-8 (3.0% pet.) at D4, and the cream itself was again positive. Twenty controls were negative to the cream and polyester-8 (1).

Cross-reactions, pseudo-cross-reactions and co-reactions

Not to octocrylene (1).

Presence in cosmetic products and chemical analyses

In the USA, in April 2017, polyester-8 was present in 2 of 56,714 cosmetic products of which the composition is known in FDA's Voluntary Cosmetic Registration Program (VCRP) (data obtained from FDA, May 2017). In April 2017, polyester-8 was present in zero of 65,434 cosmetic products of which the composition is known in EWG's Skin Deep Cosmetics Database, USA (http://www.ewg.org/skindeep/).

LITERATURE

1   Esdaile B, Cooper SM. Allergic contact dermatitis caused by polyester-8 (Polycrylene®) in a sunscreen moisturizer. Contact Dermatitis 2012;67:105-106

2.373 POLYETHYLENE

IDENTIFICATION

Description/definition	: Polyethylene is a polymer of ethylene monomers that conforms generally to the formula shown below
Chemical class(es)	: Synthetic polymers
Other names	: Coathylene®; ethylene, homopolymer
CAS registry number (s)	: 9002-88-4
Merck Index monograph	: 8957
CIR review(s)	: Int J Toxicol 2007;26(Suppl.1):115-127; Final report, June 2015 (access: www.cir-safety.org/ingredients)
Function(s) in cosmetics	: EU: abrasive; film forming; viscosity controlling. USA: abrasives; adhesives; binders; bulking agents; emulsion stabilizers; film formers; oral care agents; viscosity increasing agents - nonaqueous
Patch testing	: 10% pet. (1)
Molecular formula	: $(C_2H_4)x$

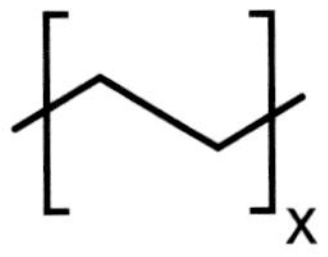

CONTACT ALLERGY

Case reports and case series

A woman had a 1-year history of a scaly eruption on both upper and lower lids of both eyes. This had begun as swelling and scaling of the upper eyelids and later spread to the lower eyelids. Personal and family history of atopy were negative. Patch tests with the European standard, a medicaments series and her personal cosmetics gave a positive reaction to a mascara. Later, the patient was tested with its ingredients and she now reacted to coathylene 10% pet. Patch testing in 15 controls was negative. Coathylene was described as a low density polyethylene (1).

Presence in cosmetic products and chemical analyses

In the USA, in April 2017, polyethylene was present in 3278 of 56,714 cosmetic products of which the composition is known in FDA's Voluntary Cosmetic Registration Program (VCRP) (data obtained from FDA, May 2017). In April 2017, polyethylene was present in 1781 of 65,434 cosmetic products of which the composition is known in EWG's Skin Deep Cosmetics Database, USA (http://www.ewg.org/skindeep/).

Irritant contact dermatitis

Polyethylene cause some irritation at temperatures above 60° C (1)

LITERATURE

1 Chowdhury MM. Allergic contact dermatitis from prime yellow carnauba wax and coathylene in mascara. Contact Dermatitis 2002;46:244

2.374   POLYGLYCERYL-10 LAURATE

IDENTIFICATION

Description/definition	: Polyglyceryl-10 laurate is an ester of lauric acid and polyglycerin-10
Chemical class(es)	: Glyceryl esters and derivatives
Chemical/IUPAC name	: 2,3-Dihydroxypropyl 2,2,3,3,4,4,5,5,6-nonakis(2,3-dihydroxypropyl)dodecanoate
Other names	: 1,2,3-Propanetriol, homopolymer, dodecanoates (1:1) (10 mol glycerol average molar ratio); decaglycerin monolaurate
CAS registry number (s)	: 34406-66-1
CIR review(s)	: Final report, September 2016 (access: www.cir-safety.org/ingredients)
Function(s) in cosmetics	: EU: skin conditioning. USA: skin-conditioning agents - miscellaneous; surfactants – emulsifying agents
Patch testing	: 1%, 0.5%, 0.1%, and 0.05% water (1)
Molecular formula	: $C_{42}H_{84}O_{22}$

CONTACT ALLERGY

Case reports and case series

A female patient had recurring pruritic erythema on her face for 3 months, which became worse despite cortico-steroid treatment. She was patch tested with her cosmetics and reacted to an 'essential gel'. Later, all ingredients of this cosmetic were tested and there was a positive reaction to polyglyceryl-10 laurate 0.5% water, which remained positive after 7 days. A dilution series was then tested with polyglyceryl-10 laurate 1%, 0.5%, 0.1%, and 0.05% in water, and she had positive reactions to all concentrations. Testing with the chemical from 3 manufacturers were all positive. Finally, the patient was patch tested with related chemicals and she reacted positively to polyglyceryl-4 laurate and polyglyceryl-6 laurate, both at 1% and 0.5% water. There were no positive reactions to polyglyceryl-10 myristate, polyglyceryl-10 isostearate, polyglyceryl-10 stearate, and polyglyceryl-10 oleate (1%, 0.5%, 0.05%, and 0.01% water). Control tests in an unspecified number of patients were negative. The dermatitis cleared and did not recur after the patient ceased using the essential gel (1).

Cross-reactions, pseudo-cross-reactions and co-reactions

Polyglyceryl-4 laurate and polyglyceryl-6 laurate (1). Not to polyglyceryl-10 myristate, polyglyceryl-10 isostearate, polyglyceryl-10 stearate, and polyglyceryl-10 oleate (1).

Presence in cosmetic products and chemical analyses

In the USA, in April 2017, polyglyceryl-10 laurate was present in 63 of 56,714 cosmetic products of which the composition is known in FDA's Voluntary Cosmetic Registration Program (VCRP) (data obtained from FDA, May 2017). In April 2017, polyglyceryl-10 laurate was present in 77 of 65,434 cosmetic products of which the composition is known in EWG's Skin Deep Cosmetics Database, USA (http://www.ewg.org/skindeep/).

LITERATURE

1   Washizaki K, Kanto H, Yazaki S, Ito M. A case of allergic contact dermatitis to polyglyceryl laurate. Contact Dermatitis 2008;58:187-188

2.375 POLYQUATERNIUM-7

IDENTIFICATION

Description/definition : Polyquaternium-7 is the polymeric quaternary ammonium salt of acrylamide and dimethyl diallyl ammonium chloride
Chemical class(es) : Quaternary ammonium compounds; synthetic polymers
Chemical/IUPAC name : Dimethyl-bis(prop-2-enyl)azanium;prop-2-enamide; chloride
Other names : Dimethyldiallyl ammonium chloride/acrylamide copolymer
CAS registry number (s) : 26590-05-6
CIR review(s) : J Am Coll Toxicol 1995;14:476-484 (access: www.cir-safety.org/ingredients)
Function(s) in cosmetics : EU: antistatic; film forming. USA: antistatic agents; film formers; hair fixatives
EU cosmetic restrictions : Regulated in Annex III/66 of the Regulation (EC) No. 1223/2009
Patch testing : 0.1-0.5-1.0% water (1)
Molecular formula : $(C_{11}H_{21}ClN_2O)_x$

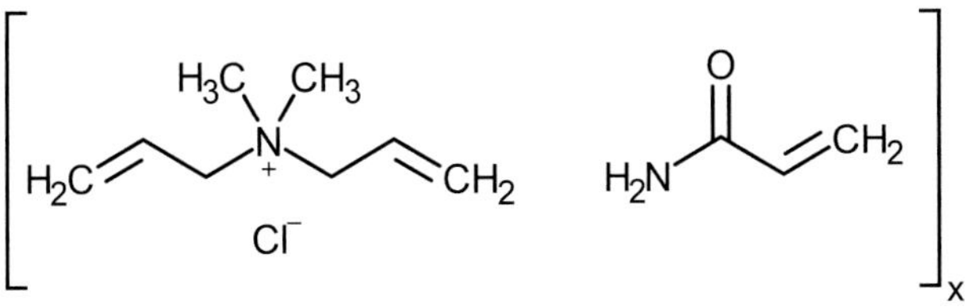

CONTACT ALLERGY

Case reports and case series

A non-atopic nurse, known to be allergic to nickel and fragrance, had a one-year history of work-related dermatitis of the hands, spreading to the arms, face, neck and V of the neck. The patient worked in an emergency hospital department, but prick tests and RAST had excluded sensitization to latex. Patch testing confirmed contact allergy to fragrances and nickel. While working on another ward there was some improvement, but her eczema had relapsed and she then started using a perfume-free moisturizing lotion several times a day. Patch tests with the Italian standard series (excluding nickel and fragrance mix), the cosmetic, corticosteroid, and rubber series and her own moisturizing lotion (tested as is), gave a positive reaction to the lotion only. Discontinuing the use of this cosmetic product resulted in clearance of the dermatitis after 3 weeks. A repeated open application test (ROAT) with the lotion was positive at D2 already.

When tested with its ingredients, the patient reacted positively to polyquaternium-7 1% water. Patch testing with a dilution series of polyquaternium-7 at 0.1%, 0.5%, and 1% resulted in positive reactions to all three concentrations, which were negative in 20 controls. Prick and patch tests with the gloves were negative, but when the nurse rubber her fingers on the inside of a particular glove, so as to pick up some powder, and then gently rubbed this onto one of her upper eyelids 1dd, within 2 days, she developed itchy erythema and edema of this eyelid. The patient was told to avoid skin-care cosmetics and other products containing fragrance, laureth-9 and polyquaternium-7 and has been free of symptoms since then. It was concluded that the patient had occupational airborne allergic contact dermatitis from an unidentified substance in glove powder and contact allergy to quaternium-7 in the moisturizing lotion (1).

Presence in cosmetic products and chemical analyses

In the USA, in April 2017, polyquaternium-7 was present in 1839 of 56,714 cosmetic products of which the composition is known in FDA's Voluntary Cosmetic Registration Program (VCRP) (data obtained from FDA, May 2017). In April 2017, polyquaternium-7 was present in 484 of 65,434 cosmetic products of which the composition is known in EWG's Skin Deep Cosmetics Database, USA (http://www.ewg.org/skindeep/).

LITERATURE

1   Gallo R, Basso M, Voltolini S, Guarrera M. Allergic contact dermatitis from laureth-9 and polyquaternium-7 in a skin-care product. Contact Dermatitis 2001;45:356-357

2.376 POLYSILICONE-15

IDENTIFICATION

Description/definition	: Polysilicone-15 is the siloxane polymer that conforms generally to the formula shown below
Chemical class(es)	: Siloxanes and silanes; synthetic polymers
Chemical/IUPAC name	: Siloxanes and silicones, dimethyl, 3-(4-(2,2-di(ethoxycarbonyl)ethenyl)phenoxy)propen-2-yl methyl, 3-(4-(2,2-di(ethoxycarbonyl)ethenyl)phenoxy)propen-1-yl methyl, trimethylsilyl terminated
Other names	: Diethylbenzylidene malonate dimethicone; dimethicodiethylbenzalmalonate; benzylidenemalonatepolysiloxane; Parsol® SLX
CAS registry number (s)	: 207574-74-1
EC number(s)	: 606-621-9
SCCS opinion(s)	: SCCS/1346/10 (12)
Function(s) in cosmetics	: EU: UV-filter. USA: light stabilizers
EU cosmetic restrictions	: Regulated in Annex VI/26 of the Regulation (EC) No. 1223/2009
Patch testing	: 10% pet. (Chemotechnique)

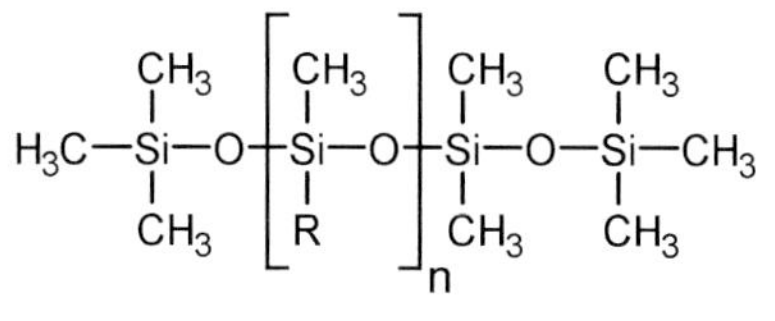

$R = \sim 92.1 - 92.5\%$ $-CH_3$

and $\sim 6\%$

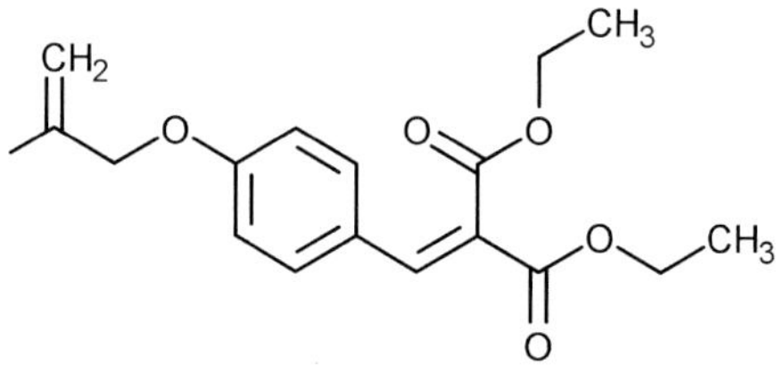

and $\sim 1.5\%$

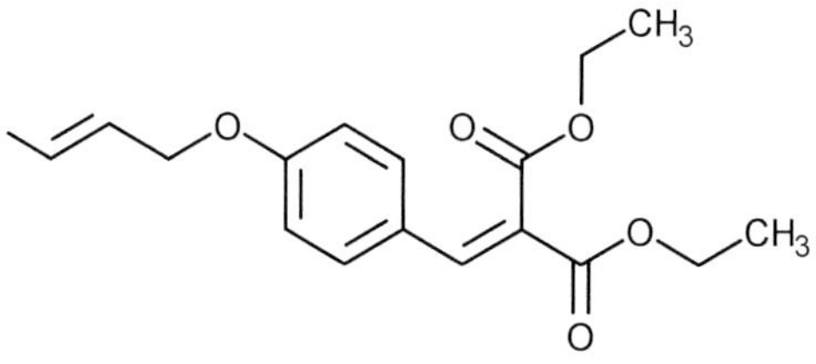

and $\sim 0.1 - 0.4\%$ $-H$

(Structural formula according to ref. 12, different from the formula given by Personal Care Products Council Ingredient Database)

GENERAL

Polysilicone-15 is a relatively new UVB filter with UV absorbance maximum (λ_{max}) at 312 nm (4,13). The literature on adverse reactions to sunscreens has been reviewed in several recent and older publications (6-11,15). A review of photocontact allergy to sunscreens was published in 2010 (14).

CONTACT ALLERGY

Case reports and case series

A young atopic girl presented with acute cheilitis. She had redness of her lips with dryness, extending around to the perioral skin. The patient had used a lipcare stick several times a day for 2 months because of chapped lips. Patch tests with the European baseline series and her own cosmetics gave positive reactions to her lipstick and to the fragrances mix I. Later, the girl was patch tested with the 10 ingredients of the stick and she reacted to the UV-filter

Parsol® SLX 10% pet. (3). An older non-atopic man was seen for acute dermatitis of the face that had started on his lips 3 weeks previously. Patch tests with the European baseline series and his cosmetics gave a positive reaction to a lipcare stick that he had been using for several weeks for the treatment of dry lips. When tested with its ingredients, the patient reacted strongly to Parsol® SLX 10% pet. In both patients, a test with a second sample of the UV-filter was again positive, whereas no reactions were seen to any UV-filter in the sunscreen series (3).

Presence in cosmetic products and chemical analyses

In the USA, in April 2017, polysilicone-15 was present in 31 of 56,714 cosmetic products of which the composition is known in FDA's Voluntary Cosmetic Registration Program (VCRP) (data obtained from FDA, May 2017). In April 2017, polysilicone-15 was present in 105 of 65,434 cosmetic products of which the composition is known in EWG's Skin Deep Cosmetics Database, USA (http://www.ewg.org/skindeep/). It should be realized that sunscreen products containing UV-filters are classified as drugs in the USA, not as cosmetics; the number mentioned here, therefore, is that of cosmetics containing the UV-filter, but it does *not* include their presence in sunscreens.

Polysilicone-15 was present in 4 (0.1%) of 4447 cosmetic products collected in Germany, 2006-2009 (2). Polysilicone-15 was an ingredient of 3% of 329 sunscreen products (incl. 21 lipstick sunscreens) marketed in the UK in 2005 (4). In a sample of 337 sunscreens marketed in the UK in 2010, polysilicone-15 was present in 10 (3%) (5).

OTHER SIDE EFFECTS

Photosensitivity

In 2008-2011, in 12 European countries, polysilicone-15 10% pet. was photopatch tested in 1031 patients with exposed site dermatitis or history of a reaction to a sunscreen or topical NSAID and 1 (0.1%) had a positive photopatch test. Its relevance was not specified, but for all photoallergic reactions together, 44% was of current and 11% of past relevance (1).

LITERATURE

1   The European Multicentre Photopatch Test Study (EMCPPTS) Taskforce. A European multicentre photopatch test study. Br J Dermatol 2012;166:1002-1009
2   Uter W, Gonçalo M, Yazar K, Kratz E-M, Mildau G, Lidén C. Coupled exposure to ingredients of cosmetic products: III. Ultraviolet filters. Contact Dermatitis 2014;71:162-169
3   Sarre, ME, Guérin-Moreau M, Lepoittevin JP, Martin L. Avenel-Audran M. Allergic contact cheilitis caused by polysilicone-15 (Parsol® SLX) in a lipcare balm. Contact Dermatitis 2014;70:119-121
4   Wahie S, Lloyd JJ, Farr PM. Sunscreen ingredients and labelling: a survey of products available in the U.K. Clin Exp Dermatol 2007;32:359-364
5   Kerr AC. A survey of the availability of sunscreen filters in the U.K. Clin Exp Dermatol 2011;36:541-543
6   Heurung AR, Raju SI, Warshaw EM. Adverse reactions to sunscreen agents: epidemiology, responsible irritants and allergens, clinical characteristics, and management. Dermatitis 2014;25:289-326
7   Heurung AR, Raju SI, Warshaw EM. Contact allergen of the year. Benzophenones. Dermatitis 2014;25:3-10 (contains many mistakes; Erratum in Dermatitis 2014;25:92-95)
8   Avenel-Audran M. Sunscreen products: finding the allergen. Eur J Dermatol 2010;20:161-166
9   Scheuer E, Warshaw E. Sunscreen allergy: a review of epidemiology, clinical characteristics, and responsible allergens. Dermatitis 2006;17:3-11
10 Funk JO, Dromgoole SH, Maibach HI. Sunscreen intolerance: contact sensitization, photocontact sensitization, and irritancy of sunscreen agents. Dermatol Clin 1995;13:473-481
11 Dromgoole SH, Maibach HI. Sunscreening agent intolerance: Contact and photocontact sensitization and contact urticaria. J Am Acad Dermatol 1990;22:1068-1078
12 SCCS (Scientific Committee on Consumer Safety). Opinion on polysilicone-15, 22 June 2010, SCCS/1346/10. Available at: http://ec.europa.eu/health/scientific_committees/consumer_safety/docs/sccs_o_024.pdf
13 Shaath NA. Ultraviolet filters. Photochem Photobiol Sci 2010;9:464-469
14 Shaw T, Simpson B, Wilson B, Oostman H, Rainey D, Storrs F. True photoallergy to sunscreens is rare despite popular belief. Dermatitis 2010;21:185-198
15 Schauder S. Survey of the literature on adverse reactions to preparations containing UV filters (1947-1989) (Literaturübersicht über Unverträglichkeitsreaktionen auf lichtfilterhaltige Produkte von 1947 bis 1989). Z Hautkr 1990;65:982-998 (article in German)

2.377 POLYSORBATE 40

IDENTIFICATION

Description/definition : Polysorbate 40 is a mixture of palmitate esters of sorbitol and sorbitol anhydrides, consisting predominantly of the monoester, condensed with approximately 20 moles of ethylene oxide. It conforms generally to the formula shown below, where w + x + y + z has an average value of 20

Chemical class(es) : Sorbitan derivatives

Chemical/IUPAC name : Sorbitan, monohexadecanoate, poly(oxy-1,2-ethanediyl) derivatives

Other names : Tween® 40; polyoxyethylene sorbitan monopalmitate

CAS registry number (s) : 9005-66-7

CIR review(s) : J Am Coll Toxicol 1984;3:1-82; Final report, June 2015 (access: www.cir-safety.org/ingredients)

Function(s) in cosmetics : EU: emulsifying; surfactant. USA: surfactants – emulsifying agents; surfactants – solubilising agents

Patch testing : 10% pet. (SmartPracticeCanada)

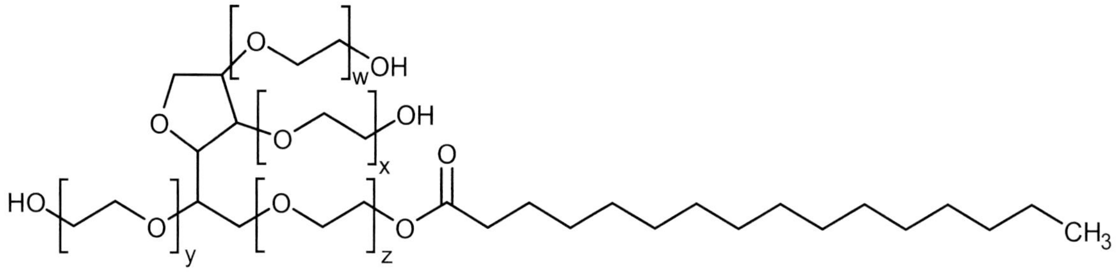

CONTACT ALLERGY

Patch testing in groups of patients

The results of patch testing in groups of patients are shown in table 2.377.1. In 1975, in Finland, 1206 consecutive patients suspected of contact dermatitis were patch tested with polysorbate 40 5% pet. mixed with polysorbate 80 5% pet. (routine testing) and there were 2 (0.2%) positive reactions. Their relevance was not specified. In two studies in which groups of *selected* patients were tested (in one the selection criteria were not specified, in the other, patients were tested who had contact dermatitis apparently related to the use of topical preparations) low rates of sensiti-zation of 0.2% and 0.7% were observed (1,3). In the Italian study, two of 5 reactions (40%) were relevant, one was related to polysorbate 40 in a cosmetic preparation and the other to a topical pharmaceutical product (1).

Table 2.377.1 Patch testing in groups of patients

Years and Country	Test conc. & vehicle	Number of patients tested	positive (%)	Selection of patients (S); Relevance (R); Comments (C)	Ref.
Routine testing					
1975 Finland	10% pet.	1206	2 (0.2%)	R: not specified; C: the test material contained 5% poly-sorbate 40 and 5% polysorbate 80	2
Testing in groups of selected patients					
1986-1989 Italy	10% pet.	737	5 (0.7%)	S: patients with contact dermatitis apparently related to the use of topical preparations; R: 2 reactions were relevant, one form a cosmetic, the other from topical medication	1
1972-1974 Finland	10% pet.	412	1 (0.2%)	S: not stated; R: not stated; C: the test substance contained 5% polysorbate 40 and 5% polysorbate 80	3

Case reports and case series

One patient had allergic contact dermatitis from polysorbate 40 in a leave-on cosmetic product, which was not specified (1).

Contact allergy to polysorbate 40 in non-cosmetic products
One patient had allergic contact dermatitis from polysorbate 40 in a topical pharmaceutical product, which was not specified (1).

Cross-reactions, pseudo-cross-reactions and co-reactions
Polysorbate 80 (1).

Presence in cosmetic products and chemical analyses
In the USA, in April 2017, polysorbate 40 was present in 101 of 56,714 cosmetic products of which the composition is known in FDA's Voluntary Cosmetic Registration Program (VCRP) (data obtained from FDA, May 2017). In April 2017, polysorbate 40 was present in 4 of 66,485 cosmetic products of which the composition is known in EWG's Skin Deep Cosmetics Database, USA (http://www.ewg.org/skindeep/).

LITERATURE
1   Tosti A, Guerra L, Morelli R, Bardazzi F. Prevalence and sources of sensitization to emulsifiers: a clinical study. Contact Dermatitis 1990;23:68-72
2   Hannuksela M, Kousa M, Pirilä V. Contact sensitivity to emulsifiers. Contact Dermatitis 1976;2:201-204
3   Hannuksela M, Kousa M, Pirilä V. Allergy to ingredients of vehicles. Contact Dermatitis 1976;2:105-110

2.378   POLYSORBATE 80

IDENTIFICATION

Description/definition   : Polysorbate 80 is a mixture of oleate esters of sorbitol and sorbitol anhydrides, consisting predominantly of the monoester, condensed with approximately 20 moles of ethylene oxide. It conforms generally to the formula shown below, where w + x + y + z has an average value of 20

Chemical class(es)   : Sorbitan derivatives

Chemical/IUPAC name   : Sorbitan, mono-9-octadecenoate, poly(oxy-1,2-ethanediyl) derivatives., (*Z*)-

Other names   : Polyoxyethylene sorbitan monooleate; Tween® 80

CAS registry number (s)   : 9005-65-6

EC number(s)   : 500-019-9

CIR review(s)   : J Amer Coll Toxicol 1984;3:1-82; Final report, June 2015 (access: www.cir-safety.org/ingredients)

Merck Index monograph   : 7582

Function(s) in cosmetics   : EU: denaturant; emulsifying; surfactant. USA: denaturants; fragrance ingredients; surfactants – emulsifying; surfactants – solubilizing

Patch testing   : 5% pet. (Chemotechnique); 10% pet. (SmartPracticeCanada)

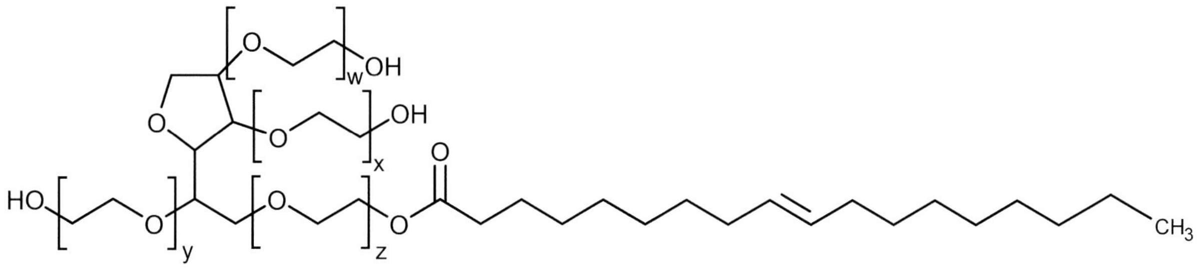

GENERAL

Polysorbate 80 is a solubilizing, emulsifying and stabilizing agent used in nutritives, creams, ointments, lotions, multiple medical injectable preparations (e.g., vitamin oils, vaccines, biologicals and anticancer agents), and industrial detergents. Experimental data have shown that polysorbate 60 is a biologically and pharmacologically active compound (16).

CONTACT ALLERGY

Patch testing in groups of patients

Results of studies patch testing polysorbate 80 in consecutive patients suspected of contact dermatitis (routine testing) and in groups of selected patients are shown in table 2.378.1. In routine testing, frequencies of sensitization in two studies were 0.2% (9) and 4.2% (5). The unlikely high percentage of 4.2 was seen in a small Chines study in 599 consecutive patients; the relevance of the positive patch tests was not mentioned (5).

In four studies patch testing polysorbate 80 in groups of *selected* patients (e.g., patients with contact dermatitis apparently related to the use of topical preparations), mostly low prevalences of sensitization of 0.2% to 0.5% were found (1,8,10,11). In a very small study of patients with allergic contact dermatitis of the eyelids, one patient (2.2%) had a relevant reaction to polysorbate 80, but the culprit product was not mentioned (6). The relevance rate ranged from 50% to 100%. In a study from the USA, all 4 positive patch test reactions were scored as relevant, but this included 'questionable' and 'past' relevance (1).

Case reports and case series

In the period 1996-2013, in a tertiary referral center in Valencia, Spain, 5419 patients were patch tested. Of these, 628 individuals had allergic contact dermatitis to cosmetics. Polysorbate 80 was the responsible allergen in one case (12). In a 4-month-period in 1996, 475 patients with contact allergy to 'cosmetic ingredients' were collected in 5 centers in Belgium, UK and Germany. There was one reaction to polysorbate 80; relevance was not stated (7). In Italy, 1986-1989, in 2 patients reacting to polysorbate 80 in a groups of 737 patients with contact dermatitis apparently related to the use of topical preparations, contact allergy was caused by cosmetic products (8).

Table 2.378.1 Patch testing in groups of patients

Years and Country	Test conc. & vehicle	Number of patients tested	positive (%)		Selection of patients (S); Relevance (R); Comments (C)	Ref.
Routine testing						
2003-2005 China		599	25	(4.2%)	R: not stated	5
1975 Finland	10% pet.	1200	2	(0.2%)	R: not specified; C: the test material contained 5% polysorbate 40 and 5% polysorbate 80	9
Testing in groups of selected patients						
2011 China	5% pet.	201	1	(0.5%)	S: healthy student volunteers 19-30 years; R: not stated	11
2000-2007 USA	5% pet.	870	4	(0.5%)	S: patients tested with a supplemental cosmetic screening series; R: 100%; C: weak study: a. high rate of macular erythema and weak reactions; b. relevance figures included 'questionable' and 'past' relevance	1
1994-2004		46	1	(2.2%)	S: patients with allergic contact dermatitis of the eyelids; R: the reaction was relevant, but the source product was not mentioned	6
1986-1989 Italy	10% pet.	737	4	(0.5%)	S: patients with contact dermatitis apparently related to the use of topical preparations; R: 2 reactions were relevant and caused by cosmetics	8
1972-1974 Finland	10% pet.	412	1	(0.2%)	S: not stated; R: not stated; C: the test substance contained 5% polysorbate 40 and 5% polysorbate 80	10

Contact allergy to polysorbate 80 in non-cosmetic products

One patient was allergic to polysorbate 80 in a corticosteroid inhaler (2). A child reacted to polysorbate 80 in a topical pharmaceutical product (3). In Switzerland, before 1994, 47 patients with chronic or recurrent (> 1 year) inflammatory skin diseases, using or having used topical preparations (23 with chronic leg ulcers, 15 with contact dermatitis, 1 with nummular eczema, 6 with psoriasis and 2 with atopic dermatitis) were tested with 10 emulsifiers including polysorbate 80 10% pet. In the group of patients with leg ulcers or contact dermatitis there were 4 positive patch test reactions to polysorbate 80. An unspecified number of these reactions was relevant, as patients had used a cold cream containing polysorbate 80 (17).

A man had allergic contact dermatitis in the groin from polysorbate 80 (and sodium sulfite and ketoconazole) in a topical antifungal cream for the treatment of tinea inguinalis (19).

Cross-reactions, pseudo-cross-reactions and co-reactions

Polysorbate 40 (8). Possibly cross-reactions to Tween® 61 (polyoxyethylene (4) sorbitan monostearate), Tween® 65 (polyoxyethylene (20) sorbitan tristearate) and Tween® 81 (polyoxyethylene (4) sorbitan monostearate) in an intradermal test (14).

Other side effects

Three patients developed large erythematous and edematous plaques 2 days after an intramuscular injection with retinyl palmitate at the injection site, which grew to plaques larger than 10 centimeter after 10 days and resembling erythema migrans. Intradermal tests showed that all three patients had delayed erythematous reactions to 0.1 ml 0.1% polysorbate 80, 7-15 mm red nodules being present at day 2 which persisted for several days. Nine other common emulsifiers related to polysorbate 80 were tested (Tween® 20 [polysorbate 20], Tween® 21 [polyoxyethylenesorbitan monolaurate], Tween® 40 [polysorbate 40, PEG-20 sorbitan monopalmitate], Tween® 60 [polysorbate 60, polyoxyethylene (20) sorbitan monostearate], Tween® 61 [polyoxyethylene (4) sorbitan monostearate], Tween® 65 [polyoxyethylene (20) sorbitan tristearate], Tween® 81 [polyoxyethylene (5) sorbitan monooleate], Tween® 85 [polyoxyethylene (20) sorbitan trioleate], and Span® 20 [sorbitan monolaurate]). One of the 3 patient had positive tests to Tween® 61, 65, and 81, which were interpreted as cross-reactions. No reactions were seen with skin tests to retinyl palmitate and the other constituents of the injectable. A patch test in one patient with polysorbate 80 was negative. Five controls had negative skin tests to all components of the retinyl palmitate injection (14).

Presence in cosmetic products and chemical analyses

In the USA, in April 2017, polysorbate 80 was present in 1097 of 56,714 cosmetic products of which the composition is known in FDA's Voluntary Cosmetic Registration Program (VCRP) (data obtained from FDA, May 2017). In January 2017, polysorbate 80 was present in 401 of 64,655 cosmetic products of which the composition is known in EWG's Skin Deep Cosmetics Database, USA (http://www.ewg.org/skindeep/).

New allergenic chemicals are formed during storage and handling of polysorbate 80, including peroxides and formaldehyde (4).

OTHER SIDE EFFECTS

Immediate-type reactions

A woman had experienced generalized urticaria with angioedema after parenteral treatment with penicillin years ago and came for allergy skin tests. She had negative prick tests but positive intradermal tests with penicilloyl-polylysine (PPL) and the minor determinant mixture (MDM, benzylpenicillin and benzylpenicilloate), but the tests with penicillins and cephalosporins yielded negative results. Later, the solvent of the PPL and MDM preparations was tested, which yielded a positive result. Skin testing was continued with the emulsifying agent polysorbate 80 contained in the solvent, causing a highly positive reaction in an intradermal test at a concentration of 0.05 mg/ml. A subsequent oral provocation test with phenoxymethylpenicillin without polysorbate 80 was well tolerated (13). A woman was investigated for an episode of anaphylactic shock reaction on intravenous infusion of a multivitamin preparation in a previous pregnancy. A few seconds after the start of the infusion, the patient had experienced dryness of the mouth, shortness of breath, bronchospasm, tachycardia, and hypotension followed by loss of consciousness. She later had a positive skin prick test to the multivitamin preparation and its ingredient polysorbate 80, and a positive basophil activation test. No drug-specific IgE antibodies were detected. Controls were negative and the authors concluded that this was a non-immunologic hypersensitivity reaction of unknown mechanism (15).

A woman developed acute angioedema of the lips and face followed by faintness when she began to eat an ice cream cone. The components were applied as 'open patch tests' (which appears to be a contradiction), which yielded a positive reaction within 10 minutes to the food consolidator Cremodan® SE 40. Its components (mono-, di- and tri-glycerides of fatty acids, sodium alginate, polysorbate 80, guar gum and carrageenan) could not be tested separately, but the author suggested 'polysorbates' as the likely causative agent (18). A man experienced wheezing from using a shampoo, possibly caused by immediate-type hypersensitivity to its ingredient polysorbate 80 (20). A girl suffered from generalized urticaria, eyelid angioedema, rhino-conjunctivitis, dyspnea and wheezing one hour after the third intramuscular administration of an HPV virus vaccine. Intradermal tests were positive to the vaccine and its constituent polysorbate 80, but the basophil activation test to polysorbate 80 was negative and no specific IgE was demonstrated (21). A woman developed generalized urticaria and intense itching each time she received an injection with a biological drug for her psoriasis. Another biological gave the same reaction. Both contained polysorbate 80. A patch test with it was negative, but a prick test with polysorbate 80 was positive after 20 minutes, whereas 10 controls were negative (22). Two women developed urticaria and angioedema from hypersensitivity to polysorbate 80 present as excipient in commercial preparations of the red cell growth hormones darbepoietin and erythropoietin (23,24).

LITERATURE

1   Wetter DA, Yiannias JA, Prakash AV, Davis MD, Farmer SA, el-Azhary RA, et al. Results of patch testing to personal care product allergens in a standard series and a supplemental cosmetic series: an analysis of 945 patients from the Mayo Clinic Contact Dermatitis Group, 2000-2007. J Am Acad Dermatol 2010;63:789-798

2   Isaksson M, Jansson L. Contact allergy to Tween 80 in an inhalation suspension. Contact Dermatitis 2002;47:312-313

3   Lucente P, Iorizzo M, Pazzaglia M. Contact sensitivity to Tween 80 in a child. Contact Dermatitis 2000;43:172

4   Bergh M, Magnusson K, Nilsson JLG, Karlberg A-T. Contact allergenic activity of Tween® 80 before and after air exposure. Contact Dermatitis 1997;37:9-18

5   Li L-F, Liu G, Wang J. Patch test in Chinese patients with cosmetic allergic contact dermatitis to common cosmetic allergens from a European cosmetic series. Contact Dermatitis 2007;57:50-54

6   Amin KA, Belsito DV. The aetiology of eyelid dermatitis: a 10-year retrospective analysis. Contact Dermatitis 2006;55:280-285

7   Goossens A, Beck MH, Haneke E, McFadden JP, Nolting S, Durupt G, Ries G. Adverse cutaneous reactions to cosmetic allergens. Contact Dermatitis 1999;40:112-113

8   Tosti A, Guerra L, Morelli R, Bardazzi F. Prevalence and sources of sensitization to emulsifiers: a clinical study. Contact Dermatitis 1990;23:68-72

9   Hannuksela M, Kousa M, Pirilä V. Contact sensitivity to emulsifiers. Contact Dermatitis 1976;2:201-204

10 Hannuksela M, Kousa M, Pirilä V. Allergy to ingredients of vehicles. Contact Dermatitis 1976;2:105-110

11 Zhao J, Li LF. Contact sensitization to cosmetic series of allergens in a general population in Beijing. J Cosmet Dermatol 2014;13:68-71

12 Zaragoza-Ninet V, Blasco Encinas R, Vilata-Corell JJ, Pérez-Ferriols A, Sierra-Talamantes C, Esteve-Martínez A, de la Cuadra-Oyanguren J. Allergic contact dermatitis due to cosmetics: A clinical and epidemiological study in a tertiary hospital. Actas Dermosifiliogr 2016;107:329-336

13 Grims RH, Kränke B, Aberer W. Pitfalls in drug allergy skin testing: false–positive reactions due to (hidden) additives. Contact Dermatitis 2006;54:290-294

14 Shelley WB, Talanin N, Shelley ED. Polysorbate 80 hypersensitivity. Lancet 1995;345 (8960):1312-1313

15 Coors EA, Seybold H, Merk HF, Mahler V. Polysorbate 80 in medical products and nonimmunologic anaphylactoid reactions. Ann Allergy Asthma Immunol 2005;95:593-599

16 Ten Tije AJ, Verweij J, Loos WJ, Sparreboom A. Pharmacological effects of formulation vehicles: implications for cancer chemotherapy. Clin Pharmacokinet 2003;42:665-685

17 Pasche-Koo F, Piletta P-A, Hunziker N, Hauser C. High sensitization rate to emulsifiers in patients with chronic leg ulcers. Contact Dermatitis 1994;31:226-228

18 Camarasa JM. Acute contact urticaria. Contact Dermatitis 1982;8:347-348

19 Garcia-Bravo B, Mazuecos J, Rodriguez-Pichardo A, Navas J, Camacho F. Hypersensitivity to ketoconazole preparations: study of 4 cases. Contact Dermatitis 1989;21:346-348

20 Yamasuji Y, Higashi Y, Sakanoue M, Katsue H, Kawai K, Arai N, Kanekura T. A case of anaphylaxis caused by polyethylene glycol analogues. Contact Dermatitis 2013;69:183-185

21 Badiu I, Geuna M, Heffler E, Rolla G. Hypersensitivity reaction to human papillomavirus vaccine due to polysorbate 80. BMJ Case Rep 2012, May 8;2012. pii: bcr0220125797. doi: 10.1136/bcr.02.2012.5797.

22 Pérez-Pérez L, García-Gavín J, Piñeiro B, Zulaica A. Biologic-induced urticaria due to polysorbate 80: usefulness of prick test. Br J Dermatol 2011;164:1119-1120

23 Steele RH, Limaye S, Cleland B, Chow J, Suranyi MG. Hypersensitivity reactions to the polysorbate contained in recombinant erythropoietin and darbepoietin. Nephrology (Carlton) 2005;10:317-320

24 Limaye S, Steele RH, Quin J, Cleland B. An allergic reaction to erythropoietin secondary to polysorbate hypersensitivity. J Allergy Clin Immunol 2002;110:530

2.379 POTASSIUM COCOYL HYDROLYZED COLLAGEN

IDENTIFICATION

Description/definition	: Potassium cocoyl hydrolyzed collagen is the potassium salt of the condensation product of coconut acid chloride and hydrolyzed collagen
Chemical class(es)	: Protein derivatives
Other names	: Potassium coco-hydrolyzed animal protein
CAS registry number (s)	: 68920-65-0
CIR review(s)	: J Am Coll Toxicol 1983;2:75-86 (access: www.cir-safety.org/ingredients)
Function(s) in cosmetics	: EU: hair conditioning; skin conditioning; surfactant. USA: hair conditioning agents; skin-conditioning agents – miscellaneous; surfactants – cleansing agents
Patch testing	: 5% water or pet. (2); 5% pet. (1)

CONTACT ALLERGY

Case reports and case series

A woman presented with itching erythematopapular to urticarial lesions on both cheeks, the pre-=auricular region and the neck, that were somewhat streaked in form. The appearance suggested allergic contact dermatitis, probably from a hair product. The patient revealed that she had regularly had itching lesions on her face, ears and neck for 2 months, possibly from a new shampoo. She also used a hair balsam, gel and styling foam. Patch tests with the European standard series, the pharmaceutical series, the cosmetics series and with her personal cosmetics revealed a strong reaction at D2 and D4 to the shampoo, tested open, as is. When tested with its ingredients, obtained from the manufacturer, the patient at D2 and D4 had positive reactions to potassium coco-hydrolyzed animal protein (INCI name: potassium cocoyl hydrolyzed collagen) as is (open test), at 30% and 5% water and at 5% pet., but there was no reaction to the material tested 2% water. Twenty controls tested with 30% and 5% water were negative.

Later, the patient was tested with TEA-coco-hydrolyzed animal protein 5% water (INCI name: TEA-cocoyl hydrolyzed collagen), TEA-abietoyl hydrolyzed animal protein 5% water, potassium undecylenoyl hydrolyzed animal protein 5% water (INCI name: potassium undecylenoyl hydrolyzed collagen) and TEA-oleylpolypeptide 5% water (INCI name TEA-oleoyl hydrolyzed collagen) and she showed positive reactions to all test materials except TEA-abietoyl hydrolyzed animal protein. The patient had probably been sensitized earlier to TEA-oleoyl hydrolyzed collagen and now cross-reacted to potassium cocoyl hydrolyzed collagen, to which she reacted at the first contact with the shampoo (2).

Cross-reactions, pseudo-cross-reactions and co-reactions

TEA-cocoyl hydrolyzed collagen (1,2); potassium undecylenoyl hydrolyzed animal protein (INCI name: potassium undecylenoyl hydrolyzed collagen) (2); TEA-oleylpolypeptide (INCI name: TEA-oleoyl hydrolyzed collagen) (2).

.

Presence in cosmetic products and chemical analyses

In the USA, in April 2017, potassium cocoyl hydrolyzed collagen was present in 48 of 56,714 cosmetic products of which the composition is known in FDA's Voluntary Cosmetic Registration Program (VCRP) (data obtained from FDA, May 2017). In April 2017, potassium cocoyl hydrolyzed collagen was present in 31 of 65,431 cosmetic products of which the composition is known in EWG's Skin Deep Cosmetics Database, USA (http://www.ewg.org/skindeep/).

LITERATURE

1   Emmett EA, Wright RC. Allergic contact dermatitis from TEA-cocohydrolyzed protein. Arch Dermatol 1976;112: 1008-1009
2   Dooms-Goossens A, Debusschère K, Dupré K, Degreef H. Can eardrops induce a shampoo dermatitis? A case study. Contact Dermatitis 1988;19:143-145

2.380 POTASSIUM PERSULFATE

IDENTIFICATION

Description/definition   : Potassium persulfate is the inorganic salt that conforms to the formula shown below
Chemical class(es)   : Inorganic salts
Chemical/IUPAC name   : Dipotassium sulfonatooxy sulfate
Other names   : Dipotassium peroxodisulfate
CAS registry number (s)   : 7727-21-1
EC number(s)   : 231-781-8
CIR review(s)   : Int J Toxicol 2001;20(Suppl.3):7-21 (access: www.cir-safety.org/ingredients)
Merck Index monograph : 9047
Function(s) in cosmetics : EU: oxidising. USA: oxidizing agents
Patch testing   : 2.5% pet. (3)
Molecular formula   : $K_2O_8S_2$

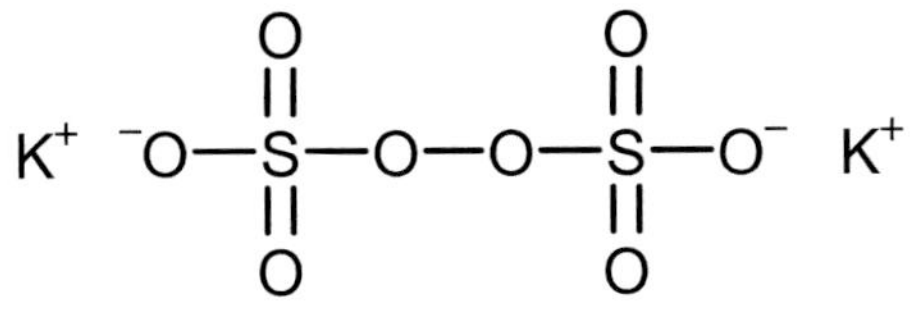

$$K^+ \quad {}^-O-\overset{\displaystyle O}{\underset{\displaystyle O}{\overset{\|}{\underset{\|}{S}}}}-O-O-\overset{\displaystyle O}{\underset{\displaystyle O}{\overset{\|}{\underset{\|}{S}}}}-O^- \quad K^+$$

GENERAL

Persulfate salts (ammonium, potassium, sodium) are strongly oxidizing inorganic salts. Persulfates are widely used in various manufacturing processes in the textile, chemical, metallurgic, pharmaceutical, photographic, food and, particularly, cosmetic industries. They are present in hair-bleaching products and hair-coloring preparations to accelerate the bleaching process, thus reducing the amount of peroxide used. Potassium persulfate is also used in paper, in the treatment of spa water (in the form of potassium monopersulfate [7]) and in analytical chemistry (1,3,5).

The persulfates can cause irritant dermatitis, allergic contact dermatitis, and immediate contact reactions including localized and generalized urticaria (rarely accompanied by anaphylactic shock) and airway problems including rhinitis and asthma. Most reactions have been caused by ammonium persulfate, sometimes concurrently by ammonium and potassium persulfate. The standard patch test material for persulfate is ammonium persulfate, which is part of most if not all 'hairdressing' series, and is tested in hairdressers with dermatitis and in individuals in who reactions to hair cosmetics are considered. Potassium persulfate itself, however, has been tested infrequently (6). Ammonium persulfate and studies in which both ammonium and potassium persulfate were tested have been fully reviewed in Chapter 2.22 Ammonium persulfate. Nearly always, it was not stated whether the incriminated products (usually hair bleaches) contained ammonium persulfate, potassium persulfate, or both, but most persulfate-sensitized patients react to both ammonium and potassium persulfate.

In this chapter, with one exception (6), only reports of dermatological reactions to potassium persulfate in products known to contain this chemical and not discussed under Ammonium persulfate are presented.

CONTACT ALLERGY

Patch testing in groups of patients: Routine testing
In the period 1986-1990, 2320 patients suspected of contact dermatitis were patch tested with potassium persulfate 2% in water in Rotterdam, The Netherlands (6). There were 16 positive reactions (0.7%). Eleven reactors were hairdressers, 5 were not; all had hand dermatitis only. Hand dermatitis in the hairdressers either greatly improved or cleared when contact with hair bleaches was avoided. In the group of non-hairdressers, an unspecified number had exacerbation of hand dermatitis when using hair bleaches (6).

Case reports and case series
A woman, when bleaching her hair, used potassium persulfate to boost the effect of hydrogen peroxide. Five hours later, she developed itching, burning and swelling of her scalp, ears and forehead and to a lesser extent of her face. The next day, the skin around her hairline was red and weeping. Patch tests were positive to 1% and 5% potassium persulfate. Scratch tests were also positive, both to potassium and to ammonium persulfate. However, the clinical picture is not consistent with an immediate-type reaction, so these tests may have been false-positive (2).

Contact allergy to potassium persulfate in non-cosmetic products

A laboratory technician in a potato-flour factory had recurrent dermatitis on the face and the fingers of both hands for 6 years. The dermatitis was only present during certain months of the year, and review of her work schedule revealed that such episodes of dermatitis coincided with the addition of potassium persulfate to certain batches of potato flour to be used in the paper industry. She did several physical and chemical analyses of the finished product in a laboratory. Patch testing revealed positive reactions to potassium persulfate at 1%, 2.5% and 5% in water and to ammonium persulfate 2.5% pet. (1). A female laboratory assistant had hand eczema that cleared on vacations. The patient was exposed daily to potassium persulfate, as it was used as an analytical agent in chemical analyses of the phosphate content of water samples from rivers, lakes and the sea. She showed positive patch test reactions to potassium and ammonium persulfate 2.5% pet. (3).

A man with a dental prosthesis had a chronic relapsing cheilitis. Patch tests were positive to the dental cleanser (10% pet.) he used for the prosthesis, which contained 20% potassium persulfate. Subsequently, he reacted positively to potassium and ammonium persulfate (5). A patient presented with a generalized scattered dermatitis from the neck down that worsened after spa use. Patch testing elicited a positive reaction to ammonium persulfate. Contact with ammonium persulfate was ruled out. However, the 'shock treatments' the patient used to eliminate organic contaminants in his hot tub water contained potassium monopersulfate (potassium peroxymonosulfate) in the form of the triple salt potassium persulfate, potassium sulfate, and potassium bisulfate (7).

Cross-reactions, pseudo-cross-reactions and co-reactions

Ammonium persulfate (1,3,5,6). Reactions to other persulfates are to be expected in potassium persulfate-sensitized patients, since the allergic reaction is due to the persulfate part (5).

Presence in cosmetic products and chemical analyses

In the USA, in April 2017, potassium persulfate was present in 73 of 56,714 cosmetic products of which the composition is known in FDA's Voluntary Cosmetic Registration Program (VCRP) (data obtained from FDA, May 2017). In January 2017, potassium persulfate was present in 41 older products of 64,655 cosmetic products of which the composition is known in EWG's Skin Deep Cosmetics Database, USA (http://www.ewg.org/skindeep/).

Immediate-type reactions

A woman developed itch and erythema of the ears, neck and forehead 15 minutes after application of a hair dye kit. Subsequently, she washed her hair, resulting in pruritus and redness of the hands. The hair dye kit applied included 3 components: cream, peroxide cream and booster, the latter being suspected by the patient. Prick tests with these 3 hair dye constituents produced a positive reaction to the booster (as is and 10%). Later, she was prick-tested with the constituents of the booster and reacted only to potassium persulfate, 4 controls being negative (4).

LITERATURE

1   Veien NK, Hattel T, Laurberg G. Contact dermatitis due to potassium persulfate. Contact Dermatitis 2001;45:176
2   Cronin E. Contact Dermatitis. Edinburgh: Churchill Livingstone, 1980:128
3   Kanerva L, Alanko K, Jolanki R, Aalto-Korte K, Estlander T. Occupational allergic contact dermatitis from potassium persulfate. Contact Dermatitis 1999;40:116-117
4   Estrada Rodríguez JL, Gozalo Reques F, Cechini Fernandez C, Rodríguez Prieto MA. Contact urticaria due to potassium persulfate. Contact Dermatitis 2001;45:177
5   Le Coz CJ, Bezard M. Allergic contact cheilitis due to effervescent dental cleanser: combined responsibilities of the allergen persulfate and prosthesis porosity. Contact Dermatitis 1999;41:268-271
6   Van Joost T, Roesyanto ID. Sensitization to persulphates in occupational and non-occupational hand dermatitis. Contact Dermatitis 1991;24:376-378
7   Yankura JA, Marks JG Jr, Anderson BE, Adams DR. Spa contact dermatitis. Dermatitis 2008;19:100-101

2.381 POTASSIUM SORBATE

IDENTIFICATION

Description/definition   : Potassium sorbate is the organic salt that conforms generally to the formula shown below
Chemical class(es)   : Organic salts
Chemical/IUPAC name   : Potassium (2E,4E)-hexa-2,4-dienoate
CAS registry number (s)   : 24634-61-5; 590-00-1
EC number(s)   : 246-376-1
CIR review(s)   : J Am Coll Toxicol 1988;7:837-880 (access: www.cir-safety.org/ingredients)
Merck Index monograph   : 10117 (sorbic acid)
Function(s) in cosmetics   : EU: preservative. USA: fragrance ingredients; preservatives
EU cosmetic restrictions   : Regulated in Annex V/14 of the Regulation (EC) No. 1223/2009
Patch testing   : 5% pet. (11)
Molecular formula   : $C_6H_8KO_2$

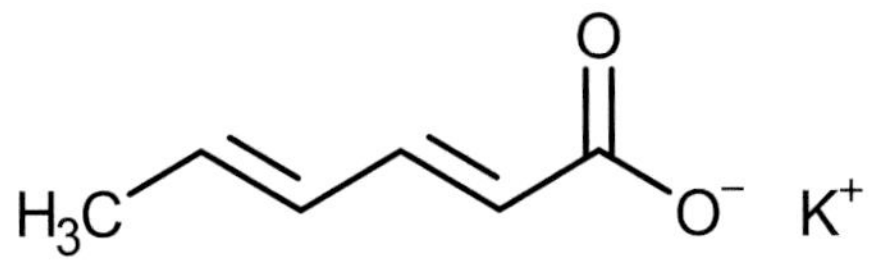

GENERAL

Sorbic acid and its salts such as potassium, calcium and sodium sorbate inhibit moulds and yeasts, and are used as preservatives to avoid further fermentation in tobacco and foods such as wines, butter, cheese, yoghurts or dried fruits. In cosmetics and pharmaceuticals, they are used mainly in fatty acids- and polyoxyethylene-based products. These chemicals also improve milling characteristics in cold rubber, and may be used in copolymerization, as intermediate for plasticizers and lubricants, in adhesives, glues, inks, paints, varnishes, tanning agents and metalworking fluids (5).

CONTACT ALLERGY

Case reports and case series

Potassium sorbate was stated to be the (or an) allergen in 2 patients in a group of 603 individuals suffering from cosmetic dermatitis, seen in the period 2010-2015 in Leuven, Belgium (6). Potassium sorbate was responsible for 2 out of 959 cases of non-fragrance cosmetic allergy where the causal allergen was identified, Belgium, 2000-2010 (2). Potassium sorbate was responsible for 2 out of 399 cases of cosmetic allergy where the causal allergen was identified in a study of the NACDG, USA, 1977-1983 (1). A woman had allergic contact dermatitis of the face from potassium sorbate in a facial makeup product (7).

Presence in cosmetic products and chemical analyses

In the USA, in April 2017, potassium sorbate was present in 3935 of 56,714 cosmetic products of which the composition is known in FDA's Voluntary Cosmetic Registration Program (VCRP) (data obtained from FDA, May 2017). In January 2017, potassium sorbate was present in 2161 of 64,655 cosmetic products of which the composition is known in EWG's Skin Deep Cosmetics Database, USA (http://www.ewg.org/skindeep/). Sorbic acid (and derivatives) were present in 70 of 178 (39%) facial wipes for which ingredient information was obtained online and from retail stores, USA, 2016 (9).

Sorbic acid and derivatives were present in 34 of 54 (63%) personal hygiene wet wipes for which ingredient information was obtained online and from retail stores, USA, 2016 (10). Sorbates (sorbic acid or potassium sorbate) were present in 261/3541 (7.0%) randomly sampled leave-on cosmetic products, Germany, 2006-2009 (3). In Germany, in 2006-2009, the labels of 4680 cosmetic products were screened for the presence of preservatives. Potassium sorbate was present in 8.4% of the products, according to labelling information (8). Potassium sorbate was present in 9% of 204 cosmetic products (92 shampoos, 61 hair conditioners, 34 liquid soaps, 17 wet tissues) in Sweden, 2008 (4).

OTHER SIDE EFFECTS

Irritant contact dermatitis
One patient had occupational irritant contact dermatitis from powdery potassium sorbate while working in a milk transformation plant (5).

LITERATURE

1   Adams RM, Maibach HI, Clendenning WE, Fisher AA, Jordan WJ, Kanof N, et al. A five-year study of cosmetic reactions. J Am Acad Dermatol 1985;13:1062-1069

2   Travassos AR, Claes L, Boey L, Drieghe J, Goossens A. Non-fragrance allergens in specific cosmetic products. Contact Dermatitis 2011;65:276-285

3   Schnuch A, Mildau G, Kratz E-M, Uter W. Risk of sensitization to preservatives estimated on the basis of patch test data and exposure, according to a sample of 3541 leave-on products. Contact Dermatitis 2011;65:167-174

4   Yazar K, Johnsson S, Lind M-L, Boman A, Lidén C. Preservatives and fragrances in selected consumer-available cosmetics and detergents. Contact Dermatitis 2011;64:265-272

5   Le Coz CJ, Abensour M. Occupational contact dermatitis from potassium sorbate in milk transformation plant. Contact Dermatitis 2005;53:176-177

6   Goossens A. Cosmetic contact allergens. Cosmetics 2016, 3, 5; doi:10.3390/cosmetics3010005

7   Fisher AA. Cutaneous reactions to sorbic acid and potassium sorbate. Cutis 1980;25:350,352,423

8   Uter W, Yazar K, Kratz EM, Mildau G, Lidén C. Coupled exposure to ingredients of cosmetic products: II. Preservatives. Contact Dermatitis 2014;70:219-226

9   Aschenbeck KA, Warshaw EM. Allergenic ingredients in facial wet wipes. Dermatitis 2017 Mar 23. doi: 10.1097/DER.0000000000000268. [Epub ahead of print]

10   Aschenbeck KA, Warshaw EM. Allergenic ingredients in personal hygiene wet wipes. Dermatitis 2017 Mar 23. doi: 10.1097/DER.0000000000000275. [Epub ahead of print]

11   De Groot AC. Patch Testing, 3rd Edition. Wapserveen, The Netherlands: acdegroot publishing, 2008 (ISBN 978-90-813233-1-4)

2.382 PPG-1-PEG-9 LAURYL GLYCOL ETHER

IDENTIFICATION

Description/definition	: PPG-1-PEG-9 lauryl glycol ether is the ethoxylated, propoxylated ether of a lauryl epoxide and ethylene glycol reaction product
Chemical class(es)	: Alkoxylated alcohols; ethers
Chemical/IUPAC name	: 2-(2-Hydroxydodecyloxy)ethanol, ethoxylated, propoxylated (9 mol EO, 1 mol PO average molar ratio)
Other names	: Eumulgin® L; polyoxyethylene (9) polyoxypropylene (1) lauryl glycol ether; polyoxypropylene (1) polyoxyethylene (9) lauryl glycol ether
CAS registry number (s)	: 154248-98-3
Function(s) in cosmetics	: EU: emulsifying; surfactant. USA: surfactants - emulsifying agents
Patch test allergens	: 10% pet. or water (1)
Molecular formula	: $C_{12}H_{26}O(C_2H_4O)_9-(C_3H_6O)$, where C_2H_4O is the ethylene oxide moiety and C_3H_6O the propylene oxide part

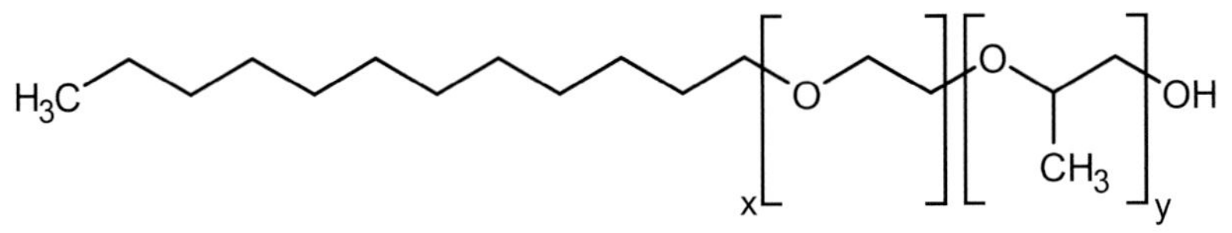

GENERAL

The description of Eumulgin L® in the publication is different from the INCI name of the current trade product Eumulgin L®, and reads as follows: cetyl stearyl alcohol 2(OP) 9(OE) is a cetyl stearyl alcohol with 2 added molecules of propylene oxide [2 (OP)] and 9 of ethylene oxide [9(OE)]. Molecular formula: $R-(C_2H_4O)_9-(C_3H_6OH)_2$, where R=cetearyl alcohol (1).

CONTACT ALLERGY

Case reports

A woman presented with an intensely itchy erythematous edematous dermatitis on the axillary folds following a few applications of a liquid deodorant. One day later, the eruption spread to the flanks and persisted for 10 days despite treatment. The dermatitis resolved with hyperpigmentation and desquamation. Patch tests with the GIRDCA standard series, preservatives, fragrance and emulsifiers series were negative. A repeated open application test (ROAT) with the deodorant, as is, on the volar forearm was positive after only 3 applications. When tested with its components, the patient reacted to the emulsifier 30% pet. NMR spectrometry revealed that the chemical nature of the emulsifier obtained was Eumulgin® L (cetyl stearylalcohol 2(OP) 9(OE)). This is of course very odd, ass NMR spectrometry cannot identify that a certain chemical has a distinctive trade name. Further patch tests with Eumulgin® L from the manufacturer of the deodorant 1% pet., 1% water, 10% pet., and 10% water were all positive. Five controls were negative (1).

Presence in cosmetic products and chemical analyses

In June 2017, PPG-1-PEG-9 lauryl glycol ether was present in 9 of 69,283 cosmetic products of which the composition is known in EWG's Skin Deep Cosmetics Database, USA (http://www.ewg.org/skindeep/). In the USA, in April 2017, PPG-1-PEG-9 lauryl glycol ether was present in 189 of 56,714 cosmetic products of which the composition is known in FDA's Voluntary Cosmetic Registration Program (VCRP) (data obtained from FDA, May 2017).

LITERATURE

1   Corazza M, Lombardi AR, Virgili A. Non-eczematous urticarioid allergic contact dermatitis due to Eumulgin® L in a deodorant. Contact Dermatitis 1997;36:159-160

2.383   PPG-2-CETEARETH-9

IDENTIFICATION

Description/definition	: PPG-2-ceteareth-9 is the polyoxypropylene, polyoxyethylene ether of cetearyl alcohol, that conforms generally to the formula shown below
hemical class(es)	: Alkoxylated alcohols
Chemical/IUPAC name	: Alcohols, C16-18, ethoxylated, propoxylated (9 mol EO, 2 mol PO average molar ratio)
Other names	: Polyoxyethylene (9) polyoxypropylene (2) cetyl/stearyl ether
CIR review(s)	: Final report, September 2013 (access: www.cir-safety.org/ingredients)
Function(s) in cosmetics	: EU: emulsifying. USA: surfactants - emulsifying agents
Patch testing	: 1% and 10% water or pet. (2)
Molecular formula:	: $R-(C_2H_4O)_9-(C_3H_6OH)_2$, where R=cetearyl alcohol

CONTACT ALLERGY

Case reports and case series

In a 4-month-period in 1996, 475 patients with contact allergy to 'cosmetic ingredients' were collected in 5 centers in Belgium, UK and Germany. There was one reaction to PPG-2-ceteareth-9; relevance was not stated (1).

A woman presented with an intensely itchy erythematous edematous dermatitis in the axillae after she had used a liquid deodorant for a few times. A day later, the eruption spread to the flanks and persisted for 10 days despite treatment with systemic and topical corticosteroids. The dermatitis healed with hyperpigmentation and desquamation. Patch tests with the GIRDCA standard series, preservatives, fragrance and emulsifiers series were negative, but a repeated open application test with the deodorant was positive after 3 applications already. Some of the components were tested but were negative. The other components were separated with extraction techniques. NMR spectrometry revealed that the chemical nature of the emulsifier obtained was Eumulgin® L (cetyl stearylalcohol 2(0P) 9(0E)) (which is rather odd, as it seems impossible to determine a trade name of a chemical with analytical investigation). A patch test with this material 30% pet. was strongly positive at D2 and D3. Later, the patient was patch tested with commercial Eumulgin® L at various concentrations and in different vehicles, and she reacted to the material tested 1% pet., 1% water, 10% pet. and 10% water. Patch tests in 5 healthy subjects were negative (2).

Presence in cosmetic products and chemical analyses

In the USA, in April 2017, PPG-2-cetereth-9 was present in 8 of 56,714 cosmetic products of which the composition is known in FDA's Voluntary Cosmetic Registration Program (VCRP) (data obtained from FDA, May 2017). In April 2017, PPG-2-ceteareth-9 was present in one of 65,434 cosmetic products of which the composition is known in EWG's Skin Deep Cosmetics Database, USA (http://www.ewg.org/skindeep/).

LITERATURE

1   Goossens A, Beck MH, Haneke E, McFadden JP, Nolting S, Durupt G, Ries G. Adverse cutaneous reactions to cosmetic allergens. Contact Dermatitis 1999;40:112-113
2   Corazza M, Lombardi AR, Virgili A. Non-eczematous urticarioid allergic contact dermatitis due to Eumulgin® L in a deodorant. Contact Dermatitis 1997;36:159-160

2.384 PROPANTHELINE BROMIDE[*]

* Not an INCI name

IDENTIFICATION

Description/definition : Propantheline bromide is the quaternary ammonium salt that conforms to the structural formula shown below
Chemical class(es) : Heterocyclic aromatic compounds; esters; quaternary ammonium salts
INCI name USA : Neither in CosIng nor in the Personal Care Products Council Ingredient Database
Chemical/IUPAC name : Methyl-di(propan-2-yl)-[2-(9H-xanthene-9-carbonyloxy)ethyl]azanium
CAS registry number (s) : 50-34-0
EC number(s) : 200-030-6
Merck Index monograph : 9189
Function(s) in cosmetics : Antiperspirant (anticholinergic drug)
Patch testing : 1% water (1); 5% water (2); 10% water (5); 5% pet. (6)
Molecular formula : $C_{23}H_{30}BrNO_3$

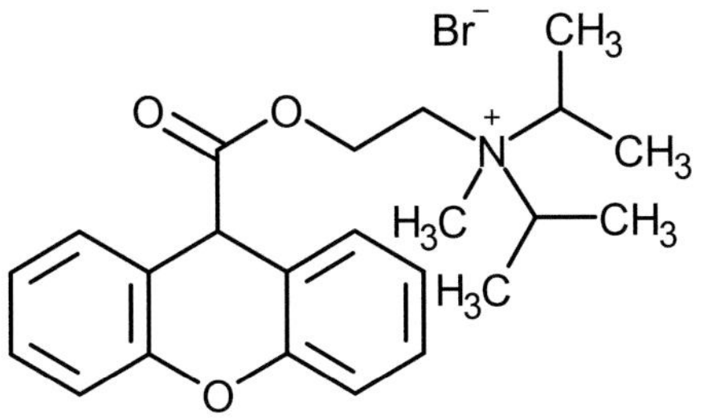

GENERAL

Discussion of side effects of this anticholinergic drug is limited to reactions caused by its presence in cosmetic products.

CONTACT ALLERGY

Case reports and case series

Three patients (1) and another 3 (7) had ACD from propantheline bromide in antiperspirants. Out of 14 patients with axillary dermatitis from an antiperspirant, 11 reacted to propantheline bromide (2). Five single case reports of contact allergy to propantheline bromide in an antiperspirant were reported in refs. 3,4,6,8,9. Of seven patients with axillary dermatitis from an antiperspirant, 6 had positive patch tests to propantheline bromide (5). All these cases of propantheline bromide contact allergy were caused by a commercial antiperspirant containing 5% propantheline bromide, 0.25% triclocarban, 90% propylene glycol and 4.75% water.

Other information

Some authors considered xanthene-9-carboxylic acid, which is a part of the propantheline bromide molecule, to be the primary sensitizer (3,6).

LITERATURE

1   Skog E. Incidence of cosmetic dermatitis. Contact Dermatitis 1980;6:449-451
2   Ågren-Jonsson S, Magnusson, B. Sensitization to propantheline bromide, trichlorocarbanilide and propylene glycol in an antiperspirant. Contact Dermatitis 1976;2:79-80
3   Fregert S, Möller H. Allergic contact dermatitis from propantheline bromide. Contact Dermatitis Newsletter 1967;1:12
4   Wereide K. Contact allergy to propantheline bromide. Contact Dermatitis Newsletter 1968;4:61
5   Hannuksela, M. Allergy to propantheline in an antiperspirant (Ercoril® lotion). Contact Dermatitis 1975;1:244
6   Osmundsen PE. Concomitant contact allergy to propantheline bromide and TCC. Contact Dermatitis 1975;1:251-252
7   Przybilla B, Schwab U, Hölzle E, Ring J. Kontaktsensibilisierung durch ein Antiperspirant mit dem Wirkstoff Propanthelinbromid. Hautarzt 1983;34:459-462
8   Fregert S, Möller H. Allergic contact dermatitis from propantheline bromide. Cont Derm Newsl 1967;1:12
9   Gall H, Kempf E. Kontaktallergie auf das lokale Antiperspirant Propanthelinbromid. Dermatosen 1982;30:55-57

2.385 PROPOLIS

PROPOLIS CERA

IDENTIFICATION

Description/definition : Propolis cera is the waxy component of the resinous material found in beehives
Chemical class(es) : Waxes (natural and synthetic)
INCI name USA : Not in the Personal Care Products Council Ingredient Database
Other names : Propolis wax (US)
CAS registry number (s) : 85665-41-4
EC number(s) : 288-130-6
Merck Index monograph : 9218 (Propolis)
Function(s) in cosmetics : EU: antiseborrhoeic; moisturising; smoothing
Patch test allergens : 10% pet. (Chemotechnique, SmartPracticeEurope, SmartPracticeCanada)

PROPOLIS WAX

IDENTIFICATION

Description/definition : Propolis wax is the material obtained from the extraction of propolis, a resinous substance found in beehives
Chemical class(es) : Waxes (natural and synthetic)
Other names : Propolis (European Pharmacopoeia); propolis cera (EU); propolis resin
CAS registry number (s) : 9009-62-5; 85665-41-4
EC number(s) : 288-130-6
Merck Index monograph : 9218 (Propolis)
Function(s) in cosmetics : EU: emollient; skin conditioning. USA: skin-conditioning agents - emollient; skin-conditioning agents - miscellaneous
Patch test allergens : 10% pet. (Chemotechnique, SmartPracticeEurope, SmartPracticeCanada)

PROPOLIS EXTRACT

IDENTIFICATION

Description/definition : Propolis extract is an extract of propolis wax
Chemical class(es) : Biological products
CAS registry number (s) : 85665-41-4
EC number(s) : 288-130-6
Merck Index monograph : 9218 (Propolis)
Function(s) in cosmetics : EU: skin conditioning. USA: Skin-conditioning agents - miscellaneous
Patch test allergens : 10% pet. (Chemotechnique, SmartPracticeEurope, SmartPracticeCanada)

This chapter discusses the material called propolis. Propolis is not an INCI name, because the raw propolis has to be chemically and/or physically modified to be suitable for use in cosmetic products. The exact nature of the materials with INCI names Propolis cera and Propolis wax as described above is not clear. Cera = wax, so both Propolis cera and Propolis wax suggest it to be beeswax, which is a constituent (approx. 30-35%) of propolis. However, there are separate entries for 'beeswax' in the EU and USA INCI nomenclature and for its synonym cera alba in the EU database. Moreover, in the EU INCI system, 'propolis' and 'propolis resin' are given as synonyms for propolis wax. Indeed, propolis, which is also termed bee *glue*, is frequently confused with bees*wax* (124). This chapter discusses the full material 'propolis' and what is termed 'propolis' in literature.

 An extensive review of properties, applications, chemical composition, contact allergy, and other adverse effects of propolis written by the author was published in 2013 (104). A smaller but useful review stems from 2005 (2). The information in this chapter is derived from the author's review article, is a summary rather than a full review and therefore has a slightly different format than the regular chapters; for a detailed account with all literature references the reader is referred to the review (104). A full list of the constituents of poplar-type propolis, written and published by De Groot et al in June 2014 (105) is available and can be downloaded from the following website: https://www.researchgate.net/profile/Anton_De_Groot2.

 In this chapter, the literature on propolis back to 1987 is presented. Older literature on contact allergy to propolis can be found in the thorough review by Hausen et al (1).

GENERAL

What is propolis?

Propolis (bee glue) is formed from a resinous material that honeybees (*Apis mellifera* L.) collect from living plants. The materials are mixed with the enzyme β-glycosidase present in the bees' saliva, partially digested and added to beeswax to form the final product (raw propolis, propolis *in natura*). Raw propolis is hard and wax-like when cool, but soft and very sticky when warm, hence the name bee glue. The material has a pleasant aromatic smell; its color varies from yellow, green, or red to dark brown, depending on its source and age. The bees use propolis in the construction and adaptation of their nests and apply it in a thin layer on the internal walls of their hive or other cavity they inhabit, e.g., to block holes and cracks, to repair combs, to strengthen the thin borders of the comb and as a thermal insulator. Propolis also has antibacterial and antimycotic properties.

Botanical sources

It is generally accepted and has been chemically demonstrated that, in temperate zones, the bud exudates of species and their hybrids of the genus *Populus* (poplars) are the main source of propolis, notably *P. nigra* L. (black poplar) and to a lesser extent *P. deltoides* L. and *P. fremontii*. Despite the honeybees' preference for these poplars, exudates are also collected from other trees, for example, eucalyptus, birch, beech, alder, oak, willow, horse chestnut, pine, various conifers and fruit trees. In tropical regions there are no poplars and birches, and bees use other plant sources of bee glue (detailed in ref. 104).

Properties and applications

Propolis has been used by humans for thousands of years for its pharmaceutical properties. Raw propolis is washed with water, solubilized in 95% ethanol and repeatedly filtered to remove the wax and organic debris, creating 'propolis balsam' or 'propolis tincture'. The balsam possesses antibacterial, antifungal and antiviral properties and is claimed to have a wide range of other beneficial biological activities (122,128,145). Propolis is widely used as a popular remedy in folk medicine (especially in the Balkan States, the former USSR, Germany and Austria), and in apitherapy, which is the medical use of honey bee products. It is also a constituent of 'biocosmetics' and is sold in many health food stores as a dietary supplement, as 'over-the-counter' products for the protection of health and prevention of diseases, and as biopharmaceuticals for self-treatment of various diseases (2,128).

Many producers of propolis claim their products to be 'all natural,' which consumers often equate with safety. However, propolis and some of its constituents, notably the caffeates, are strong sensitizers (8,9,10,11,12), and the use of propolis products not infrequently leads to sensitization and allergic contact dermatitis, both from occupational contact in beekeepers (also called apiarists) and from the use of propolis products in consumers, especially from topical administration to the skin and oral mucosae.

Chemical composition

The chemical composition of propolis is highly variable, mainly due to the variability of plant species growing around the hive, from which the bees collect the exudates. Geographic location therefore is a major determinant of the composition. Propolis from temperate regions (poplar-type propolis), for example, varies considerably from Brazilian green and red propolis (for specifics see ref. 105). In general, crude propolis is composed of 50% resin and vegetable balsam (which contains the biologically active compounds), 35% waxes (mainly beeswax, some vegetable waxes), 5-10% aromatic oils, 5% pollen, and minor other substances including organic debris.

Poplar propolis is the most widely used and the most investigated type of propolis. Over 340 constituents have been identified in this propolis from various geographical locations. They include (in sequence of declining numbers in each category): 44 aromatic acid esters; 42 terpenoids; 37 aromatic acids; 25 aliphatic fatty acids (long-chain) and their esters; 25 aliphatic hydrocarbons and wax esters; 25 amino acids; 22 flavones and flavonols; 17 aliphatic acids (short-chain); 16 glycerol derivatives; 14 flavanones; 13 aldehydes; 12 alcohols; 10 aliphatic acid esters; 9 chalcones; 9 sugars and sugar alcohols; 8 acetophenones and other ketones; 5 dihydrochalcones; 4 steroids and 7 miscellaneous ingredients. A full account can be found in ref. 105. Other reviews have recently been published (130,133).

CONTACT ALLERGY

The first description of contact dermatitis due to propolis was published in 1915. Cases of allergic contact dermatitis to propolis began to emerge with increasing frequency in the 1970s (13,14) and at that time it was already predicted that the incidence of allergy to propolis would rise with the increasing use of the strong sensitizer propolis in biocosmetics and in biopharmaceuticals for self-treatment of various diseases (9).

Occupational contact allergy to propolis in beekeepers is well known (mainly from collecting honey and cleaning hives, where contact with propolis is inevitable) and may lead to both contact dermatitis and airborne allergic contact dermatitis (8,16,17,18,19,20,21,22). Airborne contact dermatitis may sometimes also be observed in neighbors of beekeepers (23,24). Occupational contact allergy to propolis also occurs, albeit far less frequently, in musicians and people who make stringed musical instruments (25,26,27,132) and has been observed in farmers (28). A dental technician developed occupational hand dermatitis. He reacted to propolis, and the reaction was ascribed to hand-molding beeswax products in the manufacture of prosthetic components. Apparently, these authors did not know that propolis is bee *glue*, but it is possible that the beeswax was contaminated with propolis (29). A shoemaker may have reacted to beeswax contaminated with propolis (30). A worker in a retail store had contact dermatitis which was – unconvincingly - ascribed to propolis in wood varnish (31).

While formerly most cases were (thought to be) caused by occupational exposure in beekeepers, currently most are caused (or at least the cases being published) by the topical use of propolis for medicinal purposes (11,32). Thus, propolis is an important allergen in patients with leg ulcers / lower leg dermatitis (33,34,35) and the frequency of sensitization is >5% in patients with anal dermatoses (36). Other sources of sensitization to propolis include cosmetics (37), and 'biocosmetics' or 'natural cosmetics' (11). In a number of cases, a positive patch test reaction to propolis can be explained by the previous use of preparations with poplar extract (8,10). Chewing propolis or chewing gum with propolis and the use of toothpastes, lozenges, powders, mouthwashes and various remedies for intraoral uses containing propolis have been reported to cause allergic stomatitis (sometimes with ulcers), labial and oral swelling, dyspnea, cheilitis and perioral eczema (25,38,39,40,41,42,43,43,45). Oral administration of honey or propolis-containing products (capsules, tablet, powders, sprays) by patients allergic to propolis may cause generalized skin eruptions (46,47), fixed drug eruption (48), and erythroderma (49).

It should be realized that occupational contact allergy in beekeepers may still be a major problem (134). Over 3.5% of German beekeepers may suffer from it (50), with an estimated number of 2900 propolis-sensitive beekeepers in Germany. However, they do not seem to recognize the problem and continue their hobby without protecting themselves from contact with the substance. On the contrary, many use propolis as medication for other disorders. This means that very few will be seen by a dermatologist and the problem goes unrecognized (and unreported) (50). Previously, in Bologna, Italy, 5-6% of beekeepers were suspected to be allergic to propolis based on a questionnaire analysis of 153 apiarists (51).

Patch testing in groups of patients
Results of studies testing propolis in consecutive patients suspected of contact dermatitis (routine testing) back to 1987 are shown in table 2.385.1. Results of testing in groups of *selected* patients (e.g., patients with stasis dermatitis / leg ulcers, patients suspected of cosmetic intolerance, individuals with contact cheilitis, children suspected of contact dermatitis) back to 1987 are shown in table 2.385.2.

Patch testing in consecutive patients suspected of contact dermatitis: routine testing
Reports of routine testing with propolis are summarized in table 2.385.1. In the 26 studies reviewed, prevalences of positive patch test reactions ranged from 0.5% in Finland in 1995-1996 (52) to 15% in a small 2008 Polish study (55). In general, the higher frequencies were observed in mid- and eastern European countries such as Poland, Lithuania, Czech Republic, Switzerland, Austria and Germany, where the extensive use of propolis, usually for biopharmaceutical purposes, is well known (32,34,54,55,56,57). However, high frequencies of sensitization have also been observed in the USA and Canada in 2007-2008 (4.9% [58]), in the USA in 2003-2015 / 2012-2015 (3.5% [127]), in the UK in 2007 (3.5% [29]) and in Australia in 2001-2010 (3.0% [135]). Generally speaking, the studies from after 2002 show higher sensitization rates than the older ones. In fact, of the 17 reported since 2002, only four had frequencies lower than 2% (1.4% [3], 1.9% [37], 1.8% [117], 1.7% [136]), whereas seven had prevalences (far) higher than 3%.

Most recently, a prevalence of 2.48% positive reactions has been observed in a 2009-2012 study in a group of 28,474 patients in 8 European countries (125). In several of these, propolis is included in the baseline series, for example the UK (37), Germany and Poland (126). The high prevalence of positive patch test reactions might, according to the authors, warrant inclusion in the baseline series of even more European countries (125). Unfortunately, as is the case in many such studies, data on relevance of the observed positive patch test reactions were often not provided. In the studies in which was commented on relevance, percentages ranged from 24% current relevance (37) to 64% (56). In two studies of the North American Contact Dermatitis Group (NACDG), 'definite + probable relevance' was only 19% and 20% (58, 117). Incriminated products were propolis-containing pharmaceuticals (11,56), cosmetics (37) and 'biocosmetics/natural cosmetics' (11).

Patch testing in groups of selected patients
Results of testing in groups of selected patients are shown in table 2.385.2, including nurses with occupational contact dermatitis (120), patients with periorbital dermatitis (121), children (53,67,68,69), patients with fragrance allergy (70), suspected cosmetic allergy (59,71), psoriasis (72) and rosacea (73). In 18 studies, frequencies of sensitization to propolis have ranged from 0.3% to 17%. Remarkably high frequencies were observed in 2008-2009 in Polish children of 7 to 8-years old (17%), propolis being the 2nd most frequent allergen after nickel (67). Also in Italian children, high frequences of sensitization were observed (mean 5.9% in the period 1995-2002), and there was

a linear increase in the frequency of sensitization from 2% in 1995 to 13.7% in 2002 (53). In the Italian study, relevance was said to be 75%, but no details on the incriminated products were provided (53). In earlier studies in both Polish and Italian children, sensitization rates had been far lower (0.7%-1.3%) (68,69).

Table 2.385.1 Patch testing in groups of patients: Routine testing

Years and Country	Test conc. & vehicle	Number of patients tested	positive (%)	Selection of patients (S); Relevance (R); Comments (C)	Ref.
2003-2015 and 2012-2015 USA	10% pet.	3221	112 (3.5%)	R: not stated	127
2013-14 USA, Canada	10% pet.	4859	82 (1.7%)	R: definite + probable relevance: 18%	136
2011-12 USA, Canada	10% pet.	4231	76 (1.8%)	R: definite + probable relevance: 20%	117
2009-2012, 8 European countries [a]	10% pet.	28,474	(2.48%)	R: not stated; C: range per country: 0-5.7%, median 2.8%	125, 139
2007 & 2011 Lithuania	10% pet.	380	11 (2.9%)	R: 7/11 (64%) current clinical relevance from topical remedies for stasis dermatitis, leg ulcers, mycoses etc.; C: overrepresentation of patients with stasis dermatitis	56
2009-10 USA, Canada	10% pet.	4304	90 (2.1%)	R: definite + probable relevance: 35%	62
2001-2010 Australia	10% pet.	4705	143 (3.0%)	R: 14%	135
2008 Poland		275	42 (15%)	R: not stated	55
2007-8 Seven European countries [a]	10% pet.	12,350	270 (2.2%) [b]	R: not stated; C: frequencies of sensitization ranged from 0.7% (Spain) to 4.0% (Austria), median 2.2%	63
- Austria		678	(4.0%)		
- Germany		2694	(2.2%)		
- Italy		984	(1.5%)		
- Lithuania		223	(2.3%)		
- Spain		372	(0.7%)		
- Switzerland		2402	(3.8%)		
-United Kingdom		4997	(1.4%)		
2007-2008 UK	10% pet.	2828	55 (1.9%)	R: 13/55 (24%) current relevance, 4/55 (7%) past, 21/55 (38%) relevance uncertain, 17/55 (31%) due to cross-sensitivity to other allergens; C: >50% caused by cosmetics; 7% co-reactivity to beeswax, 11% to FM I, 27% to colophonium and 40% to *Myroxylon pereirae* resin	37
2007-8 USA, Canada	10% pet.	5067	248 (4.9%)	R: definite + probable relevance: 19%	58
2007 UK	10% pet.	684	24 (3.5%)	R: not stated; C: only one patient co-reacted to beeswax	29
2001-2007 Czech Rep.	10% pet.	462	35 (7.6%)	R: 9 reactions (26%) were relevant	34
1995-2005 Germany		4242	59 (1.4%)	R: not stated; C: the prevalence rose from 0.5% in 1995 to 2.0% in 2005	3
2004 Germany, Austria	10% pet.	?	(3.5%)	R: not stated	54
2000-04 Switzerland		4094	120 (2.9%)	R: not stated	118
2003 IVDK	10% pet.	1831	34 (1.9%)	R: not stated; C: frequency of propolis allergy was elevated in patients allergic to farnesol, which may be present in poplar buds	64
2002-2003, 9 European centres [a]	10% pet.	3535	(2.9%)	R: not stated; C: prevalence range per centre (n=17): 0.9-4.9%	119
2002 Austria		443	29 (6.5%)	R: not stated	57
2000-2002 Finland		5130	72 (1.4%)	R: not stated; C: rise in prevalence from 0.5% in 1995-1996 (see below in this table) to 1.4% in 2000-2002 (significant)	52
1997-2000 Austria	10% pet.	2660	35 (1.3%)	R: not stated; C: significant association with FM I, colophony and *Myroxylon pereirae* resin; probably the same population as ref. 65 (below)	60
1997-2000 Austria	10% pet.	2766	36 (1.3%)	R: not stated; C: probably the same population as ref. 60 (above)	65
1996-1999 IVDK		20,363	554 (2.7%)	R: not stated; C: there was a significant increase in the frequency of positive patch test reactions with increasing age: 60 years and younger: 2%; 71-75 years: 4.4%; >75 years: 5.3%, indicating the relevance of topical leg ulcer / lower leg dermatitis for the induction of sensitization	33
1998 Poland	10% pet.	1830	(1.4-1.8%)	R: not mentioned; C: three different samples of propolis from various parts of Poland were used for patch testing; 64-79% of patients reacting to one or more propolis samples co-reacted to *Myroxylon pereirae* resin	61
1995-1996 Finland		3885	19 (0.5%)	R: not stated	52
1988-1990 Germany	10% pet.	3199	39 (1.2%)	R: 50% had used 'biocosmetics' or 'natural cosmetics' and	11

Table 2.385.1 Patch testing in groups of patients: Routine testing (*continued*)

Years and Country	Test conc. & vehicle	Number of patients tested | positive (%)		Selection of patients (S); Relevance (R); Comments (C)	Ref.
1988 Czechoslovakia	10% alc. sol.	605	25 (4.1%)	20% had used propolis capsules R: previous contact was confirmed in 16/25 (64%), all folk remedies for various diseases; C: 52% co-reacted to *Myroxylon pereirae* resin	32
1981-7 Slowakia	5% alc.	7383	136 (1.8%)	R: not stated; C: yearly range: 0.4%-3.3%; rise in frequency in 1985-1987	66
<1987				See the review of Hausen et al (1)	1

[a] study of the ESSCA ('European Surveillance System on Contact Allergy' network)
[b] age-standardized and sex-standardized proportions
IVDK: Informationsverbund Dermatologischer Kliniken (Germany, Switzerland, Austria)

A 15% sensitization rate was found in a small UK study of 27 patients (4 positive reactions) suspected of cosmetic dermatitis. All co-reacted to the fragrance mix, which suggest that cross-sensitization from fragrance allergy may have played a role (71). In an Italian study, performed in 2011-2012, a high percentage of 11.5% positive reactions to propolis was found in a group of 122 patients tested with a botanical series, who declared having had adverse reactions to 'botanical' products (cosmetics, detergents, pharmaceutical ointments). The reactions were all considered to be relevant, but culprit products were not mentioned (144). In 42 patients with positive patch test reactions to their own shaving products/eaux de toilette/perfumes, a frequency of 7% positive patch test reactions to propolis 10% was observed; the association was statistically significant when compared with a control group with (70).

Table 2.385.2 Patch testing in groups of patients: Selected patient groups

Years and Country	Test conc. & vehicle	Number of patients tested | positive (%)		Selection of patients (S); Relevance (R); Comments (C)	Ref.
2003-2014 IVDK	10% pet.	5202	(3.8%)	S: patients with stasis dermatitis / chronic leg ulcers; R: not stated; C: percentage of reactions was not significantly higher than in a control group of routine testing	143
2009-2013 IVDK	10% pet.	13,043	481 (3.7%)	S: consecutive dermatitis patients of 65 years and older; R: not stated; C: in the group of patients <65 years, the frequency of positive patch test reactions was 2.9%	131
2011-2012 Italy	20% pet.	122	14 (11.5%)	S: patients tested with a botanical series, who declared having had adverse reactions to 'botanical' products (cosmetics, detergents, pharmaceutical ointments): R: the reactions were all considered to be relevant	144
2003-2012 IVDK		2050	49 (2.4%)	S: nurses with occupational contact dermatitis; R: not stated	120
2006-2011 IVDK	10% pet.	10,124	272 (2.9%)	S: patients suspected of cosmetic intolerance; R: not stated	138
2001-2011 USA	10% pet.	24	2 (8%)	S: patients with allergic contact cheilitis; R: 2/2 relevant	141
2000-2010 IVDK		4385	91 (2.1%)	S: patients with periorbital dermatitis; R: not stated	121
1994-2010 USA, Canada	10% pet.	?	? (?)	S: hairdressers/cosmetologists; R: in the group of 57 patients who had at least one relevant occupationally related reaction, 3 (5.3%) reacted to propolis	140
2008-2009 Poland	10% pet.	103	17 (17%)	S: consecutive children 7-8 years old with chronic recurrent eczema and atopy; R: not stated; 2nd most frequent allergen after nickel	67
		93	5 (5%)	S: consecutive adolescents 16-17 years old with chronic recurrent eczema and atopy; R: not stated; 4th most common allergen after nickel, thimerosal and cobalt	
2000-2007 USA	10% pet.	500	26 (5.2%)	S: patients tested with a supplemental cosmetic screening series; R: 100%; C: weak study: a. high rate of macular erythema and weak reactions; b. relevance figures included 'questionable' and 'past' relevance	59
2001-2006 Italy	100% pet.	129	2 (2%)	S: patients with chronic cheilitis; R: 1 reaction was relevant	142
1998-2002 IVDK	10% pet.	42	3 (7%)	S: patients with positive patch test reactions to their own shaving products / eaux de toilette / perfumes; C: statistically significant association with propolis contact allergy	70
1995-2002 Italy	20% pet.	1255	74 (5.9%)	S: consecutive children seen for patch testing aged 7 months to 12 years; R: 75% relevancy; C: linear increase in the frequency of sensitization from 2% in 1995 to 13.7% in 2002; significant association with *Myroxylon pereirae* resin	53

Table 2.385.2 Patch testing in groups of patients: Selected patient groups (*continued*)

Years and Country	Test conc. & vehicle	Number of patients tested	positive (%)		Selection of patients (S); Relevance (R); Comments (C)	Ref.
1995-2002 IVDK	10% pet.	164	5	(3.0%)	S: patients with rosacea; R: not stated; C: the frequency was significantly higher than in patients with dermatitis	73
1996-1997 UK	10% pet.	27	4	(15%)	S: patients suspected of cosmetic dermatitis; R: not specified, one had taken propolis tablets; co-reactivity to the fragrance mix in all cases	71
1996 Italy	20% pet.	305	1	(0.3%)	S: consecutive patients with psoriasis; R: not stated	72
1988-1994 Italy		670	5	(0.7%)	S: children aged 6 months – 12 years; R: not stated	69
1970-1994 Poland		626	8	(1.3%)	S: consecutive children seen for patch testing aged 3-16 years; R: not stated	68
<1987					See the review of Hausen et al (1)	1

IVDK: Informationsverbund Dermatologischer Kliniken (Germany, Switzerland, Austria)

Case reports and case series

Case series

Propolis was stated to be the (or an) allergen in 3 patients in a group of 603 individuals suffering from cosmetic dermatitis, seen in the period 2010-2015 in Leuven, Belgium (111). In the period 1996-2013, in a tertiary referral center in Valencia, Spain, 5419 patients were patch tested. Of these, 628 individuals had allergic contact dermatitis to cosmetics. Propolis was the responsible allergen in four cases (137). Propolis was responsible for 2 out of 959 cases of non-fragrance cosmetic allergy where the causal allergen was identified, Belgium, 2000-2010 (75). In a group of 119 patients with allergic contact dermatitis from cosmetics, investigated in The Netherlands in 1986-1987, one case was caused by propolis in a skin care product (112,113). In a group of 83 patients with cheilitis, seen in Bologna, Italy in the period 2001-2005, one reacted to propolis in a lip salve (114).

Case reports

Case reports of sensitization to propolis-containing products are shown in table 2.385.3 (excluding cases of occupational contact allergy in beekeepers). The relevant literature from before 1987 has been reviewed by Hausen et al (1).

Table 2.385.3 Case reports of patients allergic to propolis (adapted from ref. 104) [a]

Country	Year	Nr. pat.	Exposures and clinical data	Ref.
Sweden	2016	1	Allergic contact cheilitis from a moisturizer containing propolis and from pure (not-propolis-enriched) honey	129
Portugal	2014	1	Allergic contact dermatitis of the face from applications of honey enriched with propolis for cosmetic purposes	110
USA	2013	1	Dermatitis of the eyelids from applying a beeswax-containing lipgloss with the fingers to the lips (ectopic dermatitis) [b]	124
		1	Widespread dermatitis mimicking mycosis fungoides from beeswax used to lubricate wires for glass beading; it is uncertain whether the authors confused beeswax with bee glue (propolis) or that they assumed propolis to be present in the beeswax (but they did not mention this) [b]	
Croatia	2012	1	Lip edema with erosions in the corners of the lips, and perioral erythema caused by propolis spray used for gingival swelling	45
USA	2012	1	Fixed drug eruption from propolis food supplement	48
Korea	2011	1	Systemic contact dermatitis from oral propolis solution	46
USA	2011	1	Perioral dermatitis and eczema in a child allergic to propolis and cinnamal, improving after avoidance of topical products containing fragrances and beeswax and clearing after stopping the use of gummy multivitamins containing propolis	74
Belgium	2000-2010	2	Skin care products	75
Korea	2009	1	Cheilitis and oral mucositis from propolis solution used for the treatment of aphthous ulcers	76
Austria	2009	1	Maculopapular exanthema from propolis capsules	47
USA	2008	1	Chewable multivitamins containing beeswax [b] causing cheilitis and dermatitis	77

Table 2.385.3 Case reports of patients allergic to propolis (adapted from ref. 104) [a] (*continued*)

Country	Year	Nr. pat.	Exposures and clinical data	Ref.
UK	2007	1	Occupational contact dermatitis in a dental technician from molding Beeswax [b] products in the manufacture of prosthetic components	29
Serbia and Montenegro	2006	1	Antihemorrhoidal ointment containing propolis	78
UK	2006	1	Vulval eczema ascribed to the presence of propolis in topical corticosteroid preparations; however, these topical medications contained highly purified beeswax, unlikely to be contaminated with propolis [b]	79
Croatia	2006	1	Erosions of the lips and mouth from propolis solution	42
Korea	2006	1	Propolis ointment	80
Germany	1995-2005	19	Propolis products used for medicinal purposes	3
		1	Occupational exposure to propolis-containing ointment in a nurse	
		1	Occupational exposure to honey in a lab analyst [b]	
		1	Occupational exposure to beeswax in making candles [b]	
		1	Eating honey daily resulted in persistent exanthema [b]	
		1	Natural cosmetics provided by a beekeeper	
		1	Sunscreens containing beeswax contaminated with propolis [b]	
Canada	2004	1	Propolis ointment	81
Italy	2004	1	Contact cheilitis from eating (propolis enriched?) honey [b]	43
Spain	2004	1	Alcoholic solution of propolis used as mouthwash caused labial edema, oral pain, dysphonia and dyspnea	39
		1	Lozenge caused pain and swelling of the tongue with dyspnea	
USA	2002	1	Occupational contact dermatitis from Italian varnish in a violin maker	26
Germany	2002	1	Occupational contact dermatitis from beeswax in a shoe maker [b]	30
Germany	2002	1	Unguentum leniens containing beeswax, supposedly contaminated with propolis [b]; the authors cite 3 similar cases in two German articles (83,84)	82
Japan	2001	1	Erythroderma from oral propolis powder (patch test with the powder was negative)	49
Czechia	2000	?	Cosmetic products; 'several' patients	85
Germany	1998	1	Lip balm and an ointment caused contact cheilitis mimicking pemphigus vulgaris	86
Italy	1997-1998	2	Toothpastes containing propolis or ingredients thereof or cross-reacting substances	87
		1	Lipcream	
Italy	1997	2	Propolis (hand)cream used for psoriasis; labial edema after chewing propolis tablets in one patient	44
Italy	1996	1	Labial and oral swelling, dyspnea, oral mucosal ulcers, cheilitis and perioral dermatitis from propolis tincture	38
Spain	1990	1	Propolis ointment and tincture	88
New Zealand	1990	1	Acute oral mucositis with ulceration from propolis lozenges	41
Germany	1988	3	Propolis ointment (n=1), ointment prepared from poplar buds (n=1), Populus Fluid® (homeopathic preparation) (n=1)	10
		1	Lipstick	
Germany	1988	1	Cosmetic ointments	89
		2	Therapeutic ointment	
Germany	1987	4	Propolis ointment	8
		2	Poplar bud ointment	
		1	Cream and face lotion	
		1	'Natural products' used as cosmetics	
Netherlands	1987	1	Stomatitis and throat complaints from propolis tablet and toothpaste	90
Italy	1987	1	Allergic contact dermatitis superimposed on psoriasis from propolis containing creams	91
Netherlands	1987	1	Cosmetic cream	22
Italy	1987	1	Cheilitis and perioral eczema from 'topical and oral propolis preparations'	123

Table 2.385.3 Case reports of patients allergic to propolis (adapted from ref. 104) [a] (*continued*)

Country	Year	Nr. pat.	Exposures and clinical data	Ref.
		1	Lichenoid dermatitis of the right hand from 'topical and oral preparations containing propolis'	
		1	Hand dermatitis from propolis cream; the authors suggested that the oral application of propolis in these three patients may have enhanced sensitization	
UK	1980	1	The patient reacted to propolis in a skin care product	115
UK	1980	1	A female patient had contact dermatitis from propolis in mascara	116

[a] Cases of propolis allergy in beekeepers are not included

[b] Honey and beeswax are frequently contaminated with small amounts of propolis, but is should be realized that in no single case report, analytical investigations have been performed to verify this, so some reports may not have been accurate

It is clear that most cases are caused by the use of propolis for medicinal purposes and that cosmetics containing propolis constitute a small minority. Unusual contact dermatitis cases have included granulomatous allergic contact dermatitis accompanied by marked lymphadenopathy from the application of a 20% lotion made from Brazilian propolis to an abrasion (92) and contact cheilitis from a lip balm and an ointment mimicking pemphigus vulgaris (86).

Cross-reactions, pseudo-cross-reactions and co-reactions

Myroxylon pereirae resin

The association between positive patch test reactions to propolis and *Myroxylon pereirae* resin (balsam of Peru) has been noted for decades (1,3,10,11,32,37,53,60,61,89,93). In these studies, from 9-90% of propolis-sensitive patients also reacted to *Myroxylon pereirae* resin (mean in all studies: 43%, without a large study in children [53]: 54%; median 55%). Both substances are extremely complex materials and patch testing with (some of) their ingredients is rarely performed. At least 26 chemicals may be present in both propolis and *Myroxylon pereirae* resin (1,10,11,93,94, 95) and 9 of these have caused positive patch test reactions both in patients allergic to propolis and in patients allergic to *Myroxylon pereirae* resin: benzoic acid, benzyl benzoate, benzyl cinnamate, benzyl isoferulate, benzyl salicylate, cinnamic acid, cinnamyl alcohol, coniferyl benzoate, and cinnamyl cinnamate (105). Thus, there are ample opportunities that positive patch test reactions to both propolis and *Myroxylon pereirae* resin are caused by common ingredients.

Other co-, cross- or pseudo-cross-reactions

The fragrance mix I and propolis may have cinnamyl alcohol and eugenol in common, but in some studies there appears to be no clear relationship between the two (37,53), though in others, there is (60). Recently, in the USA, there was a 25% co-reactivity to fragrance mix I and 20% to fragrance mix II in 112 patients allergic to propolis (127). Patch tests to colophonium are overrepresented; common ingredients may include resin acids such as (dehydro)-abietic acid and certain monoterpenes (37,60,127). Most concurrent reactions to yellow beeswax (cera flava, the least purified beeswax) may conveniently be explained by contamination of the beeswax with propolis, though analytical investigations to prove this in actual cases of contact allergy have not been performed (17,37,96,97).

A high degree of co-reactivity to poplar buds and extracts is to be expected, poplar buds being the most important source of (poplar-type) propolis (1,41,66). Co-reactivity to (a number of) essential oils does not come unexpected, the highest degree being seen with clove oil (11/16 positive reactions, 69% [93]). Clove oil may contain up to 88% eugenol and 34% benzyl alcohol (98); these compounds can also be present in propolis and in *Myroxylon pereirae* resin. However, eugenol cannot explain all co-reactivity to clove oil (93).

The allergens in propolis

In a (limited) number of studies, patients allergic to propolis have been tested with a (limited) number of its ingredients. The most important sensitizers – at least of the ones that have been tested – are the esters of caffeic acid: 'LB1' (a mixture of 3-methyl-2-butenyl caffeate, 3-methyl-3-butenyl caffeate, 2-methyl-2-butenyl caffeate, phenethyl caffeate, caffeic acid and benzyl caffeate); phenethyl caffeate; benzyl caffeate; 3-methyl-2-butenyl caffeate; and geranyl caffeate. In general, the terpinoids are – conform their weak or absent sensitizing potential in animal experiments– not important sensitizers in propolis (104). This subject has been fully described in ref. 104.

Presence in cosmetic products and chemical analyses

In July 2017, propolis (as propolis, propolis extract, propolis wax, bee propolis, propolis cera, bee propolis extract) was present in 72 of 70,166 cosmetic products of which the composition is known in EWG's Skin Deep Cosmetics Database, USA (http://www.ewg.org/skindeep/). In the USA, in April 2017, propolis was present in 35 of 56,714 cosmetic products of which the composition is known in FDA's Voluntary Cosmetic Registration Program (VCRP) (data obtained from FDA, May 2017). In 2009, in the USA, the ingredient lists of 1591 facial cosmetics from one company were screened for the presence of propolis. Propolis was present in 0% of 132 blushers and 38 bronzers, in 11% of 90 concealers, in 0% of 174 eyeliners, in 5% of 304 eyeshadows, in 0% of 457 foundations, in 0% of 140 loose and pressed powders, and in 61% of 256 mascaras (106). In 2009, in the USA, the ingredient lists of 796 hair products from one company were screened for the presence of propolis. Propolis was present in 3% of 279 shampoos, in 3% of 231 conditioners, and in 2% of 286 styling products (107).

In 2009, in the USA, the ingredient lists of 730 lip cosmetics and dental care products from one company were screened for the presence of propolis. Propolis was present in 42% of 31 lip liners, in 21% of 429 lipsticks, in 61% of 92 lip moisturizers, in 0% of 153 toothpastes, and in 0% of 25 mouth washes (108). In 2009, in the USA, the ingredient lists of 657 miscellaneous cosmetics from one company were screened for the presence of propolis. Propolis was present only in 13% of 201 sunblocks (109).

OTHER SIDE EFFECTS

Immediate-type reactions

There are few documented cases of immediate reactions to propolis (99,100). A 10-year-old boy had previously suffered an immediate systemic reaction within 5 minutes after a honeybee sting. Sensitization to honeybee venom was demonstrated by skin prick test and specific serum IgE. The patient also displayed angioedema each time he had contact with beehive products (honey, propolis, beeswax, and pollen) while helping his father, a beekeeper. A prick-to-prick test was positive for propolis and negative for beeswax and honey and both IgE and IgG against propolis extract was demonstrated (99).

An 48-year-old man treated his sore throat with topical propolis. After six hours, the patient complained of dysphagia and saliva drooling. Dyspnea later occurred and he soon lost consciousness with cyanosis and a generalized seizure attack, after which the patient became apneic and developed cardiac arrest. Severe larynx angioedema resulted in difficult airway intubation. No diagnostic tests to prove the causal relationship with propolis and to demonstrate the mechanism of the reaction were performed (100).

Between 1991 and 1995, the National Poisons Information Service (London, UK), received two reports of allergic reactions to oral 'royal jelly and propolis products' with symptoms ranging from crushing chest pains to severe bronchospasm and angioneurotic edema. No skin tests were performed. Similar cases from previous investigations were cited, which concerned type-I reactions to royal jelly rather than to propolis (101).

Systemic side effects

Oral administration of propolis has been linked to seizures (4), gastrointestinal symptoms (5), and (suspicion of) acute renal failure (6,7). Chronic aspiration from instillation of propolis to the nasal mucosa was suspected to have caused a benign tumor composed of foreign bodies (52). From April 2002 to August 2007, 18 suspected adverse reactions associated with propolis-containing products were reported to the national surveillance system of natural health products, coordinated by the Italian National Health Institute. There were 4 'allergic' reactions of the airways (3 acute asthma, 1 breath impairment), 6 cases of 'allergic' skin reactions and 6 'allergic' reactions of the oral mucosa and/or uvula and/or tongue, notably edema.

Two patients had gastrointestinal problems associated with propolis preparations, one digestive difficulties with stomach ache and the other gastro-esophageal reflux with heartburn. Some of the reactions were serious: six patients were admitted to hospital or visited an emergency department and in two of these a life-threatening event was reported (102). It should be realized that a causal association between propolis and these reactions was not verified and the mechanism of action not investigated (102). Life-threatening descending necrotizing mediastinitis superimposed on concomitant aspiration pneumonia from inappropriate use of propolis has been reported; however, the causal relationship can be doubted (103).

LITERATURE

1   Hausen BM, Wollenweber E, Senf H, Post B. Propolis allergy (I). Origin, properties, usage and literature review. Contact Dermatitis 1987;17:163-170
2   Walgrave SE, Warshaw EM, Glesne LA. Allergic contact dermatitis from propolis. Dermatitis 2005;16:209-215
3   Hausen BM. Evaluation of the main contact allergens in propolis (1995 to 2005). Dermatitis 2005;16:127-129
4   Sheehy C, Hall T, Pilo K. Products derived from bees: serious adverse reactions. Can Advers Reaction Newsl 2005;15:2-3
5   Cuzzolin L, Zaffani S, Benoni G. Safety implications regarding use of phytomedicines. Eur J Clin Pharmacol 2006;62:37-42
6   Li YJ, Lin JL, Yang CW, et al. Acute renal failure induced by a Brazilian variety of propolis. Am J Kidney Dis

2005;46: e125-e129

7   Health Canada. Propolis: suspected association with renal failure. Can Advers Reaction Newsl 2009;19:3

8   Hausen BM, Wollenweber E, Senff H, Post B. Propolis allergy (II). The sensitizing properties of 1,1-dimethylallyl caffeic acid ester. Contact Dermatitis 1987;17:171-177

9   Petersen HO. Hypersensitivity to propolis. Contact Dermatitis 1977;3:278-279

10 Hausen BM, Wollenweber E. Propolis allergy. Part III. Sensitization studies with minor constituents. Contact Dermatitis 1988;19:296-303

11 Hausen BM, Evers P, Stüwe HT, et al. Propolis allergy. Part IV. Studies with further sensitizers from propolis and constituents common to propolis, poplar buds, and balsam of Peru. Contact Dermatitis 1992;26:34-44

12 Hashimoto T, Tori M, Asakawa Y, et al. Synthesis of two allergenic constituents of propolis and poplar bud excretion. Z Naturforsch C 1988;43:470-472

13 Bunney MH. Contact eczema in bee-keepers due to propolis (bee glue). Br J Dermatol 1968;80:17-23

14 Wanscher B. Contact dermatitis from propolis. Br J Dermatol 1976;94:451-455

15 Gulbahar O, Ozturk G, Erdem N, et al. Psoriasiform contact dermatitis to propolis in a beekeeper. Ann Allergy Asthma Immunol 2005;94:509-511

16 Kleinhans D. Airborne contact dermatitis due to propolis. Contact Dermatitis 1987;17:187-188

17 Garrido-Fernández S, Arroabarren-Alemán E, García-Figueroa BE, et al. Direct and airborne contact dermatitis from propolis in beekeepers. Contact Dermatitis 2004;50:320-321

18 Fernández SG, Arroabarrea Alemán E, García Figueroa BE, et al. Direct and airborne contact dermatitis from propolis in beekeepers. Contact Dermatitis 2004;50:320-321

19 Gulbahar O, Ozturk G, Efem N, et al. A. Psoriasiform contact dermatitis due to propolis in a beekeeper. Ann Allergy Asthma Immunol 2005;94:509-511

20 Cirasino L, Pisati A, Fasani F. Contact dermatitis from propolis. Contact Dermatitis 1987;16:110-111

21 Basista K. Direct and airborne contact dermatitis in a beekeeper from the Małopolska region. Int J Occupat Med Environ Health 2012;25:499-500

22 Blanken R, Koedijk FHJ, Young E. Propolis-allergie. Ned Tijdschr Geneeskd 1987;131:1121-1123

23 Tobin AM, Kirby B. Airborne contact dermatitis induced by a neighbour's beehives. Contact Dermatitis 2003;49:214-215

24 Walls AC, Silvestri DL. Prevention of airborne propolis-induced allergic contact dermatitis with barrier cream. Dermatitis 2012;23:128-129

25 Monti M, Berti E, Carminati G, Cusini M. Occupational and cosmetic dermatitis from propolis. Contact Dermatitis 1983;9:163

26 Lieberman HD, Fogelman JP, Ramsay DL, Cohen DE. Allergic contact dermatitis to propolis in a violin maker. J Am Acad Dermatol 2002;46:S30-S31

27 Lombardi C, Bottello M, Caruso A, et al. Allergy and skin diseases in musicians. Eur Ann Allergy Clin Immunol 2003;35:52-55

28 Kieć-Swierczyńska M, Krecisz B, Swierczyńska-Machura D. Most frequent causes of allergic contact dermatitis in farmers: based on material collected in the Nofer Institute of Occupational Medicine, Lodz. Med Pr 2003;54:237-243

29 Langan SM, English JS. Occupational contact dermatitis from propolis in a dental technician. Contact Dermatitis 2007;56:43

30 Henschel R, Agathos M, Breit R. Occupational contact dermatitis from propolis. Contact Dermatitis 2002;47:52

31 Downs A, Sansom J. Occupational contact dermatitis due to propolis. Contact Dermatitis 1998;38:359-360

32 Macháčková J. The incidence of allergy to propolis in 605 consecutive patients patch tested in Prague. Contact Dermatitis 1988;18:210-212

33 Uter W, Geier J, Pfahlberg A, et al.The spectrum of contact allergy in elderly patients with and without lower leg dermatitis. Dermatology 2002;204:266-272

34 Necas M, Dastychová E. Contact sensitization with lower extremity dermatitis in the South Moravian region, Czech republic. Phlebology 2010;25;132-137

35 Gallenkemper G, Rabe E, Bauer R. Contact sensitization in chronic venous insufficiency: modern wound dressings. Contact Dermatitis 1998;38:274-278

36 Bauer A, Oehme S, Geier J. Contact sensitization in the anal and genital area. Curr Probl Dermatol 2011;40:133-141

37 Rajpara S, Wilkinson MS, King CM, et al. The importance of propolis in patch testing: a multicentre survey. Contact Dermatitis 2009;61:287-290

38 Bellegrandi S, D'Offizi G, Ansotegui IJ, et al. Propolis allergy in an HIV positive patient. J Am Acad Dermatol 1996;35:644

39 Garrido Fernández S, Lasa Luaces E, Echechipía Modaz S, et al. Allergic contact stomatitis due to therapeutic propolis. Contact Dermatitis 2004;50:321

40 Kokelj F, Trevisan G. Contact dermatitis from propolis. Contact Dermatitis 1983;9:518

41 Hay KD, Greig DE. Propolis allergy: a cause of oral mucositis with ulceration. Oral Surg Oral Med Oral Pathol 1990;70:584-586

42 Brailo V, Boras VV, Alajbeg I, et al. Delayed contact sensitivity on the lips and oral mucosa due to propolis - case report. Med Oral Patol Oral Cir Bucal 2006;11:E303-304

43 Pasolini G, Semenza D, Capazora R, et al. Allergic contact cheilitis Induced by contact with propolis-enriched honey. Contact Dermatitis 2004;50:322-323

44 Silvani S, Spettoli E, Stacul F, et al. Contact dermatitis in psoriasis due to propolis. Contact Dermatitis 1997;37:48–49

45 Budimir V, Brailo V, Alajbeg I, et al. Allergic contact cheilitis and perioral dermatitis caused by propolis: case report. Acta Dermatovenerol Croat 2012;20:187-190

46 Cho E, Lee JD, Cho SH. Systemic contact dermatitis from propolis ingestion. Ann Dermatol 2011;23:85-88

47 Komericki P, Kränke B. Maculopapular exanthem from propolis: case report and review of systemic cutaneous and non-cutaneous reactions. Contact Dermatitis 2009;61:353-355

48 Ramien ML, Pratt MD. Fixed drug eruption to ingested propolis. Dermatitis 2012;23:173-175

49 Horiuchi Y. Propolis-induced erythroderma. J Dermatol 2001;28:580-581

50 Münstedt K, Hellner M, Hackethal A, et al. Contact allergy to propolis in beekeepers. Allergol Immunopathol (Madr) 2007;35:95-15

51 Tosti A, Gaspari F, Piani C, et al. propolis: Incidenza di sensibilizzazione in popolazione 'a rischio'. Giorn Ital Derm Venereol 1984;119:353-356

52 Hasan T, Rantanen T, Alanko K, et al. Patch test reactions to cosmetic allergens in 1995-1997 and 2000-2002 in Finland—a multicentre study. Contact Dermatitis 2005;53:40-45

53 Giusti F, Miglietta R, Pepe P, et al. Sensitization to propolis in 1255 children undergoing patch testing. Contact Dermatitis 2004;51:255-258

54 Hegewald J, Uter W, Aberer W, et al. The European Surveillance System of Contact Allergies (ESSCA): results of patch testing the standard series, 2004. JEADV 2008;22:174-181

55 Pietowska J, Czarnobilska E, Spiewak R. The most frequent contact sensitizers and atopic diseases among consecutive patients of a Polish patch test clinic. Allergy 2008: 63 (suppl.88):320

56 Beliauskiene A, Jankuviene E, Valiukeviciene S. Propolis – common and relevant allergen. Contact Dermatitis 2012;66 (suppl.2):60-61

57 Reider N, Komericki P, Hausen BM, et al. The seamy side of natural medicine: contact sensitisation to arnica (Arnica montana L.) and marigold (Calendula officinalis L.). Contact Dermatitis 2001;45:269-272

58 Fransway AF, Zug KA, Belsito DV, et al. North American Contact Dermatitis Group patch test results for 2007-2008. Dermatitis 2013;24:10-21

59 Wetter DA, Yiannias JA, Prakash AV, et al. Results of patch testing to personal care product allergens in a standard series and a supplemental cosmetic series: an analysis of 945 patients from the Mayo Clinic Contact Dermatitis Group, 2000-2007. J Am Acad Dermatol 2010;63:789-798

60 Wöhrl S, Hemmer W, Focke M, et al. The significance of fragrance mix, balsam of Peru, colophony and propolis as screening tools in the detection of fragrance allergy. Br J Dermatol 2001;145:268273

61 Rudzki Z, Rebandel P, Jaworski E. Comparison of the eliciting properties of 3 different propolis samples. Contact Dermatitis 1998;39:142-143

62 Warshaw EM, Belsito DV, Taylor JS, et al. North American Contact Dermatitis Group patch test results: 2009-2010. Dermatitis 2013;24:50-59

63 Uter W, Aberer W, Armario-Hita JC, et al. Current patch test results with the European baseline series and extensions to it from the 'European Surveillance System on Contact Allergy' network, 2007-2008. Contact Dermatitis 2012;67:9-19

64 Schnuch A, Uter W, Geiger J, et al. Contact allergy to farnesol in 2021 consecutively patch tested patients. Results of the IVDK. Contact Dermatitis 2004;50:117-121

65 Wöhrl S, Hemmer W, Focke M, et al. Patch testing in children, adults, and the elderly. Pediatr Dermatol 2003;20:119-123

66 Hegyi E, Suchy V, Nagy M. Zur Frage der Propolisallergie. Hautarzt 1990;41:675-679

67 Czarnobilska E, Obtulowicz K, Dyga W, et al. The most important contact sensitizers in Polish children and adolescents with atopy and chronic recurrent eczema as detected with the extended European Baseline Series. Pediatr Allergy Immunol 2011;22:252-256

68 Rudzki E, Rebandel P. Contact dermatitis in children. Contact Dermatitis 1996;34:66-67

69 Manzini BM, Ferdani G, Simonetti V, et al. Contact sensitization in children. Pediatr Dermatol 1998;15:12-17

70 Uter W, Geier J, Schnuch A, et al. Patch test results with patients'own perfumes, deodorants and shaving lotions: results of the IVDK 1998-2002. JEADV 2007;21:374-379

71 Thomson KF, Wilkinson SM. Allergic contact dermatitis to plant extracts in patients with cosmetic dermatitis. Br J Dermatol 2000;142:84-88

72 Barile M, Cozzani E, Anonide A, et al. Is contact allergy rare in psoriatics? Contact Dermatitis 1996;35:113-114

73 Jappe U, Schnuch A, Uter W. Rosacea and contact allergy to cosmetics and topical medicaments – retrospective analysis of multicenter surveillance data 1995-2002. Contact Dermatitis 2005;52:96-101

74 Matiz C, Jacob SE. Systemic contact dermatitis in children: how an avoidance diet can make a difference. Pediatr Dermatol 2011;28:368-374

75 Travassos AR, Claes L, Boey L, et al. Non-fragrance allergens in specific cosmetic products. Contact Dermatitis 2011;65:276-285

76 Kim JE, Shin H, Ro YS. A case of allergic contact dermatitis to propolis on the lips and oral mucosa. Korean J Dermatol 2009;47:199-202

77 Jacob SE, Chimento S, Castanedo-Tardan MP. Allergic contact dermatitis to propolis and carnauba wax from lip balm and chewable vitamins in a child. Contact Dermatitis 2008;58:242-243

78 Javanović M, Karadaglić D, Brkić S. Contact urticaria and allergic contact dermatitis to lidocaine in a patient sensitive to benzocaine and propolis. Contact Dermatitis 2006;54:124-126

79 Black RJ. Vulval eczema associated with propolis sensitization from topical therapies treated successfully with pimecrolimus cream. Clin Exp Dermatol 2005;30:91-92

80 Lee SY, Lee DR, You CE, et al. Autosensitization dermatitis associated with propolis-induced allergic contact dermatitis. J Drugs Dermatol 2006;5:458-460

81 Ting PT, Silver S. Allergic contact dermatitis to propolis. J Drugs Dermatol 2004;3:685-686

82 Junghans V, Geier J, Fuchs T. Allergy to propolis caused by beeswax-containing ointment. Am J Contact Dermatitis 2002;13:87

83 Panneck WB. Kontaktallergie auf Unguentum leniens. Allergologie 1990;13:183-184

84 Eichenseer M, Eisele S, Disch R. Gleichzeitiges Vorliegen von Kontaktallergien auf Propolis und Unguentum leniens. Allergologie 1994;17:265-267

85 Tumová L, Pasavová D. Allergic contact dermatitis caused by propolis. Ceska Slov Farm 2000;49:285-287 (article in Czech)

86 Thomas P, Korting HC, Przybilla B. Propolis-induced allergic contact dermatitis mimicking pemphigus vulgaris. Arch Dermatol 1998;134:511-513

87 Francalanci S, Sertoli A, Giorgini S, et al. Multicentre study of allergic contact cheilitis from toothpaste. Contact Dermatitis 2000;43:216-222

88 Ratón JA, Aguirre A, Díaz-Pérez JL. Contact dermatitis from propolis. Contact Dermatitis 1990;22:183-184

89 Schuler TM, Frosch PJ. Kontaktallergie auf propolis (Bienen-Kittharz). Hautarzt 1988;39:139-142

90 Young E. Sensitivity to propolis. Contact Dermatitis 1987;16:49-50

91 Angelini G, Vena GA, Meneghini CL. Psoriasis and contact allergy to propolis. Contact Dermatitis 1987;17:251-253

92 Teraki Y, Shiohara T. Propolis-induced granulomatous contact dermatitis accompanied by marked lymphadenopathy. Br J Dermatol 2001;144:1277-1278

93 Rudzki E, Grzywa Z. Dermatitis from propolis. Contact Dermatitis 1983;9:40-45

94 Hausen BM. Contact allergy to balsam of Peru. II. Patch test results of 102 patients with selected balsam of Peru constituents. Am J Contact Derm 2001;12:93-102

95 Hausen BM, Simatupang T, Bruhn G et al. Identification of new allergenic constituents and proof of evidence for coniferyl benzoate in Balsam of Peru. Am J Cont Derm 1995;6:199-208

96 Valsecchi R, Cainelli T. Dermatitis from propolis. Contact Dermatitis 1984;11:317

97 Jensen CD, Anderson KE. Allergic contact dermatitis from cera alba (purified propolis) in a lip balm and candy. Contact Dermatitis 2006;55:312-313

98 Chaieb K, Hajlaoui H, Zmantar T, et al. The chemical composition and biological activity of clove essential oil, Eugenia caryophyllata (Syzigium aromaticum L. Myrtaceae): a short review. Phytother Res 2007;21:501-506

99 Callejo A, Armentia A, Lombardero M, et al. Propolis, a new bee-related allergen. Allergy 2001;56:579

100 Hsu CY, Chiang WC, Weng TI, et al. Laryngeal edema and anaphylactic shock after topical propolis use for acute pharyngitis. Am J Emerg Med 2004;22:432-433

101 Shaw D, Leon C, Kolev S, et al. Traditional remedies and food supplements: a 5-year toxicological study (1991-1995). Drug Safety 1997;17:342-356

102 Menniti-Ippolito F, Mazzanti G, Vitalone A, et al. Surveillance of suspected adverse reactions to natural health products—the case of propolis. Drug Saf 2008;31:419-423

103 Wu J-Y, Hsu NY. Propolis-Induced descending necrotizing mediastinitis and aspiration pneumonia. Ann Thorac Surg 2013;95:e87-e89

104 De Groot AC. Propolis: a review of properties, applications, chemical composition, contact allergy, and other adverse effects. Dermatitis 2013;24:263-282

105 De Groot AC, Popova MP, Bankova VS. An update on the constituents of poplar-type propolis. Wapserveen, The Netherlands: acdegroot publishing, 2014. ISBN/EAN: 978-90-813233-0-7 (pdf booklet). Available at: https://www.researchgate.net/profile/Anton_De_Groot2

106 Scheman A, Jacob S, Katta R, Nedorost S, Warshaw E, Zirwas M, et al. Part 1 of a 4 part series. Facial cosmetics: trends and alternatives. Data from the American Contact Alternative Group. J Clin Aesthet Dermatol 2011;4:25-30

107 Scheman A, Jacob S, Katta R, Nedorost S, Warshaw E, Zirwas M, et al. Part 2 of a 4 part series. Hair cosmetics: trends and alternatives. Data from the American Contact Alternative Group. J Clin Aesthet Dermatol 2011;4:42-46

108 Scheman A, Jacob S, Katta R, Nedorost S, Warshaw E, Zirwas M, et al. Part 3 of a 4 part series. Lips and common Dental Care products: trends and alternatives. Data from the American Contact Alternative Group. J Clin Aesthet Dermatol 2011;4:50-53

109 Scheman A, Jacob S, Katta R, Nedorost S, Warshaw E, Zirwas M, et al. Part 4 of a 4 part series. Miscellaneous products: trends and alternatives in deodorants, antiperspirants, sunblocks, shaving products, powder, and wipes. Data from the American Contact Alternative Group. J Clin Aesthet Dermatol 2011;4:35-39

110 Matos D, Serrano P, Menezes Brandão F. A case of allergic contact dermatitis caused by propolis-enriched honey. Contact Dermatitis 2015;72:59-60

111 Goossens A. Cosmetic contact allergens. Cosmetics 2016, 3, 5; doi:10.3390/cosmetics3010005

112 De Groot AC, Bruynzeel DP, Bos JD, van der Meeren HL, van Joost T, Jagtman BA, Weyland JW. The allergens in cosmetics. Arch Dermatol 1988;124:1525-1529

113 De Groot AC. Adverse reactions to cosmetics. PhD Thesis, University of Groningen, The Netherlands: 1988, chapter 3.4, pp.105-113

114 Zoli V, Silvani S, Vincenzi C, Tosti A. Allergic contact cheilitis. Contact Dermatitis 2006;54:296-297

115 Cronin E. Contact Dermatitis. Edinburgh: Churchill Livingstone, 1980:101

116 Cronin E. Contact Dermatitis. Edinburgh: Churchill Livingstone, 1980:111

117 Warshaw EM, Maibach HI, Taylor JS, Sasseville D, DeKoven JG, Zirwas MJ, et al. North American Contact Dermatitis Group patch test results: 2011-2012. Dermatitis 2015;26:49-59

118 Janach, M, Kühne A, Seifert B, French LE, Ballmer-Weber B, Hofbauer GFL. Changing delayed-type sensitizations to the baseline series allergens over a decade at the Zurich University Hospital. Contact Dermatitis 2010;63:42-48

119 Uter W, Hegewald J, Aberer W, Ayala F, Bircher AJ, Brasch J, et al. The European standard series in 9 European countries, 2002/2003 –First results of the European Surveillance System on Contact Allergies. Contact Dermatitis 2005;53:136-145

120 Molin S, Bauer A, Schnuch A, Geier J. Occupational contact allergy in nurses: results from the Information Network of Departments of Dermatology 2003–2012. Contact Dermatitis 2015;72:164-171

121 Landeck L, John SM, Geier J. Periorbital dermatitis in 4779 patients – patch test results during a 10-year period. Contact Dermatitis 2014;70:205-212

122 Burdock GA. Review of the biological properties and toxicity of bee propolis (propolis). Food Chem Toxicol 1998;36:347-363

123 Trevisan G, Kokelj F. Contact dermatitis from propolis: role of gastrointestinal absorption. Contact Dermatitis 1987;16:48

124 Baker L, Litzner B, Le EN, Cruz PD Jr. Ectopic periorbital dermatitis and mycosis fungoides-like dermatitis due to propolis. Dermatitis 2013;24:328-329

125 Uter W, Spiewak R, Cooper SM, Wilkinson M, Sánchez Pérez J, Schnuch A, Schuttelaar M-L. Contact allergy to ingredients of topical medications: results of the European Surveillance System on Contact Allergies (ESSCA), 2009-2012. Pharmacoepidemiol Drug Saf 2016, doi: 10.1002/pds.4064.

126 Spiewak R. Alergia kontaktowa i alergiczny wyprysk kontaktowy [Contact allergy and allergic contact dermatitis]. Alergologia Polska 2014;1:150-157. doi:10.1016/j.alergo.2014.11.001 (article in Polish)

127 Shi Y, Nedorost S, Scheman L, Scheman A. Propolis, colophony, and fragrance cross-reactivity and allergic contact dermatitis. Dermatitis 2016;27:123-126

128 Sforcin JM. Biological properties and therapeutic applications of propolis. Phytother Res 2016;30:894-905

129 Nyman G, Hagvall L. A case of allergic contact cheilitis caused by propolis and honey. Contact Dermatitis 2016;74:186-187

130 Ristivojević P, Trifković J, Andrić F, Milojković-Opsenica D. Poplar-type propolis: chemical composition, botanical origin and biological activity. Nat Prod Commun 2015;10:1869-1876

131 Mahler V. Contact allergies in the elderly. Hautarzt 2015;66:665-673 (article in German)

132 Crépy MN. Skin diseases in musicians. Eur J Dermatol 2015;25:375-383

133 Huang S, Zhang CP, Wang K, Li GQ, Hu FL. Recent advances in the chemical composition of propolis. Molecules 2014;19):19610-19632

134 Münstedt K, Kalder M. Contact allergy to propolis in beekeepers. Allergol Immunopathol (Madr) 2009;37:298-301

135 Toholka R, Wang Y-S, Tate B, Tam M, Cahill J, Palmer A, Nixon R. The first Australian Baseline Series: Recommendations for patch testing in suspected contact dermatitis. Australas J Dermatol 2015;56:107-115

136 DeKoven JG, Warshaw EM, Belsito DV, Sasseville D, Maibach HI, Taylor JS, et al. North American Contact Dermatitis Group Patch Test Results: 2013-2014. Dermatitis 2017;28:33-46

137 Zaragoza-Ninet V, Blasco Encinas R, Vilata-Corell JJ, Pérez-Ferriols A, Sierra-Talamantes C, Esteve-Martínez A, de la Cuadra-Oyanguren J. Allergic contact dermatitis due to cosmetics: A clinical and epidemiological study in a tertiary hospital. Actas Dermosifiliogr 2016;107:329-336

138 Dinkloh A, Worm M, Geier J, Schnuch A, Wollenberg A. Contact sensitization in patients with suspected cosmetic intolerance: results of the IVDK 2006-2011. J Eur Acad Dermatol Venereol 2015;29:1071-1081

139 Uter W, Spiewak R, Cooper SM, Wilkinson M, Sánchez Pérez J, Schnuch A, Schuttelaar M-L. Contact allergy to ingredients of topical medications: results of the European Surveillance System on Contact Allergies (ESSCA), 2009-2012. Pharmacoepidemiol Drug Saf 2016;25:1305-1312

140 Warshaw EM, Wang MZ, Mathias CGT, Maibach HI, Belsito DV, Zug KA, et al. Occupational contact dermatitis in hairdressers/cosmetologists; retrospective analysis of North American Contact Dermatitis Group data, 1994 to 2010. Dermatitis 2012;23:258-268

141 O'Gorman SM, Torgerson RR. Contact allergy in cheilitis. Int J Dermatol 2016;55:e386-e391

142 Schena D, Fantuzzi F, Girolomoni G. Contact allergy in chronic eczematous lip dermatitis. Eur J Dermatol 2008;18:688-692

143 Erfurt-Berge C, Geier J, Mahler V. The current spectrum of contact sensitization in patients with chronic leg ulcers or stasis dermatitis - new data from the Information Network of Departments of Dermatology (IVDK). Contact Dermatitis 2017 Feb 14. doi: 10.1111/cod.12763. [Epub ahead of print]

144 Corazza M, Borghi A, Gallo R, Schena D, Pigatto P, Lauriola MM, et al. Topical botanically derived products: use, skin reactions, and usefulness of patch tests. A multicentre Italian study. Contact Dermatitis 2014;70:90-97

145 Sung SH, Choi GH, Lee NW, Shin BC. External use of propolis for oral, skin, and genital diseases: A systematic review and meta-analysis. Evid Based Complement Alternat Med 2017;2017:8025752. doi: 10.1155/2017/8025752

2.386 PROPYLENE GLYCOL

IDENTIFICATION

Description/definition   : Propylene glycol is the aliphatic alcohol that conforms generally to the formula shown below

Chemical class(es)   : Alcohols

Chemical/IUPAC name   : Propane-1,2-diol

Other names   : 1,2-Dihydroxypropane

CAS registry number (s)   : 57-55-6

EC number(s)   : 200-338-0

CIR review(s)   : J Am Coll Toxicol 1994;13:437-491; Int J Toxicol 2012;31(Suppl.2):245-260 (access: www.cir-safety.org/ingredients)

Merck Index monograph   : 7855

Function(s) in cosmetics : EU: humectants; skin conditioning; solvent; viscosity controlling. USA: fragrance ingredients; skin-conditioning agents – humectants; skin-conditioning agents – miscellaneous; solvents; viscosity decreasing agents

Patch testing   : 5% pet. (Chemotechnique, SmartPracticeEurope, SmartPracticeCanada); 10% water (Chemotechnique, SmartPracticeCanada); 20% water (SmartPracticeEurope, SmartPracticeCanada); 30% water (Chemotechnique, SmartPracticeCanada); pure (SmartPracticeCanada); the test concentrations of 20% and higher may cause irritant reactions, the lower test concentrations false-negative results

Molecular formula   : $C_3H_8O_2$

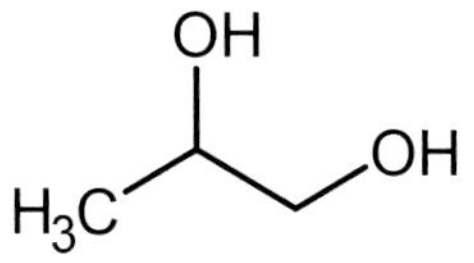

GENERAL

Propylene glycol (PG) is a viscous, colorless fluid with almost no odor and a very low toxicity (24). Of the world's production of PG, 40-45% is estimated to be used as intermediate in the synthesis of other chemicals, especially unsaturated polyester resins. The remainder of the production volume is used in a multitude of industrial products, for example as solvent in lacquers and varnishes (about 4% of the production), for certain resins and also as plasticizer, for example, in vinyl resins (about 4-10%), as component in antifreeze products, lubricants, cutting fluids, and inks (about 10-13%) (24). About 12-17% of PG is used as component in cosmetics and pharmaceutical preparations and as food additive. Other applications include household cleansers, liquid laundry detergents (about 9-15%), in animal foods (about 5%), as humectant in tobacco (about 4%) and in medical devices such as transdermal drug delivery systems (PG enhances the percutaneous penetration of many chemicals) (44) and ECG electrodes or ultrasonic contact gels. Skin exposure of consumers to PG most commonly occurs through contact with cosmetics or topical medicaments (24).

Contact allergy to propylene glycol is infrequent. Many positive patch test reactions may in fact have been irritant. Most cases of allergic contact dermatitis are caused by topical pharmaceutical preparations and conductive gels for ECG, ultrasound examinations and transcutaneous electric nerve stimulation (TENS) procedures; cosmetic allergy from PG has infrequently been observed.

The literature on propylene glycol dermatitis has been reviewed in 1991 (112,117) and again in 1994 (115).

CONTACT ALLERGY

General

Propylene glycol is a 'difficult allergen' (115). There is no test concentration known which is low enough to cause no irritation but high enough to detect all cases of sensitization. In fact, it has been stated that 'it seems impossible to define a test concentration of PG which will yield sufficient sensitivity, which does not, at the same time, cause a considerable proportion of false-positive reactions, i.e. insufficient specificity (24). Commercial PG patch tests products are available in the following concentrations and vehicles: 5% in petrolatum, 10% in water, 20% in water, 30% in water and even pure (see 'Patch testing' in the section 'Identification' above). The test concentration of 5% in petrolatum is not irritant (25), but may result in false-negative reactions (108); test concentrations of 20% (24) and higher (33,34,35,36) may cause false-positive irritant reactions.

Allergic contact dermatitis seems to be uncommon, and the clinical significance has been overestimated. In earlier studies, higher concentrations of propylene glycol may have induced many irritant patch test reactions. A diagnosis of allergic contact dermatitis should never be made on the basis of one positive patch test alone (24,115). Retesting should always be done after several weeks. Next, retests with serial dilutions down to 1% propylene glycol help in separating irritant responses from true allergic ones. A negative reaction at retesting strongly suggests a previously irritant response; a positive reaction suggests contact allergy. Repeated open application tests (ROAT) and/or provocative use tests (PUT) can be conducted to verify the allergic basis of a positive patch test result. In subjects with a negative patch test, the ROAT/PUT may also be useful as a simulation of normal application procedures.

On the basis of a thorough literature review and their experience from testing >45,000 patients with propylene glycol 20% in water, the members of the IVDK in 2005 came to the following conclusions (24):
1. neither occupation nor any special exposures are risk factors for PG contact allergy;
2. PG at 20% in water for patch testing is a slightly irritant preparation;
3. many of the weak positive reactions (i.e. + reactions), that is >80% of all positive reactions, must be interpreted as false-positive;
4. weak positive reactions may predominantly reflect individual susceptibility to a substance rather than a general property of the substance itself;
5. the majority of the remaining positive reactions, probably to be interpreted as allergic, seem to be due to exposure to PG in topical therapeutics and/or cosmetic preparations;
6. in about one-sixth of the cases, the positive reactions are correlated to leg dermatitis in chronic venous disease;
7. propylene glycol has a very low sensitizing potential;
8. the risk for sensitization to PG on uncompromised skin seems to be extremely low;
9. the diagnosis of PG contact sensitization should not be based on a positive patch test reaction alone, but only on a combination of anamnestic information and, preferably, validation tests (see above: retesting, serial dilutions, ROAT, PUT) (24).

Patch testing in groups of patients
Results of studies testing propylene glycol in consecutive patients suspected of contact dermatitis (routine testing) back to 1990 are shown in table 2.386.1. Results of testing in groups of *selected* patients (e.g., patients with periorbital dermatitis, children with dermatitis, patients with stasis dermatitis / leg ulcers, individuals suspected of cosmetic allergy or tested with a cosmetic series) back to 1996 are shown in table 2.386..

Patch testing in consecutive patients suspected of contact dermatitis: routine testing
Propylene glycol has been part of the screening series of the North American Contact Dermatitis Group (NACDG) for over 25 years. As the NACDG members publish their results biannually, there are many data on propylene glycol routine testing available from the USA and Canada. Only 2 studies published after 2000 came from other countries: a 2001-2010 study from Australia (90) and an investigation performed by the IVDK (Germany, Austria, Switzerland) in the period 1992-2002 (24).

In 20 studies in which routine testing with propylene glycol was performed, frequencies of sensitization have ranged from 0.4% to 4.2%. It should be realized that various test concentrations were used (10% pet., 10% water, 20% water, 30% water and pure), which makes comparison of the results – and their interpretation - difficult. That the test concentration is crucial is evident from a 2006-2010 USA study, in which testing with 20% water yielded 2.5% positive reactions, but testing with 10% pet. only 0.5% (77). Generally speaking, the higher rates of sensitization were observed in those studies using the higher concentration of 30% in water, as currently performed by the NACDG. Relevance rates, as defined by the sum of 'definite' and 'probable' relevance (NACDG criteria) mostly were some 40-60%. Causative products were specified in two studies only, both mentioning cosmetics and topical pharmaceuticals (24,66). In the US study (66), personal care products formed the majority, in the IVDK investigation (24) most reactions were caused by PG in topical pharmaceutical products.

Patch testing in groups of selected patients
Results of testing in groups of selected patients (e.g., patients with periorbital dermatitis, children with dermatitis, patients with stasis dermatitis / leg ulcers, individuals suspected of cosmetic allergy or tested with a cosmetic series) back to 1996 are shown in table 2.386.2. In 15 investigations, frequencies of sensitization have ranged from 0.2% in young children (102) to 11% in patients with facial allergic contact dermatitis (80) and 14% in a small group of individuals with leg ulcers (101). Because of the heterogeneity of the groups and the different test concentrations used (5% pet., 10% pet., 10%, 20% and 30% water) comparison is very difficult. Generally speaking, the higher sensitization rates were scored in groups (probably) tested with 30% in water. In the majority of the studies, no relevance data were provided. In the studies that did address the issue, 0-100% of the positive patch tests were considered to be relevant (3,80,101,102,121); culprit products were never mentioned.

Table 2.386.1 Patch testing in groups of patients: Routine testing

Years and Country	Test conc. & vehicle	Number of patients tested	positive (%)	Selection of patients (S); Relevance (R); Comments (C)	Ref.
2013-14 USA, Canada	pure	4859	137 (2.8%)	R: definite + probable relevance: 51%	92
	30% water	4859	106 (2.2%)	R: definite + probable relevance: 53%	
2011 12 USA, Canada	30% water	4232	112 (2.6%)	R: definite + probable relevance: 58%	15
2009-10 USA, Canada	30% water	4304	138 (3.2%)	R: definite + probable relevance: 25%	16
2006-2010 USA	20% water	1190	(2.5%)	R: 37%	77
	10% pet.	1905	(0.5%)	R: 33%	
2001-2010 Australia	10% water	5072	62 (1.2%)	R: 31%	90
2007-8 USA, Canada	30% water	5083	(2.1%)	R: definite + probable relevance: 60%	10
2005-6 USA, Canada	30% water	4439	(2.9%)	R: definite + probable relevance: 45%	9
1996-06 USA, Canada	30% water	23359	810 (3.5%)	R: definite + probable relevance: 43%, mostly by personal care products (54%), topical corticosteroids (18%) and other topical pharmaceutical products	66
2000-2005 USA	10% pet.	3845	(0.4%)	R: 50%	5
2003-4 USA, Canada	30% water	5143	170 (3.3%)	R: not stated	11
2001-2002 USA	30% water	4899	(4.2%)	R: definite + probable relevance: 38%	67
1992-2002 IVDK	20% water	45,138	1044 (2.3%)	R: not specified; most cases of (presumptive) sensitization were caused by topical pharmaceutical preparations and cosmetics; C: only 149 of the 1044 positive patch test reactions were ++ or +++; there were also 1083 doubtful, follicular or erythematous reactions (2.4%) and 271 explicitly irritant reactions (0.6%) to propylene glycol 20% water	24
1998-2000 USA	30% water	5804	(3.7%)	R: definite + probable relevance: 37%	68
1998-2000 USA	10% pet.	1321	(3.3%)	R: not stated	72
1998-1999 Belgium	10% water	819	8 (1.0%)	R: not specified, ascribed to cosmetics	7
1993-1999 Belgium	10% water	4277	61 (1.4%)	R: not specified, 2 probably reacted to a corticosteroid preparation	39
1996-1998 USA	30% water	4095	(3.8%)	R: definite + probable + possible relevance: 83%	69
1994-1996 USA	10% pet.	3077	(1.1%)	R: definite + probable relevance: 40%	70
1992-1994 USA	10% water	3478	(1.1%)	R: present relevance: 62%	71
1989-1990 Finland	30% water	1701	13 (0.8%)	R: not stated; C: there were 9.7% irritant reactions	36

IVDK: Information Network of Departments of Dermatology, Germany, Austria, Switzerland

Case reports and case series

Case series

Propylene glycol was stated to be the (or an) allergen in 2 patients in a group of 603 individuals suffering from cosmetic dermatitis, seen in the period 2010-2015 in Leuven, Belgium (76). In the period 1996-2013, in a tertiary referral center in Valencia, Spain, 5419 patients were patch tested. Of these, 628 individuals had allergic contact dermatitis to cosmetics. Propylene glycol was the responsible allergen in two cases (93). Propylene glycol was responsible for 18 out of 959 cases of non-fragrance cosmetic allergy where the causal allergen was identified, Belgium, 2000-2010 (2). Propylene glycol was responsible for 29 out of 399 cases of cosmetic allergy where the causal allergen was identified in a study of the NACDG, USA, 1977-1983 (4).

Table 2.386.2 Patch testing in groups of patients: Selected patient groups

Years and Country	Test conc. & vehicle	Number of patients tested	positive (%)	Selection of patients (S); Relevance (R); Comments (C)	Ref.
2013-2015 USA	30% water	818	56 (6.8%)	S: children aged 18 years or younger with dermatitis; R: 40 (71%)	121
2003-2014 IVDK	20% water	4756	(3.9%)	S: patients with stasis dermatitis / chronic leg ulcers; R: not stated	97
2002-2013 Italy	5% pet.	2614	4 (0.2%)	S: children younger than 11 suspected of contact dermatitis; R: not relevant	102
2003-2012 IVDK	20% water	1727	33 (1.9%)	S: nurses with occupational contact dermatitis; R: not stated	14
2010-2011 Korea	5% pet.	584	4 (0.7%)	S: patients suspected of allergic cosmetic dermatitis; R: not stated	75
2006-2011 IVDK	20% water	7765	(2.2%)	S: patients suspected of cosmetic intolerance and tested with an ointment base series; R: not stated	94
2006-2010 USA		100	4 (4%)	S: patients with eyelid dermatitis; R: not stated	13
2000-2010 IVDK	20% water	3447	35 (1.0%)	S: patients with periorbital dermatitis; R: not stated	18

Table 2.386.2 Patch testing in groups of patients: Selected patient groups (*continued*)

Years and Country	Test conc. & vehicle	Number of patients		Selection of patients (S); Relevance (R); Comments (C)	Ref.
		tested	positive (%)		
2004-2008 France	10% water	423	15 (3.5%)	S: patients with leg ulcers; R: not stated	74
2000-2007 USA	10% pet.	944	9 (1.0%)	S: patients tested with a supplemental cosmetic screening series; R: 89%; C: weak study: a. high rate of macular erythema and weak reactions; b. relevance figures included 'questionable' and 'past' relevance	3
<2004 USA, Canada	30% water	52	7 (14%)	S: patients with leg ulcers; R: 28% definite or probable relevance	101
2000-2002 Finland		6875	(0.2%)	S: patients tested with a cosmetic series; R: not stated	73
1995-1999 IVDK	20% water	746	(2.4%)	S: patients with allergic periorbital contact dermatitis; R: not stated	85
1995-1997 USA		57	6 (11%)	S: patients with facial allergic contact dermatitis; R: only relevant reactions were mentioned	80
1995-1996 Finland		5270	(0.3%)	S: patients tested with a cosmetic series; R: not stated	73

IVDK: Information Network of Departments of Dermatology, Germany, Austria, Switzerland

In a group of 2193 patients (1582 women, 611 men) with (presumed) cosmetic allergy, 101 reactions (5%) were caused by propylene glycol in a study of the NACDG, 2001-2004, propylene glycol ranking 14th in the list of most frequent allergens (6). Six patients out of a group of 400 routinely tested had ACD from propylene glycol. The test concentration was high (20% in water), but retesting with a lower concentration (not specified) was positive. All six had used topical pharmaceutical and/or cosmetic products containing propylene glycol (59). Out of 14 patients with axillary dermatitis from antiperspirant, one was considered to have contact allergy to propylene glycol; there were six positive patch test reactions to propylene glycol 10% in water, but only one reacted to 1% also (and even 0.1% and 0.01%). Apparently the reactions to 10% were considered to be irritant (61).

Of seven patients with axillary dermatitis from an antiperspirant, 2 had positive patch tests to propylene glycol contained in them (62). In a group of 60 patients with allergic contact cheilitis seen by the members of the NACDG between 2001 and 2004 and mostly from cosmetics, 5 (8.3%) cases were caused by propylene glycol (78).

Case reports
One patient had allergic contact cheilitis from propylene glycol in a lipstick (34). Four individuals reacted to propylene glycol in a cream (56,83). One patient was allergic to propylene glycol in a deodorant (56). A woman had a clinical history of scalp dandruff and pruritus lasting many years. She reacted to propylene glycol, which was present in various shampoos she had used. After avoiding propylene glycol, all symptoms disappeared (91). A man had dermatitis of the scalp and face mimicking seborrheic dermatitis from contact allergy to PG in shaving foam, a moisturizing cream and shampoo. The patient's 'seborrheic dermatitis' cleared after ceasing the use of these cosmetics and using preparations without PG (124).

Contact allergy to propylene glycol in non-cosmetic products
There have been numerous publications of allergic contact dermatitis from propylene glycol in non-cosmetic products. Most were the result of its presence in topical pharmaceutical products and conductive gels for ultrasound imaging, ECG, or transcutaneous electric nerve stimulation (TENS).

Topical pharmaceutical products

Corticosteroids, antifungal, antibiotic and antiviral drugs
There are several case-reports of allergic contact dermatitis from PG in topical *corticosteroid* preparations (96 [n=3], 39 [n=2], 29,42,49,109 [one patient each]). These patients may note that the eczema does not respond adequately to the steroids or that the dermatitis deteriorates under therapy (109). Three patients reacted to PG in ketoconazole *antifungal* cream (17,51,131). One individual had ACD from PG in a topical *antibiotic* pharmaceutical product (46). Contact allergy to PG in *antiviral* creams, mostly used for herpes labialis and causing allergic contact cheilitis and sometimes for herpes zoster, has been reported in three patients (108) and in single case reports (26,32,47,48,82,105).

Minoxidil lotion
Nine patients had positive patch tests to propylene glycol in a series of 11 'suspected to be allergic to minoxidil solution' containing propylene glycol; however, two reacted to a 50% concentration only, which may well cause irritant patch test reactions (38). An unknown number of patients was sensitized to PG in minoxidil solution (114). A

woman developed psoriasiform scalp dermatitis with telogen effluvium from contact allergy to PG in minoxidil solution for female pattern hair loss (129). Two more single case reports have been published (113,126).

Silver sulfadiazine cream
Four middle-aged or older women with leg ulcers and stasis dermatitis had allergic contact dermatitis from propylene glycol in silver sulfadiazine cream (104). Another four individuals with leg ulcers developed contact allergy to the same antibacterial cream and to its ingredient PG resulting in pain, worsening of the ulcers and subacute dermatitis. When retested 1-2 years later, 2 individuals had no positive patch tests anymore (118). One more case report (50).

Miscellaneous topical pharmaceuticals
One patient (22), another one (43) and two more (21) had allergic contact dermatitis from propylene glycol in a topical pharmaceutical preparation containing 5-fluorouracil to treat actinic keratoses. One patient had contact allergy to PG in an ear drop preparation containing 50% PG; the dermatitis of the ear flared 20 hours after oral provocation with 5 ml PG (30). One patient was allergic to PG in an ointment to treat psoriasis (28). Another individual had allergic contact dermatitis from propylene glycol in topical NSAID pharmaceuticals; she also reacted to brassiere gel padding inserts consisting of 100% PG (44). A woman had ACD from propylene glycol in 3 topical pharmaceutical preparations (91). Another individual reacted to propylene glycol in 4 topical pharmaceuticals (29). Six patients were diagnosed with contact allergy to propylene glycol; they all had used 'pharmaceutical and/or cosmetic preparations' containing propylene glycol (59).

Conductive gels and lubricant jellies
There have been several case reports of allergic contact dermatitis from gels used in ultrasound imaging (54 [n=2],103,119,125), ECG (31,40,41,55,56,120), and transcutaneous electric nerve stimulation (TENS) (57 [n=3],58 [n=2],29,107) examinations caused by propylene glycol. A female patient had vulvitis after exposure to PG-containing lubricant for medical examination; after receiving an intravenous injection of a diazepam preparation containing 40% PG she developed systemic contact dermatitis (27). Two female patients had vulvitis from lubricant jelly for vaginal examinations (29). A man had contact allergy to PG in a corticosteroid preparation and later developed severe dermatitis of the penis and the scrotum from PG present in the lubricant jelly used by his wife (connubial contact dermatitis) (29).

Wound dressings
Four (45), three (20), two (19), another two patients (64) and one more individual (37) reacted to propylene glycol in (hydrogel) wound dressings (37).

Miscellaneous products containing propylene glycol
A hospital cleaner had occupational allergic contact dermatitis from propylene glycol in a surface-cleaning agent (23). One patient had allergic contact dermatitis from brassiere gel padding inserts; she also reacted to propylene glycol in topical pharmaceuticals (44). A press-operative working in the printing industry had occupational ACD from propylene glycol in a fountain solution (65).

Cross-reactions, pseudo-cross-reactions and co-reactions
Hydroxypropyl cellulose (?) (48); hexylene glycol (52); propylene glycol diacetate (60). Possibly cross-reactivity to and/or from butylene glycol and hexylene glycol (36).

Presence in cosmetic products and chemical analyses
In August 2017, propylene glycol was present in 3596 of 70,166 cosmetic products of which the composition is known in EWG's Skin Deep Cosmetics Database, USA (http://www.ewg.org/skindeep/). In the USA, in April 2017, propylene glycol was present in 14,009 of 56,714 cosmetic products of which the composition is known in FDA's Voluntary Cosmetic Registration Program (VCRP) (data obtained from FDA, May 2017). Propylene glycol was present in 45 (25%) of 178 facial wipes for which ingredient information was obtained online and from retail stores, USA, 2016 (98). Propylene glycol was present in 23 (43%) of 54 personal hygiene wet wipes for which ingredient information was obtained online and from retail stores, USA, 2016 (99). In the USA, in 2015-2016, 63 diaper wipes and 41 topical diaper preparations from a large retailer were screened for the presence of potential sensitizers. Propylene glycol was found in 13/63 (21%) disposable diaper wipes and in 6/41 (15%) topical diaper preparations (100).

In 2009, in the USA, the ingredient lists of 1591 facial cosmetics from one company were screened for the presence of propylene glycol. Propylene glycol was present in 0% of 132 blushers and 38 bronzers, in 31% of 90 concealers, in 15% of 174 eyeliners, in 0% of 304 eyeshadows, in 29% of 457 foundations, in 0% of 140 loose and pressed powders, and in 43% of 256 mascaras (86). In 2009, in the USA, the ingredient lists of 796 hair products from one company were screened for the presence of propylene glycol. Propylene glycol was present in 33% of 279 shampoos, in 28% of 231 conditioners, and in 43% of 286 styling products (87). In 2009, in the USA, the ingredient lists of 730 lip cosmetics and dental care products from one company were screened for the presence of propylene glycol. Propylene glycol was present in 0% of 31 lip liners, in 6% of 429 lipsticks, in 9% of 92 lip moisturizers, in 20% of 153 toothpastes, and in 28% of 25 mouth washes (88).

In 2009, in the USA, the ingredient lists of 657 miscellaneous cosmetics from one company were screened for the presence of propylene glycol. Propylene glycol was present in 29% of 195 antiperspirants/deodorants, in 0% of 41 powders, in 0% of 167 shaving products, in 0% of 201 sunblocks, and in 47% of 53 wipes (89). Of 276 moisturizers sold in the USA in 2007, 56 (20%) contained propylene glycol (12). Propylene glycol was present in 106 out of 166 (64%) corticosteroid preparations collected in 2007, USA (79). Of 38 cosmetic products marketed for babies in the UK in 2007, 19 (50%) contained propylene glycol (81).

Miscellaneous side effects

Systemic contact dermatitis

In a woman, the ingestion of a salad dressing containing propylene glycol produced a flare of previous dermatitis of the abdomen and vulvar and rectal areas, as well as the sites of the previously positive patch test reactions to propylene glycol within 24 hours on three occasions (29). Systemic contact dermatitis from PG in foods in PG-sensitized subjects has also been reported in other publications (56,110,111). Systemic contact dermatitis may also result from propylene glycol in an injected medicaments (27) including prednisolone (130, details unknown, article not read).

In two adolescents with contact allergy to propylene glycol, (atopic) dermatitis improved dramatically after cessation of oral antihistamines containing propylene glycol. In one of them, challenge with the antihistamine syrup resulted in generalized dermatitis (122). It was previously found that 26% of oral antihistamine preparations available in the USA contain propylene glycol (123). A female patient, after receiving an intravenous injection of a diazepam preparation containing 40% PG, developed systemic contact dermatitis; previously, she had suffered from vulvitis after exposure to PG-containing lubricant for medical examination (27).

Other miscellaneous side effects

Subjective or sensory irritation, with itching, burning, or stinging sensations but no signs of inflammation, is a commonly noticed reaction among users of cosmetic products and does usually not result in visits to dermatologists (115). It is a phenomenon which apparently also occurs in volunteers after application of different concentrations of PG; no specific data were provided (115).

Two female individuals had burning mouth syndrome and contact allergy to propylene glycol; they became asymptomatic after dietary avoidance of propylene glycol (53,106; probably the same patient in two publications).

OTHER SIDE EFFECTS

Irritant contact dermatitis

Open (unoccluded) application of propylene glycol to the skin has little irritant potential (1).

Immediate-type reactions

Non-immunological contact urticaria from propylene glycol has rarely been observed (33, data cited in ref. 115). The mechanism entails micro-injury to skin. Although this does not represent a contact urticaria *sensu stricto*, it is usually categorized as such, according to the authors (115). However, in other experiments, no capability of PG to induce contact urticaria was observed (116).

Other non-eczematous contact reactions

In older literature, propylene glycol has been suspected of being comedogenic, based on rabbit ear assays (95).

Systemic side effects

An 8-month-old male infant was treated with topical silver sulfadiazine cream containing propylene glycol for a burn and complicating toxic epidermal necrolysis involving 78% of his total body surface area. Transdermal absorption of propylene glycol from the cream produced hyperosmolality with an increased osmolal gap. A peak propylene glycol concentration of 1,059 mg/dL was documented, and its osmotic effect was that predicted from its concentration. Elevated concentrations of propylene glycol may have contributed to the patient's cardiorespiratory arrest (128).

Miscellaneous side effects

'Cough or asthma crisis' has been attributed to propylene glycol (127, details unknown, article not read).

OTHER INFORMATION

A peroral challenge test with 2-15 ml of propylene glycol (PG) was performed in 38 patients with allergic-type epicutaneous test reactions to PG. Eight of 10 patients with a positive patch test reaction to 2% PG and seven of the other 28 patients with a positive epicutaneous reaction to 10-100% PG developed an exanthem 3-16 hours after ingestion of the drug. In all but one case the rash disappeared within 24-48 hours without any medication. None of 20 control patients who were not allergic to propylene glycol had any skin symptoms after oral challenge (60).

LITERATURE

1   Wahlberg JE, Nilsson G. Skin irritancy from propylene glycol. Acta Derm Venereol (Stockh) 1984;64:286-290

2   Travassos AR, Claes L, Boey L, Drieghe J, Goossens A. Non-fragrance allergens in specific cosmetic products. Contact Dermatitis 2011;65:276-285

3   Wetter DA, Yiannias JA, Prakash AV, Davis MD, Farmer SA, el-Azhary RA, et al. Results of patch testing to personal care product allergens in a standard series and a supplemental cosmetic series: an analysis of 945 patients from the Mayo Clinic Contact Dermatitis Group, 2000-2007. J Am Acad Dermatol 2010;63:789-798

4   Adams RM, Maibach HI, Clendenning WE, Fisher AA, Jordan WJ, Kanof N, et al. A five-year study of cosmetic reactions. J Am Acad Dermatol 1985;13:1062-1069

5   Davis MD, Scalf LA, Yiannias JA, Cheng JF, El-Azhary RA, Rohlinger AL, et al. Changing trends and allergens in the patch test standard series. Arch Dermatol 2008;144:67-72

6   Warshaw EM, Buchholz HJ, Belsito DV et al. Allergic patch test reactions associated with cosmetics: Retrospective analysis of cross-sectional data from the North American Contact Dermatitis Group, 2001-2004. J Am Acad Dermatol 2009;60:23-38

7   Kohl L, Blondeel A, Song M. Allergic contact dermatitis from cosmetics: retrospective analysis of 819 patch-tested patients. Dermatology 2002;204:334-337

8   Kohl L, Blondeel A, Song M. Allergic contact dermatitis from cosmetics: retrospective analysis of 819 patch-tested patients. Dermatology 2002;204:334-337

9   Zug KA, Warshaw EM, Fowler JF Jr, Maibach HI, Belsito DL, Pratt MD, et al. Patch-test results of the North American Contact Dermatitis Group 2005-2006. Dermatitis 2009;20:149-160

10   Fransway AF, Zug KA, Belsito DV, Deleo VA, Fowler JF Jr, Maibach HI, et al. North American Contact Dermatitis Group patch test results for 2007-2008. Dermatitis 2013;24:10-21

11   Warshaw EM, Belsito DV, DeLeo VA, Fowler JF Jr, Maibach HI, Marks JG, et al. North American Contact Dermatitis Group patch-test results, 2003-2004 study period. Dermatitis 2008;19:129-136

12   Zirwas MJ, Stechschulte SA. Moisturizer allergy. Diagnosis and management. J Clin Aesthetic Dermatol 2008;1:38-44

13   Wenk KS, Ehrlich AE. Fragrance series testing in eyelid dermatitis. Dermatitis 2012;23:22-26

14   Molin S, Bauer A, Schnuch A, Geier J. Occupational contact allergy in nurses: results from the Information Network of Departments of Dermatology 2003–2012. Contact Dermatitis 2015;72:164-171

15   Warshaw EM, Maibach HI, Taylor JS, Sasseville D, DeKoven JG, Zirwas MJ, et al. North American Contact Dermatitis Group patch test results: 2011-2012. Dermatitis 2015;26:49-59

16   Warshaw EM, Belsito DV, Taylor JS, Sasseville D, DeKoven JG, Zirwas MJ, et al. North American Contact Dermatitis Group patch test results: 2009 to 2010. Dermatitis 2013;24:50-59

17   Romaguera C, Ferrando J, Lecha M, Mascaro JM. Dermatitis de contacto a! propilenglicol del excipiente de un preparado de ketoconazol. Pie! 1989;4:6-8

18   Landeck L, John SM, Geier J. Periorbital dermatitis in 4779 patients – patch test results during a 10-year period. Contact Dermatitis 2014;70:205-212

19   Motolese A, Capriata S, Simonelli M. Contact sensitivity to 'advanced' wound dressings in 116 patients with leg ulcers. Contact Dermatitis 2009;60:107

20   Saap L, Fahim S, Arsenault E, Pratt M, Pierscianowski T, Falanga V, et al. Contact sensitivity in patients with leg ulcerations: a North American study. Arch Dermatol 2004;140:1241-1246

21   Meijer BUGA, De Waard-van der Spek FB. Allergic contact dermatitis because of topical use of 5-fluorouracil (Efudix® cream). Contact Dermatitis 2007;57:58-60

22   Sams WM: Untoward response with topical fluorouracil. Arch Dermatol 1968;97:14-22

23   Haj-Younes L, Sanchez-Politta S, Pasche-Koo F, Denereaz N, Bessire N, Saurat J-H, Piletta P. Occupational contact dermatitis to Mikrobac Extra™ in 8 hospital cleaners. Contact Dermatitis 2006;54:69-70

24   Lessmann H, Schnuch A, Geier J, Uter W. Skin-sensitizing and irritant properties of propylene glycol. Contact Dermatitis 2005;53:247-259

25 Wahlberg JE. Propylene glycol: search for a proper and nonirritant patch test preparation. Am J Contact Dermat 1994;5:156-159

26 Bourezane Y Girardin P, Aubin F, Vigan M, Adessi B, Humbert P H, Laurent R. Allergic contact dermatitis to Zovirax cream. Allergy 1996;51:755-759

27 Fisher AA. Systemic contact dermatitis due to intravenous Valium in a person sensitive to propylene glycol. Cutis 1995;55:327-328

28 Fisher AA. Allergic contact dermatitis to propylene glycol in calcipotriene ointment. Cutis 1997;60:43-44

29 Fisher AA, Brancaccio RR. Allergic contact sensitivity to propylene glycol in a lubricant jelly. Arch Dermatol 1979;115:1451

30 Frosch PJ, Pekar U, Enzmann H. Contact allergy to propylene glycol – do we use the appropriate test concentration. Dermatol Clin 1990;8:111-113

31 Gonzalo MA, De Argila D, Garcia JM, Alvarado MI. Allergic contact dermatitis to propylene glycol. Allergy 1999;54:82-83

32 Piletta P, Pasche-Koo F, Saurat J-H, Hauser C. Contact dermatitis to propylene glycol in topical Zovirax cream. Am J Contact Dermat 1994;5:168-169

33 Andersen AE, Storrs FJ. Hautreizungen durch Propylenglykol. Hautarzt 1982;33:12-14

34 Warshaw TG, Herrmann F. Studies of skin reactions to propylene glycol. J Invest Dermatol 1952;19:423-429

35 Nater JP, Baar AJ, Hoedemaeker PJ. Histological aspects of skin reactions to propylene glycol. Contact Dermatitis 1977;3:181-185

36 Fan W, Kinnunen T, Niinimäki A, Hannuksela M. Skin reactions to glycols used in dermatological and cosmetic vehicles. Am J Contact Dermat 1991;2:181-183

37 Lee JE, Kim S-C. Allergic contact dermatitis from a hydrogel dressing (Intrasite® Gel) in a patient with scleroderma. Contact Dermatitis 2004;50:376-377

38 Friedman ES, Friedman PM, Cohen DE, Washenik K. Allergic contact dermatitis to topical minoxidil solution: etiology and treatment. J Am Acad Dermatol 2002;46:309-312

39 Goossens A, Huygens S, Matura M, Degreef H. Fluticasone propionate: a rare contact sensitizer. Eur J Dermatol 2001;11:29-34

40 Connolly M, Buckley DA. Contact dermatitis from propylene glycol in ECG electrodes, complicated by medicament allergy. Contact Dermatitis 2004;50:42

41 Uter W, Schwanitz HJ. Contact dermatitis from propylene glycol in ECG electrode gel. Contact Dermatitis 1996:34:230-231

42 Shore BN, Shelley WB. Contact dermatitis from stearyl alcohol and propylene glycol in flucinonide cream. Arch Dermatol 1974;109:397-399

43 Farrar CW, Bell HK, King CM. Allergic contact dermatitis from propylene glycol in Efudix® cream. Contact Dermatitis 2003;48:345

44 Lamb SR, Ardley HC, Wilkinson SM. Contact allergy to propylene glycol in brassiere padding inserts. Contact Dermatitis 2003;48:224-225

45 Gallenkemper G, Rabe E, Bauer R. Contact sensitization in chronic venous insufficiency: modern wound dressings. Contact Dermatitis 1998;38:274-278

46 El Sayed F, Bayle-Lebey P, Marguery MC, Bazex J. Contact dermatitis from propylene glycol in Rifocine®. Contact Dermatitis 1995;33:127-128

47 Kim YJ, Kim J-H. Allergic contact dermatitis from propylene glycol in Zovirax cream. Contact Dermatitis 1994;30:119-120

48 Corazza M, Virgill A, Mantovani L, La Malfa W. Propylene glycol allergy from acyclovir cream with cross-reactivity to hydroxypropyl cellulose in a transdermal estradiol system?. Contact Dermatitis 1993;29:283-284

49 Aguirre A, Gardeazábal J, Izu R, Antonio Ratón J, Diaz-Pérez JL. Allergic contact dermatitis due to plant extracts in a multisensitized patient. Contact Dermatitis 1993;28:186-187

50 Stenveld HJ, Langendijk PNJ, Bruynzeel DP. Contact sensitivity to polyethylene glycols. Contact Dermatitis 1994;30:184-185

51 Eun HC, Kim YC. Propylene glycol allergy from ketoconazole cream. Contact Dermatitis 1989;21:274-275

52 Kinnunen T, Hannuksela M. Skin reactions to hexylene glycol. Contact Dermatitis 1989;21:154-158

53 Lamey P-J, Lamb AB, Forsyth A. Atypical burning mouth syndrome. Contact Dermatitis 1987;17:242-243

54 Tomb RR, Rivara G, Foussereau J. Contact dermatitis after ultrasonography and electrocardiography. Contact Dermatitis 1987;17:149-152

55 Fisher AA. Dermatologic hazards of electrocardiography. Cutis 1977;20:686 (further pages unknown, data cited in ref. 54)

56 Fisher AA. Propylene glycol dermatitis. Cutis 1978;21:166 (further pages unknown, data cited in ref. 54 and 84)

57 Fisher AA. Dermatitis associated with transcutaneous electrical nerve stimulation. Cutis 1978;21:24,33,77

58   Castelain P-Y, Chahlu G. Contact dermatitis after transcutaneous electric analgesia. Contact Dermatitis 1986;15:32-35

59   Angelini G, Meneghini CL. Contact allergy from propylene glycol. Contact Dermatitis 1981;7:197-198

60   Hannuksela M, Förström L. Reactions to peroral propylene glycol. Contact Dermatitis 1978;4:41-45

61   ÅGren-Jonsson S, Magnusson, B. Sensitization to propantheline bromide, trichlorocarbanilide and propylene glycol in an antiperspirant. Contact Dermatitis 1976;2:79-80

62   Hannuksela, M. Allergy to propantheline in an antiperspirant (Ercoril®lotion). Contact Dermatitis 1975;1:244

63   Hannuksela M, Pirilä V, Salo OP. Skin reactions to propylene glycol. Contact Dermatitis 1975;1:112-116

64   Renner R, Simon JC, Treudler R. Contact sensitization to modern wound dressings in 70 patients with chronic leg ulcers. Dermatitis 2013;24:60-63

65   Noiles K, Kudla I, deKoven J. Propylene glycol dermatitis in the printing industry: the fundamental role of a workplace visit. Dermatitis 2010;21:E1–E4

66   Warshaw EM, Botto NC, Maibach HI, Fowler JF Jr, Rietschel RL, Zug KA, et al. Positive patch-test reactions to propylene glycol: a retrospective cross-sectional analysis from the North American Contact Dermatitis Group, 1996 to 2006. Dermatitis 2009;20:14-20

67   Pratt MD, Belsito DV, DeLeo VA, Fowler JF Jr, Fransway AF, Maibach HI, et al. North American Contact Dermatitis Group patch-test results, 2001–2002 study period. Dermatitis 2004;15:176-183

68   Marks JG Jr, Belsito DV, DeLeo VA, Fowler JF Jr, Fransway AF, Maibach HI, et al. North American Contact Dermatitis Group patch-test results, 1998–2000. Am J Contact Dermat 2003;14:59-62

69   Marks JG Jr, Belsito DV, DeLeo VA, Fowler JF Jr, Fransway AF, Maibach HI, et al. North American Contact Dermatitis Group patch test results, 1996–1998. Arch Dermatol 2000;136:272-273

70   Marks JG Jr, Belsito DV, DeLeo VA, Fowler JF Jr, Fransway AF, Maibach HI,et al. North American Contact Dermatitis Group patch test results for the detection of delayed-type hypersensitivity to topical allergens. J Am Acad Dermatol 1998;38:911-918

71   Marks JG, Belsito DV, DeLeo VA, Fowler JF, Fransway AF, Maibach HI,et al. North American Contact Dermatitis Group standard tray patch test results 1992 through 1994. Am J Contact Dermatitis 1995;6:160-165

72   Wetter DA, Davis MDP, Yiannias JA, Cheng JF, Connolly SM, el-Azhary RA, et al. Patch test results from the Mayo Contact Dermatitis Group, 1998–2000. J Am Acad Dermatol 2005;53:416-421

73   Hasan T, Rantanen T, Alanko K, Harvima RJ, Jolanki R, Kalimo K, et al. Patch test reactions to cosmetic allergens in 1995–1997 and 2000–2002 in Finland –a multicentre study. Contact Dermatitis 2005;53:40-45

74   Barbaud A, Collet E, Le Coz CJ, Meaume S, Gillois P. Contact allergy in chronic leg ulcers: results of a multicentre study carried out in 423 patients and proposal for an updated series of patch tests. Contact Dermatitis 2009;60:279-287

75   Lee SS, Hong DK, Jeong NJ, Lee JH, Choi YS, Lee AY, et al. Multicenter study of preservative sensitivity in patients with suspected cosmetic contact dermatitis in Korea. J Dermatol 2012;39:677-681

76   Goossens A. Cosmetic contact allergens. Cosmetics 2016, 3, 5; doi:10.3390/cosmetics3010005

77   Wentworth AB, Yiannias JA, Keeling JH, Hall MR, Camilleri MJ, Drage LA, et al. Trends in patch-test results and allergen changes in the standard series: a Mayo Clinic 5-year retrospective review (January 1, 2006, to December 31, 2010). J Am Acad Dermatol 2014;70:269-275

78   Zug KA, Kornik R, Belsito DV, DeLeo VA, Fowler JF Jr, Maibach HI, et al. Patch-testing North American lip dermatitis patients: Data from the North American Contact Dermatitis Group, 2001 to 2004. Dermatitis 2008;19:202-208

79   Coloe J, Zirwas MJ. Allergens in corticosteroid vehicles. Dermatitis 2008;19:38-42

80   Katz AS, Sherertz EF. Facial dermatitis: Patch test results and final diagnoses. Am J Cont Dermat 1999;10:153-156

81   White JML, McFadden JP. Exposure to haptens/contact allergens in baby cosmetic products. Contact Dermatitis 2008;59:176-177

82   Özkaya E, Topkarcı Z, Özarmağǎn G. Allergic contact cheilitis from a lipstick misdiagnosed as herpes labialis: subsequent worsening due to Zovirax® contact allergy. Australas J Dermatol 2007;48:190-192

83   Fisher AA. Contact Dermatitis, 3rd Edition. Philadelphia: lea & Febiger, 1985,247

84   De Groot AC. Adverse reactions to cosmetics. PhD Thesis, Groningen, The Netherlands, 1988

85   Herbst RA, Uter W, Pirker C, Geier J, Frosch PJ. Allergic and non-allergic periorbital dermatitis: patch test results of the Information Network of the Departments of Dermatology during a 5-year period. Contact Dermatitis 2004;51:13-19

86   Scheman A, Jacob S, Katta R, Nedorost S, Warshaw E, Zirwas M, et al. Part 1 of a 4 part series. Facial cosmetics: trends and alternatives. Data from the American Contact Alternative Group. J Clin Aesthet Dermatol 2011;4:25-30

87   Scheman A, Jacob S, Katta R, Nedorost S, Warshaw E, Zirwas M, et al. Part 2 of a 4 part series. Hair cosmetics: trends and alternatives. Data from the American Contact Alternative Group. J Clin Aesthet Dermatol 2011;4:42-46

88 Scheman A, Jacob S, Katta R, Nedorost S, Warshaw E, Zirwas M, et al. Part 3 of a 4 part series. Lips and common Dental Care products: trends and alternatives. Data from the American Contact Alternative Group. J Clin Aesthet Dermatol 2011;4:50-53

89 Scheman A, Jacob S, Katta R, Nedorost S, Warshaw E, Zirwas M, et al. Part 4 of a 4 part series. Miscellaneous products: trends and alternatives in deodorants, antiperspirants, sunblocks, shaving products, powder, and wipes. Data from the American Contact Alternative Group. J Clin Aesthet Dermatol 2011;4:35-39

90 Toholka R, Wang Y-S, Tate B, Tam M, Cahill J, Palmer A, Nixon R. The first Australian Baseline Series: Recommendations for patch testing in suspected contact dermatitis. Australas J Dermatol 2015;56:107-115

91 Ortega MEG, Nieto MAP, Camacho MM, Moya AIS, Palma OA, Monné CB, et al. Allergic contact dermatitis from propylene glycol: a case with past and present relevance in relation to several owned products. Contact Dermatitis 2016;75(Suppl.1):74

92 DeKoven JG, Warshaw EM, Belsito DV, Sasseville D, Maibach HI, Taylor JS, et al. North American Contact Dermatitis Group Patch Test Results: 2013-2014. Dermatitis 2017;28:33-46

93 Zaragoza-Ninet V, Blasco Encinas R, Vilata-Corell JJ, Pérez-Ferriols A, Sierra-Talamantes C, Esteve-Martínez A, de la Cuadra-Oyanguren J. Allergic contact dermatitis due to cosmetics: A clinical and epidemiological study in a tertiary hospital. Actas Dermosifiliogr 2016;107:329-336

94 Dinkloh A, Worm M, Geier J, Schnuch A, Wollenberg A. Contact sensitization in patients with suspected cosmetic intolerance: results of the IVDK 2006-2011. J Eur Acad Dermatol Venereol 2015;29:1071-1081

95 Kligman AM, Mills OH. Acne cosmetica. Arch Dermatol 1972;106:843-850

96 Rytter M, Walther T, Süss E, Haustein UF. Allergic reactions of the immediate and delayed type following prednisolone medication (article in German). Dermatol Monatsschr 1989;175:44-48

97 Erfurt-Berge C, Geier J, Mahler V. The current spectrum of contact sensitization in patients with chronic leg ulcers or stasis dermatitis - new data from the Information Network of Departments of Dermatology (IVDK). Contact Dermatitis 2017 Feb 14. doi: 10.1111/cod.12763. [Epub ahead of print]

98 Aschenbeck KA, Warshaw EM. Allergenic ingredients in facial wet wipes. Dermatitis 2017 Mar 23. doi: 10.1097/DER.0000000000000268. [Epub ahead of print]

99 Aschenbeck KA, Warshaw EM. Allergenic ingredients in personal hygiene wet wipes. Dermatitis 2017 Mar 23. doi: 10.1097/DER.0000000000000275. [Epub ahead of print]

100 Yu J, Treat J, Chaney K, Brod B. Potential allergens in disposable diaper wipes, topical diaper preparations, and disposable diapers: under-recognized etiology of pediatric perineal dermatitis. Dermatitis 2016;27:110-118

101 Saap L, Fahim S, Arsenault E, Pratt M, Pierscianowski T, Falanga V, Pedvis-Leftick A. Contact sensitivity in patients with leg ulcerations: a North American study. Arch Dermatol 2004;140:1241-1246

102 Belloni Fortina A, Fontana E, Peserico A. Contact sensitization in children: A retrospective study of 2,614 children from a single center. Pediatr Dermatol 2016;33:399-404

103 Horiguchi Y, Honda T, Fujii S, Matsushima S, Osaki Y. A case of allergic contact dermatitis from propylene glycol in an ultrasonic gel, sensitized at a leakage skin injury due to transcatheter arterial chemoembolization for hepatocellular carcinoma. Int J Dermatol 2005;44:681-683

104 Degreef H, Dooms-Goossens A. Patch testing with silver sulfadiazine cream. Contact Dermatitis 1985;12:33-37 105

105 Hernández N, Hernández Z, Liuti F, Borrego L. Intolerance to cosmetics as key to the diagnosis in a patient with allergic contact dermatitis caused by propylene glycol contained in a topical medication. Contact Dermatitis 2017;76:246-247

106 Lamey PJ, Lamb AB, Hughes A, Milligan KA, Forsyth A. Type III burning mouth syndrome: psychological and allergic aspects. J Oral Pathol Med 1994;23:216-219

107 Zugerman C. Dermatitis from transcutaneous electric nerve stimulation. J Am Acad Dermatol 1982;6:936-939

108 Claverie F, Giordano-Labadie F, Bazex J. Contact eczema induced by propylene glycol: concentration and vehicle adapted for patch tests. Ann Dermatol Venereol 1997; 124:315-317

109 Fowler JF Jr. Contact allergy to propylene glycol in topical corticosteroids. Am J Cont Dermat 1993;4:37-38

110 Lowther A, McCormick T, Nedorost S. Systemic contact dermatitis from propylene glycol. Dermatitis 2008;19:105-108

111 Fisher AA. The management of propylene glycol-sensitive patients. Cutis 1980;25:24-6, 29-31, 44 (data cited in ref. 110)

112 Catanzaro JM, Smith JG. Propylene glycol dermatitis. J Am Acad Dermatol 1991;24:90-95

113 Van Der Willigen AH, Dutree-Meulenberg RO, Stolz E, Geursen-Reitsma AM, van Joost T. Topical minoxidil sensitization in androgenic alopecia. Contact Dermatitis 1987;17:44-45

114 Fisher AA. Use of glycerin in topical minoxidil solutions for patient allergic to propylene glycol. Cutis 1990;45:81-82

115 Funk JO, Maibach HI. Propylene glycol dermatitis: re-evaluation of an old problem. Contact Dermatitis 1994;31:236-241

116 Lahti A. Non-immunologic contact urticaria. Acta Dermato-venereol (Stockh) 1980;60(Suppl.91):1-49

117 Fransway AF. The problem of preservation in the 1990s. III. Agents with preservative function independent of formaldehyde release. Am J Contact Derm 1991;2:145-174

118 Rasmussen I. Patch test reactions to Flamazine. Contact Dermatitis 1984;11:133-134

119 Ayadi M, Martin P, Bergoend H. Contact dermatitis to a carotidian Doppler gel. Contact Dermatitis. 1987;17:118-119

120 Cochran RJ, Rosen T. Contact dermatitis caused by ECG electrode paste. South Med J 1980;73:1667-1668

121 Goldenberg A, Mousdicas N, Silverberg N, Powell D, Pelletier JL, Silverberg JI, et al. Pediatric Contact Dermatitis Registry inaugural case data. Dermatitis. 2016 Sep-Oct;27(5):293-302

122 Tocci EM, Robinson A, Belazarian L, Foley E, Wiss K, Silvestri DL. Excipients in oral antihistamines can perpetuate allergic contact dermatitis. Pediatr Dermatol 2015;32:e242-e244

123 McEnery-Stonelake M, Silvestri DL. Contact allergens in oral antihistamines. Dermatitis 2014;25:83-88

124 Kuznetsov AV, Erlenkeuser-Uebelhoer I, Thomas P. Contact allergy to propylene glycol and dodecyl gallate mimicking seborrheic dermatitis. Contact Dermatitis 2006;55:307-308

125 Eguino P, Sánchez A, Agesta N, Lasa O, Ratón JA, Díaz-Pérez JL. Allergic contact dermatitis due to propylene glycol and parabens in an ultrasonic gel. Contact Dermatitis 2003;48:290

126 Scheman AJ, West DP, Hordinksy MK, Osburn AH, West LE. Alternative formulation for patients with contact reactions to topical 2% and 5% minoxidil vehicle ingredients. Contact Dermatitis 2000;42:241

127 Spreux A, Boyer A, Baldin B, Chichmanian RM. Cough or asthma crisis induced by propylene glycol. Therapie 1996;51:561-562 (article in French)

128 Fligner CL, Jack R, Twiggs GA, Raisys VA. Hyperosmolality induced by propylene glycol. A complication of silver sulfadiazine therapy. JAMA 1985;253:1606-1609

129 La Placa M, Balestri R, Bardazzi F, Vincenzi C. Scalp psoriasiform contact dermatitis with acute telogen effluvium due to topical minoxidil treatment. Skin Appendage Disord 2016;1:141-143

130 Rytter M, Walther T, Süss E, Haustein UF. Allergic reactions of the immediate and delayed type following prednisolone medication. Dermatol Monatsschr 1989;175:44-48 (article in German).

131 Guidetti MS, Vincenzi C, Guerra L, Tosti A. Contact dermatitis due to imidazole antimycotics. Contact Dermatitis 1995;33:282

2.387 PROPYLENE GLYCOL RICINOLEATE

IDENTIFICATION

Description/definition	: Propylene glycol ricinoleate is the ester of propylene glycol and ricinoleic acid that conforms generally to the formula shown below
Chemical class(es)	: Esters
Chemical/IUPAC name	: 2-Hydroxypropyl (Z)-12-hydroxyoctadec-9-enoate
Other names	: (R)-12-Hydroxyoleic acid, monoester with propane-1,2-diol
CAS registry number (s)	: 26402-31-3; 1330-81-0
EC number(s)	: 247-669-7
Function(s) in cosmetics	: EU: emulsifying; skin conditioning; viscosity controlling. USA: dispersing agents – nonsurfactant; skin-conditioning agents – emollient; surfactants – emulsifying agents
Patch testing	: 10% pet. (1)
Molecular formula	: $C_{21}H_{40}O_4$

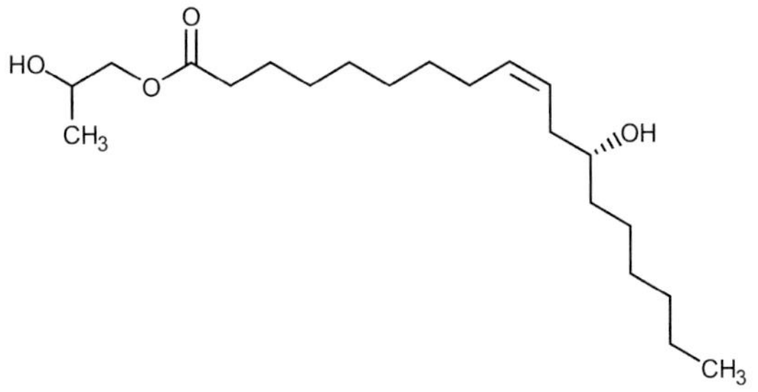

CONTACT ALLERGY

Case reports and case series

A woman had suffered from pruritic erythema and scaling on her lip for 4 months. When patch tested with 20 of her cosmetics, there was a positive reaction to one lipstick that she had been using for 6 months. Later, the patient was tested with the 17 ingredients of this cosmetic product, and a positive reaction was observed to propylene glycol ricinoleate 10% pet. There was no positive reaction to propylene glycol. Ten control subjects were negative to propylene glycol ricinoleate 10% pet. After discontinuing the use of this lipstick and avoiding other products containing propylene glycol ricinoleate, she has been free of dermatitis (1). Propylene glycol ricinoleate was present in the lipstick in a concentration of 5.5%. As the patient showed no reaction to propylene glycol 2% pet., the authors suspected that an antigenic determinant exists in the ricinoleic acid portion (1).

Cross-reactions, pseudo-cross-reactions and co-reactions

Not to propylene glycol (1); it should be appreciated that the patient was tested with 2% in petrolatum, which may well have resulted in a false-negative reaction.

Presence in cosmetic products and chemical analyses

In the USA, in April 2017, propylene glycol ricinoleate was present in 14 of 56,714 cosmetic products of which the composition is known in FDA's Voluntary Cosmetic Registration Program (VCRP) (data obtained from FDA, May 2017). In April 2017, propylene glycol ricinoleate was present in 18 of 65,434 cosmetic products of which the composition is known in EWG's Skin Deep Cosmetics Database, USA (http://www.ewg.org/skindeep/).

LITERATURE

1   Sowa J, Suzuki K, Tsuruta K, Akamatsu H, Matsunaga K. Allergic contact dermatitis from propylene glycol ricinoleate in a lipstick. Contact Dermatitis 2003;48:228-229

2.388   PROPYL GALLATE

IDENTIFICATION

Description/definition   : Propyl gallate is the aromatic ester of propyl alcohol and gallic acid, which conforms generally to the formula shown below

Chemical class(es)   : Esters; phenols

Chemical/IUPAC name   : Propyl 3,4,5-trihydroxybenzoate

CAS registry number (s) : 121-79-9

EC number(s)   : 204-498-2

CIR review(s)   : J Am Coll Toxicol 1985;4:23-64; Int J Toxicol 2007;26(Suppl.3):89-118 (access: www.cir-safety.org/ingredients)

Merck Index monograph : 9241

Function(s) in cosmetics : EU: perfuming; antioxidant. USA: antioxidants; fragrance ingredients

Patch testing   : 1% pet. (Chemotechnique); 0.5% pet. (SmartPracticeEurope, SmartPracticeCanada)

Molecular formula   : $C_{10}H_{12}O_5$

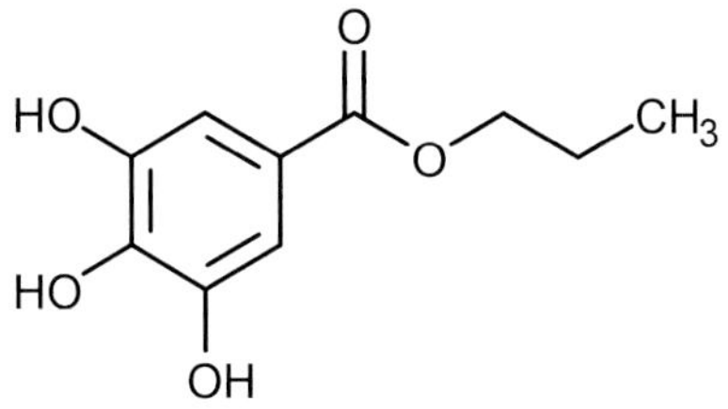

GENERAL

Gallates are antioxidants which, when added in small quantities, retard or prevent oxidation; they have been in use since 1947. The most commonly used gallic acid esters are propyl, octyl (= caprylyl) and dodecyl (= lauryl) gallate, which differ from each other in terms of the length of their side chain. Propyl gallate and other gallates are widely used as antioxidants in the cosmetic industry (creams, lotions, and lipsticks; only propyl gallate), food industry (bakery goods, frying oils, soups, sauces, chewing gum, and potato chips), and in pharmaceutical and industrial products (eardrops, suppositories, and transformer oils) (6,18). Gallates are potential allergens (moderate to strong sensitizers in animal [18,43] and human [43] experiments), but relatively few cases of contact dermatitis due to gallates have been reported to date (36). The low rates of sensitization has been explained by oral tolerance (6,43). An extensive review of the literature on contact allergy to gallates has been published in 2017 (50).

CONTACT ALLERGY

Patch testing in groups of patients

Results of studies patch testing propyl gallate in consecutive patients suspected of contact dermatitis (routine testing) and in groups of selected patients are shown in table 2.388.1. In routine testing, the frequency of sensitization in in one available study was a very high 4.1% in a UK study in 1991 (15). In this investigation, all were women and all reactions were relevant. Ten of the 13 allergic women had become sensitized to propyl gallate from its presence in a 'liposomal cream' (15).

In groups of *selected* patients (e.g., patients with chronic cheilitis, patients tested with a preservative and cosmetic series or with a bakery series, patients suspected of cosmetic dermatitis, patients tested with a face series or preservative series), rates of sensitization ranged from 0.3% to 2.6%. In the latter study, performed between 1985 and 2006 in Spain, patients were tested with a preservative and cosmetic series or with a bakery series. Of 46 patients reacting to one or more gallates (propyl, octyl, dodecyl), 35 were relevant. Twenty-nine were caused by cosmetics, of which 24 were lip products causing allergic contact cheilitis; propyl gallate was the main allergen in lipsticks (36). A 100% relevance rate was reported in a 2000-2007 US study, but this included 'questionable' and 'past' relevance (3).

Case reports and case series

Propyl gallate was stated to be the (or an) allergen in 3 patients in a group of 603 individuals suffering from cosmetic dermatitis, seen in the period 2010-2015 in Leuven, Belgium (34). In the period 1996-2013, in a tertiary referral center in Valencia, Spain, 5419 patients were patch tested. Of these, 628 individuals had allergic contact dermatitis to cosmetics. Propyl gallate was the responsible allergen in 33 cases (40). Propyl gallate was responsible for 2 out of 959 cases of non-fragrance cosmetic allergy where the causal allergen was identified, Belgium, 2000-2010 (2). In the period 2000-2007, 202 patients with allergic contact dermatitis caused by cosmetics were seen in Valencia, Spain. In this group, 16 individuals reacted to propyl gallate from its presence in lipsticks (39). Propyl gallate was responsible for 1 out of 399 cases of cosmetic allergy where the causal allergen was identified in a study of the NACDG, USA, 1977-1983 (1). Four positive patch test reactions to propyl gallate were ascribed to cosmetic allergy (4).

Table 2.388.1 Patch testing in groups of patients

Years and Country	Test conc. & vehicle	Number of patients tested | positive (%)		Selection of patients (S); Relevance (R); Comments (C)	Ref
Routine testing					
1991 UK	1% pet.	315	13 (4.1%)	R: all were considered relevant; 10/13 had used liposomal cosmetic creams containing propyl gallate; C: the frequency of sensitization in women was 5.3%; no men were sensitized; the presence of liposomes has probably enhanced the sensitizing potential	15
Testing in groups of selected patients					
1996-2013 Netherlands	0.5% pet.	231	4 (1.7%)	S: children aged 0-17 years; R: not stated	42
2000-2007 USA	1% pet.	943	7 (0.7%)	S: patients tested with a supplemental cosmetic screening series; R: 100%; C: weak study: a. high rate of macular erythema and weak reactions; b. relevance figures included 'questionable' and 'past' relevance	3
2001-2006 Italy	1% pet.	129	2 (1.6%)	S: patients with chronic cheilitis; R: both reactions were relevant	41
1985-2006 Spain	1% pet.	1173	30 (2.6%)	S: patients tested with a preservative and cosmetic series or with a bakery series (n=69); R: of 46 patients reacting to one or more gallates (propyl, octyl, dodecyl), 35 had relevant reactions; 29 were caused by cosmetics, of which 24 were lip products causing allergic contact cheilitis; there were 7 relevant reactions to octyl gallate in bakery products; propyl gallate was the main allergen in lipsticks	36
1988-2005 UK	1% pet.	9529	55 (0.6%)	S: patients tested with a face series; R: not stated; C: the prevalence rose significantly from 0.45% in the period 1988-1996 to 0.77% in the period 1997-2005	6
2001-2002 Sweden	1% pet.	1075	(0.7%)	S: patients referred for routine testing willing to participate in a study on cosmetic use and adverse reactions; R: not stated	5
1997-2000 Israel		244	3 (1.2%)	S: patients suspected of cosmetic dermatitis; R: 64% of all patch test reactions in the cosmetic series was relevant	38
1990-1994 Germany	0.5% pet.	3133	9 (0.3%)	S: patients tested with a preservative series; R: not stated	33

In a group of 146 patients patch tested for cheilitis in Amersham, UK, between 1982 and 2001, there was one positive patch test reaction to propyl gallate considered to be relevant for the lip dermatitis. Over half of the reactions in the entire group were ascribed to lipsticks and lip salves (32). Ten women had ACD from cosmetic creams containing propyl gallate in liposomes, which may have enhanced its sensitizing potency (15). Eight patients were allergic to a cosmetic lotion and reacted to its constituent propyl gallate (26). Five patients had allergic cosmetic dermatitis from propyl gallate in a baby lotion (16). A woman developed severe facial dermatitis from gallates, probably from propyl gallate, in a liposomal cream (47). A woman suffered from facial dermatitis caused by contact allergy to propyl gallate in a 'leave-on cosmetic' (10). Another female individual had chronic eyelid dermatitis from propyl gallate in a cosmetic cream (25). One patient had allergic contact cheilitis from a lip preparation used for cosmetic and sunscreening purposes (11). Another reacted to the antioxidant in a cosmetic cream (17).

A participant in the developmental testing of a cosmetic deodorant experienced an axillary dermatitis which was caused by contact allergy to propyl gallate, present in a concentration of 1% in the deodorant (22). One patient had ACD from propyl gallate in a moisturizing cream (27). A woman had allergic contact cheilitis from propyl gallate in a lip product; after avoiding the cosmetic the cheilitis healed, but flared when her husband started using the same product (connubial contact dermatitis) (36). Four women had allergic contact cheilitis from propyl gallate in lipstick (47). Single case reports of allergic contact cheilitis from propyl gallate in lipsticks have been presented in refs. 7,29,35,37, and 48. A female patient reacted to lipstick and propyl gallate but, although implied, it was not ascertained that the lipstick contained propyl gallate (13). Two patients had allergic contact cheilitis from propyl gallate in lip balms (23,31). A man had ACD from propyl gallate in an emollient cream used to treat seborrheic dermatitis (52).

Contact allergy to propyl gallate in non-cosmetic products

A man working in a plant making synthetic textile fibers developed occupational airborne allergic contact dermatitis from propyl gallate powder used as stabilizer (8). Two patients had ACD from propyl gallate in a topical corticosteroid preparation (9,14), another from the presence of the antioxidant in an antibiotic topical pharmaceutical product (12). Twelve cases of ACD from propyl gallate in antibiotic ointments and powders have been presented (19,20). Two patients had allergic contact dermatitis from propyl gallate in antibiotic ointments, of which one contained 8% propyl gallate (24). Another reacted to an antibiotic ointment containing 0.1% propyl gallate with an atypical clinical manifestation of an ulcer with an infiltrated and hyperkeratotic border (28).

Another patient developed allergic contact dermatitis from propyl gallate in a topical pharmaceutical product used to treat psoriasis (30). Another individual also reacted to propyl gallate in a topical pharmaceutical (44). One patient who was allergic to propyl gallate and dodecyl gallate developed angioedema of the lips after eating foods containing gallates (36). A 'small epidemic of contact dermatitis' from propyl gallate was observed in Italy in 1982 just a few months after a topical antibiotic, the ointment and powder base of which both contained propyl gallate, had become a rather popular remedy for treating wounds (45,46, data cited in ref. 44). One patient had ACD from propyl gallate in a topical pharmaceutical product for leg ulcers (49; this article cannot be found, data cited in ref. 18).

Cross-reactions, pseudo-cross-reactions and co-reactions

Methyl gallate, ethyl gallate, gallic acid, catechol, protocatechuic acid, and *p-tert*-butylcatechol (10). Octyl gallate (13,27,31); dodecyl gallate (27). Of 46 patients allergic to gallates, 16 (35%) reacted to more than one gallate (propyl, octyl, dodecyl) (36). In animal experiments, cross-reactions occurred when the difference between the sensitizing compound and the related gallate was 4 or less carbon atoms (18).

Presence in cosmetic products and chemical analyses

In May 2017, propyl gallate was present in 82 of 66,669 cosmetic products of which the composition is known in EWG's Skin Deep Cosmetics Database, USA (http://www.ewg.org/skindeep/). In the USA, in April 2017, propyl gallate was present in 403 of 56,714 cosmetic products of which the composition is known in FDA's Voluntary Cosmetic Registration Program (VCRP) (data obtained from FDA, May 2017).

OTHER SIDE EFFECTS

Other non-eczematous contact reactions

A woman developed contact depigmentation at several body sites after using lipstick, liquid kumkum (a coloring usually made from turmeric or saffron used for social / religious markings), and plastic or rubber slippers (flip-flops). The patient was patch test positive to propyl gallate, an ingredient common to all contact materials; the patch test site later showed depigmentation (51).

LITERATURE

1   Adams RM, Maibach HI, Clendenning WE, Fisher AA, Jordan WJ, Kanof N, et al. A five-year study of cosmetic reactions. J Am Acad Dermatol 1985;13:1062-1069
2   Travassos AR, Claes L, Boey L, Drieghe J, Goossens A. Non-fragrance allergens in specific cosmetic products. Contact Dermatitis 2011;65:276-285
3   Wetter DA, Yiannias JA, Prakash AV, Davis MD, Farmer SA, el-Azhary RA, et al. Results of patch testing to personal care product allergens in a standard series and a supplemental cosmetic series: an analysis of 945 patients from the Mayo Clinic Contact Dermatitis Group, 2000-2007. J Am Acad Dermatol 2010;63:789-798
4   Kohl L, Blondeel A, Song M. Allergic contact dermatitis from cosmetics: retrospective analysis of 819 patch-tested patients. Dermatology 2002;204:334-337
5   Lindberg M, Tammela M, Bostrom A, Fischer T, Inerot A, Sundberg K, et al. Are adverse skin reactions to cosmetics underestimated in the clinical assessment of contact dermatitis? A prospective study among 1075 patients attending Swedish patch test clinics. Acta Derm Venereol 2004;84:291-295
6   Perez A, Basketter DA, White IR, McFadden J. Positive rates to propyl gallate on patch testing: a change in trend. Contact Dermatitis 2008;58:47-48
7   Lee JH, Yoon DH, Lee JY, et al. A case of allergic contact cheilitis from propyl gallate. Korean J Dermatol 1997;35:374-378
8   Mahendran R, Quinlan RM, Wilkinson SM. Allergic contact dermatitis from occupational propyl gallate exposure. Contact Dermatitis 2002;47:122-123
9   Hernández N, Assier-Bonnet H, Terki N, Revuz J. Allergic contact dermatitis from propyl gallate in desonide cream (Locapred®). Contact Dermatitis 1997;36:111

10 Hemmer W, Focke M, Wolf-Abdolvahab S, Bracun R, Wantke F, et al. Group allergy to tri- and ortho-diphenols (catechols) in a patient sensitized by propyl gallate. Contact Dermatitis 1996;35:110-112

11 Serra-Baldrich E, Puig LL, Arnau AG, Camarasa JG. Lipstick allergic contact dermatitis from gallates. Contact Dermatitis 1995;32:359-360

12 Corazza M, Mantovani L, Roveggio C, Virgili A. Allergic contact dermatitis from propyl gallate. Contact Dermatitis 1994;31:203-204

13 Athavale NV, Srinivas CR. Contact cheilitis from propyl gallate in lipstick. Contact Dermatitis 1994;30:307

14 Wilkinson SM, Beck MH. Allergic contact dermatitis from dibutyl phthalate, propyl gallate and hydrocortisone in Timodine®. Contact Dermatitis 1992;27:197

15 Marston S. Propyl gallate on liposomes. Contact Dermatitis 1992;27:74-76

16 Fiss J, Wagner E. Allergisches Kontaktekzem durch Propylgallat. Derm Mschr 1988;174:14-19

17 Meynadier JM, Meynadier J, Colmas A, Castelain PY, Ducombs G, Chabeau G, Lacroix M, Martin P, Ngangu Z. Allergie aux conservateurs. Ann Derm Venerol (Paris) 1982;109:1017-1023

18 Hausen BM, Beyer W. The sensitizing capacity of the antioxidants propyl, octyl, and dodecyl gallate and some related gallic acid esters. Contact Dermatitis 1992;26:253-258

19 Pansera B, Valsecchi R, Tornaghi A. Dermatitis allergica da contatto a! propile gallato. Proceedings of the 3rd GIRDCA Meeting, Bergamo, 30 April 1983 (cited in ref. 21)

20 Soro A. Dermatitis allergica da contatto al propile gallato. Proceedings of the 3rd GIRDCA Meeting, Bergamo, 30 April 1983 (cited in ref. 21)

21 De Groot A C, Gerkens F. Occupational airborne contact dermatitis from octyl gallate. Contact Dermatitis 1990;23:184-186

22 Kraus AL, Stotts J, Altringer LA, Allgood GS. Allergic contact dermatitis from propyl gallate: dose response comparison using various application methods. Contact Dermatitis 1990;22:132-136

23 Wilson AG. McT., White IR, Kirby JDT. Allergic contact dermatitis from propyl gallate in a lip balm. Contact Dermatitis 1989;20:145

24 Valsecchi R, Cainelli T. Contact allergy to propyl gallate. Contact Dermatitis 1988;19:380-381

25 Bardazzi F, Misciali C, Borrello P, Capoblanco, C. Contact dermatitis due to antioxidants. Contact Dermatitis 1988;19:385-386

26 Heine A. Contact dermatitis from propyl gallate. Contact Dermatitis 1988;18:313-314

27 Bojs G, Nicklasson B, Svensson A. Allergic contact dermatitis to propyl gallate. Contact Dermatitis 1987;17:294-298

28 Pigatto PD, Boneschi V, Riva F, Altomare GF. Allergy to propylgallate, with unusual clinical and histological features. Contact Dermatitis 1984;11:43

29 Cronin E. Lipstick dermatitis due to propyl gallate. Contact Dermatitis 1980;6:213-214

30 Lidén S. Alphosyl® sensitivity and propyl gallate. Contact Dermatitis 1975;1:257-258

31 Yu Y, Scheinman PL. Lip and perioral dermatitis caused by propyl gallate. Dermatitis 2010;21:118-119

32 Strauss RM, Orton DI. Allergic contact cheilitis in the United Kingdom: a retrospective study. Am J Contact Dermat 2003;14:75-77

33 Schnuch A, Geier J, Uter W, Frosch PJ. Patch testing with preservatives, antimicrobials and industrial biocides. Results from a multicentre study. Br J Dermatol 1998;138:467-476

34 Goossens A. Cosmetic contact allergens. Cosmetics 2016, 3, 5; doi:10.3390/cosmetics3010005

35 Özkaya E, Topkarcı Z, Özarmağan G. Allergic contact cheilitis from a lipstick misdiagnosed as herpes labialis: subsequent worsening due to Zovirax® contact allergy. Australas J Dermatol 2007;48:190-192

36 García-Melgares ML, de la Cuadra J, Martín B, Laguna C, Martínez L, Alegre V. Sensitization to gallates: review of 46 cases. Actas Dermosifiliogr 2007;98:688-693

37 Pérez Ferriols A, Rodriguez Serna M, De la Cuadra Oyanguren J. Queilitis alérgicas de contacto y de fotocontacto por lápices labiales. Actas Dermosifiliogr 1994;85:545-548 (article in Spanish

38 Trattner A, Farchi Y, David M. Cosmetics patch tests: first report from Israel. Contact Dermatitis 2002;47:180-181

39 Laguna C, de la Cuadra J, Martín-González B, Zaragoza V, Martínez-Casimiro L, Alegre V. Allergic contact dermatitis to cosmetics. Actas Dermosifiliogr 2009;100:53-60

40 Zaragoza-Ninet V, Blasco Encinas R, Vilata-Corell JJ, Pérez-Ferriols A, Sierra-Talamantes C, Esteve-Martínez A, de la Cuadra-Oyanguren J. Allergic contact dermatitis due to cosmetics: A clinical and epidemiological study in a tertiary hospital. Actas Dermosifiliogr 2016;107:329-336

41 Schena D, Fantuzzi F, Girolomoni G. Contact allergy in chronic eczematous lip dermatitis. Eur J Dermatol 2008;18:688-692

42 Lubbes S, Rustemeyer T, Sillevis Smitt JH, Schuttelaar ML, Middelkamp-Hup MA. Contact sensitization in Dutch children and adolescents with and without atopic dermatitis - a retrospective analysis. Contact Dermatitis 2017;76:151-159

43   Kahn G, Phanuphak P, Klaman HN. Propyl gallate - contact sensitization and orally-induced tolerance. Arch Dermatol 1974;109:506-509

44   Cusano F, Capozzi M, Errico G. Safety of propyl gallate in topical products. J Am Acad Dermatol 1987;17(2 Pt. 1):308-310

45   Pansera B, Valsecchi R, Tornaghi A, et at. Dermatite allergica da contatto al propile gallato. Proceedings of the 3rd GIRDCA Meeting, Bergamo, April 30, 1983 (data cited in ref. 44)

46   Soro A. Dermatite allergica da contatto con propile gallato. Proceedings of the 3rd GIRDCA Meeting, Bergamo, April 30, 1983 (data cited in ref. 44)

47   Romaguera C, Vilaplana J. Contact dermatitis from gallates. Am J Cont Derm 1993;4:231-234

48   Ozkaya E, Topkarci Z, Ozarmağan G. Allergic contact cheilitis from a lipstick misdiagnosed as herpes labialis: Subsequent worsening due to Zovirax contact allergy. Australas J Dermatol 2007;48:190-192

49   Rudzki E, Baranowska E. Reactions to gallic acid esters. Contact Dermatitis 1975;1:393 (reference cannot be found, data cited in ref. 18)

50   Holcomb ZE, Van Noord MG, Atwater AR. Gallate contact dermatitis: product update and systematic review. Dermatitis 2017;28:115-127

51   Pandhi D, Vij A, Singal A. Contact depigmentation induced by propyl gallate. Clin Exp Dermatol 2011;36:366-368

52   Foti C, Bonamonte D, Cassano N, et al. Allergic contact dermatitis to propyl gallate and pentylene glycol in an emollient cream. Australas J Dermatol 2010;51:147-148

2.389 PROPYLPARABEN

IDENTIFICATION

Description/definition	: Propylparaben is the ester of *n*-propyl alcohol and *p*-hydroxybenzoic acid, which conforms to the formula shown below
Chemical class(es)	: Esters; phenols
Chemical/IUPAC name	: Propyl 4-hydroxybenzoate
CAS registry number (s)	: 94-13-3
EC number(s)	: 202-307-7
CIR review(s)	: J Am Coll Toxicol 1984;3:147-209; Int J Toxicol 2008;27(Suppl.4):1-82 (access: www.cir-safety.org/ingredients)
SCCS opinion(s)	: SCCS/1514/13 (14); SCCS/1348/10 (15); SCCS/1348/10 (16); SCCP/1183/08 (17) SCCP/1017/06 (18); SCCP/0874/05 (19)
Merck Index monograph	: 9247
Function(s) in cosmetics	: EU: perfuming; preservative. USA: fragrance ingredients; preservatives
EU cosmetic restrictions	: Regulated in Annexes V/12 and V/12 bis of the Regulation (EC) No. 1223/2009
Patch testing	: 3% pet. (Chemotechnique, SmartPracticeEurope, SmartPracticeCanada); also present in the paraben mix (see there)
Molecular formula	: $C_{10}H_{12}O_3$

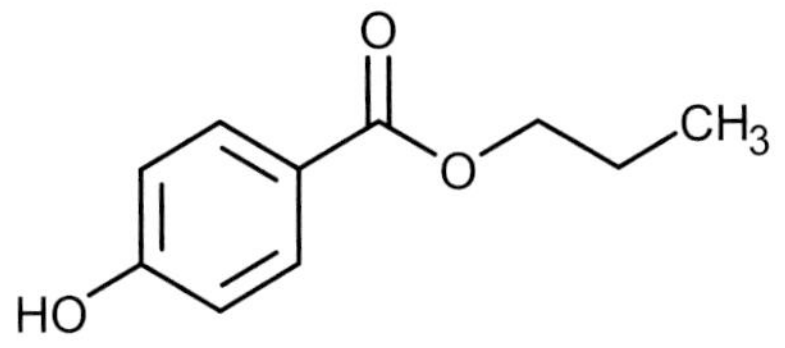

GENERAL

For general information on paraben esters see Chapter 2.333 Paraben mix. The literature on contact allergy to and other information on parabens, in which the ester is not specified ('paraben mix', 'paraben', 'parabens'), is also discussed in that chapter. The literature on contact allergy to propylparaben and other paraben esters from before 1991 has been reviewed in ref. 22. Other, more recent, useful reviews were published in 2005 (parabens) (36) and 2004 (37) and 2014 (44) (parabens and other preservatives). A safety assessment review of propylparaben has been published in ref. 43. The subject of possible endocrine effects of parabens is discussed in the section 'Systemic side effects' of Chapter 2.333 Paraben mix).

CONTACT ALLERGY

Patch testing in groups of patients

Patch testing in consecutive patients suspected of contact dermatitis: routine testing
In 1985, 627 consecutive patients suspected of contact dermatitis were patch tested with propylparaben 5% and 3 (0.5%) had a positive reaction; the relevance of these reactions was not stated (8).

Testing in groups of selected patients
Between 1971 and 1986, in Denmark, 60 patients previously reacting to the paraben mix (benzyl-, butyl-, ethyl-, methyl- and propylparaben) were tested with all five components at 5% pet. Forty (67%) reacted to one or more of the paraben-esters, most of who reacted to 2 or more. There were 21 reactions (35%) to propylparaben. The relevance of these positive patch test reactions was not mentioned (25). In India, before 1985, 100 patients suspected of ACD from topical medicaments were patch tested with propylparaben and 4 (4%) had a positive reaction; relevance was not mentioned (41).

Case reports and case series
In the period 1996-2013, in a tertiary referral center in Valencia, Spain, 5419 patients were patch tested. Of these, 628 individuals had allergic contact dermatitis to cosmetics. Propylparaben was the responsible allergen in three cases (20). In a group of 119 patients with allergic contact dermatitis from cosmetics, investigated in The Netherlands in 1986-1987, two cases were caused by propylparaben in a deodorant and in a veterinary cream used as cosmetic (1,10).

A child, known to be allergic to methyl- and propylparaben, developed vesicular hand dermatitis from a liquid soap containing parabens (5). A polysensitized HIV-patient reacted to propylparaben in a shaving foam (7). Two patients had ACD from propylparaben in skin care products (11). A woman had dermatitis of the eyelids from contact allergy to propyl- and methylparaben in a hypoallergenic eye cream (38).

A woman reported severe itching and erythema of the face and scalp with cyclic edema after using a tar shampoo for the treatment of dandruff. This happened on several occasions, she having initially tolerated the preparation. Patch testing with the European standard series, a facial series, and coal and wood tars gave positive reactions to the paraben mix and balsam of Peru. Further testing with individual components of the paraben mix showed positive results to propylparaben, ethylparaben and butylparaben. The ingredient listing of the shampoo included 'parabens'; no specific data on the esters were provided (32).

Contact allergy to propylparaben in non-cosmetic products

Topical pharmaceutical preparations

One patient reacted to propylparaben in a topical pharmaceutical product (2). One patient had allergic contact dermatitis from propylparaben in eye drops (4). Another individual developed ACD from propylparaben in an antibiotic ointment applied on stasis dermatitis (21). One patient had ACD from propylparaben and other parabens in multiple topical pharmaceutical preparations (23). Another individual was also allergic to propylparaben in a topical pharmaceutical (26). (Probably) two patients had ACD from propylparaben (and presumably also other parabens) in topical pharmaceutical products (29).

Other non-cosmetic products

One patient had ACD from propylparaben in a compress (3), another one from this preservative in Unna boots (27). A woman, who had probably been sensitized to propylparaben in topical pharmaceutical products used on a leg ulcer previously, developed generalized dermatitis after an intramuscular injection of ampicillin solution, which was preserved with propyl- and methylparaben (30). A girl had ACD of the hands from play gel. She reacted to the paraben mix. The play gel, containing methyl- and propylparaben, also gave a positive patch test. Methyl- and propylparaben were not tested separately (5). A man had ACD from propylparaben and methylparaben in an ultrasonic gel (34). One patient had severe ACD of the lower legs from contact allergy to propyl- and methylparaben in bandages (42).

Cross-reactions, pseudo-cross-reactions and co-reactions

Co-reactions with other paraben-esters are seen frequently (22,24,25). As most patients are exposed to more than one paraben, it is difficult to determine whether these co-reactions result from cross-sensitivity or from concomitant sensitization (28). Propylparaben is very often combined with methylparaben as preservative system for different products. See also this section in Chapter 2.333 Paraben mix.

Presence in cosmetic products and chemical analyses

In the USA, in April 2017, propylparaben was present in 10599 of 56,714 cosmetic products of which the composition is known in FDA's Voluntary Cosmetic Registration Program (VCRP) (data obtained from FDA, May 2017). In February 2017, propylparaben was present in 3596 of 64,482 cosmetic products of which the composition is known in EWG's Skin Deep Cosmetics Database, USA (http://www.ewg.org/skindeep/). Propylparaben was present in 9 (17%) of 54 personal hygiene wet wipes for which ingredient information was obtained online and from retail stores, USA, 2016 (46). Propylparaben was present in 38 (21%) of 178 facial wipes for which ingredient information was obtained online and from retail stores, USA, 2016 (45). Of 179 emollients available in Poland in 2014, 51 (28%) contained propylparaben (39).

In Germany, in 2006-2009, the labels of 4680 cosmetic products were screened for the presence of preservatives. Propylparaben was present in 32.9% of the products, according to labeling information (33). Propylparaben was present in 25% of 204 cosmetic products (92 shampoos, 61 hair conditioners, 34 liquid soaps, 17 wet tissues) in Sweden, 2008 (1). Propylparaben was present in 337 of 1774 (19.0%) cosmetics and toiletries in 2002 resp. in 288 of 1170 (24.6%) such products in 2005, filed in the Danish Product Register Database (PROBAS) (12). In a group of 67 samples of skin creams, randomly selected from retail outlets in Denmark in 1999, 47 (70%) contained propylparaben in a concentration range of 0.002-0.206% (13).

In the beginning of the 1990s, 215 cosmetic products (158 leave-on cosmetics and 57 rinse-off products) from 79 cosmetic-producing companies, collected in Denmark, were analysed for paraben content with high performance liquid chromatography (HPLC) (40). Of all the products investigated, 93% were found to contain paraben(s). Paraben was detected in 77% of the rinse-off products and in 99% of the leave-on products. Total paraben content in the paraben-positive cosmetics ranged from 0.01% to 0.59%, except in one sun-lotion that contained 0.87% parabens. Rinse-off cosmetics contained 0.01-0.50% parabens and the paraben content in leave-on products was 0.01-0.59%.

Propylparaben was present in 38% of the paraben-positive products in a concentration range of 0.01%-0.32% (w/w) (40).

Provocation tests

In 14 patients reacting to the paraben mix, a placebo-controlled oral challenge with a mixture of 100 mg methylparaben and 100 mg propylparaben was performed. Two of the 14 patients had flares of their usual dermatitis (which was recurrent vesicular hand dermatitis) after challenge with the paraben mix but not after the placebo. Subsequently, a diet avoiding items containing parabens did not result in improvement of their dermatitis. It was concluded that oral challenge is not a useful test procedure in patients sensitive to the paraben mix. Although specific reactions were seen in 2 paraben-sensitive patients with recurrent vesicular hand eczema, the significance of this finding remained uncertain (6).

OTHER SIDE EFFECTS

Miscellaneous side effects

A hydrocortisone preparation containing methylparaben and propylparaben provoked bronchospasm and generalized pruritus within minutes after being given intravenously to an asthmatic patient. No urticaria, angioedema or hypotension were noted. Another hydrocortisone preparation without paraben preservative did not provoke any allergic symptoms. Intradermal tests and passive transfer (Prausnitz-Küstner) skin tests for immediate hypersensitivity were positive to both parabens (31). A patient had an immediate-type reaction with generalized pruritus from allergy to propylparaben and methylparaben in a heparin solution injected intravenously (35).

LITERATURE

1   Yazar K, Johnsson S, Lind M-L, Boman A, Lidén C. Preservatives and fragrances in selected consumer-available cosmetics and detergents. Contact Dermatitis 2011;64:265-272
2   Sagara R, Nakada T, Iijima M. Paraben allergic contact dermatitis in a patient with livedo reticularis. Contact Dermatitis 2008;58:53-54
3   Oiso N, Fukai K, Ishii M. Allergic contact dermatitis caused by parabens in a compress. Contact Dermatitis 2004;50:317
4   Vilaplana J, Romaguera C. Contact dermatitis from parabens used as preservatives in eyedrops. Contact Dermatitis 2000;43:248
5   Verhaeghe I, Dooms-Goossens A. Multiple sources of allergic contact dermatitis from parabens. Contact Dermatitis 1997;36:269-270
6   Veien NK, Hattel, T, Laurberg G. Oral challenge with parabens in paraben-sensitive patients. Contact Dermatitis 1996;34:433
7   Vilaplana J, Lecha M, Romaguera C, Alsina A, Mascaro JM, Castel, T. A polysensitized HIV-positive patient. Contact Dermatitis 1993;29:101-102
8   De Groot AC, Weyland JW, Bos JD, Jagtman BA. Contact allergy to preservatives (I). Contact Dermatitis 1986;14:120-122
9   De Groot AC, Bruynzeel DP, Bos JD, van der Meeren HL, van Joost T, Jagtman BA, Weyland JW. The allergens in cosmetics. Arch Dermatol 1988;124:1525-1529
10   De Groot AC. Adverse reactions to cosmetics. PhD Thesis, University of Groningen, The Netherlands: 1988, chapter 3.4, pp.105-113
11   Cronin E. Contact Dermatitis. Edinburgh: Churchill Livingstone, 1980:670-671
12   Flyvholm, MA. Preservatives in registered chemical products. Contact Dermatitis 2005;53:27-32
13   Rastogi SC. Analytical control of preservative labelling on skin creams. Contact Dermatitis 2000;43:339-343
14   SCCS (Scientific Committee on Consumer Safety). Opinion on parabens, SCCS/1514/13, 3 May 2013. Available at: http://ec.europa.eu/health/scientific_committees/consumer_safety/docs/sccs_o_132.pdf
15   SCCS (Scientific Committee on Consumer Safety). Clarification on Opinion SCCS/1348/10 in the light of the Danish clause of safeguard banning the use of parabens in cosmetic products intended for children under three years of age, 10 October 2011. Available at: http://ec.europa.eu/health/scientific_committees/consumer_safety/docs/sccs_o_069.pdf
16   SCCS (Scientific Committee on Consumer Safety). Opinion on parabens, 14 December 2010, SCCS/1348/10. Available at: http://ec.europa.eu/health/scientific_committees/consumer_safety/docs/sccs_o_041.pdf
17   SCCP (Scientific Committee on Consumer Products). Opinion on parabens, 24 June 2008, SCCP/1183/08. Available at: http://ec.europa.eu/health/archive/ph_risk/committees/04_sccp/docs/sccp_o_138.pdf
18   SCCP (Scientific Committee on Consumer Products). Opinion on Parabens, 10 October 2006, SCCP/1017/06. Available at: http://ec.europa.eu/health/archive/ph_risk/committees/04_sccp/docs/sccp_o_074.pdf

19 SCCP (Scientific Committee on Consumer Products). Extended Opinion on Parabens, underarm cosmetics and breast cancer, 28 January 2005, SCCP/0874/05. Available at: http://ec.europa.eu/health/archive/ph_risk/committees/04_sccp/docs/sccp_o_00d.pdf

20 Zaragoza-Ninet V, Blasco Encinas R, Vilata-Corell JJ, Pérez-Ferriols A, Sierra-Talamantes C, Esteve-Martínez A, de la Cuadra-Oyanguren J. Allergic contact dermatitis due to cosmetics: A clinical and epidemiological study in a tertiary hospital. Actas Dermosifiliogr 2016;107:329-336

21 Sarkany I. Contact dermatitis from paraben. Br J Dermatol 1960;72:345-347

22 Fransway AF. The problem of preservation in the 1990s: III. Agents with preservative function independent of formaldehyde release. Am J Cont Derm 1991;2:145-174

23 Schorr WP, Mohajerin AH. Paraben sensitivity. Arch Dermatol 1966;93:721-723

24 Hjorth N, Trolle-Lassen C. Skin reactions to ointment bases. Trans St John Hosp Derm Soc 1963;49:127-140

25 Menné T, Hjorth N. Routine patch testing with paraben esters. Contact Dermatitis 1988;19:189-191

26 Schamberg IL. Allergic contact dermatitis to methyl and propyl paraben. Arch Dermatol 1967;95:626-628

27 Praditsuwan P, Taylor JS, Roenigk HH Jr. Allergy to Unna boots in four patients. J Am Acad Dermatol 1995;33(5 Pt. 2):906-908

28 Hansen J, Møllgaard B, Avnstorp C, Menné T. Paraben contact allergy: Patch testing and in vitro absorption/metabolism. Am J Cont Derm 1993;4:78-86

29 Schorr WF. Paraben allergy. A cause of intractable dermatitis. JAMA 1968;204:859-862

30 Carradori S, Peluso AM, Faccioli M. Systemic contact dermatitis due to parabens. Contact Dermatitis 1990;22:238-239

31 Nagel JE, Fuscaldo JT, Fireman P. Paraben allergy. JAMA 1977;237:1594-1595

32 Cooper SM, Shaw S. Allergic contact dermatitis from parabens in a tar shampoo. Contact Dermatitis 1998;39:140

33 Uter W, Yazar K, Kratz EM, Mildau G, Lidén C. Coupled exposure to ingredients of cosmetic products: II. Preservatives. Contact Dermatitis 2014;70:219-226

34 Eguino P, Sánchez A, Agesta N, Lasa O, Ratón JA, Diaz-Pérez JL. Allergic contact dermatitis due to propylene glycol and parabens in an ultrasonic gel. Contact Dermatitis 2003;48:290

35 Sato K, Kazama JJ, Wada Y, Maruyama H, Narita I, Gejyo F, Sugiyama K, Satoh H. Hypersensitivity to paraoxybenzoic acid esters (parabens) in a dialysis patient. Nephron 2002;92:728-729

36 Cashman AL, Warshaw EM. Parabens: A review of epidemiology, structure, allergenicity, and hormonal properties. Dermatitis 2005;16:57-66

37 Sasseville D. Hypersensitivity to preservatives. Dermatol Ther 2004;17:251-263

38 Calnan CD. Quinazoline yellow dermatitis (D&C Yellow 11) in an eye cream. Contact Dermatitis 1981;7:271

39 Osinka K, Karczmarz A, Krauze A, Feleszko W. Contact allergens in cosmetics used in atopic dermatitis: analysis of product composition. Contact Dermatitis 2016;75:241-243

40 Rastogi SC, Schouten A, de Kruijf N, Weijland JW. Contents of methyl-, ethyl-, propyl-, butyl- and benzylparaben in cosmetic products. Contact Dermatitis 1995;32:28-30

41 Bajaj AK, Chatterjee AK. Paraben contact hypersensitivity. Ind J Derm Venereol Leprol 1985;51:319-321

42 Lindner K, Cramer HJ, Köhler R. Do Varicosan bandages really rarely cause contact eczema? Case report of allergic contact dermatitis caused by propyl hydroxybenzoate following the use of Varicosan bandages. Dermatol Monatsschr 1989;175:655-657

43 Soni MG, Burdock GA, Taylor SL, Greenberg NA. Safety assessment of propyl paraben: a review of the published literature. Food Chem Toxicol 2001;39:513-532

44 Yim E, Baquerizo Nole KL, Tosti A. Contact dermatitis caused by preservatives. Dermatitis 2014;25:215-231

45 Aschenbeck KA, Warshaw EM. Allergenic ingredients in facial wet wipes. Dermatitis 2017 Mar 23. doi: 10.1097/DER.0000000000000268. [Epub ahead of print]

46 Aschenbeck KA, Warshaw EM. Allergenic ingredients in personal hygiene wet wipes. Dermatitis 2017 Mar 23. doi: 10.1097/DER.0000000000000275. [Epub ahead of print]

2.390 PRUNUS AVIUM (SWEET CHERRY) SEED OIL

IDENTIFICATION

Description/definition : Prunus avium seed oil is the fixed oil obtained from the kernels of the sweet cherry, *Prunus avium* L., Rosaceae

Chemical class(es) : Fats and oils

INCI name USA : Prunus avium (sweet cherry) seed oil

Other names : Sweet cherry seed oil; cherry pit oil

CAS registry number (s) : 85566-22-9

EC number(s) : 287-632-2

CIR review(s) : Final report March 2011 (access: www.cir-safety.org/ingredients)

Function(s) in cosmetics : EU: emollient; emulsion stabilizing; skin conditioning. USA: skin-conditioning agents – occlusive

Patch testing : No data available; suggested: 10% and 30% pet.

GENERAL

Prunus avium seed oil (= kernel oil) consists mainly of fatty acids. The amounts of the individual fatty acids depend on the cultivars used (2). In a 2016 study of the kernel oils of nine cultivars, from nine identified fatty acids, the oleic (C18:1) (40-50%), linoleic (C18:2) (31-39%), α-eleostearic (α-ESA C18:3) (7-11%) and palmitic (C16:0) (6-7%) acid together represented approximately 95% of the total detected fatty acids. Levels of 1-3% may be found for stearic (C18:0) and arachidic (C20:0) acid, values below 1% for palmitoleic (C16:1), α-linolenic (α-C18:3) and gondoic (C20:1) acid (2).

Homologues of tocopherol (α, β, γ and δ) and of tocotrienol (α and γ) may also be present. The amount of total tocochromanols in sweet cherry kernel oils is in the range of 80-110 mg/100 g oil. Carotenoids may be found in amounts of 0.4 to 0.6 mg/100 g oil. Sterols in sweet cherry kernel oils include campesterol, β-sitosterol, Δ5-avenasterol, 24-methylene-cycloartanol, cholesterol, gramisterol, Δ7-stigmasterol, Δ7-avenasterol and citrostadienol, β-sitosterol being the predominant phytosterol (200-330 mg/100 g oil), representing 75-86% of the total sterols. The total amount of sterols in sweet cherry kernel oils generally ranges from 230-420 mg/100 g (2).

CONTACT ALLERGY

Case reports and case series

'Cherry oil' was responsible for 1 out of 399 cases of cosmetic allergy where the causal allergen was identified in a study of the NACDG, USA, 1977-1983 (1).

Presence in cosmetic products and chemical analyses

In August 2017, Prunus avium (wild cherry) seed oil was present in 2 of 70,166 cosmetic products of which the composition is known in EWG's Skin Deep Cosmetics Database, USA (http://www.ewg.org/skindeep/). In the USA, in April 2017, Prunus avium (sweet cherry) seed oil was present in 2 of 56,714 cosmetic products of which the composition is known in FDA's Voluntary Cosmetic Registration Program (VCRP) (data obtained from FDA, May 2017)

LITERATURE

1   Adams RM, Maibach HI, Clendenning WE, Fisher AA, Jordan WJ, Kanof N, et al. A five-year study of cosmetic reactions. J Am Acad Dermatol 1985;13:1062-1069

2   Górnaś P, Rudzińska M, Raczyk M, Mišina I, Segliņa D. Impact of cultivar on profile and concentration of lipophilic bioactive compounds in kernel oils recovered from sweet cherry (*Prunus avium* L.) by-products. Plant Foods Hum Nutr 2016;71:158-164

2.391 PYRIDOXINE DIOCTENOATE

IDENTIFICATION

Description/definition : Pyridoxine dioctenoate is the substituted aromatic compound that conforms generally to the formula shown below
Chemical class(es) : Esters; heterocyclic compounds
Chemical/IUPAC name : Octenoic acid, 3,4-diester with 5-hydroxy-6-methyl-3,4-pyridinedimethanol
Other names : Octenoic acid, (5-hydroxy-6-methyl-3,4-pyridinediyl)bis(methylene) ester; vitamin B6 dioctenoate
CAS registry number (s) : 59599-61-0
Function(s) in cosmetics : EU: antistatic; hair conditioning; skin conditioning. USA: hair conditioning agents; skin-conditioning agents - miscellaneous
Patch testing : 1% pet.; 0.001% alc. (1) (0.01% alc. may be preferable)
Molecular formula : $C_{24}H_{35}NO_5$

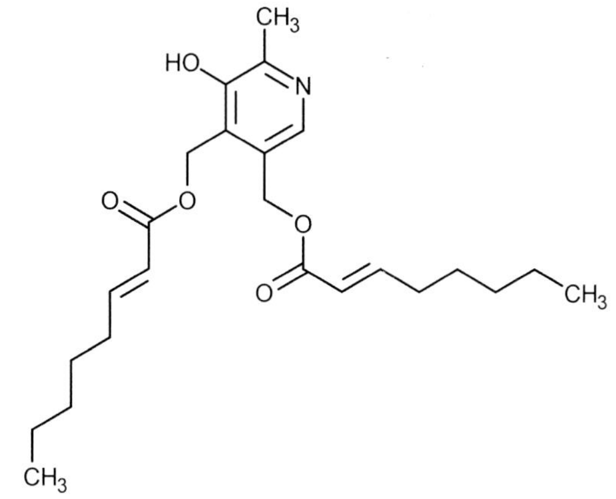

CONTACT ALLERGY

Case reports and case series

A man developed an erythematous eruption over the scalp, face, nape and back of the hands after using a hair lotion. The eruption cleared within 4 weeks with topical corticosteroid and oral antihistamine treatment. Some months later, the eruption relapsed after using the same hair liquid. The patient showed erythematous papules and desquamation over the scalp, forehead, nose, perioral region, ears, nape and back of the hands and fingers, simulating a photosensitive dermatitis. The ingredients of this cosmetic product were alcohol, propylene glycol, hinokitiol, polyoxypropylene polyoxyethylene pentaerythritol alcohol, PEG hydrogenated castor oil, pyridoxine 3,4-dioctenoate and perfume. When patch tested to its ingredients, the patient reacted to pyridoxine 3,4-dioctenoate in various concentrations and vehicles and to another ingredient, hinokitiol. The test results to pyridoxine 3,4-dioctenoate were as follows: 1% pet. +++, 0.1% pet. +, 0.01% pet. -; 0.01% alc. +++, 0.001% alc. -. There was also a positive reaction to pyridoxine hydrochloride 1% pet., but not to 0.1% pet. or 1% alc. Twenty-five controls were negative to pyridoxine 3,4-dioctenoate 1% pet. (1). Throughout this article, the incorrect name 3,4-pyridoxide dioctAnoate was used.

Cross-reactions, pseudo-cross-reactions and co-reactions

Pyridoxine hydrochloride (1).

Presence in cosmetic products and chemical analyses

In April 2017, pyridoxine dioctenoate was present in zero of 65,434 cosmetic products of which the composition is known in EWG's Skin Deep Cosmetics Database, USA (http://www.ewg.org/skindeep/).

LITERATURE

1   Fujita M, Aoki T. Allergic contact dermatitis to pyridoxine ester and hinokitiol. Contact Dermatitis 1983;9:61-65

2.392 PYROCATECHOL

IDENTIFICATION

Description/definition	: Pyrocatechol is the phenol that conforms to the formula shown below
Chemical class(es)	. Color additives – hair; phenols
Chemical/IUPAC name	: Benzene-1,2-diol
Other names	: CI 76500; catechol; 1,2-dihydroxybenzene
CAS registry number (s)	: 120-80-9
EC number(s)	: 204-427-5
CIR review(s)	: J Am Coll Toxicol 1986;5:123-165; Int J Toxicol 1997;16(Suppl.1):11-58 (access: www.cir-safety.org/ingredients)
Merck Index monograph	: 9381
Function(s) in cosmetics	: EU: formerly used for hair dyeing; delisted in 1994. USA: fragrance ingredients; hair colorants
EU cosmetic restrictions	: Regulated in Annex II/408 of the Regulation (EC) No. 1223/2009 (prohibited)
Patch testing	: 0.5% pet. (1,4)
Molecular formula	: $C_6H_6O_2$

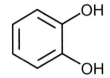

GENERAL

Pyrocatechol is a water-soluble, crystalline compound with a phenolic odor. It has been used for the preparation of dyes and medicines, photography, rubber, fur dying, specialty inks, as an agent for oxygen removal, and in the production of antioxidants for rubber and lubricating oils. It occurs in natural products such as crude wood tar, beet sugar, bituminous shale, coal, onions, cigarette smoke, wood and other plant material (1,4). The *meta-* and *para-* isomers of pyrocatechol are resorcinol and hydroquinone, respectively (4).

CONTACT ALLERGY

Case reports and case series

A young female patient developed acute contact dermatitis around her eyes after treatment of the eyelashes and eyebrows with a permanent cream dye. After her dermatitis had subsided, she was patch tested with the ICDRG standard series and the cream dye and she reacted only to the dye product, probably tested 'as is'. When tested with the ingredients of this cosmetic product, obtained from the manufacturer, the patient had positive reactions to pyrocatechol 2% pet. In a next patch test session, testing was repeated with pyrocatechol, now tested 0.1% and 0.5% pet. and the patient reacted strongly to both concentrations. She was also tested with hydroquinone and resorcinol 0.1%, 0.5% and 2% pet. and she reacted only to hydroquinone 0.5% and 2% pet.

The allergenic ingredient, pyrocatechol, was analyzed by means of nuclear magnetic resonance spectroscopy and mass spectrometry and was found to be > 99.5% pure. Commercially-available analytical-grade resorcinol and hydroquinone were used for patch testing (1).

Contact allergy to pyrocatechol in non-cosmetic products

A woman had suspected contact dermatitis of her hands since 10 years. She worked as a radiographer, developing X-ray photographs, and the dermatitis had appeared 2 years after starting the job. The lesions were hyperkeratotic, squamous and very itchy. The patient was patch tested with the ICDRG standard series and a photographic series. She showed a strongly positive reaction to pyrocatechol 2% pet. at D2 and D3. Later, patch tests were repeated with pyrocatechol, now tested 0.1% and 0.5% pet. and she reacted strongly to both concentrations. Patch tests with the related resorcinol and hydroquinone, however, were negative. (4). Quite curiously, although the title of the article was 'Occupational contact dermatitis from pyrocatechol', the authors did not mention whether the patient had come into contact with pyrocatechol and, if so, in which product(s) it was present.

Cross-reactions, pseudo-cross-reactions and co-reactions

Hydroquinone (1,2,3); resorcinol (2,3); cross-reactivity *from* resorcinol (5); not to resorcinol and hydroquinone (4).

Presence in cosmetic products and chemical analyses

In the USA, in April 2017, pyrocatechol was present in 16 of 56,714 cosmetic products of which the composition is known in FDA's Voluntary Cosmetic Registration Program (VCRP) (data obtained from FDA, May 2017). In April 2017, pyrocatechol was present in zero of 66,485 cosmetic products of which the composition is known in EWG's Skin Deep Cosmetics Database, USA (http://www.ewg.org/skindeep/).

LITERATURE

1   Andersen KE, Carisen L. Pyrocatechol contact allergy from a permanent cream dye for eyelashes and eyebrows. Contact Dermatitis 1988;18:306-307

2   Caron GA, Calnan CD. Studies in contact dermatitis. XIV. Resorcin. Trans St John's Hosp Dermatol Soc 1962;48:149-156 (data cited in ref. 1)

3   Keil H. Group reactions in contact dermatitis due to resorcinol. Arch Dermatol 1962;86:212-216 (data cited in ref. 1)

4   Morelli R, Piancastelli E, Lanzarini M, Restani S. Occupational contact dermatitis from pyrocatechol. Contact Dermatitis 1989;21:201-202

5   Barbaud A, Reichert-Penetrat S, Trechot P, Granel F, Schmutz JL. Sensitization to resorcinol in a prescription verrucide preparation: unusual systemic clinical features and prevalence. Ann Dermatol Venereol 2001;128:615-618 (Article in French)

2.393   PYROGALLOL

IDENTIFICATION

Description/definition   : Pyrogallol is the phenol that conforms to the formula shown below
Chemical class(es)   : Color additives – hair; phenols
Chemical/IUPAC name   : Benzene-1,2,3-triol
Other names   : CI 76515
CAS registry number (s)   : 87-66-1
EC number(s)   : 201-762-9
CIR review(s)   : J Am Coll Toxicol 1991;10:67-85 (access: www.cir-safety.org/ingredients)
Merck Index monograph   : 9382
Function(s) in cosmetics   : EU: formerly used for hair dyeing, delisted in 1994. USA: fragrance ingredients; hair
                             colorants
EU cosmetic restrictions   : Regulated in Annex II/409 of the Regulation (EC) No. 1223/2009 (prohibited)
Patch testing   : 1% pet. (SmartPracticeEurope, SmartPracticeCanada)
Molecular formula   : $C_6H_6O_3$

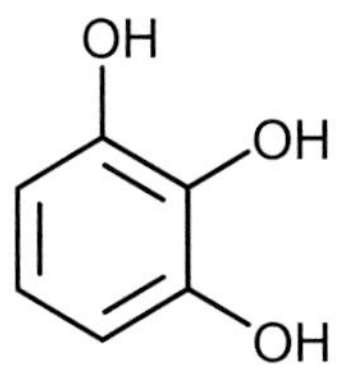

GENERAL

Pyrogallol was formerly used in in oxidative hair dying products. The chemistry of oxidative hair dying is discussed in Chapter 2.359 *p*-Phenylenediamine

CONTACT ALLERGY

Patch testing in groups of patients

Pyrogallol has not been tested in groups of consecutive patients suspected of contact dermatitis (routine testing). In many studies, though, it was patch tested in groups of *selected* patients, notably in hairdressers and in female patients in who hair cosmetics were suspected to be the cause of their dermatitis. Such patients are tested with a hairdressers' series, which contains color additives, often including pyrogallol. The results of these studies are shown in table 2.393.1. In hairdressers, rates of sensitization have ranged from 0.8% to 4.4%. In groups of patients suspected to react to hair cosmetics and patients tested with a hairdressing series, frequencies of 2.3% to 12% positive reactions have been observed.

In nearly all studies, the relevance of the observed patch test reactions was not mentioned. In one study from the USA, 68% of 19 positive patch tests to pyrogallol were considered to be relevant, despite that fact that currently not one cosmetic in the EWG's Skin Deep Cosmetics Database contains pyrogallol. As pyrogallol has been banned in the EU already 25 years ago, it may safely be assumed that most if not all positive patch tests are the result of cross-sensitivity to *p*-phenylenediamine or other para-compounds.

Table 2.393.1 Patch testing in groups of patients: Selected patient groups

Years and Country	Test conc. & vehicle	Number of patients tested | positive (%)		Selection of patients (S); Relevance (R); Comments (C)	Ref.
2007-2012 IVDK	1% pet.	712	21 (2.6%)	S: female hairdressers with current or previous occupational contact dermatitis; R: not stated	11
		1693	69 (5.3%)	S: female patients, clients of hairdressers, in who hair cosmetics were regarded as a cause of dermatitis, and who had never worked as hairdressers; R: not stated	
2000-2008 USA	1% pet.	210	19 (9.1%)	S: patients tested with a hairdresser series; R: 68%	13
1997-2007 UK	1% pet.	175	21 (12%)	S: patients suspected of hair dye allergy; R: not stated	1
2003-2006 IVDK	1% pet.	23	(3.5%)	S: female hairdressers with suspected occupational contact dermatitis; R: not stated	3
	1% pet.	613	(7.5%)	S: women with suspected reactions to hair cosmetics;	

Table 2.393.1 Patch testing in groups of patients: Selected patient groups (*continued*)

Years and Country	Test conc. & vehicle	Number of patients tested | positive (%)		Selection of patients (S); Relevance (R); Comments (C)	Ref.
1999-2004 UK		315	20 (6.4%)	R: not specified; C: probably cross-reactions S: patients tested with the hairdressing series; R: only reactions that were of current or past relevance were collected	12
1993-2003 IVDK	1% pet.	628	34 (5.4%)	S: patients with scalp dermatitis; R: not stated	4
1995-2002 IVDK		884	(4.4%)	S: female hairdressers with present or past occupational contact dermatitis; R: not specified	8
		1217	(4.6%)	S: clients of hairdressers suspected to react to hairdressing cosmetics or hair care products; R: not specified	
1988-1991, 8 European countries		781	6 (0.8%)	S: hairdressers with hand dermatitis; R: not stated	9
1985-1990 Italy	1% pet.	261	6 (2.3%)	S: patients with eczema suspected to be caused by hair dying, bleaching or permanent wave solution; R: not stated	7
1985-1990 Italy	1% pet.	302	4 (1.3%)	S: hairdressers tested with a hairdressing series; R: not stated	10

IVDK: Information Network of Departments of Dermatology, Germany, Austria, Switzerland

Case reports and case series

Pyrogallol was stated to be the (or an) allergen in 3 patients in a group of 603 individuals suffering from cosmetic dermatitis, seen in the period 2010-2015 in Leuven, Belgium (6). As pyrogallol was prohibited in the EU at least 26 years before this study started, this must have been a misinterpretation. Three positive patch test reactions to pyrogallol were ascribed to cosmetic allergy (2). In a 4-month-period in 1996, 475 patients with contact allergy to 'cosmetic ingredients' were collected in 5 centers in Belgium, UK and Germany. There was one reaction to pyrogallol; its relevance was not mentioned (5).

Cross-reactions, pseudo-cross-reactions and co-reactions

Pyrogallol may cross-react with structurally related chemicals, notably those with a para-structure. Cross-reactivity between para-compounds is discussed in Chapter 2.359 *p*-Phenylenediamine.

Presence in cosmetic products and chemical analyses

In the USA, in April 2017, pyrogallol was present in 1 of 56,714 cosmetic products of which the composition is known in FDA's Voluntary Cosmetic Registration Program (VCRP) (data obtained from FDA, May 2017). In April 2017, pyrogallol was present in zero of 64,655 cosmetic products of which the composition is known in EWG's Skin Deep Cosmetics Database, USA (http://www.ewg.org/skindeep/). Of 15 hair dyes advertised as 'hypoallergenic', 'para-phenylenediamine-free', or 'non-allergenic', purchased in South Korea in 2015, 3 (20%) proved to contain pyrogallol / gallic acid (14).

LITERATURE

1   Basketter DA, English J. Cross-reactions among hair dye allergens. Cut Ocular Toxicol 2009;28:104-106
2   Kohl L, Blondeel A, Song M. Allergic contact dermatitis from cosmetics: retrospective analysis of 819 patch-tested patients. Dermatology 2002;204:334-337
3   Uter W, Lessmann H, Geier J, Schnuch A. Contact allergy to hairdressing allergens in female hairdressers and clients – current data from the IVDK, 2003-2006. J Dtsch Dermatol Ges 2007;5:993-1001
4   Hillen U, Grabbe S, Uter W. Patch test results in patients with scalp dermatitis: analysis of data of the Information Network of Departments of Dermatology. Contact Dermatitis 2007;56:87-93
5   Goossens A, Beck MH, Haneke E, McFadden JP, Nolting S, Durupt G, Ries G. Adverse cutaneous reactions to cosmetic allergens. Contact Dermatitis 1999;40:112-113
6   Goossens A. Cosmetic contact allergens. Cosmetics 2016, 3, 5; doi:10.3390/cosmetics3010005
7   Guerra L, Bardazzi F, Tosti A. Contact dermatitis in hairdressers' clients. Contact Dermatitis 1992;26:108-111
8   Uter W, Lessmann H, Geier J, Schnuch A. Contact allergy to ingredients of hair cosmetics in female hairdressers and clients: an 8-year analysis of IVDK data. Contact Dermatitis 2003;49:236-240
9   Frosch PJ, Burrows D, Camarasa JG, Dooms-Goossens A, Ducombs G, Lahti A, et al. Allergic reactions to a hairdressers' series: results from 9 European centres. Contact Dermatitis 1993;28:180-183

10   Guerra L, Tosti A, Bardazzi F, Pigatto P, Lisi P, Santucci B, et al. Contact dermatitis in hairdressers: the Italian experience. Contact Dermatitis 1992;26:101-107

11   Uter W, Gefeller O, John SM, Schnuch A, Geier J. Contact allergy to ingredients of hair cosmetics – a comparison of female hairdressers and clients based on IVDK 2007–2012 data. Contact Dermatitis 2014;71:13-20

12   Katugampola RP, Statham BN, English JSC, Wilkinson MM, Foulds IS, Green CM, Ormerod AD, et al. A multicentre review of the hairdressing allergens tested in the UK. Contact Dermatitis 2005;53:130-132

13   Wang MZ, Farmer SA, Richardson DM, Davis MD. Patch-testing with hairdressing chemicals. Dermatitis 2011;22:16-26

14   Lee HJ, Kim WJ, Kim JY, Kim HS, Kim BS, Kim MB, Ko HC. Patch tests with commercial hair dye products in patients with allergic contact dermatitis to para-phenylenediamine. Indian J Dermatol Venereol Leprol 2016;82:645-650

2.394 QUATERNIUM-15

IDENTIFICATION

Description/definition	: Quaternium-15 is the quaternary ammonium salt that conforms to the formula shown below
Chemical class(es)	: Quaternary ammonium compounds; halogen compounds; heterocyclic compounds
Chemical/IUPAC name	: Methenamine 3-chloroallylochloride
Other names	: *N*-(3-Chloroallyl)hexaminium chloride; hexamethylenetetramine chloroallyl chloride; Dowicil® 200
CAS registry number (s)	: 4080-31-3; 51229-78-8
EC number(s)	: 223-805-0; 426-020-3
CIR review(s)	: J Am Coll Toxicol 1986;5:61-101; Int J Toxicol 2010;29(Suppl.2):98-114 (access: www.cir-safety.org/ingredients)
SCCS opinion(s)	: SCCS/1344/10 (*cis*-isomer) (75)
Merck Index monograph	: 9413
Function(s) in cosmetics	: EU: preservative. USA: antistatic agents; pesticides; preservatives
EU cosmetic restrictions	: Regulated in Annex V/31 of the Regulation (EC) No. 1223/2009
Patch testing	: 1.0% pet. (Chemotechnique, SmartPracticeCanada); 2.0% pet. (Chemotechnique, SmartPracticeEurope, SmartPracticeCanada)
Molecular formula	: $C_9H_{16}Cl_2N_4$

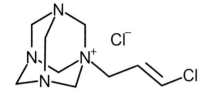

GENERAL

Quaternium-15 is an odorless, colorless, water-soluble formaldehyde-releasing preservative. At typical use levels of 0.05-0.2%, quaternium-15 is a highly active, broad- spectrum preservative providing effective antimicrobial activity against bacteria (particularly effective against *Pseudomonas* species), yeast, and molds. It was formerly frequently used in cosmetics, buts its use is strongly declining. Quaternium-15 may also be present in non-cosmetic applications including metalworking fluids, detergents, floor waxes and polishes, inks, latex-based paints, laundry starch, paper and pulp products, textile finishing solutions, spinning emulsions, printing pastes, joint cements, and photocopier toner (37,102).

The literature on formaldehyde-releasers in cosmetic products including quaternium-15 up to 2009-2010 has been reviewed by the author (37,105). The literature on contact allergy to quaternium-15 and other formaldehyde-releasers up to 1990 has been reviewed in refs. 103 and 104. Other useful preservative allergy reviews have appeared in 2014 (110) and 2004 (102).

CONTACT ALLERGY

Quaternium-15 1% in petrolatum has been part of the European baseline series for over 3 decades. Because in European countries, with exception of the UK, rates of positive reactions are mostly below 1%, over half of the reactions are already detected by formaldehyde sensitivity, and neither common occurrence in the environment nor a high percentage of relevant reactions has been ascertained, is has been argued that quaternium-15 does not deserve its place in the European baseline series and could be incorporated in a cosmetic screening series or preservative series instead. In the United Kingdom, however, routine testing should be continued (92).

Patch testing in the general population and in subgroups

There have been several investigations in some European countries, notably in Denmark, in which random samples of the population of certain age groups have been patch tested with quaternium-15 (table 2.394.1). Frequencies of sensi-tization have ranged from 0.2% to 0.4% (29,60,62,63,64). In three Danish studies finding low rates of 0.2%, the patch tests were read only at day 2, which may have resulted in underestimation of the actual rate of sensitization (29,62, 63). In a group of 8th grade Danish schoolchildren, aged 12-16 years, a prevalence of 0.2% was found in 1995-1996 (27,28). When this group was again tested 15 years later, the frequency of sensitization to quaternium-15 had risen slightly to 0.5% (in women from 0.2% to 0.7%) (61), but the groups were small.

Estimates of the 10-year prevalence of contact allergy to quaternium-15 in the general population of Denmark based on the CE-DUR method ranged from 0.26% to 0.35% (59).

Table 2.394.1   Contact allergy in the general population and subgroups

Year and country	Selection and number tested	Prevalence of contact allergy			Comments	Ref.
		Total	Women	Men		
General population						
2008-11 five European countries	general population, random sample, 18-74 years; n=3119	0.4%	0.4%	0.4%		60
2008 Denmark	general population, random sample, 15-41 years; n=469		0.4%	0%	patch tests were read on day 2 only	29
2006 Denmark	general population, random sample, 18-69 years; n=3460	0.2%	0.2%	0.2%	patch tests were read on day 2 only	62
2005 Norway	general population, random sample, 18-69 years; n=1236	0.4%	0.3%	0.5%		64
1990 Denmark	general population, random sample, 18-69 years; n=543	0.2%	0%	0.2%	patch tests were read on day 2 only; data from 15-17 years old are excluded in the data presented here	63
Subgroups						
2011 China	volunteer healthy Chinese students, 19-30 years; n=201	0.5%	0%	1.6%	one positive reaction in 60 men	113
2010 Denmark	unselected population of 8th grade schoolchildren in Denmark, 15 years later; n=442	0.5%	0.7%	0%	follow-up study	61
1995-1996 Denmark	8th grade schoolchildren, 12-16 years; n=1146	0.2%	0.2%	0.2%		27, 28

Patch testing in groups of patients

Results of testing quaternium-15 in consecutive patients suspected of contact dermatitis (routine testing) back to 2000 are shown in table 2.394.2. Results of testing in groups of *selected* patients (e.g., patients with eyelid dermatitis, individuals suspected of cosmetic allergy, health care workers) back to 1997 are shown in table 2.394.3.

Patch testing in consecutive patients suspected of contact dermatitis: routine testing

Quaternium-15 has been present in the European baseline series, the screening series of the North American Contact Dermatitis Group (NACDG) and most other national routine test series for several decades. The NACDG uses a test concentration of 2% (in petrolatum), other investigators employ a 1% pet. patch test material. No comparative investigations appear to have been performed with both the 1% and 2% test preparations. The results of the NACDG have been published biannually (table 2.394.2). In these North American studies, frequencies of sensitization have ranged from 4.8% to 10.3%, with a gradual decline from >8.4% in the period 1998-2008 to 5.8%, 6.4% and 4.8% in the 2009-2014 study periods (13,15,16,30,31,43,50,114). Similar results were obtained in other US centers (6,55).

In European countries, however, prevalences have been consistently lower, ranging from 0.7% to 1.9% , with a mean (unadjusted for sample size) of 1.1% and a median of 1.2% (1,2,10,14,38,39,42,44,45,46,47,48,83). Equally low sensitization rates were found in non-European countries such as Singapore (1.4% [56]), Israel (0.8% [40]; 0.6% [49]) and Turkey (0.8% [41]), whereas Australia holds a middle position with rates of 3.4% (79) and 2.9% (80). The frequencies of sensitization have been consistently higher in women than in men.

In many investigations, no relevance data were provided. In the NACDG studies, 'definite' + 'probable' relevance has ranged from 28% to 38% (mean 31%) (13,15,30,31,43,50,114). In other studies, there were higher relevance scores, ranging from 47% to 90% (6,46,55,79,80). The implicated products were never mentioned, but contact allergy to quaternium-15 is nearly always the result of its presence in cosmetic products (81,101). The reasons for the large differences in rates of sensitization to quaternium-15 between the USA and Europe are unknown, but may include stricter selection of patients in the USA for patch testing (the members of the NACDG all work in tertiary referral centers), patch testing with a higher concentration of quaternium-15 (2% in the USA, 1% in Europe), the (far) higher prevalence of formaldehyde allergy in USA studies (resulting in more pseudo-cross-reactions to quaternium-15), more frequent and widespread use of cosmetics in the USA and the use of higher concentrations of quaternium-15 in these products compared to those in products produced and marketed in the EU (37).

Table 2.394.2 Patch testing in groups of patients: Routine testing

Years and Country	Test conc. & vehicle	Number of patients tested	positive (%)	Selection of patients (S); Relevance (R); Comments (C)	Ref.
2013-14 USA, Canada	2% pet.	4856	235 (4.8%)	R: definite + probable relevance: 20%	114
2013-2014 [b] 12 European countries, 46 departments	1% pet.	18404	(0.8%)	R: not stated; C: results of 6 occupational dermatology clinics and one pediatric clinic not included in these figures; range of positive reactions: 0%-2.9%	124
2011-12 USA, Canada	2% pet.	4235	273 (6.4%)	R: definite + probable relevance: 28%	30
2009-2012, 12 European countries [b]	1% pet.	39,342	(0.9%) [a]	R: not stated	119
2011 Sweden	1% pet.	2122	18 (0.8%)	R: not stated; C: 13/18 (72%) co-reacted to formaldehyde	83
2006-2011 Singapore	1% pet.	3150	45 (1.4%)	R: not stated; C: prevalence was 0.9% in men, 1.9% in women	56
2009-10 USA, Canada	2% pet.	4302	250 (5.8%)	R: definite + probable relevance: 30%	31
2009-2010 , 10 European countries + USA	1% pet.	3591	25 (0.7%)	R: not stated; C: 21/25 co-reacted to formaldehyde 1% and/or 2% in water	14
2006-2010 USA	1% pet.	3091	(8.9%)	R: 64%	55
2001-2010 Australia	1% pet.	5139	176 (3.4%)	R: 47%	79
2005-2009 Spain	1% pet.	7838	69 (0.9%)	R: not specified	2
2009 Sweden	1% pet.	3112	(1.4%)	R: not stated	51
2007-2008, 8 European countries [b]	1% pet.	18,145	268 (1.5%) [a]	R: not stated; C: prevalence rates ranged from 0.1% (Italy) to 3.2% (Finland)	1
2007-8 USA, Canada	2% pet.	5081	(8.6%)	R: definite + probable relevance: 36%	15
2005-6 USA, Canada	2% pet.	4446	(10.3%)	R: definite + probable relevance: 38%	13
2005-6 10 European countries [b]	1% pet.	14,062	220 (1.6%)	R: not stated; C: prevalences in the four regions (Central, West, Northeast and South Europe) ranged from 0.8 to 1.9%	116
1993-2006 Australia	1% pet.	6845	(2.9%)	R: 49%	80
2004-2005 UK	1% pet.	6958	(1.9%)	R: not stated; C: prevalence 2.2% in women, 1.1% in men	39
2000-2005 USA	1% pet.	3841	(8.1%)	R: 76%	6
1985-2005 Denmark	1% pet.	14,993	(0.9%)	R: not stated; C: prevalence 1.1% in women, 0.5% in men	38
2004, 11 European countries [b]	1% pet.	7454	102 (1.4%) [a]	R: not stated; C: range positives per center: 0.2%- 4.2%	10
2003-4 USA, Canada	2% pet.	5139	460 (8.9%)	R: not stated	16
1998-2004 Israel	1% pet.	2156	(0.8%)	R: not stated	40
1992-2004 Turkey	1% pet.	1038	(0.8%)	R: not stated; C: prevalence in women 1.2%, in men 0%	41
2002-2003 Europe [b]	1% pet.	5845	(1.2%)	R: not stated; C: 17 centers in nine European countries	42
2001-2 USA, Canada	2% pet.	4910	(8.4%)	R: definite + probable relevance: 29%	43
2000-2002 Finland	1% pet.	11,802	(0.8%)	R: not stated	44
1997-2001 Czech Republic	1% pet.	7642	(0.7%)	R: not stated; C: prevalence in women 0.8%, in men 0.5%	45
2000 United Kingdom	1% pet.	3063	(1.3%)	R: 90% (current and past relevance given in one center)	46
2000 Sweden	1% pet.	3790	(1.2%)	R: not stated	47
1998-2000 USA	2% pet.	408	(5.1%)	R: not stated	25
1999-2000 Israel	1% pet.	943	(0.6%)	R: not stated; C: prevalence in women 0.7%, in men 0.5%	49
1998-00 USA, Canada	2% pet.	5832	(9.2%)	R: definite + probable relevance: 35%	50
1996-2000 Europe	1% pet.	26,210	(1.3%)	R: not stated; C: prevalence in women 1.5%, in men 1.0%; ten centers, seven countries, EECDRG study	48

[a] age-standardized and sex-standardized proportions
[b] study of the ESSCA (European Surveillance System on Contact Allergy network)
EECDRG: European Environmental and Contact Dermatitis Research group

Patch testing in groups of selected patients

Results of patch testing quaternium-15 in groups of selected patients (e.g., patients with eyelid dermatitis, individuals suspected of cosmetic allergy, health care workers) back to 1997 are shown in table 2.394.3. It was found that patients with atopic dermatitis as a subgroup of consecutive patients suspected of contact dermatitis had a significantly higher rate of sensitization (11.1%) than the control group (7.2%) (111). Selection for eyelid dermatitis and suspicion of cosmetic allergy resulted in sensitization frequencies of 3.3% to 9% (18,26,52,53,57). Quaternium-15 was found to be an important contact allergen in hairdressers and cosmetologists (17).

In the majority of the investigations, no data on relevance of the positive patch test reactions were provided. In the studies that did address this issue, relevance scores were mostly very high, up to 100% (or only relevant reactions were recorded) (4,26,52,57,81), but causative products were mentioned in one study only: cosmetics, cleansers, a disinfectant and a medical device were the sources of sensitization in 11 health care workers with occupational allergic contact dermatitis (81).

Table 2.394.3 Patch testing in groups of patients: Selected patient groups

Years and Country	Test conc. & vehicle	Number of patients tested	positive (%)		Selection of patients (S); Relevance (R); Comments (C)	Ref.
1996-2013 Netherlands	1% pet.	995	9	(0.9%)	S: children aged 0-17 years; R: not stated	120
1994-2013 USA		342	38	(11.1%)	S: patients with atopic dermatitis as subgroup of 2453 successive patients suspected of contact dermatitis; R: not stated; C: in the non-atopic group, the frequency was 7.2%; it was significantly higher in atopic dermatitis patients	111
2003-2012 IVDK		1735	28	(1.6%)	S: nurses with occupational contact dermatitis; R: not stated	23
2010-2011 Korea	1% pet.	584	19	(3.3%)	S: patients suspected of allergic cosmetic dermatitis; R: not stated	53
2002-2011 Denmark		399	4	(1.0%)	S: hairdressers with contact dermatitis; R: not stated	117
2006-2010 USA	2% pet.	100	4	(4%)	S: patients with eyelid dermatitis; R: not stated	18
1994-2010 USA, Canada	2% pet.	432	?	(?)	S: hairdressers/cosmetologists; R: in the group of 184 patients who had at least one relevant occupationally related reaction, 37 (20%) reacted to quaternium-15	17
1996-2009 IVDK	1% pet.	79,745	510	(0.7%) [a]	S: not specified; R: not specified	8
2000-2007 USA	1% pet.	942	71	(7.5%)	S: patients tested with a supplemental cosmetic screening series; R: 96%; C: weak study: a. high rate of macular erythema and weak reactions; b. relevance figures included 'questionable' and 'past' relevance	4
1998-04 USA, Canada	2% pet.	1254	11	(0.9%)	S: health care workers; R: only occupation-related (=relevant) reactions were recorded; C: because of this selection, the frequency of sensitization is low; the frequency was significantly higher than the rate of occupation-related reactions in non-healthcare workers (0.4%); the causative products were cosmetics, cleansers, a disinfectant and a medical device	81
1994-2004 USA	2% pet.	46	4	(8.7%)	S: patients with eyelid dermatitis; R: all were relevant	52
1994-1998 UK	1% pet.	232	11	(4.7%)	S: patients with eyelid dermatitis; R: 10 were currently relevant	26
1995-1997 USA		57	5	(9%)	S: patients with facial allergic contact dermatitis; R: only relevant reactions were mentioned	57

[a] age-standardized and sex-standardized proportions
IVDK: Information Network of Departments of Dermatology, Germany, Austria, Switzerland

Case reports and case series

Case series

Quaternium-15 was stated to be the (or an) allergen in 18 patients in a group of 603 individuals suffering from cosmetic dermatitis, seen in the period 2010-2015 in Leuven, Belgium (54). In the period 1996-2013, in a tertiary referral center in Valencia, Spain, 5419 patients were patch tested. Of these, 628 individuals had allergic contact dermatitis to cosmetics. Quaternium-15 was the responsible allergen in twelve case (115, overlap with ref. 76). Quaternium-15 was responsible for 2 out of 959 cases of non-fragrance cosmetic allergy where the causal allergen was identified, Belgium, 2000-2010 (3). In the period 2000-2007, 202 patients with allergic contact dermatitis caused by cosmetics were seen in Valencia, Spain. In this group, five individuals reacted to quaternium-15 from its presence in shampoo (n=2), in moisturizing cream (n=1), in gel/soap (n=1), and in deodorant (n=1) (76, overlap with ref. 115). In a group of 2193 patients (1582 women, 611 men) with (presumed) cosmetic allergy, 485 reactions (22%) were caused by quaternium-15 in a study of the NACDG, 2001-2004, quaternium-15 ranking first in the list of most frequent allergens (7).

Quaternium-15 was responsible for 65 out of 399 (16.3%) cases of cosmetic allergy where the causal allergen was identified in a study of the NACDG, USA, 1977-1983 (5). In a group of 119 patients with allergic contact dermatitis from cosmetics, investigated in The Netherlands in 1986-1987, three cases were caused by quaternium-15 in skin care products (67,68). In a group of 75 patients allergic to cosmetic products, seen in a private practice in The Netherlands in the period 1981-1986, two cases were caused by quaternium-15 in skin care products (69).

In Cleveland, USA, in the period 1983-1987, 1408 consecutive patients suspected of contact dermatitis were patch tested with quaternium-15 2% in petrolatum (and sometimes also 2% in water); 89 (6.3%) had a positive patch test to the preservative (101). In 39 patients (44%), the reaction was of current relevance and in 19 (21%) of past relevance. The causative products were moisturizers (in 46 patients), non-coloring hair preparations (19 patients), face makeup (n=4), eye makeup (n=3), deodorants (n=2), baby products (n=2), hair color (n=1) and a barrier cream (n=1). Three of the patients had occupational ACD caused by quaternium-15; two were beauticians who reacted to hair dye products and the third was a tool and dye maker who had extensive dermatitis from contact allergy to quaternium-15 in a barrier cream (101).

In 3 clinics in Belgium, in the period 1978-1985, 279 patients with allergic contact dermatitis exclusively caused by cosmetics were seen. In this group, there were 2 reactions to quaternium-15. It was implied that this was the cause of the allergic reaction (78). Nine patients had allergic contact dermatitis from baby towelettes. They all had hand dermatitis, one also perianal eczema. Five individuals used the towelettes for their children's hygiene, two were occupationally exposed (a nurse and a machine repairman working in the factory where the towelettes were produced), the others used them on their person. In this group of nine, 7 reacted to quaternium-15. Six of these 7 co-reacted to formaldehyde. It was suggested that preservatives are the main allergens (sometimes combined with fragrances) in these products, but the composition of the culprit towelettes was not provided (82). Of 28 patients with allergic reactions to quaternium-15 seen in one center of the UK, 6 recalled using a particular brand of moisturizing cream often used for atopic dermatitis preserved with quaternium-15. Of these 6, five reported worsening of their skin condition after use. However, the cream itself was probably not tested (95).

Case reports
A man had allergic contact dermatitis of the buttock, gluteal cleft, perianal skin and scrotum caused by quaternium-15 present in baby wipes (12). One patient had ACD from quaternium-15 in a hand and body lotion (33). Another individual developed ACD from quaternium-15 in a sunscreen cream (34). In a Finnish occupational contact dermatitis clinic, in a period of 6.5 year, only one case of occupational ACD from quaternium-15 was seen, a hairdresser who reacted to the preservative in many products (77). A woman had lymphomatoid allergic contact dermatitis of the buttocks, perineum and the groins, which later spread to the arms, from quaternium-15 in baby wipes (90).

Another female individual had contact dermatitis around her eyes from contact allergy to quaternium-15 in a baby body lotion (91). Two hairdressers had occupational allergic contact dermatitis of the hands from quaternium-15 present 'in certain of their rinse-off products' (98). A man had ACD of the face from quaternium-15 present in a baby lotion (99). A woman had dermatitis of the arms and legs from contact allergy to quaternium-15 in a hand and body lotion (100). A nurse developed occupational ACD from quaternium-15 in a moisturizing lotion which is frequently used in Australian hospitals; the manufacturer of the lotion soon after the publication replaced quaternium-15 with another preservative system (112).

Contact allergy to quaternium-15 in non-cosmetic products
A man had occupational airborne contact dermatitis from contact allergy to formaldehyde released by quaternium-15 in a photocopier toner (84). One patient allergic to formaldehyde and quaternium-15 developed extensive and severe dermatitis requiring hospitalization from exposure to a water-based paint containing 0.15% quaternium-15 (85). An engineer involved in the maintenance of machinery in a chicken processing plant developed painful nail dystrophy with thickened and discolored nails, subungual hyperkeratosis and onycholysis, later followed by eczema of the fingertips and interdigital spaces. The cause proved to be contact allergy to quaternium-15 in an industrial cleanser (96). A neurophysiology technician had occupational ACD of the periorbital skin and hands from quaternium-15 in an electrode gel used for EEG examinations (97). A tool and dye maker had extensive dermatitis from contact allergy to quaternium-15 in a barrier cream (101). In a Finnish occupational contact dermatitis clinic, in a period of 6.5 year, only one case of occupational contact dermatitis was seen, a maintenance man reacting to quaternium-15 in a protecting cream (77).

Cross-reactions, pseudo-cross-reactions and co-reactions
Quaternium-15 is a formaldehyde-releaser. In a number of patients, contact allergy to the preservative is the result of sensitivity to formaldehyde. In these cases, pseudo-cross-reactions may be observed to formaldehyde and to other formaldehyde-releasers including diazolidinyl urea, DMDM hydantoin, imidazolidinyl urea, and − to a lesser degree − 2-bromo-2-nitropropane-1,3-diol (8,14,19, 87,89,101,125).

Over half to up to 84% of the patients reacting to quaternium-15 are also allergic to formaldehyde (14,19,24,83). This means that patients react to both formaldehyde and quaternium-15, and the reaction to quaternium-15 can be explained by the presence and release of formaldehyde in the quaternium-15 patch test material (24). In a study on the relationship between the two chemicals, investigating the role of the strength of the positive patch test reactions, over 80% of women with contact allergy to formaldehyde (TRUE test) also reacted to quaternium-15, and stronger patch test reactivity to formaldehyde increased the likelihood of positive quaternium-15 co-reactions. The strength of the reaction to formaldehyde also closely correlated with the strength of the quaternium-15 patch tests. These data − albeit not reproduced in a USA study (19) - are in favor of a very important causative role for formaldehyde allergy in positive quaternium-15 patch test reactions. For unknown reasons, the correlation between formaldehyde and quaternium-15 in men was substantially less (24).

It is often stated that contact allergy to quaternium-15 can result from sensitivity to formaldehyde, to the entire molecule or to the combination of both (19,25,26,27,28,102). However, the concept of quaternium-15 allergy being caused *by the entire molecule* has never been proven , but was only concluded from negative reactions to formaldehyde. A maximum of six formaldehyde molecules/mole quaternium-15 can be split off, and it is well known that it releases formaldehyde readily in aqueous environment, depending on the pH and temperature (21,106). Although the kinetics of the passage of quaternium 15 from the patch test material into and through the skin is unknown, it is very likely that most 'entire' quaternium-15 molecules will lose one or more methylol groups from hydrolysis in the skin. Also, quaternium-15 sensitivity probably results from the use of cosmetic products in the majority of cases. The cosmetics and personal care products that need preservation all contain water and in such products, formaldehyde-release by hydrolysis is highly likely and indeed – for reasons of antimicrobial activity – desirable. This means that the concept of allergy to the *entire* quaternium-15 molecule, with its six methylol groups intact, is rather unlikely (24).

The subject of the relationship between patch tests to formaldehyde-releasers and formaldehyde contact allergy is summarized in Chapter 2.188 Formaldehyde and discussed in detail in a review article by the author (105). Co-reactivity to the formaldehyde-releaser methenamine may be the result of formaldehyde sensitivity (pseudo-cross-reactions), but may also be caused by true cross-sensitivity (independent of formaldehyde allergy) (94). Contact allergies to quaternium-15 and to the preservative methylchloroisothiazolinone/methylisothiazolinone have been observed to be significantly associated. This probably results from concomitant or successive sensitization to these chemicals in the same or different products rather than from cross-reactivity (87,125).

Presence of quaternium-15 in cosmetic products

In July 2017, quaternium-15 was present in 190 of 69,542 (0.3%) cosmetic products of which the composition is known in EWG's Skin Deep Cosmetics Database, USA (http://www.ewg.org/skindeep/). In 2010, the preservative had been listed in the same database as ingredient in 1.4% of 41,113 products, but none of 6614 moisturizers contained quaternium-15 at that time (37). In the USA, in April 2017, quaternium-15 was present in 217 of 56,714 cosmetic products of which the composition is known in FDA's Voluntary Cosmetic Registration Program (VCRP) (data obtained from FDA, May 2017). Quaternium-15 was present in 32 of 4737 (0.7%) commonly used cosmetic products of which the full composition was known in 2016 in The Contact Allergen Management Program (CAMP) database of the American Contact Dermatitis Society (121).

In the USA, in 2015-2016, 63 diaper wipes and 41 topical diaper preparations from a large retailer were screened for the presence of potential sensitizers. Quaternium-15 was found in 1/63 (2%) disposable diaper wipes and in none of 41 topical diaper preparations (122). In 2014, in Thailand, the labels of 1000 cosmetic products (593 leave-on, 407 rinse-off products) were examined for the presence of preservatives. These were partly purchased in shops and on markets and partly brought in by patients. Quaternioum-15 was present in 2 products (0.02%); in the leave-on products, the percentage was zero and in the rinse-off products 0.5 (123).

In 2013, 60 cosmetic products manufactured and purchased in Israel (40 stay-on and 20 rinse-off products) were investigated for preservatives. According to the labelling, 1 (2%) cosmetics contained quaternium-15. In the stay-on products (hand and body creams), the percentage was zero, whereas one of the 20 shampoos and soaps (5%) was preserved with quaternium-15 (88). In 2009, in the USA, the ingredient lists of 1591 facial cosmetics from one company were screened for the presence of quaternium-15. Quaternium-15 was present in 0% of 132 blushers and 38 bronzers, in 0% of 90 concealers, in 0% of 174 eyeliners, in 0% of 304 eyeshadows, in 1% of 457 foundations, in 19% of 140 loose and pressed powders, and in 5% of 256 mascaras (72).

In 2009, in the USA, the ingredient lists of 796 hair products from one company were screened for the presence of quaternium-15. Quaternium-15 was present in 1% of 279 shampoos, in 0% of 231 conditioners, and in 1% of 286 styling products (73). In 2009, in the USA, the ingredient lists of 657 miscellaneous cosmetics from one company were screened for the presence of quaternium-15. Quaternium-15 was present in 0% of 195 antiperspirants/deodorants, in 0% of 41 powders, in 1% of 167 shaving products, in 1% of 201 sunblocks, and in 4% of 53 wipes (74).

Quaternium-15 was present in only 0.2% of 4133 stay-on products purchased in Germany, 2006-2009 (9). In Germany, in 2006-2009, the labels of 4680 cosmetic products were screened for the presence of preservatives. Quaternium-15 was present in 0.1% of the products, according to labelling information (118). The preservative was present in 1% of 204 cosmetic products (92 shampoos, 61 hair conditioners, 34 liquid soaps, 17 wet tissues) in Sweden, 2008 (11). In 2008, 19.5% of 33,212 cosmetics and toiletries registered in the USA Food and Drug Administration (FDA) Voluntary Cosmetic Registration Database contained a formaldehyde-releaser. They were more frequently used in rinse-off products (27.3%) than in stay-on cosmetics (16.9%). Quaternium-15 was present in 1.4% of all products; in stay-on cosmetics, the percentage was 1.0 and in rinse-off products 2.8 (35).

In the same period, of 496 stay-on cosmetic products present in a local drugstore in The Netherlands and investigated by checking the ingredient labelling, zero products proved to contain this preservative. Any formaldehyde-releaser was found in 122 of this group of stay-on products (24.6%) (35). Of 38 cosmetic products marketed for babies in the UK in 2007, 6 (16%) contained quaternium-15 (66). Quaternium-15 was present in 16 of 1774 (0.9%) cosmetics and toiletries in 2002 and in 13 of 1170 (1.1%) such products in 2005 filed in the Danish Product Register Database (PROBAS) (70). In 1998, 100 moisturizers sold in Sweden were analyzed for the presence and amount of preservatives. Thirty-five products contained a formaldehyde-releaser, of which one contained quaternium-15 (65). In 1996, in the USA, quaternium-15 was present in 3.7% of approximately 20,000 formulae voluntarily registered by cosmetic companies in the FDA Voluntary Cosmetic Registration Database (36).

Amounts of free formaldehyde released by quaternium-15 and chemical analyses

Quaternium-15 can release 6 moles of formaldehyde per mole quaternium-15 and has been shown to do so in 3 minutes in a shampoo heated to steam bath temperatures (106). The actual amount of free formaldehyde that will be released depends on the concentration of quaternium-15, the pH of the product, the temperature (the higher the temperature, the more formaldehyde is present in solution after constant time) (107), the age of the product (upon storage increased levels of formaldehyde will be released), the level of microbial contamination, and the other constituents of the products containing the releaser (20, 107,108,109). The pH may greatly influence the release of formaldehyde. Indeed, in a 0.1% quaternium-15 solution, the amount of formaldehyde was strongly dependent on the pH: <200 ppm formaldehyde at pH >9, 250-300 ppm at pH 7 and 600 ppm at pH 3 (21) (table 2.394.4). Other ingredients in a product may also influence the amount of free formaldehyde. In a protein-free shampoo, 0.1% quaternium-15 released 482 ppm formaldehyde, but in a shampoo with protein only 122 ppm was found. (table 2.394.4). Presumably, the protein forms complexes with released formaldehyde (106). In recent experiments, quaternium-15 in cosmetics released about the same amount of formaldehyde as DMDM hydantoin and imidazolidinyl urea, less than paraformaldehyde and diazolidinyl urea, but more than methenamine and 2-bromo-2-nitropropane-1,3-diol (86).

Examples of reports of free formaldehyde concentrations in products containing quaternium-15 are shown in table 2.394.4. Results of analyses of free formaldehyde in quaternium-15 patch test preparations are presented in Chapter 2.188 Formaldehyde (32). A 1% aqueous solution prepared by a supplier of patch test materials at pH 5.5 contained 0.11% (1100 ppm) free formaldehyde and a 2% solution with pH 4.5 0.21% (2100 ppm) (32).

Table 2.394.4 Reports of free formaldehyde released from products containing quaternium-15 (adapted from [105])

Product	Conc. of quaternium-15		Free formaldehyde (ppm)	Ref.
Bath foam	0.2%		398	21
Cleansing milk	0.2%		482	21
Eye cream	0.2%		266	107
Eyeliner	0.2%		286	107
Lotion	0.2%		525	21
Preservative buffer solution	0.1%		700	22
Preservative solution	0.1%	−pH >9	<200	21
		−pH 7	250-300	
		−pH 3	600	
Product not specified	0.1%		100	103
Shampoo	0.2%		310	21
Shampoo	0.2%		265	107
Shampoo containing protein	0.1%		122	106
	0.2%		187	
	0.4%		237	
	0.8%		278	
Shampoo *not* containing protein	0.1%		482	106
	0.2%		546	
	0.4%		731	
	0.8%		777	
Sunscreen emulsion	0.2%		406	21

Other information

In one study, positive quaternium-15 patch tests in 6 patients were associated with the presence of specific anti-NMBA IgE in their serum. NMBAs are curare-like quaternary ammonium salt neuromuscular blocking agents used for general anesthesia, including suxamethonium, atracurium, vecuronium and pancuronium. NMBAs are responsible for >50% of all anaphylactic reactions during surgery. The main limit of this study was the absence of clinical relevance: none of the patients had previously suffered from anesthetic anaphylaxis (93).

Patch testing and use testing with tretinoin cream and its vehicle containing an unspecified concentration of quaternium-15 in patients allergic to this preservative were negative in 5/6 individuals (58).

OTHER SIDE EFFECTS

Immediate-type reactions

In a group of 664 patch tested patients, there was one (0.2%) immediate contact reactions to quaternium-15 as shown by 'well distinguished erythema' after 30 minutes (71).

Other non-eczematous contact reactions

An engineer involved in the maintenance of machinery in a chicken processing plant developed painful nail dystrophy with thickened and discolored nails, subungual hyperkeratosis and onycholysis (later followed by eczema of the fingertips and interdigital spaces). The cause proved to be contact allergy to quaternium-15 in an industrial cleanser (96).

LITERATURE

1   Uter W, Aberer W, Armario-Hita JC, , Fernandez-Vozmediano JM, Ayala F, Balato A, et al. Current patch test results with the European baseline series and extensions to it from the 'European Surveillance System on Contact Allergy' network, 2007-2008. Contact Dermatitis 2012;67:9-19

2   Latorre N, Borrego L, Fernández-Redondo V, García-Bravo B, Giménez-Arnau AM, Sánchez J, et al. Patch testing with formaldehyde and formaldehyde-releasers: multicenter study in Spain (2005-2009). Contact Dermatitis 2011;65:286-292

3   Travassos AR, Claes L, Boey L, Drieghe J, Goossens A. Non-fragrance allergens in specific cosmetic products. Contact Dermatitis 2011;65:276-285

4   Wetter DA, Yiannias JA, Prakash AV, Davis MD, Farmer SA, el-Azhary RA, et al. Results of patch testing to personal care product allergens in a standard series and a supplemental cosmetic series: an analysis of 945 patients from the Mayo Clinic Contact Dermatitis Group, 2000-2007. J Am Acad Dermatol 2010;63:789-798

5   Adams RM, Maibach HI, Clendenning WE, Fisher AA, Jordan WJ, Kanof N, et al. A five-year study of cosmetic reactions. J Am Acad Dermatol 1985;13:1062-1069

6   Davis MD, Scalf LA, Yiannias JA, Cheng JF, El-Azhary RA, Rohlinger AL, et al. Changing trends and allergens in the patch test standard series. Arch Dermatol 2008;144:67-72

7   Warshaw EM, Buchholz HJ, Belsito DV et al. Allergic patch test reactions associated with cosmetics: Retrospective analysis of cross-sectional data from the North American Contact Dermatitis Group, 2001-2004. J Am Acad Dermatol 2009;60:23-38

8   Schnuch A, Lessmann H, Geier J, Uter W. Contact allergy to preservatives. Analysis of IVDK data 1996-2009. Br J Dermatol 2011;164:1316-1325

9   Mildau G. INCI Labelling of fragrances and preservatives on 5451 randomly selected cosmetic products in Germany, 2006 to 2009. Karlsruhe: Chemisches und Veterinär-Untersuchungsamt, 2010

10 ESSCA Writing Group. The European Surveillance System of Contact Allergies (ESSCA): results of patch testing the standard series, 2004. J Eur Acad Dermatol Venereol 2008;22:174-181

11 Yazar K, Johnsson S, Lind M-L, Boman A, Lidén C. Preservatives and fragrances in selected consumer-available cosmetics and detergents. Contact Dermatitis 2011;64:265-272

12 Fields KS, Nelson T, Powell D. Contact dermatitis caused by baby wipes. J Am Acad Dermatol 2006;54:S230-S232

13 Zug KA, Warshaw EM, Fowler JF Jr, Maibach HI, Belsito DL, Pratt MD, et al. Patch-test results of the North American Contact Dermatitis Group 2005-2006. Dermatitis 2009;20:149-160

14 Pontén A, Aalto-Korte K, Agner T, Andersen KE, Giménez-Arnau AM, Gonçalo M. Patch testing with 2.0% (0.60 mg/cm^2) formaldehyde instead of 1.0% (0.30 mg/cm^2) detects significantly more contact allergy. Contact Dermatitis 2013;68:50-53

15 Fransway AF, Zug KA, Belsito DV, Deleo VA, Fowler JF Jr, Maibach HI, et al. North American Contact Dermatitis Group patch test results for 2007-2008. Dermatitis 2013;24:10-21

16 Warshaw EM, Belsito DV, DeLeo VA, Fowler JF Jr, Maibach HI, Marks JG, et al. North American Contact Dermatitis Group patch-test results, 2003-2004 study period. Dermatitis 2008;19:129-136

17 Warshaw EM, Wang MZ, Mathias CGT, Maibach HI, Belsito DV, Zug KA, et al. Occupational contact dermatitis in hairdressers/cosmetologists; retrospective analysis of North American Contact Dermatitis Group data, 1994 to 2010. Dermatitis 2012;23:258-268

18 Wenk KS, Ehrlich AE. Fragrance series testing in eyelid dermatitis. Dermatitis 2012;23:22-26

19 Odhav A, Belsito DV. Is quaternium-15 a formaldehyde releaser? Correlation between positive patch test reactions to formaldehyde and quaternium-15. Dermatitis 2012;23:39-43

20 Geier J, Lessmann H, Schuch A, Fuchs Th. Kontaktallergien durch formaldehydabspaltende Biozide. Allergologie 1997;20:215-224

21 Benassi CA, Semenzato A, Zaccaria F, Bettero A. High performance liquid chromatographic determination of free formaldehyde in cosmetics preserved with Dowicil 200. J Chromatogr 1990;502:193-200

22 Kijami K, Takeda M, Okaya Y, Takamatsu T, Murase M, Sawamura K, et al. A study on release of formaldehyde from its donor type preservatives. Anal Sci 1991;7(Suppl):913-916

23 Molin S, Bauer A, Schnuch A, Geier J. Occupational contact allergy in nurses: results from the Information Network of Departments of Dermatology 2003–2012. Contact Dermatitis 2015;72:164-171

24 De Groot AC, Blok J, Coenraads P-J. Relationship between formaldehyde and quaternium-15 contact allergy. Influence of strength of patch test reactions. Contact Dermatitis 2010;63:187-191

25 Wetter DA, Davis MDP, Yiannias JA, Cheng JF, Connolly SM, el-Azhary RA, et al. Patch test results from the Mayo Contact Dermatitis Group, 1998–2000. J Am Acad Dermatol 2005;53:416-421

26 Cooper SM, Shaw S. Eyelid dermatitis: an evaluation of 232 patch test patients over 5 years. Contact Dermatitis 2000: 42;291-293

27 Mortz CG, Lauritsen JM, Bindslev-Jensen C, Andersen KE. Prevalence of atopic dermatitis, asthma, allergic rhinitis, and hand and contact dermatitis in adolescents. The Odense Adolescence Cohort Study on Atopic Diseases and Dermatitis. Br J Dermatol 2001;144:523-532

28 Mortz CG, Lauritsen JM, Bindslev-Jensen C, Andersen KE. Contact allergy and allergic contact dermatitis in adolescents: prevalence measures and associations. Acta Derm Venereol 2002;82:352-358

29 Nielsen NH, Linneberg A, Menné T, Madsen F, Frølund L, Dirksen A, et al. Allergic contact sensitization in an adult Danish population: two cross-sectional surveys eight years apart (the Copenhagen Allergy Study). Acta Derm Venereol 2001;81:31-34

30 Warshaw EM, Maibach HI, Taylor JS, Sasseville D, DeKoven JG, Zirwas MJ, et al. North American Contact Dermatitis Group patch test results: 2011-2012. Dermatitis 2015;26:49-59

31 Warshaw EM, Belsito DV, Taylor JS, Sasseville D, DeKoven JG, Zirwas MJ, et al. North American Contact Dermatitis Group patch test results: 2009 to 2010. Dermatitis 2013;24:50-59

32 Emeis D, De Groot AC, Brinkmann J. Determination of formaldehyde in formaldehyde-releaser patch test preparations. Contact Dermatitis 2010;63:57-62

33 Neill SM, Vivier A. Contact dermatitis to trilaureth phosphate. Contact Dermatitis 1984;11:30-31

34 Freeman S, Frederiksen P. Sunscreen allergy. Am J Cont Derm 1990;1:240-243

35 De Groot AC, Veenstra M. Formaldehyde-releasers in cosmetics in the USA and in Europe. Contact Dermatitis 2010;62:221-224

36 Steinberg D. Frequency of use of preservatives in the United States. Paper given at Preservatech, Paris, 1996. www.creative-developments.co.uk/papers/Preservatives%201999.htm (last accessed 20-3-2009).

37 De Groot AC, White IR, Flyvholm M-A, Lensen G, Coenraads P-J. Formaldehyde-releasers in cosmetics: relationship to formaldehyde contact allergy. Part 1. Characterization, frequency and relevance of sensitization, and frequency of use in cosmetics. Contact Dermatitis 2010;62:2-17

38 Carlsen BC, Menné T, Johansen JD. 20 years of standard patch testing in an eczema population with focus on patients with multiple contact allergies. Contact Dermatitis 2007;57:76-83

39 Jong CT, Statham BN, Green CM, King CM, Gawkrodger DJ, Sansom JE, et al. Contact sensitivity to preservatives in the UK 2004–2005: results of a multicenter study. Contact Dermatitis 2007;57:165-168

40 Lazarov A. European Standard Series patch test results from a contact dermatitis clinic in Israel during the 7-year period from 1998 to 2004. Contact Dermatitis 2006;55:73-76

41 Akyol A, Boyvat A, Peksari Y, Gurgey E. Contact sensitivity to standard series allergens in 1038 patients with contact dermatitis in Turkey. Contact Dermatitis 2005;52:333-337

42 Uter W, Hegewald J, Aberer W, Ayala F, Bircher AJ, Brasch J, et al. The European standard series in 9 European countries, 2002/2003 –First results of the European Surveillance System on Contact Allergies. Contact Dermatitis 2005;53:136-145

43 Pratt MD, Belsito DV, DeLeo VA, Fowler JF Jr, Fransway AF, Maibach HI, et al. North American Contact Dermatitis Group patch-test results, 2001–2002 study period. Dermatitis 2004;15:176-183

44 Hasan T, Rantanen T, Alanko K, Harvima RJ, Jolanki R, Kalimo K, et al. Patch test reactions to cosmetic allergens in 1995–1997 and 2000–2002 in Finland –a multicentre study. Contact Dermatitis 2005;53:40-45

45 Machovcova A, Dastychova E, Kostalova D, et al. Common contact sensitizers in the Czech Republic. Patch test results in 12,058 patients with suspected contact dermatitis. Contact Dermatitis 2005;53:162-166

46 Britton JE, Wilkinson SM, English JSC, Gawkrodger DJ, Ormerod AD, Sansom JE, et al. The British standard series of contact dermatitis allergens: validation in clinical practice and value for clinical governance. Br J Dermatol 2003;148:259-264

47 Lindberg M, Edman B, Fischer T, Stenberg B. Time trends in Swedish patch test data from 1992 to 2000. A multi-centre study based on age- and sex-adjusted results of the Swedish standard series. Contact Dermatitis 2007;56:205-210

48 Bruynzeel DP, Diepgen TL, Andersen KE, Brandão FM, Bruze M, Frosch PJ, et al (EECDRG). Monitoring the European Standard Series in 10 centres 1996–2000. Contact Dermatitis 2005;53:146-152

49 Freireich-Astman M, David M, Trattner A. Standard patch test results in patients with contact dermatitis in Israel: age and sex differences. Contact Dermatitis 2007;56:103-107

50 Marks JG Jr, Belsito DV, DeLeo VA, Fowler JF Jr, Fransway AF, Maibach HI, et al. North American Contact Dermatitis Group patch-test results, 1998–2000. Am J Contact Dermat 2003;14:59-68

51 Fall S, Bruze M, Isaksson M, Lidén C, Matura M, Stenberg B, Lindberg M. Contact allergy trends in Sweden – a retrospective comparison of patch test data from 1992, 2000, and 2009. Contact Dermatitis 2015;72:297-304

52 Amin KA, Belsito DV. The aetiology of eyelid dermatitis: a 10-year retrospective analysis. Contact Dermatitis 2006;55:280-285

53 Lee SS, Hong DK, Jeong NJ, Lee JH, Choi YS, Lee AY, et al. Multicenter study of preservative sensitivity in patients with suspected cosmetic contact dermatitis in Korea. J Dermatol 2012;39:677-681

54 Goossens A. Cosmetic contact allergens. Cosmetics 2016, 3, 5; doi:10.3390/cosmetics3010005

55 Wentworth AB, Yiannias JA, Keeling JH, Hall MR, Camilleri MJ, Drage LA, et al. Trends in patch-test results and allergen changes in the standard series: a Mayo Clinic 5-year retrospective review (January 1, 2006, to December 31, 2010). J Am Acad Dermatol 2014;70:269-275

56 Cheng S, Leow YH, Goh CL, Goon A. contact sensitivity to preservatives in Singapore: frequency of sensitization to 11 common preservatives 2006–2011. Dermatitis 2014;25:77-82

57 Katz AS, Sherertz EF. Facial dermatitis: Patch test results and final diagnoses. Am J Cont Dermat 1999;10:153-156

58 Skinner SL, Marks JG. Allergic contact dermatitis to preservatives in topical medicaments. Am J Cont Dermatit 1998;9:199-201

59 Thyssen JP, Uter W, Schnuch A, Linneberg A, Johansen JD. 10-year prevalence of contact allergy in the general population in Denmark estimated through the CE-DUR method. Contact Dermatitis 2007;57:265-272

60 Diepgen TL, Ofenloch RF, Bruze M, Bertuccio P, Cazzaniga S, Coenraads P-J, et al. Prevalence of contact allergy in the general population in different European regions. Br J Dermatol 2016;174:319-329

61 Mortz CG, Bindslev-Jensen C, Andersen KE. Prevalence, incidence rates and persistence of contact allergy and allergic contact dermatitis in The Odense Adolescence Cohort Study: a 15-year follow-up. Brit J Dermatol 2013;168:318-325

62 Thyssen JP, Linneberg A, Menné T, Nielsen NH, Johansen JD. Contact allergy to allergens of the TRUE-test (panels 1 and 2) has decreased modestly in the general population. Br J Dermatol 2009;161:1124-1129

63 Nielsen SH, Menné T. Allergic contact sensitization in an unselected Danish population. The Glostrup Allergy Study, Denmark. Acta Derm Venereol 1992;72:456-460

64 Dotterud LK, Smith-Sivertsen T. Allergic contact sensitization in the general adult population: a population-based study from Northern Norway. Contact Dermatitis 2007;56:10-15

65 Gruvberger B, Bruze M, Tammela M. Preservatives in moisturizers on the Swedish market. Acta Derm Venereol 1998;78:52-56

66 White JML, McFadden JP. Exposure to haptens/contact allergens in baby cosmetic products. Contact Dermatitis 2008;59:176-177

67 De Groot AC, Bruynzeel DP, Bos JD, van der Meeren HL, van Joost T, Jagtman BA, Weyland JW. The allergens in cosmetics. Arch Dermatol 1988;124:1525-1529

68 De Groot AC. Adverse reactions to cosmetics. PhD Thesis, University of Groningen, The Netherlands: 1988, chapter 3.4, pp.105-113

69 De Groot AC. Contact allergy to cosmetics: Causative ingredients. Contact Dermatitis 1987;17:26-34

70 Flyvholm, MA. Preservatives in registered chemical products. Contact Dermatitis 2005;53:27-32

71 Katsarou A, Armenaka M, Ale I, Koufou V, Kalogeromitros, D. Frequency of immediate reactions to the European standard series. Contact Dermatitis 1999;41:276-279

72 Scheman A, Jacob S, Katta R, Nedorost S, Warshaw E, Zirwas M, et al. Part 1 of a 4 part series. Facial cosmetics: trends and alternatives. Data from the American Contact Alternative Group. J Clin Aesthet Dermatol 2011;4:25-30

73 Scheman A, Jacob S, Katta R, Nedorost S, Warshaw E, Zirwas M, et al. Part 2 of a 4 part series. Hair cosmetics: trends and alternatives. Data from the American Contact Alternative Group. J Clin Aesthet Dermatol 2011;4:42-46

74 Scheman A, Jacob S, Katta R, Nedorost S, Warshaw E, Zirwas M, et al. Part 4 of a 4 part series. Miscellaneous products: trends and alternatives in deodorants, antiperspirants, sunblocks, shaving products, powder, and wipes. Data from the American Contact Alternative Group. J Clin Aesthet Dermatol 2011;4:35-39

75   SCCS (Scientific Committee on Consumer Safety). Opinion on quaternium-15, 13-14 December 2011, SCCS/1344/10. Available at: http://ec.europa.eu/health/scientific_committees/consumer_safety/docs/sccs_o_077.pdf

76   Laguna C, de la Cuadra J, Martín-González B, Zaragoza V, Martínez-Casimiro L, Alegre V. Allergic contact dermatitis to cosmetics. Actas Dermosifiliogr 2009;100:53-60

77   Aalto-Korte K, Kuuliala O, Suuronen K, Alanko K. Occupational contact allergy to formaldehyde and formaldehyde releasers. Contact Dermatitis 2008;59:280-289

78   Dooms-Goossens A, de Boulle K, Dooms M, Degreef H. Imidazolidinyl urea dermatitis. Contact Dermatitis 1986;14:322-324

79   Toholka R, Wang Y-S, Tate B, Tam M, Cahill J, Palmer A, Nixon R. The first Australian Baseline Series: Recommendations for patch testing in suspected contact dermatitis. Australas J Dermatol 2015;56:107-115

80   Chow ET, Avolio AM, Lee A, Nixon R. Frequency of positive patch test reactions to preservatives: The Australian experience. Australas J Dermatol 2013;54:31-35

81   Warshaw EM, Schram SE, Maibach HI, Belsito DV, Marks JG Jr, Fowler JF Jr, et al. Occupation-related contact dermatitis in North American health care workers referred for patch testing: cross-sectional data, 1998 to 2004. Dermatitis 2008;19:261-274

82   Guin JD, Kincannon J, Church FL. Baby-wipe dermatitis: preservative-induced hand eczema in parents and persons using moist towelettes. Am J Cont Derm 2001;12:189-192

83   Isaksson M, Bråred-Christensson J, Engfeldt M, Lindberg M, Matura M, Möller H, et al. Swedish Contact Dermatitis Research Group. Patch testing with formaldehyde 2.0% in parallel with 1.0% by the Swedish contact dermatitis research group. Acta Derm Venereol 2014;94:408-410

84   Zina AM, Fanan E, Bundino S. Allergic contact dermatitis from formaldehyde and quaternium-15 in photocopier toner. Contact Dermatitis 2000;43:241

85   Flyholm M-A, Menné T. Allergic contact dermatitis from formaldehyde. Contact Dermatitis 1992;27:27-36

86   Lv C, Hou J, Xie W, Cheng H. Investigation on formaldehyde release from preservatives in cosmetics. Int J Cosm Sci 2015;37:474-478

87   Statham BN, Smith EV, Bodger OG, Green CM, King CM, Ormerod AD, et al. Concomitant contact allergy to methylchloroisothiazolinone/ methylisothiazolinone and formaldehyde-releasing preservatives. Contact Dermatitis 2010;62:56-57

88   Horev L, Isaksson M, Engfeldt M, Persson L, Ingber A, Bruze M. Preservatives in cosmetics in the Israeli market conform well to the EU legislation. J Eur Acad Dermatol Venereol 2015;29:761-766

89   Landeck L, González E, Baden L, Neumann K, Schalock P. Positive concomitant test reactions to allergens in the standard patch test series. Int J Dermatol 2010;49:517-519

90   Mendese G, Beckford A, Demierre M F. Lymphomatoid contact dermatitis to baby wipes. Arch Dermatol 2010;146:934-935

91   De Groot AC, Liem DH. Contact allergy to oleamidopropyl dimethylamine. Contact Dermatitis 1984;11:298-301

92   De Groot AC, Coenraads P-J. Twenty-five years quaternium-15 in the European baseline series: does it deserve its place there? Contact Dermatitis 2010;62:210-220

93   Osdoit S, Guillet M-H, Guillet G. Contact sensitization to quaternium-15 acting as a warning sign for curare allergy. Contact Dermatitis 2011;65:120-122

94   Aalto-Korte K. Simultaneous allergic reactions to quaternium-15 and methenamine. Contact Dermatitis 2000;42:365

95   Boffa MJ, Beck MH. Allergic contact dermatitis from quaternium 15 in Oilatum cream. Contact Dermatitis 1996;35:45-46

96   Marren P, de Berker D, Dawber RPR, Powell S. Occupational contact dermatitis due to quaternium 15 presenting as nail dystrophy. Contact Dermatitis 1991;25:253-255

97   Finch TM, Prais L, Foulds IS. Occupational allergic contact dermatitis from quaternium-15 in an electroencephalography skin preparation gel. Contact Dermatitis 2001;44:44-45

98   Tosti A, Piraccini B, Bardazzo F. Occupational contact dermatitis due to quaternium 15. Contact Dermatitis 1990;23:41-42

99   Cronin E. Photosensitivity to musk ambrette. Contact Dermatitis 1984;11:88-92

100 Neill SM, Du Vivier A. Contact dermatitis to trilaureth phosphate. Contact Dermatitis 1984;11:130-131

101 Parker LU, Taylor JS. A 5-year study of contact allergy to quaternium-15. Am J Contact Dermatitis 1991;2:231-234

102 Sasseville D. Hypersensitivity to preservatives. Dermatol Ther 2004;17:251-263

103 Fransway AF. The problem of preservation in the 1990s: I. Statement of the problem. Solution(s) of the industry, and the current use of formaldehyde and formaldehyde-releasing biocides. Am J Contact Dermatitis 1991;2:6-23

104 Fransway AF, Schmitz NA. The problem of preservation in the 1990s: II. Formaldehyde and formaldehyde-releasing biocides: incidences of cross-reactivity and the significance of the positive response to formaldehyde. Am J Contact Dermatitis 1991;2:78-88

105 De Groot AC, White IR, Flyvholm M-A, Lensen G, Coenraads P-J. Formaldehyde-releasers in cosmetics: relationship to formaldehyde contact allergy. Part 2. Patch test relationship to formaldehyde contact allergy, experimental provocation tests, amount of formaldehyde released and assessment of risk to consumers allergic to formaldehyde. Contact Dermatitis 2010;62:18-31

106 Rosen M, McFarland A. Free formaldehyde in anionic shampoos. J Soc Cosmet Chem 1984;35:157-169

107 Engelhardt H, Klinkner R. Determination of free formaldehyde in the presence of donators in cosmetics by HPLC and post-column derivation. Chromatographia 1985;20:559-565

108 Geier J, Lessmann H, Schnuch A, Uter W. Contact sensitizations in metalworkers with occupational dermatitis exposed to water-based metalworking fluids: results of the research project 'FaSt'. Int Arch Occup Environ Health 2004;77:543-551

109 Geier J, Lessmann H, Becker D, et al. Formaldehydabspalter. Dermatologie in Beruf und Umwelt 2008;56:34-36

110 Yim E, Baquerizo Nole KL, Tosti A. Contact dermatitis caused by preservatives. Dermatitis 2014;25:215-231

111 Shaughnessy CN, Malajian D, Belsito DV. Cutaneous delayed-type hypersensitivity in patients with atopic dermatitis: reactivity to topical preservatives. J Am Acad Dermatol 2014;70:102-107

112 Cahill J, Nixon R. Allergic contact dermatitis to quaternium 15 in a moisturizing lotion. Australas J Dermatol 2005;46:284-285

113 Zhao J, Li LF. Contact sensitization to cosmetic series of allergens in a general population in Beijing. J Cosmet Dermatol 2014;13:68-71

114 DeKoven JG, Warshaw EM, Belsito DV, Sasseville D, Maibach HI, Taylor JS, et al. North American Contact Dermatitis Group Patch Test Results: 2013-2014. Dermatitis 2017;28:33-46

115 Zaragoza-Ninet V, Blasco Encinas R, Vilata-Corell JJ, Pérez-Ferriols A, Sierra-Talamantes C, Esteve-Martínez A, de la Cuadra-Oyanguren J. Allergic contact dermatitis due to cosmetics: A clinical and epidemiological study in a tertiary hospital. Actas Dermosifiliogr 2016;107:329-336

116 Uter W, Rämsch C, Aberer, W, Ayala F, Balato A, Beliauskiene A, et al. The European baseline series in 10 European Countries, 2005/2006 – Results of the European Surveillance System on Contact Allergies (ESSCA). Contact Dermatitis 2009;61:31-38

117 Schwensen JF, Johansen JD, Veien NK, Funding AT, Avnstorp C, Østerballe M, et al. Occupational contact dermatitis in hairdressers: an analysis of patch test data from the Danish Contact Dermatitis Group, 2002–2011. Contact Dermatitis 2014;70:233-237

118 Uter W, Yazar K, Kratz EM, Mildau G, Lidén C. Coupled exposure to ingredients of cosmetic products: II. Preservatives. Contact Dermatitis 2014;70:219-226

119 Giménez-Arnau AM, Deza G, Bauer A, Johnston GA, Mahler V, Schuttelaar ML, et al. Contact allergy to preservatives: ESSCA* results with the baseline series, 2009-2012. J Eur Acad Dermatol Venereol 2017;31:664-671

120 Lubbes S, Rustemeyer T, Sillevis Smitt JH, Schuttelaar ML, Middelkamp-Hup MA. Contact sensitization in Dutch children and adolescents with and without atopic dermatitis - a retrospective analysis. Contact Dermatitis 2017;76:151-159

121 Beene KM, Scheman A, Severson D, Reeder MJ. Prevalence of preservatives across all product types in the Contact Allergen Management Program. Dermatitis 2017;28:81-87

122 Yu J, Treat J, Chaney K, Brod B. Potential allergens in disposable diaper wipes, topical diaper preparations, and disposable diapers: under-recognized etiology of pediatric perineal dermatitis. Dermatitis 2016;27:110-118

123 Bunyavaree M, Kasemsarn P, Boonchai W. Cosmetic preservative labelling on the Thai market. Contact Dermatitis 2016;74:217-221

124 Uter W, Amario-Hita JC, Balato A, Ballmer-Weber B, Bauer A, Belloni Fortina A, et al. European Surveillance System on Contact Allergies (ESSCA): results with the European baseline series, 2013/14. J Eur Acad Dermatol Venereol. 2017 Jun 19. doi: 10.1111/jdv.14423. [Epub ahead of print]

125 Lynch MD, White JM, McFadden JP, Wang Y, White IR, Banerjee P. A dynamic landscape of allergen associations in delayed-type cutaneous hypersensitivity. Br J Dermatol 2017;176:184-196

2.395 QUATERNIUM-22

IDENTIFICATION

Description/definition   : Quaternium-22 is the quaternary ammonium salt reported to conform generally to the formula shown below
Chemical class(es)   : Carbohydrates; quaternary ammonium compounds
Chemical/IUPAC name   : 2-Hydroxyethyl-dimethyl-[3-[[(2R,3S,4R,5R)-2,3,4,5,6-pentahydroxyhexanoyl]-amino]propyl]azanium;chloride
Other names   : 3-(D-Gluconoylamino)propyl(2-hydroxyethyl)dimethylammonium chloride
CAS registry number (s)   : 51812-80-7; 82970-95-4
EC number(s)   : 257-440-3
CIR review(s)   : J Am Coll Toxicol 1995;14:485-497 (access: www.cir-safety.org/ingredients)
Function(s) in cosmetics : EU: antistatic; film forming; hair conditioning. USA: antistatic agents; film formers
Patch testing   : 0.1% and 0.01% water (1,2)
Molecular formula   : $C_{13}H_{29}ClN_2O_7$

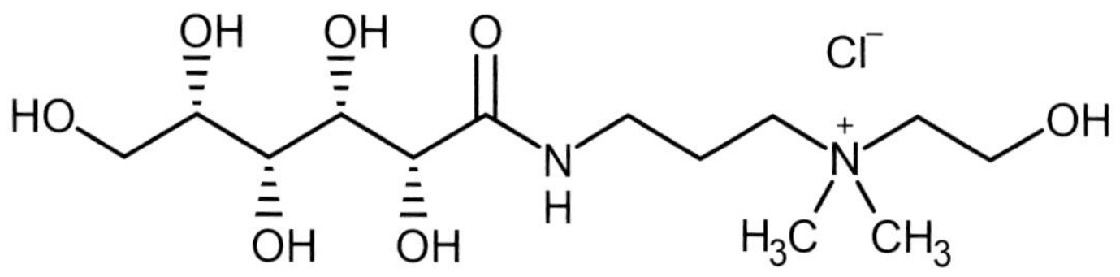

CONTACT ALLERGY

Case reports and case series

A woman presented with a 9-month history of swelling and itching of the upper eyelids, always appearing within 2 days of using a particular mascara, purchased just before the onset of her symptoms. She could wear other eye make-up (including both eyeshadow and mascaras) without any problem. Patch tests with the standard series, a cosmetics series and the mascara gave a positive reaction to the mascara and a non-relevant reaction to nickel. When tested with the ingredients of this cosmetic product, obtained from the manufacturer, there were positive reactions to quaternium-22 0.1% and 0.01% in water and to another ingredient, shellac. Control testing in 23 patients with quaternium-22 0.01% and 0.1% in water was negative. After stopping the use of this mascara, the patient's problem has disappeared and did not recur (2).

A woman had consulted several practitioners for a recurrent itchy dermatitis of her eyelids, which she related to a newly bought mascara. Patch tests with the ICDRG standard series, additional allergens and the patient's own topical products and cosmetics gave a positive reaction to the suspected mascara. When tested with its ingredients, there were positive reactions to quaternium-22 0.1% and 0.01% in water (but negative to 0.001% water) and to another ingredient, shellac. Quaternium-22 was retested in a third session, which confirmed contact allergy to it (1).

Presence in cosmetic products and chemical analyses

In the USA, in April 2017, quaternium-22 was present in 35 of 56,714 cosmetic products of which the composition is known in FDA's Voluntary Cosmetic Registration Program (VCRP) (data obtained from FDA, May 2017). In April 2017, quaternium-22 was present in 18 of 65,434 cosmetic products of which the composition is known in EWG's Skin Deep Cosmetics Database, USA (http://www.ewg.org/skindeep/).

LITERATURE

1   Le Coz CJ, Leclere JM, Arnoult E, Raison-Peyron N, Pons-Guiraud A, Vigan M. Allergic contact dermatitis from shellac in mascara. Contact Dermatitis 2002;46:149-152
2   Scheman AJ. Contact allergy to quaternium-22 and shellac in mascara. Contact Dermatitis 1998;38:342-343

2.396   QUININE

IDENTIFICATION

Description/definition	: Quinine is an alkaloid from the bark of *Cinchona officinalis,* which conforms to the formula shown below
Chemical class(es)	: Amines; heterocyclic compounds
Chemical/IUPAC name	: (R)-[(2S,4S,5R)-5-Ethenyl-1-azabicyclo[2.2.2]octan-2-yl]-(6-methoxyquinolin-4-yl)methanol
Other names	: Chininum; cinchonan-9-ol, 6'-methoxy-, (8α,9R)-; 6'-methoxycinchonan-9-ol
CAS registry number (s)	: 130-95-0
EC number(s)	: 205-003-2
Merck Index monograph	: 9447
Function(s) in cosmetics	: EU: denaturant; hair conditioning; masking. USA: denaturants; fragrance ingredients; hair conditioning agents
EU cosmetic restrictions	: Regulated in Annex III/21 of the Regulation (EC) No. 1223/2009
Patch testing	: Quinine sulfate 1% pet. (Chemotechnique)
Molecular formula	: $C_{20}H_{24}N_2O_2$

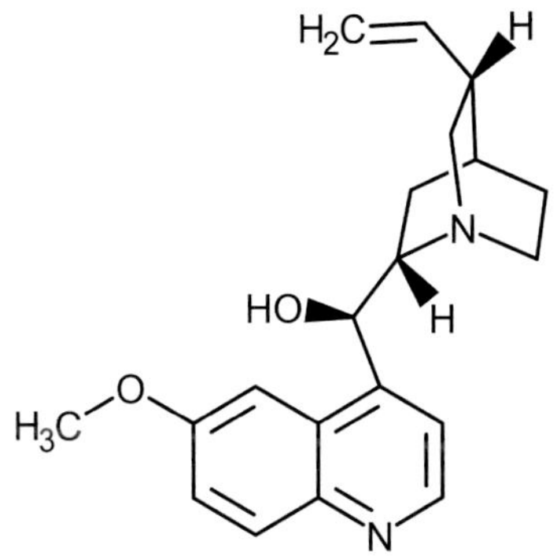

GENERAL

Quinine is an alkaloid obtained from the bark of various species of *Cinchona* trees. Sensitization to quinine is well-recognized, though is now rarely seen. Sensitization used to occur frequently from contraceptives containing quinine as a spermicidal agent (2), or from quinine-containing hair lotions (1,2), even today (22). It is still widely used in the pharmaceutical industry (e.g., for the treatment of muscle cramps) and by food manufacturers, mainly for tonic water and bitter lemon (3). Systemic contact dermatitis with a generalized rash or recurrence of previous dermatitis from drinking tonic or bitter lemon may be observed in sensitized patients (1,2), as may immediate-type reactions with urticaria (24). The literature on quinine allergy from before 1960 is reviewed in ref. 2. The more recent literature is reviewed in this chapter only briefly and not complete. A systematic review of adverse reactions to quinine, with focus on acute, immune-mediated reactions, has been published in 2016 (13).

CONTACT ALLERGY

Case reports and case series
In the period 1996-2013, in a tertiary referral center in Valencia, Spain, 5419 patients were patch tested. Of these, 628 individuals had allergic contact dermatitis to cosmetics. Quinine was the responsible allergen in one case (11). One patient had ACD from quinine in a hair lotion; the dermatitis exacerbated after drinking tonic water (1).

Another patient also reacted to quinine in hair lotion; he was previously sensitized by his wife's quinine-containing contraceptive pessary (2). A woman had ACD from quinine in a hair lotion used to treat androgenetic alopecia (22). The literature on quinine allergy from hair tonics older than 1960 is reviewed in ref. 2.

Contact allergy to quinine in non-cosmetic products
Three men had connubial (or 'consort') ACD from quinine in their wives' contraceptive pessary (2). Another patient had generalized itching and a macular eruption from allergy to quinine in bitter lemon drink; he had probably previously been sensitized by quinine in a hair lotion (2). A child reacted to quinine in a topical pharmaceutical product (3). A man working in a factory producing quinine had a dermatitis resembling atopic dermatitis, which exacerbated each time he came in contact with quinine; there was a positive patch test to 1% quinine sulfate (9). The literature on quinine allergy from non-cosmetic sources older than 1960 is reviewed in ref. 2

Cross-reactions, pseudo-cross-reactions and co-reactions
Photo-cross-sensitivity to quinidine (4); photo-cross-sensitivity to quindoxin (12).

Other information
In a systematic literature review, 142 patients with immune-mediated adverse reactions to quinine were identified up to 2015. Forty-four of these patients had dermatological manifestations: photosensitive dermatitis/eczema (n=12), photosensitive erythema (n=3), photosensitive vasculitis (n=1), photosensitive lichen planus (n=1), fixed drug eruption (n=9), contact dermatitis/eczema (n=9), lichen planus (n=2), systemic erythematous rash (n=3), urticaria (n=1), toxic epidermal necrolysis (n=1), exfoliative dermatitis (n=1), and photosensitive mycosis fungoides-like eruption (n=1 [10]) (13). Fixed drug eruptions from oral quinine have been reviewed in 2014 (14). Patients with such reactions, often from drinking tonic water, have been reported in refs. 15-20 (examples). Patch tests were either positive (19), negative (20) or not performed. Other drug eruptions from quinine reported include a photodistributed lichenoid drug eruption (21).

Presence in cosmetic products and chemical analyses
In the USA, in April 2017, quinine was present in 2 of 56,714 cosmetic products of which the composition is known in FDA's Voluntary Cosmetic Registration Program (VCRP) (data obtained from FDA, May 2017). In August 2017, quinine was present in zero of 70,704 cosmetic products of which the composition is known in EWG's Skin Deep Cosmetics Database, USA (http://www.ewg.org/skindeep/).

OTHER SIDE EFFECTS

Irritant contact dermatitis
Many workers in a factory producing quinine suffered from irritant contact dermatitis (9).

Photosensitivity
A woman developed an eczematous photodistributed skin eruption while taking oral quinine hydrochloride. Phototesting revealed normal erythema thresholds for UV-A and UV-B light, but a drastically lowered threshold for UV-A light after the patient had been taking oral quinine for 10 days. According to the authors, the clinical picture, the results of the phototests, and the histopathology suggested a photoallergic mechanism, but, unfortunately, photopatch tests were not performed (5). A man developed an eczematous eruption on the face and dorsal aspects of the hands after 3 weeks' oral treatment with quinine. The photoreaction cleared within a week of quinine being stopped. UVA and UVB erythema threshold determinations were normal. A photopatch test was positive for irradiated quinine down to a concentration of 0.01% and for unirradiated quinine to 0.5%. There was a photo-cross-reaction to the isomer quinidine down to a concentration of 0.01% (4). A patient working in a factory producing quinine had occupational photoallergic contact dermatitis from quinine (9).

Other patients with photosensitivity of an eczematous type to systemically administered quinine (often for muscle cramps) have been reported in refs. 6,7, 8 and 23 (examples). Only in some of these patients were photo-patch tests performed and positive (8,23). An industrial chemist had photoallergic contact dermatitis from quinine. The photopatch test was positive and he showed a photo-cross-reaction to quindoxin (12).

Immediate-type reactions
A woman experienced, 15 minutes after drinking a glass of 'Schweppes', sneezing, urticaria, respiratory discomfort, and a feeling of chest oppression. Prick tests were positive to the drink and to its ingredient quinine (24). Immediate-type reactions to quinine have been described in a few publications (25,26,27).

LITERATURE
1   Tapadinhas C, Dias M, Conchon I, Pereira F, Cardoso J. Contact dermatitis due to quinine-containing hair lotion. Contact Dermatitis 1994;31:127
2   Calnan CD, Caron GA. Quinine sensitivity. Br Med J 1961;ii(5269):1750-1752
3   Dias M, Conchon I, Vale, T. Allergic contact dermatitis from quinine. Contact Dermatitis 1994;30:121-122
4   Liunggren B, Hindsén M, Isaksson M. Systemic quinine photosensitivity with photoepicutaneous cross-reactivity to quinidine. Contact Dermatitis 1992;26:1-4
5   Ljunggren B, Sjovall P. Systemic quinine photosensitivity. Arch Dermatol 1986;122:909-911
6   Ferguson J, Addo HA, Johnson BE, Frain-Bell W. Quinine-induced photosensitivity: clinical and experimental studies. Br J Dermatol 1987;117:631-640
7   Diffey BL, Farr PM, Adams SJ. The action spectrum in quinine photosensitivity. Br J Dermatol 1988:118:679-685
8   Guzzo C, Kaidbey K. Persistent light reactivity from systemic quinine. Photodermatol Photoimmunol

Photomed 1990;7:166-168

9   Hardie RA, Savin JA, White DA, Pumford S. Quinine dermatitis: Investigation of a factory outbreak. Contact Dermatitis 1978;4:121-124

10   Okun MM, Henner M, Paulson C. A quinine-induced drug reaction of photosensitive distribution with histological features mimicking mycosis fungoides. Clin Exp Dermatol 1994;19:246-248

11   Zaragoza-Ninet V, Blasco Encinas R, Vilata-Corell JJ, Pérez-Ferriols A, Sierra-Talamantes C, Esteve-Martínez A, de la Cuadra-Oyanguren J. Allergic contact dermatitis due to cosmetics: A clinical and epidemiological study in a tertiary hospital. Actas Dermosifiliogr 2016;107:329-336

12   Johnson BE, Zaynoun S, Gardiner JM, Frain-Bell W. A study of persistent light reaction in quindoxin and quinine photosensitivity. Br J Dermatol 1975;93(Suppl.11):21-22

13   Liles NW, Page EE, Liles AL, Vesely SK, Raskob GE, George JN. Diversity and severity of adverse reactions to quinine: A systematic review. Am J Hematol 2016;91:461-466

14   Genest G, Thomson DM. Fixed drug eruption to quinine: a case report and review of the literature. J Allergy Clin Immunol Pract 2014;2:469-470

15   Lonsdale-Eccles E, Wallett A, Ward AM. A case of fixed drug eruption secondary to quinine in tonic water presenting to a sexual health clinic. Sex Transm Infect 2014;90:356-357

16   Ohira A, Yamaguchi S, Miyagi T, Yamamoto Y, Yamada S, Shiohira H, et al. Fixed eruption due to quinine in tonic water: a case report with high-performance liquid chromatography and ultraviolet A analyses. J Dermatol 2013;40:629-631

17   Asero R. Fixed drug eruptions caused by tonic water. J Allergy Clin Immunol 2003;111:198-199

18   Muso Y, Kentarou O, Itami S, Yoshikawa K. Fixed eruption due to quinine: report of two cases. J Dermatol 2007;34:385-386

19   Bel B, Jeudy G, Bouilly D Dalac S, Vabres P, Collet E. Fixed eruption due to quinine contained in tonic water: positive patch-testing. Contact Dermatitis 2009;61:242-244

20   Gázquez V, Gómez C, Daimau G, Gaig P, Landeyo J. A case of fixed drug eruption due to quinine. Clin Exp Dermatol 2009;34:95-97

21   Natkunarajah J, Stitson RN, Harland CC. A florid rash during summer. Photodistributed lichenoid drug eruption (LDE) secondary to quinine. Clin Exp Dermatol 2010;35:e83-84

22   Hernández-Bel P, de la Cuadra-Oyanguren J, Martínez L, López J, Agustí A, Alegre V. Contact allergic dermatitis to quinine in an anti-hair loss lotion. Actas Dermosifiliogr 2010;101:373-375

23   Hickey JR, Dunnill GS, Sansom JE. Photoallergic reaction to systemic quinine sulphate. Contact Dermatitis 2007;57:384-386

24   Kanny G, Flabbée J, Morisset M, Moneret Vautrin DA. Allergy to quinine and tonic water. Eur J Intern Med 2003;14:395-396

25   Cundall R. Idiosyncrasy to quinine in bitter lemon. Br Med J 1964;20:1638

26   González R, Merchán R, Crespo JF, Rodríguez J. Allergic urticaria from tonic water. Allergy 2002;57:52

27   Pin I, Dor P, Vervloet D, Senft M, Charpin J. Immediate hypersensitivity to quinine. Presse Med 1985;14:967-969

2.397   RESORCINOL

IDENTIFICATION

Description/definition	: Resorcinol is the phenol that conforms to the formula shown below
Chemical class(es)	: Color additives - hair; phenols
Chemical/IUPAC name	: Benzene-1,3-diol
Other names	: CI 76505; 1,3-benzenediol
CAS registry number (s)	: 108-46-3
EC number(s)	: 203-585-2
CIR review(s)	: J Am Coll Toxicol 1986;5:167-203 (access: www.cir-safety.org/ingredients)
SCCS opinion(s)	: SCCS/1270/09 (24); SCCP/1117/07 (25)
Merck Index monograph	: 9546
Function(s) in cosmetics	: EU: hair dyeing; masking. USA: antioxidants; denaturants; external analgesics; fragrance ingredients; hair colorants
EU cosmetic restrictions	: Regulated in Annex III/22 of the Regulation (EC) No. 1223/2009
Patch testing	: 1% pet. (Chemotechnique, SmartPracticeCanada); 2% pet. (SmartPracticeEurope, SmartPracticeCanada)
Molecular formula	: $C_6H_6O_2$

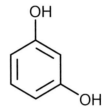

GENERAL

Resorcinol is a simple aromatic chemical (1,3-benzenediol) that has widespread use as a coupler in hair dyes, in food (for example as an anti-browning agent in crustaceans), and formally, because of its (alleged) itch relieving, keratolytic and antifungal properties, in anti-acne preparations, anti-wart ointments, antipsoriatic creams, exfoliative preparations, suppositories, eye drops and Castellani's paint. It is also used in radiotherapy dyes or patch test marking ink (43), dyes, celluloid, tanning, plastic, rubber, explosives industries, photoduplicating inks and photographic developers (70).

Resorcinol has been classified as a moderate (44) and strong (45) sensitizer. Despite this, contact allergy to this chemical was (52) and is very infrequent. Most cases have been caused in the past by Castellani paint, anti-wart treatments in France and Belgium, topical anti-acne preparations and a few cases by its presence as a coupler in hair dye. For the chemistry of hair dying see Chapter 2.359 *p*-Phenylenediamine.

In older literature, some cases of intoxication caused by percutaneous absorption of resorcinol from topical products containing resorcinol (2%-40%) with methemoglobinemia or thyroid dysfunction have been described.

CONTACT ALLERGY

Patch testing in groups of patients

Results of studies patch testing resorcinol in consecutive patients suspected of contact dermatitis (routine testing) and in groups of *selected* patients (e.g., hairdressers, patients tested with a hairdressing series, patients suspected of hair dye allergy) are shown in table 2.397.1. In three studies in which routine testing was performed, low rates of sensitization of 0.1% to 0.5% were found (10,29,46). Most sensitizations were caused by topical medicaments, including anti-wart treatments (10,46).

Results of studies patch testing resorcinol in groups of *selected* patients are shown in table 2.397.1. In 12 investigations, frequencies of sensitization have ranged from 0.4% to 6.3%, but 7 scored lower than 1% and 9 lower than 2% positive patch test reactions. The highest frequency (6.3%) was observed in a group of 175 patients from the UK suspected of hair dye allergy, but the relevance of the 11 positive patch tests was not mentioned (1). Other high frequencies of sensitization of 5% resp. 4.7% were found in a very small study of 42 patients with allergic contact cheilitis, in which there were 2 positive patch tests to resorcinol (36) and in a group of 106 hairdressers with contact dermatitis (35). In the former study (36), one of 2 reactions was relevant but the causative product was not mentioned; in the latter investigation (35), the issue of relevance was not addressed. In fact, relevance was not discussed at all or not specified for resorcinol in the majority of the studies. In a recent Belgian publication describing 5 resorcinol-allergic patients, 2 reactions were caused by hair dye, one by a topical pharmaceutical, one by a skin marker and the fifth was a cross-reaction from resorcinol monobenzoate sensitization causing dermatitis in spectacle frames (43).

Table 2.397.1 Patch testing in groups of patients

Years and Country	Test conc. & vehicle	Number of patients tested	positive (%)		Selection of patients (S); Relevance (R); Comments (C)	Ref.
Routine testing						
2007-2008, 9 European countries [a]	1% pet.	2939	3	(0.1%)	R: not specified	29
1999-2000 France		983	5	(0.5%)	R: most were caused by anti-wart treatments	46
1989-1990 Portugal		5911	6	(0.1%)	R: all were caused by topical medicaments	10
Testing in groups of selected patients						
1990-2015 Belgium	1% pet.	1187	5	(0.4%)	S: patients tested with the hairdressers' series, patients who had used resorcinol topically, or patients investigated for cross-reactivity; R: 2 reactions were caused by hair dye, one by a topical pharmaceutical, one from a skin marker and the fifth was a cross-reaction from resorcinol monobenzoate sensitization causing dermatitis in spectacle frames	43
2002-2011 Denmark		283	1	(0.4%)	S: hairdressers with contact dermatitis; R: not stated	32
2001-2011 USA	1% pet.	41	2	(5%)	S: patients with allergic contact cheilitis; R: 1 of 2 relevant	36
2000-2008 USA	1% pet.	209		(1.9%)	S: patients tested with a hairdresser's series; R: 50%	21
1997-2007 UK	1% pet.	175	11	(6.3%)	S: patients suspected of hair dye allergy; R: not stated	1
1999-2004 UK		501	2	(0.4%)	S: patients tested with the hairdressing series; R: only reactions that were of current or past relevance were collected	34
2000-2002 Finland		478		(0.4%)	S: patients tested with a hairdressing series; R: not stated	19
1990-1999 Italy	1% pet.	209	2	(0.9%)	S: hairdressers with contact dermatitis; R: not specified	3
1995-1996 Finland		443		(0.7%)	S: patients tested with a hairdressing series; R: not stated	19
1985-1994 Greece	2% pet.	106	5	(4.7%)	S: hairdressers with contact dermatitis; R: not specified	35
1988-1991, 8 European countries [a]		354	2	(0.6%)	S: hairdressers with hand dermatitis; R: not stated	22
1985-1990 Italy	2% pet.	302	4	(1.3%)	S: hairdressers with contact dermatitis; R: not specified	23

[a] Study by the ESSCA (European Surveillance System on Contact Allergies)

Case reports and case series

Resorcinol was responsible for 3 out of 399 cases of cosmetic allergy where the causal allergen was identified in a study of the NACDG, USA, 1977-1983 (2). In a 4-month-period in 1996, 475 patients with contact allergy to 'cosmetic ingredients' were collected in 5 centers in Belgium, UK and Germany. There was one reaction to resorcinol; relevance was not stated (20). Two individuals developed allergic contact dermatitis from hair dyes caused by resorcinol (43). A hairdresser developed occupational hand dermatitis after being sensitized to resorcinol from dyeing her own hair (11). An unknown number of patients was cited to have developed allergic contact dermatitis from resorcinol used as a dye coupler (39,40, data cited in ref. 41).

Contact allergy to resorcinol in non-cosmetic products

Topical pharmaceutical preparations

Of eight early cases of contact allergy to resorcinol, 5 were caused by topical medicaments and one by resorcinol in eye drops; in two patients, the allergy was probably of past relevance from previous use of resorcinol-containing topical drugs (5). In France, in the period 1992-1999, contact sensitization to resorcinol was found in 24 patients, who all but one had previously used an anti-wart ointment containing resorcinol. All developed contact dermatitis at the site of application of the ointment, with generalized urticaria (4 cases), pompholyx (1 case), and generalized papulovesicular rash with pompholyx (6 cases) (46,70). Four patients from the Netherlands had allergic contact dermatitis from resorcinol. Two were sensitized by an anti-acne cream and one by a suppository containing resorcinol and causing perianal dermatitis; the fourth patient probably had been primarily sensitized by oral hexylresorcinol and later developed facial dermatitis from a cream containing resorcinol (68).

A man developed a bullous allergic contact dermatitis of the legs from contact allergy to resorcinol in an anti-wart ointment used by his wife on the soles of her feet (connubial contact dermatitis, contact dermatitis by proxy). Because of cold feet, the woman would habitually rub her feet against the legs of her husband in bed. The patient had suffered from allergic contact dermatitis as a child from a topical anti-wart treatment (69). One patient had periorbital and eyelid ACD from resorcinol in a pharmaceutical eye ointment (7). Resorcinol in an anti-acne product caused ACD in one patient (8). Resorcinol ointment caused ACD in another individual superimposed on psoriasis (16).

A woman developed allergic contact dermatitis from resorcinol in an anti-wart treatment (43). Two patients had anal dermatitis from contact allergy to resorcinol in anal suppositories (54). Three young women became sensitized to resorcinol from their anti-acne medication containing 2% resorcinol (66). During 1975 and 1976, three cases of contact allergy to resorcinol in Castellani paint have been observed in one clinic in London, UK (50). Several single case reports of contact allergy to resorcinol in Castellani paint have been published (17,47,48,49).

Other products

Two patients reacted to resorcinol in Castellani paint used as radiotherapy marker dye (9,18). Two patients (15) and another two (43) had allergic contact dermatitis from resorcinol in Castellani paint used as marker for patch tests. A young boy developed an allergic reaction to a black henna tattoo. When patch tested, he reacted only to resorcinol, not to PPD or other para-dyes which are known to cause allergic reactions to henna tattoos. The authors present the case as ACD from resorcinol in the henna tattoo, but the used henna ink was not analyzed and, therefore, the possible role of resorcinol in it remained uncertain (76).

Cross-reactions, pseudo-cross-reactions and co-reactions

(Possible) cross-reactions are summarized in table 2.397.2.

Table 2.397.2 Possible cross-reactions to / from resorcinol

Chemical	Frequency of cross-reactions and references [a]
Catechol	4, cited in ref. 6
Hexylresorcinol	2/7 cases (5); 68; *not* to hexylresorcinol (46)
Hydroquinone	6/17 cases (46); 4/8 cases (5); 1/3 cases (70); 13; 54; 4, cited in ref. 6
Hydroxyhydroquinone	1/4 cases (5)
Orcinol	4/8 cases (5)
Phenol	3/8 cases (5); 9
p-Phenylenediamine	28
Phloroglucinol	1/5 cases (5)
Pyrocatechol	7/14 cases (46); 3/8 cases (5); 4/4 cases (70); 13; 54
Pyrogallol	5/8 cases (5); 9/19 cases (46)
Resorcinol acetate	7/8 cases (5); 68
Resorcinol benzoate	6/6 cases (70); 15/19 cases (46); 8; 43
Salicylaldehyde	1/2 cases (70); 2/17 cases (46)

[a] if only references are given, the number of cross-reactions is either one or unknown

Presence in cosmetic products and chemical analyses

In July 2017, resorcinol was present in 175 of 69,542 cosmetic products of which the composition is known in EWG's Skin Deep Cosmetics Database, USA (http://www.ewg.org/skindeep/). In the USA, in April 2017, resorcinol was present in 1649 of 56,714 cosmetic products of which the composition is known in FDA's Voluntary Cosmetic Registration Program (VCRP) (data obtained from FDA, May 2017). In 2016, in Sweden, the labels of 26 oxidative hair dye products advertised with the signal words organic, natural or similar, or sold/used at a hair dressing salon advertised with the same terminology, were screened for the presence of known contact allergens. Resorcinol was present in 10 (38%) products (27). Of 15 hair dyes advertised as 'hypoallergenic', 'para-phenylenediamine-free', or 'non-allergenic', purchased in South Korea in 2015, 9 (60%) proved to contain resorcinol (75). In 2013-2014, labeled ingredient information from 252 home use and professional hair dye products (210 permanent and 42 non-permanent dyes) from 48 brands sold in Bangkok, Thailand, was collected to identify the type and frequency of potent contact sensitizers. Resorcinol was present in 161 (64%) products (26).

In southern Germany, in 2013-2014, the labels of 924 permanent oxidative hair dyes were checked for the presence of hair dye components. There were 334 retail products (of seven different brands) and 590 professional products (of six different brands). The 924 products analyzed revealed a total of 58 different hair dye components, with retail products containing 32 and professional products 52. Resorcinol was present in 78% of the 924 products (31).

In 2013, in Korea, the labels of 99 oxidative hair dyes produced by Korean domestic manufacturers were examined for potent skin sensitizers. Resorcinol was found to be present in 77 (77%) of the hair dyes (42). In the USA, in 2012, ingredient labels of 107 different consumer oxidative hair dyes from 10 different companies were assessed in stores across the city of Phoenix, Arizona. Resorcinol was present in 89% of the products (33). In 2011, labels and other information on 365 hair dye products (282 permanent dyes, 79 semi-permanent dyes, 4 direct dyes) available on the Danish market (159 hair dyes for private use, 206 for professional use by hairdressers) were collected to identify the presence of sensitizers. Resorcinol was present in 218 (60%) products (30).

In April 2010, in Spain, 111 consumer-available oxidative hair dye products of 19 brands were purchased to check the labeling for sensitizers. A systematic selection of products to be purchased from each hair dye brand was applied, including the darkest blonde shade available, one 'regular' light brown shade, one 'regular' dark brown shade, one 'regular' black shade, and two further shades with different colours (red, blue, purple, etc.). In this group of 111 hair dyes, resorcinol was present in 81% of the products (38). In the period August - October 2008, the labels of 122 oxidative hair dye products on the Swedish market were examined for the presence of hair dye substances categorized as potent skin sensitizers. Resorcinol was present in 100 (82%) of these products (37).

OTHER SIDE EFFECTS

Irritant contact dermatitis
Resorcinol may cause dose-dependent irritation of the skin or irritant contact dermatitis.

Other non-eczematous contact reactions
In several (review) articles on exogenous ochronosis caused by hydroquinone, it has been stated that this reaction can also be induced by topical resorcinol (14,51,55,56,57,58). The author has been able to locate only one original report of possible exogenous ochronosis by resorcinol (59). A woman had treated extensive leg ulceration for 13 years with an ointment containing 12.5% resorcinol as an antiseptic. Pigmentation was observed around the areas where the drug had been applied but also far apart in the skin and cartilage of the ears and in the sclerae. The urine was dark; the authors assumed that this resulted from a polymer of resorcinol. Histological study was not carried out, however, which means that a definitive diagnosis of exogenous ochronosis from resorcinol lacks an important diagnostic criterion (59). More information on exogenous ochronosis can be found in Chapter 2.238 Hydroquinone.

A rusty red pigmentation of various color intensities and dimensions, mainly in the thenar and hypothenar eminences, on the pulps of all the fingers, and in some cases on the flexor surface of the fingers and on the palms of both hands in tire makers was ascribed to contact with resorcinol (incorrectly called resorcinAl throughout the article) (67).

Systemic side effects
Resorcinol has an antithyroid activity. As the drug can penetrate the skin, some cases of hypothyroidism and myxedema have been described from topical application of resorcinol, especially on ulcerated surfaces. All symptoms disappeared after discontinuation of treatment with resorcinol (59,60,74). In children, methemoglobine-mia has been observed caused by the absorption of resorcinol, in some cases applied to wounds (62,63,72). In another infant, the application of an ointment containing 12.5% resorcinol to the napkin area produced cyanosis, a maculopapular eruption, hemolytic anemia and hemoglobinuria. The author of that article in literature found seven cases of acute poisoning in babies, as a consequence of topical resorcinol application, in some instances to limited areas; five fatalities were recorded (64). Two young adults treated once daily with a peeling paste containing 40% resorcinol for pustular acne after three to four weeks developed adverse reactions consisting of pallor, dizziness, cold sweat, tremors, collapse and violet-black urine (65).

The literature on systemic side effects has been reviewed in refs. 61 and 73.

Miscellaneous side effects
Resorcinol may have caused urticaria (71, no data available, article not read).

LITERATURE
1   Basketter DA, English J. Cross-reactions among hair dye allergens. Cut Ocular Toxicol 2009;28:104-106
2   Adams RM, Maibach HI, Clendenning WE, Fisher AA, Jordan WJ, Kanof N, et al. A five-year study of cosmetic reactions. J Am Acad Dermatol 1985;13:1062-1069
3   Iorizzo M, Parente G, Vincenzi C, Pazzaglia M, Tosti A. Allergic contact dermatitis in hairdressers; frequency and source of sensitization. Eur J Dermatol 2002;12:179-182
4   Bloch B. Ekzem Pathogenese. Arch Derm Syph (Berl.) 1924;145:34-82
5   Keil H. Group reactions in contact dermatitis due to resorcinol. Arch Dermatol 1962;86:212-216
6   Hemmer W, Focke M, Wolf-Abdolvahab S, Bracun R, Wantke F, et al. Group allergy to tri- and ortho-diphenols (catechols) in a patient sensitized by propyl gallate. Contact Dermatitis 1996;35:110-112

7   Massone L, Anonide A, Borghi S, Usiglio D. Contact dermatitis of the eyelids from resorcinol in an ophthalmic ointment. Contact Dermatitis 1993;29:49

8   Nakagawa M, Kawai K, Kawai K. Cross-sensitivity between resorcinol, resorcinol monobenzoate and phenyl salicylate. Contact Dermatitis 1992;27:199

9   Pecegueiro M. Contact dermatitis due to resorcinol in a radiotherapy dye. Contact Dermatitis 1992;26:273

10 Estatica do GPEDC. Boletim Informativo 1991, no. 5 (cited in ref. 9)

11 Vilaplana J, Romaguera C, Grimalt F. Contact dermatitis from resorcinol in a hair dye. Contact Dermatitis 1991;24:151-152

12 Andersen KE, Carisen L. Pyrocatechol contact allergy from a permanent cream dye for eyelashes and eyebrows. Contact Dermatitis 1988;18:306-307

13 Caron GA, Calnan CD. Studies in contact dermatitis. XIV. Resorcin. Trans St John's Hosp Dermatol Soc 1962;48:149-156 (data cited in ref. 12)

14 Tan SK. Exogenous ochronosis--a diagnostic challenge. J Cosmet Dermatol 2010;9:313-317

15 Langeland T, Braathen LR. Allergic contact dermatitis from resorcinol. Contact Dermatitis 1987;17:126

16 Waddell MM, Finn DA. Sensitivity to resorcin. Contact Dermatitis 1981;7:216

17 Cronin E. Resorcin in Castellani's paint. Contact Dermatitis Newsletter 1973;14:401

18 Marks JG, West GW. Allergic contact dermatitis to radiotherapy dye. Contact Dermatitis 1978;4:1-2

19 Hasan T, Rantanen T, Alanko K, Harvima RJ, Jolanki R, Kalimo K, et al. Patch test reactions to cosmetic allergens in 1995–1997 and 2000–2002 in Finland –a multicentre study. Contact Dermatitis 2005;53:40-45

20 Goossens A, Beck MH, Haneke E, McFadden JP, Nolting S, Durupt G, Ries G. Adverse cutaneous reactions to cosmetic allergens. Contact Dermatitis 1999;40:112-113

21 Wang MZ, Farmer SA, Richardson DM, Davis MDP. Patch-testing with hairdressing chemicals. Dermatitis 2011;22:16-26

22 Frosch PJ, Burrows D, Camarasa JG, Dooms-Goossens A, Ducombs G, Lahti A, et al. Allergic reactions to a hairdressers' series: results from 9 European centres. Contact Dermatitis 1993;28:180-183

23 Guerra L, Tosti A, Bardazzi F, Pigatto P, Lisi P, Santucci B, et al. Contact dermatitis in hairdressers: the Italian experience. Contact Dermatitis 1992;26:101-107

24 SCCS (Scientific Committee on Consumer Safety). Opinion on resorcinol, 23 March 2010, SCCS/1270/09. Available at: http://ec.europa.eu/health/scientific_committees/consumer_safety/docs/sccs_o_015.pdf

25 SCCP (Scientific Committee on Consumer Products). Opinion on resorcinol, 15 April 2008, SCCP/1117/07. Available at: http://ec.europa.eu/health/archive/ph_risk/committees/04_sccp/docs/sccp_o_124.pdf

26 Boonchai W, Bunyavaree M, Winayanuwattikun W, Kasemsarn P. Contact sensitizers in commercial hair dye products sold in Thailand. Contact Dermatitis 2016;74:222-229

27 Thorén S, Yazar K. Contact allergens in 'natural' hair dyes. Contact Dermatitis 2016;74:302-304

28 Basketter DA, English J. Cross-reactions among hair dye allergens. Cut Ocular Toxicol 2009;28:104-106

29 Søsted H, Rustemeyer T, Gonçalo M, Bruze M, Goossens A, Giménez-Arnau AM, et al. Contact allergy to common ingredients in hair dyes. Contact Dermatitis 2013;69:32-39

30 The Danish Environmental Protection Agency. Survey and occurrence of PPD, PTD and other allergenic hair dye substances in hair dyes. Copenhagen, Denmark: The Danish Environmental Protection Agency, 2013 (ISBN 978-87-92903-92-1). Available at: http://www2.mst.dk/Udgiv/publications/2013/02/978-87-92903-92-1.pdf

31 Kirchlecher S, Hübner A, Uter W. Survey of sensitizing constituents of oxidative hair dyes (retail and professional products) in Germany. J Dtsch Dermatol Ges 2016;14:707-715

32 Schwensen JF, Johansen JD, Veien NK, Funding AT, Avnstorp C, Østerballe M, et al. Occupational contact dermatitis in hairdressers: an analysis of patch test data from the Danish Contact Dermatitis Group, 2002–2011. Contact Dermatitis 2014;70:233-237

33 Hamann D, Yazar K, Hamann CR, Thyssen JP, Lidén C. p-Phenylenediamine and other allergens in hair dye products in the United States: a consumer exposure study. Contact Dermatitis 2014;70:213-218

34 Katugampola RP, Statham BN, English JSC, Wilkinson MM, Foulds IS, Green CM, Ormerod AD, et al. A multicentre review of the hairdressing allergens tested in the UK. Contact Dermatitis 2005;53:130-132

35 Katsarou A, Koufou B, Takou K, Kalogeromitros D, Papanayiotou G, Vareltzidis A. Patch test results in hairdressers with contact dermatitis in Greece (1985-1994). Contact Dermatitis 1995;33:347-348

36 O'Gorman SM, Torgerson RR. Contact allergy in cheilitis. Int J Dermatol 2016;55:e386-e391

37 Yazar K, Boman A, Lidén C. Potent skin sensitizers in oxidative hair dye products on the Swedish market. Contact Dermatitis 2009;61:269-275

38 Yazar K, Boman A, Lidén C. p-Phenylenediamine and other hair dye sensitizers in Spain. Contact Dermatitis 2012;66:27-32

39 Borelli S. Die Verträglichkeit gebrauchlicher Haarfärbungspraparate, Farbstoffsgrundsubstanzen und verwandter chemischer Verbindungen. Hautarzt 1958;9:19-25 (data cited in ref. 41)

40 Connor DS, Ritz HL, Ampulski RS, Kowollik HG, Lim P, Thomas DW, Parkhurst R. Identification of certain sultones as the sensitizers in alkyl ethoxy sulfate. Fette, Seifen, Anstrichmittel 1975;77:25-29 (data cited in ref. 41, possibly incorrect)

41 Eskelinen A, Molitor C, Kanerva L. Allergic contact dermatitis from 2,7-dihydroxynaphthalene in hair dye. Contact Dermatitis 1997;36:312-313

42 Kim H, Kim K. Prevalence of potent skin sensitizers in oxidative hair dye products in Korea. Cutan Ocul Toxicol 2016;35:204-207

43 Darcis J, Goossens A. Resorcinol: a strong sensitizer but a rare contact allergen in the clinic. Contact Dermatitis 2016;74:310-312

44 Kern PS, Gerberick F, Ryan CA, Kimber I, Aptula A, Basketter DA. Local lymph node data for the evaluation of skin sensitization alternatives: a second compilation. Dermatitis 2010;21:8-32

45 SCCS (Scientific Committee on Consumer Safety). Opinion on: Resorcinol (A11), 23 March 2010. Available at: https://ec.europa.eu/health/scientific_committees/consumer_safety/docs/sccs_o_015.pdf

46 Barbaud A, Reichert-Penetrat S, Trechot P et al. Sensitization to resorcinol in a prescription verrucide preparation: unusual systemic clinical features and prevalence. Ann Dermatol Venereol 2001;128:615-618

47 Komericki P, Kränke B, Aberer W. Allergische Kontaktdermatitis auf die Epikutantest-Markierungslösung Solutio Castellani. Dermatologie in Beruf und Umwelt (Dermatosen) 1997;45:176-178

48 Foti C, Romita P, Ettorre G, Angelini, G, Bonamonte D. Allergic contact dermatitis caused by resorcinol and sodium dehydroacetate in a patient with leg ulcers. Contact Dermatitis 2016;74:383-384

49 Dave VK. Contact dermatitis due to resorcin in Castellani's paint. Contact Dermatitis Newsletter 1973;13:384

50 Cronin E. Contact Dermatitis. Edinburgh: Churchill Livingstone, 1980:265

51 Bhattar PA, Zawar VP, Godse KV, Patil SP, Nadkarni NJ, Gautam MM. Exogenous ochronosis. Indian J Dermatol 2015;60:537-543

52 Fisher AA. Resorcinol, a rare sensitizer. Cutis 1982;29:331-332

53 Knight TE, Boll P, Epstein WL, Prasad AK. Resorcinols and catechols: A clinical study of cross-sensitivity. Am J Cont Derm 1996;7:138-145

54 Mitchell JH. Resorcin anal dermatitis due to resorcin in anusol suppositories. JAMA 1933;101:1067

55 Levin CY, Maibach H. Exogenous ochronosis. An update on clinical features, causative agents and treatment options. Am J Clin Dermatol 2001;2:213-217

56 Romero SA, Pereira PM, Mariano AV, Francesconi F, Francesconi VA. Use of dermoscopy for diagnosis of exogenous ochronosis. An Bras Dermatol 2011;86(4 Suppl.1):S31-34

57 Ribas J, Schettini AP, Cavalcante M de S. Exogenous ochronosis hydroquinone induced: a report of four cases. An Bras Dermatol 2010;85:699-703

58 Lawrence N, Bligard CA, Reed R, Perret WJ. Exogenous ochronosis in the United States. J Am Acad Dermatol 1988;18(5 Pt.2):1207-1211

59 Thomas AE, Gisburn MA. Exogenous ochronosis and oedema from resorcinol. Br J Dermatol 1961;73:378-381

60 Berthezène F, Fournier M, Bernier E, mornex R. L'Hypothyroidie induite par la résorcine. Lyon Med 1973;230:319 (data cited in ref. 61

61 De Groot AC, Weyland JW, Nater JP. Unwanted effects of cosmetics and drugs used in dermatology, 3rd Edition. Amsterdam – London – New York – Tokyo: Elsevier, 1994:259-260

62 Flandin C, Rabeau H, Ukrainczyk M. Intolérance à la résorcine. Test cutané. Soc Derm Syph 1953;12:1804 (data cited in ref. 61)

63 Murray MC. Analysis of sixty cases of drug poisoning. Arch Pediat 1926;43:193 (data cited in ref. 61)

64 Cunningham AA. Resorcin poisoning. Arch Dis Childh 1956;31:173 (data cited in ref. 61).

65 Wuthrich B, Zabrodsky S, Storck H. Percutaneous poisoning by resorcinol, salicylic acid and ammoniated mercury. Pharm Acta Helv 1972;45:453 (data cited in ref. 61).

66 Serrano G, Fortea JM, Millan F, Botella R, Latasa JM. Contact allergy to resorcinol in acne medications: report of three cases. J Am Acad Dermatol 1992;26(3 Pt.2):502-504

67 Abbate C, Polito I, Puglisi A, Brecciaroli R, Tanzariello A, Germano D. Dermatosis from resorcinal in tyre makers. Br J Ind Med 1989;46:212-214

68 Van Ketel WG. Allergic contact eczema caused by resorcinol. Ned Tijdschr Geneeskd 1970;114:905-907 (article in Dutch)

69 Kanny G, Blanchard N, Morisset M, Nominé V, Moneret-Vautrin DA. Bullous skin eruption to resorcin by proxy. Rev Med Interne 2004;25:324-327 (article in French)

70 Barbaud A, Modiano P, Cocciale M, Reichert S, Schmutz JL. The topical application of resorcinol can provoke a systemic allergic reaction. Br J Dermatol 1996;135:1014-1015

71 Wachters DH. Resorcinol-urticaria. Ned Tijdschr Geneeskd 1961;105:1402-1404 (article in Dutch)

72 Gasser C. Peracute hemolytic Heinz body anemia with methemoglobinemia after treatment of infant eczema with resorcin.Helv Paediatr Acta 1954;9:285-297 (article in German)

73 Pascher F. Systemic reactions to topically applied drugs. Int J Dermatol 1978;17:768-775

74 Bull GM, Fraser R. Myxedema from resorcinol ointment applied to leg ulcers. Lancet 1950;1 (6610):851-855

75 Lee HJ, Kim WJ, Kim JY, Kim HS, Kim BS, Kim MB, Ko HC. Patch tests with commercial hair dye products in patients with allergic contact dermatitis to para-phenylenediamine. Indian J Dermatol Venereol Leprol 2016;82:645-650

76 Ormerod E, Hughes TM, Stone N. Allergic contact dermatitis caused by resorcinol following a temporary black henna tattoo. Contact Dermatitis 2017;77:187-188

2.398 RESVERATROL

IDENTIFICATION

Description/definition	: Resveratrol is the organic compound that conforms to the formula shown below
Chemical class(es)	: Phenols
Chemical/IUPAC name	: 1,3-Benzenediol, 5-[(1E)-2-(4-hydroxyphenyl)ethenyl]-
Other names	: 3,5,4'-$trans$-Trihydroxystilbene
CAS registry number (s)	: 501-36-0
Merck Index monograph	: 9549
Function(s) in cosmetics	: EU: antioxidant; skin protecting. USA: antioxidants; skin protectants
Patch testing	: 5% pet. (1)
Molecular formula	: $C_{14}H_{12}O_3$

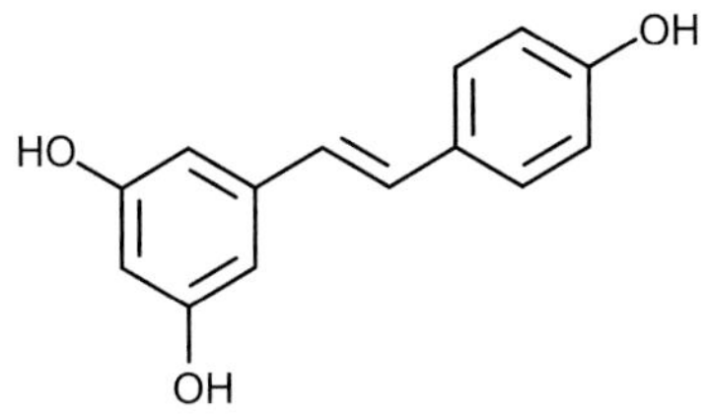

GENERAL

Resveratrol (3,5,4'-$trans$-trihydroxystilbene) is a phenolic phytoalexin produced naturally in red grape skin and in the leaf epidermis of various plants, as a stress metabolite protecting against fungal attack. In recent years, it has been reported to have anticarcinogenic, antioxidant, anti-inflammatory, phytoestrogenic and cardioprotective activities (1). Because of its wide spectrum of alleged beneficial properties, it is becoming more and more popular as a nutritional supplement. The literature reports scanty data concerning its possible topical applications (1).

CONTACT ALLERGY

Case reports and case series

A man had a 6-month history of recurrent scaling erythematous dermatitis localized to his groins and axillae. He was prescribed a resveratrol-containing emollient cream. Within 14 days, the dermatitis flared, became exudative and intensely itchy and spread to the upper legs. After the emollient cream was discontinued, the dermatitis slowly cleared. Patch tests with the SIDAPA standard series, a cosmetics series, and the emollient cream 'as is' showed a positive reaction to the cosmetic product only. When tested with its ingredients 4 months later, the patient weakly reacted to resveratrol 10%, 1% and 0.1% alcohol and strongly to pentylene glycol. Of 10 controls, one, who had irritable skin, showed mild erythema to both resveratrol and pentylene glycol. To clarify the nature of the patient's reaction to resveratrol, it was tested again, but now in concentrations of 5%, 1% and 0.1% in petrolatum. The patient reacted at D2 and D3 to resveratrol 5% pet. only, but 10 controls were negative. (1)

A woman had developed dermatitis of the face from using a resveratrol-containing cream for several weeks. The eczema cleared after she stopped using the cream, but would immediately recur when she applied it again. A repeated open application test gave a positive reaction within 2 days. Patch testing with the Italian baseline series, the cosmetic series and the patient's own products gave a positive reaction to the cream, tested 'as is'. Later, when tested with the ingredients of the product, the patient showed positive reactions at D2 and D3 to resveratrol 1% pet. and to another ingredient, Scutellaria baicalensis extract. After avoiding products containing these chemicals, the dermatitis has not recurred (2).

Presence in cosmetic products and chemical analyses

In the USA, in April 2017, resveratrol was present in 91 of 56,714 cosmetic products of which the composition is known in FDA's Voluntary Cosmetic Registration Program (VCRP) (data obtained from FDA, May 2017). In April 2017, resveratrol was present in 60 of 65,434 cosmetic products of which the composition is known in EWG's Skin Deep Cosmetics Database, USA (http://www.ewg.org/skindeep/).

LITERATURE

1   Gallo R, Viglizzo G, Vecchio F, Parodi A. Allergic contact dermatitis from pentylene glycol in an emollient cream, with possible co-sensitization to resveratrol. Contact Dermatitis 2003;48:176-177

2   Gallo R, Pastorino C, Gasparini G, Ciccarese G, Parodi A. Scutellaria baicalensis extract: a novel botanical allergen in cosmetic products? Contact Dermatitis 2016;75:387-388

2.399   RETINOL

IDENTIFICATION

Description/definition   : Retinol is the organic compound that conforms to the formula shown below
Chemical class(es)   : Alcohols
Chemical/IUPAC name   : (2E,4E,6E,8E)-3,7-Dimethyl-9-(2,6,6-trimethylcyclohexen-1-yl)nona-2,4,6,8-tetraen-1-ol
Other names   : Vitamin A
CAS registry number (s)   : 68-26-8; 11103-57-4
EC number(s)   : 200-683-7; 234-328-2
CIR review(s)   : J Am Coll Toxicol 1987;6:279-320 (access: www.cir-safety.org/ingredients)
SCCS opinion(s)   : SCCS/1576/16 (3)
Merck Index monograph : 11481
Function(s) in cosmetics   : EU: skin conditioning. USA: skin-conditioning agents - miscellaneous
Patch testing   : 1% and 10% acet. (1)
Molecular formula   : $C_{20}H_{30}O$

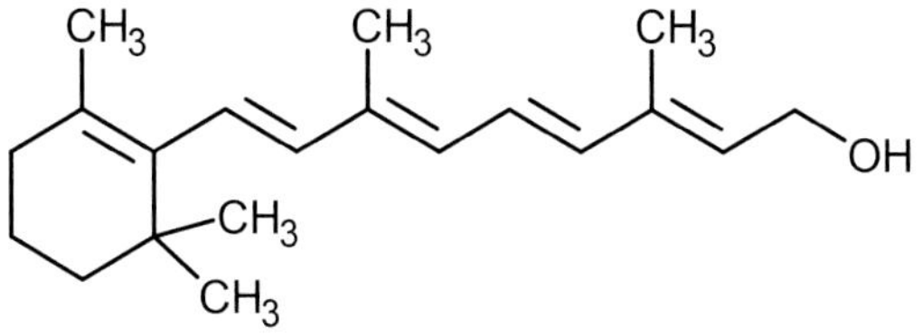

GENERAL

Discussion of adverse reactions to retinol (vitamin A) in this chapter is limited to contact allergy from its presence in cosmetics and topical pharmaceuticals.

CONTACT ALLERGY

Case reports and case series

A young boy had atopic dermatitis on the face and was intermittently treated with a corticosteroid and an emollient cream. After 3 weeks, erythemato-vesicular, intensely pruritic papules and patches developed on his cheeks. When patch tested with its ingredients, the patient reacted to retinol 1% and 10% in acetone, but not to retinol 0.1% pet. (1). In another report from the same authors on the same product, it is suggested that the allergenic ingredient is not retinol but retinyl palmitate (2).

Contact allergy to retinol in non-cosmetic products

A woman developed ACD from a pharmaceutical cream containing vitamin A (retinol) 100,000 IU, vitamin E (tocopherol) 5% and urea 10%. She reacted to the cream, and to retinol 200,000 IU/100 g corn oil and tocopherol 2.5% pet. on two occasions, while 4 controls were negative (4).

Presence in cosmetic products and chemical analyses

In the USA, in April 2017, retinol was present in 279 of 56,714 cosmetic products of which the composition is known in FDA's Voluntary Cosmetic Registration Program (VCRP) (data obtained from FDA, May 2017). In April 2017, retinol was present in 150 of 65,434 cosmetic products of which the composition is known in EWG's Skin Deep Cosmetics Database, USA (http://www.ewg.org/skindeep/).

LITERATURE

1   De Galdeano CS, Aguirre A, Ratón JA, Zabala R, Landa N, Díaz-Perez JL. Contact dermatitis from a moisturizing cream. Contact Dermatitis 1994;30:50-51
2   Manzano D, Aguirre A, Gardeazabal J, Eizaguirre X, Pérez J LD. Allergic contact dermatitis form tocopheryl acetate (vitamin E) and retinol palmitate (vitamin A) in a moisturizing cream. Contact Dermatitis 1994;31:324
3   SCCS (Scientific Committee on Consumer Safety). Opinion on Vitamin A (Retinol, Retinyl Acetate, Retinyl Palmitate), SCCS/1576/16, 20 April 2016. Available at:
    http://ec.europa.eu/health/scientific_committees/consumer_safety/docs/sccs_o_199.pdf
4   Bazzano C, de Angeles S, Kleist G, Macedo N. Allergic contact dermatitis from topical vitamins A and E. Contact Dermatitis 1996;35:261-262

2.400 RETINYL PALMITATE

IDENTIFICATION

Description/definition	: Retinyl palmitate is the ester of retinol (vitamin A) and palmitic acid
Chemical class(es)	: Esters
Chemical/IUPAC name	: [(2E,4E,6E,8E)-3,7-Dimethyl-9-(2,6,6-trimethylcyclohexen-1-yl)nona-2,4,6,8-tetraenyl] hexadecanoate
Other names	: Retinol palmitate; vitamin A palmitate; retinol, hexadecanoate
CAS registry number (s)	: 79-81-2
EC number(s)	: 201-228-5
CIR review(s)	: J Am Coll Toxicol 1987;6:279-320 (access: www.cir-safety.org/ingredients)
SCCS opinion(s)	: SCCS/1576/16 (5)
Merck Index monograph	: 11481 (vitamin A, retinol)
Function(s) in cosmetics	: EU: skin conditioning. USA: skin-conditioning agents - miscellaneous
Patch test allergens	: 5% pet. (1); this concentration may cause occasional irritant reactions (1); 1% and 10% MEK (methyl ethyl ketone) (2)
Molecular formula	: $C_{36}H_{60}O_2$

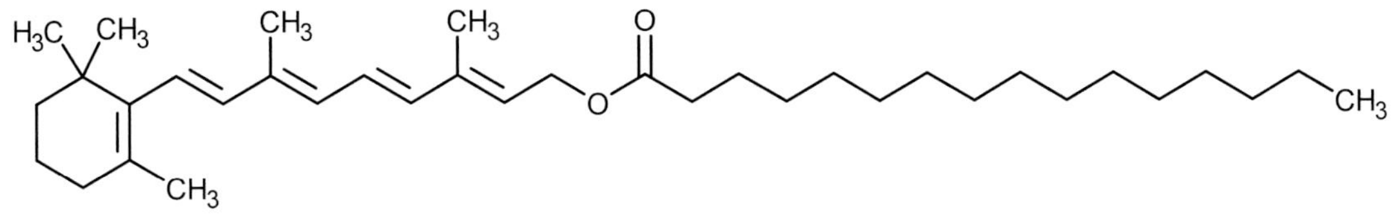

CONTACT ALLERGY

Case reports and case series

A woman developed dermatitis of the face after a few days use of a new anti-wrinkle cream. She performed a use test on the forearm with subsequent development of itchy erythema. Patch tests with the standard series, her personal products and selected cosmetic ingredients showed a positive reaction to the cream. A ROAT became positive after 5 applications. Testing with the ingredients of the cosmetic product showed a strong positive reaction to a retinyl palmitate - polycaprolactone (PCL) complex. Subsequent patch tests with retinyl palmitate 5% pet. and PCL 5% pet. gave a positive reaction to retinyl palmitate but negative result to PCL. A ROAT with retinyl palmitate 5% pet. was positive. In 27 controls, there were 3 ?+ reactions on D3, but the reactions had disappeared by D7 (1). This patient reacted to retinyl palmitate in the complex with polycaprolactone (PCL). PCL is a biodegradable polyester used in skin care formulations as part of so called solid lipid nanoparticles. By coating the active ingredient, PCL enhances its penetration into the skin (1).

One patient had contact dermatitis from allergy to retinyl palmitate in a moisturizing cream (2). In another publication from the same authors on the same product, it was suggested that it contains retinol rather than retinyl palmitate (4).

Contact allergy to retinyl palmitate in non-cosmetic products

One patient reacted to retinyl palmitate in a topical pharmaceutical product (magistral preparation) (3). A woman was given intramuscular water soluble retinyl palmitate injections for lichen sclerosus et atrophicus. Two weeks after receiving a second injection (50,000 IU) she noted a red itchy area on her right buttock over the injection site. This grew into an oval erythematous scaly plaque with a size of 7.5 x 9.0 cm and a hemorrhagic component; it slowly disappeared over three weeks. An intradermal skin test to retinyl palmitate (0.1%) was positive at 48 hours, showing a red nodule of 1.2 cm. Similar intradermal tests with all other constituents of the water soluble retinol injection gave negative results. Five control patients tested with the same material showed no reaction. A retinol patch test gave negative results and oral challenge with vitamin A was without incident (6).

Presence in cosmetic products and chemical analyses

In the USA, in April 2017, retinyl palmitate was present in 2795 of 56,714 cosmetic products of which the composition is known in FDA's Voluntary Cosmetic Registration Program (VCRP) (data obtained from FDA, May 2017). In April 2017, retinyl palmitate was present in 1407 of 65,434 cosmetic products of which the composition is known in EWG's Skin Deep Cosmetics Database, USA (http://www.ewg.org/skindeep/).

LITERATURE

1   Clemmensen A, Thormann J, Andersen, KE. Allergic contact dermatitis from retinyl palmitate in polycaprolactone. Contact Dermatitis 2007;56:288-289
2   Manzano D, Aguirre A, Gardeazabal J, Eizaguirre X, Pérez J LD. Allergic contact dermatitis form tocopheryl acetate (vitamin E) and retinol palmitate (vitamin A) in a moisturizing cream. Contact Dermatitis 1994;31:324
3   Blondeel A. Contact allergy to vitamin A. Contact Dermatitis 1984;11:191-192
4   De Galdeano CS, Aguirre A, Ratón JA, Zabala R, Landa N, Díaz-Perez JL. Contact dermatitis from a moisturizing cream. Contact Dermatitis 1994;30:50-51
5   SCCS (Scientific Committee on Consumer Safety). Opinion on Vitamin A (Retinol, Retinyl Acetate, Retinyl Palmitate), SCCS/1576/16, 20 April 2016. Available at: http://ec.europa.eu/health/scientific_committees/consumer_safety/docs/sccs_o_199.pdf
6   Shelley WB, Shelley ED, Talanin NY. Hypersensitivity to retinol palmitate injection. BMJ 1995;311(6999):232

2.401 RICINOLEIC ACID

IDENTIFICATION

Description/definition	: Ricinoleic acid is the unsaturated fatty acid that conforms generally to the formula shown below
Chemical class(es)	: Fatty acids
Chemical/IUPAC name	: (Z,12R)-12-Hydroxyoctadec-9-enoic acid
Other names	: 12-Hydroxyoleic acid; ricinic acid; ricinolic acid; 12-hydroxy-9-octadecenoic acid
CAS registry number (s)	: 141-22-0; 7431-95-0
EC number(s)	: 205-470-2
CIR review(s)	: Int J Toxicol 2007;26(Suppl.3):31-77 (access: www.cir-safety.org/ingredients)
Merck Index monograph	: 9605
Function(s) in cosmetics	: EU: cleansing; emollient; emulsifying; surfactant. USA: surfactants - cleansing agents
Patch testing	: 10% pet. (1); 30% pet. (3,4), which concentration may be slightly irritant (8)
Molecular formula	: $C_{18}H_{34}O_3$

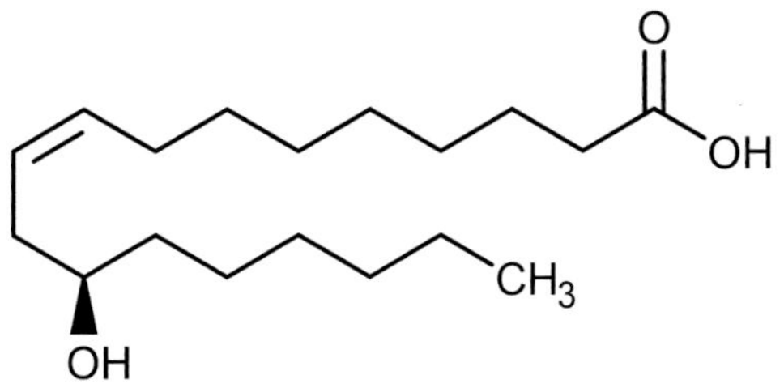

GENERAL

Ricinoleic acid is the main constituent of Ricinus communis seed oil (castor oil) (Chapter 2.402). It accounts for about 90% of the glyceride fatty acids of castor oil. Ricinoleic acid is used in textile finishes, in dry cleaning soaps, and as a spermicide in contraceptive jellies. Ricinoleates (zinc ricinoleate, magnesium ricinoleate, and glyceryl ricinoleate) are (metal) soaps of ricinoleic acid. They are used in adhesives, corrosion inhibitors, cosmetics, greases, varnishes, print pigments, and for deodorizing various products (12).

CONTACT ALLERGY

Testing in groups of patients

Of 202 patients with primary symptoms and signs of eczematous cheilitis seen in Singapore in the period 1996-1999, there were 29 positive patch test reactions to ricinoleic acid, of which 22 (11% of the total population) were relevant from its presence in lipsticks and possibly other lip cosmetics (6).

Case reports and case series

A patient had allergic contact dermatitis from lipstick that contained castor oil; castor oil itself was negative upon patch testing, but a test with ricinoleic acid 10% pet., the main ingredient of castor oil, was positive (1). It was suggested that the concentration of ricinoleic acid in castor oil was too low to elicit a positive response (1). A female individual had allergic contact cheilitis from Ricinus communis seed oil (castor oil) present in many lipsticks and lip creams. She reacted to 13 of 15 products, that were patch tested. These cosmetics (3 lip creams, 10 lipsticks) contained 10-67% castor oil (3). This patient was later tested with the main ingredient of castor oil, ricinoleic acid, and she had positive patch tests to it at 30% pet. and pure. In addition, she reacted positively to a purified castor oil (2).

A woman had pigmented allergic cosmetic cheilitis from ricinoleic acid in lipsticks; the positive patch test to one of the lipsticks also showed hyperpigmentation (4). Seven patients from Japan were reported to have allergic contact cheilitis from ricinoleic acid in lipsticks; clinical details are missing, but apparently, patch tests to castor oil were negative (article not read, in Japanese) (5). In a group of 27 patients with cheilitis, seen in a center in Singapore from 1989 to 1991, one had allergic contact cheilitis from ricinoleic acid in lipstick (7). Two women had allergic contact cheilitis from a lipstick. They had positive patch tests to the lipstick and later to castor oil that it contained and to its main ingredient ricinoleic acid (8,10). An unknown number of patients with allergic contact dermatitis caused by castor oil in lipsticks, presumably from its main ingredient ricinoleic acid (9).

Contact allergy to ricinoleic acid in non-cosmetic products
An army recruit had suffered from rashes on two occasions after applying camouflage with a camouflage stick. A mildly pruritic vesicular eruption over the neck, chin, face and hands appeared one day after applying the camouflage, associated with eyelid swelling and lasting for 3-4 days. The camouflage stick was a stick of wax in a military green color, looking otherwise very much like lipstick. Patch testing was performed to the standard series, the camouflage stick and suspected substances in it and there were positive reactions to the camouflage product and to ricinoleic acid 30% pet. The main component of the camouflage stick turned out to be castor oil (47.1% w/w), of which ricinoleic acid is the main constituent. However, its other ingredients were not tested (11).

Cross-reactions, pseudo-cross-reactions and co-reactions
Not to linoleic, oleic, palmitic, or stearic acids (2). Castor oil (Rinicus communis seed oil), of which ricinoleic acid is the main ingredient, may (8,10) or may not (1,5) co-react (which would be pseudo-cross-sensitivity). Alleged cross-sensitivity with oleyl alcohol (10).

Presence in cosmetic products and chemical analyses
In the USA, in April 2017, ricinoleic acid was present in 6 of 56,714 cosmetic products of which the composition is known in FDA's Voluntary Cosmetic Registration Program (VCRP) (data obtained from FDA, May 2017). In April 2017, ricinoleic acid was present in zero of 66,485 cosmetic products of which the composition is known in EWG's Skin Deep Cosmetics Database, USA (http://www.ewg.org/skindeep/). However, 1783 of these products contain castor oil, and, consequently, ricinoleic acid.

LITERATURE

1   Inoue A, Shoji A, Aso S. Allergic lipstick cheilitis due to ester gum and ricinoleic acid. Contact Dermatitis 1998;39:39
2   Sai S. Lipstick dermatitis caused by ricinoleic acid. Contact Dermatitis 1983;9:524
3   Sai S. Lipstick dermatitis caused by castor oil. Contact Dermatitis 1983;9:75
4   Leow YH, Tan SH, Ng SK. Pigmented contact cheilitis from ricinoleic acid in lipsticks. Contact Dermatitis 2003;49:48-49
5   Hayashi C, Shoji A, Inoue A, Akai I, Taniguchi S. Seven cases of lipstick cheilitis with positive patch test reactions to ricinoleic acid but negative to castor oil. Environ Dermatol 1998;5:101-105 (in Japanese)
6   Lim SW, Goh CL. Epidemiology of eczematous cheilitis at a tertiary dermatological referral centre in Singapore. Contact Dermatitis 2000;43:322-326
7   Lim JTE, Ng SK, Goh CL. Contact cheilitis in Singapore. Contact Dermatitis 1992;27:263-264
8   Andersen KE, Nielsen R. Lipstick dermatitis related to castor oil. Contact Dermatitis 1984;11:253-254
9   Fisher AA. Allergic cheilitis due castor oil in lipsticks. Cutis 1991;47:389-390
10 Tan BB, Noble AL, Roberts ME, Lear JT, English JSC. Allergic contact dermatitis from oleyl alcohol in lipstick cross-reacting with ricinoleic acid in castor oil and lanolin. Contact Dermatitis 1997;37:41-42
11 Goon AT-J, Ng PP-L, Ng SK. Allergic contact dermatitis from military camouflage. Contact Dermatitis 1999;40:290-291
12 Kalavala M, Hughes TM, Stone NM. Allergic contact dermatitis to polyethylene glycol-7 hydrogenated castor oil. Contact Dermatitis 2007;56:287-288

2.402 RICINUS COMMUNIS (CASTOR) SEED OIL

IDENTIFICATION

Description/definition : Ricinus communis seed oil is the fixed oil obtained from the seeds of castor, *Ricinus communis*, Euphorbiaceae
Chemical class(es) : Fats and oils
INCI name USA : Ricinus communis (castor) seed oil
Other names : Castor oil; ricinus oil; oleum ricini; oil of Palma Christi (6)
CAS registry number (s) : 8001-79-4
EC number(s) : 232-293-8
CIR review(s) : Int J Toxicol 2007;26(Suppl.3):31-77 (access: www.cir-safety.org/ingredients)
Merck Index monograph : 3168
Function(s) in cosmetics : EU: emollient; masking; moisturising; skin conditioning; smoothing; solvent. USA: fragrance ingredients; skin-conditioning agents - occlusive
Patch testing : Pure (3,8,19)

GENERAL

Ricinus communis seed oil (from here on termed 'castor oil') is a yellowish fixed (vegetable) oil extracted from the seeds of *Ricinus communis* L. It is a triglyceride, in which the main fatty acids are ricinoleic acid (90%), oleic acid, linoleic acid, palmitic acid, and stearic acid. The oil is widely used in cosmetics such as lipsticks, sunscreens, deodorants, moisturizers, nail lacquer removers and soaps for its emollient properties, resistance to rancidness, and ready solubility in alcohol. Castor oil is used in most lipsticks: it renders the pigment soluble, and its high viscosity delays the settling of pigments from the molten lipstick and lessens the tendency to smear and run off (6). It is also used in pharmaceuticals (e.g., in laxatives), as biofuel, as a lubricant, in cutting fluids and for food flavoring (19).

CONTACT ALLERGY

Testing in groups of patients

There are no studies in which castor oil has been patch tested in consecutive patients suspected of contact dermatitis (routine testing). In an Italian study performed in 2001-2006, 129 patients with chronic cheilitis were patch tested with castor oil 100% and there was one (1%) reaction, which was, however, not relevant (17).

Case reports and case series

Castor oil was stated to be the (or an) allergen in one patient in a group of 603 individuals suffering from cosmetic dermatitis, seen in the period 2010-2015 in Leuven, Belgium (15). One patient had allergic contact cheilitis from castor oil in a large number of lipsticks (3); later testing (13) revealed that she was allergic to ricinoleic acid, the main constituent of castor oil. A woman had recurrent dermatitis and cheilitis from castor oil present in a moisturizing lotion, 3 lipsticks and 4 lip balms (6).

Two patients had contact allergy to castor oil in a lipstick; they also reacted to ricinoleic acid, the main constituent of the oil (7,12). One patient reacted to castor oil in a make-up remover (14). Two patients (16) and one more (5) had allergic contact cheilitis from castor oil in lipsticks. Two women (19) and another female patient (4) had perioral eczema from contact allergy to castor oil in lip balms (19).

Contact allergy to Ricinus communis seed oil in non-cosmetic products

Allergic contact dermatitis of the ear canal and palpebral edema developed in a patient from contact allergy to castor oil in a cerumenolytic product (1). Angioedema-like allergic contact dermatitis from castor oil in a cerumenolytic has also been observed (2). One patient had allergic contact dermatitis from castor oil in 'zinc and castor oil cream' (8). Another two individuals reacted to castor oil in a wart remover (9,10). A man had anogenital dermatitis from contact allergy to castor oil in an antihemorrhoidal cream (18).

Cross-reactions, pseudo-cross-reactions and co-reactions

Pseudo-cross-reaction to ricinoleic acid, the main constituent of castor oil (7,12). Hydrogenated castor oil, sulfated castor oil, glyceryl ricinoleate, PEG-400 ricinoleate (INCI name: PEG-8 ricinoleate), zinc ricinoleate and sodium sulforicinate (11). *Not* to hydrogenated castor oil (19).

Presence in cosmetic products and chemical analyses

In June 2017, castor oil was present in 1799 of 69,510 cosmetic products of which the composition is known in EWG's Skin Deep Cosmetics Database, USA (http://www.ewg.org/skindeep/). In the USA, in April 2017, Ricinus communis (castor) seed oil was present in 2312 of 56,714 cosmetic products of which the composition is known in FDA's Voluntary Cosmetic Registration Program (VCRP) (data obtained from FDA, May 2017).

LITERATURE

1   Caralli ME, Rodríguez MS, Rojas Pérez-Ezquerra P, Pelta Fernández R, De Barrio Fernández M. Palpebral angioedema and allergic contact dermatitis caused by a cerumenolytic. Contact Dermatitis 2015;73:376-377
2   Sánchez-Guerrero IM, Huertas AJ, López MP, Carreño A, Ramírez M, Pajarón, M. Angioedema-like allergic contact dermatitis to castor oil. Contact Dermatitis 2010;62:318-319
3   Sai S. Lipstick dermatitis caused by castor oil. Contact Dermatitis 1983;9:75
4   Sasseville D, Desjardins M, Almutawa F. Allergic contact dermatitis caused by glycyrrhetinic acid and castor oil. Contact Dermatitis 2011;64,168-169
5   Yojiro K. A case of allergic contact dermatitis to castor oil in lipstick. Skin Res 1991;33 (Suppl. 11):245-249 (in Japanese)
6   Le Coz C-J, Ball C. Recurrent allergic contact dermatitis and cheilitis due to castor oil. Contact Dermatitis 2000;42:114-115
7   Tan BB, Noble AL, Roberts ME, Lear JT, English JSC. Allergic contact dermatitis from oleyl alcohol in lipstick cross-reacting with ricinoleic acid in castor oil and lanolin. Contact Dermatitis 1997;37:41-42
8   Wakelin SH, Harris AJ, Shaw S. Contact dermatitis from castor oil in zinc and castor oil cream. Contact Dermatitis 1996;35:259
9   Tabar AI, Muro MD, Quirce S, Olaguibel JM. Contact dermatitis due to sensitization to lactic acid and castor oil in a wart remover solution. Contact Dermatitis 1993;29:49-50
10   Lodi A, Leuchi S, Mancini L, Chiarelli G, Crosti C. Allergy to castor oil and colophony in a wart remover. Contact Dermatitis 1992;26:266-267
11   Dooms-Goossens A, Dupré K, Borghijs A, Swinnen C, Dooms M, Degreef H. Zinc ricinoleate: sensitizer in deodorants. Contact Dermatitis 1987;16:292-294
12   Andersen KE, Nielsen R. Lipstick dermatitis related to castor oil. Contact Dermatitis 1984;11:253-254
13   Sai S. Lipstick dermatitis caused by ricinoleic acid. Contact Dermatitis 1983;9:524
14   Brändle I, Boujnah-Khouadja A, Foussereau J. Allergy to castor oil. Contact Dermatitis 1983;9:424-425
15   Goossens A. Cosmetic contact allergens. Cosmetics 2016, 3, 5; doi:10.3390/cosmetics3010005
16   Fisher AA. Allergic cheilitis due castor oil in lipsticks. Cutis 1991;47:389-390
17   Schena D, Fantuzzi F, Girolomoni G. Contact allergy in chronic eczematous lip dermatitis. Eur J Dermatol 2008;18:688-692
18   Leysen J, Goossens A, Lambert J, Aerts O. Polyhexamethylene biguanide is a relevant sensitizer in wet wipes. Contact Dermatitis 2014: 70: 323-325
19   Verheyden M, Rombouts S, Lambert J, Aerts O. Contact allergy to castor oil, but not to castor wax. Cosmetics 2017, 4, 5; doi:10.3390/cosmetics4010005

2.403   RUSCOGENIN

IDENTIFICATION

Description/definition	: Ruscogenin is the sterol that conforms to the formula shown below
Chemical class(es)	: Sterols
Chemical/IUPAC name	: (25R)-Spirost-5-ene-1β,3β-diol
Other names	: (1β,3β,25R)-Spirost-5-ene-1,3-diol
CAS registry number (s)	: 472-11-7
EC number(s)	: 207-447-2
Function(s) in cosmetics	: EU: skin conditioning. USA: skin-conditioning agents - miscellaneous
Patch testing	: 1% pet. (5)
Molecular formula	: $C_{27}H_{42}O_4$

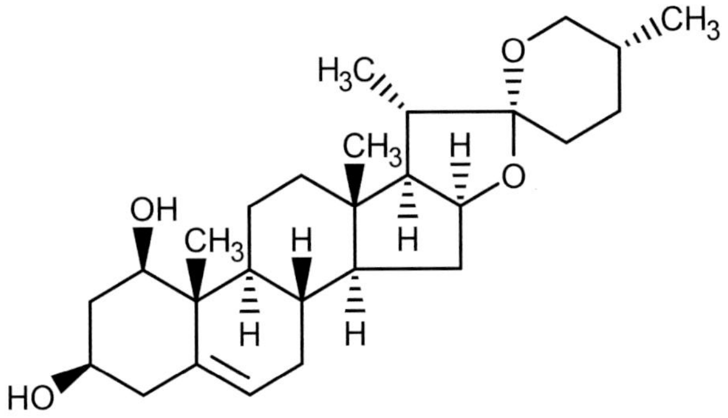

GENERAL

Ruscogenin is an important component of the plant Butcher's broom (*Ruscus aculeatus*). This is an evergreen shrub, native to Mediterranean Europe and Africa, and is widely distributed in Europe. It is also cultivated by hobby gardeners and grown for the florist trade. The rhizome is the part of the plant used medicinally. Its main constituents are steroidal (or, more precisely, spirostanol) saponins based on the aglycones ruscogenin and neoruscogenin, and include ruscin, neoruscin, deglucoruscin, and ruscoside, with their various sulfated and acetylated derivatives, ruscozepines A and B, aculeosides A and B, and others. Coumarins, including esculin and esculetin, triterpenes, and flavonoids, are also present. Possibly, the active substances in *R. aculeatus* rhizome are the spirostanol saponins ruscin and deglucoruscin, and the coumarin glucoside esculin (3).

Butcher's broom has a vasoconstrictive effect which may improve capillary flow and vascular tone. Vasoconstriction following oral or topical use of Butcher's broom extracts has improved symptoms such as heaviness or discomfort of legs associated with venous insufficiency and gave symptomatic relief of itching and burning associated with hemorrhoids (1,3). Not the plant itself, but topical products labeled as containing ruscogenins or *R. aculeatus* extract and sold as hemorrhoid treatments, anti-cellulite creams, and local treatments for varices, may cause allergic reactions (3).

The traditional uses of *Ruscus* spp., the current knowledge of the chemistry of this genus, and the pharmacological studies carried out on *Ruscus* spp. extracts have been reviewed in 2016 (6).

CONTACT ALLERGY

Case reports and case series
A woman presented with pruritic erythematous lesions following the local application of an antihemorrhoidal cream. She had developed a cutaneous rash consisting of eczematous plaques located on the perianal region which cleared within several days of ceasing the cream's use. Several months later, the patient had a generalized eczematous cutaneous eruption, one day after topical application of a cosmetic anti-cellulite product on the legs. Patch tests with these 2 creams were both positive. Later, the patient was patch tested with their ingredients and now she had positive reactions to ruscogenins (test concentration and vehicle not mentioned), which was present in both products. Twenty controls were negative (1).

Contact allergy to ruscogenin in non-cosmetic products
A woman had allergic contact dermatitis of the perianal region from ruscogenin in an antihemorrhoidal preparation (1). One patient had allergic contact dermatitis from *Ruscus aculeatus* (extract) in a vasoconstrictor cream, but

ruscogenins were not tested separately (2). Similar cases of contact sensitivity to *R. aculeatus* extract and/or to ruscogenins have been reported from France (4).

A man presented with pruritic erythematous lesions on the perianal area and buttocks five days after initiating the local application of a cream for hemorrhoids. The lesions spread within a day to the trunk and both legs. The antihemorrhoidal cream contained ruscogenin, a local anesthetic and a corticosteroid as active principles. Patch testing with GEIDAC (Spanish Group of Investigation of Contact Dermatitis) standard series, local anesthetics series and the cream as is yielded positive reactions to the cream, tixocortol pivalate and local anesthetics. Later, patch testing with the cream confirmed sensitivity to it and testing with its ingredients gave positive reactions to ruscogenin 1% pet. and the local anesthetic at D2 and D4. Five controls were negative to ruscogenin 1% pet. (5).

Presence in cosmetic products and chemical analyses
In the USA, in April 2017, ruscogenin was present in 15 of 56,714 cosmetic products of which the composition is known in FDA's Voluntary Cosmetic Registration Program (VCRP) (data obtained from FDA, May 2017). In April 2017, ruscogenin was present in zero of 66,485 cosmetic products of which the composition is known in EWG's Skin Deep Cosmetics Database, USA (http://www.ewg.org/skindeep/). However, 27 products contained Ruscus aculeatus (box holly) root extract.

LITERATURE

1   Ramírez-Hernández M, García-Sellés J, Mérida-Fernández C, Martínez-Escribano JA. Allergic contact dermatitis to ruscogenins. Contact Dermatitis 2006;54:60
2   Landa N, Aguirre A, Goday J, Ratón JA, Díaz-Pérez JL. Allergic contact dermatitis from a vasoconstrictor cream. Contact Dermatitis 1990;22:290-291
3   Calapai G, Minciullo PL, Miroddi M, Chinou I, Gangemi S, Schmidt RJ. Contact dermatitis as an adverse reaction to some topically used European herbal medicinal products – Part 3: *Mentha × piperita – Solanum dulcamara*. Contact Dermatitis 2016;74:131-144
4   Elbadir S, El Ayed F, Renaud F, Bazex J. L'allergie de contact aux ruscogénines. [Contact allergy to ruscogenins]. Revue Française d'Allergologie et d'Immunologie Clinique 1998;38:37-40 (article in French)
5   Córdoba S, Martínez-Moràn C, Hernàndez-Nuñez A, Borbujo J. Contact dermatitis from an anti-haemorroidal cream containing ruscogenin. Eur J Dermatol 2009;19:276-277
6   Masullo M, Pizza C, Piacente S. Ruscus genus: a rich source of bioactive steroidal saponins. Planta Med 2016;82:1513-1524

2.404   SALVIA OFFICINALIS (SAGE) EXTRACT

IDENTIFICATION

Description/definition	: Salvia officinalis extract is an extract of the whole plant the sage, *Salvia officinalis* L., Lamiaceae
Chemical class(es)	: Botanical products and botanical derivatives
INCI name USA	: Salvia officinalis (sage) extract
CAS registry number (s)	: 8022-56-8; 84082-79-1
EC number(s)	: 282-025-9; 282-025-9
Merck Index monograph	: 9750 (Salvia)
Function(s) in cosmetics	: EU: antidandruff; antimicrobial; antioxidant; adstringent; cleansing; deodorant; skin conditioning; skin protecting; soothing; tonic. USA: skin-conditioning agents – miscellaneous
Patch testing	: As is in water and pet. (not further specified [1])

GENERAL

Salvia officinalis L. is a perennial, evergreen subshrub, up to 60 cm tall, with a woody base, soft gray-green oval leaves and a mass of blue or violet inflorescences The name Salvia comes from the Latin salvere, which means 'to be well, to be in good health', indicating the (perceived) medical value of the plant. The Dalmatian sage is native to south-eastern Europe and is now widely cultivated in many (warm)-temperate regions of the world, mainly to obtain dried leaves to be used as a raw material in medicine, perfumery, and the food industry .The leaves and extracts of *Salvia officinalis* L. are used as spices and for healing of different diseases. In folk medicine, Dalmatian sage is used to treat inflamed throat and gingivitis (by gargling), cure laryngitis and hoarse voice, reduce sweat gland activity, treat fevers, reduce digestive tract disturbances, stimulate micturition, purify the colon and liver, and to strengthen the nervous system.

The essential oil of sage, which is obtained by steam-distillation of the flowering tops or the leaves, is used in traditional medicine and by the pharmaceutical, perfumery, liqueur and food industry. Essential oils of sage and their preparations are externally used for inflammations and infections of the mucous membranes of throat and mouth (stomatitis, gingivitis and pharyngitis). Internally, they are used for dyspeptic symptoms and excessive perspiration. It is also employed in incense and for aromatherapy, though it often considered too toxic for that practice because of the high thujone content (2).

CONTACT ALLERGY

Case reports and case series
A woman had suffered from swelling and redness of the lips and surrounding area, followed by tightness and a burning sensation in the involved area for three months. Previously, she had started applying a natural lip balm to prevent her lips from drying and cracking. Patch tests with the European baseline, cosmetic and bakery series, and with the lip balm gave a positive reaction to the lip balm, tested 'as is' only. Later, the patient was tested with its ingredients and she now reacted to Salvia extract (*S. officinalis*), tested as is in water and pet. (what does this mean?). Patch tests with the lip balm and with Salvia extract in water and pet. were negative in 20 controls (1).

Presence in cosmetic products and chemical analyses
In the USA, in April 2017, Salvia officinalis (sage) leaf was present in 8 of 56,714 cosmetic products of which the composition is known in FDA's Voluntary Cosmetic Registration Program (VCRP) (data obtained from FDA, May 2017). In April 2017, Salvia officinalis extract was present in 70 (extract) and 317 (leaf extract) products of 66,485 cosmetic products of which the composition is known in EWG's Skin Deep Cosmetics Database, USA (http://www.ewg.org/skindeep/).

LITERATURE
1   Mayer E, Gescheidt-Shoshany H, Weltfriend S. Allergic contact dermatitis caused by *Salvia officinalis* extract. Contact Dermatitis 2011;64:237-238
2   De Groot AC, Schmidt E. Essential oils: contact allergy and chemical composition. Boca Raton, Fl., USA: CRC Press, Taylor and Francis Group, 2016:731-743 (ISBN 9781482246407)

2.405   SCUTELLARIA BAICALENSIS EXTRACT

IDENTIFICATION

Description/definition   : Scutellaria baicalensis extract is the extract of the whole plant, *Scutellaria baicalensis*,
                            Lamiaceae
Chemical class(es)   : Botanical products and botanical derivatives
CAS registry number (s)   : 94279-99-9
EC number(s)   : 304-845-9
Function(s) in cosmetics : EU: antimicrobial. USA: antimicrobial agents
Patch testing   : 0.5% water (1)

GENERAL

Scutellaria baicalensis is a widely used traditional herbal remedy that contains several active flavonoids, including baicalin and baicalein, with anti-inflammatory, antioxidant and possibly anti-allergic properties (2,3).

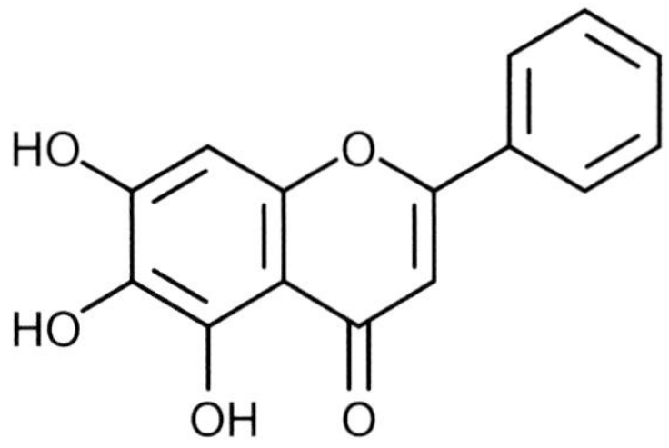

Structural formula of baicalein

CONTACT ALLERGY

Case reports and case series

A woman had developed dermatitis of the face from using a cosmetic cream for several weeks. The eczema cleared after she stopped using the cream, but would immediately recur when she applied it again. A repeated open application test gave a positive reaction within 2 days. Patch testing with the Italian baseline series, the cosmetic series and the patient's own products gave a positive reaction to the cream, tested 'as is'. Later, when tested with the ingredients of the product, the patient showed positive reactions at D2 and D3 to Scutellaria baicalensis extract 0.5% in water and to another ingredient, resveratrol. Fifteen controls tested with the two test materials were negative. After avoiding products containing these chemicals, the dermatitis has not recurred (1).

Presence in cosmetic products and chemical analyses

In the USA, in April 2017, Scutellaria baicalensis extract was present in 106 of 56,714 cosmetic products of which the composition is known in FDA's Voluntary Cosmetic Registration Program (VCRP) (data obtained from FDA, May 2017). In April 2017, Scutellaria baicalensis extract was present in 3 of 65,434 cosmetic products of which the composition is known in EWG's Skin Deep Cosmetics Database, USA (http://www.ewg.org/skindeep/). Much more often used is the extract of the root: Scutellaria baicalensis (Baikal skullcap) root extract (158 products).

LITERATURE

1   Gallo R, Pastorino C, Gasparini G, Ciccarese G, Parodi A. *Scutellaria baicalensis* extract: a novel botanical allergen in cosmetic products? Contact Dermatitis 2016;75:387-388
2   Jung HS, Kim MH, Gwak NG, et al. Antiallergic effects of *Scutellaria baicalensis* on inflammation *in vivo* and *in vitro*. J Ethnopharmacol 2012;14: 345-349
3   Kim TW, Choi JM, Kim MS, Son HY, Lim JH. Topical application of *Scutellaria baicalensis* suppresses 2,4-dinitrochlorobenzene-induced contact dermatitis. Nat Prod Res 2016;30:705-709

2.406 SELENIUM SULFIDE

IDENTIFICATION

Description/definition : Selenium sulfide is the inorganic salt that conforms to the formula shown below
Chemical class(es) : Inorganic salts
Other names : Selenium disulfide
CAS registry number (s) : 7488-56-4
EC number(s) : 231-303-8
Merck Index monograph : 9843 (Selenium sulfides)
Function(s) in cosmetics : EU: antidandruff; hair conditioning. USA: antidandruff agents; hair conditioning agents
EU cosmetic restrictions : Regulated in Annex III/49 of the Regulation (EC) No. 1223/2009
Patch testing : 2% pet. (13); 3% pet. may cause irritant reactions, so 2% pet. may be too high (13)
Molecular formula : S_2Se

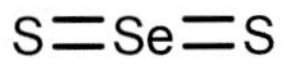

$$S = Se = S$$

GENERAL

Topical selenium sulfide has been used for decades in the treatment of seborrheic dermatitis and tinea versicolor. Selenium sulfide is available in various topical formulations including shampoo, lotion, cream, foam, and suspension. Several publications have reported side effects of selenium sulfide shampoo, suspension or other products, but in most, the causative role of their component selenium sulfide was not established beyond doubt and, in fact, the causal relationship between the product and the effect it allegedly caused, was not always clear.

CONTACT ALLERGY

Case reports and case series

In a group of 119 patients with allergic contact dermatitis from cosmetics, investigated in The Netherlands in 1986-1987, one case was caused by selenium sulfide in a shampoo (1,2). Three patients had contact dermatitis of the earlobes, external auditory canal and one of them also the neck, from the use of selenium sulfide shampoo. The symptoms were reproduced by application of undiluted or 'properly' diluted selenium sulfide shampoo. It was not specified whether patch tests have been performed with the shampoo, but certainly not with the active ingredient selenium sulfide; thus, contact allergy to selenium sulfide was not proven. With proper attention to plugging the ears and thorough rinsing of the scalp and ears after use of the preparation, the patients were able to continue using selenium sulfide once every three weeks (4).

Presence in cosmetic products and chemical analyses

In April 2017, selenium sulfide was present in 9 of 66,485 cosmetic products of which the composition is known in EWG's Skin Deep Cosmetics Database, USA (http://www.ewg.org/skindeep/).

OTHER SIDE EFFECTS

Other non-eczematous contact reactions

Several patients have developed orange to red-brown scalp discoloration after application of selenium sulfide-containing shampoos. In all of the cases, the discoloration resolved shortly after discontinuing the selenium sulfide. Lightly swabbing with isopropyl alcohol facilitated removal of the discoloration and therefore, may serve as a painless diagnostic method to prevent unnecessary evaluation with a biopsy (5).

Other discolorations of the skin and cutaneous appendages reported to be caused by selenium sulfide applications include brown discoloration of the distal fingernails (7), green hair (8), white hair turning yellow (xanthotrichia) (9,12), patchy hyperpigmentation (10), lightening of the hair (11), and orange staining of the scalp (11).

Systemic side effects

A woman who had been shampooing her hair with selenium sulfide shampoo 2 or 3 times weekly for 8 months may have developed systemic effects with generalized tremor, perspiration, pain in the lower abdomen, lethargy and anorexia with occasional vomiting. The patient had a 5 by 12 centimeter excoriated lesion on the scalp, which may have promoted absorption of selenium (3).

A lactating woman had tinea versicolor which was treated with selenium sulfide suspension one hour before bathing. This was to be done once a week for 3 weeks. On the second day after the initial application of the medicine, she noticed sudden suppression of lactation. It was discontinued for 1 week. Repeat application of the selenium sulfide suspension the next week gave the same result. The mechanism of this suppression of lactation, which was ascribed to selenium sulfide, was not clear (6).

LITERATURE

1 De Groot AC, Bruynzeel DP, Bos JD, van der Meeren HI, van Joost T, Jagtman BA, Weyland JW. The allergens in cosmetics. Arch Dermatol 1988;124:1525-1529
2 De Groot AC. Adverse reactions to cosmetics. PhD Thesis, University of Groningen, The Netherlands: 1988, chapter 3.4, pp.105-113
3 Ransone JW, Scott NM, Knobloch EC. Selenium sulfide intoxication. New Engl J Med 1961;264:384-385
4 Eisenberg BC. Contact dermatitis from selenium sulfide shampoo. Arch Derm Syph 1955;72:71-72
5 Gilbertson K, Jarrett R, Bayliss SJ, Berk DR. Scalp discoloration from selenium sulfide shampoo: a case series and review of the literature. Pediatr Dermatol 2012;29:84-88
6 Sugathan P, Riyaz N. Suppression of lactation by selenium disulfide. Int J Dermatol 1990;29:232-233
7 Wolf R, Perluk C, Krakowski A. Nail pigmentation resulting from selenium sulfide and copper. Int J Dermatol 1989;28:556-557
8 Fitzgerald EA, Purcell SM, Goldman HM. Green hair discoloration due to selenium sulfide. Int J Dermatol 1997;36:238-239
9 Prevost N, English JC III. Xanthotrichia (yellow hair) due to selenium sulfide and dihydroxyacetone. J Drugs Dermatol 2008;7:689-691
10 Gillum RF. Hyperpigmentation associated with selenium sulfide lotion. J Natl Med Assoc 1996;88:551
11 Danby FW, Maddin WS, Margesson LJ, Rosenthal D. A randomized, double-blind placebo-controlled trial of ketoconazole shampoo versus selenium sulfide 2.5% shampoo in the treatment of moderate to severe dandruff. J Am Acad Dermatol 1993;29:1008-1012
12 Crowley CS, Cohen PR. Yellow hair following sequential application of bacitracin zinc and selenium sulfide: Report of acquired xanthotrichosis and review of yellow hair discoloration. Dermatol Online J 2016 Jun 15;22(6)
13 De Groot AC. Patch Testing, 3rd Edition. Wapserveen, The Netherlands: acdegroot publishing, 2008 (ISBN 978-90-813233-1-4)

2.407 SESAMUM INDICUM (SESAME) SEED OIL

IDENTIFICATION

Description/definition : Sesamum indicum seed oil is the oil obtained from the seed of the sesame, *Sesamum indicum* L., Pedaliaceae

Chemical class(es) : Fats and oils

INCI name USA : Sesamum indicum (sesame) seed oil

Other names : Sesame oil

CAS registry number (s) : 8008-74-0

EC number(s) : 232-370-6

RIFM monograph/review : J Am Coll Toxicol 1993;12:261-277; Final report, March 2011; Int J Toxicol 2011; 30(Suppl.1):40-53 (access: www.cir-safety.org/ingredients)

Merck Index monograph : 8978

Patch testing : Undiluted (1,2,5)

Function(s) in cosmetics : EU: emollient; hair conditioning; masking; skin conditioning. USA: fragrance ingredients; skin-conditioning agents - occlusive

GENERAL

Sesame oil is a vegetable oil produced from the seeds of the sesame, *Sesamum indicum* L., Pedaliaceae. The oil is used in the production of perfumes, ointments, cosmetics, traditional Chinese topical medicines used for skin disorders (1), insecticides (synergist for pyrethrum insecticides), paints, varnishes, as a mild laxative, topical drug preparations, as a solvent for intramuscular injections and as a salad and cooking oil (13). Sesame oil is an unsaturated type vegetable oil which contains mainly the fatty acids oleic C18:1 (35-50%) and linoleic C18:2 (35-50%). The oil is classified in the oleic-linoleic acid group. It has a high unsaponifiable matters content (1.8%) (11). Sesame oil has remarkable stability to oxidation which may be due to the presence of the lignins sesamol, sesamolin and sesamin (12).

Contact allergy to sesame oil appears to be rare and has mainly been observed in patients with leg ulcers/stasis dermatitis treated with ointments containing sesame oil. Allergenic ingredients are sesamin and sesamolin (2,4,5,6). Sesamol has also been suspected as an allergen in sesame oil (4), but other authors reported negative patch test reactions to sesamol in sesame oil-allergic patients (2,5,6).

Immediate-type reactions to sesame oil in cosmetics (7-10) (contact urticaria) and from foods containing sesame oil (15-17) have been observed sporadically. Immediate hypersensitivity to sesame *seeds*, however, often resulting in anaphylaxis, is far from rare (18,19,22), and is estimated to affect 0.1-0.2% of the population (18), in areas where the food is available, but allergy to the seeds is not discussed in this chapter.

CONTACT ALLERGY

Case reports and case series

A woman had allergic contact cheilitis from contact allergy to sesame oil in a lipstick; she also reacted to its ingredients sesamin (0.1%-5% pet.) and sesamolin (0.5%-5%), but not to sesamol (2).

Contact allergy to Sesamum indicum seed oil in non-cosmetic products

Fifteen cases of allergic contact dermatitis from sesame oil in a group of 98 patients with leg ulcer and stasis dermatitis have been described. All 15 patients had been treated for long periods with ointments and creams containing sesame oil, and were positive on patch testing to sesame oil (3,24). Thirteen of these patients were investigated further and tested with three ingredients that were identified as sesamol, sesamin and sesamolin in crude and purified (pharmaceutical) sesame oil by the Baudovin color reaction method. Eight of the thirteen patients had positive patch test reactions to sesamol, 12 to sesamolin and 12 to sesamin. Patch tests with the pure substances on thin-layer sheets were inconclusive as to any difference between these chemicals (4). In another Dutch study, 14 of 81 patients with venous leg ulcers, that were more acute, extensive or more painful than could be expected, and who were patch tested, reacted to 100% olive oil (25).

A woman with palmoplantar pustulosis presented with severe pruritic erythematous macules, vesicles, pustules and crusts on the soles and palms, where she had applied an over-the-counter topical Chinese medicine, *shi-un-ko*. The lesions spread to the arms and legs and the patient had a fever from secondary erysipelas of the leg. The topical drug was composed of sesame oil as a solvent (60%) and of *Angelica acutiloba, Lithospermum erythrorhizon*, beeswax and lard. Patch tests were positive to *shi-un-ko*, undiluted and, in a second test session with its ingredients, to undiluted sesame oil, which was negative in 20 healthy volunteer controls (1).

Another woman treated a deep burn on her arm with the same ointment 'Shiunkoh' (pronounced Zi-Yun-Gao in Chinese). After 10 days of application, allergic contact dermatitis with erythema, edema and vesicles appeared around the wound. Patch tests showed positive reactions to 'Shiunkoh' (undiluted and 50%, 10%, 1% pet.), sesame oil (undiluted and 60%, 10% in petrolatum), sesamin 1% pet. and sesamolin 1% pet. (10 controls were negative to these substances). The patient had negative reactions to sesamol 1% pet., rapeseed oil (Brassica napus seed oil) 10% pet., and olive oil (Olea Europaea fruit oil) 10% pet. (5).

Cross-reactions, pseudo-cross-reactions and co-reactions

Not to rapeseed oil (Brassica napus seed oil) (5), olive oil (Olea Europaea fruit oil) (3,5) or peanut (Arachis hypogaea) oil (3).

Presence in cosmetic products and chemical analyses

In the USA, in April 2017, Sesamum indicum (sesame) seed oil was present in 755 of 56,714 cosmetic products of which the composition is known in FDA's Voluntary Cosmetic Registration Program (VCRP) (data obtained from FDA, May 2017). In January 2017, Sesamum indicum (sesame) seed oil was present in 468 of 64,655 cosmetic products of which the composition is known in EWG's Skin Deep Cosmetics Database, USA (http://www.ewg.org/skindeep/).

OTHER SIDE EFFECTS

Immediate-type reactions

Two patients had contact urticaria from sesame oil in cosmetics. One reacted to a cream and lipstick of his wife (connubial contact urticaria, consort contact urticaria), the other to a body oil. Eating foods with sesame seeds resulted in generalized urticaria (7). A woman with known sesame allergy developed contact urticaria from the application of a foundation cream containing sesame oil. Prick tests to the cream and sesame seed were positive (8,9). One patient had contact urticaria from sesame oil in a cosmetic (10). A review of contact urticaria caused by ingredients of cosmetics has been provided in ref 14.

A man had recurrent bouts of severe food reactions for 18 years. He found that many of the reactions could be attributed to ingestion of sesame products, particularly sesame oil. During these attacks, he would first experience a pin-and-needle sensation on his face, to be followed shortly by onset of chills, shakiness, and abdominal cramps after eating. On several occasions, he also experienced vomiting, fecal incontinence, and fainting. On other occasions, he would experience only a pin-and-needle sensation on his face, flushing, pruritic welts, and occasionally facial and lip swelling. Skin testing revealed a strongly positive response to whole commercial sesame seed oil. RAST was only marginally positive to sesame seed oil, commercial SSA (sesame seed antigen), and whole sesame seed. However, basophil histamine release tests revealed significant histamine release with SSA (90%), cooked sesame seed extract (80%), commercial sesame seed oil (40%), and intact sesame seed (70%) (15).

Another male patient suffered from urticaria but progressively more severe reactions with angioedema, bronchospasm, hypotension and shock after eating sesame seeds or foodstuffs containing sesame oil. Basophil activation tests were positive to both the seeds and the oil (16). Two similar patients with anaphylaxis from sesame oil are presented in ref. 17. A male individual had an 8-year history of several urticarial and angioedematous reactions within 30 minutes after ingesting sesame-containing foods, such as bread, crackers, and products cooked in sesame oil. Skin prick tests with sesame were negative. No sesame-specific IgE was detected. An open application test with sesame oil on the volar aspect of the forearm, however, was strongly positive. Oral provocation tests with increasing doses of sesame seeds (0.05, 0.5, 1, 5, and 10 gram) every 30 minutes gave a positive reaction with urticarial lesions 15 minutes after the dose of 1 gram. No oral provocation test with sesame oil was performed (23).

Other side effects

A man experienced subcutaneous nodules 9 months after self-injection of sesame seed oil into the pectoral area for muscle augmentation, a procedure apparently frequently performed in the body-building and fitness scene. Ultrasound imaging showed multiple, low reflecting round nodular areas of up to 1 centimeter in diameter in both breasts. Excision of a representative nodule revealed a cyst filled with oily material, surrounded by granulomatous tissue (subcutaneous oleomas) (20). Two patients developed exogenous lipoid pneumonia caused by repeated sesame oil 'pulling' via nasal or mouth washing and sometimes aspiration for several months (21).

LITERATURE

1   Oiso N, Yamadori Y, Higashimori N, Kawara S, Kawada A. Allergic contact dermatitis caused by sesame oil in a topical Chinese medicine, shi-un-ko. Contact Dermatitis 2008;58:109
2   Hayakawa R, Matsunaga K, Suzuki M, Hosokawa K, Arima Y, Shin C S, Yoshida M. Is sesamol present in sesame oil? Contact Dermatitis 1987;17:133-135

3   Dijk E van, Neering H, Vitanyi BEJ. Contact hypersensitivity to sesame oil in patients with ulcers and eczema. Acta Dermato-Venereol 1973;53:133-135

4   Neering H, Vitanyi BEJ, Malten KE, Ketel WG van, Dijk E van. Allergens in sesame oil contact dermatitis. Acta Dermato-venereol 1975;55:31-34

5   Kubo Y, Nonaka S, Yoshida H. Contact sensitivity to unsaponifiable substances in sesame oil. Contact Dermatitis 1986;15:215-217

6   Yoshida M, Hashimoto T. Determination of sesamolin, sesamin and sesamol in sesame oil by high performance liquid chromatography. J Food Hyg Soc Japan 1982;23:142-148

7   Pecquet C, Leynadier F, Saïag P. Immediate hypersensitivity to sesame in foods and cosmetics. Contact Dermatitis 1998;39:313

8   Dezfoulian B, De la brassinne M. urticaire de contact par application d'un fond de teint contenant de l'huile de sésame. Alim'inter 2002;7:no.6

9   Codreanu F, Morisset M, Cordebar V, Kanny G, Moneret-Vautrin DA. Risk of allergy to food proteins in topical medicinal agents and cosmetics. Eur Ann Allergy Clin Immunol 2006;38:126-130

10 Birnbaum J, Porri F, Castelain M, Vervloet D. Sesame seed and oil anaphylaxis. J Allergy Clin Immunol 1997;99:587 (data cited in ref. 2, article cannot be found)

11 Nzikou JM, Matos L, Bouanga-Kalou G, Ndangui CB, Pambou-Tobi NPG, Kimbonguila A, et al. Chemical composition on the seeds and oil of sesame (*Sesamum indicum* L.) grown in Congo-Brazzaville. Adv J Food Sc Technol 2009;1: 6-11

12 Lee J, Lee Y, Choe E. Effects of sesamol, sesamin and sesamolin extracted from roasted sesame oil on the thermal oxidation of methyl linoleate. LWT Food Sci Tech 2008;41:1871-1875

13 Mohammed MI, Hamza ZU. Physicochemical properties of oil extract from *Sesamum indicum* L. seeds grown in Jigawa state, Nigeria. J Appl Sci Environ Manage 2008;12:99-101

14 Verhulst L, Goossens A. Cosmetic components causing contact urticaria: a review and update. Contact Dermatitis 2016;75:333-344

15 Chiu JT, Haydik IB. Sesame seed oil anaphylaxis. J Allergy Clin Immunol 1991;88(3 Part 1):414-415

16 Stevens WJ, Ebo DG, Bridts CH, De Clerck LS. Anaphylaxis to sesame (*Sesamum indicum*) seed and sesame oil. J Allergy Clin Immunol 2002;109(Suppl.1):S217

17 Kanny G, De Hauteclocque C, Moneret-Vautrin DA. Sesame seed and sesame seed oil contain masked allergens of growing importance. Allergy 1996;51:952-957

18 Dalal I, Goldberg M, Katz Y. Sesame seed food allergy. Curr Allergy Asthma Rep 2012;12:339-345

19 Cianferoni A, Muraro A. Food-induced anaphylaxis. Immunol Allergy Clin North Am 2012;32:165-195

20 Darsow U, Bruckbauer H, Worret WI, Hofmann H, Ring J. Subcutaneous oleomas induced by self-injection of sesame seed oil for muscle augmentation. J Am Acad Dermatol 2000;42(2 Pt.1):292-294

21 Kuroyama M, Kagawa H, Kitada S, Maekura R, Mori M, Hirano H. Exogenous lipoid pneumonia caused by repeated sesame oil pulling: a report of two cases. BMC Pulm Med 2015;15:135

22 Gangur V, Kelly C, Navuluri L. Sesame allergy: a growing food allergy of global proportions? Ann Allergy Asthma Immunol 2005;95:4-11

23 Alonzi C, Campi P, Gaeta F, Pineda F, Romano A. Diagnosing IgE-mediated hypersensitivity to sesame by an immediate-reading 'contact test' with sesame oil. J Allergy Clin Immunol 2011;127:1627-1629

24 Van Dijk E, Neering H, Vitányi BE. Contactovergevoeligheid voor in zinkolie verwerkte Oleum Sesami. Ned Tijdschr Geneeskd 1972;116:2255-2259 (article in Dutch)

25 Malten KE, Kuiper JP. Contact cutaneous allergy in 100 cases of varicose ulcers. Phlebologie 1974;27:417-420 (article in French)

2.408   SHELLAC

IDENTIFICATION

Description/definition	: Shellac is the resinous secretion of the insect *Laccifer (Tachardia) lacca,* Coccidae
Chemical class(es)	: Biological products
Other names	: Lacca; lac resin; gum lac
CAS registry number (s)	: 9000-59-3
EC number(s)	: 232-549-9
CIR review(s)	: J Am Coll Toxicol 1986;5:309-327; Int J Toxicol 2011;30(Suppl.2):73-127 (access: www.cir-safety.org/ingredients)
Merck Index monograph	: 9887
Function(s) in cosmetics	: EU: binding; emollient; film forming; hair fixing; viscosity controlling. USA: binders; film formers; hair fixatives
Patch testing	: 20% alc. (Chemotechnique, SmartPracticeCanada)

GENERAL

Shellac is the purified form of a resin produced by the female insect *Laccifer (Tachardia) lacca,* which parasitically grows on some types of trees such as the jujube tree (*Zizyphus mauritiana*), the kusum tree (*Schleichera oleosa*), the plassey tree (*Butea monosperma*), the ghont tree (*Zizyphus xyloporus*) or the sacred fig tree (*Ficus religiosa*), which may be found in India, Thailand, Myanmar, and the south area of China (22). These insects voraciously consume tree sap while secreting viscous gummy resin (the metabolized byproduct) through their pores. The resin upon exposure to air dries to a substance called lac, which forms a protective barrier that encases the larvae and ultimately cocoons the immobilized adult insects as well. The resin forms thick encrustations on the twigs. The life cycle of the insects is approximately 6 months. After the swarming of the young insects, the resin, which is called sticklac, is scraped off the twigs and is further processed. By crushing the raw sticklac and then sieving, followed by water washing, seedlac is prepared. From seedlac, shellac is obtained through further purification by dissolving seedlac in methanol, then filtering, and evaporating the solvent (16). The chemical composition, the properties, and the color of shellac depend on the insect strain or insect species, the host trees, the environmental conditions as well as the process used for refining (3,12,16).

Composition

Seedlac consists of 70-80% resin, 6-7% wax, 4-8% coloring matter and 15-25% other materials, such as debris and moisture (16). The resin portion that constitutes the backbone of shellac is a complex mixture of polyesters consisting of a number of closely related sesquiterpenic acids of the cedrene skeleton (mainly jalaric acid and laccijalaric acid) and hydroxy fatty acids (mainly aleuritic acid), which can be separated into about 30% soft resin (single ester) and about 70% hard resin (polyesters consisting of several resin acid components) (16). The structural formulas of aleuritic acid and the terpenic acids are shown in Figure 1.

Figure 1. Structural formulas of aleuritic acid and terpenic acids in seedlac *

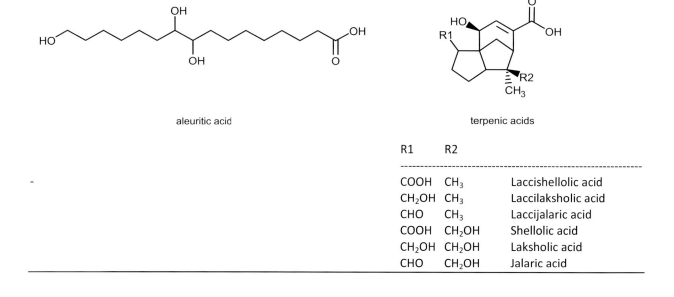

aleuritic acid   terpenic acids

R1	R2	
COOH	CH₃	Laccishellolic acid
CH₂OH	CH₃	Laccilaksholic acid
CHO	CH₃	Laccijalaric acid
COOH	CH₂OH	Shellolic acid
CH₂OH	CH₂OH	Laksholic acid
CHO	CH₂OH	Jalaric acid

Figure 1. Structural formulas of aleuritic acid and terpenic acids in seedlac * (*continued*)

* Adapted with permission from Wang L, Ishida Y, Ohtani H, Tsuge S, Nakayama T. Characterization of natural resin shellac by reactive pyrolysis-gas chromatography in the presence of organic alkali. Anal Chem 1999;71:1316-1322. Copyright 1999 American Chemical Society

The (average) amounts (mole percentages) of the acidic components of shellac determined in 4 Indian and 4 Thai shellac samples are shown in table 2.408.1. The wax part of shellac was found to contain a.o. C28 alcohol (octacosanol; CAS 67905-27-5), C30 alcohol (myricyl alcohol, triacontanol; CAS 67905-26-4), C32 alcohol (dotriacontanol; CAS 79554-32-8), and C34 alcohol (tetratriacontanol, carnatyl alcohol; CAS 28484-70-0) (16).

Table 2.408.1 Shellac: constituents of the acidic fraction of Indian and Thai shellac samples (adapted from ref. 16)

Constituent	Synonyms	CAS	Aver. amount (mole percent)
Terpenic acids (52 mole percent)			
Jalaric acid		24205-55-8	31.4 - 35.4
Laccijalaric acid			7.0 - 10.4
Shellolic acid	10β,13-dihydroxycedr-8-ene-12,15-dioic acid	4448-95-7	5.0 - 5.8
Laksholic acid		24205-56-9	2.0 - 2.3
Laccilaksholic acid		33051-49-9	0.9 - 1.4
Laccishellolic acid		24393-95-1	0.6 - 1.4
Aleuritic acid (34 mole percent)	9,10,16-Trihydroxyhexadecanoic acid	18951-77-4	33.6 - 34.8
Other fatty acids (14 mole percent)			
9,10-Dihydroxyhexadecanoic acid	9,10-Dihydroxypalmitic acid	29242-09-9	3.4 - 7.7
6-Hydroxytetradecanoic acid	Butolic acid	24205-54-7	1.3 - 4.3
16-Hydroxyhexadec-9-enoic acid	Epiambrettolic acid	17278-80-7	3.0 - 3.5
9,10-Dihydroxytetradecanoic acid	9,10-Dihydroxymyristic acid		1.2 - 1.4
Hexadecanoic acid	Palmitic acid	67701-02-4	0.1 - 0.4
Tetradecanoic acid	Myristic acid	32112-52-0	0.1 - 0.4
Hexadecenoic acid	Gaidic acid	25447-95-4	0.1 - 0.2

Aver.: Average

Uses

Shellac has been used as thermoplastics, adhesives, sealants, insulating materials, and coating materials in various fields such as industrial materials, medicine (15) and food ingredients (fruit, candy) due to its various unique properties such as thermoplasticity, oil resistibility, cohesiveness, and insulating ability along with its nonpoisonous nature. Other applications include wood varnishes, shoe polish, floor wax, and in cosmetics. Its emollient film–forming nature and ability to control viscosity make shellac (and shellac wax) particularly suitable for cosmetics such as eyeliners, mascaras, lipsticks, and hair dyes (as curling agent), nail lacquers and hair sprays (5,22).

CONTACT ALLERGY

Allergic contact dermatitis to shellac is uncommon and should be considered when patients are suffering from cheilitis or eyelid dermatitis. Some 30 cases have been reported, mostly from mascara, lipstick or other lip products, and eyeliner. The haptens responsible for contact sensitivity are unknown (3).

Patch testing in groups of patients

Results of testing shellac in groups of consecutive patients suspected of contact dermatitis (routine testing) and in *selected* patient groups are shown in table 2.408.2.

Routine testing

Shellac was part of the NACDG screening series in the period 2009-2012. In two of their biannual reports, the members of the NACDG found rates of sensitization of 1.6% and 1.7% (17,18). Probably because relevance rates were low (definite + probable relevance 12% in 2009-2010 and 35% in 2011-2012), shellac was thereafter removed from the screening series.

Testing in groups of selected patients

In a small group of 201 Chinese healthy student volunteers aged 19-30 years tested with shellac, there were 6 (3.0%) positive reactions, but their relevance was not mentioned (20).

Table 2.408.2 Patch testing in groups of patients

Years and Country	Test conc. & vehicle	Number of patients tested	positive (%)	Selection of patients (S); Relevance (R); Comments (C)	Ref.
Routine testing					
2011-12 USA, Canada	20% alc.	4231	66 (1.6%)	R: definite + probable relevance: 35%	17
2009-10 USA, Canada	20% alc.	4301	73 (1.7%)	R: definite + probable relevance: 12%	18
Testing in groups of selected patients					
2011 China	20% alc.	201	6 (3.0%)	S: healthy student volunteers 19-30 years; R: not stated	20

Case reports and case series

Shellac was responsible for 2 out of 959 cases of non-fragrance cosmetic allergy where the causal allergen was identified, Belgium, 2000-2010 (2). Shellac was responsible for 1 out of 399 cases of cosmetic allergy where the causal allergen was identified in a study of the NACDG, USA, 1977-1983 (1). In a group of 22 patients with allergic contact cheilitis seen in the period 1982-2001 in a tertiary referral center in the UK, 4 (18%) cases were caused by shellac (8). Single case reports of allergic contact dermatitis caused by shellac in mascara have been presented in refs. 9,10,19. Case series of three (14), four (5) and six (4) patients with contact allergic eyelid dermatitis from shellac in mascaras have also been published. One patient reacted to shellac in an eyeliner (11), another had allergic contact cheilitis from shellac in lipstick sealant (6) and five individuals reacted to shellac in lip care products (7).

Contact allergy to shellac in non-cosmetic products

A man had a large black tattoo over his left leg, in which numerous pruritic papules, 1-3 mm in size, had arisen a few weeks after tattooing. Patch tests showed positive reactions to shellac (20% alcohol) and to the original black tattoo ink. The diagnosis was allergic contact dermatitis caused by a tattoo ink in a patient with hypersensitivity to shellac. Shellac is often used as a binding agent in black tattoo ink, but whether the ink actually contained shellac, remained unknown (21).

Presence in cosmetic products and chemical analyses

In the USA, in April 2017, shellac was present in 49 of 56,714 cosmetic products of which the composition is known in FDA's Voluntary Cosmetic Registration Program (VCRP) (data obtained from FDA, May 2017). In April 2017, shellac was present in 20 of 66,485 cosmetic products of which the composition is known in EWG's Skin Deep Cosmetics Database, USA (http://www.ewg.org/skindeep/).

OTHER SIDE EFFECTS

Systemic side effects

Shellac in hair sprays has been linked to the development of thesaurosis in hairdressers (13).

LITERATURE

1   Adams RM, Maibach HI, Clendenning WE, Fisher AA, Jordan WJ, Kanof N, et al. A five-year study of cosmetic reactions. J Am Acad Dermatol 1985;13:1062-1069
2   Travassos AR, Claes L, Boey L, Drieghe J, Goossens A. Non-fragrance allergens in specific cosmetic products. Contact Dermatitis 2011;65:276-285
3   Das S, Jacob SE. Shellac. Dermatitis 2011;22:220-222
4   Le Coz CJ, Leclere JM, Arnoult E, Raison-Peyron N, Pons-Guiraud A, Vigan M. Allergic contact dermatitis from shellac in mascara. Contact Dermatitis 2002;46:149-152
5   Shaw T, Oostman H, Rainey D, Storrs F. A rare eyelid dermatitis allergen: shellac in a popular mascara. Dermatitis 2009;20:341-345
6   Rademaker M, Kirby JD, White IR. Contact cheilitis to shellac, Lanpol 5 and colophony. Contact Dermatitis 1986;15:307-308
7   Orton DI, Salim A, Shaw S. Allergic contact cheilitis due to shellac. Contact Dermatitis 2001;44:250
8   Strauss RM, Orton DI. Allergic contact cheilitis in the United Kingdom: a retrospective study. Am J Contact Dermat 2003;14:75-77
9   Scheman AJ. Contact allergy to quaternium-22 and shellac in mascara. Contact Dermatitis 1998;38:342-343

10 Gallo R, Marro I, Pavesi A. Allergic contact dermatitis from shellac in mascara. Contact Dermatitis 2005;53:238-239

11 Magerl A, Pirker C, Frosch PJ. Allergic contact eczema from shellac and 1,3-butylene glycol in an eyeliner. J Dtsch Dermatol Ges 2003;1:300-302

12 Pascoe D, Moreau L, Sasseville D. Emergent and unusual allergens in cosmetics. Dermatitis 2010;21:127-137

13 McLaughlin AI, Bidstrup PL, Konstam M. The effects of hair lacquer sprays on the lungs. Food Cosmet Toxicol (Oxford) 1963;1:171-188

14 McDonnell J, Taylor J, Evey P. Contact allergy to shellac in mascara. Am J Contact Dermat 2001;12:124

15 Henning S, Leick S, Kott M, Rehage H, Suter D. Sealing liquid-filled pectinate capsules with a shellac coating. J Microencapsul 2012;29:147-155

16 Wang L, Ishida Y, Ohtani H, Tsuge S, Nakayama T. Characterization of natural resin shellac by reactive pyrolysis-gas chromatography in the presence of organic alkali. Anal Chem 1999;71:1316-1322

17 Warshaw EM, Maibach HI, Taylor JS, Sasseville D, DeKoven JG, Zirwas MJ, et al. North American Contact Dermatitis Group patch test results: 2011-2012. Dermatitis 2015;26:49-59

18 Warshaw EM, Belsito DV, Taylor JS, Sasseville D, DeKoven JG, Zirwas MJ, et al. North American Contact Dermatitis Group patch test results: 2009 to 2010. Dermatitis 2013;24:50-59

19 Fisher AA. Contact Dermatitis, 3rd Edition. Philadelphia: Lea & Febiger, 1986:669

20 Zhao J, Li LF. Contact sensitization to cosmetic series of allergens in a general population in Beijing. J Cosmet Dermatol 2014;13:68-71

21 González-Villanueva, I, Hispán Ocete P, Silvestre Salvador JF. Allergic contact dermatitis caused by a black tattoo ink in a patient allergic to shellac. Contact Dermatitis 2016;75:247-248

22 Pecquet C. Allergic reactions to insect secretions. Eur J Dermatol 2013;23:767-773

2.409   SIMMONDSIA CHINENSIS (JOJOBA) SEED OIL

IDENTIFICATION

Description/definition	: Simmondsia chinensis seed oil is the fixed oil expressed or extracted from seeds of the desert shrub, jojoba, *Simmondsia chinensis*, Buxaceae
Chemical class(es)	: Botanical products and botanical derivatives
INCI name USA	: Simmondsia chinensis (jojoba) seed oil
Other names	: Buxus chinensis oil; jojoba seed oil
CAS registry number (s)	: 90045-98-0; 61789-91-1
EC number(s)	: 289-964-3
CIR review(s)	: J Am Coll Toxicol 1992;11:57-74; Final report, September 2008 (access: www.cir-safety.org/ingredients)
Merck Index monograph	: 6584 (jojoba)
Function(s) in cosmetics	: EU: emollient; hair conditioning; skin conditioning. USA: hair conditioning agents; skin-conditioning agents - occlusive
Patch testing	: 20% pet.

GENERAL

Jojoba (Simmondsia chinensis) is an arid perennial woody shrub grown in several American and African countries. Jojoba seeds, which are rich in liquid wax, were used in folk medicine for diverse ailments. Now, their products are frequently used in cosmetics, particularly body creams and hair care products (3). A review of jojoba products, their properties and (possible) applications have been reviewed (4) (Italian journal, but article in English).

CONTACT ALLERGY

Case reports and case series

Six patients had allergic contact dermatitis from jojoba oil in shampoo, hair conditioner, in creams or from pure oil.Five of them developed erythema or erythema and vesicles on their forearms to covered patch tests with jojoba oil 20% in olive oil and in liquid paraffin. The sixth individual, suspected of being sensitive to jojoba oil used as a hair conditioner, did not develop any reaction on his forearm to these patch tests. However, on two subsequent 'usage tests' of applying pure jojoba oil as a hair dressing, he again developed contact dermatitis on his scalp on both occasions. Twenty-eight control patients did not react to pure jojoba oil (1).

A woman had applied a moisturizing cream daily to her face for at least 5 years. For the past 3 months, itching had occurred a few hours after application, and for the past 2 weeks there had been dermatitis on her face. Patch testing with the European standard series, an ointment series, and her own cosmetics gave a positive reaction to one of the cosmetic creams. Later, she was tested again to the cream and with its 23 individual ingredients and positive reactions were seen to the cream itself (tested 'as is'), to jojoba oil 1.5% and to two other ingredients. Twenty controls were negative. However, when the patient was retested a year later, the reaction to jojoba oil 1.5% was negative (2).

Presence in cosmetic products and chemical analyses

In the USA, in April 2017, Simmondsia chinensis (jojoba) seed oil was present in 3452 of 56,714 cosmetic products of which the composition is known in FDA's Voluntary Cosmetic Registration Program (VCRP) (data obtained from FDA, May 2017). In April 2017, Simmondsia chinensis (jojoba) seed oil was present in 3287 of 65,434 cosmetic products of which the composition is known in EWG's Skin Deep Cosmetics Database, USA (http://www.ewg.org/skindeep/).

LITERATURE

1   Scott MJ, Scott MJ Jr. Jojoba oil. J Am Acad Dermatol 1982;6:545
2   Wantke F, Hemmer W, Gotz M, Jarisch R. Contact dermatitis from jojoba oil and myristyl lactate/maleated soybean oil. Contact Dermatitis 1996;34:71-72
3   Di Berardino L, Di Berardino F, Castelli A, Della Torre F. A case of contact dermatitis from jojoba. Contact Dermatitis 2006;55:57-58
4   Pazyar N, Yaghoobi R, Ghassemi MR, Kazerouni A, Rafeie E, Jamshydian N. Jojoba in dermatology: a succinct review. G Ital Dermatol Venereol 2013;148:687-691

2.410 SIMMONDSIA CHINENSIS (JOJOBA) SEED POWDER

IDENTIFICATION

Description/definition : Simmondsia chinensis seed powder is a powder obtained from the dried, ground seeds of the jojoba, *Simmondsia chinensis*, Buxaceae
Chemical class(es) : Botanical products and botanical derivatives
INCI name USA : Simmondsia chinensis (jojoba) seed powder
Other names : Jojoba powder; jojoba seed powder; Buxus chinensis powder
CAS registry number (s) : 90045-98-0
EC number(s) : 289-964-3
Merck Index monograph : 6584 (jojoba)
Function(s) in cosmetics : EU: skin conditioning. USA: skin-conditioning agents - miscellaneous
Patch testing : 15% pet. (1)

GENERAL

jojoba (*Simmondsia chinensis*) is an arid perennial woody shrub grown in several American and African countries. Jojoba seeds, which are rich in liquid wax, were used in folk medicine for diverse ailments. Now, their products are frequently used in cosmetics, particularly body creams and hair care products (1). A review of jojoba products, their properties and (possible) applications have been reviewed (2) (Italian journal, but article in English).

CONTACT ALLERGY

Case reports and case series

A female atopic patient presented with erythematous lesions spread all over the body, particularly on the abdomen and forearms. The day before, she had applied a cosmetic body cream. The dermatitis quickly healed with oral corticosteroid treatment. Patch tests were performed with all ingredients of the cosmetic product and the patient reacted to Simmondsia chinensis (jojoba) seed powder 15% pet. with erythema, edema and vesicles at D3. One control tested with this material was negative. Four months later the test with Simmondsia chinensis (jojoba) seed powder 15% pet. was repeated, and the existence of contact allergy was confirmed by a positive patch test. Another five control patients gave no positive reactions to the test material (1).

Presence in cosmetic products and chemical analyses

In the USA, in April 2017, Simmondsia chinensis (jojoba) seed powder was present in 16 of 56,714 cosmetic products of which the composition is known in FDA's Voluntary Cosmetic Registration Program (VCRP) (data obtained from FDA, May 2017). In April 2017, Simmondsia chinensis seed powder was present in 5 of 65,434 cosmetic products of which the composition is known in EWG's Skin Deep Cosmetics Database, USA (http://www.ewg.org/skindeep/).

LITERATURE

1 Di Berardino L, Di Berardino F, Castelli A, Della Torre F. A case of contact dermatitis from jojoba. Contact Dermatitis 2006;55:57-58
2 Pazyar N, Yaghoobi R, Ghassemi MR, Kazerouni A, Rafeie E, Jamshydian N. Jojoba in dermatology: a succinct review. G Ital Dermatol Venereol 2013;148:687-691

2.411 SODIUM BENZOATE

IDENTIFICATION

Description/definition   : Sodium benzoate is the sodium salt of benzoic acid that conforms to the formula shown below

Chemical class(es)   : Organic salts

Chemical/IUPAC name   : Sodium;benzoate

Other name(s)   : E211

CAS registry number (s)   : 532-32-1

EC number(s)   : 208-534-8

CIR review(s)   : Int J Toxicol 2001;20(Suppl.3):23-50; Final report, October 2011 (access: www.cir-safety.org/ingredients)

SCCS opinion(s)   : SCCP/0891/05 (18); SCCNFP/0532/01 (19)

Merck Index monograph   : 9988

Function(s) in cosmetics   : EU: anticorrosive; masking; preservative. USA: corrosion inhibitors; fragrance ingredients; preservatives

EU cosmetic restrictions   : Regulated in Annex V/1 of the Regulation (EC) No. 1223/2009

Patch testing   : 2% pet. (SmartPracticeEurope, SmartPracticeCanada); 5% pet. (Chemotechnique, SmartPracticeCanada); the test concentration/vehicle of the 5% pet. material needs improvement, as many positive reactions are weak and difficult to differentiate from non-allergic (irritant) patch test reactions (5)

Molecular formula   : $C_7H_6NaO_2$

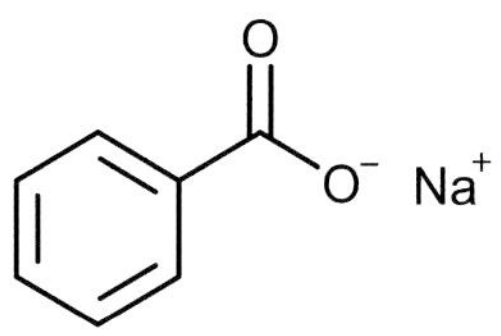

GENERAL

Sodium benzoate is widely used by the food industry to preserve soft drinks, wines, canned fish, mayonnaise, dressings, cheese, fruit juices, and even some fresh foods (banana, plum, blueberry) (36). It is also used in cosmetics (particularly toothpaste and mouthwash) and pharmaceutical products for preservation purposes. Numerous cases of adverse reactions to sodium benzoate have been recorded, but most of the studies that have been conducted lacked proper placebo controls or blinding. Cases of urticaria, asthma, rhinitis, dermatitis or anaphylactic shock have been reported following oral, dermal or inhalation exposure to sodium benzoate. Sodium benzoate may occasionally aggravate chronic urticaria, but is not thought to be the cause (33). The exact mechanism of such reactions is unknown, but does not appear to involve immunological mechanisms.

CONTACT ALLERGY

Patch testing in groups of patients

There have been no studies in which sodium benzoate was tested in consecutive patients suspected of contact dermatitis (routine testing). Sodium benzoate has been added to the North American Contact Dermatitis Group (NACDG) screening series in 2017. Results of studies patch testing sodium benzoate in groups of selected patients are shown in table 2.411.1. A high prevalence of sensitization (3.1%) was found in a study from the USA performed in patients tested with a supplemental cosmetic screening series, and 93% of the 27 positive patch test reactions were considered to be relevant (1), but this investigation had certain weaknesses. In other groups of selected patients (e.g., female hairdressers, female clients of hairdressers suspected of contact dermatitis, patients suspected of reactions to cosmetics), rates of sensitization to sodium benzoate ranged from 0.3% to 2%, the latter being one patient with ACD of the eyelids in a very small group of 46 such patients (15). Relevance was not mentioned or specified in any of the other studies (2,15,20,21,22).

Table 2.411.1 Patch testing in groups of patients: Selected patient groups

Years and Country	Test conc. & vehicle	Number of patients tested	positive (%)		Selection of patients (S); Relevance (R); Comments (C)	Ref.
2007-2012 IVDK	5% pet.	655	1	(0.3%)	S: female hairdressers with current or previous occupational contact dermatitis; R: not stated	21
		1431	8	(0.6%)	S: female patients, clients of hairdressers, in who hair cosmetics were regarded as a cause of dermatitis, and who had never worked as hairdressers; R: not stated	
2006-2011 IVDK	5% pet.	6934		(0.5%)	S: patients suspected of cosmetic intolerance and tested with a preservative series (selection procedure not stated); R: not stated	20
1996-2009 IVDK	5% pet.	79046	512	(0.7%) [a]	S: not specified; R: not specified; C: test substance slightly irritant, may result in false-positive reactions; increase in prevalence of sensitization	2
2000-2007 USA	5% pet.	868	27	(3.1%)	S: patients tested with a supplemental cosmetic screening series; R: 93%; C: weak study: a. high rate of macular erythema and weak reactions; b. relevance figures included 'questionable' and 'past' relevance	1
1994-2004 USA		46	1	(2%)	S: patients with allergic contact dermatitis of the eyelids; R: the reaction was relevant, but the culprit product was not mentioned	15
1981 France	5% pet.	465	9	(1.9%)	S: patients suspected of allergy to cosmetics, drugs, industrial products, or clothes; R: not stated	22

IVDK: Information Network of Departments of Dermatology, Germany, Austria, Switzerland
[a] standardized for sex and age

Case reports and case series

A patient had edematous cheilitis from contact allergy to sodium benzoate in toothpaste. He had positive patch test reactions to the toothpaste and to its ingredient sodium benzoate, tested 1% and 2% in both water and petrolatum. As the cheilitis got worse during brushing, non-immunological contact urticaria probably also played a role. The cheilitis also worsened from intake of a mucolytic drug containing sodium benzoate. Stopping the use of the toothpaste resulted in clinical improvement (14).

Presence in cosmetic products and chemical analyses

In the USA, in April 2017, sodium benzoate was present in 3662 of 56,714 cosmetic products of which the composition is known in FDA's Voluntary Cosmetic Registration Program (VCRP) (data obtained from FDA, May 2017). In January 2017, sodium benzoate was present in 2296 of 64,655 cosmetic products of which the composition is known in EWG's Skin Deep Cosmetics Database, USA (http://www.ewg.org/skindeep/). Sodium benzoate was present in 43 (24%) of 178 facial wipes for which ingredient information was obtained online and from retail stores, USA, 2016 (25). Sodium benzoate was present in 19 (35%) of 54 personal hygiene wet wipes for which ingredient information was obtained online and from retail stores, USA, 2016 (26). In 2009, in the USA, the ingredient lists of 796 hair products from one company were screened for the presence of sodium benzoate. Sodium benzoate was present in 30% of 279 shampoos, in 2% of 231 conditioners, and in 7% of 286 styling products (16).

In 2009, in the USA, the ingredient lists of 730 lip cosmetics and dental care products from one company were screened for the presence of sodium benzoate. Sodium benzoate was present in 0% of 31 lip liners, in 0% of 429 lipsticks, in 0% of 92 lip moisturizers, in 16% of 153 toothpastes, and in 60% of 25 mouth washes (17). In Germany, in 2006-2009, the labels of 4680 cosmetic products were screened for the presence of preservatives. Sodium benzoate was present in 10.6% of the products, according to labelling information (23). Benzoates (benzoid acid or sodium benzoate) were present in 250/3541 (6.7%) randomly sampled leave-on cosmetic products, Germany, 2006-2009 (3). Sodium benzoate was present in 34% of 204 cosmetic products (92 shampoos, 61 hair conditioners, 34 liquid soaps, 17 wet tissues) in Sweden, 2008 (4).

Miscellaneous allergic side effects

One patient had a fixed drug eruption from contact allergy to sodium benzoate in a syrup; the eruption was reproduced by oral provocation. A patch test with sodium benzoate was positive on uninvolved, but not involved skin (6).

OTHER SIDE EFFECTS

Immediate-type reactions

Three patients had airborne contact urticaria from sodium benzoate that they worked with occupationally in a pharmaceutical manufacturing plant (11). Another patient probably also had occupational airborne contact urticaria from sodium benzoate. This man, employed as an operator at a pharmaceutical plant for 3 years, recently started a new role within the plant. He was sieving sodium benzoate while wearing a hairnet, mask and nitrile gloves in a dusty environment. Within minutes of starting the procedure he became hot and red and quickly moved outside. His face and neck became red; the reaction settled over 1.5 hours (29). One patient had an anaphylactoid reaction to general anesthesia caused by intolerance to sodium benzoate (details unknown, article not read [37]). Non-immunological contact urticaria from sodium benzoate was seen in a child from toothpaste (perioral erythema) and a cream (13). A review of contact urticaria caused by ingredients of cosmetics has been provided in 2016 (10).

Miscellaneous side effects

Sodium benzoate has been incriminated in acute leucocytoclastic vasculitis (7) and in asthmatic crises (8) from its presence in some foods and drinks. A severe systemic reaction in a young woman with flush, angioedema, dyspnea, and severe hypotension (systolic blood pressure under 50 mm Hg) was ascribed to the presence of sodium benzoate in mustard and cheese (9). Sodium benzoate and other additives in foods and drugs have been held responsible for exacerbations of chronic idiopathic urticaria by some authors (27,28). A recent study in 100 such patients, who were challenged with 11 additives including sodium benzoate, showed with 95% confidence intervals, that sensitivity to any of the 11 food and drug additives occurs in fewer than 1% of patients with chronic idiopathic urticaria (24).

Another recent study with double-blind, placebo-controlled challenge tests also showed that that the percentage of repeated episodes of acute urticaria/angioedema reactions induced by sodium benzoate is very low (33).

Oral provocation with sodium benzoate has resulted in flare of atopic dermatitis in some children (12). Persistent non-atopic rhinitis has been ascribed to hypersensitivity to sodium benzoate present in foods (31,34,35). Some (especially urticarial) drug eruptions from amoxicillin-clavulanic acid in children may be related to hypersensitivity to the drug's excipient sodium benzoate (32). A woman had generalized pruritus without skin symptoms, very likely caused by intolerance to sodium benzoate (36).

LITERATURE

1   Wetter DA, Yiannias JA, Prakash AV, Davis MD, Farmer SA, el-Azhary RA, et al. Results of patch testing to personal care product allergens in a standard series and a supplemental cosmetic series: an analysis of 945 patients from the Mayo Clinic Contact Dermatitis Group, 2000-2007. J Am Acad Dermatol 2010;63:789-798
2   Schnuch A, Lessmann H, Geier J, Uter W. Contact allergy to preservatives. Analysis of IVDK data 1996-2009. Br J Dermatol 2011;164:1316-1325
3   Schnuch A, Mildau G, Kratz E-M, Uter W. Risk of sensitization to preservatives estimated on the basis of patch test data and exposure, according to a sample of 3541 leave-on products. Contact Dermatitis 2011;65:167-174
4   Yazar K, Johnsson S, Lind M-L, Boman A, Lidén C. Preservatives and fragrances in selected consumer-available cosmetics and detergents. Contact Dermatitis 2011;64:265-272
5   Brasch J, Uter W; Information Network of Departments of Dermatology (IVDK); German Contact Dermatitis Group (DKG). Characteristics of patch test reactions to common preservatives incorporated in petrolatum and water, respectively. Contact Dermatitis 2011;64:43-48
6   Vilaplana J, Romaguera C. Fixed drug eruption from sodium benzoate. Contact Dermatitis 2003;49:290-291
7   Vogt T, Landthaler M, Stolz W. Sodium benzoate-induced acute leukocytoclastic vasculitis with unusual clinical appearance. Arch Dermatol 1999;135:726-727
8   Petrus M, Bonaz S, Causse E, Rhabbour M, Moulie N, Netter JC, Bildstein G. Asthma and intolerance to benzoates. Arch Pediatr 1996;3:984-987
9   Michils A, Vandermoten G, Duchateau J, Yernault JC. Anaphylaxis with sodium benzoate. Lancet 1991;337(8754):1424-1425
10 Verhulst L, Goossens A. Cosmetic components causing contact urticaria: a review and update. Contact Dermatitis 2016;75:333-344
11 Nethercott JR, Lawrence MJ, Roy AM, Gibson BL. Airborne contact urticaria due to sodium benzoate in a pharmaceutical manufacturing plant. J Occup Med 1984;26:734-736
12 Van Bever HP, Docx M, Stevens WJ. Food and food additives in severe atopic dermatitis. Allergy 1989;44:588-594
13 Muñoz FJ, Bellido J, Moyano JC, Alvarez M, Fonseca JL. Perioral contact urticaria from sodium benzoate in a toothpaste. Contact Dermatitis 1996;35:51
14 Aguirre A, Izu R, Gardeazabal J, Diaz-Pérez JL. Edematous allergic contact cheilitis from a toothpaste. Contact Dermatitis 1993;28:42

15 Amin KA, Belsito DV. The aetiology of eyelid dermatitis: a 10-year retrospective analysis. Contact Dermatitis 2006;55:280-285

16 Scheman A, Jacob S, Katta R, Nedorost S, Warshaw E, Zirwas M, et al. Part 2 of a 4 part series. Hair cosmetics: trends and alternatives. Data from the American Contact Alternative Group. J Clin Aesthet Dermatol 2011;4:42-46

17 Scheman A, Jacob S, Katta R, Nedorost S, Warshaw E, Zirwas M, et al. Part 3 of a 4 part series. Lips and common Dental Care products: trends and alternatives. Data from the American Contact Alternative Group. J Clin Aesthet Dermatol 2011;4:50-53

18 SCCP (Scientific Committee on Consumer Products). Opinion on Benzoic Acid and Sodium Benzoate, 21 June 2005, SCCP/0891/05. Available at:
http://ec.europa.eu/health/archive/ph_risk/committees/04_sccp/docs/sccp_o_015.pdf

19 SCCNFP (Scientific Committee on Cosmetics and Non Food Products). Opinion concerning benzoic acid and sodium benzoate, 4 June 2002, SCCNFP/0532/01. Available at:
http://ec.europa.eu/health/archive/ph_risk/committees/sccp/documents/out166_en.pdf

20 Dinkloh A, Worm M, Geier J, Schnuch A, Wollenberg A. Contact sensitization in patients with suspected cosmetic intolerance: results of the IVDK 2006-2011. J Eur Acad Dermatol Venereol 2015;29:1071-1081

21 Uter W, Gefeller O, John SM, Schnuch A, Geier J. Contact allergy to ingredients of hair cosmetics – a comparison of female hairdressers and clients based on IVDK 2007–2012 data. Contact Dermatitis 2014;71:13-20

22 Meynadier JM, Meynadier J, Colmas A, Castelain PY, Ducombs G, Chabeau G, et al. Allergy to preservatives. Ann Dermatol Venereol 1982;109:1017-1023

23 Uter W, Yazar K, Kratz EM, Mildau G, Lidén C. Coupled exposure to ingredients of cosmetic products: II. Preservatives. Contact Dermatitis 2014;70:219-226

24 Rajan JP, Simon RA, Bosso JV. Prevalence of sensitivity to food and drug additives in patients with chronic idiopathic urticaria. J Allergy Clin Immunol Pract 2014;2:168-171

25 Aschenbeck KA, Warshaw EM. Allergenic ingredients in facial wet wipes. Dermatitis 2017 Mar 23. doi: 10.1097/DER.0000000000000268. [Epub ahead of print]

26 Aschenbeck KA, Warshaw EM. Allergenic ingredients in personal hygiene wet wipes. Dermatitis 2017 Mar 23. doi: 10.1097/DER.0000000000000275. [Epub ahead of print]

27 Juhlin L. Recurrent urticaria: clinical investigation of 330 patients. Br J Dermatol 1981;104:369-381

28 Supramaniam G, Warner JO. Artificial food additives intolerance in patients with angioedema and urticaria. Lancet 1986; ii:907-909

29 O'Connor R, McCarthy S, Murphy M, Bourke J. Airborne contact urticaria resulting from occupational exposure to sodium benzoate. Contact Dermatitis 2016;75(Suppl.1):101

30 Schalock PC, Dunnick CA, Nedorost S, Brod B, Warshaw E, Mowad C. American Contact Dermatitis Society Core Allergen Series: 2017 Update. Dermatitis 2017;28:141-143

31 Pacor ML, Di Lorenzo G, Martinelli N, Mansueto P, Rini GB, Corrocher R. Monosodium benzoate hypersensitivity in subjects with persistent rhinitis. Allergy 2004;59:192-197

32 Mori F, Barni S, Pucci N, Rossi ME, de Martino M, Novembre E. Cutaneous adverse reactions to amoxicillin-clavulanic acid suspension in children: the role of sodium benzoate. Curr Drug Saf 2012;7:87-91

33 Nettis E, Colanardi MC, Ferrannini A, Tursi A. Sodium benzoate-induced repeated episodes of acute urticaria/angio-oedema: randomized controlled trial. Br J Dermatol 2004;151:898-902

34 Asero R. Multiple intolerance to food additives. J Allergy Clin Immunol 2002;110:531-532

35 Asero R. Perennial rhinitis induced by benzoate intolerance. J Allergy Clin Immunol 2001;107:197

36 Asero R. Sodium benzoate-induced pruritus. Allergy 2006;61:1240-1241

37 Moneret-Vautrin DA, Moeller R, Malingrey L, Laxenaire MC. Anaphylactoid reaction to general anaesthesia: a case of intolerance to sodium benzoate. Anaesth Intensive Care 1982;10:156-157

2.412　SODIUM BISULFITE

IDENTIFICATION

Description/definition　　　: Sodium bisulfite is the inorganic salt that conforms to the formula shown below
Chemical class(es)　　　　: Inorganic salts
Chemical/IUPAC name　　 : Sodium hydrogen sulfite
CAS registry number (s)　 : 7631-90-5
EC number(s)　　　　　　 : 231-548-0
CIR review(s)　　　　　　 : Int J Toxicol 2003;22(Suppl.2):63-88 (access: www.cir-safety.org/ingredients)
Merck Index monograph : 9994
Function(s) in cosmetics　 : EU: antioxidant; preservative; reducing. USA: antioxidants; hair waving/straightening
　　　　　　　　　　　　　 agents; reducing agents
EU cosmetic restrictions　 : Regulated in Annexes III/99 and V/9 of the Regulation (EC) No. 1223/2009
Patch testing　　　　　　 : 1% pet. (SmartPracticeEurope, SmartPracticeCanada)
Molecular formula　　　　 : HO_3NaS

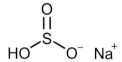

GENERAL

General information on (the adverse reactions to) sulfites can be found in Chapter 2.422 Sodium metabisulfite. The literature on contact allergy to sodium bisulfite, sodium sulfite, sodium metabisulfite, and some other sulfites (ammonium bisulfite, potassium metabisulfite and sodium hyposulfite [sodium thiosulfate]) has been reviewed in 2012 (3).

CONTACT ALLERGY

Patch testing in groups of patients

In 1995-1999, in a study by the IVDK (Germany, Austria, Switzerland), 579 patients with allergic periorbital contact dermatitis were patch tested with sodium bisulfite 1% pet. and 27 patients (4.7%) had a positive reaction; their relevance was not mentioned (7).

Case reports and case series

Sodium bisulfite was responsible for 1 out of 399 cases of cosmetic allergy where the causal allergen was identified in a study of the NACDG, USA, 1977-1983 (1).

Contact allergy to sodium bisulfite in non-cosmetic products

A woman had been treated daily with two types of eye drops for senile cataract for over two years. At one time, she developed edema, swelling, erythema, and vesicles on her eyelids. Patch tests gave a positive reaction to one of the eye drops and later to its ingredient sodium bisulfite 1% and 0.2% in water. The eye drops contained 0.2% sodium bisulfite. Ten controls were negative to the 1% patch test solution. However, when she was retested with sodium bisulfite, this time in a concentration of 2% in water, the reaction was negative. In spite of this, the authors suggested that the patient had allergic contact dermatitis (2). One patient had allergic contact dermatitis from sodium bisulfite in ketoconazole cream (5). A salad maker reacted to sodium bisulfite in foods (6).

　　A woman was referred because of a systemic skin eruption. Because she had difficulty with food intake due to decreased bowel movement resulting from myasthenia gravis, she had started a high-calorie infusion 10 days previously. Three days after the start of infusion, small red pruritic papules developed over most of the patient's body, indicative of a drug eruption. Topical steroid treatment did not improve the eruption, and the infusion was discontinued, after which the eruption gradually disappeared. Of the additives in the infusion, sodium bisulfite, present in a concentration of 0.04%, was suspected. Patch tests were positive to sodium bisulfite 0.1% and 1% pet., and the patient indicated itching at the patch test site of the infusion, despite her using 10 mg prednisolone per day. The patient was diagnosed with systemic contact dermatitis from sodium bisulfite (8).

Cross-reactions, pseudo-cross-reactions and co-reactions
Not to sodium sulfite (2); cross-reactivity from sodium metabisulfite (4). Sodium sulfite, sodium metabisulfite, and sodium bisulfite, when dissolved in water, exist in pH-dependent equilibrium with each other (see Chapter 2.412 Sodium bisulfite).

Presence in cosmetic products and chemical analyses
In the USA, in April 2017, sodium bisulfite was present in 65 of 56,714 cosmetic products of which the composition is known in FDA's Voluntary Cosmetic Registration Program (VCRP) (data obtained from FDA, May 2017). In April 2017, sodium bisulfite was present in 9 of 66,485 cosmetic products of which the composition is known in EWG's Skin Deep Cosmetics Database, USA (http://www.ewg.org/skindeep/).

OTHER SIDE EFFECTS

Immediate-type reactions
A man had episodes of bronchospasm requiring hospital admission after handling sodium bisulfite at the job. Skin tests with sodium *meta*bisulfite in a concentration of 10 mg/ml were negative. However, single-blind oral provocation tests with 1,5,20 and 50 mg sodium *meta*bisulfite in acid medium were positive at the 50-mg dose, eliciting bronchial and nasal symptoms (10). In a female asthmatic patient, wheezing and dyspnea became worse after an injection of betamethasone containing sodium bisulfite. An intradermal test revealed an immediate positive reaction to sodium bisulfite at a concentration of 100 mg/L. Challenge tests with increasing amounts of sodium bisulfite caused bronchospasm (11).

A young asthmatic woman had recurrent episodes of wheezing from certain foods. Later, she had an episode of diffuse pruritus, bright erythematous flushing, and acute wheezing after receiving an intravenous drug; inhalation of another drug resulted in respiratory arrest. Both pharmaceuticals contained sodium bisulfite. Skin testing for immediate hypersensitivity was positive and double-blind oral provocation tests with sodium *meta*bisulfite resulted in acute wheezing and flushing without urticaria within 10 minutes after receiving the *meta*bisulfite but not with placebo (12). Another individual had anaphylaxis after ingestion of sodium bisulfite (clinical details unknown) (13).

Miscellaneous side effects
A woman developed localized periorbital erythema and edema around the left eye after an intramuscular injection of dexamethasone containing 1 mg sodium bisulfite. The patient's sulfite sensitivity was confirmed by a sulfite oral provocation test: periorbital edema on the same site developed 12 hours after ingestion of 200 mg sodium bisulfite. An allergy skin prick test with 100 mg/ml sodium bisulfite showed a negative result. Patch tests were not performed and the pathogenesis of this reaction remained uncertain (9).

LITERATURE
1 Adams RM, Maibach HI, Clendenning WE, Fisher AA, Jordan WJ, Kanof N, et al. A five-year study of cosmetic reactions. J Am Acad Dermatol 1985;13:1062-1069
2 Nagayama H, Hatamochi A, Shinkai H. A case of contact dermatitis due to sodium bisulfite in an ophthalmic solution. J Dermatol 1997;24:675-677
3 Garcia-Gavin J, Parente J, Goossens A. Allergic contact dermatitis caused by sodium metabisulfite: a challenging allergen. A case series and literature review. Contact Dermatitis 2012;67:260-269
4 Vena GA, Foti C, Angelini G. Sulphite contact allergy. Contact Dermatitis 1994;31:172-175
5 Köhler A, Gall H. Kontaktallergisches Ekzem auf Natriumdisulfit in einer antimykotischen Ketoconazol-creme. Dermatosen Beruf Umwelt 2000;48:11-12
6 Epstein E. Sodium bisulfite. Contact Dermatitis Newsletter 1970;7:55
7 Herbst RA, Uter W, Pirker C, Geier J, Frosch PJ. Allergic and non-allergic periorbital dermatitis: patch test results of the Information Network of the Departments of Dermatology during a 5-year period. Contact Dermatitis 2004;51:13-19
8 Honda T, Kitoh A, Miyachi Y, Kabashima K. Drug eruption following high-calorie infusion: a possible systemic type IV allergic reaction to sulphites. Acta Derm Venereol 2015;95:854-855
9 Park HS, Nahm D. Localized periorbital edema as a clinical manifestation of sulfite sensitivity. J Korean Med Sci 1996;11:356-357

10 Valero AL, Bescos M, Amat P, Malet A. Bronchial asthma caused by occupational sulfite exposure. Allergol Immunopathol (Madr) 1993;21:221-224 (Article in Spanish)

11 Yoshikawa T, Fujiuchi S, Inaba S, Nagai T, Terai T. A case of asthma exacerbated by sulfite contained in betamethasone. Nihon Kyobu Shikkan Gakkai Zasshi 1990;28:895-899 (Article in Japanese)

12 Twarog FJ, Leung DY. Anaphylaxis to a component of isoetharine (sodium bisulfite). JAMA 1982;248:2030-2031

13 Prenner BM, Stevens JJ. Anaphylaxis after ingestion of sodium bisulfite. Ann Allergy 1976;37:180-182

2.413 SODIUM CHONDROITIN SULFATE

IDENTIFICATION

Description/definition : Sodium chondroitin sulfate is a derivative of a natural mucopolysaccharide
Chemical class(es) : Biological polymers and their derivatives; sulfuric acid esters
Other names : Chondroitin, hydrogen sulfate
CAS registry number (s) : 9007-28-7; 9082-07-9
EC number(s) : 232-696-9
Function(s) in cosmetics : EU: antistatic; hair conditioning; skin conditioning. USA: hair conditioning agents; skin-conditioning agents - miscellaneous
Patch testing : 1% pet. (1)

GENERAL

Sodium chondroitin sulfate is an oligosaccharide used in cosmetic products for its antistatic, hair conditioning and skin-conditioning properties, and as an emollient; it is also claimed to have 'anti-aging' properties. It is manufactured from fish cartilage or from cartilage from other animals. In France, and possibly in other countries, sodium chondroitin sulfate, taken by mouth, is also used to reduce osteoarthritis pain. It can be used in food supplements, and there is some concern that chondroitin sulfate might make asthma worse. Some cutaneous adverse reactions to sodium chondroitin sulfate in cosmetics have been reported to the manufacturer of these products, but patch testing was not performed (1).

CONTACT ALLERGY

Case reports and case series

A non-atopic woman was seen with erythematous, sharply demarcated dermatitis affecting her face, particularly the lower eyelids, chin, and neck. The eruption had been present for 7 months and was resistant to various treatments. Patch tests with the European baseline, fragrance and cosmetic series and with the patient's personal hygiene, cosmetic, and topical pharmaceutical products gave a positive reaction to a night cream. A repeated open application test (ROAT) with this cream in the left elbow induced an eczematous reaction after 3 days. Further tests (open test and patch test, read at D2 and D4) were performed later with all ingredients, provided by the manufacturer and there was a positive reaction to sodium chondroitin sulfate 1% pet. at D2 and D4. On D2, a flare-up of her previous dermatitis was evident. Fifty control patients were tested with chondroitin sulfate 1% pet. and there were no positive reactions.

Presence in cosmetic products and chemical analyses

In the USA, in April 2017, sodium chondroitin sulfate was present in 228 of 56,714 cosmetic products of which the composition is known in FDA's Voluntary Cosmetic Registration Program (VCRP) (data obtained from FDA, May 2017). In April 2017, sodium chondroitin sulfate was present in 134 of 65,434 cosmetic products of which the composition is known in EWG's Skin Deep Cosmetics Database, USA (http://www.ewg.org/skindeep/).

LITERATURE

1   Vigan M. Allergic contact dermatitis caused by sodium chondroitin sulfate contained in a cosmetic cream. Contact Dermatitis 2014;70:383-384

2.414   SODIUM COCOAMPHOACETATE

IDENTIFICATION

Description/definition : Sodium cocoamphoacetate is the amphoteric organic compound that conforms generally to the formula shown below, where RCO- represents the fatty acids derived from coconut oil

Chemical class(es) : Alkylamido alkylamines

Other names : Glycine, *N*-(2-aminoethyl)-*N*-(2-hydroxyethyl)-, *N*-coco-acyl derivatives, monosodium salts; cocoamphoglycinate

CAS registry number (s) : 90387-76-1; 68334-21-4

EC number(s) : 291-352-6; 269-819-0

CIR review(s) : J Am Coll Toxicol 1990;9:121-142; Int J Toxicol 2008;27(Suppl.1):77-142 (access: www.cir-safety.org/ingredients)

Function(s) in cosmetics : EU: cleansing; foaming; hair conditioning; surfactant. USA: hair conditioning agents; surfactants - cleansing agents; surfactants – foam boosters

Patch testing : 1% and 2% water (2); 2% water is slightly irritant

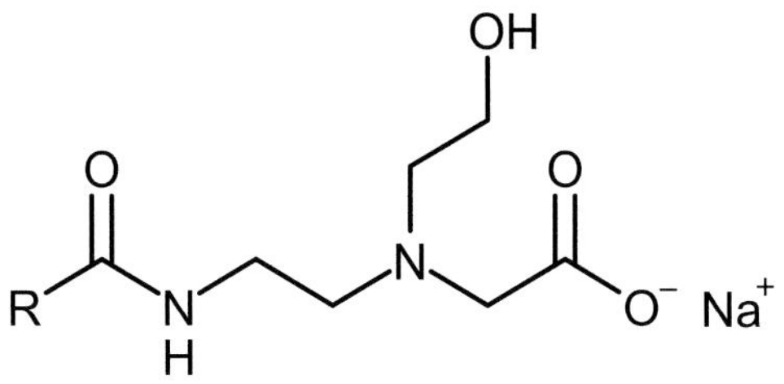

GENERAL

Sodium cocoamphoacetate is an amphoteric surfactant that belongs to the alkylamido alkylamides. Chemically related surfactants are lauroamphoacetate, coco- and lauroamphodiacetate, coco- and lauro-amphopropionate, and lauro- and cocoamphodipropionate (3), which are all obtained by the condensation reaction between fatty acids and aminoethyl ethanolamines. They are widely used in skin and hair cleansing products, hair conditioning products, and in hair dyes, in concentrations ranging from 0.1% to 50%. Apart from cosmetics, they are also used in pharmaceutical products for the treatment of glaucoma and hemorrhoids, in disinfectants for contact lenses, in materials for bandages, and for household and industrial applications such as in dishwashing and laundry detergents and paints (2).

CONTACT ALLERGY

Case reports and case series

Sodium cocoamphoacetate was responsible for 3 out of 959 cases of non-fragrance cosmetic allergy where the causal allergen was identified, Belgium, 2000-2010 (1).

An atopic woman suffered from longstanding hand dermatitis and was shown to be allergic to MCI/MI, methyldibromo glutaronitrile, 2-bromo-2-nitropropane-1,3-diol, fragrance mix, dihydroxyacetone, and the rubber additives thiuram mix and mercaptobenzothiazole. One day, she developed dermatitis of the face following the application of an eye make-up remover, which did not contain any of the known contact allergens. She had already performed a ROAT that had produced a strong positive reaction. Patch testing confirmed most previous results and there was a positive reaction to the eye makeup remover at D2 and D4. Chemical analysis of the product did not show methyldibromo glutaronitrile to be present in it. The manufacturer provided all ingredients and the patient had a positive reaction to sodium cocoamphoacetate 2% water with induration, many papules, and some vesicles, spreading outside the patch test area at D2 and D4 and still visible at D7. The patient had a weaker, but still positive reaction to a 1% test preparation. Thirty-three control subjects were tested with both concentrations and 'some' weak irritant reactions were seen in 'some' subjects tested with sodium cocoamphoacetate 2% water, but the 1% dilution did not evoke any responses. After withdrawal of the causative product and treatment with a local corticosteroid and emollient, the dermatitis of the face cleared (2). This individual probably was one of the three patients mentioned in ref. 1 (above).

Cross-reactions, pseudo-cross-reactions and co-reactions

Sodium lauroamphoacetate, disodium cocoamphodipropionate, sodium cocoamphopropionate (4). It remains to be clarified whether these amphoacetate products share a common impurity that might represent the actual allergen (4).

Presence in cosmetic products and chemical analyses

In the USA, in April 2017, sodium cocoamphoacetate was present in 200 of 56,714 cosmetic products of which the composition is known in FDA's Voluntary Cosmetic Registration Program (VCRP) (data obtained from FDA, May 2017). In April 2017, sodium cocoamphoacetate was present in 117 of 65,434 cosmetic products of which the composition is known in EWG's Skin Deep Cosmetics Database, USA (http://www.ewg.org/skindeep/).

LITERATURE

1   Travassos AR, Claes L, Boey L, Drieghe J, Goossens A. Non-fragrance allergens in specific cosmetic products. Contact Dermatitis 2011;65:276-285
2   Goossens A, Bruze M, Gruvberger B, Gielen K, Stoskute L. Contact allergy to sodium cocoamphoacetate present in an eye make-up remover. Contact Dermatitis 2006;55:302-304
3   De Groot AC, Weijland JW. Contact allergy to disodium cocoamhodipropionate. Contact Dermatitis 1996;35:248-249
4   Pesonen M, Suomela S, Kuuliala O, Aalto-Korte K. Occupational contact allergy to sodium cocoamphopropionate in a hand cleanser. Contact Dermatitis 2016;74:246-248

2.415 SODIUM COCOAMPHOPROPIONATE

IDENTIFICATION

Description/definition	: Sodium cocoamphopropionate is the amphoteric organic compound that conforms generally to the formula shown below, where RCO- represents the fatty acids derived from coconut oil
Chemical class(es)	: Alkylamido alkylamines
Other names	: Fatty acids, coco, reaction products with 2-((2-aminoethyl)amino)ethanol, mono(2-carboxyethyl) derivs., monosodium salts
CAS registry number (s)	: 132647-08-6; 93820-52-1
EC number(s)	: 298-632-7
CIR review(s)	: J Am Coll Toxicol 1990;9:121-142 (access: www.cir-safety.org/ingredients)
Function(s) in cosmetics	: EU: cleansing; foam boosting; foaming; hair conditioning; surfactant. USA: hair conditioning agents; surfactants - cleansing agents; surfactants - foam boosters; surfactants - hydrotropes
Patch testing	: 1% water (1); 10% pet. (2); 20 controls were negative to 10% pet. (3)

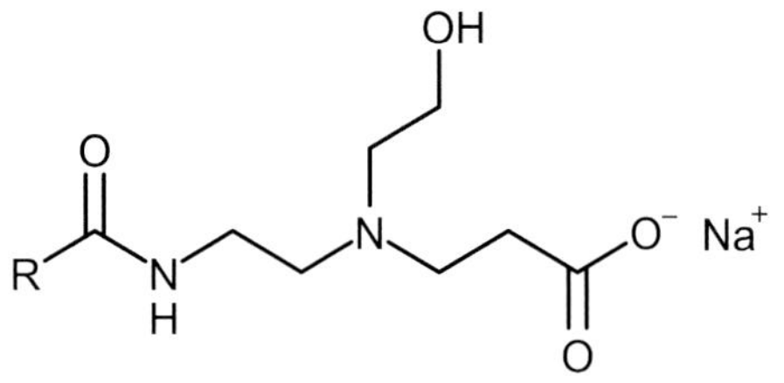

GENERAL

Sodium cocoamphopropionate is an amphoteric surfactant used as a foaming and cleansing agent in skin cleansers, shampoos and hair conditioners.

CONTACT ALLERGY

Case reports and case series

Two patients had occupational allergic contact dermatitis from cocoamphopropionate in a disinfectant soap (1). Eight patients developed occupational allergic contact dermatitis caused by sodium cocoamphopropionate in the same disinfectant hand cleanser containing 2% of the surfactant. Seven of them were employees of an international fast-food restaurant chain, and one was a nurse in a surgical department. The affected restaurant workers were young adults. They developed hand eczema a few months after beginning restaurant work, in which frequent hand washing with this particular hand cleanser was required as part of the hygiene routines. Patch tests were positive to the hand cleanser in a dilution series and to sodium cocoamphoacetate 10% in petrolatum; twenty controls were negative (2,3). The actual allergen in the sodium cocoamphopropionate product remains to be defined.

Cross-reactions, pseudo-cross-reactions and co-reactions

Possibly cross-reactivity between ethylenediamine and ethanolamine derivatives present as by-products, intermediates or reactants in the surfactant (1). Sodium cocoamphoacetate, sodium lauroamphoacetate and disodium cocoamphodipropionate (3). It remains to be clarified whether these amphoacetate products share a common impurity that might represent the actual allergen (3).

Presence in cosmetic products and chemical analyses

In the USA, in April 2017, sodium cocoamphopropionate was present in 78 of 56,714 cosmetic products of which the composition is known in FDA's Voluntary Cosmetic Registration Program (VCRP) (data obtained from FDA, May 2017). In April 2017, sodium cocoamphopropionate was present in 12 of 66,485 cosmetic products of which the composition is known in EWG's Skin Deep Cosmetics Database, USA (http://www.ewg.org/skindeep/).

LITERATURE

1   Hagvall L, Bråred-Christensson J, Inerot A. Occupational contact dermatitis caused by sodium cocoampho-propionate in a liquid soap used in fast-food restaurants. Contact Dermatitis 2014;71:122-124

2   Pesonen M, Kuuliala O, Suomela S, Aalto-Korte K. Epidemic of occupational contact dermatitis caused by sodium cocoamphopropionate in a hand cleanser among fast-food restaurant workers. Contact Dermatitis 2016;75(Suppl.1):37

3   Pesonen M, Suomela S, Kuuliala O, Aalto-Korte K. Occupational contact allergy to sodium cocoamphopropionate in a hand cleanser. Contact Dermatitis 2016;74:246-248

2.416   SODIUM DIHYDROXYCETYL PHOSPHATE

IDENTIFICATION

Description/definition : Sodium dihydroxycetyl phosphate is the sodium salt of a complex mixture of phosphate esters of dihydroxycetyl alcohol
Chemical class(es)   : Phosphorus compounds
Chemical/IUPAC name   : Sodium;bis(2-hydroxyhexadecyl) phosphate
Other names   : Sodium bis(2-hydroxyhexadecyl) phosphate; sodium 1-(2-hydroxyhexadecoxy-oxido-phosphoryl)oxyhexadecan-2-ol
CAS registry number (s) : 94277-32-4
EC number(s)   : 304-615-8
Function(s) in cosmetics : EU: emulsifying; surfactant. USA: surfactants - emulsifying agents
Patch testing   : 0.5%-2% water; 5% pet. (1); especially 5% pet. may induce irritant reactions (1)
Molecular formula   : $C_{32}H_{66}NaO_6P$

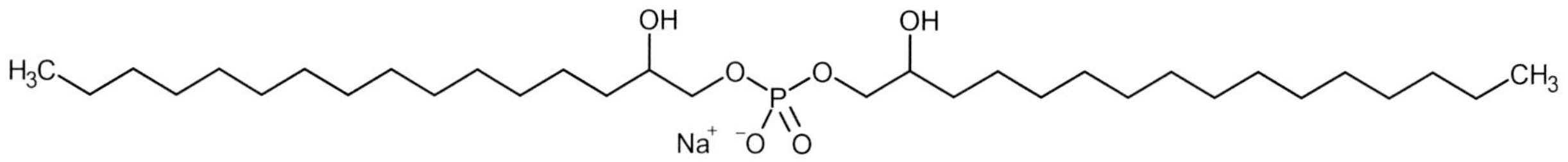

CONTACT ALLERGY

Case reports and case series

A woman, with previous atopic dermatitis, had acute severe confluent edematous dermatitis of the face, neck and hands. She was treated with systemic prednisolone. Patch tests, performed after healing of the dermatitis, gave a positive reaction to one of three herbal moisturizing creams, that the patient had used before the onset of dermatitis. Later, when patch tested with its ingredients, she showed a positive reaction to sodium dihydroxycetyl phosphate (SDP) 5% pet. This emulsifier was present in the cream 'in the range of one to 5%'. In a second patch test session, this reaction was reproduced and the patient also reacted with many positives to an aqueous dilution series down to 0.1%. A repeated open application test with 1% aqueous sodium dihydroxycetyl phosphate was strongly positive already after three applications, accompanied by a flare of the dermatitis of the face. Later, the patient was tested with an ethanol extract of the commercial sodium dihydroxycetyl phosphate (Dragophos S 2/918501), four of its fractions, and its components, as identified by gas chromatography – mass spectrometric (GC-MS) analysis. The SDP extract contained 1-hexadecene, hexadecan-2-one, isopropyl myristate, hexadecane-1,2-diol, and an unknown substance, possibly isopropyl ether of hexadecane-1,2-diol. The patient reacted to the extract, to 3 of the fractions and to hexadecane-1,2-diol 3% in alcohol. However, as the latter reaction was much weaker than previous patch tests, it was suggested that the unidentified chemical, possibly the isopropyl ether of hexane-1,2-diol, was the actual allergenic component (1). Of 20 controls tested with sodium dihydroxycetyl phosphate 5% pet., 8 (40%) had a ?+ reaction, indicating an irritant potential of SDP in this test concentration and vehicle.

A man started applying a cosmetic 12% ammonium lactate lotion twice daily for xerosis on the anterior left leg. Five days later, a very pruriginous erythema developed, which then became eczematous. After discontinuing application of the lotion, and with the administration of topical corticosteroids, the dermatitis resolved in a couple of days. Patch test with the GEIDC standard series and the lotion, tested as is, gave a positive reaction to the cosmetic product. When tested with its ingredients, the patient reacted to the emulsifier Dragophos® S 5% and 1% in water. Fifteen controls carried out with the lotion and Dragophos® S 5% water were negative. The emulsifier was described as sodium dihydroxycetyl phosphate isopropyl hydroxycetyl ether (3).

Cross-reactions, pseudo-cross-reactions and co-reactions

DEA-hydroxypalmitylether and palmityl phosphate mixture (1).

Presence in cosmetic products and chemical analyses

In the USA, in April 2017, sodium dihydroxycetyl phosphate was present in 12 of 56,714 cosmetic products of which the composition is known in FDA's Voluntary Cosmetic Registration Program (VCRP) (data obtained from FDA, May 2017). In April 2017, sodium dihydroxycetyl phosphate was present in 16 of 65,522 cosmetic products of which the composition is known in EWG's Skin Deep Cosmetics Database, USA (http://www.ewg.org/skindeep/).

Other information

Seven patients, known to be allergic to Arnica, were patch tested with various cosmetic preparations containing Arnica extract. Three reacted to an Arnica herbal hand cream preparation, which contains sodium dihydroxycetyl phosphate (SDP). The patients were tested with sodium dihydroxycetyl phosphate 5% pet. as well as the commercial emulsifier containing SDP (trade name Dragophos S 2/918501) 1% pet. Two individuals had doubtful positive patch tests to Dragophos S 2/918501; one of these was also doubtful positive to SDP, while the other had a positive patch test to SDP. The third person was positive to SDP but had a negative reaction to Dragophos S 2/918501 (2). It is difficult to interpret these data, but as the test concentration of 5% pet. for sodium dihydroxycetyl phosphate induces irritant responses in 40% of controls (1), a proper test concentration for the commercial Dragophos is unknown and the three patients had many other positive patch tests (risk of excited skin syndrome), it is likely that some or may be all reactions to SDP have been irritant rather than allergic.

LITERATURE

1   Lomholt H, Rastogi SC, Andersen KE. Allergic contact dermatitis from sodium dihydroxycetyl phosphate, a new cosmetic allergen?. Contact Dermatitis 2001;45:143-145
2   Paulsen E, Christensen LP, Andersen KA. Cosmetics and herbal remedies with Compositae plant extracts – are they tolerated by Compositae-allergic patients? Contact Dermatitis 2008;58:15-23
3   Goday Bujan JJ, Bayona IY, Güemes MG, Lorentzen RI, Arechavala RS. Allergic contact dermatitis from Dragophos S, a new emulsifier. Contact Dermatitis 1996;34:158

2.417   SODIUM HYDROXYMETHYLGLYCINATE

IDENTIFICATION

Description/definition   : Sodium hydroxymethylglycinate is the sodium salt of the substituted amino acid that
                             conforms to the formula shown below
Chemical class(es)   : Alkyl-substituted amino acids
Chemical/IUPAC name   : Sodium;2-(hydroxymethylamino)acetate
Other names   : Glycine, *N*-(hydroxymethyl)-, monosodium salt
CAS registry number (s)   : 70161-44-3
EC number(s)   : 274-357-8
Function(s) in cosmetics   : EU: hair conditioning; preservative. USA: hair conditioning agents; preservatives
EU cosmetic restrictions   : Regulated in Annex V/51 of the Regulation (EC) No. 1223/2009
Patch testing   : No data available
Molecular formula   : $C_3H_7NaNO_3$

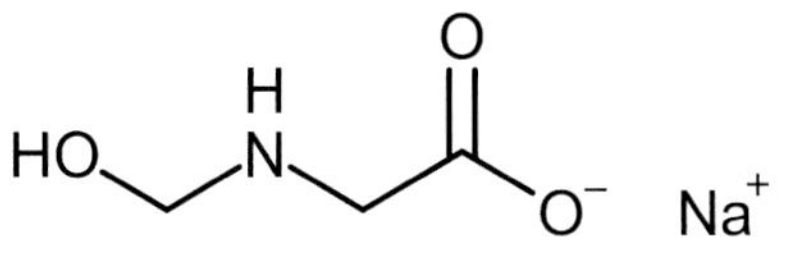

GENERAL

Sodium hydroxymethylglycinate (SHMG) is formed from synthetic glycine reacting with sodium hydroxide in water and formaldehyde. SHMG has antimicrobial activity against gram-negative and gram-positive organisms, yeasts, and molds. Generally, it is used at concentrations of 0.1% to 0.5% and may be employed in cosmetics such as shampoos, conditioners, soaps, moisturizers, body sprays, and baby wipes (8). SHMG may also be used as preservative in a variety of non-cosmetic products, including surface coatings, adhesives, as neutralizing agent for acids/acrylics polymers, in cleaning/washing agents, room sprays, in rinsing agents, pesticides and in artificial tears (5,7,8). Notably, SHMG is used in many products marketed as being 'natural' or 'organic' (5,8).

CONTACT ALLERGY

Case reports and case series

Two children may have reacted to sodium hydroxymethylglycinate in baby wipes and one in a cosmetic cream. All three patients had positive patch tests to formaldehyde. However, neither the products nor their ingredients have been patch tested and the causal relationship was mainly based on clinical data of improvement of dermatitis after avoidance of the products (1).

Cross-reactions, pseudo-cross-reactions and co-reactions

As sodium hydroxymethylglycinate is a formaldehyde-releaser, pseudo-cross-reactivity with formaldehyde is to be expected.

Presence of sodium hydroxymethylglycinate in cosmetic products

In May 2017, sodium hydroxymethylglycinate was present in 104 of 66,923 cosmetic products of which the composition is known in EWG's Skin Deep Cosmetics Database, USA (http://www.ewg.org/skindeep/). In the USA, in April 2017, sodium hydroxymethylglycinate was present in 113 of 56,714 cosmetic products of which the composition is known in FDA's Voluntary Cosmetic Registration Program (VCRP) (data obtained from FDA, May 2017). In 2010, the preservative had been listed in the same database as ingredient in 0.5% of 41,113 products (5).

In 2008, 19.5% of 33,212 cosmetics and toiletries registered in the USA Food and Drug Administration (FDA) Voluntary Cosmetic Registration Database contained a formaldehyde-releaser. They were more frequently used in rinse-off products (27.3%) than in stay-on cosmetics (16.9%). Sodium hydroxymethylglycinate was present in 0.2% of all products; in stay-on cosmetics, the percentage was 0.1 and in rinse-off products 0.6 (4). In the same period, of 496 stay-on cosmetic products present in a local drugstore in The Netherlands and investigated by checking the ingredient labelling, not one single product proved to contain this preservative (4).

Amounts of free formaldehyde released by sodium hydroxymethylglycinate and chemical analyses

Sodium hydroxymethylglycinate is a formaldehyde-releaser, synthesized by reacting glycine with sodium hydroxide in water and formaldehyde. SHMG decomposes very rapidly and releases formaldehyde when dissolved in water or polar solvents. It theoretically releases all of the formaldehyde it contains upon decomposition, translating to one mole of formaldehyde per mole of SHMG and resulting in a total free formaldehyde content of 0.118% (1180 ppm) in a product containing 0.5% SHMG (the maximum concentration allowed in the EU) (2,3). A 0.5 wt% preservative solution of SHMG at pH 8.5 was found to contain 0.12 wt% (1200 ppm) of free formaldehyde (6).

LITERATURE

1 Jacob SE, Hsu JW. Sodium hydroxymethylglycinate: a potential formaldehyde-releasing preservative in child products. Dermatitis 2009;20:347-349

2 Scientific Committee on Cosmetic Products and Non-Food Products Intended for Consumers. Opinion concerning the determination of certain formaldehyde releasers in cosmetic products. SCCNFP/586/02, final. Adopted by the SCCNFP during the 22nd plenary meeting of 17 December 2002. Available at: http://ec.europa.eu/health/ph_risk/committees/sccp/documents/outl88_en.pdf

3 Scientific Committee on Cosmetic Products and Non-Food Products Intended for Consumers. Opinion concerning a clarification on the formaldehyde and para-formaldehyde entry in Directive 76/768/EEC on cosmetic products. SCCNFP/587/02, final. Adopted by the SCCNFP during the 22nd plenary meeting of 17 December 2002. Available at: http://ec.europa.eu/health/ph_risk/committees/sccp/documents/outl87_en.pdf

4 De Groot AC, Veenstra M. Formaldehyde-releasers in cosmetics in the USA and in Europe. Contact Dermatitis 2010;62:221-224

5 De Groot AC, White IR, Flyvholm M-A, Lensen G, Coenraads P-J. Formaldehyde-releasers in cosmetics: relationship to formaldehyde contact allergy. Part 1. Characterization, frequency and relevance of sensitization, and frequency of use in cosmetics. Contact Dermatitis 2010;62:2-17

6 Emeis D, Anker W, Wittern K-P. Quantitative ^{13}C NMR spectroscopic studies on the equilibrium of formaldehyde with its releasing preservatives. Anal Chem 2007;79:2096-2100

7 Ghelardi E, Celandroni F, Gueye SA, Salvetti S, Campa M, Senesi S. Antimicrobial activity of a new preservative for multiuse ophthalmic solutions. J Ocul Pharmacol Ther 2013;29:586-590

8 Russell K, Jacob SE. Sodium hydroxymethylglycinate. Dermatitis 2010;21:109-110

2.418   SODIUM LAURETH SULFATE

IDENTIFICATION

Description/definition	: Sodium laureth sulfate is the sodium salt of sulfated ethoxylated lauryl alcohol that conforms generally to the formula shown below, where n averages between 1 and 4
Chemical class(es)	: Alkyl ether sulfates
Chemical/IUPAC name	: Poly(oxy-1,2-ethanediyl),α-sulfo-ω-(dodecyloxy)-, sodium salt (1-4 mol EO average molar ratio)
Other names	: Dodecyl sodium sulfate; PEG-(1-4) lauryl ether sulfate, sodium salt; sodium 2-(2-dodecyloxyethoxy)ethyl sulfate; sodium polyoxyethylene lauryl ether sulfate; sodium lauryl ether sulfate
CAS registry number (s)	: 3088-31-1; 9004-82-4; 68891-38-3; 1335-72-4; 68585-34-2; 91648-56-5
EC number(s)	: 221-416-0; 500-234-8; 500-223-8; 293-918-8
CIR review(s)	: J Am Coll Toxicol 1983;2:1-34; Int J Toxicol 2010;29(Suppl.3):151-161 (access: www.cir-safety.org/ingredients)
Function(s) in cosmetics	: EU: cleansing; emulsifying; foaming; surfactant. USA: surfactants - cleansing agents; surfactants – emulsifying agents
Patch testing	: 2% water (1); 1% water (2)
Molecular formula	: $CH_3(CH_2)_{11}(OCH_2CH_2)_nOSO_3Na$

CONTACT ALLERGY

Case reports and case series

A woman presented with a red, swollen face with weeping eczematous lesions. There were also red, oozing and crusted acute lesions on her shoulders and scalp. Two days previously, the patient had washed her hair with a new shampoo. Patch tests with the standard series and the shampoo gave a positive reaction to the shampoo, both in an open test (undiluted) and in a patch test with the product 2% water. When the ingredients of this cosmetic product were tested separately, the patient reacted to sodium lauryl ethyl sulfate 2% water. Three controls were negative. The symptoms cleared when she changed to a shampoo with a saponine base (1).

Contact allergy to sodium laureth sulfate in non-cosmetic products

Lauryl ether sulfate (LES) is a synthetic detergent with very low sensitizing and irritant properties often used in shampoos, bath foams, shower gels, and dishwashing products. Contact allergy to these agents has been reported (3,5,6) but this was mainly due to highly allergenic contaminants, which were sometimes formed during the production process (notably unsaturated sultones and 2-chlorosultones) (3,7,8). Thus, single batches of the finished product sold in one locality were allergenic, while no harmful effects from the use of the same brand were observed elsewhere (4,5). LES used for dishwashing, shampooing, or cleaning has caused several outbreaks of contact dermatitis in Norway (5) and Sweden (4).

In Denmark, 6 out of 12 women cleaning for 7 hours per day at a boarding-school developed an itching eruption within 2 months after the introduction of a new liquid detergent for dish-washing and general cleaning. They reacted to the batch of LES used in the product, but not to other 'normal' batches (2). LES itself was not tested, but the product diluted to obtain a 1% LES concentration. The other ingredients were tested separately and were negative. The allergenic impurity was not identified (2).

Presence in cosmetic products and chemical analyses

In the USA, in April 2017, sodium laureth sulfate was present in 4560 of 56,714 cosmetic products of which the composition is known in FDA's Voluntary Cosmetic Registration Program (VCRP) (data obtained from FDA, May 2017). In April 2017, sodium laureth sulfate was present in 1815 of 66,485 cosmetic products of which the composition is known in EWG's Skin Deep Cosmetics Database, USA (http://www.ewg.org/skindeep/).

LITERATURE

1   Van Haute N, Dooms-Goossens A. Shampoo dermatitis due to cocobetaine and sodium lauryl ether sulphate. Contact Dermatitis 1983;9:169

2   Sylvest B, Hjorth N, Magnusson B. Lauryl ether sulphate dermatitis in Denmark. Contact Dermatitis 1975;1:359-362

3   Walker AP, Ashforth GK, Davies RE, Newman EA, Ritz HL. Some characteristics of the sensitizer in alkyl ethoxy sulphate. Acta Dermatovener (Stockholm) 1973;53:141-144

4   Fregert S, Magnusson B. Personal communication (cited in ref. 3)

5   Magnusson B, Gilje O. Allergic contact dermatitis from a dish-washing liquid containing laury! ether sulphate. Acta Dermatovener (Stockholm) 1973;53:136-140
6   Gloxhuber C, Potokar M, Braig S, et al. Untersuchungen über das Vorkommen eines sensibilisierenden Bestandteils in einem technischen Alkyläthersulfat. Fette-Seifen-Anstrichmittel 1974;76:126-129
7   Lindup WE, Nowell PT. Role of sultone contaminants in an outbreak of allergic contact dermatitis caused by alkylethoxysulphates: A review. Food Cosmet Toxicol 1978;16:59-62
8   Connor DS, Ritz HL, Ampulski RS, et al. Identification of certain sultones as the sensitizers in an alkyl ethoxy sulfate. Fette-Seifen-Anstrichmittel 1975;77:25-29

2.419   SODIUM LAUROAMPHOACETATE

IDENTIFICATION

Description/definition   : Sodium lauroamphoacetate is the amphoteric organic compound that conforms
                          to the formula shown below
Chemical class(es)   : Alkylamido alkylamines
Chemical/IUPAC name   : Sodium;2-[2-(dodecanoylamino)ethyl-(2-hydroxyethyl)amino]acetate
Other names   : Glycine, N-(2-hydroxyethyl)-N-[2-(1-oxododecylamino)ethyl]-, monosodium salt;
                          lauroamphoglycinate
CAS registry number (s)   : 66161-62-4; 156028-14-7
EC number(s)   : 266-197-2
Function(s) in cosmetics : EU: cleansing; foam boosting; foaming; hair conditioning; surfactant. USA: hair
                          conditioning agents; surfactants - cleansing agents; surfactants - foam boosters
Patch testing   : Commercial solution containing 35% sodium lauroamphoacetate 10%, 5% and 1%
                          in water (1)
Molecular formula   : $C_{18}H_{35}N_2NaO_4$

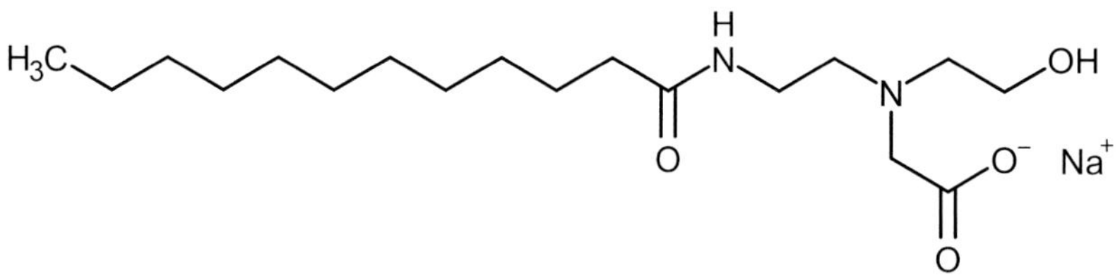

CONTACT ALLERGY

Case reports and case series

A non-atopic woman presented with dermatitis of the face of 3 weeks duration. She attributed her symptoms to the use of a face wash containing sodium lauroamphoacetate. Another female patient developed severe dermatitis on the face after using a face wash containing sodium lauroamphoacetate. Patch tests were performed with the European standard series, sodium lauroamphoacetate solution containing 35% active ingredients (tested pure, 10% water, 5% water, 1% water) and aminoethylethanolamine (AEE) 1% in various vehicles including water and alcohol and in a dilution series down to 0.005%. Both patients showed positive reactions to sodium lauroamphoacetate at all the tested concentrations and to AEE 1% in all vehicles. Of 20 controls, 6 had irritant reactions to the undiluted sodium lauroamphoacetate, but there were no reactions to any other dilution or to AEE. The undiluted sodium lauroamphoacetate test material contained 1130 ppm AEE. As aminoethylethanolamine has known sensitizing capacity, the authors suggested this may have been be the actual allergen by its presence as an impurity in sodium lauroamphoacetate (1).

Contact allergy to sodium lauroamphoacetate in non-cosmetic products

Two patients had allergic contact dermatitis from lauroamphoacetate in detergents; the patients also reacted to aminoethylethanolamine, a reagent used in the synthesis of commercial lauroamphoacetate. As aminoethylethanol-amine was shown to be present in the commercial lauroamphoacetate solution and it has known sensitizing capacity, the authors suggested this may have been the actual allergen by its presence as an impurity (1).

Cross-reactions, pseudo-cross-reactions and co-reactions

Sodium cocoamphoacetate, disodium cocoamphodipropionate, sodium cocoamphopropionate (2). It remains to be clarified whether these amphoacetate products share a common impurity that might represent the actual allergen (2).

Presence in cosmetic products and chemical analyses

In the USA, in April 2017, sodium lauroamphoacetate was present in 264 of 56,714 cosmetic products of which the composition is known in FDA's Voluntary Cosmetic Registration Program (VCRP) (data obtained from FDA, May 2017). In April 2017, sodium lauroamphoacetate was present in 123 of 65,434 cosmetic products of which the composition is known in EWG's Skin Deep Cosmetics Database, USA (http://www.ewg.org/skindeep/).

LITERATURE

1 Foti C, Bonamonte D, Mascolo G, Tiravanti G, Rigano L, Angelini G. Aminoethylethanolamine: a new allergen in cosmetics? Contact Dermatitis 2001;45:129-133

2 Pesonen M, Suomela S, Kuuliala O, Aalto-Korte K. Occupational contact allergy to sodium cocoamphopropionate in a hand cleanser. Contact Dermatitis 2016;74:246-248

2.420 SODIUM LAUROYL SARCOSINATE

IDENTIFICATION

Description/definition	: Sodium lauroyl sarcosinate is the sodium salt of lauroyl sarcosine, which conforms generally to the formula shown below
Chemical class(es)	: Sarcosinates and sarcosine derivatives
Chemical/IUPAC name	: Sodium;2-[dodecanoyl(methyl)amino]acetate
Other names	: *N*-Dodecanoylsarcosine sodium salt; sodium *N*-lauroylsarcosinate; *N*-methyl-*N*-(1-oxododecyl)glycine, sodium salt
CAS registry number (s)	: 137-16-6
EC number(s)	: 205-281-5
CIR review(s)	: Int J Toxicol 2001;20(Suppl.1):1-14; Final report, April 2016 (access: www.cir-safety.org/ingredients)
Merck Index monograph	: 5671 (Gardol®)
Function(s) in cosmetics	: EU: antistatic; cleansing; emulsifying; foaming; hair conditioning; skin conditioning; surfactant; viscosity controlling. USA: hair conditioning agents; surfactants – cleansing agents
Patch testing	: 30% water (1); this test concentration is likely to be irritant, only 2 controls were performed; 1% water, to which 10 controls were negative (2)
Molecular formula	: $C_{15}H_{28}NNaO_3$

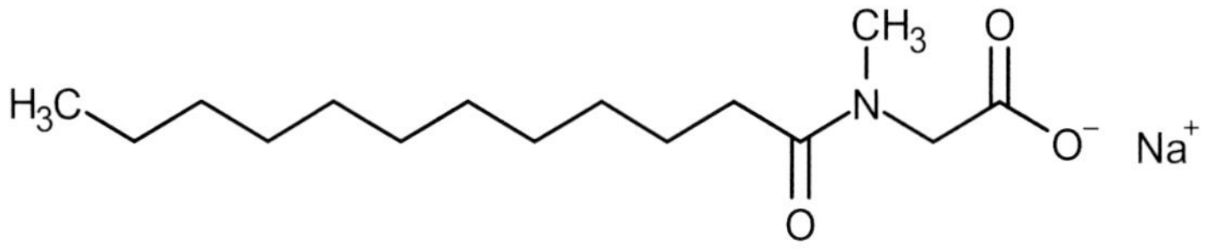

CONTACT ALLERGY

In 2015-2016, in the USA, 47 patients who had previously reacted to one or more surfactants present in the NACDG screening series were patch tested with sodium lauroyl sarcosinate 0.5% and 1% water and 3 (6.4%) had positive reactions. The relevance of these reactions was not mentioned. There were also 10 doubtful reactions, which may indicate that these concentrations (or at least the higher one) are marginally irritant (4).

Case reports and case series

A nurse had occupational allergic contact dermatitis from sodium lauroyl sarcosinate in a hand soap (1). A massage therapist had occupational ACD from sodium lauroyl sarcosinate in a liquid hand cleanser she used for her hands (2). This same patient was probably again presented in an Abstract one year later (3).

Cross-reactions, pseudo-cross-reactions and co-reactions

Oleamidopropyl dimethylamine (2); cocamidopropyl betaine (2); the authors suggested cross-sensitivity, but another likely explanation is pseudo-cross-reactivity to common ingredients in these amide-type surfactants. Co-reactions with chemically related surfactants (cocamidopropyl dimethylamine [amidoamine], oleamidopropyl dimethylamine, cocamidopropyl betaine, isostearamidopropyl morpholine lactate, disodium lauroamphodiacetate) have been observed (4).

Presence in cosmetic products and chemical analyses

In the USA, in April 2017, sodium lauroyl sarcosinate was present in 589 of 56,714 cosmetic products of which the composition is known in FDA's Voluntary Cosmetic Registration Program (VCRP) (data obtained from FDA, May 2017). In April 2017, sodium lauroyl sarcosinate was present in 223 of 65,434 cosmetic products of which the composition is known in EWG's Skin Deep Cosmetics Database, USA (http://www.ewg.org/skindeep/).

LITERATURE

1   Zemtsov A, Fett D. Occupational allergic contact dermatitis to sodium lauroyl sarcosinate in the liquid soap. Contact Dermatitis 2005;52:166-167
2   Hanson JL, Warshaw EM. Contact allergy to surfactants in a hypoallergenic liquid cleanser. Dermatitis 2015;26:284-286
3   Hanson JL, Warshaw EM. Contact allergy to surfactants in a liquid cleanser. Dermatitis 2016;27(5):e2
4   Grey KR, Hanson J, Hagen SL, Hylwa SA, Warshaw EM. Epidemiology and co-reactivity of novel surfactant allergens: a double-blind randomized controlled study. Dermatitis 2016;27:348-354

2.421   SODIUM LAURYL SULFATE

IDENTIFICATION

Description/definition	: Sodium lauryl sulfate is the sodium salt of lauryl sulfate that conforms to the formula shown below
Chemical class(es)	: Alkyl sulfates
Chemical/IUPAC name	: Sodium dodecyl sulfate
Other name(s)	: Sodium lauryl sulphate
CAS registry number (s)	: 151-21-3
EC number(s)	: 205-788-1
CIR review(s)	: J Am Coll Toxicol 1983;2:127-181 (access: www.cir-safety.org/ingredients)
Merck Index monograph	: 10038
Function(s) in cosmetics	: EU: cleansing; denaturant; emulsifying; foaming; surfactant. USA: denaturants; surfactants – cleansing agents
Patch testing	: 0.25% water (Chemotechnique, SmartPracticeEurope, SmartPracticeCanada); 0.5% pet. (SmartPracticeCanada)
Molecular formula	: $C_{12}H_{26}NaO_4S$

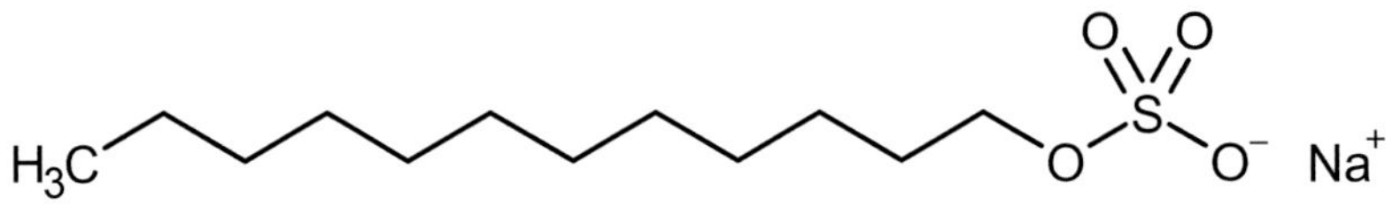

GENERAL

Sodium lauryl sulfate (SLS) is with sodium lauryl sarcosinate the most commonly used surface-active agent. SLS is used in hard surface cleansing products, dishwashing liquids, grease cleaners, car washing detergents, personal hygiene products such as shampoos, shower gels, bath foams, face cleansing soaps and toothpastes, as detergents and foaming agents (9). Contact allergy to SLS – if it exists at all (well-documented and proven cases of contact allergy have not been reported) – is extremely rare. The commercial preparations available for patch testing (0.25% water from Chemotechnique, SmartPracticeEurope, and SmartPracticeCanada and 0.5% pet. from SmartPractice Canada) are not meant to demonstrate contact allergy to SLS, as these concentrations result in 20-35% irritant patch test reactions (8). However, irritability to SLS has been found to be related to irritability to certain allergens.

Therefore, routine patch testing with the irritant sodium lauryl sulfate, supplemental to diagnostic patch testing with allergens, has been advocated as an aid to the interpretation of certain erythematous, possibly infiltrated allergen patch test reactions as presumably irritant (in case of an irritant reaction to SLS) or probably allergic (if no reaction to SLS was observed) at the time of patch test reading (8,12). In other words, the patch test may be used to form an idea of the individual's susceptibility to irritation of the skin. In one large study, the risk of an irritant reaction to SLS was significantly increased in males and in older patients (and with 2 days application time), but other studies have presented different results (8). Such irritancy studies are not discussed here.

CONTACT ALLERGY

Patch testing in groups of patients
In Italy, in 2001-2006, 129 patients with chronic cheilitis were patch tested with sodium lauryl sulfate 1% in water and one (0.8%) had a positive reaction which was considered to be relevant. The culprit product was not mentioned and the test concentration was obviously far too high (3).

Case reports and case series
In the period 1996-2013, in a tertiary referral center in Valencia, Spain, 5419 patients were patch tested. Of these, 628 individuals had allergic contact dermatitis to cosmetics. Sodium lauryl sulfate was the responsible allergen in one individual (2). Two patients had allergic contact cheilitis and perioral dermatitis from sodium lauryl sulfate present in toothpaste. The first patient had positive reactions to a toothpaste 2% in water and later reacted strongly to its ingredient SLS, both at 1% and at 0.1% in water. The other allergic individual reacted weakly to a toothpaste 1% water and had a strong reaction to SLS 1% and a weakly positive reaction to SLS 0.1% water at D4. It was not mentioned whether the skin eruption disappeared after avoidance of SLS-containing products and no control tests were performed with SLS 1% and 0.1% water (1).

Contact allergy to sodium lauryl sulfate in non-cosmetic products

A woman had allergic contact dermatitis from hydrocortisone ointment. When patch tested with its ingredients, there were positive reactions at D2 to sodium lauryl sulfate and 'self-emulsifying wax'. The test concentrations were not mentioned. The self-emulsifying wax was a partially sulfated (approximately 10%) fatty alcohol mixture in the 12- to 18-carbon-atom range. Sodium lauryl sulfate is a 12-carbon-atom sulfated lauryl alcohol, which means that the wax may have contained sodium lauryl sulfate (7) A woman had allergic contact cheilitis from a lip salve and from a topical pharmaceutical preparation to treat herpes labialis. When patch tested, she reacted to both products. The allergen in the lip salve was mandelic acid (Chapter 2.284 Mandelic acid). When tested with the ingredients of the topical pharmaceutical preparation, the patient had positive reactions to acyclovir and to sodium lauryl sulfate 0.5% water (D2 +++, D3 ++). The authors suggested this to be an irritant patch test reaction, but no explanatory information was provided and no repeat test with SLS was performed (6).

In experiments with SLS 5% in water as an irritant in wetting tests in 495 patients with occupational contact dermatitis, cumulative insult dermatitis and healthy control persons, irritant reactions were seen in 52% of the patients with eczema and in 12% of control subjects. In 12 patients (11 with contact and cumulative insult dermatitis) crescendo reactions were noted in the wetting tests. The histories of these persons showed that they had been exposed to SLS-containing substances in detergents, dishwashing agents, and cosmetics. The lymphocyte transformation test with SLS was positive in 10 of 12 patients with an eczematous reaction to the SLS wetting test. There was no increased DNA synthesis in patients with cumulative insult dermatitis. These results were, according to the authors, an almost certain sign of sensitization. Patch tests with SLS 0.1% water were, however, positive in only two of 12 wetting test positive subjects with an eczematous reaction. Unfortunately, it was not mentioned what the causative products were and whether the dermatitis healed or improved after avoiding them. Control tests with SLS 0.1% water were not performed (5).

Presence in cosmetic products and chemical analyses

In the USA, in April 2017, sodium lauryl sulfate was present in 2511 of 56,714 cosmetic products of which the composition is known in FDA's Voluntary Cosmetic Registration Program (VCRP) (data obtained from FDA, May 2017). In January 2017, sodium lauryl sulfate was present in 661 of 64,655 cosmetic products of which the composition is known in EWG's Skin Deep Cosmetics Database, USA (http://www.ewg.org/skindeep/).

OTHER SIDE EFFECTS

Immediate-type reactions

A man indicated that he was unable to brush his teeth with toothpaste, because it would result in abdominal gas, bloating, cramps, and diarrhea occurring after brushing using toothpaste. Blind tests with 2 toothpastes containing SLS and one without it resulted in the usual gastrointestinal symptoms with the 2 SLS-containing toothpastes, whereas he had no trouble when using the product without sodium lauryl sulfate. A prick test with 0.001 mg/ml SLS solution resulted in a wheal of 6 mm (same as the positive histamine control) and a flare of 30 mm, which proved, according to the authors, the existence of allergy to SLS. Control prick tests were not performed. The patient has been using SLS-free toothpaste for nearly one year without any adverse reactions (9).

Other non-eczematous contact reactions

In patients with recurrent aphthous ulcers, the number of ulcers decreased significantly when switching from a SLS-containing toothpaste to a toothpaste free of SLS. It was suggested that the denaturing effect of SLS on the oral mucin layer, with exposure of the underlying epithelium, induces an increased incidence of recurrent aphthous ulcers (10,11). In (somewhat) older literature, sodium lauryl sulfate has been suspected of being comedogenic in 'people with more sensitive complexions or acne-prone problems', based on rabbit ear assays (4).

LITERATURE

1   Lee A-Y, Yoo S-H, Oh J-G, Kim Y-G. 2 Cases of allergic contact cheilitis from sodium lauryl sulfate in toothpaste. Contact Dermatitis 2000;42:111
2   Zaragoza-Ninet V, Blasco Encinas R, Vilata-Corell JJ, Pérez-Ferriols A, Sierra-Talamantes C, Esteve-Martínez A, de la Cuadra-Oyanguren J. Allergic contact dermatitis due to cosmetics: A clinical and epidemiological study in a tertiary hospital. Actas Dermosifiliogr 2016;107:329-336
3   Schena D, Fantuzzi F, Girolomoni G. Contact allergy in chronic eczematous lip dermatitis. Eur J Dermatol 2008;18:688-692
4   Fulton JE Jr, Pay SR, Fulton JE 3rd. Comedogenicity of current therapeutic products, cosmetics, and ingredients in the rabbit ear. J Am Acad Dermatol 1984;10:96-105
5   Prater E, Goring HD, Schubert H. Sodium lauryl sulfate. A contact allergen. Contact Dermatitis 1978;4:242-243

6   Aguirre A, Manzano D, Izu R, Gardeazabal J, Pérez JLD. Allergic contact cheilitis from mandelic acid. Contact Dermatitis 1994;31:133-134

7   Sams WM, Smith G. Contact dermatitis due to hydrocortisone ointment. Report of a case of sensitivity to emulsifying agents in a hydrophilic ointment base. JAMA 1957;164:1212-1213

8   Uter W, Geier J, Becker D, Brasch J, Löffler H and for the German Contact Dermatitis Research Group (DKG) and the Information Network of Departments of Dermatology (IVDK). The MOAHLFA index of irritant sodium lauryl sulfate reactions: first results of a multicentre study on routine sodium lauryl sulfate patch testing. Contact Dermatitis 2004;51:259-262

9   Ersoy M, Tanalp J, Ozel E, Cengizlier R, Soyman M. The allergy of toothpaste: a case report. Allergol Immunopathol (Madr) 2008;36:368-370

10   Benta H, Barkvoll P. Sodium lauryl sulfate and recurrent aphthous ulcers: A preliminary study. Acta Odontol Scand 1994;52:257-259

11   Benta H, Barkvoll P. The effect of two toothpaste detergents on the frequency of recurrent aphthous ulcers. Acta Odontol Scand 1996;54:150-153

12   Löffler H, Becker D, Brasch J, Geier J, German Contact Dermatitis Research Group (DKG). Simultaneous sodium lauryl sulphate testing improves the diagnostic validity of allergic patch tests. Results from a prospective multicentre study of the German Contact Dermatitis Research Group (Deutsche Kontaktallergie-Gruppe, DKG). Br J Dermatol 2005;152:709-719

2.422 SODIUM METABISULFITE

IDENTIFICATION

Description/definition   : Sodium metabisulfite is the inorganic salt that conforms to the formula shown below
Chemical class(es)   : Inorganic salts
Chemical/IUPAC name   : Disodium disultite
Other names   : Sodium pyrosulfite
CAS registry number (s)   : 7681-57-4; 7757-74-6
EC number(s)   : 231-673-0
CIR review(s)   : Int J Toxicol 2003;22(Suppl.2):63-88 (access: www.cir-safety.org/ingredients)
Merck Index monograph : 10040
Function(s) in cosmetics   : EU: antioxidant; preservative; reducing. USA: antioxidants; reducing agents
EU cosmetic restrictions   : Regulated in Annexes III/99 and V/9 of the Regulation (EC) No. 1223/2009
Patch testing   : 1% pet. (Chemotechnique)
Molecular formula   : $H_2Na_2O_5S_2$

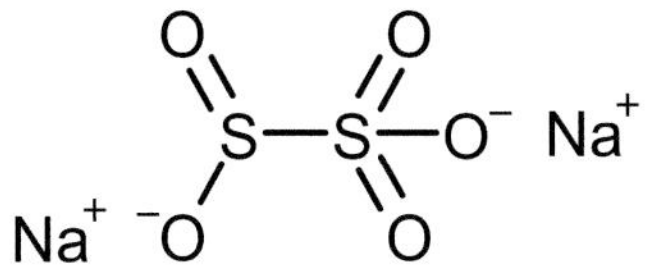

GENERAL

Sulfites are a ubiquitous group of sulfur-based compounds that contain the sulfite ion SO_3^{2-}. To this group belong sodium sulfite, sodium bisulfite, sodium metabisulfite, and potassium metabisulfite, which are widely used in the cosmetic, pharmaceutical, leather and textile, glass, wood pulp and paper, chemical, photographic, rubber, food and drink industries and in cleaning and laundry products, water and sewage treatment and in swimming pool water products for their preservative, bleaching, reducing and antioxidant properties (5,6,43).

Sulfites occur naturally in some foods and beverages, as a result of fermentation, whereas others are of synthetic origin. Sodium, potassium and calcium salts are used as food additives; sodium, potassium and ammonium sulfite salts are approved for use in cosmetics (table 2.422.1). Although the apparent safety of the sulfite additives has led to their widespread use, an increasing number of adverse reactions began to appear in the 1970s. Even minimal oral, parenteral, respiratory or cutaneous exposure in subjects with intolerance may provoke various types of reactions, such as asthma, rhinoconjunctivitis, and even anaphylaxis leading to death. Malaise, dizziness, confusion, abdominal pain and diarrhea have also been described (2). These manifestations have been well documented and are common. Cutaneous manifestations of sulfite reactions include (a) flushing, urticarial or anaphylactoid reactions following ingestion and/or parenteral exposure, and (b) allergic contact dermatitis. These reactions may occur simultaneously, in various combinations, and with varying degrees of severity in some susceptible individuals (5). Contact allergy is being reported with increasing frequency and sodium metabisulfite appears to be more relevant as a contact allergen than previously thought (5).

The literature on contact allergy to sodium metabisulfite, sodium sulfite and some other sulfites (ammonium bisulfite, sodium bisulfite, potassium metabisulfite and sodium hyposulfite (sodium thiosulfate) has been reviewed in 2012 (5). Foods that contain sulfites are summarized in refs. 5,7 and 43. Commercially available sulfites (with molecular formula, CAS number and E-number) and their presence or absence in foods and cosmetics are shown in table 2.422.1 (5).

Table 2.422.1 Commercially available sulfites and their presence in foods and cosmetics (5)

	Molecular formula	CAS number	E-number	Food	Cosmetics
Sodium sulfite	Na_2SO_3	7757-83-7	E221	Yes	Yes
Sodium bisulfite	$NaHSO_3$	7631-90-5	E222	Yes	Yes
Sodium metabisulfite	$Na_2S_2O_5$	7681-57-4	E223	Yes	Yes
Potassium sulfite	K_2SO_3	10117-38-1	E225	Yes	Yes
Potassium bisulfite	$KHSO_3$	7773-03-7	E228	Yes	Yes
Potassium metabisulfite	$K_2S_2O_5$	16731-55-8	E224	Yes	Yes
Calcium sulfite	$CaSO_3$	10257-55-3	E226	Yes	No
Calcium bisulfite	$Ca(HSO_3)_2$	13780-03-5	E227	Yes	No
Ammonium bisulfite	NH_4HSO_3	10192-30-0	-	No	Yes
Ammonium sulfite	$(NH_4)_2SO_3$	7026-44-7	-	No	Yes

CONTACT ALLERGY

Patch testing in groups of patients

Results of studies testing sodium metabisulfite in consecutive patients suspected of contact dermatitis (routine testing) back to 1994 are shown in table 2.422.2. Results of testing in groups of *selected* patients (e.g., patients with periorbital dermatitis, patients tested with a pharmaceutical or cosmetic series, patients with leg ulcers) back to 2007 are shown in table 2.422.3.

Patch testing in consecutive patients suspected of contact dermatitis: routine testing

In 8 studies in which routine testing with sodium metabisulfite was performed, frequencies of sensitization have ranged from 1.4% to 7.0%. Since 1998, rates have not been lower than 3.1%. Relevance data have varied widely. In some investigations, only a small minority of the positive patch test reactions were relevant or even 'possibly clinically relevant' (9,45). In others, however, 34% (43) and 47% (14) were currently relevant. Most reactions have been caused by cosmetics and topical medicaments (14,43), but occupational allergic contact dermatitis was also observed (9,15).

Table 2 Patch testing in groups of patients: Routine testing

Years and Country	Test conc. & vehicle	Number of patients tested	positive (%)	Selection of patients (S); Relevance (R); Comments (C)	Ref.
2009-2013 Ireland	1% pet.	996	70 (7.0%)	R: 24 (34%) currently relevant, 14 (20%) possibly relevant or past relevance, 32 (46%) unknown relevance; C: most reactions were caused by cosmetics and by topical medications; the patients were also tested with sodium metabisulfite 0.1% and 0.01% pet., but the 1% test substance was considered to be adequate; in the prospective part of the study, 10/14 reactions (70%) proved to be relevant	43
2009-2012 12 European countries, ESSCA	1% pet.	16,485	(3.1%)	R: not specified	41
2010 UK	1% pet.	946	39 (4.1%)	R: 7 reactions (18%) were 'possibly clinically relevant'	45
2009 UK	1% pet.	183	10 (5.5%)	R: 8 were of possible (n=5) or past (n=3) relevance	1
1998-2007 Sweden	2% pet.	1518	51 (3.4%)	R: 2 current relevance, 1 from a photo-developing chemical and another from a skin cleanser	9
<2007 UK	1% pet.	1751	71 (4.1%)	R: 33 (47%) were relevant; most were caused by a cortico-steroid-antifungal preparation; there were 2 cases caused by cosmetics, one by a 'false tan lotion' and one by a hair dye	14
<1997 Italy	1% pet.	980	14 (1.4%)	R: not stated	33
<1994 Italy	1% pet.	2894	50 (1.7%)	R: there were 7 relevant occupational cases (14%) and 5 patients with dermatitis from non-occupational exposure to topical preparations; C: 100% co-reactivity to potassium metabisulfite and sodium bisulfite, but only 4% co-reactions to sodium sulfite	15

ESSCA: European Surveillance System on Contact Allergy' network

Patch testing in groups of selected patients

Results of testing in groups of selected patients (e.g., patients with periorbital dermatitis, patients tested with a pharmaceutical or cosmetic series, patients with leg ulcers) back to 2007 are shown in table 3. In 4 investigations, frequencies of sensitization have ranged from 3.1% to 6.8%, which is – despite the selection procedure – not significantly higher than in routine testing (table 2). In 2 studies, no relevance data were provided; in the other 2, current relevance was 50% in one (32) and 58% in the other (5). Most reactions were caused by cosmetics (often hair dyes) and topical medicaments (antifungal creams) (5). In the case of the topical medicaments, these products actually contained sodium sulfite and the allergy was discovered by the positive patch test reactions to sodium metabisulfite (5) (see also the section 'Cross-reactions, pseudo-cross-reactions and co-reactions' below).

Case reports and case series

Sodium metabisulfite was stated to be the (or an) allergen in 17 patients in a group of 603 individuals suffering from cosmetic dermatitis, seen in the period 2010-2015 in Leuven, Belgium (40). In a group of 14 patients with positive reactions to sodium metabisulfite seen in Ireland in 2011-2013, six had allergic contact dermatitis from cosmetic products: moisturizing cream (n=4), eyebrow tint (n=2), bleaching shampoo (n=1) and baby powder (n=1) (2 patients reacted to 2 products) (43). Sodium metabisulfite was responsible for 4 out of 959 cases of non-fragrance cosmetic allergy where the causal allergen was identified, Belgium, 2000-2010 (3). In a group of 60 patients with positive patch tests to sodium metabisulfite, the dermatitis in 31 cases was considered to have been caused by cosmetics (5). Twenty-six patients had used leave-on products containing the allergen (hair dyes 18, facial cleanser 3, body emollient 2, unspecified 3) and 5 had used rinse-off products (shampoo 3, hand cleaner 1, toothpaste 1) (5, overlap with refs. 3 and 40).

Table 2.422.3 Patch testing in groups of patients: Selected patient groups

Years and Country	Test conc. & vehicle	Number of patients tested	positive (%)	Selection of patients (S); Relevance (R); Comments (C)	Ref.
2000-2010 IVDK		1996	76 (3.8%)	S: patients with periorbital dermatitis; R: not stated	38
1990-2010 Belgium	2% pet., later 1% pet.	2763	124 (4.5%)	S: patients tested with a pharmaceutical or cosmetic series and patients exposed to sulfites; R: 58% present relevance, 6% past relevance; 26 cases (21%) were caused by an antifungal cream, 34 (27%) were related to cosmetics, of which 22 (18%) to metabisulfite in hair dyes	5
2004-2008 France	1% pet.	423	13 (3.1%)	S: patients with leg ulcers; R: not stated	39
<2007 Ireland	1% pet.	117	8 (6.8%)	S: patients tested with a bases + preservative series: R: four patients (50%); one was allergic to cosmetic creams containing sodium sulfite, other products were not specified	32

IVDK: Information Network of Departments of Dermatology, Germany, Austria, Switzerland

Four positive patch test reactions to sodium metabisulfite were ascribed to cosmetic allergy (4). Four hairdressers had occupational allergic contact dermatitis from hair dyes and a nurse was sensitized to sodium metabisulfite in a hand cleaner (5). Another hairdresser was also allergic to sodium metabisulfite in hair dye (12). Three patients had facial dermatitis from sodium metabisulfite in a hydroquinone-containing bleaching cream (23,37,47). One individual was allergic to a 'false tan lotion' (14), another to a hair dye (14) containing sodium metabisulfite.

Contact allergy to sodium metabisulfite in non-cosmetic products
Many cases of contact allergy to and allergic contact dermatitis from sodium metabisulfite in products other than cosmetics have been reported, usually in the form of case-reports or small case series. Some patients had occupational allergic contact dermatitis, notably from contact with foods (5,10,13,14,20,21,22) or photographic chemicals (5,9,18,19,43) (in some of these cases their role was not proven but highly likely). Other products containing sodium metabisulfite causing occupational contact dermatitis have included a skin cleanser (9), an acidifying agent in the tannery industry (34), a cleaning product (43), and pickling in tanneries (48).

Non-occupational allergic contact dermatitis is most often caused by topical pharmaceutical products including topical antifungals (5,19), topical steroids (5), a combination of a steroid and an antifungal (14,26,28), topical anesthetics (5), local anesthetics (5,19,25), topical antibiotic preparations (27,30,42), mesalazine cream (31), eye drops (5,24,35) and unspecified topical medications (43). In a particular topical antifungal product (containing ketoconazole, Nizoral® cream) causing many reactions in patients sensitized to sodium metabisulfite, the allergenic ingredient was sodium sulfite, not sodium metabisulfite (cross- or pseudo-cross-reaction, see the section 'Cross-reactions, pseudo-cross-reactions and co-reactions' below) (5,19). Patients reacting to the corticosteroid-antifungal preparations often had perianal dermatitis (14,27,28). Other products responsible for non-occupational allergic contact dermatitis from sodium metabisulfite have included blue jeans (sulfites used for bleaching purposes [8]), swimming pool water (14), and a gel for urinary catheterization (44).

In sodium metabisulfite-sensitized individuals, an injection with a sulfite-containing local anesthetic may cause anaphylactoid reactions (5). Systemic contact dermatitis has occasionally been observed from high dietary intake of sulfites (6). Burning mouth syndrome has been linked to hypersensitivity to sodium metabisulfite (probably in food, article not read [52]).

Cross-reactions, pseudo-cross-reactions and co-reactions
Sodium sulfite (1,15); potassium metabisulfite (11,15); sodium bisulfite (15). Sodium metabisulfite, sodium sulfite, and sodium bisulfite, when dissolved in water, exist in pH-dependent equilibrium with each other (2). The buffering capacity of skin would result in a similar mixture of sodium sulfite, sodium metabisulfite, and sodium bisulfite, whichever compound is applied (1).

Patch test sensitization
In performing assays for cumulative irritancy of topical corticosteroid formulations, 2 out of a panel of 50 participants were actively sensitized to sodium metabisulfite. The formulations were 1% hydrocortisone (for over-the-counter distribution) in which metabisulfite was included at an unstated concentration (29).

Presence in cosmetic products and chemical analyses

In July 2017, sodium metabisulfite was present in 114 of 70,166 cosmetic products of which the composition is known in EWG's Skin Deep Cosmetics Database, USA (http://www.ewg.org/skindeep/). In the USA, in April 2017, sodium metabisulfite was present in 844 of 56,714 cosmetic products of which the composition is known in FDA's Voluntary Cosmetic Registration Program (VCRP) (data obtained from FDA, May 2017).

OTHER SIDE EFFECTS

Immediate-type reactions

Immediate reactions such as urticaria, angioedema, asthma, rhinoconjunctivitis and anaphylaxis from sodium metabisulfite in foods, drinks, medications and other products are well recognized (2,16,17,22,36,50,51) (see also under GENERAL). In such cases, scratch or prick tests have rarely been positive, which seems to exclude type I immediate hypersensitivity in most cases of immediate reactions (intolerance) (2); however, some cases with IgE-mediated mechanisms have been described (53).

It has been suggested that some of the immediate reactions may actually be the result of delayed hypersensitivity (5). Combined immediate and delayed-type reaction from sodium metabisulfite in injected local anesthetic has been observed (19). The literature on Immediate type reactions to sulfites from before 1984 has been reviewed (46).

Miscellaneous side effects

No flare-up of dermatitis or of patch tests were provoked by oral challenge with 30 and 50 mg doses of sodium metabisulfite in 5 patients with positive patch tests (15).

OTHER INFORMATION

The potential *in cutaneo* reaction chemistry of sodium metabisulfite leading to contact allergy has been investigated (49).

LITERATURE

1. Oliphant T, Mitra A, Wilkinson M. Contact allergy to sodium sulfite and its relationship to sodium metabisulfite. Contact Dermatitis 2012;66:128-130
2. Vally H, Misso NLA, Madan V. Clinical effects of sulphite additives. Clin Exp Allergy 2009;39;1643-1651
3. Travassos AR, Claes L, Boey L, Drieghe J, Goossens A. Non-fragrance allergens in specific cosmetic products. Contact Dermatitis 2011;65:276-285
4. Kohl L, Blondeel A, Song M. Allergic contact dermatitis from cosmetics: retrospective analysis of 819 patch-tested patients. Dermatology 2002;204:334-337
5. Garcia-Gavin J, Parente J, Goossens A. Allergic contact dermatitis caused by sodium metabisulfite: a challenging allergen. A case series and literature review. Contact Dermatitis 2012;67:260-269
6. Cussans A, McFadden J, Ostlere L. Systemic sodium metabisulfite allergy. Contact Dermatitis 2015;73:316-317
7. Australasian Society of Clinical Immunology and Allergy. Sulfite sensitivity. 2014. Available at: http://www.allergy.org.au/patients/product-allergy/sulfite-allergy
8. Aerts O, Duchateau N, Lambert J, Bechtold T. Sodium metabisulfite in blue jeans: an unexpected cause of textile contact dermatitis. Contact Dermatitis 2014;70:190-192
9. Kaaman A-C, Boman A, Wrangsjö K, Matura M. Contact allergy to sodium metabisulfite: an occupational problem. Contact Dermatitis 2010;63:110-112
10. Sasseville D, El-Helou T. Occupational allergic contact dermatitis from sodium metabisulfite. Contact Dermatitis 2009;61:244-245
11. Stingeni L, Bianchi L, Lisi P. Occupational airborne allergic contact dermatitis from potassium metabisulfite. Contact Dermatitis 2009;60:52-53
12. Aalto-Korte K, Suuronen K, Alanko K. Sodium metabisulfite – a contact allergen? Contact Dermatitis 2009;60:115-117
13. Lee A, Nixon R. Contact dermatitis from sodium metabisulfite in a baker. Contact Dermatitis 2001;44:127-128
14. Madan V, Walker SL, Beck MH. Sodium metabisulfite allergy is common but is it relevant? Contact Dermatitis 2007;57:173-176
15. Vena GA, Foti C, Angelini G. Sulphite contact allergy. Contact Dermatitis 1994;31:172-175
16. Jamieson DM, Guill MF, Wray BB, May JR. Metabisulfite sensitivity: case report and literature review. Ann Allergy 1985;54:115-121
17. Merget R, Korn M. Metabisulphite-induced occupational asthma in a radiographer. Eur Respir J 2005;25:386-388

18 Jacobs MC, Rycroft RJ. Contact dermatitis and asthma from sodium metabisulfite in a photographic technician. Contact Dermatitis 1995;33:65-66

19 Dooms-Goossens A, de Alam AG, Degreef H, Kochuyt A. Local anesthetic intolerance due to metabisulfite. Contact Dermatitis 1989;20:124-126

20 Apetato M, Marques MS. Contact dermatitis caused by sodium metabisulphite. Contact Dermatitis 1986;14:194

21 Epstein E. Sodium bisulfite. Contact Dermatitis Newsl 1970;7:155

22 Fisher AA. Reactions to sulfites in foods: delayed eczematous and immediate urticarial, anaphylactoid, and asthmatic reactions. Part III. Cutis 1989;44:187-190

23 Huang PY, Chu CY. Allergic contact dermatitis due to sodium metabisulfite in a bleaching cream. Contact Dermatitis 2007;56:123-124

24 Seitz CS, Bröcker EB, Trautmann A. Eyelid dermatitis due to sodium metabisulfite. Contact Dermatitis 2006;55:249-250

25 Riemersma WA, Schuttelaar ML, Coenraads PJ. Type IV hypersensitivity to sodium metabisulfite in local anaesthetic. Contact Dermatitis 2004;51:148

26 Harrison DA, Smith AG. Concomitant sensitivity to sodium metabisulfite and clobetasone butyrate in trimovate cream. Contact Dermatitis 2002;46:310

27 Sánchez-Pérez J, Abajo P, Córdoba S, García-Díez A. Allergic contact dermatitis from sodium metabisulfite in an antihemorrhoidal cream. Contact Dermatitis 2000;42:176-177

28 Tucker SC, Yell JA, Beck MH. Allergic contact dermatitis from sodium metabisulfite in trimovate cream. Contact Dermatitis 1999;40:164

29 Heshmati S, Maibach HI. Active sensitization to sodium metabisulfite in hydrocortisone cream. Contact Dermatitis 1999;41:166-167

30 Giorgini S, Brusi C, Melle MC, Sertoli A. Contact dermatitis by sodium metabisulfite. Med Staff Dermatol 1998;44:16-17

31 Vestergaard L, Andersen KE. Allergic contact dermatitis from sodium metabisulfite in a topical preparation. Am J Contact Dermat 1995;6:174-175

32 Malik MM, Hegarty MA, Bourke JF. Sodium metabisulfite – a marker for cosmetic allergy? Contact Dermatitis 2007;56:241-242

33 Angelini G, Vena GA, Foti C, Grandolfo M. Contact allergy to preservatives and perfumed compounds used in skin care products. J Appl Cosmet 1997;15:49-57

34 Febriana SA, Jungbauer F, Soebono H, Coenraads P-J. Occupational allergic contact dermatitis and patch test results of leather workers at two Indonesian tanneries. Contact Dermatitis 2012;67:277-283

35 Veramme J, de Zaeytijd J, LamberTJ. and Lapeere H. Contact dermatitis in patients undergoing serial intravitreal injections. Contact Dermatitis 2016;74:18-21

36 Schwartz HJ, Sher TH. Bisulfite sensitivity manifesting as allergy to local dental anesthesia. J Allergy Clin Immunol 1985;75:525-527

37 Laureano A, Amaro C, Vieira R, Cardoso J. Allergic contact dermatitis due to sodium metabisulfite in bleaching cream. Contact Dermatitis 2012;66 (Suppl. 2):19

38 Landeck L, John SM, Geier J. Periorbital dermatitis in 4779 patients – patch test results during a 10-year period. Contact Dermatitis 2014;70:205-212

39 Barbaud A, Collet E, Le Coz CJ, Meaume S, Gillois P. Contact allergy in chronic leg ulcers: results of a multicentre study carried out in 423 patients and proposal for an updated series of patch tests. Contact Dermatitis 2009;60:279-287

40 Goossens A. Cosmetic contact allergens. Cosmetics 2016, 3, 5; doi:10.3390/cosmetics3010005

41 Uter W, Spiewak R, Cooper SM, Wilkinson M, Sánchez Pérez J, Schnuch A, Schuttelaar M-L. Contact allergy to ingredients of topical medications: results of the European Surveillance System on Contact Allergies (ESSCA), 2009-2012. Pharmacoepidemiol Drug Saf 2016;25:1305-1312

42 Milpied B, Wassenhove LV, Larousse C, Barriere H. Contact dermatitis from rifamycin. Contact Dermatitis 1986;14:252-253

43 Ralph N, Verma S, Merry S. What is the relevance of contact allergy to sodium metabisulfite and which concentration of the allergen should we use? Dermatitis 2015;26:162-165

44 Grosch E, Mahler V. Allergic contact dermatitis caused by a catheter system containing sodium metabisulfite. Contact Dermatitis 2017;76:186-187

45 Pink A, Banerjee P, White IR. Contact allergy to sodium metabisulphite: a red herring? Br J Dermatol 2011;165(Suppl.1):71

46 Settipane GA. Adverse reactions to sulfites in drugs and foods. J Am Acad Dermatol 1984;10:1077-1080

47 Oliveira A, Amaro C, Cardoso J. Allergic contact dermatitis caused by sodium metabisulphite in a cosmetic bleaching cream. Australas J Dermatol 2015;56:144-145

48 Febriana SA, Jungbauer F, Soebono H, Coenraads PJ. Occupational allergic contact dermatitis and patch test results of leather workers at two Indonesian tanneries. Contact Dermatitis 2012;67:277-2 83

49 Roberts DW, Basketter D, Kimber I, White J, McFadden J, White IR. Sodium metabisulfite as a contact allergen-- an example of a rare chemical mechanism for protein modification. Contact Dermatitis 2012;66:123-127

50 Gall H, Boehncke WH, Gietzen K. Intolerance to sodium metabisulfite in beer. Allergy 1996;51:516-517

51 Bellido J, Alvarez MJ, Moyano JC, Fonseca JL, Muñoz FJ. Adverse reaction to sodium metabisulfite from fresh fish. Allergy 1996;51:196-197

52 Levanti C, Ricciardi L, Isola S, Cilia M, Guarneri F, Purello D'Ambrosio F. Burning mouth syndrome: hypersensitivity to sodium metabisulfite. Acta Derm Venereol 1996;76:158-159

53 Sokol WN, Hydick IB.Nasal congestion, urticaria, and angioedema caused by an IgE-mediated reaction to sodium metabisulfite. Ann Allergy 1990;65:233-238

2.423 SODIUM MYRISTOYL SARCOSINATE

IDENTIFICATION

Description/definition	: Sodium myristoyl sarcosinate is the sodium salt of myristoyl sarcosine, which conforms to the formula shown below
Chemical class(es)	: Sarcosinates and sarcosine derivatives
Chemical/IUPAC name	: Sodium;2-[methyl(tetradecanoyl)amino]acetate
Other names	: Sodium N-methyl-N-(1-oxotetradecyl)aminoacetate; glycine, N-methyl-N-(1-oxotetradecyl)-, sodium salt; sodium myristoylmethyl glycinate
CAS registry number (s)	: 30364-51-3
EC number(s)	: 250-151-3
CIR review(s)	: Int J Toxicol 2001;20(Suppl.1):1-14; Final, April 2016 (access: www.cir-safety.org/ingredients)
Function(s) in cosmetics	: EU: antistatic; cleansing; foaming; hair conditioning; surfactant; viscosity controlling. USA: hair conditioning agents; surfactants - cleansing agents
Patch testing	: 1% water (commercial solution used in cosmetic product, containing 30% sodium myristoyl sarcosinate and up to 2% sodium myristoate (1)
Molecular formula	: $C_{17}H_{32}NNaO_3$

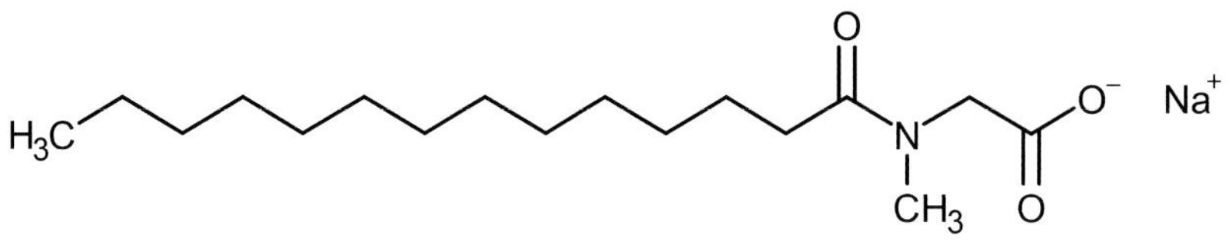

CONTACT ALLERGY

Case reports and case series

A woman had occasionally suffered from eczema of the face in a period of 6 months. One day, she again developed facial dermatitis, starting on the upper lip, and spreading to the forehead and cheeks, after which her eyelids became swollen. She recalled having used a 'gentle foaming facewash' on her face before the dermatitis appeared. She had used it according to the instructions, applying the product to her face at night and then washing it off. Patch tests with the European standard series, with lichens and sesquiterpene lactones, the gentle foaming facewash 1% water and with seven other cosmetic products that she had recently used on her face showed a positive reaction to the facewash 1% water only with erythematous infiltration at D4. A repeated open application test was then performed on the lower arm, using it according to the instructions on the product. It irritated the skin in the area of application to such a degree that the test was stopped at D3. Later, the patient was patch tested with the ingredients of the cosmetic product in the same concentrations as in the product itself and she showed positivity to sodium myristoyl sarcosinate (SMS) 1% in water. Twelve controls were negative. The 1% SMS in water turned out to be in fact a 1% dilution of a solution which contained 30% sodium myristoyl sarcosinate and up to 2% sodium myristoate. Thus, the patch test material contained 0.3% of sodium myristoyl sarcosinate and up to 0.02% of sodium myristoate. The chemicals could not be tested separately (1).

Presence in cosmetic products and chemical analyses

In the USA, in April 2017, sodium myristoyl sarcosinate was present in 40 of 56,714 cosmetic products of which the composition is known in FDA's Voluntary Cosmetic Registration Program (VCRP) (data obtained from FDA, May 2017). In April 2017, sodium myristoyl sarcosinate was present in 34 of 65,434 cosmetic products of which the composition is known in EWG's Skin Deep Cosmetics Database, USA (http://www.ewg.org/skindeep/).

LITERATURE

1   Malanin KEN. Allergic contact dermatitis caused by a mixture of sodium myristoyl sarcosinate and sodium myristoate in a cosmetic product. Contact Dermatitis 2002;47:50

2.424 SODIUM PCA

IDENTIFICATION

Description/definition : Sodium PCA is the sodium salt of PCA (Pyrrolidone Carboxylic Acid) that conforms to the formula shown below
Chemical class(es) : Amides; heterocyclic compounds; organic salts
Chemical/IUPAC name : Sodium;(2S)-5-oxopyrrolidine-2-carboxylate
Other names : Sodium 5-oxo-2-pyrrolidinecarboxylate; sodium pyroglutamate
CAS registry number (s) : 28874-51-3
EC number(s) : 249-277-1
CIR review(s) : Int J Toxicol 1999;18(Suppl.2):25-34; Final report, December 2014 (access: www.cir-safety.org/ingredients)
Function(s) in cosmetics : EU: antistatic; hair conditioning; humectant; skin conditioning. USA: hair conditioning agents; humectants; skin-conditioning agents - humectant
Patch testing : No data available
Molecular formula : $C_5H_6NNaO_3$

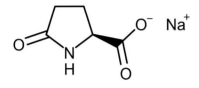

CONTACT ALLERGY

Case reports and case series
In a group of 119 patients with allergic contact dermatitis from cosmetics, investigated in The Netherlands in 1986-1987, one case was caused by sodium PCA in a skin care product (1,2).

Presence in cosmetic products and chemical analyses
In the USA, in April 2017, sodium PCA was present in 1750 of 56,714 cosmetic products of which the composition is known in FDA's Voluntary Cosmetic Registration Program (VCRP) (data obtained from FDA, May 2017). In April 2017, sodium PCA was present in 598 of 65,434 cosmetic products of which the composition is known in EWG's Skin Deep Cosmetics Database, USA (http://www.ewg.org/skindeep/).

OTHER SIDE EFFECTS

Immediate-type reactions
Under experimental conditions, sodium PCA was shown to cause immediate contact reactions of unknown mechanism. Quite curiously, these reactions appeared on the back, but not on the – generally more sensitive - skin of the cheek, neck and forehead (3).

LITERATURE
1 De Groot AC, Bruynzeel DP, Bos JD, van der Meeren HL, van Joost T, Jagtman BA, Weyland JW. The allergens in cosmetics. Arch Dermatol 1988;124:1525-1529
2 De Groot AC. Adverse reactions to cosmetics. PhD Thesis, University of Groningen, The Netherlands: 1988, chapter 3.4, pp.105-113
3 Larmi E, Lahti A, Hannuksela M. Immediate contact reactions to benzoic acid and the sodium salt of pyrrolidone carboxylic acid. Comparison of various skin sites. Contact Dermatitis 1989;20:38-40

2.425   SODIUM PYRITHIONE

IDENTIFICATION

Description/definition	: Sodium pyrithione is the organic compound that conforms to the formula shown below
Chemical class(es)	: Heterocyclic compounds; organic salts; thio compounds
Chemical/IUPAC name	: Sodium 1-oxidopyridine-2-thione
Other names	: Sodium omadine; sodium-2-pyridinethiol-1-oxide
CAS registry number (s)	: 3811-73-2
EC number(s)	: 223-296-5
Function(s) in cosmetics	: EU: formerly used as preservative; delisted in 1989. USA: preservatives
EU cosmetic restrictions	: Regulated in Annex II/369 of the Regulation (EC) No. 1223/2009 (prohibited)
Patch testing	: 0.1% water (SmartPracticeEurope, SmartPracticeCanada)
Molecular formula	: C_5H_5NaNOS

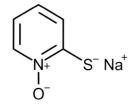

GENERAL

Sodium pyrithione has antibacterial activity and germicidal activity against a wide spectrum of yeasts and fungi. Sodium pyrithione is utilized in the metallurgical industry as a component of water-based metalworking fluids (soluble, semi-synthetic and synthetic oils). It is also used as component of aceto-polyvinyl lattices, water-based printer's ink, lubricants for synthetic fibers and anti-dandruff shampoos (9).

CONTACT ALLERGY

Patch testing in groups of patients

The results of patch testing with sodium pyrithione in consecutive patients suspected of contact dermatitis (routine testing) and testing in groups of selected patients are shown in table 2.425.1. In routine testing in one (very) small study from Turkey, the frequency of sensitization was 1% (6). In four studies testing groups of selected patient groups (healthy student volunteers, patients suspected of cosmetic dermatitis, patients tested with an industrial biocide series), rates of sensitization ranged from 0.3% in patients tested with an industrial biocide series (2) to 1.9% in patient suspected of allergic cosmetic dermatitis (3). The relevance of the observed reactions was mentioned in one US study only: all 8 reactions were considered to be relevant, but relevancy included 'questionable' and 'past' relevance (1).

Table 2.425.1 Patch testing in groups of patients

Years and Country	Test conc. & vehicle	Number of patients tested	positive (%)		Selection of patients (S); Relevance (R); Comments (C)	Ref.
Routine testing						
2005-2006 Turkey		93	1	(1%)	R: the reaction was considered not to be relevant	6
Testing in groups of selected patients						
2011 China	1% pet.	201	1	(0.5%)	S: healthy student volunteers 19-30 years; R: not stated	5
2010-2011 Korea	0.1% pet.	584	11	(1.9%)	S: patients suspected of allergic cosmetic dermatitis; R: not stated	3
2000-2007 USA	0.1% water	939	8	(0.9%)	S: patients tested with a supplemental cosmetic screening series; R: 100%; C: weak study: a. high rate of macular erythema and weak reactions; b. relevance figures included 'questionable' and 'past' relevance	1
1990-1994 Germany	0.1% water	1696	5	(0.3%)	S: patients tested with an industrial biocide series; R: not stated	2

Case reports and case series

Sodium pyrithione was stated to be the (or an) allergen in one patient in a group of 603 individuals suffering from cosmetic dermatitis, seen in the period 2010-2015 in Leuven, Belgium (4).

Contact allergy to pyrithione sodium in non-cosmetic products

A machinist was seen because of an itchy dermatitis on the back of his left hand, present for 4 years during work, but clearing on holidays and when he had sick leave. In his work, the patient was exposed to a water-based metalworking fluid (MWF). When patch tested, he reacted to the metalworking fluid concentrate 5% in acid buffer and to its ingredient sodium pyrithione 0.1% water, the latter on two occasions. Sodium pyrithione was present in the MWF in a concentration of 0.1% to 1.0%. Zinc pyrithione was also tested, but was negative (7). The author mentioned having seen two other patients with contact allergy to sodium pyrithione, which reactions were considered to be of past relevance (causative products not mentioned) (7). Two similar cases of contact allergy to sodium pyrithione in metalworking fluids had previously been reported (8,9).

Cross-reactions, pseudo-cross-reactions and co-reactions

Not to zinc pyrithione (7), although the hapten is said to be the pyrithione moiety (8).

Presence in cosmetic products and chemical analyses

In the USA, in April 2017, sodium pyrithione was present in zero of 56,714 cosmetic products of which the composition is known in FDA's Voluntary Cosmetic Registration Program (VCRP) (data obtained from FDA, May 2017). In April 2017, sodium pyrithione sodium was present in zero of 66,485 cosmetic products of which the composition is known in EWG's Skin Deep Cosmetics Database, USA (http://www.ewg.org/skindeep/).

LITERATURE

1   Wetter DA, Yiannias JA, Prakash AV, Davis MD, Farmer SA, el-Azhary RA, et al. Results of patch testing to personal care product allergens in a standard series and a supplemental cosmetic series: an analysis of 945 patients from the Mayo Clinic Contact Dermatitis Group, 2000-2007. J Am Acad Dermatol 2010;63:789-798
2   Schnuch A, Geier J, Uter W, Frosch PJ. Patch testing with preservatives, antimicrobials and industrial biocides. Results from a multicentre study. Br J Dermatol 1998;138:467-476
3   Lee SS, Hong DK, Jeong NJ, Lee JH, Choi YS, Lee AY, et al. Multicenter study of preservative sensitivity in patients with suspected cosmetic contact dermatitis in Korea. J Dermatol 2012;39:677-681
4   Goossens A. Cosmetic contact allergens. Cosmetics 2016, 3, 5; doi:10.3390/cosmetics3010005
5   Zhao J, Li LF. Contact sensitization to cosmetic series of allergens in a general population in Beijing. J Cosmet Dermatol 2014;13:68-71
6   Ada S, Seçkin D. Patch testing in allergic contact dermatitis: is it useful to perform the cosmetic series in addition to the European standard series? J Eur Acad Dermatol Venereol 2010;24:1192-1196
7   Isaksson M. Delayed diagnosis of occupational contact dermatitis from sodium pyrithione in a metalworking fluid. Contact Dermatitis 2002;47:248-249
8   Le Coz CJ. Allergic contact dermatitis from sodium pyrithione in metalworking fluid. Contact Dermatitis 2001;45:58-59
9   Tosti A, Piraccini B, Brasile GP. Occupational contact dermatitis due to sodium pyrithione. Contact Dermatitis 1990;22:118-119

2.426   SODIUM STEARATE

IDENTIFICATION

Description/definition	: Sodium stearate is the sodium salt of stearic acid that conforms generally to the formula shown below
Chemical class(es)	: Soaps
Chemical/IUPAC name	: Sodium octadecanoate
Other names	: Octadecanoic acid, sodium salt; stearic acid, sodium salt
CAS registry number (s)	: 822-16-2
EC number(s)	: 212-490-5
CIR review(s)	: J Am Coll Toxicol 1982;1:143-177 (access: www.cir-safety.org/ingredients)
Merck Index monograph	: 10076
Function(s) in cosmetics	: EU: cleaning; emulsifying; surfactant; viscosity controlling. USA: surfactants – cleansing agents; surfactants - emulsifying agents; viscosity increasing agents
Patch testing	: 1% water (1)
Molecular formula	: $C_{18}H_{35}NaO_2$

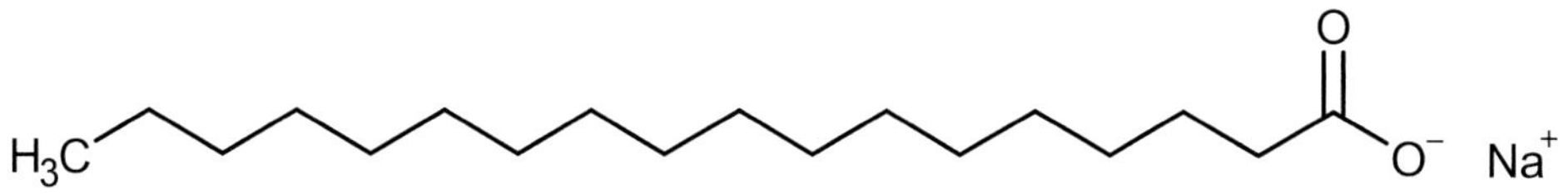

CONTACT ALLERGY

Case reports and case series

A man had dermatitis of the face which he ascribed to a facial moisturizer that he had been using for one week. When patch tested, the patient reacted to *Myroxylon pereirae*, fragrance-mix I, formaldehyde, and the cream, tested as is. When tested later with all the ingredients of the cream, obtained from the manufacturer, he reacted to sodium stearate 1% water and stearic acid 5% pet. On withdrawal of the moisturizer, the dermatitis disappeared. Twenty-five controls were negative to sodium stearate 1% water and stearic acid 5% pet. (1).

Cross-reactions, pseudo-cross-reactions and co-reactions

Stearic acid (1).

Presence in cosmetic products and chemical analyses

In the USA, in April 2017, sodium stearate was present in 544 of 56,714 cosmetic products of which the composition is known in FDA's Voluntary Cosmetic Registration Program (VCRP) (data obtained from FDA, May 2017). In April 2017, sodium stearate was present in 159 of 65,434 cosmetic products of which the composition is known in EWG's Skin Deep Cosmetics Database, USA (http://www.ewg.org/skindeep/).

LITERATURE

1   De Groot AC, van der Meeren HLM, Weyland JW. Cosmetic allergy from stearic acid and glyceryl stearate. Contact Dermatitis 1988;19:77-78

2.427 SODIUM STEAROYL LACTYLATE

IDENTIFICATION

Description/definition : Sodium stearoyl lactylate is the sodium salt of the stearic acid ester of lactyl lactate
Chemical class(es) : Esters; organic salts
Chemical/IUPAC name : Sodium;2-(2-octadecanoyloxypropanoyloxy)propanoate
Other names : Sodium 2-stearoyllactate; sodium 2-(stearoyloxy) propionate
CAS registry number (s) : 25383-99-7; 18200-72-1
EC number(s) : 246-929-7; 242-090-6
Function(s) in cosmetics : EU: emulsifying. USA: surfactants - emulsifying agents
Patch testing : 2% and 5% in petrolatum; both concentrations may cause irritant reactions (1)
Molecular formula : $C_{24}H_{43}NaO_6$

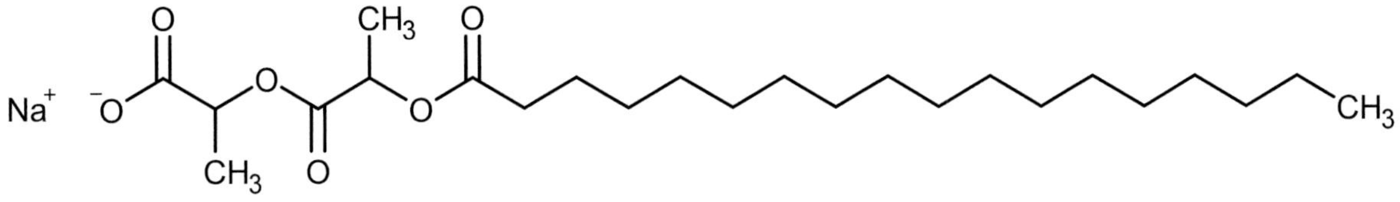

GENERAL

Sodium stearoyl lactylate (SSL) is made by combining lactic acid and stearic acid, and subsequent reaction with sodium hydroxide makes the sodium salt. SSL is used in foods as a dough conditioner to improve the texture of baked goods, as a stabilizer and whipping agent in egg whites and artificial whipped cream and as an emulsifying agent in salad dressings, soups and coffee whiteners. It is used in cosmetics for its emulsifying properties (1).

CONTACT ALLERGY

Case reports and case series

A woman had a 20-year history of palmoplantar pustulosis and chronic hand and foot dermatitis. One day, she had an acute deterioration and spreading of her dermatitis, for which she was admitted to hospital. After symptomatic treatment, she was patch tested with her own cosmetic products, and one of them, an 'oil cream' produced a strong positive reaction. The ingredients were later tested, which yielded a positive reaction to sodium stearoyl lactylate (SLL) 5% in petrolatum. Subsequently, the patient was patch tested with the chemical 2% pet. which was also positive. A repeated open application test on the lower arm with of SLL 5% pet. showed small papules and itching after a few days and was clearly positive on D18. To exclude irritancy, 25 controls were tested with 2% SLL pet. and 26 with 5% SLL in petrolatum. The 2% preparation produced ten doubtful responses, which were probably irritant. The 5% preparation induced 14 doubtful reactions and one positive reaction on D3. Although the authors admit that 'SLL has irritant potential', they considered the reproducible patch test and use test reactions to be of allergic nature, because of the clinical picture, patient history and patch tests in controls (1). This is rather curious, as patch tests were not performed twice with the same concentration and therefore not reproducible, and the results of control testing with many doubtful reactions can hardly be evidence of the allergic nature of the reactions in their patient, quite the opposite!

Presence in cosmetic products and chemical analyses

In the USA, in April 2017, sodium stearoyl lactylate was present in 293 of 56,714 cosmetic products of which the composition is known in FDA's Voluntary Cosmetic Registration Program (VCRP) (data obtained from FDA, May 2017). In April 2017, sodium stearoyl lactylate was present in 213 of 65,434 cosmetic products of which the composition is known in EWG's Skin Deep Cosmetics Database, USA (http://www.ewg.org/skindeep/).

LITERATURE

1   Jensen CD, Andersen KE. Allergic contact dermatitis from sodium stearoyl lactylate, an emulsifier commonly used in food products. Contact Dermatitis 2005;53:116

2.428   SODIUM SULFITE

IDENTIFICATION

Description/definition   : Sodium sulfite is the inorganic salt that conforms to the formula shown below
chemical class(es)   : Inorganic salts
chemical/iupac name   : Disodium sulfite
CAS registry number (s)   : 7757-83-7
EC number(s)   : 231-821-4
CIR review(s)   : Int J Toxicol 2003;22(Suppl.2):63-88 (access: www.cir-safety.org/ingredients)
Merck Index monograph   : 10081
Function(s) in cosmetics   : EU: hair waving or straightening; preservative. USA: antioxidants; hair
                                waving/straightening agents; reducing agents
EU cosmetic restrictions   : Regulated in Annexes III/99 and V/9 of the Regulation (EC) No. 1223/2009
Patch testing   : 1% pet. (1); 5% pet. (4)
Molecular formula   : Na_2O_3S

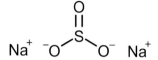

GENERAL

General information on (the adverse reactions to) sulfites is discussed in Chapter 2.422 Sodium metabisulfite. The literature on contact allergy to sodium sulfite, sodium metabisulfite, and some other sulfites (ammonium bisulfite, sodium bisulfite, potassium metabisulfite and sodium hyposulfite (sodium thiosulfate) has been reviewed in 2012 (3).

CONTACT ALLERGY

Patch testing in groups of patients

In 2009, in the UK, 183 consecutive patients suspected of contact dermatitis were patch tested with sodium sulfite 1% pet. (routine testing) and 7 (3.8%) had a positive patch test. One of these reactions was of current relevance, the patient had used a hair dye containing sodium sulfite (1). In the period 1989-1991, in Denmark, routine testing with sodium sulfite 1% pet. was performed in 1762 patients and 25 (1.4%) had a positive reaction. Three of these patients used or had used ketoconazole cream containing sodium sulfite, but patch tests to the cream itself were negative. In the others, no relevance was found (6).

Case reports and case series

A woman developed dermatitis of the face and lips the day after she applied a cosmetic package comprising day and night creams. Patch tests with the British Contact Dermatitis Society standard series, a bases, preservatives and cosmetic series and the patient's own products gave a positive reaction to both creams and to sodium metabisulfite 1% pet. When tested with the individual ingredients of the cosmetic products, there was a positive reaction to sodium sulfite 5% pet., which was present in both creams. Control testing was not performed (4). A man had dermatitis of the scalp from contact allergy to sodium sulfite in a hair dye (1).

Contact allergy to sodium sulfite in non-cosmetic products

In the period 1990-2010, in a tertiary referral center in Belgium, over 25 patients had contact allergy to the antifungal preparation ketoconazole cream containing sodium sulfite; these were detected by positive patch tests to sodium metabisulfite (3). Three patients may have been sensitized to sodium sulfite in ketoconazole cream (6). One (7), two (8), two (10) and three (9) individuals had allergic contact dermatitis from sodium sulfite in (ketoconazole) antifungal cream.

Cross-reactions, pseudo-cross-reactions and co-reactions

Patients allergic to sodium sulfite almost always react to sodium metabisulfite (1,4). Conversely, only a few reactions to sodium sulfite are observed in patients allergic to sodium metabisulfite (5). Sodium sulfite, sodium metabisulfite, and sodium bisulfite, when dissolved in water, exist in pH-dependent equilibrium with each other (2). The buffering capacity of skin would result in a similar mixture of sodium sulfite, sodium metabisulfite, and sodium bisulfite, whichever compound is applied (1).

Presence in cosmetic products and chemical analyses
In the USA, in April 2017, sodium sulfite was present in 1787 of 56,714 cosmetic products of which the composition is known in FDA's Voluntary Cosmetic Registration Program (VCRP) (data obtained from FDA, May 2017). In April 2017, sodium sulfite was present in 153 of 66,485 cosmetic products of which the composition is known in EWG's Skin Deep Cosmetics Database, USA (http://www.ewg.org/skindeep/).

LITERATURE

1   Oliphant T, Mitra A, Wilkinson M. Contact allergy to sodium sulfite and its relationship to sodium metabisulfite. Contact Dermatitis 2012;66:128-130
2   Vally H, Misso NLA, Madan V. Clinical effects of sulphite additives. Clin Exp Allergy 2009;39:1643-1651
3   Garcia-Gavin J, Parente J, Goossens A. Allergic contact dermatitis caused by sodium metabisulfite: a challenging allergen. A case series and literature review. Contact Dermatitis 2012;67:260-269
4   Malik MM, Hegarty MA, Bourke JF. Sodium metabisulfite – a marker for cosmetic allergy? Contact Dermatitis 2007;56:241-242
5   Vena GA, Foti C, Angelini G. Sulfite contact allergy. Contact Dermatitis 1994;31:172-175
6   Petersen CS, Menné T. Consecutive patch testing with sodium sulphite in eczema patients. Contact Dermatitis 1992;27:344-345
7   Vissers-Croughs KJM, Van der K!ey AMJ, Vulto AG, Hulsmans RFHJ. Allergic contact dermatitis from sodium sulfite. Contact Dermatitis 1988;18:252-253
8   Garcia-Bravo B, Mazuecos J, Rodriguez-Pichardo A, Navas J, Camacho F. Hypersensitivity to ketoconazole preparations: study of 4 cases. Contact Dermatitis 1989;21:346-348
9   Lodi A, Chiarelli G, Mancini LL, Crosti C. Contact allergy to sodium sulfite contained in an antifungal preparation. Contact Dermatitis 1993;29:97
10 Ikehata K, KatoJ, Kuwano A, Mita T, Sugai T. Two cases of allergic contact dermatitis caused by sodium sulfite in the vehicle of antifungal cream. Skin Research 1996;38:198-202 (in Japanese)
11 Guidetti MS, Vincenzi C, Guerra L, Tosti A. Contact dermatitis due to imidazole antimycotics. Contact Dermatitis 1995;33:282

2.429   SOLVENT YELLOW 44

IDENTIFICATION

Description/definition   : Solvent yellow 44 is an aminoketone color, which conforms to the formula shown
                              below
Chemical class(es)   : Color additives - miscellaneous
Chemical/IUPAC name   : 6-Amino-2-(2,4-dimethylphenyl)-1*H*-benz[de]isoquinoline-1,3[2*H*]-dione
Other names   : CI 56200; disperse yellow 11; FD&C yellow 11
CAS registry number (s)   : 2478-20-8
EC number(s)   : 219-607-9
Function(s) in cosmetics   : EU: formerly used for hair dyeing; delisted in 2008. USA: colorants
EU cosmetic restrictions   : Regulated in Annex II/127 of the Regulation (EC) No. 1223/2009 (prohibited)
Patch testing   : No data available; suggested: 1% pet.
Molecular formula   : $C_{20}H_{16}N_2O_2$

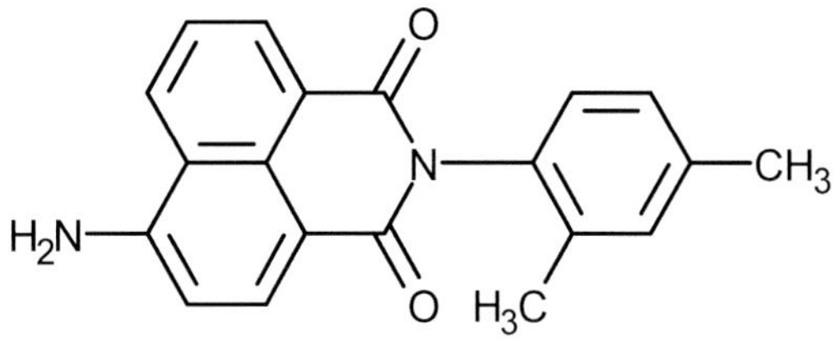

CONTACT ALLERGY

Case reports and case series

A woman complained of soreness at the angle of her mouth. Her mouth, face and eyelids became swollen and she was treated with systemic steroids. The condition recurred four times in a month. She had recently bought a new shade of lipstick (of her regular brand) and used it as rouge on her cheeks. Initial patch tests to the standard series and to eosin (50%) and the rest of her cosmetic preparations, including one of her two lipsticks, were all negative. Only later was she tested with her second lipstick and this was strongly positive. The manufacturer supplied all the ingredients which were tested separately. It contained two colors: FD&C Yellow 11 (Solvent yellow 44) and Red 17. The yellow color gave a positive reaction, the red one was negative, as were the other ingredients of the incrimi-nated lipstick. It was not mentioned what concentration had been used for patch testing (1). The patient cited by Fisher (2) may have been the same.

Presence in cosmetic products and chemical analyses

In the USA, in April 2017, solvent yellow 44 was present in zero of 56,714 cosmetic products of which the compo-sition is known in FDA's Voluntary Cosmetic Registration Program (VCRP) (data obtained from FDA, May 2017). In April 2017, solvent yellow 44 was present in zero of 65,434 cosmetic products of which the composition is known in EWG's Skin Deep Cosmetics Database, USA (http://www.ewg.org/skindeep/).

LITERATURE

1   Calnan CD. FD & C Yellow 11 in lipstick. Contact Dermatitis 1975;1:121
2   Calnan CD, cited by Fisher AA. Highlights of the First International Symposium on Contact Dermatitis. Cutis 1976;18:645-662

2.430   SORBIC ACID

Description/definition   : Sorbic acid is the organic acid that conforms to the formula shown below
Chemical class(es)   : Carboxylic acids
Chemical/IUPAC name   : (2E,4E)-Hexa-2,4-dienoic acid
CAS registry number (s)   : 110-44-1
EC number(s)   : 203-768-7
CIR review(s)   : J Am Coll Toxicol 1988;7:837-880 (access: www.cir-safety.org/ingredients)
Merck Index monograph : 10117
Function(s) in cosmetics : EU: preservative. USA: preservatives; fragrance ingredients
EU cosmetic restrictions : Regulated in Annex V/4 of the Regulation (EC) No. 1223/2009
Patch testing   : 2% pet. (Chemotechnique, SmartPracticeEurope, SmartPracticeCanada); 2% alc.
                               (SmartPracticeCanada)
Molecular formula   : $C_6H_8O_2$

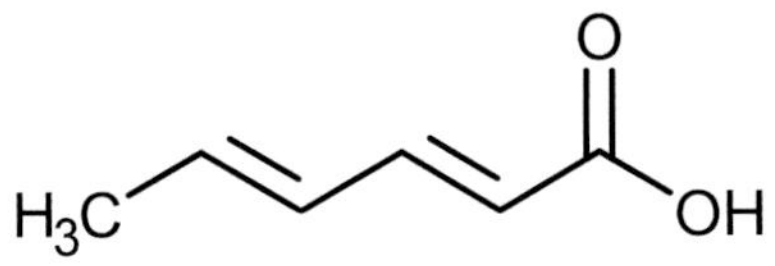

GENERAL

Sorbic acid is present naturally in several red fruits including cranberries, strawberries, and currants and may be synthesized. Sorbic acid and its salts such as potassium, calcium and sodium inhibit molds and yeasts, and are used as preservatives to avoid further fermentation in tobacco and foods (as E200 in the EU) such as wines, butter, cheese, yoghurts or dried fruits. In cosmetics and pharmaceuticals, they are used mainly in fatty acids and polyoxyethylene-based products. These chemicals also improve milling characteristics in cold rubber, and may be used in copolymerization, as intermediate for plasticizers and lubricants, in adhesives, glues, inks, paints, varnishes, tanning agents and metalworking fluids (57). Contact allergy to sorbic acid is infrequent, but it is a well-known cause of non-immunologic immediate contact reactions (11-14,27-29). The literature on sorbic acid up to 1991 has been reviewed in ref. 58.

CONTACT ALLERGY

Patch testing in groups of patients

Results of studies testing sorbic acid in consecutive patients suspected of contact dermatitis (routine testing) are shown in table 2.430.1. Results of testing in groups of selected patients (e.g., patients suspected of cosmetic dermatitis, patients with leg ulcers, individuals tested with a cosmetic or preservative series) back to 1992 are shown in table 2.430.2.

Patch testing in consecutive patients suspected of contact dermatitis: routine testing

In four studies in which routine testing with sorbic acid was performed, rates of sensitization have been consistently low, ranging from 0.3% to 0.8% (31,32,36,40). In two studies in which relevance was addressed, 10 of 25 resp. 4 of 10 positive patch test reactions (both 40%) were scored as relevant, but culprit products were not mentioned (31,40).

Table 2.430.1 Patch testing in groups of patients: Routine testing

Years and Country	Test conc. & vehicle	Number of patients tested	positive (%)	Selection of patients (S); Relevance (R); Comments (C)	Ref.
2006-2010 USA	2% pet.	3084	25 (0.8%)	R: 40%	40
2003-2005 China		599	4 (0.7%)	R: not stated	36
1998-2000 USA	2% pet.	610	(0.3%)	R: not stated	32
1992-1994 USA	2% pet.	3476	10 (0.3%)	R: present relevance: 40%	31

Patch testing in groups of selected patients

Results of studies patch testing sorbic acid in groups of selected patients (e.g., patients suspected of cosmetic dermatitis, patients with leg ulcers, individuals tested with a cosmetic or preservative series) back to 1992 are shown in table 2.430.2. In 10 investigations, frequencies of sensitization have ranged from 0.2% to 2.1%, but 7/10 scored lower than 1%. The highest 2.1% frequency was found in a Korean study among 584 patients suspected of allergic cosmetic dermatitis; however, the relevance of the positive patch tests was not mentioned and neither were causative products (37). In fact, the issue of relevance was addressed in two studies only (2,21). In a study from the USA, all 8 positive reactions were scored as relevant, but this study had certain weaknesses. In a Danish investigation, 7 of 10 reactions were relevant, 6 from a moisturizing cream and one from the presence of sorbic acid in a topical corticosteroid preparation (21).

Table 2.430.2 Patch testing in groups of patients: Selected patient groups

Years and Country	Test conc. & vehicle	Number of patients tested	positive (%)		Selection of patients (S); Relevance (R); Comments (C)	Ref.
2007-2012 IVDK	2% pet.	1369	3	(0.2%)	S: female patients, clients of hairdressers, in who hair cos-metics were regarded as a cause of dermatitis, and who had never worked as hairdressers; R: not stated	48
2010-2011 Korea	2% pet.	584	12	(2.1%)	S: patients suspected of allergic cosmetic dermatitis; R: not stated	37
2006-2011 IVDK	2% pet.	6978		(0.7%)	S: patients suspected of cosmetic intolerance and tested with a preservative series; R: not stated	47
1996-2009 IVDK	2% pet.	77,708	519	(0.6%) [a]	S: not specified; R: not specified	4
2004-2008 France	2% pet.	423	5	(1.2%)	S: patients with leg ulcers; R: not stated	35
2000-2007 USA	2% pet.	871	8	(0.9%)	S: patients tested with a supplemental cosmetic screening series; R: 100%; C: weak study: a. high rate of macular erythema and weak reactions; b. relevance figures included 'questionable' and 'past' relevance	2
2000-2002 Finland		6037		(0.1%)	S: patients tested with a cosmetic series; R: not stated	33
1995-1996 Finland		3744		(0.3%)	S: patients tested with a cosmetic series; R: not stated	33
1990-1994 Germany	2% pet.	11,437	85	(0.7%)	S: patients tested with a preservative series; R: not stated	34
1988-1992 Denmark	2% pet.	718	10	(1.4%)	S: patients tested with a medicament and cosmetics series; R: 7 were relevant, 6 from a moisturizing cream and 1 from a topical corticosteroid preparation	21

[a] standardized for sex and age
IVDK: Information Network of Departments of Dermatology, Germany, Austria, Switzerland

Case reports and case series
Sorbic acid was stated to be the (or an) allergen in one patient in a group of 603 individuals suffering from cosmetic dermatitis, seen in the period 2010-2015 in Leuven, Belgium (38). Of 10 patients reacting to sorbic acid seen in one hospital in Denmark in the period 1988-1992, 6 were caused by the use of a moisturizer containing 0.15% sorbic acid (21). In 3 clinics in Belgium, in the period 1978-1985, 279 patients with allergic contact dermatitis exclusively caused by cosmetics were seen. In this group, there were 3 reactions to sorbic acid. It was implied that this was the cause of the allergic reaction (46).

Sorbic acid was responsible for 6 out of 399 cases of cosmetic allergy where the causal allergen was identified in a study of the NACDG, USA, 1977-1983 (1). In one hospital in Sweden, 17 cases of contact allergy to sorbic acid in 'Unguentum Merck', an ointment base widely used as moisturizer have been observed in the period 1973-1980 (9). Three more patients reacted to sorbic acid in 'Unguentum Merck' (6,7,8). Five cases of sorbic acid sensitivity in this ointment had been reported to the manufacturer up to 1981 (cited in ref. 7). A child had contact dermatitis from sorbic acid in moist toilet tissues (20). One positive patch test reaction to sorbic acid was ascribed to cosmetic allergy (3).

Contact allergy to sorbic acid in non-cosmetic products
Two patients had allergic contact dermatitis from sorbic acid in a topical pharmaceutical product (15,19). In both, dermatitis resolved after a 15 days sorbic acid-free diet (15,19). A child had contact dermatitis from allergy to sorbic acid in a corticosteroid cream (20). Another patient also reacted to a corticosteroid topical pharmaceutical product (21). Three patients had periocular allergic contact dermatitis from sorbic acid in ophthalmic preparations (22). One individual presented with allergic contact conjunctivitis from sorbic acid in a contact lens solution (23).

A man had allergic contact dermatitis from sorbic acid in a topical pharmaceutical preparation and in tobacco (59). Another male individual became sensitized to sorbic acid from its presence in a pharmaceutical preparation to treat a hypertrophic scar on the back of his left hand (56).

Cross-reactions, pseudo-cross-reactions and co-reactions
Potassium sorbate (25,57).

Presence in cosmetic products and chemical analyses

In July 2017, sorbic acid was present in 763 of 69,548 cosmetic products of which the composition is known in EWG's Skin Deep Cosmetics Database, USA (http://www.ewg.org/skindeep/). In the USA, in April 2017, sorbic acid was present in 2006 of 56,714 cosmetic products of which the composition is known in FDA's Voluntary Cosmetic Registration Program (VCRP) (data obtained from FDA, May 2017). Sorbic acid was present in 391 of 4737 (8.3%) commonly used cosmetic products of which the full composition was known in 2016 in The Contact Allergen Management Program (CAMP) database of the American Contact Dermatitis Society (52). Sorbic acid (and derivatives) were present in 70 (39%) of 178 facial wipes for which ingredient information was obtained online and from retail stores, USA, 2016 (50). Sorbic acid and derivatives were present in 34 (63%) of 54 personal hygiene wet wipes for which ingredient information was obtained online and from retail stores, USA, 2016 (51). In 2009, in the USA, the ingredient lists of 1591 facial cosmetics from one company were screened for the presence of sorbic acid. Sorbic acid was present in 22% of 132 blushers and 38 bronzers, in 0% of 90 concealers, in 12% of 174 eyeliners, in 17% of 304 eyeshadows, in 4% of 457 foundations, in 20% of 140 loose and pressed powders, and in 0% of 256 mascaras (42). In 2009, in the USA, the ingredient lists of 796 hair products from one company were screened for the presence of sorbic acid. Sorbic acid was present in 4% of 279 shampoos, in 0% of 231 conditioners, and in 0% of 286 styling products (43).

In 2009, in the USA, the ingredient lists of 730 lip cosmetics and dental care products from one company were screened for the presence of sorbic acid. Sorbic acid was present in 32% of 31 lip liners, in 5% of 429 lipsticks, in 1 of 92 lip moisturizers, in 0 of 153 toothpastes, and in 8% of 25 mouth washes (44). In 2009, in the USA, the ingredient lists of 657 miscellaneous cosmetics from one company were screened for the presence of sorbic acid. Sorbic acid was present in 0% of 195 antiperspirants/deodorants, in 0% of 41 powders, in 0% of 167 shaving products, in 1of 201 sunblocks, and in 7% of 53 wipes (45). Sorbates (sorbic acid or potassium sorbate) were present in 261/3541 (7.0%) randomly sampled leave-on cosmetic products, Germany, 2006-2009 (5). In Germany, in 2006-2009, the labels of 4680 cosmetic products were screened for the presence of preservatives. Sorbic acid was present in 1.5% of the products, according to labelling information (49). In a group of 67 samples of skin creams, randomly selected from retail outlets in Denmark in 1999, 4 (6%) contained sorbic acid in a concentration range of 0.015-0.219%. In one product it was present but not declared (41).

Other information

In a patient with dermatitis and contact allergy to sorbic acid, lasting improvement was noticed after 15 days on a sorbic acid-free diet, with reappearance on reintroduction of foods containing sorbic acid, such as yoghurt with prunes and strawberries and margarine (15). Exacerbation of eczema after eating cheese labelled as containing sorbic acid has previously been noted in a patient sensitized to sorbic acid (16). However, other authors (17,18) found that in patients who were allergic to sorbic acid, no reaction could be provoked orally (17,18). In one patient dermatitis that was caused by sorbic acid in a topical pharmaceutical product did not disappear after discontinuing its application; however, a 15 days sorbic acid-free diet cured the dermatitis permanently (19).

OTHER SIDE EFFECTS

Immediate-type reactions

The capability of sorbic acid, down to a concentration of 0.1%, to induce erythema and wheals in a large percentage of test persons (non-immunologic contact urticaria) is well known (11,12,13,14,27).). Sorbic acid in topical products has long been known to cause such immediate contact reactions (28,29). Contact urticaria to sorbic acid in a topical pharmaceutical was observed in one patient; when 20 controls were tested with sorbic acid, 3 had a similar reaction indicative of non-immunologic immediate contact reaction (10). Two patients with 'contact lens intolerance' had contact urticaria from sorbic acid in the lens solution (24). In a kindergarten, 18 of 20 children developed perioral contact urticaria from sorbic acid in a mayonnaise-containing salad dressing (27). A woman had contact urticaria of the face from washing her hair with a sorbic acid-containing shampoo; when the patient smelled her shampoo directly from the bottle, nasal itching and sneezing commenced; open testing with sorbic acid reproduced the immediate contact reactions (30). Another female individual with burning mouth syndrome and contact urticaria to sorbic acid upon patch testing, became asymptomatic after dietary avoidance of sorbic acid (54). A review of contact urticaria caused by ingredients of cosmetics has been provided in 2016 (53).

Other non-eczematous contact reactions

Burning mouth syndrome was (unconvincingly) ascribed to contact allergy to sorbic acid in food (25). A woman with burning mouth syndrome became asymptomatic when avoiding sorbic acid, to which she was contact allergic, in foods (26). In the past, sorbic acid has been considered a contributing factor in some patients with recurrent chronic urticaria on the basis of positive oral provocation tests (55).

LITERATURE

1 Adams RM, Maibach HI, Clendenning WE, Fisher AA, Jordan WJ, Kanof N, et al. A five-year study of cosmetic reactions. J Am Acad Dermatol 1985;13:1062-1069

2 Wetter DA, Yiannias JA, Prakash AV, Davis MD, Farmer SA, el-Azhary RA, et al. Results of patch testing to personal care product allergens in a standard series and a supplemental cosmetic series: an analysis of 945 patients from the Mayo Clinic Contact Dermatitis Group, 2000-2007. J Am Acad Dermatol 2010;63:789-798

3 Kohl L, Blondeel A, Song M. Allergic contact dermatitis from cosmetics: retrospective analysis of 819 patch-tested patients. Dermatology 2002;204:334-337

4 Schnuch A, Lessmann H, Geier J, Uter W. Contact allergy to preservatives. Analysis of IVDK data 1996-2009. Br J Dermatol 2011;164:1316-1325

5 Schnuch A, Mildau G, Kratz E-M, Uter W. Risk of sensitization to preservatives estimated on the basis of patch test data and exposure, according to a sample of 3541 leave-on products. Contact Dermatitis 2011;65:167-174

6 Saihan EM, Harman RM. Contact sensitivity to sorbic acid in 'Unguentum Merck'. Br J Dermatol 1978;99:583-584

7 Coyle HE, Miller E, Chapman RS. Sorbic acid sensitivity from Unguentum Merck. Contact Dermatitis 1981;7:56-57

8 Brown R. Another case of sorbic acid sensitivity. Contact Dermatitis 1979;5:268

9 Göransson K, Lidén S. Contact allergy to sorbic acid and Unguentum Merck. Contact Dermatitis 1981;7:277

10 Peréz RG, Gortzaiez M, Gonzalez R, Soloeta R. Clinically relevant contact urticaria caused by Thrombocid® ointment. Contact Dermatitis 2003;48:225-226

11 Lahti A. Non-immunologic contact urticaria. Acta Derm-Venereol 1989;60 (Suppl. 91):8-49

12 Soschin D, Leyden JJ. Sorbic acid-induced erythema and edema. J Am Acad Dermatol 1986:14:234-241

13 Kligman AM. The spectrum of contact urticaria. Dermatol Clin 1990;8:57-60

14 Fisher AA. Sorbic acid: a cause of immediate nonallergic facial erythema. An Update. Cutis 1998;61:17

15 Dejobert Y, Delaporte E, Piette F, Thomas P. Vesicular eczema and systemic contact dermatitis from sorbic acid. Contact Dermatitis 2001;45:291

16 Grater W C. Hypersensitive skin reactions to F.D. and C. dyes. Cutis 1976;17:1163-1165

17 Klaschka F, Beiersdorff HU. Allergic eczematous reaction from sorbic acid used as a preservative in external medicaments. Hautklin Munch Med Wschr 1965;107:185

18 Fisher AA. Cutaneous reactions to sorbic acid and potassium sorbate. Cutis 1980;25:350,352,423

19 Giordano Labadie F, Pech-Ormieres C, Bazex J. Systemic contact dermatitis from sorbic acid. Contact Dermatitis 1996;34:61-62

20 Raison-Peyron N, Meynadier JM, Meynadier J. Sorbic acid: an unusual cause of systemic contact dermatitis in an infant. Contact Dermatitis 2000;43:247-248

21 Ramsing DW, Menné T. Contact sensitivity to sorbic acid. Contact Dermatitis 1993;28:124-125

22 Maucher OM. Periorbitalekzem als iatrogene Erkrankung. Klin Monatsbl Augenheilkd 1974;164:350-356

23 Fisher AA. Allergic reactions to contact lens solutions. Cutis 1985;85:209-211

24 Podmore P and Storrs FJ. Contact lens intolerance; allergic conjunctivitis?. Contact Dermatitis 1989;20:98-103

25 Haustein U-F. Burning mouth syndrome due to nicotinic acid esters and sorbic acid. Contact Dermatitis 1988;19:225-226

26 Lamey P-J, Lamb AB, Forsyth A. Atypical burning mouth syndrome. Contact Dermatitis 1987;17:242-243

27 Clemmensen O, Hjorth N. Perioral contact urticaria from sorbic acid and benzoic acid in a salad dressing. Contact Dermatitis 1982;8:1-6

28 Fryklöf L-B. Irritant properties of sorbic acid in ointments and creams. J Pharm Pharmacol 1958;10:719 (data cited in ref. 27)

29 Hjorth N, Trolle-Lassen C. Skin reactions to preservatives in creams. American Perfumer 1962;77:43-46 (data cited in ref. 27).

30 Rietschel RL. Contact urticaria from synthetic cassia oil and sorbic acid limited to the face. Contact Dermatitis 1978;4:347-349

31 Marks JG, Belsito DV, DeLeo VA, Fowler JF, Fransway AF, Maibach HI,et al. North American Contact Dermatitis Group standard tray patch test results 1992 through 1994. Am J Contact Dermatitis 1995;6:160-165

32 Wetter DA, Davis MDP, Yiannias JA, Cheng JF, Connolly SM, el-Azhary RA, et al. Patch test results from the Mayo Contact Dermatitis Group, 1998–2000. J Am Acad Dermatol 2005;53:416-421

33 Hasan T, Rantanen T, Alanko K, Harvima RJ, Jolanki R, Kalimo K, et al. Patch test reactions to cosmetic allergens in 1995–1997 and 2000–2002 in Finland –a multicentre study. Contact Dermatitis 2005;53:40-45

34 Schnuch A, Geier J, Uter W, Frosch PJ. Patch testing with preservatives, antimicrobials and industrial biocides. Results from a multicentre study. Br J Dermatol 1998;138:467-476

35 Barbaud A, Collet E, Le Coz CJ, Meaume S, Gillois P. Contact allergy in chronic leg ulcers: results of a multicentre study carried out in 423 patients and proposal for an updated series of patch tests. Contact Dermatitis 2009;60:279-287

36 Li L-F, Liu G, Wang J. Patch test in Chinese patients with cosmetic allergic contact dermatitis to common cosmetic allergens from a European cosmetic series. Contact Dermatitis 2007;57:50-54

37 Lee SS, Hong DK, Jeong NJ, Lee JH, Choi YS, Lee AY, et al. Multicenter study of preservative sensitivity in patients with suspected cosmetic contact dermatitis in Korea. J Dermatol 2012;39:677-681

38 Goossens A. Cosmetic contact allergens. Cosmetics 2016, 3, 5; doi:10.3390/cosmetics3010005

39 Rudner EJ. North American Group Results. Contact Dermatitis 1977;3:208-209

40 Wentworth AB, Yiannias JA, Keeling JH, Hall MR, Camilleri MJ, Drage LA, et al. Trends in patch-test results and allergen changes in the standard series: a Mayo Clinic 5-year retrospective review (January 1, 2006, to December 31, 2010). J Am Acad Dermatol 2014;70:269-275

41 Rastogi SC. Analytical control of preservative labelling on skin creams. Contact Dermatitis 2000;43:339-343

42 Scheman A, Jacob S, Katta R, Nedorost S, Warshaw E, Zirwas M, et al. Part 1 of a 4 part series. Facial cosmetics: trends and alternatives. Data from the American Contact Alternative Group. J Clin Aesthet Dermatol 2011;4:25-30

43 Scheman A, Jacob S, Katta R, Nedorost S, Warshaw E, Zirwas M, et al. Part 2 of a 4 part series. Hair cosmetics: trends and alternatives. Data from the American Contact Alternative Group. J Clin Aesthet Dermatol 2011;4:42-46

44 Scheman A, Jacob S, Katta R, Nedorost S, Warshaw E, Zirwas M, et al. Part 3 of a 4 part series. Lips and common Dental Care products: trends and alternatives. Data from the American Contact Alternative Group. J Clin Aesthet Dermatol 2011;4:50-53

45 Scheman A, Jacob S, Katta R, Nedorost S, Warshaw E, Zirwas M, et al. Part 4 of a 4 part series. Miscellaneous products: trends and alternatives in deodorants, antiperspirants, sunblocks, shaving products, powder, and wipes. Data from the American Contact Alternative Group. J Clin Aesthet Dermatol 2011;4:35-39

46 Dooms-Goossens A, de Boulle K, Dooms M, Degreef H. Imidazolidinyl urea dermatitis. Contact Dermatitis 1986;14:322-324

47 Dinkloh A, Worm M, Geier J, Schnuch A, Wollenberg A. Contact sensitization in patients with suspected cosmetic intolerance: results of the IVDK 2006-2011. J Eur Acad Dermatol Venereol 2015;29:1071-1081

48 Uter W, Gefeller O, John SM, Schnuch A, Geier J. Contact allergy to ingredients of hair cosmetics – a comparison of female hairdressers and clients based on IVDK 2007–2012 data. Contact Dermatitis 2014;71:13-20

49 Uter W, Yazar K, Kratz EM, Mildau G, Lidén C. Coupled exposure to ingredients of cosmetic products: II. Preservatives. Contact Dermatitis 2014;70:219-226

50 Aschenbeck KA, Warshaw EM. Allergenic ingredients in facial wet wipes. Dermatitis 2017 Mar 23. doi: 10.1097/DER.0000000000000268. [Epub ahead of print]

51 Aschenbeck KA, Warshaw EM. Allergenic ingredients in personal hygiene wet wipes. Dermatitis 2017 Mar 23. doi: 10.1097/DER.0000000000000275. [Epub ahead of print]

52 Beene KM, Scheman A, Severson D, Reeder MJ. Prevalence of preservatives across all product types in the Contact Allergen Management Program. Dermatitis 2017;28:81-87

53 Verhulst L, Goossens A. Cosmetic components causing contact urticaria: a review and update. Contact Dermatitis 2016;75:333-344

54 Lamey PJ, Lamb AB, Hughes A, Milligan KA, Forsyth A. Type III burning mouth syndrome: psychological and allergic aspects. J Oral Pathol Med 1994;23:216-219

55 Juhlin L. Recurrent urticaria: clinical investigation of 330 patients. Br J Dermatol 1981;104:369-381

56 Patrizi A, Orlandi C, Vincenzi C, Bardazzi F. Allergic contact dermatitis caused by sorbic acid: rare occurrence. Am J Contact Dermat 1999;10:52

57 Le Coz CJ, Abensour M. Occupational contact dermatitis from potassium sorbate in milk transformation plant. Contact Dermatitis 2005;53:176-177

58 Fransway AF. The problem of preservation in the 1990s. III. Agents with preservative function independent of formaldehyde release. Am J Contact Derm 1991;2:145-174

59 Grange-Prunier A, Bezier M, Perceau G, Bernard P. Tobacco contact dermatitis caused by sensitivity to sorbic acid. Ann Dermatol Venereol 2008;135:135-138 (article in French)

2.431   SORBITAN OLEATE

IDENTIFICATION

Description/definition   : Sorbitan oleate is the monoester of oleic acid and hexitol anhydrides derived from sorbitol. It conforms generally to the formula shown below
Chemical class(es)   : Sorbitan derivatives
Chemical/IUPAC name   : [2-(3,4-Dihydroxyoxolan-2-yl)-2-hydroxyethyl] octadec-9-enoate
Other names   : Sorbitan monooleate; Span® 80
CAS registry number (s)   : 1338-43-8; 37318-79-9
EC number(s)   : 215-665-4
Merck Index monograph   : 10120 (Sorbitan esters)
CIR review(s)   : J Am Coll Toxicol 1985;4:65-121; Final report, December 2014 (access: www.cir-safety.org/ingredients)
Function(s) in cosmetics   : EU: emulsifying. USA: fragrance ingredients; surfactants – emulsifying agents
Patch testing   : 5% pet. (Chemotechnique, SmartPracticeCanada)
Molecular formula   : $C_{24}H_{44}O_6$

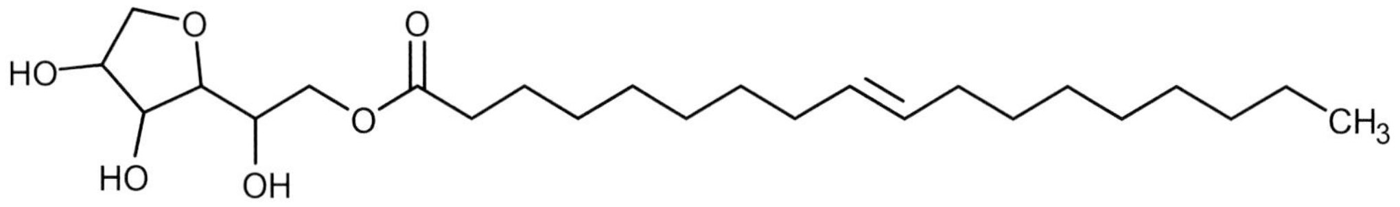

CONTACT ALLERGY

Patch testing in groups of patients
Results of patch testing sorbitan oleate in consecutive patients suspected of contact dermatitis (routine testing) and of testing groups of *selected* patients (e.g., patients suspected of cosmetic dermatitis, patients with chronic or recurrent inflammatory skin diseases, using or having used topical preparations) are shown in table 2.431.1. In 5 studies performing routine testing, rates of sensitization have ranged from 0.4% to 7.8%, but 3/5 scored 1% or lower. The high percentage of 7.8 was found in a Chinese study, in which 11.8% of the group of patients ultimately diagnosed with cosmetic allergy reacted to sorbitan oleate, versus 7.1% in the others, who did not react to cosmetic products. The relevance of the reactions was not mentioned (8).

In studies patch testing groups of *selected* patients, (e.g., patients suspected of cosmetic dermatitis, patients with chronic or recurrent (> 1 year) inflammatory skin diseases, using or having used topical preparations), frequencies of sensitization ranged from 0.4% (12) to 8.5% (10). In the latter study, a small but very heterogeneous group of 47 individuals (23 with chronic leg ulcers, 15 with contact dermatitis, 1 with nummular eczema, 6 with psoriasis, 2 with atopic dermatitis), there were 4 positive patch test reactions to sorbitan oleate. The relevance of these reactions was not specified, but some of the patients were sensitized to the emulsifier in cold cream (10).

Case reports and case series
Sorbitan oleate was responsible for 2 out of 959 cases of non-fragrance cosmetic allergy where the causal allergen was identified, Belgium, 2000-2010 (1). In a 4-month-period in 1996, 475 patients with contact allergy to 'cosmetic ingredients' were collected in 5 centers in Belgium, UK and Germany. There was one reaction to sorbitan oleate; relevance was not stated (9).

Contact allergy to sorbitan oleate in an emollient worsened existing irritant contact hand dermatitis in a metal turner (7). An unknown number of individuals with chronic or recurrent inflammatory skin diseases (probably 1-3) reacted to sorbitan oleate in cold cream (10). One patient had relevant positive patch test reactions to a moisturizer and to its ingredient sorbitan oleate (14).

Contact allergy to sorbitan oleate in non-cosmetic products
One patient reacted to sorbitan oleate in a topical pharmaceutical preparation containing 5-fluorouracil for the treatment of actinic keratoses. A patch test with the commercial cream itself was negative, but there was a weak positive reaction to sorbitan oleate 5% pet. on two occasions (4). Three patients reacted to sorbitan oleate in paste bandages. All suffered from leg ulcers and had multiple sensitizations (polysensitization) (6).

Table 2.431.1 Patch testing in groups of patients

Years and Country	Test conc. & vehicle	Number of patients tested	positive (%)		Selection of patients (S); Relevance (R); Comments (C)	Ref.
Routine testing						
2008-1010 USA	5% pet.	591	5	(0.8%)	R: not specified; C: 4/5 also reacted to sorbitan sesquioleate	3
2006-2007 USA	5% pet.	112	3	(2.7%)	R: all three used products containing sorbitan derivatives or sorbitol	17
2005-2006 Turkey		93	1	(1%)	R: the reaction was considered to be relevant	15
2003-2005 China		599	47	(7.8%)	R: not stated; C: in patients with cosmetic allergy, 11.8% reacted to sorbitan oleate, versus 7.1% in the group without reactions to cosmetics	8
1975 Finland	10% pet.	1206	5	(0.4%)	R: not specified; C: the test material contained 5% sorbitan oleate and 5% sorbitan stearate	11
Testing in groups of selected patients						
2000-2007 USA	5% pet.	945	7	(0.7%)	S: patients tested with a supplemental cosmetic screening series; R: 86%; C: weak study: a. high rate of macular erythema and weak reactions; b. relevance figures included 'questionable' and 'past' relevance	2
<2005 India	2% pet.	50	2	(4%)	S: patients suspected of cosmetic dermatitis; R: not stated	13
<1993 Switzerland	10% pet.	47	4	(8.5%)	S: patients with chronic or recurrent (> 1 year) inflammatory skin diseases, using or having used topical preparations (23 chronic leg ulcers, 15 contact dermatitis, 1 nummular eczema, 6 psoriasis, 2 atopic dermatitis); unspecified number of patients had used cold cream containing sorbitan oleate	10
1972-1974 Finland	10% pet.	486	2	(0.4%)	S: not stated; R: not stated; C: the test substance contained 5% sorbitan oleate and 5% sorbitan stearate	12

Cross-reactions, pseudo-cross-reactions and co-reactions
Sorbitan sesquioleate (3,5,6,10,18).

Presence in cosmetic products and chemical analyses
In the USA, in April 2017, sorbitan oleate was present in 377 of 56,714 cosmetic products of which the composition is known in FDA's Voluntary Cosmetic Registration Program (VCRP) (data obtained from FDA, May 2017). In January 2017, sorbitan oleate was present in 270 of 64,655 cosmetic products of which the composition is known in EWG's Skin Deep Cosmetics Database, USA (http://www.ewg.org/skindeep/).

OTHER SIDE EFFECTS

Other non-eczematous contact reactions
In (somewhat) older literature, sorbitan oleate has been suspected of being comedogenic, based on the rabbit ear assay (16).

LITERATURE

1   Travassos AR, Claes L, Boey L, Drieghe J, Goossens A. Non-fragrance allergens in specific cosmetic products. Contact Dermatitis 2011;65:276-285
2   Wetter DA, Yiannias JA, Prakash AV, Davis MD, Farmer SA, el-Azhary RA, et al. Results of patch testing to personal care product allergens in a standard series and a supplemental cosmetic series: an analysis of 945 patients from the Mayo Clinic Contact Dermatitis Group, 2000-2007. J Am Acad Dermatol 2010;63:789-798
3   Cressey BD, Kumar N, Scheinman PL. Contact allergy to sorbitans: A follow-up study. Dermatitis 2012;23:158-161
4   Meijer BUGA, De Waard-van der Spek FB. Allergic contact dermatitis because of topical use of 5-fluorouracil (Efudix® cream). Contact Dermatitis 2007;57:58-60
5   Pereira F, Cunha H, Dias M. Contact dermatitis due to emulsifiers. Contact Dermatitis 1997;36:114
6   Wakelin SH, Cooper S, Marren P, Shaw S. Sorbitan mono-oleate: a potential allergen in paste bandages. Contact Dermatitis 1996;35:377
7   Austad J. Allergic contact dermatitis to sorbitan monooleate (Span 80). Contact Dermatitis 19823;8:426
8   Li L-F, Liu G, Wang J. Patch test in Chinese patients with cosmetic allergic contact dermatitis to common cosmetic allergens from a European cosmetic series. Contact Dermatitis 2007;57:50-54
9   Goossens A, Beck MH, Haneke E, McFadden JP, Nolting S, Durupt G, Ries G. Adverse cutaneous reactions to cosmetic allergens. Contact Dermatitis 1999;40:112-113

10 Pasche-Koo F, Piletta P-A, Hunziker N, Hauser C. High sensitization rate to emulsifiers in patients with chronic leg ulcers. Contact Dermatitis 1994;31:226-228

11 Hannuksela M, Kousa M, Pirilä V. Contact sensitivity to emulsifiers. Contact Dermatitis 1976;2:201-204

12 Hannuksela M, Kousa M, Pirilä V. Allergy to ingredients of vehicles. Contact Dermatitis 1976;2:105-110

13 Tomar J, Jain VK, Aggarwal K, Dayal S, Guptaet S. Contact allergies to cosmetics: testing with 52 cosmetic ingredients and personal products. J Dermatol 2005;32:951-955

14 Held E, Johansen JD, Agner T, Menné T. Contact allergy to cosmetics: testing with patients' own products. Contact Dermatitis 1999;40:310-315

15 Ada S, Seçkin D. Patch testing in allergic contact dermatitis: is it useful to perform the cosmetic series in addition to the European standard series? J Eur Acad Dermatol Venereol 2010;24:1192-1196

16 Lanzet M. Comedogenic effects of cosmetic raw materials. Cosmetics & Toiletries 1986;101:63-72

17 Asarch A, Scheinman PL. Sorbitan sesquioleate, a common emulsifier in topical corticosteroids, is an important contact allergen. Dermatitis 2008;19:323-327

18 Mallon E, Powell SM. Sorbitan sesquioleate—a potential allergen in leg ulcer patients. Contact Dermatitis 1994;30:180-181

2.432 SORBITAN SESQUIOLEATE

IDENTIFICATION

Description/definition : Sorbitan sesquioleate is a mixture of mono- and diesters of oleic acid and hexitol anhydrides derived from sorbitol

Chemical class(es) : Sorbitan derivatives

Chemical/IUPAC name : (2R,3R,4R,5S)-Hexane-1,2,3,4,5,6-hexol; (Z)-octadec-9-enoic acid

Other names : Arlacel® C

CAS registry number (s) : 8007-43-0

EC number(s) : 232-360-1

CIR review(s) : J Am Coll Toxicol 1985;4:65-121; Final report, December 2014 (access: www.cir-safety.org/ingredients)

Function(s) in cosmetics : EU: emulsifying. USA: surfactants - emulsifying agents

Patch testing : 20% pet. (Chemotechnique, SmartPracticeEurope, SmartPracticeCanada)

Molecular formula : $C_{66}H_{126}O_{16}$

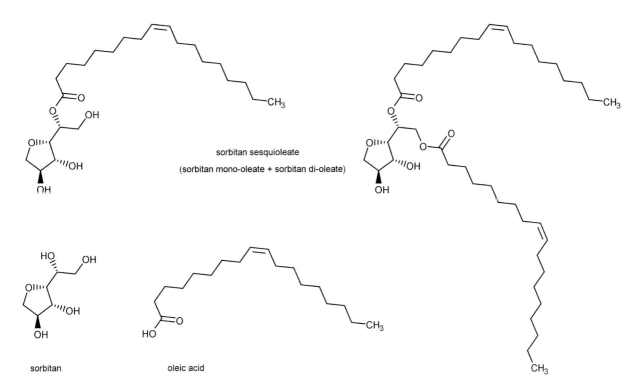

sorbitan sesquioleate

(sorbitan mono-oleate + sorbitan di-oleate)

sorbitan   oleic acid

GENERAL

Sorbitan sesquioleate (SSO) is a fatty acid ester derived from a mixture of mono- and diesters of oleic acid and hexitol anhydrides of sorbitol. It is an oil-soluble, water-dispersible, non-ionic surfactant, which functions as a water-in-oil emulsifier, increasing skin permeability and changing the physicochemical characteristics of other compounds. It is used widely in many skin care products, pharmaceutical preparations including topical corticosteroid ointments and creams, topical antibiotic and antifungal creams, wound dressings, diapers and oral hygiene products including toothpastes. It also has applications in agrochemicals, inks, paints and metalworking applications (9,36,39,42).

Sorbitan sesquioleate has been added to several patch test substances of some providers as an emulsifier in order to ensure a stable, homogeneous distribution of the chemicals. In the products of Chemotechnique www.che-motechnique.se) these are decyl glucoside, DMDM hydantoin, ethylene urea, melamine formaldehyde mix, formaldehyde (1% pet.), fragrance mix I (FM 1), glutaraldehyde, MCI/MI (in pet.), melamine formaldehyde, *Myroxylon pereirae* resin (Balsam of Peru), oakmoss absolute and the perfume mix. This means that positive reactions to these substances may be misinterpreted in patients allergic to the emulsifier. Reactivity to SSO can, for instance, result in a positive patch test reaction to the fragrance mix I in the European baseline series in patients who are *not* allergic to fragrances.

Indeed, in a recent IVDK study, of 2952 patients allergic to the FM 1, 154 (5.2%) co-reacted to sorbitan sesquioleate. Only a few of these reactions to the fragrance mix were clinically relevant, i.e. that the patients had a history of fragrance sensitivity. Therefore, sorbitan sesquioleate 20% pet. should ideally be included in the baseline series

(6,41). In a 2016 Danish study, however, only 6 of 426 (1.4%) patients reacting to the FM mix I co-reacted to SSO 20% pet. (36) and also in an earlier study of the EECDRG, there were very few co-reactions to SSO (41).

Whether the other major providers of patch test materials (SmartPractice Canada [www.smartpractcanada.com] and SmartPractice Europe [www.smartpracticeeurope.com]) use sorbitan sesquioleate in their products and, if yes, in which, cannot be found on their websites. However, in refs. 8 and 36, the individual components of the fragrance mix of SmartPractice Europe (formerly Almirall Hermal, Reinbek, Germany) are stated to contain sorbitan sesquioleate, 1% for all except oakmoss absolute, which contains 5% sorbitan sesquioleate (36).

The literature on contact allergy to sorbitan sesquioleate from before 1987 is cited in ref. 1.

CONTACT ALLERGY

Patch testing in groups of patients
Results of studies testing sorbitan sesquioleate in consecutive patients suspected of contact dermatitis (routine testing) back to 1975 are shown in table 2.432.1. Results of testing sorbitan sesquioleate in groups of *selected* patients (e.g., patients suspected of cosmetic allergy, patients reacting to the fragrance mix I, individuals with leg ulcers, patients tested with a cosmetic or ointment series) back to 1974 are shown in table 2.432.2.

Patch testing in consecutive patients suspected of contact dermatitis: routine testing
In eleven studies in which routine testing with sorbitan sesquioleate was performed, rates of sensitization have ranged from 0.2% to 10.7% (table 2.432.1). The highest rate of sensitization (10.7%) was found in a USA study in a very small group of 112 consecutive patients suspected of contact dermatitis, of who 12 reacted to SSO (38). This is a surprisingly – if not unrealistically - high frequency. All reactions were considered to be relevant, as the patients used topical corticosteroids, antifungal preparations or other, unspecified, products containing 'sorbitol or sorbitan derivatives'. However, the derivatives were not specified and cross- or pseudo-cross-reactivity to sorbitol has been suggested (5,9), but not proven with patch testing. Some 40% of the patients reacting to SSO had at least 5 positive patch test reactions, which increases the risk of false-positives from excited skin syndrome. Such high frequencies of sensitization to SSO have not been observed in any study afterwards, including a 2008-2010 study from the same center, where the rate had dropped from 10.7% to 3.9% (5). An explanation was not provided (5).

Table 2.432.1 Patch testing in groups of patients: Routine testing

Years and Country	Test conc. & vehicle	Number of patients tested	positive (%)	Selection of patients (S); Relevance (R); Comments (C)	Ref.
2000-2014 Denmark	20% pet.	4637	9 (0.2%)	R: 3 relevant from leave-on cosmetic products (n=2) and a topical steroid ointment (n=1); one patient past relevance	36
2008-2010 USA	20% pet.	591	23 (3.9%)	R: over half were relevant; C: 4/23 (17%) also reacted to sorbitan oleate; 50% reacted to *Myroxylon pereirae* and 46% to fragrance mix I, which both contain 5% sorbitan sesquioleate; significant association with reactions to lanolin alcohol and Amerchol® L 101	5
2006-2007 USA	20% pet.	112	12 (10.7%)	R: all 12 used products (topical corticosteroids, antifungals, non-specified products) containing sorbitol or sorbitan derivatives; C: surprisingly high frequency of sensitization; 5/13 patients (the 13th reacted to sorbitan oleate) had at least 5 positive reactions: risk of false-positives from excited skin syndrome; 8/13 (62%) co-reacted to fragrance mix 1 (which contains 5% sorbitan sesquioleate)	38
1998-2000 USA	20% pet.	610	(3.3%)	R: not stated	18
1998-1999 Belgium	20% pet.	819	24 (2.9%)	R: not specified, ascribed to topical medicaments and cosmetics (?)	4
1997-1999 Belgium	20% pet.	1441	75 (5.2%)	R: not stated	12
<1995 EECDRG	20% pet.	709	5 (0.7%)	R: not stated	41
1992-1994 USA	20% pet.	3469	(0.2%)	R: present relevance: 17%	17
1986-1987 Finland	20% pet.	1374	10 (0.7%)	R: three patients had widespread dermatitis from SSO in a moisturizing cream	1
1979-1983 Finland	20% pet.	3095	15 (0.5%)	R: not mentioned	1
1975 Finland	20% pet.	1206	6 (0.5%)	R: not specified, one patient reacted to SSO in 'various ointments'	24

EECDRG: European Environmental and Contact Dermatitis Research Group

Nevertheless, relatively high rates of sensitization of 3.3% and 5.2% were also found in other studies from the USA (18) and from Belgium (12), but the relevance of the observed positive patch test reactions was not mentioned. In studies that did address the relevance issue, relevance rates ranged from 17% to 100%, but the study with 100% relevance had certain weaknesses (38). Culprit products appear to be mostly topical pharmaceutical products and cosmetics (1,4,24,38).

Patch testing in groups of selected patients
Results of testing sorbitan sesquioleate in groups of *selected* patients (e.g., patients suspected of cosmetic allergy, patients reacting to the fragrance mix I, individuals with leg ulcers, patients tested with a cosmetic or ointment series) back to 1974 are shown in table 2.432.2. In 12 investigations, frequencies of sensitization have ranged from 0.4% to 5.2%, but in 7, the rates were below 1%. The highest frequency was seen in patients with a positive reaction to the fragrance mix I, which contains 5% sorbitan sesquioleate as emulsifier (6). Relevance was rarely mentioned and in the few studies that specified causative products they were topical medicaments (16,23).

Table 2.432.2 Patch testing in groups of patients: Selected patient groups

Years and Country	Test conc. & vehicle	Number of patients tested	positive (%)	Selection of patients (S); Relevance (R); Comments (C)	Ref.
1998-2013 IVDK	20% pet.	2952	154 (5.2%)	S: patients reacting to the fragrance mix I; causes positive patch test reactions to the FM I and individual components; R: in only a few patients reacting to SSO was clinical *fragrance* relevance documented, indicating that the reaction to the mix was caused by SSO allergy	6
1996-2013 Netherlands	20% pet.	339	9 (2.7%)	S: children aged 0-17 years; R: not stated	34
2011 China	20% pet.	201	1 (0.5%)	S: healthy student volunteers 19-30 years; R: not stated	31
2006-2011 IVDK	20% pet.	3211	(1.6%)	S: patients suspected of cosmetic intolerance and tested with an ointment base series; R: not stated	33
2004-2008 France	20% pet.	423	14 (4.0%)	S: patients with leg ulcers; R: not stated	20
2000-2007 USA	20% pet.	870	8 (0.9%)	S: patients tested with a supplemental cosmetic screening series; R: 75%; C: weak study: a. high rate of macular erythema and weak reactions; b. relevance figures included 'questionable' and 'past' relevance	3
2000-2002 Finland		4424	(0.6%)	S: patients tested with a cosmetic series; R: not stated	19
1995-1996 Finland		9332	(0.5%)	S: patients tested with a cosmetic series; R: not stated	19
1989-1993 UK		340	5 (1.5%)	S: patients with leg ulcers; R: 1 patient, who was allergic to a corticosteroid ointment containing SSO	16
1990-1991 IVDK	20% pet.	1872	7 (0.4%)	S: patients tested with an 'ointment series'; also 2.4% doubtful positive reactions; R: unknown, article not read	7
1986-1989 Italy	20% pet.	737	7 (0.9%)	S: patients with contact dermatitis apparently related to the use of topical preparations; R: 2 reactions were relevant and caused by topical medicaments	23
1972-1974 Finland	20% pet.	486	2 (0.4%)	S: not stated; R: not stated	25

IVDK: Information Network of Departments of Dermatology, Germany, Austria, Switzerland

Case reports and case series
In the period 1996-2013, in a tertiary referral center in Valencia, Spain, 5419 patients were patch tested. Of these, 628 individuals had allergic contact dermatitis to cosmetics. Sorbitan sesquioleate was the responsible allergen in one case (32). Sorbitan sesquioleate was responsible for 4 out of 959 cases of non-fragrance cosmetic allergy where the causal allergen was identified, Belgium, 2000-2010 (2). In a 4-month-period in 1996, 475 patients with contact allergy to 'cosmetic ingredients' were collected in 5 centers in Belgium, UK and Germany. There were 3 reactions to sorbitan sesquioleate; relevance was not mentioned (21).

Six children had recalcitrant dermatitis from sorbitan sesquioleate in cosmetic products such as diaper rash ointment, baby oil or skin cream; some had positive provocation tests with corticosteroid preparations containing either SSO or sorbitol (9). One patient had axillary dermatitis from sorbitan sesquioleate in a deodorant (5).

Contact allergy to sorbitan sesquioleate in non-cosmetic products
A female patient had allergic contact dermatitis from sorbitan sesquioleate in a corticosteroid ointment and liver oil ointment (8). Three patients were contact allergic to SSO in non-adhering wound dressings (11). One more patient had allergic contact dermatitis from dressings with sorbitan sesquioleate (14). In another study, an unknown number of patients (probably 1-3) were found to react to sorbitan sesquioleate in a wound dressing (22). Two patients (12) and another one (16) were allergic to sorbitan sesquioleate from its presence in a corticosteroid preparation (12). A

woman had allergic contact dermatitis from SSO present in a corticosteroid ointment used to treat stasis dermatitis (40).

Cross-reactions, pseudo-cross-reactions and co-reactions

Sorbitan oleate (5,14,16,38). Possibly to sorbitol, which may be present in SSO, but sorbitol was not patch tested (9). Pseudo-cross-reactivity to sorbitan sesquioleate containing test substances including fragrance-mix I (5,13,14,38) and *Myroxylon pereirae* (Balsam of Peru) (5). Significant co-reactivity with wool alcohols, from independent sensitization, not from cross-reactivity (5,16).

Presence in cosmetic products and chemical analyses

In July 2017, sorbitan sesquioleate was present in 293 of 69,548 cosmetic products of which the composition is known in EWG's Skin Deep Cosmetics Database, USA (http://www.ewg.org/skindeep/). In the USA, in April 2017, sorbitan sesquioleate was present in 534 of 56,714 cosmetic products of which the composition is known in FDA's Voluntary Cosmetic Registration Program (VCRP) (data obtained from FDA, May 2017). In the USA, in 2015-2016, 63 diaper wipes and 41 topical diaper preparations from a large retailer were screened for the presence of potential sensitizers. Sorbitan sesquioleate (and derivatives) was found in none of 63 disposable diaper wipes and in 6/41 (15%) topical diaper preparations (35). In 2009, in the USA, the ingredient lists of 1591 facial cosmetics from one company were screened for the presence of sorbitan sesquioleate. Sorbitan sesquioleate was present in 31% of 132 blushers and 38 bronzers, in 53% of 90 concealers, in 0% of 174 eyeliners, in 21% of 304 eyeshadows, in 34% of 457 foundations, in 21% of 140 loose and pressed powders, and in 26% of 256 mascaras (27).

In 2009, in the USA, the ingredient lists of 796 hair products from one company were screened for the presence of sorbitan sesquioleate. Sorbitan sesquioleate was present in 15% of 279 shampoos, in 29% of 231 conditioners, and in 22% of 286 styling products (28). In 2009, in the USA, the ingredient lists of 730 lip cosmetics and dental care products from one company were screened for the presence of sorbitan sesquioleate. Sorbitan sesquioleate was present in 32% of 31 lip liners, in 7% of 429 lipsticks, in 4% of 92 lip moisturizers, in 61% of 153 toothpastes, and in 36% of 25 mouth washes (29). In 2009, in the USA, the ingredient lists of 657 miscellaneous cosmetics from one company were screened for the presence of sorbitan sesquioleate (derivatives). These were present in 3% of 195 antiperspirants/deodorants, in 5% of 41 powders, in 36% of 167 shaving products, in 18% of 201 sunblocks, and in 75% of 53 wipes (30). Sorbitan sesquioleate was present in 47 out of 166 (28%) corticosteroid preparations collected in 2007, USA (26).

OTHER SIDE EFFECTS

Immediate-type reactions

A woman had contact urticaria and wheezing from sorbitan sesquioleate in a corticosteroid preparation (15,43).

OTHER INFORMATION

Dubious positive (?+) patch test reactions to sorbitan sesquioleate may represent (real) contact allergic reactions, as shown by a positive repeated open application test (ROAT) with the patch test material (37).

LITERATURE

1   Hannuksela M. Skin contact allergy to emulsifiers. Int J Cosmet Sci 1988;10:9-14
2   Travassos AR, Claes L, Boey L, Drieghe J, Goossens A. Non-fragrance allergens in specific cosmetic products. Contact Dermatitis 2011;65:276-285
3   Wetter DA, Yiannias JA, Prakash AV, Davis MD, Farmer SA, el-Azhary RA, et al. Results of patch testing to personal care product allergens in a standard series and a supplemental cosmetic series: an analysis of 945 patients from the Mayo Clinic Contact Dermatitis Group, 2000-2007. J Am Acad Dermatol 2010;63:789-798
4   Kohl L, Blondeel A, Song M. Allergic contact dermatitis from cosmetics: retrospective analysis of 819 patch-tested patients. Dermatology 2002;204:334-337
5   Cressey BD, Kumar N, Scheinman PL. Contact allergy to sorbitans: A follow-up study. Dermatitis 2012;23:158-161
6   Geier J, Schnuch A, Lessmann H, Uter W. Reactivity to sorbitan sesquioleate affects reactivity to fragrance mix I. Contact Dermatitis 2015;73:296-304
7   Schnuch A, Arnold R, Bahmer F, et al. Epikutantestung mit der Salbengrundlagenreihe – Ergebnisse des 'Informationsverbundes Dermatologischer Kliniken' (IVDK). Derm Beruf Umwelt 1993;41:176-183
8   Hald M, Menné T, Johansen JD, Zachariae C. Allergic contact dermatitis caused by sorbitan sesquioleate imitating severe glove dermatitis in a patient with filaggrin mutation. Contact Dermatitis 2013;69:313-315
9   Castanedo-Tardan MP, Jacob SE. Allergic contact dermatitis to sorbitan sesquioleate in children. Contact Dermatitis 2008;58:171-172

10 Lanigan RS, Torill A, Yamarik TA. Final report on the safety assessment of sorbitan caprylate, sorbitan cocoate, sorbitan diisostearate, sorbitan dioleate, sorbitan distearate, sorbitan isostearate, sorbitan olivate, sorbitan sesquiisostearate, sorbitan sesquistearate, and sorbitan triisostearate. Int J Toxicol 2002;21 (Suppl. 1):93-112

11 De Waard-van der Spek FB, Devillers ACA, Oranje AP. Allergic contact dermatitis to sorbitan sesquioleate in Adaptic® wound dressing. Contact Dermatitis 2007;57:54-56

12 Goossens A, Huygens S, Matura M, Degreef H. Fluticasone propionate: a rare contact sensitizer. Eur J Dermatol 2001;11:29-34

13 Orton DI, Shaw S, Sorbitan sesquioleate as an allergen. Contact Dermatitis 2001;44:190-191

14 Pereira F, Cunha H, Dias M. Contact dermatitis due to emulsifiers. Contact Dermatitis 1997;36:114

15 Hardy M, Maribach HI. Contact urticaria syndrome from sorbitan sesquioleate in a corticosteroid ointment. Contact Dermatitis, 1995;32:360-361

16 Mallon E, Powell SM. Sorbitan sesquioleate – a potential allergen in leg ulcer patients. Contact Dermatitis1994;30:180

17 Marks JG, Belsito DV, DeLeo VA, Fowler JF, Fransway AF, Maibach HI,et al. North American Contact Dermatitis Group standard tray patch test results 1992 through 1994. Am J Contact Dermatitis 1995;6:160-165

18 Wetter DA, Davis MDP, Yiannias JA, Cheng JF, Connolly SM, el-Azhary RA, et al. Patch test results from the Mayo Contact Dermatitis Group, 1998–2000. J Am Acad Dermatol 2005;53:416-421

19 Hasan T, Rantanen T, Alanko K, Harvima RJ, Jolanki R, Kalimo K, et al. Patch test reactions to cosmetic allergens in 1995–1997 and 2000–2002 in Finland –a multicentre study. Contact Dermatitis 2005;53:40-45

20 Barbaud A, Collet E, Le Coz CJ, Meaume S, Gillois P. Contact allergy in chronic leg ulcers: results of a multicentre study carried out in 423 patients and proposal for an updated series of patch tests. Contact Dermatitis 2009;60:279-287

21 Goossens A, Beck MH, Haneke E, McFadden JP, Nolting S, Durupt G, Ries G. Adverse cutaneous reactions to cosmetic allergens. Contact Dermatitis 1999;40:112-113

22 Pasche-Koo F, Piletta P-A, Hunziker N, Hauser C. High sensitization rate to emulsifiers in patients with chronic leg ulcers. Contact Dermatitis 1994;31:226-228

23 Tosti A, Guerra L, Morelli R, Bardazzi F. Prevalence and sources of sensitization to emulsifiers: a clinical study. Contact Dermatitis 1990;23:68-72

24 Hannuksela M, Kousa M, Pirilä V. Contact sensitivity to emulsifiers. Contact Dermatitis 1976;2:201-204

25 Hannuksela M, Kousa M, Pirilä V. Allergy to ingredients of vehicles. Contact Dermatitis 1976;2:105-110

26 Coloe J, Zirwas MJ. Allergens in corticosteroid vehicles. Dermatitis 2008;19:38-42

27 Scheman A, Jacob S, Katta R, Nedorost S, Warshaw E, Zirwas M, et al. Part 1 of a 4 part series. Facial cosmetics: trends and alternatives. Data from the American Contact Alternative Group. J Clin Aesthet Dermatol 2011;4:25-30

28 Scheman A, Jacob S, Katta R, Nedorost S, Warshaw E, Zirwas M, et al. Part 2 of a 4 part series. Hair cosmetics: trends and alternatives. Data from the American Contact Alternative Group. J Clin Aesthet Dermatol 2011;4:42-46

29 Scheman A, Jacob S, Katta R, Nedorost S, Warshaw E, Zirwas M, et al. Part 3 of a 4 part series. Lips and common Dental Care products: trends and alternatives. Data from the American Contact Alternative Group. J Clin Aesthet Dermatol 2011;4:50-53

30 Scheman A, Jacob S, Katta R, Nedorost S, Warshaw E, Zirwas M, et al. Part 4 of a 4 part series. Miscellaneous products: trends and alternatives in deodorants, antiperspirants, sunblocks, shaving products, powder, and wipes. Data from the American Contact Alternative Group. J Clin Aesthet Dermatol 2011;4:35-39

31 Zhao J, Li LF. Contact sensitization to cosmetic series of allergens in a general population in Beijing. J Cosmet Dermatol 2014;13:68-71

32 Zaragoza-Ninet V, Blasco Encinas R, Vilata-Corell JJ, Pérez-Ferriols A, Sierra-Talamantes C, Esteve-Martínez A, de la Cuadra-Oyanguren J. Allergic contact dermatitis due to cosmetics: A clinical and epidemiological study in a tertiary hospital. Actas Dermosifiliogr 2016;107:329-336

33 Dinkloh A, Worm M, Geier J, Schnuch A, Wollenberg A. Contact sensitization in patients with suspected cosmetic intolerance: results of the IVDK 2006-2011. J Eur Acad Dermatol Venereol 2015;29:1071-1081

34 Lubbes S, Rustemeyer T, Sillevis Smitt JH, Schuttelaar ML, Middelkamp-Hup MA. Contact sensitization in Dutch children and adolescents with and without atopic dermatitis - a retrospective analysis. Contact Dermatitis 2017;76:151-159

35 Yu J, Treat J, Chaney K, Brod B. Potential allergens in disposable diaper wipes, topical diaper preparations, and disposable diapers: under-recognized etiology of pediatric perineal dermatitis. Dermatitis 2016;27:110-118

36 Bennike NH, Johansen JD. Sorbitan sesquioleate; a rare cause of contact allergy in consecutively patch tested dermatitis patients. Contact Dermatitis 2016;74:242-245

37 Hannuksela M, Salo H. The repeated open application test (ROAT). Contact Dermatitis 1986;14:221-227

38 Asarch A, Scheinman PL. Sorbitan sesquioleate, a common emulsifier in topical corticosteroids, is an important contact allergen. Dermatitis 2008;19:323-327

39 Asarch A, Scheinman PL. Sorbitan sesquioleate: An emerging contact allergen. Dermatitis 2008;19:339-341

40 Green C, Kenicer KJ. A case of 'contact allergy to corticosteroid'. Contact Dermatitis 1993;28:39-40

41 Frosch PJ, Pilz B, Burrows D, Camarasa J G, Lachapelle J M, Lahti A, Menne T, Wilkinson J D. Testing with fragrance mix. Is the addition of sorbitan sesquioleate to the constituents useful? Results of a multicentre trial of the European Environmental and Contact Dermatitis Research Group (EECDRG). Contact Dermatitis 1995;32:266-272

42 Castanedo-Tardan MP, Jacob SE. Sorbitan sesquioleate. Dermatitis 2008;19(4):E22-23

43 Hardy MP, Maibach HI. Contact urticaria syndrome from sorbitan sesquioleate in a corticosteroid ointment. Contact Dermatitis 1995;32:114

2.433 SORBITAN TRISTEARATE

IDENTIFICATION

Description/definition	: Sorbitan tristearate is the triester of stearic acid and hexitol anhydrides derived from sorbitol
Chemical class(es)	: Sorbitan derivatives
Chemical/IUPAC name	: [2-[(2R,3S,4R)-4-Hydroxy-3-octadecanoyloxyoxolan-2-yl]-2-octadecanoyloxyethyl] octadecanoate
Other names	: Anhydrosorbitol tristearate; sorbitan, trioctadecanoate; Span® 65
CAS registry number (s)	: 26658-19-5
EC number(s)	: 247-891-4
CIR review(s)	: J Am Coll Toxicol 1985;4:65-121; Final report, December 2014 (access: www.cir-safety.org/ingredients)
Function(s) in cosmetics	: EU: emulsifying. USA: surfactants - emulsifying agents
Patch testing	: 5% pet. (1).
Molecular formula	: $C_{60}H_{114}O_8$

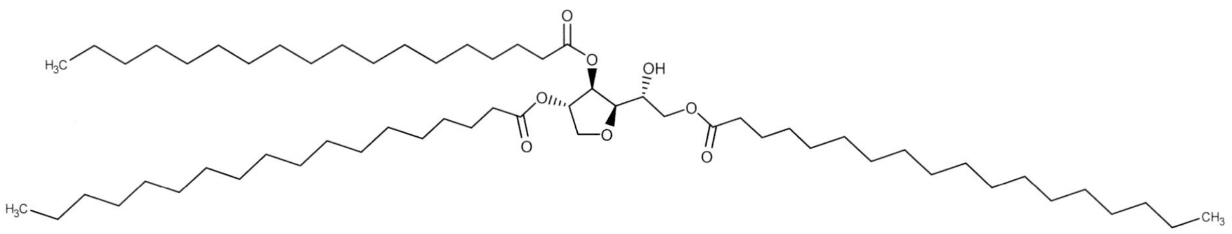

CONTACT ALLERGY

Case reports and case series

A woman presented with dermatitis of the face that had started 6 months earlier. Previously, the patient had experienced a facial eruption several times. Patch tests with the European baseline series, a cosmetic series, and her personal cosmetic products gave various positive reactions including to fragrances and a night cream. Later, the patient was again patch tested with this cosmetic product and with its ingredients. The night cream again gave positive reactions, as did 4 ingredients including sorbitan stearate 5% in mineral oil, but the patient did not react to the fragrance of this product. She has remained free of dermatitis after stopping the use of the night cream and avoiding other products containing the allergens to which she reacted. Due to lack of cooperation of the manufacturer, control testing or repeat testing could not be performed (1).

Presence in cosmetic products and chemical analyses

In the USA, in April 2017, sorbitan tristearate was present in 135 of 56,714 cosmetic products of which the composition is known in FDA's Voluntary Cosmetic Registration Program (VCRP) (data obtained from FDA, May 2017). In April 2017, sorbitan tristearate was present in 41 of 65,434 cosmetic products of which the composition is known in EWG's Skin Deep Cosmetics Database, USA (http://www.ewg.org/skindeep/).

LITERATURE

1   De Groot AC, Rustemeyer T, Hissink D, Bakker M. Contact allergy to capryloyl salicylic acid. Contact Dermatitis 2014;71:185-187

2.434 SORBITOL

IDENTIFICATION

Description/definition   : Sorbitol is the hexahydric alcohol that conforms to the formula shown below
Chemical class(es)   : Polyols
Chemical/IUPAC name   : (2R,3R,4R,5S)-Hexane-1,2,3,4,5,6-hexol
Other names   : Sorbitolum; D-glucitol
CAS registry number (s)   : 50-70-4
EC number(s)   : 200-061-5
Merck Index monograph   : 10121
Function(s) in cosmetics   : EU: humectant; plasticiser; skin conditioning. USA: flavoring agents; fragrance ingredients; humectants; skin-conditioning agents - humectant
Patch testing   : 10% water (1)
Molecular formula   : $C_6H_{14}O_6$

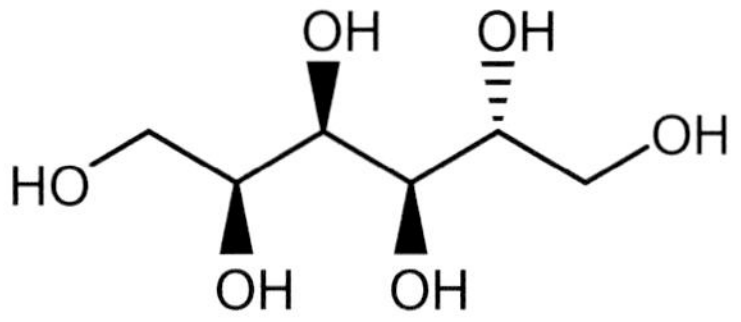

CONTACT ALLERGY

Case reports and case series
A man had suffered from intense outbreaks of seborrheic dermatitis, which improved with topical corticosteroids and ketoconazole but recurred on ceasing medication. For the past 3 months, papular, erythematous, intensely pruriginous lesions had been appearing on sun-exposed areas of the face, neck and hands. Patch tests and photopatch tests with the standard series were negative at 2 and 4 days, as were his cosmetics and toiletries with the single exception of a shaving foam, as is, which gave a strongly positive patch test reaction at both readings. Patch and photopatch tests were then carried out with the ingredients of this product supplied by the manufacturer and he had positive patch test reactions to 6 ingredients including sorbitol 10% in water. There were no positive reactions in 25 controls. The patient was retested 7 months later to all 6 allergens previously positive and reacted again at 2 and 4 days to sorbitol (1).

Presence in cosmetic products and chemical analyses
In the USA, in April 2017, sorbitol was present in 1957 of 56,714 cosmetic products of which the composition is known in FDA's Voluntary Cosmetic Registration Program (VCRP) (data obtained from FDA, May 2017). In April 2017, sorbitol was present in 1030 of 65,434 cosmetic products of which the composition is known in EWG's Skin Deep Cosmetics Database, USA (http://www.ewg.org/skindeep/).

LITERATURE
1   Vilaplana J, Lecha M, Romaguera C, Alsina A, Mascaro JM, Castel, T. A polysensitized HIV-positive patient. Contact Dermatitis 1993;29:101-102

2.435   STANNOUS FLUORIDE

IDENTIFICATION

Description/definition   : Stannous fluoride is the inorganic salt that conforms to the formula shown below
Chemical class(es)   : Inorganic salts
Chemical/IUPAC name   : Difluorotin
Other names   : Tin difluoride
CAS registry number (s)   : 7783-47-3
EC number(s)   : 231-999-3
Merck Index monograph   : 10181
Function(s) in cosmetics : EU: antiplaque; oral care. USA: anticaries agents; oral care agents; oral health care
                            drugs
EU cosmetic restrictions : Regulated in Annex III/35 of the Regulation (EC) No. 1223/2009
Patch testing   : Tin 50% pet. (Chemotechnique)
Molecular formula   : SnF_2; F_2Sn

CONTACT ALLERGY

Case reports and case series

A female patient presented with recurrent idiopathic urticaria and cheilitis. Her symptoms had started following dental work, with recurrent lip swelling and daily hives occurring over 10 months. She received oral prednisone courses on eight occasions during this time, and her symptoms ultimately disappeared. One month before presentation, the patient again had dental work done. Local anesthesia with lidocaine was well tolerated. Six hours later, the patient had developed lip and oral swelling. In the weeks thereafter, she continued to experience intermittent lip swelling, facial dermatitis, and urticaria. Skin prick testing and intradermal testing with lidocaine, mepivacaine, and proparacaine yielded negative results. Patch tests showed positive reactions to methyldibromo-glutaronitrile, lidocaine, dodecyl gallate, and to tin. Lidocaine was relevant to her episode of oral swelling occurring hours after her dental procedure. It was considered possible that the reaction to tin was relevant to the patient's symptoms.

Her exposures included prior amalgam dental fillings (which typically contain mercury, silver, copper, and tin) and a toothpaste with the active ingredient stannous fluoride (tin (II) fluoride). Upon discontinuation of this toothpaste, the patient's recurrent lip edema and hives resolved. She was symptom-free for 8 weeks, when an inadvertent re-exposure to the same toothpaste was associated with recurrence of urticaria and lip swelling within a few hours. After subsequent avoidance of the toothpaste, she again became and remained symptom-free. It was postulated by the authors that the stannous fluoride in the toothpaste may be the cause of the urticaria of this patient (1). The toothpaste itself, however, was not tested. In addition, the picture of the 'positive' patch test reaction to tin only showed isolated papules, which can, as an isolated and one-time observation, hardly be considered to be adequate proof of contact allergy.

Presence in cosmetic products and chemical analyses

In the USA, in April 2017, stannous fluoride was present in zero of 56,714 cosmetic products of which the composition is known in FDA's Voluntary Cosmetic Registration Program (VCRP) (data obtained from FDA, May 2017). In April 2017, stannous fluoride was present in 7 of 65,434 cosmetic products of which the composition is known in EWG's Skin Deep Cosmetics Database, USA (http://www.ewg.org/skindeep/).

LITERATURE

1   Enamandram M, Das S, Chaney KS. Cheilitis and urticaria associated with stannous fluoride in toothpaste. J Am Acad Dermatol 2014;71:e75-76

2.436 STEARAMIDOETHYL DIETHYLAMINE PHOSPHATE

IDENTIFICATION

Description/definition   : Stearamidoethyl diethylamine phosphate is a complex mixture of phosphoric acid and stearamidoethyl diethylamine

Chemical class(es)   : Amines; phosphorus compounds

Chemical/IUPAC name : N-[2-(Diethylamino)ethyl]octadecanamide; phosphoric acid

Other names   : Diethylaminoethyl stearamide phosphate; octadecanamide, N-[2-(diethylamino)ethyl]-, phosphate; N-[2-(Diethylamino)ethyl]stearamide phosphate

CAS registry number (s) : 68133-34-6

EC number(s)   : 268-677-7

Function(s) in cosmetics : EU: antistatic; hair conditioning. USA: antistatic agents; hair conditioning agents

Patch testing   : 0.4% water (1)

Molecular formula   : $C_{24}H_{53}N_2O_5P$

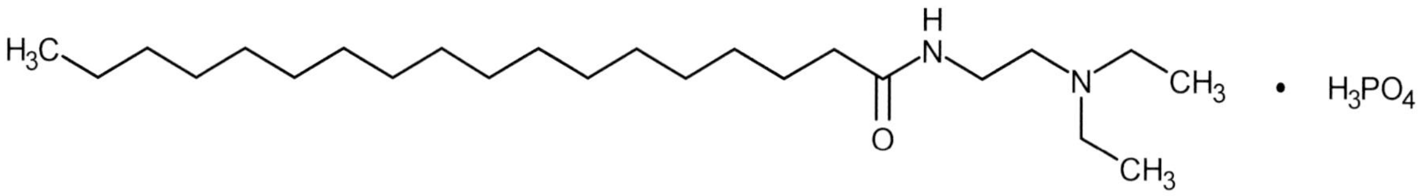

CONTACT ALLERGY

Case reports and case series

An atopic woman was seen with an acute eczematous dermatitis on her left leg which had developed following the application of a dry skin lotion. She also had chronic eczema on the hands. Another female patient with a 6-year history of recurrent dermatitis on the arms and legs, and currently using the same dry skin lotion, was referred for patch testing. A third patient had applied the lotion to her chest, shoulder, and neck area to prevent dryness of the skin. After approximately one month's use of this product, a dermatitis developed; a diffuse, macular, papular eruption predominately over the neck and anterior chest. She sought medical attention within 3 days of the eruption because of the pruritus. All three patients were tested with the NACDG screening series and their personal products and all reacted to the dry skin lotion. When tested with its ingredients, a positive reaction to stearamidoethyl diethylamine phosphate 0.4% water was observed (1). After these findings, the manufacturer of the dry skin lotion decided to change the composition of the cosmetic product by replacing stearamidoethyl diethylamine phosphate with quaternium-7.

A fourth female individual developed an acute vesicular dermatitis in the periaxillary area after she had used a deodorant for at least one moth. The allergenic culprit was stearamidoethyl diethylamine phosphate. One of the authors tested the material in the routine series for one year, but saw no positive reactions, excluding irritancy (1).

Presence in cosmetic products and chemical analyses

In the USA, in April 2017, stearamidoethyl diethylamine phosphate was present in zero of 56,714 cosmetic products of which the composition is known in FDA's Voluntary Cosmetic Registration Program (VCRP) (data obtained from FDA, May 2017). In April 2017, stearamidoethyl diethylamine phosphate was present in zero of 65,434 cosmetic products of which the composition is known in EWG's Skin Deep Cosmetics Database, USA (http://www.ewg.org/skindeep/).

LITERATURE

1   Taylor JS, Jordan WP, Maibach HI. Allergic contact dermatitis from stearamidoethyl diethylamine phosphate: a cosmetic emulsifier. Contact Dermatitis 1984;10:74-76

2.437   STEARETH-10

IDENTIFICATION

Description/definition	: Steareth-10 is the polyethylene glycol ether of stearyl alcohol that conforms to the formula shown below, where n has an average value of 10
Chemical class(es)	: Alkoxylated alcohols
Chemical/IUPAC name	: Poly(oxy-1,2-ethanediyl),α-octadecyl-ω-hydroxy
Other names	: 3,6,9,12,15,18,21,24,27,30-Decaoxaoctatetracontan-1-ol; PEG-10 stearyl ether; polyethylene glycol 500 stearyl ether; polyoxyethylene (10) stearyl ether
CAS registry number (s)	: 9005-00-9 (generic); 13149-86-5
CIR review(s)	: J Am Coll Toxicol 1988;7:881-910; Int J Toxicol 2012;31(Suppl.2):169-244 (access: www.cir-safety.org/ingredients)
Merck Index monograph	: 8967 (Polyoxyethylene alcohols)
Function(s) in cosmetics	: EU: emulsifying; refatting; surfactant. USA: surfactants - emulsifying agents
Patch testing	: 5% water (2,3)
Molecular formula	: $C_{38}H_{78}O_{11}$
Structural formula (linear): $CH_3(CH_2)_{17}(OCH_2CH_2)_nOH$	

CONTACT ALLERGY

Case reports and case series
A woman had allergic contact dermatitis of the face from cetearyl alcohol in multiple cosmetics she used. She had a positive ROAT and a positive use test to a makeup remover wet wipe. Patch tests with the ingredients revealed a positive reaction to steareth-10 5% water; the patient also reacted weakly to stearyl alcohol 10% pet. The presence of stearyl alcohol, which is used in the manufacture of steareth-10, was shown by chemical analyses, including gas chromatography–mass spectrometry both in the wet wipe and in the steareth-10 solution. The authors concluded that, apart from steareth-10 as the actual culprit allergen, hidden, low amounts of stearyl alcohol (or impurities originating from this allergen), used as a primary chemical to produce steareth-10, may also have contributed to the patient's dermatitis; furthermore, that a byproduct of the production of steareth-10 other than stearyl alcohol might have been responsible (1,3).

Cross-reactions, pseudo-cross-reactions and co-reactions
Pseudo-cross-reaction to stearyl alcohol (1).

Presence in cosmetic products and chemical analyses
In the USA, in April 2017, steareth-10 was present in 48 of 56,714 cosmetic products of which the composition is known in FDA's Voluntary Cosmetic Registration Program (VCRP) (data obtained from FDA, May 2017). In April 2017, steareth-10 was present in 13 of 65,434 cosmetic products of which the composition is known in EWG's Skin Deep Cosmetics Database, USA (http://www.ewg.org/skindeep/).

LITERATURE

1   Aerts O, Leysen J, Naessens T, Dandelooy J, Apers S, Lambert J. Steareths may sometimes prove problematic in patients contact allergic to cetostearyl alcohol: an example. Contact Dermatitis 2016;75(Suppl.1):54-55
2   De Groot AC. Patch Testing, 3rd Edition. Wapserveen, The Netherlands: acdegroot publishing, 2008 (ISBN 978-90-813233-1-4)
3   Aerts O, Naessens T, Dandelooy J, Leysen J, Lambert J, Apers S. Allergic contact dermatitis caused by wet wipes containing steareth-10: Is stearyl alcohol to blame? Contact Dermatitis 2017;77:117-119

2.438   STEARIC ACID

IDENTIFICATION

Description/definition   : Stearic acid is the fatty acid that conforms generally to the formula shown below
Chemical class(es)   : Fatty acids
Chemical/IUPAC name   : Octadecanoic acid
CAS registry number (s)   : 57-11-4
EC number(s)   : 200-313-4
CIR review(s)   : J Am Coll Toxicol 1987;6:321-401 (access: www.cir-safety.org/ingredients)
Merck Index monograph : 10200
Function(s) in cosmetics : EU: cleansing; emulsifying; emulsion stabilising; masking; refatting; surfactant. USA:
                            fragrance ingredients; surfactants - cleansing agents; surfactants – emulsifying agents
Patch testing   : 3.4% and 5% pet. (2); 5% pet. (3)
Molecular formula   : $C_{18}H_{36}O_2$

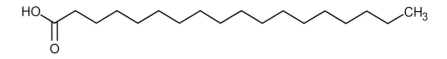

CONTACT ALLERGY

Case reports and case series
Stearic acid was responsible for 1 out of 399 cases of cosmetic allergy where the causal allergen was identified in a study of the NACDG, USA, 1977-1983 (1). Two patients (2) and one individual (3) had contact allergy to stearic acid present in a moisturizing cream. In a group of 119 patients with allergic contact dermatitis from cosmetics, investigated in The Netherlands in 1986-1987, one case was caused by stearic acid in a skin care product and in soap (4,5, same patient as in ref. 3).

Cross-reactions, pseudo-cross-reactions and co-reactions
Sodium stearate (3).

Presence in cosmetic products and chemical analyses
In the USA, in April 2017, stearic acid was present in 6097 of 56,714 cosmetic products of which the composition is known in FDA's Voluntary Cosmetic Registration Program (VCRP) (data obtained from FDA, May 2017). In April 2017, stearic acid was present in 2650 of 65,434 cosmetic products of which the composition is known in EWG's Skin Deep Cosmetics Database, USA (http://www.ewg.org/skindeep/). In 1984, stearic acid was present in 2336 of approximately 19,000 cosmetic formulas on file with the FDA (3).

OTHER SIDE EFFECTS

Other non-eczematous contact reactions
In older literature, stearic acid has been suspected of being comedogenic, based on rabbit ear assays (6).

LITERATURE
1   Adams RM, Maibach HI, Clendenning WE, Fisher AA, Jordan WJ, Kanof N, et al. A five-year study of cosmetic reactions. J Am Acad Dermatol 1985;13:1062-1069
2   Batten, TL, Wakeel RA, Douglas WS, Evans C, White MI, Moody R, Ormerod AD. Contact dermatitis from the old formula E45 cream. Contact Dermatitis 1994;30:159-161
3   De Groot AC, van der Meeren HLM, Weyland JW. Cosmetic allergy from stearic acid and glyceryl stearate. Contact Dermatitis 1988;19:77-78
4   De Groot AC, Bruynzeel DP, Bos JD, van der Meeren HL, van Joost T, Jagtman BA, Weyland JW. The allergens in cosmetics. Arch Dermatol 1988;124:1525-1529
5   De Groot AC. Adverse reactions to cosmetics. PhD Thesis, University of Groningen, The Netherlands: 1988, chapter 3.4, pp.105-113
6   Kligman AM, Mills OH. Acne cosmetica. Arch Dermatol 1972;106:843-850

2.439 STEARYL ALCOHOL

IDENTIFICATION

Description/definition	: Stearyl alcohol is the fatty alcohol that conforms generally to the formula shown below
Chemical class(es)	: Fatty alcohols
Chemical/IUPAC name	: Octadecan 1 ol
Other names	: Octadecyl alcohol
CAS registry number (s)	: 112-92-5
EC number(s)	: 204-017-6
CIR review(s)	: J Am Coll Toxicol 1985;4:1-29 (access: www.cir-safety.org/ingredients)
Merck Index monograph	: 10202
Function(s) in cosmetics	: EU: emollient; emulsifying; emulsion stabilizing; foam boosting; masking; opacifying; refatting; surfactant; viscosity controlling. USA: emulsion stabilizers; fragrance ingredients; surfactants – emulsifying agents; surfactants – foam boosters; viscosity increasing agents – aqueous / nonaqueous
Patch testing	: 30% pet. (Chemotechnique, SmartPracticeCanada)
Molecular formula	: $C_{18}H_{38}O$

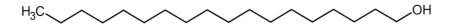

GENERAL

Stearyl alcohol is a rare allergen in cosmetic products. Most cases of sensitization have been caused by its presence in topical pharmaceutical products. See also Chapter 2.83 Cetearyl alcohol (cetearyl alcohol is as mixture of cetyl alcohol and stearyl alcohol).

CONTACT ALLERGY

Patch testing in groups of patients

Results of patch testing in consecutive patients suspected of contact dermatitis (routine testing) and of testing groups of selected patients are shown in table 2.439.1. In 3 studies from the USA, frequencies of sensitization were all 0.3% (2,16,18). Relevance was given as 22% to 44%; causative products were not mentioned.

In groups of *selected* patients (e.g., patients suspected of cosmetic dermatitis, patients suspected to react to topical preparations), frequencies of sensitization ranged from 0.8% to 5%. The highest percentages (4% [20] and 5% [25]) were found in small studies of 50 and 69 patients suspected to suffer from allergic contact dermatitis to cosmetics or topical preparations. Relevance of the positive patch test reactions and culprit products were not mentioned (20,25). In a study from the USA, all 6 positive patch test reactions were scored as relevant, but this included 'questionable' and 'past' relevance (1).

Table 2.439.1 Patch testing in groups of patients

Years and Country	Test conc. & vehicle	Number of patients tested | positive (%)		Selection of patients (S); Relevance (R); Comments (C)	Ref.
Routine testing					
2006-2010 USA	30% pet.	3087	(0.3%)	R: 22%	18
2000-2005 USA	30% pet.	3844	(0.3%)	R: 42%	2
1998-2000 USA	30% pet.	711	(0.3%)	R: not stated	16
Testing in groups of selected patients					
2000-2007 USA	30% pet.	944	6 (0.6%)	S: patients tested with a supplemental cosmetic screening series; R: 100%; C: weak study: a. high rate of macular erythema and weak reactions; b. relevance figures included 'questionable' and 'past' relevance	1
<2005 India	30% pet.	50	2 (4%)	S: patients suspected of cosmetic dermatitis; R: not stated	20
1997-2000 Israel		244	2 (0.8%)	S: patients suspected of cosmetic dermatitis; R: 64% of all patch test reactions in the cosmetic series were relevant	21
1992-1995 Italy	30% pet.	146	2 (1.4%)	S: patients suspected of contact allergy to cosmetics or topical pharmaceutical products; R: not specified; C: the purity of stearyl alcohol was >99%	12

Table 2.439.1 Patch testing in groups of patients (*continued*)

Years and Country	Test conc. & vehicle	Number of patients tested | positive (%)			Selection of patients (S); Relevance (R); Comments (C)	Ref.
<1990 India	30% pet.	69	3	(5%)	S: patients, with features suggestive of allergic contact dermatitis and histories of prolonged use of numerous topical preparations, or of exacerbation or spread of derma- titis following the use of such preparations; R: not stated	25
1975-6 USA, Canada	30% pet.	172		(1.2%)	S: not stated; R: not stated	17

Case reports and case series

In the period 1996-2013, in a tertiary referral center in Valencia, Spain, 5419 patients were patch tested. Of these, 628 individuals had allergic contact dermatitis to cosmetics. Stearyl alcohol was the responsible allergen in one case (23).

One patient had ACD from stearyl alcohol in a moisturizing cream (5). A woman had facial dermatitis from contact allergy to makeup remover wet wipes. She had a positive ROAT to the wipes, a positive reaction to its ingredient steareth-10 and a dubious positive reaction to stearyl alcohol. The presence of stearyl alcohol, which is used in the manufacture of steareth-10, was shown by chemical analyses, including gas chromatography–mass spectrometry. It was concluded that stearyl alcohol was the actual allergenic culprit in steareth-10 in this case (22).

Contact allergy to stearyl alcohol in non-cosmetic products

A man, suffering from psoriasis, developed ACD to stearyl alcohol present in hydrocortisone cream (5). A young woman developed ACD superimposed on psoriasis from stearyl alcohol in a corticosteroid preparation that she applied under plastic occlusion (15). Another female individual reacted to stearyl alcohol in fluocinonide cream applied under occlusion for linear scleroderma. The patch test to commercial stearyl alcohol was positive, but she did not react to pure stearyl alcohol. It was concluded that the allergens must have been an impurity (8,27). A female individual had ACD from stearyl alcohol in aqueous cream, evening primrose oil cream and a corticosteroid cream (10).

Three patients had allergic contact dermatitis from stearyl alcohol in a cream containing 5-fluorouracil used to treat actinic keratoses (6). Three more patients became sensitized to stearyl alcohol in the same product, used in two cases for the treatment of Bowen's disease and in the third for actinic keratoses (9). A woman also reacted to stearyl alcohol in this cream (10). In all patients, the inflammatory reaction, that is normally seen with 5-fluorouracil cream treatment, was far worse than expected. It is suggested that the normal inflammatory response promotes penetration of potential allergens and subsequent sensitization (6,9,10).

One patient reacted to stearyl alcohol (and alcohol, and cetyl alcohol) present in a topical antimycotic lotion; she did not react to pure cetyl alcohol and stearyl alcohol, but had positive patch test reactions to oleyl alcohol and *n*-decyl alcohol, which are known impurities in stearyl and cetyl alcohol (13). A woman had urticarial-like allergic contact dermatitis from a topical pharmaceutical preparation (probably a corticosteroid) used to treat dermatitis from a green tent canvas (7). Six leg ulcer patients had contact allergy to a pharmaceutical cream containing cetearyl alcohol; (at least) 2 reacted to stearyl alcohol 30% pet., (at least) 2 reacted to cetearyl alcohol 20% pet., and (at least) one to cetyl alcohol 5% pet. (14). A woman had allergic contact dermatitis of the left upper eyelid from stearyl alcohol and cetyl alcohol in an antifungal preparation used to treat seborrheic dermatitis (29). A man had allergic contact dermatitis from stearyl alcohol in a moisturizing coating on the inside of a rubber glove (3).

Cross-reactions, pseudo-cross-reactions and co-reactions

Possibly from or to ceteareth-2 and/or ceteareth-3, which are cetearyl alcohols with a variable number of ethoxylene molecules (4); cetearyl alcohol (4); lanolin; Emulgator E2155 ® (stearyl alcohol, steareth-7, steareth-10) (5). Catyl alcohol (28). Cetyl alcohol used in cosmetics often contains 30-35% stearyl alcohol (C18) (11). Oleyl alcohol (19); panthenol (cited in ref. 19).

Presence in cosmetic products and chemical analyses

In May 2017, stearyl alcohol was present in 1533 of 68,675 cosmetic products of which the composition is known in EWG's Skin Deep Cosmetics Database, USA (http://www.ewg.org/skindeep/). In the USA, in April 2017, stearyl alcohol was present in 2416 of 56,714 cosmetic products of which the composition is known in FDA's Voluntary Cosmetic Registration Program (VCRP) (data obtained from FDA, May 2017).

Other information
Oleyl alcohol and *n*-decyl alcohol, present in cosmetic grade stearyl alcohol, may be the true sensitizers in some cases of stearyl alcohol sensitization (13).

OTHER SIDE EFFECTS

Other non-eczematous contact reactions
In (somewhat) older literature (24), stearyl alcohol has been suspected of being comedogenic in 'people with more sensitive complexions or acne-prone problems', based on rabbit ear assays. More recent research, also with rabbit ear assays, could not reproduce these findings (26).

LITERATURE

1   Wetter DA, Yiannias JA, Prakash AV, Davis MD, Farmer SA, el-Azhary RA, et al. Results of patch testing to personal care product allergens in a standard series and a supplemental cosmetic series: an analysis of 945 patients from the Mayo Clinic Contact Dermatitis Group, 2000-2007. J Am Acad Dermatol 2010;63:789-798

2   Davis MD, Scalf LA, Yiannias JA, Cheng JF, El-Azhary RA, Rohlinger AL, et al. Changing trends and allergens in the patch test standard series. Arch Dermatol 2008;144:67-72

3   Vanden Broecke K, Zimerson E, Bruze M, Goossens A. Severe allergic contact dermatitis caused by a rubber glove coated with a moisturizer. Contact Dermatitis 2014;71:117-119

4   Corazza M, Zauli S, Bianchi A, Benetti S, Borghi A, Virgili A. Contact dermatitis caused by fatty alcohols: may polyethoxylation of the fatty alcohols influence their sensitizing potential?. Contact Dermatitis 2013;68:189-190

5   Thormann H, Kollander M, Andersen KE. Allergic contact dermatitis from dichlorobenzyl alcohol in a patient with multiple contact allergies. Contact Dermatitis 2009;60:295-296

6   Meijer BUGA, De Waard-van der Spek FB. Allergic contact dermatitis because of topical use of 5-fluorouracil (Efudix® cream). Contact Dermatitis 2007;57:58-60

7   Gaul LE. Dermatitis from cetyl and stearyl alcohols. Arch Dermatol 1969;99:593

8   Shore BN, Shelley WB. Contact dermatitis from stearyl alcohol and propylene glycol in flucinonide cream. Arch Dermatol 1974;109:397-399

9   Yesudian PD, King CM. Allergic contact dermatitis from stearyl alcohol in Efudix® cream. Contact Dermatitis 2001;45:313-314

10 DeBerker D, Marren P, Powell SM, Ryan TJ. Contact sensitivity to the stearyl alcohol in Efudix cream (5-fluorouracil). Contact Dermatitis 1992;26:138

11 Kscomamura H, Dor T, Inui S, Yoshikawa K. A case of contact dermatitis due to impurities of cetyl alcohol. Contact Dermatitis 1997;36:44-46

12 Tosti A, Vincenzi C, Guerra L, Andrisano E. Contact dermatitis from fatty alcohols. Contact Dermatitis 1996;35:287-289

13 Ishiguro N, Kawashima M. Contact dermatitis from impurities in alcohol. Contact Dermatitis 1991;25:257

14 Dissanayke M, Powell SM. Hioxyl® sensitivity. Contact Dermatitis 1990;22:242-243

15 Black H. Contact dermatitis from stearyl alcohol in Metosyn (Fluocinonide) Cream. Contact Dermatitis 1975;1:125

16 Wetter DA, Davis MDP, Yiannias JA, Cheng JF, Connolly SM, el-Azhary RA, et al. Patch test results from the Mayo Contact Dermatitis Group, 1998–2000. J Am Acad Dermatol 2005;53:416-421

17 Rudner EJ. North American Group Results. Contact Dermatitis 1977;3:208-209

18 Wentworth AB, Yiannias JA, Keeling JH, Hall MR, Camilleri MJ, Drage LA, et al. Trends in patch-test results and allergen changes in the standard series: a Mayo Clinic 5-year retrospective review (January 1, 2006, to December 31, 2010). J Am Acad Dermatol 2014;70:269-275

19 Fisher AA. Contact dermatitis from stearyl alcohol and propylene glycol. Arch Derm 1974;110:636

20 Tomar J, Jain VK, Aggarwal K, Dayal S, Guptaet S. Contact allergies to cosmetics: testing with 52 cosmetic ingredients and personal products. J Dermatol 2005;32:951-955

21 Trattner A, Farchi Y, David M. Cosmetics patch tests: first report from Israel. Contact Dermatitis 2002;47:180-181

22 Aerts O, Leysen J, Naessens T, Dandelooy J, Apers S, Lambert J. Steareths may sometimes prove problematic in patients contact allergic to cetostearyl alcohol: an example. Contact Dermatitis 2016;75(Suppl.1):54-55

23 Zaragoza-Ninet V, Blasco Encinas R, Vilata-Corell JJ, Pérez-Ferriols A, Sierra-Talamantes C, Esteve-Martínez A, de la Cuadra-Oyanguren J. Allergic contact dermatitis due to cosmetics: A clinical and epidemiological study in a tertiary hospital. Actas Dermosifiliogr 2016;107:329-336

24 Fulton JE Jr, Pay SR, Fulton JE 3rd. Comedogenicity of current therapeutic products, cosmetics, and ingredients in the rabbit ear. J Am Acad Dermatol 1984;10:96-105

25 George ND, Srinivas CR, Balachandran C, Shenoi SD. Sensitivity to various ingredients of topical preparations following prolonged use. Contact Dermatitis 1990;23:367-368

26 Nguyen SH, Dang TP, Maibach HI. Comedogenicity in rabbit: some cosmetic ingredients/vehicles. Cutan Ocul Toxicol 2007;26:287-292

27 Shore RN, Shelley WB. Contact dermatitis from stearyl alcohol and propylene glycol. Arch Derm 1974;110:636

28 Degreef H, Dooms-Goossens A. Patch testing with silver sulfadiazine cream. Contact Dermatitis 1985;12:33-37

29 Kang H, Choi J, Lee A Y. Allergic contact dermatitis to white petrolatum. J Dermatol 2004;31:428-430

2.440   STYRAX BENZOIN GUM

IDENTIFICATION

Description/definition	: Styrax benzoin gum is a balsamic resin obtained from the benzoin, *Styrax benzoin*, Styracaceae. It is a product which may contain resin acids and their esters, terpenes, and oxidation or polymerization products of these terpenes
Chemical class(es)	: Gums, hydrophilic colloids and derivatives
Other names	: Benzoin gum; gum benzoin; benzoin
CAS registry number (s)	: 9000-05-9; 9000-72-0
EC number(s)	: 232-523-7; 232-556-7
Merck Index monograph	: 5885 (Gum benzoin)
Function(s) in cosmetics	: EU: film forming; masking; perfuming; skin conditioning. USA: adhesives; film formers; fragrance ingredients; skin-conditioning agents - miscellaneous
Patch testing	: Benzoin 10% alc.

GENERAL

Styrax benzoin gum may be used in cosmetics as film former, skin conditioning agent and as fragrance. In non-cosmetic products, Styrax benzoin gum is an important component of 'compound tincture of benzoin' (CTB), which was commonly used to increase adherence of adhesive tape to skin after surgical skin incisions. CTB has also been used to prevent blister formation on the feet in areas of friction, on fissured nipples, under plaster casts, as an adhesive to increase the tackiness of dressings, as a dressing support for rhinoplasty, as palliation of pruritus ani and as an antiseptic (5,7, see Case reports and case series). The compound tincture of benzoin is composed of benzoin 10%, styrax 8%, balsam of Tolu (*Myroxylon toluiferum*) 4% and aloe 2% in an alcoholic vehicle (7). *Tincture* of benzoin consists of 10% benzoin in alcohol (5). Benzoin may also be or have been used in nail polish, expectorant, Arning's tincture, throat lozenges, water-repellent barrier creams, benzoinated lard, cuticle removers, adhesives and ink (7).

In this chapter, allergic reactions to benzoin are presented, but also those caused by compound tincture of benzoin and by tincture of benzoin. Styrax benzoin (benzoin) should not be confused with styrax (synonym: storax), which is a fragrant balsam obtained from the bark of trees of the genus *Liquidambar*, most often *Liquidambar orientalis*. *Styrax* is also a large genus of shrubs and trees (the type genus of the family Styracaceae).

CONTACT ALLERGY

Testing in groups of patients

In 1999, in a tertiary referral center in Melbourne, Australia, 477 consecutive patients suspected of contact dermatitis were patch tested (routine testing) with compound tincture of benzoin (CTB). There were 45 positive reaction (9.4%), which made it the third most common allergen. Of these 45 patients, 14 had strong positive reactions, but only two definitely recalled exposure to compound tincture of benzoin and these were clinically relevant. Twenty-eight patients had co-reacted with allergens such as the fragrance mix, *Myroxylon pereirae* resin, colophonium and tea tree oil. Co-reactivity was seen especially in patients with strong reactions to compound tincture of benzoin. Cross-reactivity *from* these allergens (fragrance mix, *Myroxylon pereirae* resin, colophonium, tea tree oil) was suggested to be the explanation for the high frequency of reactions to compound tincture of benzoin (although it may be argued that strong reactions are less likely to be cross-reactions than weaker ones). The individual ingredients of compound tincture of benzoin were not tested (7).

Case reports and case series

'Benzoin' was responsible for 2 out of 399 cases of cosmetic allergy where the causal allergen was identified in a study of the NACDG, USA, 1977-1983 (2). One patient had allergic contact dermatitis from benzoin resin in a hair lacquer and (as cited in ref. 27) rose water (3). A woman had eczema of the fingers, exacerbated by contact with detergents, perfumed products and orange peel. She had noticed that the use of a cream to soften and smoothen the hands caused a flare-up of the eczema on 3 occasions. Patch tests with the standard series, the cream and some of its constituents (it contained a perfume and Sumatra benzoin) showed positive reactions to the fragrance mix, *Myroxylon pereirae* resin, the cream itself, benzoin 1% and 10% in alcohol and eugenol (27).

Contact allergy to Styrax benzoin gum in non-cosmetic products

Fixation of tapes, dressings et cetera

In 1930, the ingredients of compound tincture of benzoin were obtained for the first time and closed patch testing to CTB was performed in a patient sensitized to CTB under adhesive tape (9). Seven patients had allergic contact dermatitis from compound tincture of benzoin from its use in surgery, but its ingredients were not tested separately (4). A woman had postoperative allergic contact dermatitis from a product containing benzoin and colophonium before applying a wound dressing; she had a positive patch test to tincture of benzoin, the causative product itself was not tested (5). Of 26 patients who were treated with tincture of benzoin under tape for fissures of the feet, two became sensitized as shown by positive patch tests with compound tincture of benzoin (6). A patient developed necrotizing contact dermatitis after a single topical application of tincture of benzoin and a pressure bandage following enucleation of an eye; this may have been either allergic or irritant contact dermatitis, patch tests were not performed (10). Two patients had ACD from benzoin in skin adhesive spray (11). One patient had ACD from benzoin painted postoperatively as benzoin solution (14). Another individual developed ACD from benzoin present in a supportive dressing following rhinoplasty (15). A football player had ACD of the leg with dissemination from benzoin in a spray applied to the leg under tape (17).

A patient developed acute hemorrhagic contact dermatitis to compound benzoin tincture sprayed under a cast. Patch tests with the product, benzoin 3% and 10% alc. and styrax 2.2% were strongly positive (18). A student developed acute eczematous contact dermatitis in response to the application of tincture of benzoin to the skin under a cast. This was followed within 2 days by the appearance of a generalized non-eczematous rash. The authors suggested that absorption of benzoin through the skin was responsible for the rash. Patch tests demonstrated contact allergy to benzoin, tincture of benzoin and other gums (myrrh, locust, galbanum, gamboge, olibanum) (20). Three patients had ACD to CTB used to increase tackiness of wound dressings. Two were tested with the components and both showed positive reactions benzoin 10% alc., styrax 8% alc., balsam of Tolu 4% alc. and aloe 2% alc. One of these patients inhaled compound tincture of benzoin because of a sore throat and the next day she developed a pruritic skin rash and frontal headache (22). A woman probably became sensitized to tincture of benzoin applied during rhinoplasty and developed ACD a month later (24). A man developed ACD from tincture of benzoin aerosol sprayed to fixate a bandage; patch tests were not performed. This was incorrectly stated to be occupational allergic contact dermatitis. The patient was an anesthesiologist who used the benzoin spray for a laceration on his own hand, it was not a compound that he worked with while exercising his occupation (25).

Other applications of benzoin, tincture of benzoin and compound tincture of benzoin
In the period 1978-2008, in a tertiary referral center in Belgium, among 3378 patients suffering from iatrogenic allergic contact dermatitis, 127 were found to react to 48 specific pharmaceutical products; in eighteen cases, 'benzoin' was one of the responsible allergens, used in those products as fragrance (1). Approximately 4,500 army cadets were exposed to CTB for the prevention of blister formation during a 3-year period (1979-1981). Sixteen patients (0.4%) had allergic contact dermatitis severe enough to render them unfit for duty. There were three patients with generalized rashes complicating acute local allergic reactions. Thirteen of the sixteen patients were challenged with open testing on the forearm to CTB. All showed positive reactions. Five representative patients had closed patch tests on the back to the components of CTB. All had positive patch tests to benzoin 10% pet., styrax 2% pet., and to balsam of Tolu 1% and 4% in alcohol; none reacted to aloe 10% pet. The patients were also tested with Mastisol® (containing styrax) and 4 had positive reactions (12). The authors also presented 2 additional non-army patients with contact allergy to CTB used to aid securing tape or gauze (12).

Three women had allergic contact dermatitis from compound tincture of benzoin applied to the breasts as treatment of fissured nipples macerated by breast-feeding. Two were patch tested with the material and their ingredients; one reacted only to benzoin and the second only to styrax (13). Two patients had ACD of the face from benzoin in greasepaint makeup (16). A man had ACD from benzoin painted on the skin for pruritus ani (17). A man had ACD from tincture of benzoin present in Arning's tincture, a topical product formerly used for treatment of skin diseases, e.g., eczema (26).

Cross-reactions, pseudo-cross-reactions and co-reactions
Fragrance mix I, fragrance mix II, *Myroxylon pereirae* resin (balsam of Peru), various essential oils, various fragrances (especially cinnamic acid, esters and derivatives, substituted cinnamic acids [e.g., benzoic acid], vanillin, eugenol), colophonium, styrax, Compositae mix (4,5,7). Benzoin contains cinnamic acids and their esters, which are also present in the fragrance mix I and balsam of Peru. Mastisol® , which is composed of gum mastic and styrax (which is also part of compound tincture of benzoin) (5,12,23). Other gums (myrrh, locust, galbanum, gamboge, olibanum) (20). Of patients allergic to *Myroxylon pereirae*, some 80% also react to benzoin (21).

Presence in cosmetic products and topical pharmaceutical preparations and chemical analyses
In the USA, in April 2017, Styrax benzoin gum was present in 16 of 56,714 cosmetic products of which the composition is known in FDA's Voluntary Cosmetic Registration Program (VCRP) (data obtained from FDA, May 2017). In April 2017, 'benzoin gum' was present in 40 of 66,485 cosmetic products of which the composition is known in EWG's Skin Deep Cosmetics Database, USA (http://www.ewg.org/skindeep/). In the period 1978-2008, in a tertiary

referral center in Belgium, information was collected on the composition of 370 topical pharmaceutical preparations. Ten of these (2.7%) contained Styrax benzoin gum (benzoin) (1).

Other information
Apparently, some benzoin sprays may contain colophonium, which are sometimes the allergenic culprit in cases of ACD to benzoin spray (28).

OTHER SIDE EFFECTS

Other non-eczematous reactions
In one patient, contact allergy to compound tincture of benzoin applied under post-operative adhesive tape may have exacerbated a form of pemphigus (pemphigus erythematosus) (19).

Systemic reactions
The first case of benzoin allergy is usually cited to have been reported in 1874, in a patient who developed a purpuric eruption after inhaling a vapor containing compound tincture of benzoin (8). A student developed acute eczematous contact dermatitis in response to the application of tincture of benzoin to the skin under a cast. This was followed within 2 days by the appearance of a generalized non-eczematous rash. The authors suggested that absorption of benzoin through the skin was responsible for the rash (systemic contact dermatitis) (20). One patient known to be allergic to benzoin inhaled compound tincture of benzoin because of a sore throat and the next day she developed a pruritic skin rash and frontal headache (22).

LITERATURE

1   Nardelli A, D'Hooge E, Drieghe J, Dooms M, Goossens A. Allergic contact dermatitis from fragrance components in specific topical pharmaceutical products in Belgium. Contact Dermatitis 2009;60:303-313
2   Adams RM, Maibach HI, Clendenning WE, Fisher AA, Jordan WJ, Kanof N, et al. A five-year study of cosmetic reactions. J Am Acad Dermatol 1985;13:1062-1069
3   Garnier MG. Dermite bulleuse par un fixateur d'ondulations. Bull Soc Franç Derm Syph 1950;57:397
4   Fettig J, Taylor J, Sood A. Post-surgical allergic contact dermatitis to compound tincture of benzoin and association with reactions to fragrances and essential oils. Dermatitis 2014;25:211-212
5   Sasseville D, Saber M, Lessard L. Allergic contact dermatitis from tincture of benzoin with multiple concomitant reactions. Contact Dermatitis 2009;61:358-360
6   Lakshmi C, Srinivas CR. Contact dermatitis to compound tincture of benzoin applied under occlusion. Indian J Dermatol Venereol Leprol 2006;72:62-63
7   Scardamaglia L, Nixon R, Fewings J. Compound tincture of benzoin: a common contact allergen? Australas J Dermatol 2005;44:180-184
8   Fox T. Purpura urticaria produced by inhalation of Friars' balsam. Lancet 1874;1:195
9   James BM. Dermatitis produced by compound tincture of benzoin. J Med Soc NJ 1930;27:596-599
10 Tripathi RC, Fekrat-Polascik S, Tripathi BJ, Ernest JT. An unusual necrotizing dermatitis after a single application of topical benzoin and pressure bandage for enucleation of an eye. Lens Eye Toxic Res 1990;7:173-178
11 Rademaker M, Kirby JD. Contact dermatitis to a skin adhesive. Contact Dermatitis 1987;16:297-298
12 James WD, White SW, Yanklowitz B. Allergic contact dermatitis to compound tincture of benzoin. J Am Acad Dermatol 1984;11(5 part 1):847-850
13 Eades MF. Dermatitis of the breasts caused by compound tincture of benzoin. N Engl J Med 1934;211:632-634
14 Marks JG Jr, Rainey MA. Cutaneous reactions to surgical preparations and dressings. Contact Dermatitis. 1984;10:1-5
15 Luria PP, Lawrence LI. Allergic reaction to tincture of benzoin compound. Eye Ear Nose Throat Mon 1967;46:224-227
16 Hoffman TE, Adams RM. Contact dermatitis to benzoin in greasepaint makeup. Contact Dermatitis 1978;4:379-380
17 Coskey RJ. Contact dermatitis owing to tincture of benzoin. Arch Dermatol 1978;114:128
18 Cullen SI, Tonkin A, May FE. Allergic contact dermatitis to compound tincture of benzoin spray. J Trauma 1974;14:348-350
19 Lynfield YL, Pertshuk LP, Zimmerman A. Pemphigus erythematosus provoked by allergic contact dermatitis. Arch Dermatol 1973;108:690-693
20 Spott DA, Shelley WB. Exanthem due to contact allergen (benzoin) absorbed through skin. J Amer Med Assoc 1970;214:1881-1882
21 Hjorth N. Eczematous allergy to balsams. Acta Derm Venereol (Stockh) 1961;46(Suppl):1-216

22 Steiner K, Leifer W. Investigation of contact-type dermatitis due to compound tincture of benzoin. J Invest
    Dermatol 1949;13:351-359
23 Worsnop F, Affleck A, Varma S, English J. Allergic contact dermatitis from Mastisol mistaken for cellulitis. Contact
    Dermatitis 2007;56:357-358
24 Rajabian MH, Sodaify M, Aghaei S. Severe facial dermatitis as a late complication of aesthetic rhinoplasty; a case
    report. BMC Dermatol 2004;4:1
25 Klein TG, Woehlck HJ, Pagel PS. Severe allergic contact dermatitis resulting from occupational exposure to
    tincture of benzoin aerosol spray in an anesthesiologist. J Anesth 2009;23:292-294
26 Keller-Melchior R, Bräuninger W. Allergic contact dermatitis from anthrarobin. Contact Dermatitis 1995;33:361
27 Mann RJ. Benzoin sensitivity. Contact Dermatitis 1982;8:263
28 Han JS, Jung JM, Lee WJ, Won CH, Jang YJ, Chang SE, Lee MW, Choi JH, Moon KC. Benzoin spray: cause of allergic
    contact dermatitis due to its rosin content. Ann Dermatol 2014;26:524-525

2.441   SULFATED CASTOR OIL

IDENTIFICATION

Description/definition	: Sulfated castor oil is the oil that consists primarily of the sodium salt of the sulfated triglyceride of castor oil
Chemical class(es)	: Glyceryl esters and derivatives; sulfuric acid esters
Other names	: Castor oil, sulfated; turkey-red oil
CAS registry number (s)	: 8002-33-3
EC number(s)	: 232-306-7
Function(s) in cosmetics	: EU: cleansing; emulsifying; humectant; surfactant. USA: surfactants - cleansing agents
Patch testing	: 1% olive oil (3)

CONTACT ALLERGY

Case reports and case series
Twelve cases of allergic contact dermatitis from a hair conditioner spray were reported (to the manufacturer?) (1). The reactions were ascribed to sulfated castor oil, but the patients were probably not patch tested with it and no clinical descriptions were presented. In a modified Draize repeated insult patch test, 4 of 53 normal test individuals became allergic to sulfated castor oil (1).

Presence in cosmetic products and chemical analyses
In the USA, in April 2017, sulfated castor oil was present in 22 of 56,714 cosmetic products of which the composition is known in FDA's Voluntary Cosmetic Registration Program (VCRP) (data obtained from FDA, May 2017). In April 2017, sulfated castor oil was present in 33 of 65,434 cosmetic products of which the composition is known in EWG's Skin Deep Cosmetics Database, USA (http://www.ewg.org/skindeep/).

OTHER SIDE EFFECTS

Other non-eczematous contact reactions
In (somewhat) older literature, sulfated castor oil has been suspected of being comedogenic in 'people with more sensitive complexions or acne-prone problems', based on rabbit ear assays (2).

LITERATURE
1   Fisher LB, Berman B. Contact allergy to sulfonated castor oil. Contact Dermatitis 1981;7:339-340
2   Fulton JE Jr, Pay SR, Fulton JE 3rd. Comedogenicity of current therapeutic products, cosmetics, and ingredients in the rabbit ear. J Am Acad Dermatol 1984;10:96-105
3   De Groot AC. Patch Testing, 3rd Edition. Wapserveen, The Netherlands: acdegroot publishing, 2008 (ISBN 978-90-813233-1-4)

2.442   SULFIRAM*

Not an INCI name

IDENTIFICATION

Description/definition   : Sulfiram is the thiocarbamoyl sulfide that corresponds to the structural formula shown
                               below
Chemical class(es)   : Organic sulfur compounds; carbamothioates
INCI name EU & USA   : Neither in CosIng nor in the Personal Care Products Council Ingredient Database
Chemical/IUPAC name   : Diethylcarbamothioyl *N,N*-diethylcarbamodithioate
Other names   : Monosulfiram; tetraethylthiuram monosulfide
CAS registry number (s)   : 95-05-6
EC number(s)   : 202-387-3
Merck Index monograph   : 10350
Patch testing   : 1% pet. (2)
Molecular formula   : $C_{10}H_{20}N_2S_3$

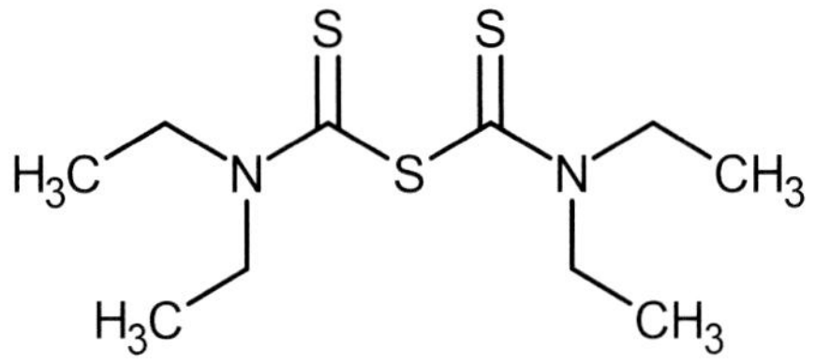

GENERAL

The discussion of sulfiram is limited to allergic contact dermatitis from its presence in cosmetic products.

CONTACT ALLERGY

Case reports and case series

A woman developed swelling of the lips and periorbital tissues within a day of washing her hands and face with monosulfiram soap. Over the next 2 days she developed eczematous patches on her face and neck while the swelling on her face became worse so that she was unable to open her eyes. The patient gave a history of suspender dermatitis in the past and for the preceding 6 years had suffered from recurrent dermatitis of the hands. A few weeks after her facial eruption had healed by corticosteroid therapy, patch tests gave positive reactions to nickel, colophonium, carba-mix, thiuram-mix and tetramethylthiuramdisulphide (TMTD). The patient's rubber gloves probably contained a thiuram compound in the inner layer. She was advised not to wear rubber gloves and to wear PVC gloves instead both at home and at work. This gave a dramatic improvement in her hand dermatitis. The authors believed that their patient had acute contact dermatitis shortly after a single exposure to monosulfiram soap because she had acquired thiuram sensitivity from contact with rubber. However, sulfiram nor the soap itself nor other constituents of the soap were patch tested (1).

Presence in cosmetic products and chemical analyses

In May 2017, sulfiram was present in zero of 66,975 cosmetic products of which the composition is known in EWG's Skin Deep Cosmetics Database, USA (http://www.ewg.org/skindeep/). In the USA, in April 2017, sulfiram was present in zero of 56,714 cosmetic products of which the composition is known in FDA's Voluntary Cosmetic Registration Program (VCRP) (data obtained from FDA, May 2017).

LITERATURE

1   Dick DC, Adams RH. Allergic contact dermatitis from monosulfiram (Tetmosol) soap. Contact Dermatitis 1979;5:199
2   De Groot AC. Patch Testing, 3rd Edition. Wapserveen, The Netherlands: acdegroot publishing, 2008 (ISBN 978-90-813233-1-4)

2.443   TANACETUM PARTHENIUM (FEVERFEW) EXTRACT

IDENTIFICATION

Description/definition	: Chrysanthemum parthenium extract is the extract of the herb of the feverfew, *Chrysanthemum parthenium*, Asteraceae (Asteraceae is the old name for Compositae)
Chemical class(es)	: Botanical products and botanical derivatives
INCI name USA	: Chrysanthemum parthenium (feverfew) extract
Other names	: Feverfew extract; Matricaria parthenium extract; Tanacetum parthenium extract
CAS registry number (s)	: 89997-65-9
EC number(s)	: 289-701-2
Merck Index monograph	: 5366 (Feverfew)
Function(s) in cosmetics	: EU: skin conditioning. USA: skin-conditioning agents - miscellaneous
Patch testing	: Chrysanthemum parthenium extract 1% pet.; parthenolide 0.1% pet. (Chemotechnique)

The accepted scientific name for *Chrysanthemum parthenium*, as incorrectly used in the INCI nomenclature, is *Tanacetum parthenium.*

GENERAL

Feverfew (*Tanacetum parthenium* L.) (Compositae) is a plant, which has a long history of use in traditional and folk medicine, especially among Greek and other early European herbalists. It is traditionally used for the treatment of fevers, migraine headaches, rheumatoid arthritis, stomach aches, toothaches, insect bites, infertility, and problems with menstruation and labor during childbirth (hence the colloquial name 'mother herb' [8]). Feverfew has also been employed in the treatment of psoriasis, allergies, asthma, tinnitus, dizziness, nausea, and vomiting. The plant is perceived to have multiple pharmacologic properties, such as anticancer, anti-inflammatory, cardiotonic, antispasmodic, and emmenagogue (menstruation stimulating) (3). More recently, feverfew has become popular for prevention of migraine headache attacks, but the evidence for its efficacy is weak (12).

   Tanacetum parthenium contains a large number of chemicals, but the active principles probably include one or more of its sesquiterpene lactones; other potentially active constituents include flavonoid glycosides and pinenes. Chrysanthemum parthenium extract contains a variety of sesquiterpene lactones, representing three major structural groups, namely the eudesmanolides, the guaianolides, and the germacranolides. In western Europe, the germacranolide parthenolide is the main sesquiterpene lactone (85% of the total sesquiterpene lactone component) and also the major cause of contact allergy to feverfew (6,7); indeed, parthenolide is a very strong sensitizer (13). At the same time, It is likely that a large proportion of the positive reactions to feverfew are due to primary chrysanthemum sensitization (1,7,8).

   Discussion of adverse effects to *Tanacetum parthenium* in this chapter is limited to its extracts and products containing them.

CONTACT ALLERGY

Testing in groups of patients

There are no studies in which consecutive patients suspected of contact dermatitis have been patch tested with Tanacetum parthenium extract (routine testing). Results of testing the extract in groups of *selected* patients are shown in table 2.443.1. In most investigations, patients sensitive to Compositae and/or previously reacting to the Compositae mix were patch tested with its ingredients including feverfew extract. Rates of reactions to feverfew in these patient groups have ranged from 53% to 91% (1,6,7,11). In a very small study of 27 patients suspected of cosmetic dermatitis, 3 (11%) reacted to feverfew; all also had positive patch tests to the fragrance mix, and the feverfew reactions were probably due to cross-sensitivity (4). Relevance was sometimes not stated or related to the reactions to the Compositae mix, but was never specified for feverfew.

Case reports and case series

A patient who was allergic to the sesquiterpene lactone mix, the sesquiterpene(s) (iso)alantolactone and the plant *Matricaria parthenium* (= *Tanacetum parthenium*) had allergic contact dermatitis from Tanacetum parthenium extract in a make-up cosmetic product used by his girlfriend ('consort dermatitis', 'connubial dermatitis') (5). A woman presented with erythematous scaly plaques throughout the scalp, on the forehead, cheeks, chin, and periorbital area, neck, and behind the ears. She suffered from a seasonal eruption on the face and scalp compatible with an allergic airborne dermatitis. The eruption was apparently exacerbated after the use of a calming moisturizer containing feverfew. The patient was patch tested with the standard series, a cosmetic and a plant series, her own products, including the calming moisturizer, and a moisturizer, made by the same company, with a very similar chemical composition but without feverfew. The patient had positive reactions to the sesquiterpene lactone mix (SL mix), the Compositae mix, Achillea millefolium (yarrow) extract, parthenolide, Tanacetum vulgare (tansy) extract, and the calming moisturizer with feverfew (tested as is). She had negative reactions to all other tested allergens, including the similar moisturizer not containing feverfew (9). *Comment*: Although the extract of *Tanacetum parthenium* itself was apparently not tested (apart from being present in the Compositae mix), the causal role of the extract is highly likely, as the patient did not react to the same moisturizer without feverfew and because of the reactions to other Compositae extracts (yarrow, tansy) and to the sesquiterpene lactones SL-mix, Compositae mix and parthenolide, the latter being the main sensitizer in both *Tanacetum parthenium* and *Tanacetum vulgare*.

Table 2.443.1 Patch testing in groups of patients: Selected patient groups

Years and Country	Test conc. & vehicle	Number of patients tested | positive (%)		Selection of patients (S); Relevance (R); Comments (C)	Ref.
2000-2004 Denmark	1% pet.	76	56 (74%)	S: patients reacting to the Compositae mix 6% (Trolab); R: 80% of positive reactions to all allergens were considered of current and/or past relevance	1
1996-1999 Germany	?	39	20 (51%)	C: article not read	2
1990-1998 Denmark	1% pet.	129	104 (81%)	S: patients sensitive to Compositae; R: not stated	7
1996-1997 UK	1% pet.	27	3 (11%)	S: patients suspected of cosmetic dermatitis; R: not specified; co-reactivity to the fragrance mix in all cases	4
1990 Denmark	1% pet.	22	20 (91%)	S: patients reacting to the Compositae mix; R: 75% for 32 patients sensitized to the Compositae mix, not specified for its ingredients including feverfew	6
1985-1990 Germany	1% pet.	85	45 (53%)	S: patients reacting to the Compositae mix; R: nearly all reactions to the Compositae mix were relevant and were most often caused by contact with plants, some by 'natural' cosmetics; thirty-three (28%) patients were occupationally sensitized (e.g., florists, gardeners) and 11 (9.3%) had airborne allergic contact dermatitis. The relevance of the reactions to the individual ingredients of the Compositae mix including feverfew was not specified	11

A woman presented with a 1-month history of intense pruritus, redness, and swelling in the periorbital areas. She reported having started using a new eye cream containing feverfew a few weeks before her symptoms began. Physical examination revealed eczematous weeping areas and edema on the upper and lower eyelids bilaterally, with extension onto the cheeks. The patient was tested with the standard series, selected cosmetic allergens, and her personal products, including the implicated feverfew-containing moisturizer. She had positive reactions to the Compositae mix, sesquiterpene lactone mix and the feverfew-containing moisturizer (tested as is). After treatment and avoidance measures, the dermatitis cleared and no recurrences were noted (9). *Comment*: The causative role of feverfew extract is not proven, but given the positive reactions to the sesquiterpene lactone mix and the Compositae mix, the latter of which containing extracts of *Tanacetum parthenium* and other Compositae plant which frequently cross-react, very likely (9).

In a German study performed between 1985 and 1990, a group of 118 patients reacted to the Compositae mix consisting of five ingredients: arnica (*Arnica montana* L.), German chamomile (*Chamomilla recutita*), feverfew (*Tanacetum parthenium*), tansy (*Tanacetum vulgare*) and yarrow (*Achillea millefolium*). In 4 patients, the sensitization was caused by 'natural cosmetics', in 3 by 'natural ointments', in one by a herbal massage oil and in one (probably) by a herbal shampoo, soap and ointment. However, it was not specified, which of the 5 plant extracts was/were the actual sensitizer(s) in these products (11).

One out of 959 cases of non-fragrance cosmetic allergy where the causal allergen was identified, Belgium, 2000-2010, was caused by 'Chrysanthemum extract'. Whether this was *Chrysanthemum parthenium* (the incorrect INCI name for *Tanacetum parthenium*) is unknown (10).

Cross-reactions, pseudo-cross-reactions and co-reactions
Cross-reactions between Compositae plants and extracts are frequent (7). It is likely that a large proportion of the positive reactions to feverfew are due to primary chrysanthemum sensitization (1,7). Fragrance mix I (4,14).

Provocation tests
Of seven patients allergic to the extract of *Tanacetum parthenium*, 4 had a positive and one a dubious positive patch test reaction to a cosmetic cream containing a parthenolide-depleted feverfew extract. These 5 were all also allergic

to parthenolide. The cream was analysed about 2 years later, and no parthenolide was detected, probably because of degradation of the compound over time (14).

Presence in cosmetic products and chemical analyses

In the USA, in April 2017, Chrysanthemum parthenium (feverfew) extract was present in 30 of 56,714 cosmetic products of which the composition is known in FDA's Voluntary Cosmetic Registration Program (VCRP) (data obtained from FDA, May 2017). In February 2017, Chrysanthemum parthenium (feverfew) extract was present in 9 (extract) and 18 (flower extract) products of 64,480 cosmetic products of which the composition is known in EWG's Skin Deep Cosmetics Database, USA (http://www.ewg.org/skindeep/).

LITERATURE

1   Paulsen E, Andersen KE. Patch testing with constituents of Compositae mixes. Contact Dermatitis 2012;66:241-246

2   Geier J, Hausen BM. Epikutantesting mit dem Kompositen-mix. Allergologie 2000;23:334-341

3   Pareek A, Suthar M, Rathore GS, Bansal V. Feverfew (*Tanacetum parthenium* L.): a systematic review. Pharmacogn Rev 2011;5:103-110

4   Thomson KF, Wilkinson SM. Allergic contact dermatitis to plant extracts in patients with cosmetic dermatitis. Br J Dermatol 2000;142:84-88

5   Bernedo N, Audicana MT, Uriel O, Velasco M, Gastaminza G, Fernández E, Muñoz D. Allergic contact dermatitis from cosmetics applied by the patient's girlfriend. Contact Dermatitis 2004;50:252-253

6   Paulsen E, Andersen KE, Hausen BM. Compositae dermatitis in a Danish dermatology department in one year. Contact Dermatitis 1993;29:6-10

7   Paulsen E, Andersen KE, Hausen BM. Sensitization and cross-reaction patterns in Danish Compositae-allergic patients. Contact Dermatitis 2001;45:197-204

8   Aberer W. Contact allergy and medicinal herbs. J Dtsch Dermatol Ges 2008;6:15-24

9   Killoran CE, Crawford GH, Pedvis-Leftick A. Two cases of Compositae dermatitis exacerbated by moisturizer containing feverfew. Dermatitis 2007;18:225-229

10 Travassos AR, Claes L, Boey L, Drieghe J, Goossens A. Non-fragrance allergens in specific cosmetic products. Contact Dermatitis 2011;65:276-285

11 Hausen BM. A 6-year experience with Compositae mix. Am J Contact Dermatitis 1996;7:94-99

12 Wider B, Pittler MH, Ernst E. Feverfew for preventing migraine. Cochrane Database Syst Rev 2015;20;4:CD002286

13 Paulsen E, Christensen LP, Andersen KE. Compositae dermatitis from airborne parthenolide. Br J Dermatol 2007;156:510-515

14 Paulsen E, Christensen LP, Fretté XC, Andersen KE. Patch test reactivity to feverfew-containing creams in feverfew-allergic patients. Contact Dermatitis 2010;63:146-150

2.444 TANACETUM VULGARE (TANSY) EXTRACT

IDENTIFICATION

Description/definition	: Tanacetum vulgare extract is an extract of the herb, flowers and seeds of the tansy, *Tanacetum vulgare* L., Compositae
Chemical class(es)	: Botanical products and botanical derivatives
Other names	: Tansy extract; Chrysanthemum vulgare extract
CAS registry number (s)	: 84961-64-8
EC number(s)	: 284-653-9
Function(s) in cosmetics	: EU: skin conditioning. USA: skin-conditioning agents - miscellaneous
Patch testing	: 1% pet. (Chemotechnique); also present in the Compositae mix II (Chemotechnique)

GENERAL

Tanacetum vulgare L. (synonym: *Chrysanthemum vulgare* (L.) Bernh.), in Europe commonly known as tansy, is a perennial herb of the Compositae family, adapted to the northern climate and growing widely in Europe, Asia, and North America. It is traditionally used in the preparation of food, cosmetics, dyes, insecticides, preservatives, acaricides and medicines in many countries (7). The aerial parts of this plant are popularly used to treat migraine, neuralgia, and rheumatism, and as an anthelmintic and insect repellent (9). Studies have indicated that the essential oil and extract of tansy exhibits anti-inflammatory, antibacterial and antifungal activities (7). However, the plant also causes allergic contact dermatitis, mainly from the presence of parthenolide, which is a very strong sensitizer (5,8). Alternatively, It is likely that a large proportion of the positive reactions to tansy are due to primary chrysanthemum sensitivity (5,6).

Discussion of adverse effects to *Tanacetum vulgare* in this chapter is limited to its extracts and products containing them.

CONTACT ALLERGY

Testing in groups of patients

There are no studies in which consecutive patients suspected of contact dermatitis have been patch tested with Tanacetum vulgare extract (routine testing). Results of testing the extract in groups of *selected* patients are shown in table 2.444.1. In most investigations, patients sensitive to Compositae and/or previously reacting to the Compositae mix were patch tested with its ingredients including tansy. Rates of reactions to tansy in these patient groups have ranged from 54% to 77% (1,3,4,5). Relevance was sometimes not stated or related to the reactions to the Compositae mix, but was never specified for tansy.

Table 2.444.2 Patch testing in groups of patients: Selected patient groups

Years and Country	Test conc. & vehicle	Number of patients tested | positive (%)		Selection of patients (S); Relevance (R); Comments (C)	Ref.
2006-2011 Denmark	1% pet.	29	21 (72%)	S: patients reacting to the Compositae mix 5% (Chemotechnique); R: 80% of positive reactions to all allergens were considered of current and/or past relevance	1
2000-2004 Denmark	1% pet.	76	53 (70%)	S: patients reacting to the Compositae mix 6% (Trolab); R: 80% of positive reactions to all allergens were consi-dered of current and/or pastrelevance	1
1996-1999 Germany	?	39	19 (49%)	C: article not read	2
1990-1998 Denmark	1% pet.	129	99 (77%)	S: patients sensitive to Compositae; R: not stated	5
1990 Denmark	1% pet.	24	13 (54%)	S: patients reacting to the Compositae mix; R: 75% for 32 patients sensitized to the Compositae mix, not specified for its ingredients including tansy	3
1985-1990 Germany	1% pet.	56	34 (61%)	S: patients reacting to the Compositae mix; R: nearly all reactions to the Compositae mix were relevant and were most often caused by contact with plants, some by 'natural' cosmetics; thirty-three (28%) patients were occupationally sensitized (e.g., florists, gardeners) and 11 (9.3%) had air-borne allergic contact dermatitis. The relevance of the reactions to the individual ingredients of the Compositae mix including tansy was not specified	4

Case reports and case series

In a German study performed between 1985 and 1990, a group of 118 patients reacted to the Compositae mix consisting of five ingredients: arnica (*Arnica montana* L.), German chamomile (*Chamomilla recutita*), feverfew (*Tanacetum parthenium*), tansy (*Tanacetum vulgare*) and yarrow (*Achillea millefolium*). In 4 patients, the sensitization was caused by 'natural cosmetics', in 3 by 'natural ointments', in one by a herbal massage oil and in one (probably) by a herbal shampoo, soap and ointment. However, it was not specified, which of the 5 plant extracts was/were the actual sensitizer(s) in these products (4).

Cross-reactions, pseudo-cross-reactions and co-reactions

Cross-sensitization between Compositae plants and extracts is frequent (5). It is likely that a large proportion of the positive reactions to tansy are due to primary chrysanthemum sensitivity (5,6).

Presence in cosmetic products and chemical analyses

In the USA, in April 2017, Tanacetum vulgare extract was present in 7 of 56,714 cosmetic products of which the composition is known in FDA's Voluntary Cosmetic Registration Program (VCRP) (data obtained from FDA, May 2017). In February 2017, Tanacetum vulgare (extract) was present in 3 products of 64,480 cosmetic products of which the composition is known in EWG's Skin Deep Cosmetics Database, USA (http://www.ewg.org/skindeep/).

OTHER SIDE EFFECTS

Photosensitivity

Photopatch testing in groups of patients

Photopatch testing with Tanacetum vulgare extract has been performed in two small studies of selected patients (table 2.444.2) (10,11). A high frequency of photocontact allergy of 7% was seen in a group of 30 patients with chronic actinic dermatitis, in which disease photocontact allergy and contact allergic reactions are frequent. Two patients had positive photopatch tests to *Tanacetum vulgare*, but their relevance was not mentioned (10).

Table 2.444.2 Photopatch testing in groups of patients

Years and Country	Test conc. & vehicle	Number of patients tested	positive (%)	Selection of patients (S); Relevance (R); Comments (C)	Ref.
1993-2009 USA	1% pet.	30	2 (7%)	S: patients with chronic actinic dermatitis; R: not stated	10
1993-2006 USA	1% pet.	76	1 (1%)	S: not stated; R: not specified	11

LITERATURE

1 Paulsen E, Andersen KE. Patch testing with constituents of Compositae mixes. Contact Dermatitis 2012;66:241-46

2 Geier J, Hausen BM. Epikutantesting mit dem Kompositen-mix. Allergologie 2000;23:334-341

3 Paulsen E, Andersen KE, Hausen BM. Compositae dermatitis in a Danish dermatology department in one year. Contact Dermatitis 1993;29:6-10

4 Hausen BM. A 6-year experience with Compositae mix. Am J Cont Derm 1996;7:94-99

5 Paulsen E, Andersen KE, Hausen BM. Sensitization and cross-reaction patterns in Danish Compositae-allergic patients. Contact Dermatitis 2001;45:197-204

6 Hausen BM. The sensitizing capacity of Compositae plants. III. Test results and cross-reactions in Compositae-sensitive patients. Dermatologica 1979;159:1-11

7 Piras A, Falconieri D, Bagdonaite E, Maxia A, Gonçalves MJ, Cavaleiro C, et al. Chemical composition and antifungal activity of supercritical extract and essential oil of *Tanacetum vulgare* growing wild in Lithuania. Nat Prod Res 2014;28:1906-1909

8 Paulsen E, Christensen LP, Andersen KE. Compositae dermatitis from airborne parthenolide. Br J Dermatol 2007; 156:510-515

9 Onozato T, Nakamura CV, Garcia Cortez DA, Dias Filho BP, Ueda-Nakamura T. *Tanacetum vulgare*: antiherpes virus activity of crude extract and the purified compound parthenolide. Phytother Res 2009;23:791-796

10 Que SK, Brauer JA, Soter NA, Cohen DE. Chronic actinic dermatitis: an analysis at a single institution over 25 years. Dermatitis 2011;22:147-154

11 Victor FC, Cohen DE, Soter NA. A 20-year analysis of previous and emerging allergens that elicit photoallergic contact dermatitis. J Am Acad Dermatol 2010;62:605-610

2.445 TBHQ

IDENTIFICATION

Description/definition	: TBHQ is the phenol that conforms to the formula shown below
Chemical class(es)	: Phenols
Chemical/IUPAC name	: 2-*tert*-Butylbenzene-1,4-diol
Other names	: *t*-Butyl hydroquinone
CAS registry number (s)	: 1948-33-0
EC number(s)	: 217-752-2
CIR review(s)	: J Am Coll Toxicol 1986;5:329-351; J Am Coll Toxicol 1991;10:1-7 (access: www.cir-safety.org/ingredients)
Functions in cosmetics	: EU: antioxidant; masking; perfuming. USA: antioxidants; fragrance ingredients
Patch testing	: 1.0% pet. (Chemotechnique, SmartPracticeCanada)
Molecular formula	: $C_{10}H_{14}O_2$

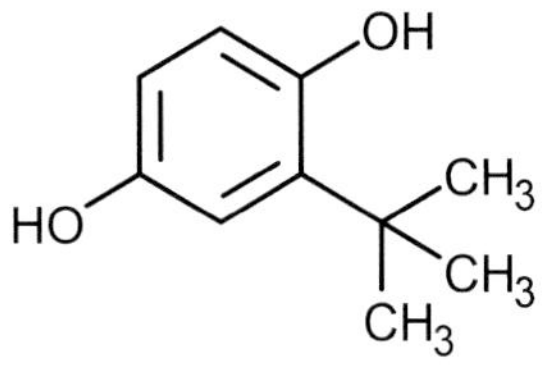

GENERAL

TBHQ is an antioxidant used in cosmetics and foods. In industry, it is used as a chemical stabilizer and retarder of polymerization of polyesters (2). TBHQ is considered to be a weak sensitizer (19).

CONTACT ALLERGY

Patch testing in groups of patients

There have been no studies in which TBHQ was tested in consecutive patients suspected of contact dermatitis (routine testing). Results of patch testing with TBHQ in groups of *selected* patients (patients suspected of cosmetic dermatitis, patients with facial, periorbital or scalp dermatitis, patients with stasis dermatitis/leg ulcers) are shown in table 2.445.1. Frequencies of sensitization have ranged from 0.5% to 8.7%. In all but three, the frequencies were below 2%. In most studies, no data on relevance were provided or specified. In an early UK study, 2 of 5 positive patch test reactions (40%) were relevant: the patients had been exposed to cosmetic products containing TBHQ (3). A high rate of 8% positive reactions was found in a study from India, in which 4 of 50 patients suspected of cosmetic dermatitis reacted to TBHQ 1% pet. The relevance of these reactions was not mentioned (15).

An even higher rate of 8.7% was found in patients with stasis dermatitis / leg ulcers. Here also, relevance was not mentioned (20). In one study from the USA, 21 of 22 positive reactions (96%) were considered to be relevant, but this percentage included 'questionable' and 'past' relevance. Also, there were many reactions consisting of macular erythema, which were counted as positive, which is not consistent with international guidelines (1).

Case reports and case series

In a group of 119 patients with allergic contact dermatitis from cosmetics, investigated in The Netherlands in 1986-1987, one case was caused by TBHQ in a lip cream (13,14). In a 4-month-period in 1996, 475 patients with contact allergy to 'cosmetic ingredients' were collected in 5 centers in Belgium, UK and Germany. There were 6 reactions to TBHQ; the relevance of these positive patch tests was not mentioned (12).

A woman presented with a history of recurrent edema of the face and irritation of the scalp after using hair dyes. Patch tests with the British Contact Dermatitis Society standard series and the hairdressing series were negative. Later, she was tested with constituents of her hair product, and to the bases, preservatives, and cosmetics series, and the patient now showed a positive reaction to TBHQ. She also had a positive reaction to laureth-12 in the hair dye and to BHA, which was not present in any of her products (5). A woman had developed an itchy inflammatory edema of her scalp and face, with occipital lymph node swelling, one day after the second application of a new hair-coloring preparation. She had regularly used hair dyes for several years, but with transient local discomfort only. Patch tests with the European standard series and a hairdressers series were negative, but semi-open tests showed a weakly positive reaction to the coloring solution. When the patient was tested with its ingredients, there was a strongly positive reaction to TBHQ 0.3% alc./water 50/50. In a subsequent test session, the patient reacted to BHA and BHT, which was considered to indicate cross-sensitivity (8). Two patients had contact allergy to TBHQ in cosmetics, one from lipstick, the other from eyeshadow (3). One patient reacted to TBHQ in a lipstick (6), another had allergic contact cheilitis from TBHQ present in lip gloss (7).

Table 2.445.1 Patch testing in groups of patients: Selected patient groups

Years and Country	Test conc. & vehicle	Number of patients tested	positive (%)		Selection of patients (S); Relevance (R); Comments (C)	Ref.
2003-2014 IVDK	1% pet.	4756		(8.7%)	S: patients with stasis dermatitis/ chronic leg ulcers; R: not stated	20
2011 China	1% pet.	201	1	(0.5%)	S: healthy student volunteers 19-30 years; R: not stated	17
2006-2011 IVDK	1% pet.	7769		(1.9%)	S: patients suspected of cosmetic intolerance and tested with an ointment base series (selection procedure not stated); R: not stated	18
2000-2010 IVDK		3449	52	(1.5%)	S: patients with periorbital dermatitis; R: not stated	4
2000-2007 USA	1% pet.	937	22	(2.3%)	S: patients tested with a supplemental cosmetic screening series; R: 96%; C: weak study: a. high rate of macular erythema and weak reactions; b. relevance figures included 'questionable' and 'past' relevance	1
<2005 India	1% pet.	50	4	(8%)	S: patients suspected of cosmetic dermatitis; R: not stated	15
1993-2003 IVDK	1% pet.	802	16	(2.0%)	S: patients with scalp dermatitis; R: not stated	11
1997-2000 Israel		244	4	(1.6%)	S: patients suspected of cosmetic dermatitis; R: 64% of all patch test reactions in the cosmetic series was relevant	16
1982-1983 UK	1% pet.	1096	5	(0.5%)	S: patients tested with facial dermatitis; 2 reactions were relevant, one from lipstick, the other from eyeshadow	3

IVDK: Information Network of Departments of Dermatology, Germany, Austria, Switzerland

Contact allergy to TBHQ in non-cosmetic products
A turner had occupational allergic contact dermatitis from TBHQ present in a vegetable hydraulic oil (2). A metalworker had occupational allergic contact dermatitis from TBHQ in a cutting oil (9). Another male individual, producing synthetic rubber, had occupational contact allergy to TBHQ (10).

Cross-reactions, pseudo-cross-reactions and co-reactions
BHA (2,3,5,8); BHT (3,8).

Presence in cosmetic products and chemical analyses
In the USA, in April 2017, *tert*-butylhydroquinone was present in 37 of 56,714 cosmetic products of which the composition is known in FDA's Voluntary Cosmetic Registration Program (VCRP) (data obtained from FDA, May 2017). In April 2017, TBHQ was present in 27 of 66,485 cosmetic products of which the composition is known in EWG's Skin Deep Cosmetics Database, USA (http://www.ewg.org/skindeep/).

LITERATURE

1   Wetter DA, Yiannias JA, Prakash AV, Davis MD, Farmer SA, el-Azhary RA, et al. Results of patch testing to personal care product allergens in a standard series and a supplemental cosmetic series: an analysis of 945 patients from the Mayo Clinic Contact Dermatitis Group, 2000-2007. J Am Acad Dermatol 2010;63:789-798
2   Aalto-Korte K. Allergic contact dermatitis from tertiary-butylhydroquinone (TBHQ) in a vegetable hydraulic oil. Contact Dermatitis 2000;43:303
3   White IR, Lovell CR, Cronin E. Antioxidants in cosmetics. Contact Dermatitis 1984;11:265-267
4   Landeck L, John SM, Geier J. Periorbital dermatitis in 4779 patients – patch test results during a 10-year period. Contact Dermatitis 2014;70:205-212
5   Field S, Hazelwood E, Bourke B, Bourke JF. Allergic contact dermatitis from tertiary-butylhydroquinone and Laureth 12 in a hair dye. Contact Dermatitis 2007;56:116
6   Calnan CD. Monotertiary butyl hydroquinone in lipstick. Contact Dermatitis 1981;7:280-281
7   Van Joost T, Liem DH, Stolz E. Allergic contact dermatitis to mono tertiary butyl hydroquinone in lip gloss. Contact Dermatitis 1984;10:189-190
8   Le Coz CJ, Schneider GA. Contact dermatitis from tertiary-butylhydroquinone in a hair dye, with cross-sensitivity to BHA and BHT. Contact Dermatitis 1998;39:39-40
9   Meding B. Occupational contact dermatitis from tertiarybutylhydroquinone (TBHQ) in a cutting fluid. Contact Dermatitis 1996;34:224
10 Higashi N, Matsumura T. A case of occupational contact dermatitis from peroxide curing agents for rubber. Skin Res 1987;29:563-567 (in Japanese, cited in ref. 9)

11 Hillen U, Grabbe S, Uter W. Patch test results in patients with scalp dermatitis: analysis of data of the Information Network of Departments of Dermatology. Contact Dermatitis 2007;56:87-93

12 Goossens A, Beck MH, Haneke E, McFadden JP, Nolting S, Durupt G, Ries G. Adverse cutaneous reactions to cosmetic allergens. Contact Dermatitis 1999;40:112-113

13 De Groot AC, Bruynzeel DP, Bos JD, van der Meeren HL, van Joost T, Jagtman BA, Weyland JW. The allergens in cosmetics. Arch Dermatol 1988;124:1525-1529

14 De Groot AC. Adverse reactions to cosmetics. PhD Thesis, University of Groningen, The Netherlands: 1988, chapter 3.4, pp.105-113

15 Tomar J, Jain VK, Aggarwal K, Dayal S, Guptaet S. Contact allergies to cosmetics: testing with 52 cosmetic ingredients and personal products. J Dermatol 2005;32:951-955

16 Trattner A, Farchi Y, David M. Cosmetics patch tests: first report from Israel. Contact Dermatitis 2002;47:180-181

17 Zhao J, Li LF. Contact sensitization to cosmetic series of allergens in a general population in Beijing. J Cosmet Dermatol 2014;13:68-71

18 Dinkloh A, Worm M, Geier J, Schnuch A, Wollenberg A. Contact sensitization in patients with suspected cosmetic intolerance: results of the IVDK 2006-2011. J Eur Acad Dermatol Venereol 2015;29:1071-1081

19 Deyo JA, Dyer WM Jr, Maibach HI. Induction of contact sensitization to monotertiary butyl hydroquinone. Contact Dermatitis 1997;37:92-93

20 Erfurt-Berge C, Geier J, Mahler V. The current spectrum of contact sensitization in patients with chronic leg ulcers or stasis dermatitis - new data from the Information Network of Departments of Dermatology (IVDK). Contact Dermatitis 2017;77:151-158

2.446   TEA-COCOYL HYDROLYZED COLLAGEN

IDENTIFICATION

Description/definition	: TEA-cocoyl hydrolyzed collagen is the triethanolamine salt of the condensation product of coconut acid chloride and hydrolyzed collagen
Chemical class(es)	: Protein derivatives
Chemical/IUPAC name	: Acid chlorides, coco, reaction products with protein hydrolyzates, compds. with triethanolamine
Other names	: TEA-coco hydrolyzed animal protein
CAS registry number (s)	: 68952-16-9
CIR review(s)	: J Am Coll Toxicol 1983;2:75-86 (access: www.cir-safety.org/ingredients)
Function(s) in cosmetics	: EU: antistatic; cleansing; hair conditioning; skin conditioning; surfactant. USA: hair conditioning agents; skin-conditioning agents – miscellaneous; surfactants – cleansing agents
EU cosmetic restrictions	: Regulated in Annex III/62 of the Regulation (EC) No. 1223/2009
Patch testing	: 5% water (2); 5% water and 5% pet. (1)

CONTACT ALLERGY

Case reports and case series

A young non-atopic woman used a proprietary skin cleanser once daily for three consecutive days. On the third day she developed a pruritic area of dermatitis on the right cheek. Within four hours the eruption had extended to the chin, and within 24 hours it involved the entire face, at which time she stopped using the skin cleanser. At this time she had a weeping eruption around the mouth and severe periorbital edema, and a mildly erythematous papular eruption developed on the extensor surfaces of both forearms. Two weeks after her dermatitis had disappeared on therapy, she applied a moisturizing cream that she had used in the past without difficulty. Within an hour she noticed pruritus and erythema of facial areas on which the cream had been used. Over the next few months similar reactions were noted to occur following the use of various moisturizing lotions and several soaps.

Patch testing was performed with the full-strength proprietary skin cleanser to which the patient attributed her reaction. A severe vesicular eruption spreading several centimeter beyond the area of application was noted. Patch testing with the ingredients of the skin cleanser gave strongly positive reactions TEA-coco hydrolyzed protein at aqueous concentrations of 5% and 50%, but no reactions were observed to the other components. Four healthy controls were negative to these test substances. Further testing was performed with triethanolamine, diethanolamine, monoethanolamine and a variety of protein hydrolysate preparations (1). Positive reactions can be found in the section Cross-reactions, pseudo-cross-reactions and co-reactions below.

Contact allergy to TEA-cocoyl hydrolyzed collagen in non-cosmetic products
One patient reacted to TEA-cocoyl hydrolyzed collagen in an ECG contact gel (3).

Cross-reactions, pseudo-cross-reactions and co-reactions
Sodium cocoyl hydrolyzed collagen; potassium cocoyl hydrolyzed collagen; sodium soy hydrolyzed collagen; potassium undecylenoyl hydrolyzed collagen (1). TEA-oleoyl hydrolyzed collagen ('TEA oleyl polypeptide') (2,3).

Presence in cosmetic products and chemical analyses
In the USA, in April 2017, TEA-cocoyl hydrolyzed collagen was present in 1 of 56,714 cosmetic products of which the composition is known in FDA's Voluntary Cosmetic Registration Program (VCRP) (data obtained from FDA, May 2017). In April 2017, TEA-cocoyl hydrolyzed collagen was present in one of 65,434 cosmetic products of which the composition is known in EWG's Skin Deep Cosmetics Database, USA (http://www.ewg.org/skindeep/).

LITERATURE

1   Emmett EA, Wright RC. Allergic contact dermatitis from TEA-cocohydrolysed protein. Arch Dermatol 1976;112: 1008-1009
2   Dooms-Goossens A, Blockeel I. Allergic contact dermatitis and photoallergic contact dermatitis due to soaps and detergents. Clin Dermatol 1996;14: 67-76
3   Gall H, Rodermund OE. Allergisches Kontaktekzem auf Eiweiss-Fetsäure-Kondensate. Dermatosen 1980;28:19-22

2.447   TEA-PEG-3 COCAMIDE SULFATE

IDENTIFICATION

Description/definition   : TEA-PEG-3 cocamide sulfate is the triethanolamine salt of a mixture of sulfated esters of
                             PEG-3 cocamide
Chemical class(es)   : Alkoxylated amides; alkyl ether sulfates
Chemical/IUPAC name   : Ethanol, 2,2',2''-nitrilotris-, compds. with polyethylene glycol hydrogen sulfate 2-(coco
                             acylamino)ethyl ether
CAS registry number (s)   : 73246-94-3
CIR review(s)   : Int J Toxicol 2013;32(Suppl.1):59-83 (access: www.cir-safety.org/ingredients)
Function(s) in cosmetics   : EU: cleansing; emulsifying; foaming; hydrotrope; surfactant. USA: surfactants -
                             cleansing agents; surfactants - hydrotropes
EU cosmetic restrictions   : Regulated in Annex III/62 of the Regulation (EC) No. 1223/2009
Patch testing   : 1% water (1)

CONTACT ALLERGY

Patch testing in groups of patients
In 2002, in the USA, 12 patients previously reacting to cocamidopropyl betaine (CAPB) were retested with CAPB and with a number of coconut oil derivatives including TEA-PEG-3 cocamide sulfate 10% water (2). Only 3 patients had positive reactions to CAPB on retesting, and all were doubtful. However, there were 5 doubtful reactions to TEA-PEG-3 cocamide sulfate and 2 weak positive reactions. Obviously, this strongly points at irritancy of the test material. Quite curiously, none of 10 controls reacted to the material, and the tests had been performed in a double-blind manner. Nevertheless, the authors also offer the possibility that this 10% water concentration may have been irritant (2).

Case reports and case series
Two patients complained of itchy, burning papules on the scalp after the use of a shampoo, which they suspected to be the cause. The scalp symptoms disappeared after discontinuing the use of the shampoo, and reappeared within a day after renewed use. One of the patients also had face, neck and hand dermatitis related to use of the shampoo. Patch tests with the European standard series and the shampoo 1% in water yielded positive reactions to the shampoos. Later, they were patch tested with the ingredients of the cosmetic products, supplied by the manufacturer and both showed positive reactions to TEA-PEG-3 cocamide sulfate 1% water and cocamidopropyl betaine. Further details are lacking (article only partially accessible on-line) (1).

Cross-reactions, pseudo-cross-reactions and co-reactions
Cocamidopropyl betaine (1)

Presence in cosmetic products and chemical analyses
In the USA, in April 2017, TEA-PEG-3 cocamide sulfate was present in zero of 56,714 cosmetic products of which the composition is known in FDA's Voluntary Cosmetic Registration Program (VCRP) (data obtained from FDA, May 2017). In April 2017, TEA-PEG-3 cocamide sulfate was present in one of 65,434 cosmetic products of which the composition is known in EWG's Skin Deep Cosmetics Database, USA (http://www.ewg.org/skindeep/).

LITERATURE
1   Andersen KE, Roed-Petersen J, Kamp P. Contact allergy related to TEA-PEG-3 cocamide sulfate and
    cocamidopropyl betaine in a shampoo. Contact Dermatitis 1984;11:192
2   Shaffer KK, Jaimes JP, Hordinsky MK, Zielke GR, Warshaw EM. Allergenicity and cross-reactivity of coconut oil
    derivatives: A double-blind randomized controlled pilot study. Dermatitis 2006;17:71-76

2.448   TEA-STEARATE

IDENTIFICATION

Description/definition	: TEA-stearate is the triethanolamine salt of stearic acid that conforms generally to the formula shown below
Chemical class(es)	: Soaps
Chemical/IUPAC name	: Octadecanoate; tris(2-hydroxyethyl)azanium
Other names	: Triethanolamine stearate; stearic acid, compound with 2,2',2''-nitrilotriethanol (1:1)
CAS registry number (s)	: 4568-28-9
EC number(s)	: 224-945-5
CIR review(s)	: J Am Coll Toxicol 1995;14:240-248; Int J Toxicol 2013;32(Suppl.1):59-83 (access: www.cir-safety.org/ingredients)
Function(s) in cosmetics	: EU: cleansing; emulsifying; surfactant. USA: surfactants – cleansing agents; surfactants – emulsifying agents
EU cosmetic restrictions	: Regulated in Annex III/62 of the Regulation (EC) No. 1223/2009
Patch testing	: 5% pet. (3); this test concentration was found to induce irritant reactions in 25% of patients and controls tested in another study (4); a 10% concentration caused 74% irritant reactions and all of 23 individuals had irritant patch test reactions from TEA-stearate 20% pet. (4)
Molecular formula	: $C_{24}H_{51}NO_5$

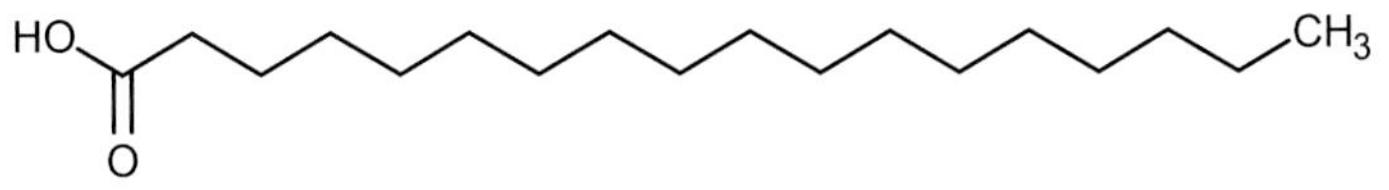

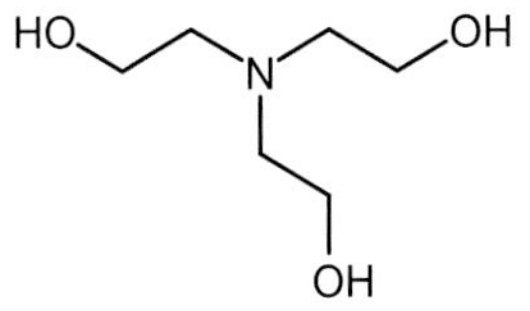

CONTACT ALLERGY

Patch testing in groups of patients

In Finland, in 1972-1974, 412 selected patients (selection criteria not mentioned) were patch tested with triethanolamine stearate 5% pet. and one (0.2%) had a positive reaction; its relevance was not mentioned (3). A patient with leprosy has been described who had an allergic reaction to a moisturizing cream. When patch tested with its ingredients, there was a positive reaction to triethanolamine, and this was, considering the title of the publication, the causative allergen. However, the manufacturer was quoted to state that only 0.5% triethanolamine is used along with stearic acid to neutralize it completely and to form triethanolamine stearate soap which acts as the chief emulsifying agent for the product. Thus, there was no free triethanolamine in the cream (5).

Case reports and case series

TEA-stearate was responsible for 1 out of 399 cases of cosmetic allergy where the causal allergen was identified in a study of the NACDG, USA, 1977-1983 (1). One patient had allergic contact dermatitis from TEA-stearate in a sunscreen (2).

Presence in cosmetic products and chemical analyses

In the USA, in April 2017, TEA-stearate was present in 98 of 56,714 cosmetic products of which the composition is known in FDA's Voluntary Cosmetic Registration Program (VCRP) (data obtained from FDA, May 2017). In April 2017, TEA-stearate was present in 13 of 65,434 cosmetic products of which the composition is known in EWG's Skin Deep Cosmetics Database, USA (http://www.ewg.org/skindeep/).

LITERATURE

1   Adams RM, Maibach HI, Clendenning WE, Fisher AA, Jordan WJ, Kanof N, et al. A five-year study of cosmetic reactions. J Am Acad Dermatol 1985;13:1062-1069
2   Edwards EK Jr, Edwards E K. Allergic reactions to triethanolamine stearate in a sunscreen. Cutis 1983;31:195-196
3   Hannuksela M, Kousa M, Pirilä V. Allergy to ingredients of vehicles. Contact Dermatitis 1976;2:105-110
4   Batten TL, Wakeel RA, Douglas WS, Evans C, White MI, Moody R, Ormerod AD. Contact dermatitis from the old formula E45 cream. Contact Dermatitis 1994;30:159-161
5   Srinivas CR, Padhee A, George ND. Triethanolamine-induced allergic contact dermatitis over a tuberculoid leprosy lesion. Int J Lepr Other Mycobact Dis 1990;58:382-384

2.449   TEREPHTHALYLIDENE DICAMPHOR SULFONIC ACID

IDENTIFICATION

Description/definition   : Terephthalylidene dicamphor sulfonic acid is the organic compound that conforms to the formula shown below
Chemical class(es)   : Sulfonic acids
Chemical/IUPAC name   : 3,3'-(1,4-Phenylenedimethylene)bis[7,7-dimethyl-2-oxo-bicyclo[2.2.1]heptane-1-methanesulfonic acid]
Other names   : Ecamsule
CAS registry number (s)   : 92761-26-7; 90457-82-2
EC number(s)   : 410-960-6
Function(s) in cosmetics   : EU: UV-absorber; UV-filter. USA: light stabilizers
EU cosmetic restrictions   : Regulated in Annex VI/7 of the Regulation (EC) No. 1223/2009
Patch testing   : 10% water (3); a petrolatum-based test material may be preferable
Molecular formula   : $C_{28}H_{34}O_8S_2$

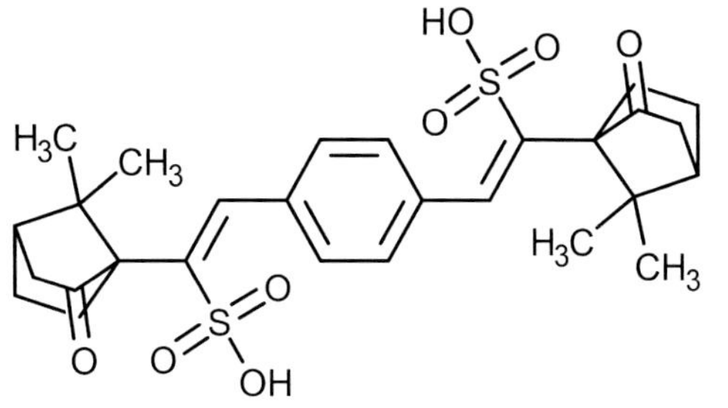

GENERAL

Terephthalylidene dicamphor sulfonic acid is a relatively new UVA filter with UV absorbance maximum (λ_{max}) at 345 nm (6,16,17). The literature on adverse reactions to sunscreens has been reviewed in several recent and older publications (8-13,18). A review of photocontact allergy to sunscreens was published in 2010 (15).

CONTACT ALLERGY

Patch testing in groups of patients

In the period 2008-2011, in 12 European countries, 1031 patients with exposed site dermatitis or history of a reaction to a sunscreen or topical NSAID were patch tested and photopatch tested with terephthalylidene dicamphor sulfonic acid 10% water and there were 4 (0.4%) positive patch test reactions. The relevance of these reactions was not specified (3).

Case reports and case series

Terephthalylidene dicamphor sulfonic acid was responsible for 1 out of 959 cases of non-fragrance cosmetic allergy where the causal allergen was identified, Belgium, 2000-2010 (2).

Presence in cosmetic products and chemical analyses

In the USA, in April 2017, terephthalylidene dicamphor sulfonic acid was present in 3 of 56,714 cosmetic products of which the composition is known in FDA's Voluntary Cosmetic Registration Program (VCRP) (data obtained from FDA, May 2017). In April 2017, terephthalylidene dicamphor sulfonic acid was present in 5 of 66,485 cosmetic products of which the composition is known in EWG's Skin Deep Cosmetics Database, USA (http://www.ewg.org/skindeep/). It should be appreciated that sunscreen products containing UV-filters are classified as drugs in the USA, not as cosmetics; the number mentioned here, therefore, is that of cosmetics containing the UV-filter, but it does *not* include their presence in sunscreens. In 2012, in Switzerland, 116 cosmetics from seven widely used leave-on product categories (19 lip care products, 8 lipsticks, 29 face creams, 11 liquid makeup foundations, 3 aftershaves, 7 hand creams and 39 sunscreens) were investigated to determine the frequency of occurrence and concentrations of 22 organic UV filters in these products. Terephthalylidene dicamphor sulfonic acid was found in 5% of the products in a concentration range of 0.25-1.43%, mean 0.81% (14).

In a sample of 337 sunscreens marketed in the UK in 2010, terephthalylidene dicamphor sulfonic acid was present in 14% (7). Terephthalylidene dicamphor sulfonic acid was present in 6.1% of 4447 cosmetic products collected in Germany, 2006-2009 (4). Terephthalylidene dicamphor sulfonic acid was present in 15% of 329 sunscreen products (incl. 21 lipstick sunscreens) marketed in the UK in 2005 (6). Terephthalylidene dicamphor sulfonic acid and its salts were present in 16 of 75 (21%) sunscreen creams and lotions from 30 European and US producers purchased in Denmark in 2001 in a concentration range of 0.02-3.8% (5).

OTHER SIDE EFFECTS

Photosensitivity

Photopatch test testing in groups of patients
In the period 2008-2011, in 12 European countries, 1031 patients with exposed site dermatitis or history of a reaction to a sunscreen or topical NSAID were patch tested and photopatch tested with terephthalylidene dicamphor sulfonic acid 10% water and there were 4 (0.4%) positive photopatch test reactions. The relevance of these reactions was not specified, but of all photoallergens together, 44% of the positive photopatch tests had current and 11% past relevance (3).

Case reports and case series
One patient had photocontact allergy to terephthalylidene dicamphor sulfonic acid (1, article not read).

LITERATURE

1   Léonard F, Kalis B, Adamski H, et al. The new standard battery for photopatchtests in France. Nouv Dermatol 1996;15:243-248
2   Travassos AR, Claes L, Boey L, Drieghe J, Goossens A. Non-fragrance allergens in specific cosmetic products. Contact Dermatitis 2011;65:276-285
3   The European Multicentre Photopatch Test Study (EMCPPTS) Taskforce. A European multicentre photopatch test study. Br J Dermatol 2012;166:1002-1009
4   Uter W, Gonçalo M, Yazar K, Kratz E-M, Mildau G, Lidén C. Coupled exposure to ingredients of cosmetic products: III. Ultraviolet filters. Contact Dermatitis 2014;71:162-169
5   Rastogi SC. UV filters in sunscreen products – a survey. Contact Dermatitis 2002;46:348-351
6   Wahie S, Lloyd JJ, Farr PM. Sunscreen ingredients and labelling: a survey of products available in the U.K. Clin Exp Dermatol 2007;32:359-364
7   Kerr AC. A survey of the availability of sunscreen filters in the U.K. Clin Exp Dermatol 2011;36:541-543
8   Heurung AR, Raju SI, Warshaw EM. Adverse reactions to sunscreen agents: epidemiology, responsible irritants and allergens, clinical characteristics, and management. Dermatitis 2014;25:289-326
9   Heurung AR, Raju SI, Warshaw EM. Contact allergen of the year. Benzophenones. Dermatitis 2014;25:3-10 (contains many mistakes; Erratum in Dermatitis 2014;25:92-95)
10 Avenel-Audran M. Sunscreen products: finding the allergen. Eur J Dermatol 2010;20:161-166
11 Scheuer E, Warshaw E. Sunscreen allergy: a review of epidemiology, clinical characteristics, and responsible allergens. Dermatitis 2006;17:3-11
12 Funk JO, Dromgoole SH, Maibach HI. Sunscreen intolerance: contact sensitization, photocontact sensitization, and irritancy of sunscreen agents. Dermatol Clin 1995;13:473-481
13 Dromgoole SH, Maibach HI. Sunscreening agent intolerance: Contact and photocontact sensitization and contact urticaria. J Am Acad Dermatol 1990;22:1068-1078
14 Manová E, von Goetz N, Hauri U, Bogdal C, Hungerbühler K. Organic UV filters in personal care products in Switzerland: A survey of occurrence and concentrations. Int J Hyg Environ Health 2013;216:508-514
15 Shaw T, Simpson B, Wilson B, Oostman H, Rainey D, Storrs F. True photoallergy to sunscreens is rare despite popular belief. Dermatitis 2010;21:185-198
16 D'Souza G, Evans GR; Plastic Surgery Educational Foundation Technology Assessment Committee. Mexoryl: a review of an ultraviolet a filter. Plast Reconstr Surg 2007;120:1071-1075
17 Shaath NA. Ultraviolet filters. Photochem Photobiol Sci 2010;9:464-469
18 Schauder S. Survey of the literature on adverse reactions to preparations containing UV filters (1947-1989) (Literaturübersicht über Unverträglichkeitsreaktionen auf lichtfilterhaltige Produkte von 1947 bis 1989). Z Hautkr 1990;65:982-998 (article in German)

2.450   TETRACHLOROSALICYLANILIDES[*]

Not an INCI name

GENERAL INTRODUCTION TO THE HALOGENATED SALICYLANILIDES AND HALOGENATED PHENOLIC COMPOUNDS

In the beginning of the 1960s, the halogenated salicylanilide tetrachlorosalicylanilide caused virtually an epidemic (an estimated 10,000 patients) of photoallergic reactions in the United Kingdom (1,2,9,10,11,12,13,14,15). A number of other halogenated salicylanilides (3,4',5-tribromosalicylanilide, 4',5-dibromosalicylanilide, 5-bromo-4'-chloro-salicylanilide) and related halogenated phenolic compounds (bithionol, fenticlor [see Chapter 2.457 2,2'-Thiobis(4-chlorophenol)], hexachlorophene, dichlorophene) were also incorporated in soaps and other cleansers to combat infection (molds and bacteria), to counter the formation of unpleasant body orders, and to function as preservatives. Some were also used in other products such as cosmetics, antiseptic creams (e.g., hexachlorophene, bithionol) and antifungal creams (e.g., bithionol, 5-bromo-4'-chlorosalicylanilide [Multifungin]). Contact but more often photo-contact allergic reactions, not infrequently with persistent light sensitivity (32), were induced by many of these agents in the UK, Denmark (especially tribromosalicylanilide), Australia and the USA (15) (especially the brominated salicylanilides and bithionol).

Most reactions were caused by tribromosalicylanilide (4,7,8,16,17,20,31,32), dibromosalicylanilide (4,20,21,22, 32) and bithionol (3,4,7,23,24,25,30,31,32). Fewer cases of (photo)sensitization were reported from fenticlor (8,18,26), hexachlorophene (4,7,16,23,25) and dichlorophene (4,27,28,29,32), and rare reactions have been observed to 5-bromo-4'-chlorosalicylanilide (18,33). (Photo)cross-reactions between the different halogenated salicylanilides were very frequent (e.g., 32), between these and bithionol (e.g., 32) and fenticlor common, and were - to a (far) lesser degree – also seen with hexachlorophene and dichlorophene. When assessing the data from these early studies, and notably in the distinction between contact allergy and photocontact allergy, it should be realized that, in those days, experience with photopatch tests was limited and such tests may not always have been reliable.

Since 1968, there has been a rapid reduction in the induction of photoallergic reactions by halogenated salicylanilides and related structures in the USA (34) and other countries, which is likely the result of the removal of the more powerful sensitizers by manufacturers from the market. Tetrachlorosalicylanilide was already withdrawn in 1960 before the epidemic emerged, but the eruptions were mostly caused by products containing tetra-chlorosalicylanilide that had already been sold or were later sold by wholesalers and retailers from their stocks. Bithionol was officially excluded in the USA from incorporation into cosmetic and antibacterial preparations in June 1968. Subsequently, the dibrominated compounds (1972) and tribromosalicylanilide (1974) were eliminated from such use (34).

In the decades following the 1970s, occasional positive photopatch test reactions to the various chemicals discussed here have been observed in routine photopatch testing, some of which were deemed relevant. However, no convincing cases of photoallergic contact dermatitis were presented with the exception of a 1992 report from France, a case of photocontact allergy to fenticlor present in a liquid hand soap used in industry (6).

Currently, the use of the halogenated salicylanilides and bithionol in cosmetics is prohibited in both the USA and the EU. Dichlorophene and fenticlor are still allowed in both the EU and the USA. Hexachlorophene is prohibited in the EU but , under strict provisions, allowed in the US. However, hexachlorophene, dichlorophene nor fenticlor were present in any of 56,714 cosmetic products of which the composition is known in FDA's Voluntary Cosmetic Registration Program (VCRP) in April 2017 (data obtained from FDA, May 2017) nor in any of 64,655 cosmetic products of which the composition is known in EWG's Skin Deep Cosmetics Database, USA (http://www.ewg.org/skindeep/) in 2017.

LITERATURE OF THE GENERAL INTRODUCTION

1   Wilkinson DS. Photodermatitis due to tetrachlorsalicylanilide. Br J Dermatol 1961;73:213-219
2   Calnan CD. Photo-contact dermatitis from soaps. J Soc Cosmet Chem 1962;13:187-192
3   Epstein S. Photocontact dermatitis from bithionol. Arch Dermatol 1965;92:591
4   Epstein JH, Wuepper KD, Maibach HI. Photocontact dermatitis to halogenated salicylanilides and related compounds: A clinical and histologic review of 26 patients. Arch Dermatol 1968;97:236-244
5   Horio T. Actinic reticuloid via persistent light reaction from photoallergic contact dermatitis. Arch Dermatol 1982;118:339-342
6   Jeanmougin M, Manciet JR, Dubertret L. Photoallergie de contact au Fenticlor present dans un savon d'hygiene pour les mains. Ann Dermatol Venereol 1992;119:983-985 (article in French)
7   Freeman RG, Knox JM. The action spectrum of photocontact dermatitis caused by halogenated salicylanilide and related compounds. Arch Dermatol 1968;97:130-136
8   Osmundsen PE. Contact photodermatitis due to tribromsalicylanilide. Br J Dermatol 1968;80:228-234
9   Anderson I. Photodermatitis due to toilet soap. Trans St John's Hosp Derm Soc 1963;49:54

10 Calnan CD, Harmon BRM, Wells GC. Photodermatitis from soap. Brit Med J 1961;11:1266

11 Wilkinson DS. Further experiences with halogenated salicylanilides. Br J Dermatol 1962;74:245-301

12 Calnan CD. Photodermatitis due to tetrachlorsalicylanilide. Proc R Soc Med 1961;54:819-820

13 Wells GC, Harman RR. Two cases of photodermatitis due to tetrachlorsalicylanilide. Proc R Soc Med 1961;54:819

14 Wilkinson DS. Two cases of photodermatitis due to tetrachlorsalicylanilide (TCSA). Proc R Soc Med 1961;54:817-818

15 Burry JN. The hazards of modern soap: a review of photo-contact dermatitis from halogenated phenolic compounds in the United Kingdom, the United States of America, Denmark and Australia Med J Aust 1968;35:1114-1115

16 Burry JN, Donald GF. Photo-contact dermatitis from soap. Br J Dermatol 1968;80:711-718

17 Osmundsen PE. Photocontact dermatitis caused by tribromosalicylanilide in toilet soap. Ugeskr Laeger 1967;129:1607-1610 (article in Danish).

18 Burry J. Photoallergies to fenticlor and multifungin. Arch Dermatol 1967;95:287-291

19 Burry JN. Photo-allergic contact dermatitis from halogenated phenolic compounds. Australas J Dermatol 1967;9:142-149

20 Epstein S. Photosensitizers in soaps. JAMA 1966;195:878

21 Molloy JF, Mayer JA. Photodermatitis from dibromsalan. Arch Dermatol 1966;93:329-331

22 Behrbohm P, Schzunke E. Arbeitsbedingtes Ekzem durch 5,4'-Dibromsalicylanilid in Haarkosmetische Präparaten. Berufsdermatosen 1966;14:169 (article in German)

23 Gaul LE. Sensitivity to bithionol. Arch Dermatol 1960;81:600

24 Gaul LE. Sensitivity to bithionol. Arch Dermatol 1963;87:383

25 O'Quinn S, Kennedy D, Isbell K. Contact photodermatitis due to bithionol and related compounds. JAMA 1967;199:89-92

26 Ramsay CA, Crow KD. Personal communication, cited in: Burry JN. Fenticlor, actinic reticuloid, and antihistamines. Br Med J 1974;2(5918):556-557

27 Schorr WF. Dichlorophene (G-4) allergy. Arch Dermatol 1970;102;515-520

28 Gaul LE, Underwood GB. The cutaneous toxicity of dihydroxydichlordiphenylmethane: A new fungicide for athlete's foot. J Indiana Med Assoc 1949;42:22-24

29 Epstein E. Dichlorophene allergy. Ann Allergy 1966;24:437-439

30 Baughman RD. Contact photodermatitis from bithionol. II. Cross-sensitivities to hexachlorophene and salicylanilides. Arch Dermatol 1964;90:153-157

31 Harber LC, Harris H, Baer RL. Photoallergic contact dermatitis due to halogenated salicylanilides and related compounds. Arch Dermatol 1966;94:255-262

32 Harber LC, Targovnik SE, Baer RL. Contact photosensitivity patterns to halogenated salicylanilides in man and guinea pigs. Arch Dermatol 1967;96:646-656

33 Buckley DB. Allergic contact dermatitis to bromsalicylchloranilide. Contact Dermatitis 1986;14:319

34 Smith SZ, Epstein JH. Photocontact dermatitis to halogenated salicylanilides and related compounds. Our experience between 1967 and 1975. Arch Dermatol 1977;113:1372-1374

3,3',4',5-TETRACHLOROSALICYLANILIDE[*]

Not an INCI name

IDENTIFICATION

Description/definition	: 3,3',4',5-Tetrachlorosalicylanilide is the chlorinated aromatic amide that conforms to the structural formula shown below
Chemical class(es)	: Organochlorine compounds; aromatic compounds; amides
INCI name USA	: Neither in CosIng nor in the Personal Care Products Council Ingredient Database
Chemical/IUPAC name	: 3,5-Dichloro-N-(3,4-dichlorophenyl)-2-hydroxybenzamide
Other names	: 3,5-Dichlorosalicyl 3,4-dichloroanilide
CAS registry number (s)	: **1154-59-2**
EC number(s)	: 214-576-8
Merck Index monograph	: 10606
Function(s) in cosmetics	: EU: 'tetrachlorosalicylanilides' are prohibited since 1976; formerly used as antimicrobials, especially in the UK
EU cosmetic restrictions	: Regulated in Annex II/348 of the Regulation (EC) No. 1223/2009 (prohibited)
USA cosmetic restrictions	: Prohibited (FDA)
Patch testing	: 0.1% pet. (Chemotechnique)
Molecular formula	: $C_{13}H_7Cl_4NO_2$

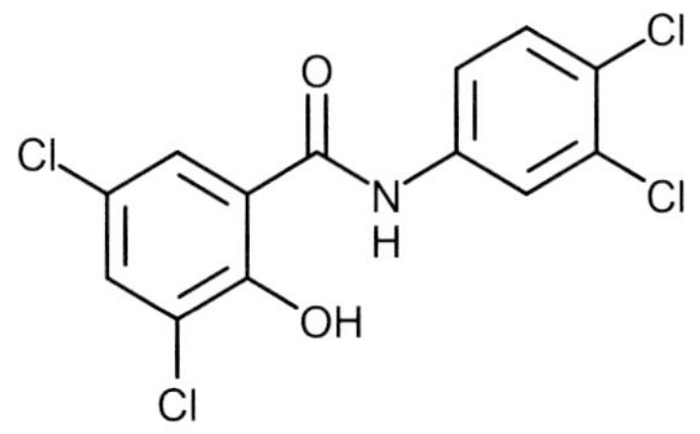

TETRACHLOROSALICYLANILIDE[*]

Not an INCI name

IDENTIFICATION

Description/definition	: Tetrachlorosalicylanilide is the chlorinated aromatic amide that conform to the structural formula shown below
Chemical class(es)	: Organochlorine compounds; aromatic compounds; amides
INCI name USA	: Neither in CosIng nor in the Personal Care Products Council Ingredient Database
Chemical/IUPAC name	: 2,3,4,5-Tetrachloro-6-hydroxy-N-phenylbenzamide
CAS registry number (s)	: 7426-07-5
Merck Index monograph	: 9191
Function(s) in cosmetics	: EU: 'tetrachlorosalicylanilides' are prohibited since 1976; formerly used as antimicrobials, especially in the UK
EU cosmetic restrictions	: Regulated in Annex II/348 of the Regulation (EC) No. 1223/2009 (prohibited)
USA cosmetic restrictions	: Prohibited (FDA)
Patch testing	: 0.1%-1% alc. or pet.
Molecular formula	: $C_{13}H_7Cl_4NO_2$

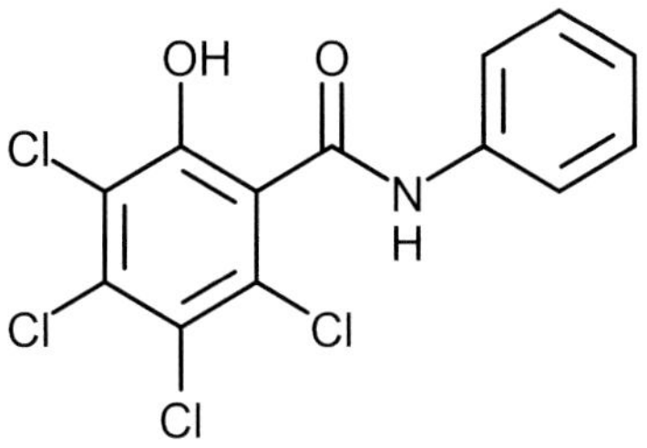

GENERAL

Tetrachlorosalicylanilide (TCSA) is a halogenated salicylanilide which was widely used in the late 1950s and early 1960s as an antimicrobial agent in germicidal soaps, especially in the United Kingdom, where it was responsible for an estimated 10,000 cases of photocontact allergy. The TCSA had already been replaced in the soap before the 'epidemic' was discovered, but the eruptions were caused by soaps containing TCSA that had already been sold or were in stock with wholesalers and retailers at that time and were sold afterwards (20). The United States Food and Drug Administration (FDA) prohibited the use of halogenated salicylanilides in cosmetics 1975 (35) and one year later it was banned in Europe. It may be assumed that tetrachlorosalicylanilide is not in use anymore.

A general introduction to the halogenated salicylanilides and related chemicals (halogenated phenols) is described above (see 'General introduction to halogenated salicylanilides and related chemicals'). In assessing the data from early studies, and notably in the distinction between contact allergy and photocontact allergy, it should be realized that, in those days, experience with photopatch tests was limited and such tests may not always have been reliable.

CONTACT ALLERGY

Patch testing in groups of patients

There are no studies in which tetrachlorosalicylanilide (TCSA) has been tested in consecutive patients suspected of contact dermatitis (routine testing). Results of patch testing TCSA in groups of *selected* patients (patients suspected of photosensitivity) are shown in table 2.450.1. In four studies, rates of positive reactions ranged from 0.5% to 1.1%. No relevant reactions were reported (6,8,11,12).

Table 2.450.1 Patch testing in groups of patients: Selected patient groups

Years and Country	Test conc. & vehicle	Number of patients tested	positive (%)	Selection of patients (S); Relevance (R); Comments (C)	Ref.
2005-2014 China	0.1% pet.	5031	53 (1.1%)	S: patients suspected of photodermatoses; R: not stated	6
2000-2005 USA	1% pet.	179	1 (0.6%)	S: patients photopatch tested for suspected photodermatitis; R: not relevant	12
1985-1990 USA	1% pet.	176	1 (0.6%)	S: patients with a history of photosensitivity; R: not relevant	8
1980-1981 4 Scandinavian countries	0.1% pet.	745	4 (0.5%)	S: patients suspected of sun-related skin disease; R: not stated	11

Case reports and case series

In the last two months of 1960 and the beginning of 1961, a dermatologist in Buckinghamshire, UK, saw 53 cases of acute photodermatitis of the face, neck and sometimes the backs of the hands, which was attributed to tetrachlorosalicylanilide in soap. Twenty-four of these were seen in hospital and 29 occurred in a factory, where workers were heavy users of the soap because of dirty work. Patch tests were performed with TCSA 0.1% -1% in 22 patients and were positive in 19. Few photopatch tests were performed; no negative reactions in patch tests became positive in the photopatch test. In a postscript, the author mentioned having seen 11 new cases. The TCSA had already been replaced in the soap before the 'epidemic' was discovered, but the eruptions were caused by soaps containing TCSA that had been sold already or were in stock with wholesalers and retailers at that time and were sold afterwards (20). Another 50 patients with photodermatitis caused by TSCA in soaps were seen by the same author up to April 1962. Some 75% had contact allergy to TCSA and 25% photocontact allergy (26).

In 1960 and 1961, in a center in London, UK, patch tests were performed on 102 patients (87 men and 15 women) with the clinical picture of soap photodermatitis. Ninety gave positive patch tests and 12 were negative. About 1/3 had plain contact allergy and 2/3 photocontact allergy. In most, the eruption subsided when the soap was avoided, but some became persistent light reactors (25). Later, some authors have assumed that these positive conventional patch tests in photosensitive individuals were actually so-called "masked" photopatch tests in which the test site received a sufficient quantity of light during application of the patch, through the patch itself, or during removal of the patch to cause a reaction (22,23). Indeed, the author of the original publication (20) later found that some patients only reacted to photopatch tests (26) and stated that 'There is some evidence, that the strength of the reaction is determined by the presence of light at the time of application of the test' (27). However, other authors have disputed the concept of 'masked photopatch tests' (28). Probably, there were cases of contact allergy, photocontact allergy and photoaggravated contact allergy.

Tetrachlorosalicylanilide was responsible for 1 out of 399 cases of cosmetic allergy where the causal allergen was identified in a study of the NACDG, USA, 1977-1983 (1).

Cross-reactions, pseudo-cross-reactions and co-reactions (also photoreactions)

(Photo)cross-reactions from tetrachlorosalicylanilide

Patients with photosensitization to tetrachlorosalicylanilide may photocross-react to tribromosalicylanilide (20,26, 27,30; frequent), dibromosalicylanilide (26,27), bithionol (30) and hexachlorophene (photocross-reaction: 27,30; plain contact allergy cross-reaction: 4 [both infrequent]). Photocross-reactions have also been observed to 5-chlorosalicylic acid (27), 3,5-dibromo-3',4'-dichlorosalicylanilide (19), 3,4-dichloroaniline (27), 3,5-dichlorosalicylic acid (28), 3,3',4',5-tetrabromosalicylanilide (19), 3,3',5-tribromosalicylanilide (19), trichlorosalicylanilide (27), 3,3',5-trichlorosalicylanilide (19), and 3,4',5-trichlorosalicylanilide (19). No photocross-reactivity and limited contact allergic cross-sensitivity to triclocarban from primary halogenated salicylanilides photosensitization (4).

(Photo)cross-reactions to tetrachlorosalicylanilide

Primary photosensitization to tribromosalicylanilide almost invariably leads to TCSA photo-cross-reactivity and in 50% to plain TCSA contact allergy (16, 21). (Photo)cross-reactions from dibromosalicylanilide to TCSA may be observed (21). Many patients with photocontact allergy to bithionol have photocross-sensitivity (and some plain contact allergic cross-sensitivity) to tetrachlorosalicylanilide (24). In a group of 18 patients photosensitized to ketoprofen, 5 (28%) had positive photopatch tests to tetrachlorosalicylanilide. As there were also many photoreactions to fenticlor (n=12, 67%) (see Chapter 2.457 2,2'-Thiobis(4-chlorophenol)), tribromosalicylanilide (n=2, 11%), triclosan (n=3, 17%), and bithionol (n=2, 11%) with no clinical relevance, the authors raised the question of hyperphotosusceptibility to non-relevant photoallergens induced by photosensitivity to ketoprofen (32). In another group of 35 patients photoallergic to ketoprofen from Sweden, simultaneous photoallergy to tetrachlorosalicylanilide was seen in 40%, to fenticlor in 74%, to triclosan in 9% and to bithionol, tribromosalicylanilide and hexachlorophene in 6% of the patients. No explanation for these co-reactivities was offered (33). In a French study, of 11 patients with photocontact allergy to ketoprofen, 9 had positive photopatch tests to fenticlor and 4 to tetrachlorosalicylanilide (34).

Presence in cosmetic products and chemical analyses

In May 2017, tetrachlorosalicylanilide was present in zero of 66,975 cosmetic products of which the composition is known in EWG's Skin Deep Cosmetics Database, USA (http://www.ewg.org/skindeep/). In the USA, in April 2017, tetrachlorosalicylanilides was present in zero of 56,714 cosmetic products of which the composition is known in FDA's Voluntary Cosmetic Registration Program (VCRP) (data obtained from FDA, May 2017).

OTHER SIDE EFFECTS

Photosensitivity

Photopatch testing in groups of patients

Results of photopatch testing with tetrachlorosalicylanilide in groups of selected patients (e.g., patients suspected of photosensitivity, patients with persistent light reaction, patients with an eruption involving sun-exposed areas) are shown in table 2.450.2. In 13 studies, rates of photosensitization have ranged from 0.4% to 22%, but were 3% or less in 10 of the thirteen investigations (table 2.450.2). The highest frequencies were found in a very small study of 18 patients with persistent light reactions (10) and in an older study from the USA, when TCSA may have been in use there (31; probably most, if not all, positive photopatch tests were photocross-reactions to tribromosalicylanilide). Only two reactions have been scored as relevant (12); in 12 of the 13 studies, relevance was either not mentioned or not specified for tetrachlorosalicylanilide.

Table 2.450.2 Patch testing in groups of patients: Selected patient groups

Years and Country	Test conc. & vehicle	Number of patients tested | positive (%)		Selection of patients (S); Relevance (R); Comments (C)	Ref.
2005-2014 China	0.1% pet.	5031	113 (2.3%)	S: patients suspected of photodermatoses; R: not stated	6
2006-2012 China	0.1% pet	3717	72 (1.9%)	S: patients with suspected photodermatoses; R: not stated	5
1992-2006 Greece	0.1% pet.	207	2 (1.0%)	S: patients suspected of photosensitivity; R: not stated	13
2000-2005 USA	1% pet.	179	4 (2.2%)	S: patients photopatch tested for suspected photodermatitis; R: 2 reactions were relevant	12
1994-1999 NL	0.1% pet.	55	1 (2%)	S: patients suspected of photosensitivity disorders; R: not stated	15
1991-97 Ger, Au, Swi	0.1% pet.	1261	(0.4%)	S: patients suspected of photosensitivity; R: not stated	14
1985-1994 Italy		1050	11 (1.0%)	S: patients with histories or clinical pictures suggestive of allergic contact photodermatitis; R: 78% for all photoallergens together	2
1991-1993 Singapore	0.1% pet.	62	2 (3%)	S: patients with clinical features suggestive of photosensitivity; R: not stated	7
1980-85 Ger, Au, Swi	2% pet.	1129	6 (0.5%)	S: patients suspected of photoallergy, polymorphic light eruption, phototoxicity and skin problems with photodistribution; R: not stated	3
1980-1985 USA	1% pet.	70	3 (4%)	S: not stated; R: not stated	9
<1984 Norway	0.1% pet.	18	4 (22%)	S: patients with persistent light reactions; R: not stated	10
1980-1981 4 Scandinavian countries	0.1% pet.	745	4 (0.5%)	S: patients suspected of sun-related skin disease; R: not stated	11
1967-1975 USA		239	34 (14.2%)	S: patients with a history suggestive of a photosensitivity problem or an eruption involving sun-exposed areas; R: not stated	31

AU: Austria; Ger: Germany; NL: Netherlands; Swi: Switzerland

Case reports and case series

Approximately 50 (additional, see ref. 20) patients with photodermatitis caused by TSCA in soaps were seen in Buckinghamshire, UK, up to April 1962. Some 75% had contact allergy to TCSA and 25% photocontact allergy (26). Of 19 patients with the clinical picture of soap photocontact dermatitis (mostly sharply demarcated erythematous and lichenoid eruption limited to sun-exposed areas of the body, such as the face, neck, hands, and forearms), 16 photoreacted to tetrachlorosalicylanilide. Most patients had a definite history of exposure to a soap containing the offending photosensitizing agent (17).

In a period of 1.5 year (1966-1967), in a university center in San Francisco, USA, 26 patients suspected of photosensitivity were investigated with photopatch tests with halogenated salicylanilides and related compounds.

TCSA was the most frequent photosensitizer (21/22 tested), followed by bithionol (10/26), tribromosalicylanilide (9/22), hexachlorophene (n=4), triclocarban (n=3) and dichlorophene (n=3). Six patients became persistent light reactors. The relevance of the reactions was not specified. In fact, the authors stated that it was generally impossible to determine which was the original photosensitizer and which positive photopatch tests were the result of photocross-sensitivity (18).

In 1960 and 1961, in a center in London, UK, patch tests were performed on 102 patients (87 men and 15 women) with the clinical picture of soap photodermatitis. Ninety gave positive patch tests and 12 were negative. About 1/3 had plain contact allergy and 2/3 photocontact allergy. In most, the eruption subsided when the soap was avoided, but some became persistent light reactors (25). Eight individuals suffered from photoallergic contact dermatitis from tetrachlorosalicylanilide in soap bars (19). One patient had photocontact dermatitis from TCSA in soap (29).

LITERATURE

1   Adams RM, Maibach HI, Clendenning WE, Fisher AA, Jordan WJ, Kanof N, et al. A five-year study of cosmetic reactions. J Am Acad Dermatol 1985;13:1062-1069

2   Pigatto PD, Legori A, Bigardi AS, Guarrera M, Tosti A, Santucci B, et al. Gruppo Italiano recerca dermatiti da contatto ed ambientali Italian multicenter study of allergic contact photodermatitis: epidemiological aspects. Am J Contact Dermatitis 1996;17:158-163

3   Hölzle E, Neumann N, Hausen B, Przybilla B, Schauder S, Hönigsmann H, et al. Photopatch testing: the 5-year experience of the German, Austrian and Swiss Photopatch Test Group. J Am Acad Dermatol 1991;25:59-68

4   Harber LC, Targovnik SE, Baer RL. Studies on contact photosensitivity to hexachlorophene and trichlorocarbanilide in guinea pigs and man. J Invest Dermatol 1968; 51:373-377

5   Gao L, Hu Y, Ni C, Xu Y, Ma L, Yan S, Dou X. Retrospective study of photopatch testing in a Chinese population during a 7-year period. Dermatitis 2014;25:22-26

6   Hu Y, Wang D, Shen Y, Tang H. Photopatch testing in Chinese patients over 10 years. Dermatitis 2016;27:137-142

7   Leow YH, Wong WK, Ng SK, Goh CL. 2 years experience of photopatch testing in Singapore. Contact Dermatitis 1994;31:181-182

8   DeLeo VA, Suarez SM, Maso MJ. Photoallergic contact dermatitis. Results of photopatch testing in New York, 1985 to 1990. Arch Dermatol 1992;128:1513-1518

9   Menz J, Muller SA, Connolly SM. Photopatch testing: a 6-year experience. J Am Acad Dermatol 1988;18:1044-1047

10 Thune P, Eeg-Larsen T. Contact and photocontact allergy in persistent light reactivity. Contact Dermatitis 1984;11:98-107

11 Wennersten G, Thune P, Brodthagen H, Jansen C, Rystedt I, Crames M, et al. The Scandinavian multicenter photopatch study. Contact Dermatitis 1984;10:305-309

12 Scalf LA, Davis MDP, Rohlinger AL, Connolly SM. Photopatch testing of 182 patients: A 6-year experience at the Mayo Clinic. Dermatitis 2009;20:44-52

13 Katsarou A, Makris M, Zarafonitis G, Lagogianni E, Gregoriou S, Kalogeromitros D. Photoallergic contact dermatitis: the 15-year experience of a tertiary referral center in a sunny Mediterranean city. Int J Immunopathol Pharmacol 2008;21:725-727

14 Neumann NJ, Hölzle E, Plewig G, Schwarz T, Panizzon RG, Breit R, et al. Photopatch testing: The 12-year experience of the German, Austrian and Swiss Photopatch Test Group. J Am Acad Dermatol 2000;42:183-192

15 Bakkum RS, Heule F. Results of photopatch testing in Rotterdam during a 10-year period. Br J Dermatol 2002;146:275-279

16 Osmundsen PE. Contact photodermatitis due to tribromsalicylanilide. Br J Dermatol 1968;80:228-234

17 Freeman RG, Knox JM. The action spectrum of photocontact dermatitis caused by halogenated salicylanilide and related compounds. Arch Dermatol 1968;97:130-136

18 Epstein JH, Wuepper KD, Maibach HI. Photocontact dermatitis to halogenated salicylanilides and related compounds: A clinical and histologic review of 26 patients. Arch Dermatol 1968;97:236-244

19 Vinson LJ, Flatt RS. Photosensitization by tetrachlorosalicylanilide. J Invest Dermatol 1962;38:327-328

20 Wilkinson DS. Photodermatitis due to tetrachlorsalicylanilide. Br J Dermatol 1961;73:213-219

21 Epstein S. Photosensitizers in soaps. JAMA 1966;195:878

22 Epstein S. "Masked" photopatch tests. J Invest Dermatol 1963;41:369-370

23 Anderson I. Photodermatitis due to toilet soap. Trans St. John Hosp Derm Soc 1963;49:54

24 Baughman RD. Contact photodermatitis from bithionol. II. Cross-sensitivities to hexachlorophene and salicylanilides. Arch Dermatol 1964;90:153-157

25 Calnan CD, Harmon BRM, Wells GC. Photodermatitis from soap. Brit Med J 1961;2(5262):1266

26   Wilkinson DS. Further experiences with halogenated salicylanilides. Br J Dermatol 1962;74:295-301

27   Wilkinson DS. Patch test reactions to certain halogenated salicylanilides. Br J Dermatol 1962;74:302-306

28 Harber LC, Harris H, Baer RL. Photoallergic contact dermatitis due to halogenated salicylanilides and related compounds. Arch Dermatol 1966;94:255-262

29 Epstein S. Photocontact dermatitis from TCSA (tetrachlorosalicylanilide) and chlorpromazine. Arch Dermatol 1965;92:591

30 Crow KD, Wilkinson DS, Osmundsen PE. A review of photoreactions to halogenated salicylanilides. Br J Dermatol 1969;81:180-185

31 Smith SZ, Epstein JH. Photocontact dermatitis to halogenated salicylanilides and related compounds. Our experience between 1967 and 1975. Arch Dermatol 1977;113:1372-1374

32 Durbize E, Vigan M, Puzenat E, Girardin P, Adessi B, Desprez PH, Humbert PH, Laurent R, Aubin F. Spectrum of cross-photosensitization in 18 consecutive patients with contact photoallergy to ketoprofen: associated photoallergies to non-benzophenone-containing molecules. Contact Dermatitis 2003;48:144-149

33 Hindsén M, Zimerson E, Bruze M. Photoallergic contact dermatitis from ketoprofen in southern Sweden. Contact Dermatitis 2006;54:150-157

34 Vigan M, Girardin P, Desprez P, Adessi B, Aubin F, Laurent R. Photoallergie au kétoprofène et photosensibilisations au tétrachlorosalicylanide et au Fentichlor. Ann Dermatol Venereol 2002;129:1125-1127 (a

35 Wolverton JE, Soter NA, Cohen DE. Fentichlor photocontact dermatitis: A persistent enigma. Dermatitis 2013;24:77-81

2.451   TETRAHYDROCURCUMIN

GENERAL

There are two case reports that may relate to contact allergy to tetrahydrocurcumin (1,2). In one (2), the allergen was termed 'tetrahydrocurcuminoid', despite the fact that the authors used the word tetrahydrocurcumin in the title of their article and they show a structural formula of 'tetrahydrocurcuminoid' that of tetrahydrocurcumin as identified in ChemIDplus, CAS 36062-04-1; http://chem.sis.nlm.nih.gov/chemidplus/rn/36062-04-1) (an extra methyl group was added in the article, but that was most likely a mistake).

In the other case report (1), the term tetrahydracurcumin is used, which appears not to exist. These authors state: 'Tetrahydracurcumin is a colourless hydrogenated derivative of the natural yellow curcuminoids, which are extracts of the root of the *Curcuma longa* plant also known as turmeric. It appears in cosmetic products as its three sub-ingredients: tetrahydrodiferuloylmethane, tetrahydrodemethoxycurcumin, and tetrahydrobisdemethoxycurcumin (1).

Tetrahydrocurcumin itself is not present in CosIng (INCI EU) or of the Personal Care Products Council (INCI USA), only its diacetate. However, the abovementioned chemicals are present in CosIng under their INCI names: tetrahydrodiferuloylmethane, tetrahydrodemethoxydiferuloylmethane and tetrahydrobisdemethoxydiferuloylmethane (diferuloylmethane = curcumin). Also, in the Personal Care Products Council a commercial product 'Tetrahydrocurcuminoids GC' was found, that is composed of these same ingredients: (http://online.personal carecouncil.org/jsp/ MixtureDetailPage.jsp?ID=378725&type=M; subscription only). Some information on these chemicals is given below. What the exact contact allergen has been in the two case reports remains unknown (1,2). The same goes for the exact nature of the patch test materials ('tetrahydrocurcumin'; 'tetrahydrocurcuminoid'), which were both tested at 1% in petrolatum (1,2).

TETRAHYDRODIFERULOYLMETHANE

IDENTIFICATION

Description/definition	: Tetrahydrodiferuloylmethane is the organic compound that conforms to the formula shown below
Chemical class(es)	: Ethers; ketones
Chemical/IUPAC name	: 1,7-Bis(4-hydroxy-3-methoxyphenyl)heptane-3,5-dione
Other names	: Tetrahydrocurcumin; 3,5-Heptanedione, 1,7-bis(4-hydroxy-3-methoxyphenyl)
CAS registry number (s)	: 36062-04-1
Function(s) in cosmetics	: EU: antioxidant. USA: antioxidants
Patch testing	: Tetrahydrocurcumin 1% pet. (1)
Molecular formula	: $C_{21}H_{24}O_6$

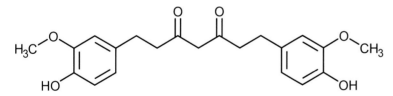

TETRAHYDRODEMETHOXYDIFERULOYLMETHANE

IDENTIFICATION

Description/definition	: Tetrahydrodemethoxydiferuloylmethane is the organic compound that conforms to the formula shown below
Chemical class(es)	: Ethers; ketones; phenols
Chemical/IUPAC name	: 1-(4-Hydroxy-3-methoxyphenyl)-7-(4-hydroxyphenyl)heptane-3,5-dione
Other names	: Tetrahydrodemethoxycurcumin
CAS registry number (s)	: 149579-07-7
Function(s) in cosmetics	: EU: antioxidant; oral care; skin conditioning. USA: antioxidants; oral care agents; skin-conditioning agents - miscellaneous
Patch testing	: Tetrahydrocurcumin 1% pet. (1)
Molecular formula	: $C_{20}H_{22}O_5$

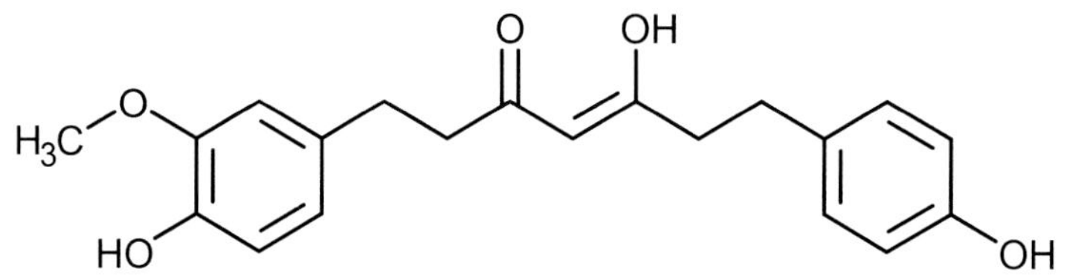

TETRAHYDROBISDEMETHOXYDIFERULOYLMETHANE

IDENTIFICATION

Description/definition   : Tetrahydrobisdemethoxydiferuloylmethane is the organic compound that conforms to the formula shown below
Chemical class(es)   : Ketones; phenols
Chemical/IUPAC name   : 1,7-Bis(4-hydroxyphenyl)heptane-3,5-dione
Other names   : Tetrahydrobisdemethoxycurcumin
CAS registry number (s)   : 113482-94-3
Function(s) in cosmetics   : EU: antioxidant; oral care; skin conditioning. USA: antioxidants; oral care agents; skin-conditioning agents - miscellaneous
Patch testing   : Tetrahydrocurcumin 1% pet. (1)
Molecular formula   : $C_{19}H_{20}O_4$

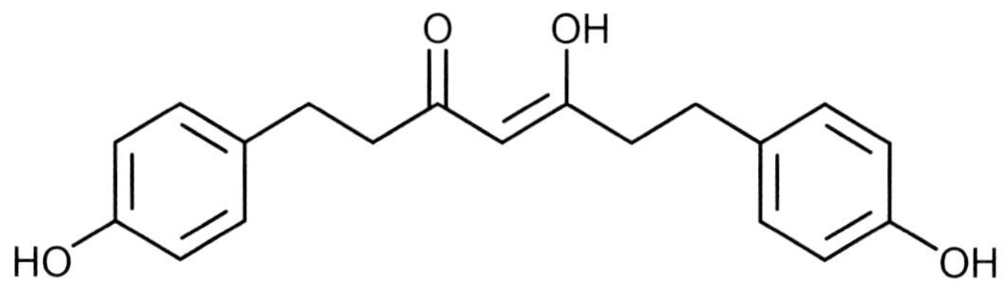

CONTACT ALLERGY

Case reports and case series
A woman presented with a 12-month history of intermittent episodes of swelling of the face and the eyelids associated with a red, scaly, itchy rash that lasted for 2 weeks on each occasion. She only used a cosmetic 'age block cream'. Patch testing with the European standard series and her own products gave a positive reaction to the cosmetic product, tested 'as is', at D2 and D4. Later, the 26 ingredients of the product, obtained from the manufacturer, were tested separately, and the patient now reacted to the compound tetrahydracurcumin (should be tetrahydrocurcumin) 1% pet. All other ingredients were negative. Ten controls had no reaction to the patch test material. After discontinuing the use of the age block cream, the patient had not had any skin reactions anymore (1).

Another female patient developed an eczematous reaction to the same cosmetic product as used by the previous patient. Open application on her arm with the same cream caused a similar response. Patch tests with the British standard series and a facial series were negative, but the sunblock cream itself gave a positive reaction at D2 and D4. Ten controls were negative to the cream. Later, the individual ingredients of the cream were patch tested, and the patient now reacted to 'tetrahydrocurcuminoid' 1% pet. at D2 and D4; none of the other ingredients gave a positive reaction. The tetrahydrocurcuminoid patch test material was tested in 20 controls, who all showed negative results (2).

Contact allergy to tetrahydrocurcumin in non-cosmetic products
Some cases of allergic contact dermatitis *from the related* curcumin have been reported among workers who dye animal furs (8), in a worker at a pasta factory (5), in an Indian spice miller (3), from use of the Chinese herbal cream Chuu-ou-kou (4) and from the use of yellow chlorhexidine solution (6). These are merely some examples, not a full review has been performed.

Presence in cosmetic products and chemical analyses
In the USA, in April 2017, tetrahydrocurcumin was present in 3 of 56,714 cosmetic products of which the composition is known in FDA's Voluntary Cosmetic Registration Program (VCRP) (data obtained from FDA, May 2017). In April 2017, tetrahydrocurcumin was present in 3, tetrahydrodiferuloylmethane in 8, tetrahydrode-

methoxydiferuloylmethane in 5 and tetrahydrobisdemethoxydiferuloylmethane in 5 of 66,485 cosmetic products of which the composition is known in EWG's Skin Deep Cosmetics Database, USA (http://www.ewg.org/skindeep/).

OTHER SIDE EFFECTS

Immediate-type reactions
Two patients had contact urticaria from *the related* curcumin. They both had positive prick tests. For some mysterious reason, one of the reactions was considered to be non-immunological and the other immunological (7).

LITERATURE

1   Thompson DA, Tan BB. Tetrahydracurcumin-related allergic contact dermatitis. Contact Dermatitis 2006;55:254-255

2   Lamb SR, Wilkinson SM. Contact allergy to tetrahydrocurcumin. Contact Dermatitis 2003;48:227

3   Goh CL, Ng SK. Allergic contact dermatitis to *Curcuma longa* (turmeric). Contact Dermatitis 1987;17:186

4   Hata M, Sasaki E, Ota M, Fujimoto K, Yajima J. Shichida T, Honda M. Allergic contact dermatitis from curcumin (turmeric). Contact Dermatitis 1997;36:107-108

5   Kiec-Swierczynska M, Krecisz B. Occupational allergic contact dermatitis due to curcumin food colour in a pasta factory worker. Contact Dermatitis 1998;39:30-31

6   Fischer LA, Agner T. Curcumin allergy in relation to yellow chlorhexidine solution used for skin disinfection prior to surgery. Contact Dermatitis 2004;51:39-40

7   Liddle M, Hull C, Liu C, Douglas P. Contact urticaria from curcumin. Dermatitis 2006;17:196-197

8   Swartz L, Tulipan L, Birmingham DJ. Occupational diseases of the skin. Philadelphia: Lea & Febiger; 1957: 472

2.452 TETRAHYDROFURFURYL METHACRYLATE

IDENTIFICATION

Description/definition	: Tetrahydrofurfuryl methacrylate is the heterocyclic compound that conforms to the formula shown below
Chemical class(es)	: Esters; heterocyclic compounds
Chemical/IUPAC name	: Oxolan-2-ylmethyl 2-methylprop-2-enoate
Other names	: 2-Propenoic acid, 2-methyl-, (tetrahydro-2-furanyl)methyl ester
CAS registry number (s)	: 2455-24-5
EC number(s)	: 219-529-5
CIR review(s)	: Int J Toxicol 2005;24(Suppl.5):53-100 (access: www.cir-safety.org/ingredients)
Function(s) in cosmetics	: EU: film forming. USA: film formers
Patch testing	: 2% pet. (Chemotechnique, SmartPracticeEurope, SmartPracticeCanada)
Molecular formula	: $C_9H_{14}O_3$

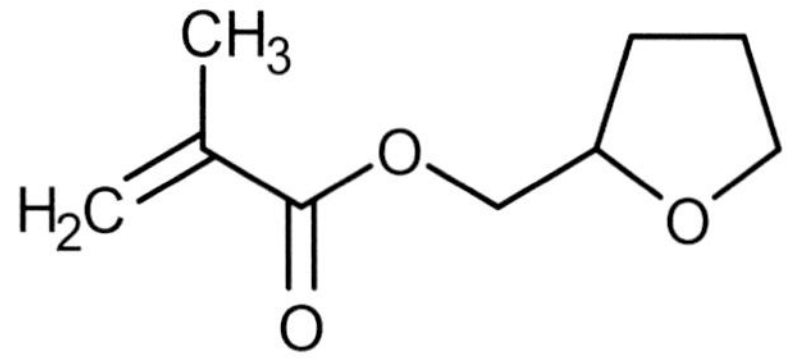

GENERAL

Discussion of contact allergy to (meth)acrylates *from non-cosmetic sources* is considered to fall outside the scope of this book. Therefore, only contact allergy from their presence in cosmetics is presented, which virtually always is from artificial nails. There are many reports of contact allergy to artificial nails, but the specific sensitizers have rarely been identified and – consequently - such publications are not presented in this and other acrylate and methacrylate monographs. Discussion is limited to publications in which the culprit (meth)acrylates have been identified, e.g., from information found in Material Data Safety Sheets, data obtained from the manufacturer or from chemical analyses.

Patients often react to many (meth)acrylates on patch testing. Primary sensitization to methacrylates may result in both methacrylate and acrylate cross-sensitization. Conversely, patients sensitized to acrylates are unlikely to show cross-sensitization to methacrylates (3).

General aspects of acrylates and methacrylates are presented in Chapter 2.219 HEMA (hydroxyethyl methacrylate). A discussion of general aspects of artificial nails, contact allergy to these products, the clinical picture of allergic contact dermatitis and other side effects of sculptured nails can also be found there. A very useful review of contact sensitization to allergens in nail cosmetics, with emphasis on acrylic manicures, was published in 2017 (5).

CONTACT ALLERGY

Patch testing in groups of patients

Studies in which consecutive patients suspected of contact dermatitis have been tested with tetrahydrofurfuryl methacrylate (routine testing) and studies testing groups of selected patients are planned to be discussed in a future publication.

Case reports and case series

Tetrahydrofurfuryl methacrylate was responsible for 1 out of 399 cases of cosmetic allergy where the causal allergen was identified in a study of the NACDG, USA, 1977-1983 (1). A group of 55 female patients presenting with hand eczema and who had contact with artificial nails, were patch tested with a series of acrylates in one center in Israel, 2001-2004. Twenty-one had one or more positive reactions, of who 14 were professional beauticians specializing in nail sculpturing. All reactions, including 6 to tetrahydrofurfuryl methacrylate, were stated to be of current relevance (2). Because of the general lack of information on the composition of artificial nail materials, the fact that the author did no analyses of these products and the frequent occurrence of cross-reactivity among acrylates, one may wonder whether this statement can be accepted as entirely correct.

Between 2013 and 2016, in 4 dermatology departments in Spain, forty-three patients were diagnosed with ACD caused by (meth)acrylates in long-lasting nail polish. All were female, and all had hand dermatitis. Patients were mostly less than 40 years old and had an occupational cause of their dermatitis (93%, beauticians), which developed ~10 months after they had started to use the technique of applying long-lasting nail polish in their clients. The most frequently reacting patch test allergens were 2-hydroxypropyl methacrylate (41/43 [95%]), 2-hydroxyethyl methacrylate (HEMA) (39/43 [91%]), and tetrahydrofurfuryl methacrylate (31/39 [79%]). These three allergens were also the (meth)acrylate compounds most frequently identified on the labels of the patients' products (6).

One patient had painful onychia and paronychia from contact allergy to tetrahydrofurfuryl methacrylate in a nail extender (cold-curing artificial nails) (4).

Presence in cosmetic products and chemical analyses

In the USA, in April 2017, tetrahydrofurfuryl methacrylate was present in 72 of 50,714 cosmetic products of which the composition is known in FDA's Voluntary Cosmetic Registration Program (VCRP) (data obtained from FDA, May 2017). In February 2017, tetrahydrofurfuryl methacrylate was present in 7 of 64,480 cosmetic products of which the composition is known in EWG's Skin Deep Cosmetics Database, USA (http://www.ewg.org/skindeep/).

LITERATURE

1   Adams RM, Maibach HI, Clendenning WE, Fisher AA, Jordan WJ, Kanof N, et al. A five-year study of cosmetic reactions. J Am Acad Dermatol 1985;13:1062-1069
2   Lazarov A. Sensitization to acrylates is a common adverse reaction to artificial fingernails. J Eur Acad Derm Venereol 2007;21:169-174
3   Aalto-Korte K, Henriks-Eckerman M-L, Kuuliala O, Jolanki R. Occupational methacrylate and acrylate allergy – cross-reactions and possible screening allergens. Contact Dermatitis 2010;63:301-312
4   Fisher AA. Cross reactions between methyl methacrylate monomer and acrylic monomers presently used in acrylic nail preparations. Contact Dermatitis 1980;6:345-347
5   Chou M, Dhingra N, Strugar TL. Contact sensitization to allergens in nail cosmetics. Dermatitis 2017;28:231-240
6   Gatica-Ortega ME, Pastor-Nieto MA, Mercader-García P, Silvestre-Salvador JF. Allergic contact dermatitis caused by (meth)acrylates in long-lasting nail polish - are we facing a new epidemic in the beauty industry? Contact Dermatitis 2017 Jun 27. doi: 10.1111/cod.12827. [Epub ahead of print]

2.453   TETRAHYDROMAGNOLOL

IDENTIFICATION

Description/definition   : Tetrahydromagnolol is the organic compound that conforms to the formula shown
                            below
Chemical class(es)   : Phenols
Chemical/IUPAC name   : 2-(2-Hydroxy-5-propylphenyl)-4-propylphenol
Other names   : [1,1'-Biphenyl]-2,2'-diol, 5,5'-dipropyl-; 5,5'-dipropylbiphenyl-2,2'-diol
CAS registry number (s)   : 20601-85-8
Function(s) in cosmetics : EU: skin conditioning. USA: skin-conditioning agents - miscellaneous
Patch testing   : 0.5% pet. (1,3); 1% pet. (2)
Molecular formula   : $C_{18}H_{22}O_2$

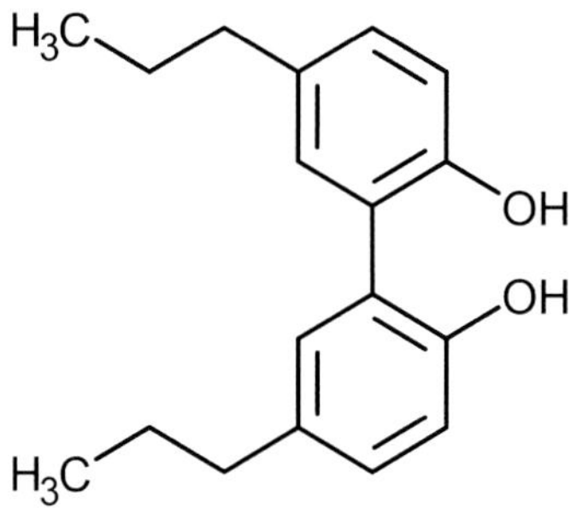

GENERAL

Tetrahydromagnolol is a biphenyl derivative, that downregulates melanin synthesis by inhibiting tyrosinase maturation, leading to accelerated tyrosinase degradation. It is used in Japan since 2006 as a skin lightening agent (1). It has been suggested that the sensitization potential results from oxidation of tetrahydromagnolol into a quinone-like derivative (4). All patients sensitized to tetrahydromagnolol thus far came from Japan (1,2,3)

CONTACT ALLERGY

Case reports and case series

A woman had suffered from an itchy erythematous rash on her cheek and neck for two months. She had treated the eruption with a corticosteroid, but as cosmetic dermatitis was not suspected, she had continued to use her cosmetics, which resulted in gradual worsening of the symptoms. She was advised to stop the use of all cosmetics and was treated with topical and oral steroids and an oral antihistamine. After healing of the dermatitis, patch tests were performed with her personal cosmetics and a cosmetic series, which yielded positive reactions to a cream and a beauty essence. Later, the ingredients of both products were tested, and the patient reacted to 5,5-dipropylbiphe-nyl-2,2-diol (tetrahydromagnolol) 0.5% pet., which was present in both the cream and the beauty essence as a skin-lightening agent. The skin did not lighten over the area of the patch test with this chemical. Four controls were negative to the test material (1).

A woman had facial dermatitis from contact allergy to tetrahydromagnolol present in a skin-lightening lotion (3). First reported case of contact allergy to tetrahydromagnolol with a positive patch test to the chemical 1% pet. (2, article not read).

Presence in cosmetic products and chemical analyses

In the USA, in April 2017, tetrahydromagnolol was present in zero of 56,714 cosmetic products of which the composition is known in FDA's Voluntary Cosmetic Registration Program (VCRP) (data obtained from FDA, May 2017). In April 2017, tetrahydromagnolol was present in zero of 65,434 cosmetic products of which the composition is known in EWG's Skin Deep Cosmetics Database, USA (http://www.ewg.org/skindeep/).

LITERATURE

1   Suzuki K, Yagami A, Matsunaga K. Allergic contact dermatitis caused by a skin lightening agent, 5,5'-dipropylbiphenyl-2,2'-diol. Contact Dermatitis 2012;66:51-52
2   Tsuruta K, Inaba Y, Nkagawa M, Matsunaga K. Allergic contact dermatitis from 5,5'-dipropylbiphenyl-2,2'-diol. J Environ Dermatol Cutan Allergol 2009;3:368 (in Japanese).

3   Yagami A, Suzuki K, Sano A, et al. Rhododendrol-induced leukoderma accompanied by allergic contact dermatitis caused by a non-rhododendrol skin-lightening agent, 5,5'-dipropylbiphenyl-2,2'-diol. J Dermatol 2015;42:739-740

4   Roberts DW, Aptula AO. Allergic contact dermatitis caused by a skin-lightening agent, 5,5'-dipropylbiphenyl-2,2'-diol. A comment. Contact Dermatitis 2012;66:357-359

2.454 TETRAHYDROXYPROPYL ETHYLENEDIAMINE

IDENTIFICATION

Description/definition   : Tetrahydroxypropyl ethylenediamine is the substituted amine that conforms to the formula shown below
Chemical class(es)   : Amines
Chemical/IUPAC name   : 1-[2-[bis(2-Hydroxypropyl)amino]ethyl-(2-hydroxypropyl)amino]propan-2-ol
Other names   : Edetol; 1,1',1'',1'''-ethylenedinitrilotetrapropan-2-ol; Entprol
CAS registry number (s)   : 102-60-3
EC number(s)   : 203-041-4
Merck Index monograph   : 4923
Function(s) in cosmetics   : EU: chelating. USA: chelating agents
Patch testing   : 1% pet (2); 10% pet. (3)
Molecular formula   : $C_{14}H_{32}N_2O_4$

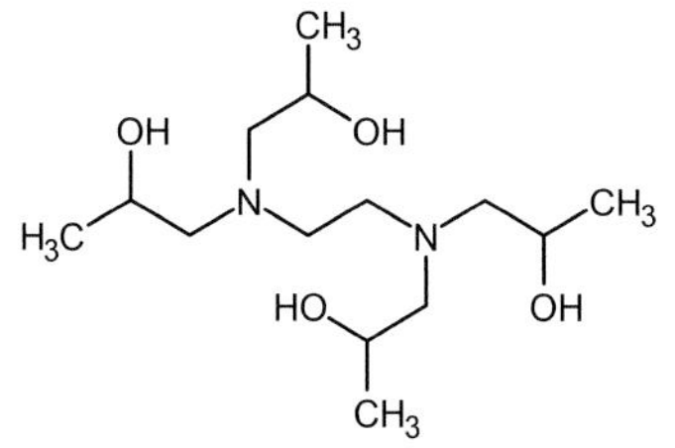

CONTACT ALLERGY

Case reports and case series

Tetrahydroxypropyl ethylenediamine was stated to be the (or an) allergen in 2 patients in a group of 603 individuals suffering from cosmetic dermatitis, seen in the period 2010-2015 in Leuven, Belgium (4). Tetrahydroxypropyl ethylenediamine was responsible for 5 out of 959 cases of non-fragrance cosmetic allergy where the causal allergen was identified, Belgium, 2000-2010 (1). These 5 cases were presented in detail (2). In 4, the chelating agent had been present in hand cream (2 patients), anti-aging creams and skin lotion; in the fifth, a patient who had been tested with tetrahydroxypropyl ethylenediamine as a control, the relevance was unknown (2). A woman had with a 3-year history of an itchy eruption on the exposed skin of her arms, which spread to the lower legs. She was seen with an acute exacerbation following sun exposure, during which she had used a proprietary SPF 25 sunscreen. Patch testing with an extended European standard series, facial and preservative series, plant series and photopatch series and her sunscreen gave a positive reaction to the cosmetic product. She was subsequently tested to the constituents of the sunscreen and was positive at D2 and D4 to tetrahydroxypropyl ethylenediamine 10% pet.; twenty controls were negative (3).

Cross-reactions, pseudo-cross-reactions and co-reactions
Not to ethylenediamine (3).

Presence in cosmetic products and chemical analyses
In the USA, in April 2017, tetrahydroxypropyl ethylenediamine was present in 70 of 56,714 cosmetic products of which the composition is known in FDA's Voluntary Cosmetic Registration Program (VCRP) (data obtained from FDA, May 2017). In April 2017, tetrahydroxypropyl ethylenediamine was present in 33 of 65,434 cosmetic products of which the composition is known in EWG's Skin Deep Cosmetics Database, USA (http://www.ewg.org/skindeep/).

LITERATURE
1   Travassos AR, Claes L, Boey L, Drieghe J, Goossens A. Non-fragrance allergens in specific cosmetic products. Contact Dermatitis 2011;65:276-285
2   Goossens A, Baret I, Swevers A. Allergic contact dermatitis caused by tetrahydroxypropyl ethylenediamine in cosmetic products. Contact Dermatitis 2011;64:161-164
3   Kirkup ME, Sansom JE. Contact sensitivity to tetrahydroxypropyl ethylenediamine in a sunscreen, without cross-sensitivity to ethylenediamine. Contact Dermatitis 2000;43:121-122
4   Goossens A. Cosmetic contact allergens. Cosmetics 2016, 3, 5; doi:10.3390/cosmetics3010005

2.455   TETRASODIUM EDTA

IDENTIFICATION

Description/definition   : Tetrasodium EDTA is the substituted amine that conforms to the formula shown below
Chemical class(es)   : Alkyl-substituted amino acids; amines; organic salts
Chemical/IUPAC name   : Tetrasodium ethylenediaminetetraacetate
Other names   : Edetate sodium
CAS registry number (s)   : 64-02-8
EC number(s)   : 200-573-9
CIR review(s)   : Int J Toxicol 2002;21(Suppl.2):95-142 (access: www.cir-safety.org/ingredients)
Merck Index monograph   : 4835 (EDTA)
Function(s) in cosmetics   : EU: chelating. USA: chelating agents
Patch testing   : 1% pet. (SmartPracticeEurope); 0.2% water (1)
Molecular formula   : $C_{10}H_{12}Na_4N_2O_8$

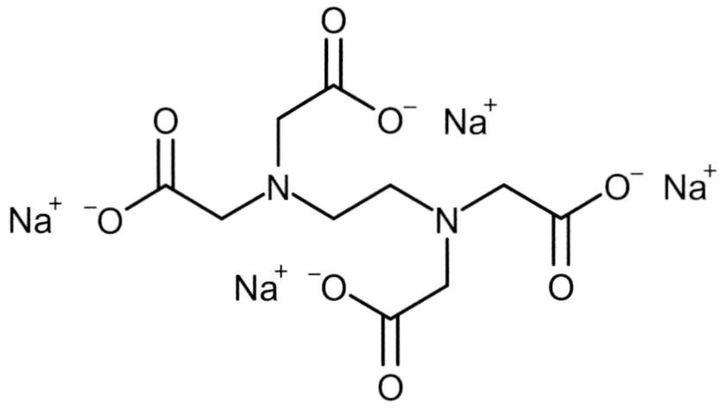

GENERAL

EDTA and its salts are used as preservatives and antioxidant agents in eye, nose and ear drops, and in cosmetic creams. Although its antibacterial activity is low, EDTA increases the antibacterial properties of benzalkonium chloride, chlorobutanol and thimerosal in ophthalmic solutions. As a chelating agent, it shows strong affinity for metallic ions, such as nickel, calcium, magnesium and lead, and has been used in the treatment of urinary calculi, corneal deposits, hypercalcemia and lead poisoning. EDTA is also a stabilizer of certain solutions, including those of ascorbic acid, hydrogen peroxide, formaldehyde, folic acid and hyaluronidase (1).

CONTACT ALLERGY

Case reports and case series

A man, who was treated for several malignant epithelial tumors of the skin, was prescribed a sunscreen SPF50+ cream. After 10 months of using the product, the patient presented with dermatitis at the sites where the sunscreen had been applied: face, neck and back of hands. Patch testing with the standard series of GEIDAC (Spanish Contact Dermatitis and Cutaneous Allergy Research Group), a sunscreen series and the sunscreen cream gave a positive reaction to the cosmetic product only. When tested with its 24 individual ingredients, tetrasodium ethylenediamine-tetraacetate (tetrasodium EDTA) 0.2% in water was positive; five controls subjects had negative reactions to the test substance. The patient's dermatitis resolved once the use of the sunscreen was stopped (1).

Cross-reactions, pseudo-cross-reactions and co-reactions

Not to ethylenediamine (1); trisodium EDTA (2); disodium EDTA (2).

Presence in cosmetic products and chemical analyses

In the USA, in April 2017, tetrasodium EDTA was present in 7374 of 56,714 cosmetic products of which the composition is known in FDA's Voluntary Cosmetic Registration Program (VCRP) (data obtained from FDA, May 2017). In April 2017, tetrasodium EDTA was present in 1909 of 65,434 cosmetic products of which the composition is known in EWG's Skin Deep Cosmetics Database, USA (http://www.ewg.org/skindeep/).

OTHER SIDE EFFECTS

Other side effects

Detergents and disinfectants containing tetrasodium EDTA may cause occupational rhinitis and/or asthma in (mostly) cleaners and healthcare workers, using spray formulations of cleaning products. An irritant mechanism is unlikely and it is unknown whether the respiratory effects are caused by an immunoallergic or a pharmacological mechanism (3).

LITERATURE

1 Sánchez-Pedreño P, García-Bravo B, Frías-Iniesta J. Contact allergy to tetrasodium EDTA in a sunscreen. Contact Dermatitis 2009;61:125-126
2 Kimura M, Kawada A. Contact dermatitis due to trisodium ethylenediaminetetra-acetic acid (EDTA) in a cosmetic lotion. Contact Dermatitis 1999: 41: 341
3 Laborde-Castérot H, Villa AF, Rosenberg N, Dupont P, Lee HM, Garnier R. Occupational rhinitis and asthma due to EDTA-containing detergents or disinfectants. Am J Ind Med 2012;55:677-682

2.456 THIMEROSAL

IDENTIFICATION

Description/definition	: Thimerosal is the metallo-organic compound that conforms to the formula shown below
Chemical class(es)	: Organic salts
Chemical/IUPAC name	: Sodium (2-carboxylatophenyl)sulfanyl-ethylmercury
Other names	: Thiomersal; merthiolate; sodium ethylmercurythiosalicylate
CAS registry number (s)	: 54-64-8
EC number(s)	: 200-210-4
Merck Index monograph	: 10740
Function(s) in cosmetics	: EU: preservative. USA: preservatives
EU cosmetic restrictions	: Regulated in Annex V/16 of the Regulation (EC) No. 1223/2009
Patch testing	: 0.1% pet. (Chemotechnique, SmartPracticeEurope, SmartPracticeCanada); 1% pet. (SmartPracticeCanada); the 1% test substance will certainly cause many irritant reactions, but these may also occur with thimerosal 0.1% pet. (48)
Molecular formula	: $C_9H_9NaHgO_2S$

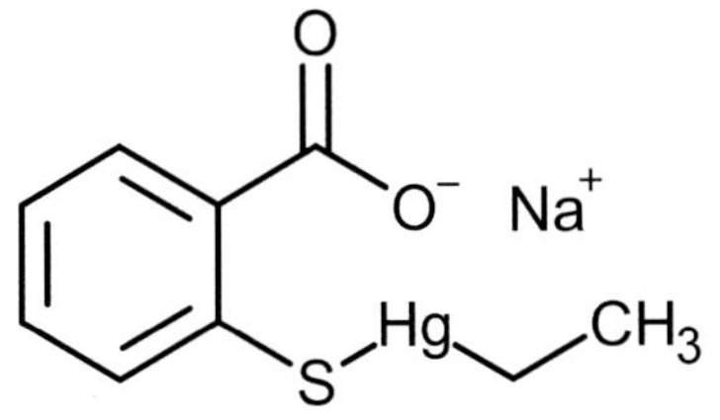

GENERAL

Thimerosal is an anionic organic mercurial synthesized from ethylmercuric chloride and thiosalicylic acid. It is a cream-colored crystalline powder soluble in water and alcohol, which is stabilized in aqueous solutions using chemicals such as EDTA (ethylenediamine tetraacetate). Thimerosal exhibits antimicrobial activity against gram-positive and particularly against gram-negative bacteria including *Pseudomonas aeruginosa*, *Acinobacter* species, *Serratia* species and *Escherichia coli*. It may be used as preservative in ophthalmological preparations, contact lens solutions, vaccines, allergen extracts, and immunoglobulin preparations (42,61,70). Thimerosal may also be used in (other) topical medicaments, in tattoo ink (75) and is said to be sold in some countries as an over-the-counter skin disinfectant (70). It is allowed in cosmetics in the USA and the EU.

Soon after its introduction it was found that thimerosal is a strong sensitizer, especially from its use in topical medicaments (44-47). Various patterns of sensitization have been described (58,93). In general, a positive patch test with thimerosal is not a marker for mercury allergy, neither the metal as such, nor inorganic mercury salts being positive in the majority of cases. Thiosalicylic acid, one thimerosal building brick, has attracted particular interest because of early reports of frequent co-reactivity between thimerosal and this compound. In later studies, however, only a few patients with thimerosal allergy reacted to thiosalicylic acid, which seems to rule out this part of the thimerosal molecule as a major allergenic determinant. In animal experiments, however, there seems to be full cross-sensitivity between the 2 compounds (70). Instead, the other building brick of thimerosal, ethylmercuric chloride, appears to be a potent sensitizing agent and has been reported to be the most frequent responsible agent in thimerosal hypersensitivity (59,60,66).

Positive patch test reactions to thimerosal are frequent, even in healthy subjects, with prevalences up to 5% in a general population and up to nearly 11% in consecutive patients patch tested because of suspected contact dermatitis (routine testing), depending on the country (tables 2.456.1 and 2.456.2). This world-wide sensitization to thimerosal, found even in infants, has been explained as an iatrogenic consequence of mandatory parenteral vaccinations (49,54,55,62). Health care workers are over-represented among thimerosal-sensitized patients, most likely not from relevant exposures, but from higher vaccination rates in this group, who are recommended to have protective vaccinations against infectious diseases such as influenza and hepatitis (79,82).

However, allergic contact dermatitis due to thimerosal is very infrequent and most positive patch test reactions to this preservative are clinically irrelevant (70,84,86). Possibly, a number of positive patch test reactions to thimerosal have in fact been false-positive, irritant reactions (48), although arguments have been brought forward that testify to the allergic nature of positive patch tests (70). Most clinical allergic reactions were caused in the 1980s and 1990s by thimerosal in contact lens solutions and pharmaceutical eye drops causing conjunctivitis, irritation, ocular redness, contact lens intolerance and sometimes (also) eyelid dermatitis. In those days, such reactions were far from rare. There are case series of 36 (94), 27 (8), 27 (40) and 4 (10) patients with allergic eye and/or periorbital reactions from thimerosal in contact lens solutions and eye drops. Also, in a period of 1 year, two of 29 patients starting wearing contact lenses wetted with thimerosal-containing solutions and patch test negative at the beginning, developed clinical hypersensitivity reactions during the one-year study period (91). Some allergic reactions have been caused by vaccines and immunoglobulins, but patients allergic to thimerosal in >90% tolerate injections of vaccines without problems, only some having mild local reactions (52,59,62). Subcutaneous injection far more often caused (in experimental conditions)local allergic reactions in thimerosal-sensitive individuals (93). Clinically relevant allergic reactions have hardly been reported in the last 10 years (75,83), which may be the result of decrease of thimerosal use as preservative or reflect non-publication bias because the effects are well-known.

Cosmetic allergy from thimerosal is extremely rare. In fact, there are only two case reports from the 1980s here atients had allergic contact dermatitis of the eyelids from thimerosal in an eyeshadow (13) and from an eye cream (95). It appears that, currently, thimerosal is hardly, if at all, used in cosmetic products (see the section 'Presence in cosmetic products and chemical analyses' below).

The literature on contact allergy to thimerosal and other preservatives up to 1991 has been reviewed in ref. 42 and literature up to 1994 in ref. 58. Literature speculating that thimerosal is related to autism is not discussed.

CONTACT ALLERGY

General population and subgroups

In several studies, the frequency of sensitization to thimerosal in the general population and in subgroups has been studies; their results are shown in table 2.456.1. In a recent 2008-2011 study in 5 European countries (Sweden, The Netherlands, Germany, Italy and Portugal), 5.0% of a sample of adult individuals from the general population (women 5.5%, men 4.3%) had contact allergy to thimerosal. The rate was lowest in Sweden (1.0%) and The Netherlands (1.2%) and highest in Germany (7.3%) (16). Lower frequencies were found in Denmark in 2008 and 2006 (18,21). In 1990, 3.5% of individuals from the Danish general population had been sensitized (19). The lower frequencies 16 and 18 years later may be related to a reduction of exposure to thimerosal in vaccination materials. In subgroups of the general population (table 2.456.1), Germany again had high rates of contact allergy to thimerosal (4.7% [23,26]) as had Italy with a 4.7% prevalence in male soldiers without skin disease in 1989 (25). An exceptionally high percentage of 19.4 was seen in a group of 201 healthy student volunteers in a 2011 study from China (29).

Table 2.456.1 Contact allergy in the general population and in subgroups

Year and country	Selection and number tested	Prevalence of contact allergy			Comments	Ref.
		Total	Women	Men		
General population						
2008-11 five European countries	general population, random sample, 18-74 years, n=3119	5.0%	5.5%	4.3%		16
2008 Denmark	general population, random sample, 15-41 year, n=469		1.8%	2.6%	patch tests were read on day 2 only	21
2006 Denmark	general population, random sample, 18-69 years, n=3460	0.5%	0.6%	0.4%	patch tests were read on day 2 only	18
2005 Norway	general population, random sample, 18-69 years, n=1236	1.8%	1.7%	1.8%		20
1990 Denmark	general population, random sample, 18-69 years, n=543	3.5%	3.3%	3.7%	patch tests were read on day 2 only; data from 15-17 years old were excluded in the data presented here	19
Subgroups						
2011 China	healthy student volunteers 19-30 years; n=201	19.4%				29
2010 Denmark	unselected population of 8th grade schoolchildren in Denmark, 15 years later, n=442	1.4%	0.7%	2.4%	follow-up study	17
1997-1998 Germany	adults 28-78 years, with a large percentage (>50%) of atopic individuals, n=1141	4.7%	6.0%	3.4%		23, 26
1995-1996 Denmark	8th grade school children, 12-16 years, n=1146	1.0%	1.0%	1.1%		22, 24
1989 Italy	male soldiers without skin disease, 18-28 years, n=593	4.7%				25

Results of testing in groups of patients without skin disease in studies from before 1990 have been summarized in 1995 (70). In recruits, twins, medical students and schoolchildren from different countries, rates of sensitization ranging from 2% to 16% have been found. The highest frequencies were observed in Southern Sweden in the beginning of the 1970s, for which later a reasonable explanation was found: sensitization by tuberculin injections (70).

Patch testing in groups of patients

Up to 2003, thimerosal was tested routinely in the USA, being part of the screening series of the North American Contact Dermatitis Group (NACDG). Thimerosal gave high frequencies of sensitization of around 10%; nevertheless, it was removed from the NACDG screening series because of very low relevance rates (53,76). Thimerosal was removed from the Spanish standard series in 2016, but the preservative was never part of the European baseline (previously: standard) series. Results of studies testing thimerosal in consecutive patients suspected of contact dermatitis (routine testing) back to 1990 are shown in table 2.456.2. Results of testing in groups of *selected* patients (e.g., children suspected of contact dermatitis, patients with periorbital dermatitis, individuals suspected of cosmetic dermatitis, patients tested with a preservative series) back to 1992 are shown in table 2.456.3.

Patch testing in consecutive patients suspected of contact dermatitis: routine testing

In eleven studies in which routine testing with thimerosal was performed, rates of sensitization have ranged from 3% (30) to 10.9% (101). In the USA, rates have been very constant, varying between 9.3% and 10.9%. In other countries (Turkey, Israel, Switzerland), the frequencies of sensitization were far lower: 3% (30, very small population tested), 3.7% (6) and 4.2% (12). In the NACDG studies, relevance rates were invariably low. In some others, relevance was scored between 28% and 67% (2 out of 3 reactions) (3,6,30,38), but in not a single study were culprit products mentioned.

Table 2.456.2 Patch testing in groups of patients: Routine testing (limited review)

Years and Country	Test conc. & vehicle	Number of patients tested | positive (%)		Selection of patients (S); Relevance (R); Comments (C)	Ref.
2005-2006 Turkey		93	3 (3%)	R: 2/3 reactions were considered to be relevant	30
2000-2005 USA	0.1% pet.	1747	(10.5%)	R: 40%	3
2004 Israel	0.1% pet.	508	19 (3.7%)	R: 32% definite relevance and 42% probable relevance; C: the causative products were not mentioned	6
2001-2002 USA	0.1% pet.	4899	(10.2%)	R: definite + probable relevance: 1.8%	99
1998-2000 USA	0.1% pet.	5795	(10.8%)	R: definite + probable relevance: 18%	100
1998–2000 USA	0.1% pet.	1319	(9.3%)	R: not stated	104
1997-1999 Greece	0.1% pet.	895	68 (7.6%)	R: 28% was 'relevant to a history either of occupational exposure or wearing contact lenses'	38
1996-1998 USA	0.1% pet.	4087	(10.9%)	R: definite + probable + possible relevance: 17%	101
1994-1996 USA	0.1% pet.	3075	(10.4%)	R: definite + probable relevance: 6%	102
1992-1994 USA	0.1% pet.	3472	(10.6%)	R: present relevance: 12%	103
1989-90 Switzerland	0.1% pet.	2295	(4.2%)	R: not stated	12

Patch testing in groups of selected patients

Results of testing in groups of selected patients (e.g., children suspected of contact dermatitis, patients with periorbital dermatitis, individuals suspected of cosmetic dermatitis, patients tested with a preservative series) back to 1992 are shown in table 2.456.3. In 12 investigations, frequencies of sensitization have ranged from 1.1% to 13.6%. The highest rate (13.6%) was seen in study from the USA in a group of patients tested with a supplemental cosmetic screening series (1), but this study had certain weaknesses. The lowest frequencies of positive patch test reactions to thimerosal were found in The Netherlands (1.1% and 1.3% [33,58]) and the higher ones in the studies of the IVDK (Germany, Austria, Switzerland) (4,27,32), Korea (15) and Israel (56). In two IVDK studies, high frequencies were seen in patients with periorbital dermatitis, but the relevance of the reactions was not mentioned and in one, this frequency was not higher than in a control group (27,32). In 9/12 investigations, relevance was not mentioned. In the studies that did address the issue of relevance, the rates ranged from 12% to 89%, but the latter figure is unbelievable, as it included 'questionable' and 'past' relevance (1). Culprit products were mentioned in one study only: eye medication (n=2) and pesticides (n=1) (58).

Case reports and case series

Thimerosal was responsible for 1 out of 399 cases of cosmetic allergy where the causal allergen was identified in a study of the NACDG, USA, 1977-1983 (2). One patient with periorbital eczema had contact allergy to thimerosal in an eyeshadow (13). A woman had eyelid contact dermatitis from thimerosal in an eye cream; she had previously been sensitized to thimerosal by a contact lens solution (95). In 3 clinics in Belgium, in the period 1978-1985, 279 patients with allergic contact dermatitis exclusively caused by cosmetics were seen. In this group, there were 11 reactions to thimerosal. It was implied that this was the cause of the allergic reaction (34).

Table 2.456.3 Patch testing in groups of patients: Selected patient groups (limited review)

Years and Country	Test conc. & vehicle	Number of patients tested | positive (%)		Selection of patients (S); Relevance (R); Comments (C)	Ref.
2002-2013 Italy	0.1% pet.	2614	110 (4.2%)	S: children younger than 11 suspected of contact dermatitis; R: 13 (12%); C: the prevalence was very low in the youngest age group, which was attributed to the recent limitation of its use as a preservative in vaccines	81
1996-2013 Nether-lands	0.1% pet.	661	7 (1.1%)	S: children aged 0-17 years with eczema; R: not stated	33
2010-2011 Korea	0.1% pet.	584	58 (9.9%)	S: patients suspected of allergic cosmetic dermatitis; R: not stated	15
2000-2010 IVDK		2490	179 (7.2%)	S: patients with periorbital dermatitis; R: not stated	4
2000-2007 USA	0.1% pet.	942	129 (13.6%)	S: patients tested with a supplemental cosmetic screening series; R: 89%; C: weak study: a. high rate of macular erythema and weak reactions; b. relevance figures included 'questionable' and 'past' relevance	1
2000-2002 Finland		6527	(3.8%)	S: patients tested with a cosmetic series; R: not stated	105
1997-2000 Israel		244	21 (8.6%)	S: patients suspected of allergic cosmetic dermatitis; R: not stated	56
1995-1999 IVDK	0.1% pet.	1013	(10.2%)	S: patients with allergic periorbital contact dermatitis; R: not stated	27
1995-1996 Finland		3743	(4.2%)	S: patients tested with a cosmetic series; R: not stated	105
1990-1994 IVDK		590	56 (9.5%)	S: patients with periorbital eczema; R: not often relevant; C: the frequency of sensitization was not significantly higher than in a control group of patients not having periorbital dermatitis	32
1990-1994 Germany	0.1% pet. 0.05% pet.	3619 9361	241 (6.7%) 440 (4.7%)	S: patients tested with a preservative series; R: not stated S: patients tested with a preservative series; R: not stated	106
1987-1992 Nether-lands	0.1% pet.	2461	32 (1.3%)	S: patients tested with an 'additional series', approximately ¾ of all patients seen with dermatitis; R: 3 reactions (10%) were relevant, 2 from eye medication, one from pesticides	58

IVDK: Information Network of Departments of Dermatology, Germany, Austria, Switzerland

Contact allergy to thimerosal in non-cosmetic products

Contact lens solutions and eye drops
Thirty-six patients with thimerosal-induced allergic follicular contact conjunctivitis were reported from Italy (94). Many of them also had periorbital dermatitis, and most had used eye drops containing thimerosal for various eye problems (sometimes prescribed by the ophthalmologist) or contact lens solutions; patch tests with the eye drops and contact lens solutions themselves were nearly always negative (94). Of 38 patients who were using soft contact lenses and had unexplained conjunctivitis or keratitis, 31 had positive ocular provocation tests to a thimerosal-preserved (0.004%) artificial tears solution. Delayed hypersensitivity to thimerosal was demonstrated by positive patch tests in 27 patients. Avoidance of thimerosal and the use of unit-dose sterile saline solutions resulted in complete resolution of ocular symptoms (40). In another study, twenty-seven patients with allergic contact conjunctivitis from thimerosal in contact lens solutions were presented (8).

One patient reacted to thimerosal in dexamethasone eye drops (7). Another individual was allergic to thimerosal in an ophthalmic drug and had several ill-defined symptoms (11). A man had dermatitis of the eyelids from contact allergy to thimerosal in eye drops (74). Another man had conjunctivitis and eyelid dermatitis from contact allergy to thimerosal in eye drops, which was mistaken for hay fever (88). Another 4 suffered from periorbital ACD caused by thimerosal in contact lens solutions (10). Two patients with 'contact lens intolerance' had contact allergy to thimerosal in the lens solution (13). Two of 15 patients with conjunctivitis related to soft contact lenses reacted to thimerosal; it was implied but not verified that the lens solutions used contained thimerosal (96). A woman had contact allergy to thimerosal in contact lens fluids; interestingly, she did not have eye problems, but localized vesicular dermatitis on the hands at the site of contact with the lens fluids (97). In a female patient, exacerbation of rosacea with erythema, scaling and intense itching may have been caused by contact allergy to thimerosal, present in eye drops she used to treat rosacea blepharitis (36).

A man had bullous dermatitis on the back of his hands and occasional conjunctivitis and dermatitis of the eye lids from thimerosal in eye drops. It is hard to imagine how this could cause bullous dermatitis of the back of the hands, but, nevertheless, according to the authors, both ocular and dermatological symptoms permanently disappeared after the use of the eye drops was discontinued (72). A man had recurrent conjunctivitis from contact allergy to thimerosal. He had noted that he would only get the symptoms when he used the contact lens wetting solution of his wife (which contained thimerosal), but he tolerated his own thimerosal-free preparation without problems ('connubial contact dermatitis'). The patient had probably been sensitized from a hepatitis B vaccination two years previously, which had caused local erythema, induration and pain (77). There have been several other single case reports of patients with conjunctivitis and/or dermatitis of the eyelids from thimerosal allergy in contact lens solutions (9,39,98).

Vaccines and immunoglobulins

Approximately 24 hours after receiving a single intramuscular dose (300 µg) of RhoGAM as antepartum prophylaxis for Rh iso-immunization, a woman noted that the injection site became warm, indurated (to 10 × 10 cm), and pruritic. She had no signs of immediate reactivity. The site remained unchanged for about 10 days and then began to resolve. Patch testing revealed strong contact allergy to thimerosal, present in the Rho(D) immunoglobulin (89). A nurse had occupational allergic contact dermatitis from thimerosal caused by vaccinating babies. When she started wearing gloves, the dermatitis disappeared (83). Another nurse, who had probably previously been sensitized to thimerosal from a vaccination against viral hepatitis, also developed allergic contact dermatitis of the hands from vaccinating schoolchildren with thimerosal-containing vaccines (37). A child had acute episodes of vesiculation and weeping at the site of previous vaccinations, but she also developed dermatitis in an atopic distribution, suggestive of systemic contact dermatitis. She had positive patch tests to thimerosal and aluminum, both of which were present in the vaccines used (41). A man had a 'severe local reaction' from contact allergy to thimerosal in hepatis B vaccine (90).

Other products

A woman had dermatitis from bindi on the forehead. A ROAT with the bindi material was positive. Patch tests were positive to thimerosal and the gallate mix, which were pointed out as the culprit allergens in this case, but without checking the composition of the bindi material (85). A woman had auricular allergic contact dermatitis from thimerosal in an otic suspension (75). A hospital laboratory technician had occupational allergic symmetrical vesicular eczema of the sides of the fingers and fingertips from thimerosal in an electrophoresis gel she worked with in the laboratory (73). A male patient had laryngeal obstruction developing within hours necessitating an emergency tracheotomy. He had treated his slightly sore throat with a thimerosal first aid spray. Patch testing revealed an extreme spreading reaction to thimerosal. The author suggested that the acute laryngeal obstruction was caused by delayed hypersensitivity to this first aid spray (67).

A woman developed allergic contact dermatitis of the legs, spreading to the entire skin, from thimerosal (and the active ingredient *Ruscus aculeatus*) in a vasoconstrictor cream she used for treatment of varices (35). In a group of 46 patients with allergic contact dermatitis of the eyelids seen in Kansas City, USA, between 1994 and 2004, two cases (4.3%) were caused by contact allergy to thimerosal, but the source products were not mentioned) (14).

Cross-reactions, pseudo-cross-reactions and co-reactions

Patients allergic to thimerosal may (52) or may – more frequently - not cross-react to other organic or inorganic mercurial compounds. Pseudo-cross-reactions to ethylmercuric chloride, possibly the most important sensitizer in thimerosal (59,60,66); methylmercuric chloride (66).

Photocontact allergy to piroxicam is very often associated with contact allergy to thimerosal (57). Conversely, the majority of patients sensitized to thimerosal (notably those sensitized to thiosalicylic acid) have positive photopatch tests to piroxicam, also in the absence of a history of photoallergic reactions (63,87). After UVA exposure of piroxicam, photoproducts may be formed that are responsible for the induction of contact allergy to thimerosal as well as to thiosalicylic acid. The relationship between contact allergy to thimerosal and thiosalicylic acid on the one hand, and photoallergy to piroxicam, on the other, has been demonstrated (in both directions) in animal experiments (71).

Presence in cosmetic products and chemical analyses

In July 2017, thimerosal was present in 8 older products of 69,751 cosmetic products of which the composition is known in EWG's Skin Deep Cosmetics Database, USA (http://www.ewg.org/skindeep/). In the USA, in April 2017, thimerosal was present in zero of 56,714 cosmetic products of which the composition is known in FDA's Voluntary Cosmetic Registration Program (VCRP) (data obtained from FDA, May 2017).

Other side effects: systemic contact dermatitis

A woman developed a generalized maculopapular eruption after receiving a thimerosal-containing influenza vaccine. Patch testing with thimerosal was positive. She had a history of previous eyelid dermatitis from thimerosal-containing contact lens solution (51). Two children had systemic contact dermatitis from daily oral resp. nasal doses of anti-pneumococcal vaccines containing thimerosal (64). Two other patients allergic to thimerosal developed urticaria 1-3 days after having received a vaccination containing thimerosal as a preservative; a third individual developed a generalized exanthematic eruption 2 days after receiving tetanus immunoglobulins containing 0.1% thimerosal (65).

A woman developed widespread dermatitis from contact allergy to thimerosal in hepatitis B vaccinations (68). Hypersensitivity to thimerosal in hepatitis B vaccine has also caused a lichen striatus type reaction in one patient and eczematous urticarial reactions in another (69, article not read). A female sanitation department worker developed generalized dermatitis after receiving an intramuscular injection of a hepatitis B vaccination following an accidental prick from a needle in garbage. The vaccine contained 0.05% thimerosal to which the patient had a strongly positive patch test reaction (78).

OTHER SIDE EFFECTS

Photosensitivity

In China, in one center, thimerosal has been photopatch tested in patients suspected of photodermatoses in two overlapping studies (28,31). An unbelievable 8.9% and 9.8% of the patients apparently had positive photopatch test reactions. Whether these were relevant was not mentioned (28,31). The results are summarized in table 2.456.4.

Table 2.456.4 Photopatch testing in groups of patients

Years and Country	Test conc. & vehicle	Number of patients tested	positive (%)	Selection of patients (S); Relevance (R); Comments (C)	Ref.
2005-2014 China	0.1% pet.	5622	551 (9.8%)	S: patients suspected of photodermatoses; R: not stated; C: same center as in ref. 28	31
2006-2012 China	0.1% pet	4331	387 (8.9%)	S: patients with suspected photodermatoses; R: not stated; C: same center as in ref. 31	28

Immediate-type reactions

A patient, who had a history of eyelid pain and erythema after use of thimerosal-containing contact lens solutions but who tolerated solutions without thimerosal well, developed wheals and an anaphylactic response with pruritus, throat tightness, cough, and shortness of breath within 20 minutes of a skin prick test using the full-strength adult influenza vaccine containing 50 µg of thimerosal per 0.5-mL dose. Later, a prick test with the pediatric influenza vaccine *without* thimerosal was negative. Thimerosal itself was not tested (50).

Within 30 minutes of hepatitis B vaccine injection, generalized pruritus, dyspnea, urticaria and infraorbital edema developed in a woman vaccinated because she was working in a high-risk occupation. The reaction was ascribed to thimerosal, but this was on the basis of literature data; no tests to prove the assumption were performed (92).

LITERATURE

1   Wetter DA, Yiannias JA, Prakash AV, Davis MD, Farmer SA, el-Azhary RA, et al. Results of patch testing to personal care product allergens in a standard series and a supplemental cosmetic series: an analysis of 945 patients from the Mayo Clinic Contact Dermatitis Group, 2000-2007. J Am Acad Dermatol 2010;63:789-798

2   Adams RM, Maibach HI, Clendenning WE, Fisher AA, Jordan WJ, Kanof N, et al. A five-year study of cosmetic reactions. J Am Acad Dermatol 1985;13:1062-1069

3   Davis MD, Scalf LA, Yiannias JA, Cheng JF, El-Azhary RA, Rohlinger AL, et al. Changing trends and allergens in the patch test standard series. Arch Dermatol 2008;144:67-72

4   Landeck L, John SM, Geier J. Periorbital dermatitis in 4779 patients – patch test results during a 10-year period. Contact Dermatitis 2014;70:205-212

5   Özkaya E, Mirzoyeva L, Ötkür B. Mercury-induced systemic allergic dermatitis caused by 'white precipitate' in a skin lightening cream. Contact Dermatitis 2009;60:61-63

6   Slodownik D, Ingber A. Thimerosal – Is it really irrelevant? Contact Dermatitis 2005;53:324-326

7   Tabar AI, García BE, Rodríguez A, Quirce S, Olaguibel JM. Etiologic agents in allergic contact dermatitis caused by eyedrops. Contact Dermatitis 1993;29:50-51

8   Wilson LA, McNatt I, Rietschel R. Delayed hypersensitivity to thimerosal in soft contact lens wearers. Ophthalmol 1981;88:804-809

9   Pedersen NB. Allergy to chemical solutions for soft contact lenses. Lancet 1976;12:1363

10 Fisher AA. Allergic reactions to contact lens solutions. Cutis 1985;85:209-211 (bibliography probably incorrect)

11 Frosch PJ, Weickel R, Schmitt T, Krastel H. Nebenwirkungen von ophthalmologischen Externa. Z Hautkr 1988;63:126-136

12 Perrenoud D, Bircher A, Hunziker T, Suter H, Bruckner-Tuderman L, Stäger J, et al. Frequency of sensitization to 13 common preservatives in Switzerland. Contact Dermatitis 1994;30:276-279

13 Podmore P, Storrs FJ. Contact lens intolerance; allergic conjunctivitis? Contact Dermatitis 1989;20:98-103

14 Amin KA, Belsito DV. The aetiology of eyelid dermatitis: a 10-year retrospective analysis. Contact Dermatitis 2006;55:280-285

15 Lee SS, Hong DK, Jeong NJ, Lee JH, Choi YS, Lee AY, et al. Multicenter study of preservative sensitivity in patients with suspected cosmetic contact dermatitis in Korea. J Dermatol 2012;39:677-681

16 Diepgen TL, Ofenloch RF, Bruze M, Bertuccio P, Cazzaniga S, Coenraads P-J, et al. Prevalence of contact allergy in the general population in different European regions. Br J Dermatol 2016;174:319-329

17 Mortz CG, Bindslev-Jensen C, Andersen KE. Prevalence, incidence rates and persistence of contact allergy and allergic contact dermatitis in The Odense Adolescence Cohort Study: a 15-year follow-up. Brit J Dermatol 2013;168:318-325

18 Thyssen JP, Linneberg A, Menné T, Nielsen NH, Johansen JD. Contact allergy to allergens of the TRUE-test (panels 1 and 2) has decreased modestly in the general population. Br J Dermatol 2009;161:1124-1129

19 Nielsen SH, Menné T. Allergic contact sensitization in an unselected Danish population. The Glostrup Allergy Study, Denmark. Acta Derm Venereol 1992;72:456-460

20 Dotterud LK, Smith-Sivertsen T. Allergic contact sensitization in the general adult population: a population-based study from Northern Norway. Contact Dermatitis 2007;56:10-15

21 Nielsen NH, Linneberg A, Menné T, Madsen F, Frølund L, Dirksen A, et al. Allergic contact sensitization in an adult Danish population: two cross-sectional surveys eight years apart (the Copenhagen Allergy Study). Acta Derm Venereol 2001;81:31-34

22 Mortz CG, Lauritsen JM, Bindslev-Jensen C, Andersen KE. Contact allergy and allergic contact dermatitis in adolescents: prevalence measures and associations. Acta Derm Venereol 2002;82:352-358

23 Schäfer T, Böhler E, Ruhdorfer S, Weigl L, Wessner D, Filipiak B, et al. Epidemiology of contact allergy in adults. Allergy 2001;56:1192-1196

24 Mortz CG, Lauritsen JM, Bindslev-Jensen C, Andersen KE. Prevalence of atopic dermatitis, asthma, allergic rhinitis, and hand and contact dermatitis in adolescents. The Odense Adolescence Cohort Study on Atopic Diseases and Dermatitis. Br J Dermatol 2001;144:523-532

25 Seidenari S, Manzini BM, Danese P, Motolese A. Patch and prick test study of 593 healthy subjects. Contact Dermatitis 1990; 23:162-167

26 Uter W, Ludwig A, Balda BR, Schnuch A, Pfahlberg A, Schäfer T, Wichmann HE, Ring J. The prevalence of contact allergy differed between population-based data and clinic–based data. J Clin Epidemiol 2004;57:627-632

27 Herbst RA, Uter W, Pirker C, Geier J, Frosch PJ. Allergic and non-allergic periorbital dermatitis: patch test results of the Information Network of the Departments of Dermatology during a 5-year period. Contact Dermatitis 2004;51:13-19

28 Gao L, Hu Y, Ni C, Xu Y, Ma L, Yan S, Dou X. Retrospective study of photopatch testing in a Chinese population during a 7-year period. Dermatitis 2014;25:22-26

29 Zhao J, Li LF. Contact sensitization to cosmetic series of allergens in a general population in Beijing. J Cosmet Dermatol 2014;13:68-71

30 Ada S, Seçkin D. Patch testing in allergic contact dermatitis: is it useful to perform the cosmetic series in addition to the European standard series? J Eur Acad Dermatol Venereol 2010;24:1192-1196

31 Hu Y, Wang D, Shen Y, Tang H. Photopatch testing in Chinese patients over 10 years. Dermatitis 2016;27:137-142

32 Ockenfels H, Seemann U, Goos M. Contact allergy in patients with periorbital eczema: an analysis of allergens. Dermatology 1997;195:119-124

33 Lubbes S, Rustemeyer T, Sillevis Smitt JH, Schuttelaar ML, Middelkamp-Hup MA. Contact sensitization in Dutch children and adolescents with and without atopic dermatitis - a retrospective analysis. Contact Dermatitis 2017;76:151-159

34 Dooms-Goossens A, de Boulle K, Dooms M, Degreef H. Imidazolidinyl urea dermatitis. Contact Dermatitis 1986;14:322-324

35 Landa N, Aguirre A, Goday J, Ratón JA, Díaz-Pérez JL. Allergic contact dermatitis from a vasoconstrictor cream. Contact Dermatitis 1990;22:290-291

36 Bardazzi F, Manuzzi P, Riguzzi G, Veronesi S. Contact dermatitis with rosacea. Contact Dermatitis 1987;16:298

37 Kiec-Swierczynska M, Krecisz B, Swierczynska-Machura D. Occupational allergic contact dermatitis due to thimerosal. Contact Dermatitis 2003;48:337-338

38 Katsarou A, Lambrinopoulou K, Armenaka M. The positivity of thimerosal in Greece. Contact Dermatitis 1999;41:291-292

39 Sertoli A, Lombardi P, Palleschi GM, Gola M, Giorgini S. Tegobetaine in contact lens solutions. Contact Dermatitis 1987;16:111-112

40 Rietschel RL, Wilson LA. Ocular inflammation in patients using soft contact lenses. Arch Dermatol1982;118:147-149

41 Cox NH, Moss C, Forsyth A. Allergy to non-toxoid constituents of vaccines and implications for patch testing. Contact Dermatitis 1988;18:143-146

42 Fransway AF. The problem of preservation in the 1990s. III. Agents with preservative function independent of formaldehyde release. Am J Contact Derm 1991;2:145-174

43 Leventhal JS, Berger EM, Brauer JA, Cohen DE. Hypersensitivity reactions to vaccine constituents: a case series and review of the literature. Dermatitis 2012;23:102-109

44 Ellis FA. The sensitizing factor in merthiolate. J Allergy 1947;18:212-213

45 Gaul LE. Sensitizing component in thiosalicylic acid. J Invest Dermatol 1958;31:91-92

46 Lipson L. Sensitivity to tincture of merthiolate. N Engl J Med 1946;234:441

47 Reisman RE. Delayed hypersensitivity to merthiolate preservative. J Allergy 1969;43:245-248

48 Lisi P, Perno P, Ottaviani M, Morelli P. Minimum eliciting patch test concentration of thimerosal. Contact Dermatitis 1991;24:22-26

49 Bruckner AL, Weston WL, Morelli JG. Does sensitization to contact allergens begin in infancy? Pediatrics 2000;105:e3

50 Zheng W, Dreskin SC. Thimerosal in influenza vaccine: an immediate hypersensitivity reaction. Ann Allergy Asthma Immunol 2007;99:574-575

51 Lee-Wong M, Resnick D, Chong K. A generalized reaction to thimerosal from an influenza vaccine. Ann Allergy Asthma Immunol 2005;94:90-94

52 Audicana MT, Munoz D, del Pozo MD, Fernández E, Gastaminza G, Fernández de Corres L. Allergic contact dermatitis from mercury antiseptics and derivatives: study protocol of tolerance to intramuscular injections of thimerosal. Am J Contact Dermat 2002;13:3-9

53 Belsito DV. Thimerosal: contact (non) allergen of the year. Am J Contact Dermat 2002;13:1-2

54 Schäfer T, Enders F, Przybilla B. Sensitization to thimerosal and previous vaccination. Contact Dermatitis 1995;32:114-116

55 Osawa J, Kitamura K, Ikezawa Z, Nakajima H. A probable role for vaccines containing thimerosal in thimerosal hypersensitivity. Contact Dermatitis 1991;24:178-182

56 Trattner A, Farchi Y, David M. Cosmetics patch tests: first report from Israel. Contact Dermatitis 2002;47:180-181

57 McKerrow KJ, Greig DB. Piroxicam-induced photosensitive dermatitis. J Am Acad Dermatol 1986;15:1237-1241

58 Van 't Veen AJ, Van Joost Th. Sensitization to thimerosal (Merthiolate) is still present today. Contact Dermatitis 1994;31:293-298

59 Wantke F, Demmer CM, Götz M, Jarisch R. Contact dermatitis from thimerosal. Contact Dermatitis 1994;30:115-117

60 Pirker C, Möslinger T, Wantke F, Götz M, Jarisch R. Ethylmercuric chloride: the responsible agent in thimerosal hypersensitivity. Contact Dermatitis 1993;29:152-154

61 Tosti A, Guerra L, Bardazzi F. Hyposensitizing therapy with standard antigenic extracts: an important source of thimerosal sensitization. Contact Dermatitis 1989;20:173-176

62 Aberer W. Vaccination despite thimerosal sensitivity. Contact Dermatitis 1991;24:6-10

63 Cirne de Castro JL, Freitas JP, Brandão FM, Themido R. Sensitivity to thimerosal and photosensitivity to piroxicam. Contact Dermatitis 1991;24:187-192

64 Zenarola P, Gimma A, Lomuto M. Systemic contact dermatitis from thimerosal. Contact Dermatitis 1995;32:107-108

65 Tosti A, Melino M, Bardazzi F. Systemic reaction due to thimerosal. Contact Dermatitis 1986;15:187-188

66 Santucci B, Cannistraci C, Cristaudo A, Camera E, Picardo M. Thimerosal positivities: the role of organomercury alkyl compounds. Contact Dermatitis 1998;38:325-328

67 Maibach H. Acute laryngeal obstruction presumed secondary to thiomersal (merthiolate) delayed hypersensitivity. Contact Dermatitis 1975;1:221-222

68 McKenna KE. Eczematous reaction to hepatitis B vaccine. Contact Dermatitis 1999;40:158-159

69 Rietschel RL, Adams RM. Reactions to thimerosal in hepatitis B vaccines. Dermatol Clin 1990;8:161-164

70 Möller H. All these positive tests to thimerosal. Contact Dermatitis 1994;31:209-213

71 Ikezawa Z, Kitamura K, Osawa J, Hariya T. Photosensitivity to piroxicam is induced by sensitization to thimerosal and thiosalicylate. J Invest Dermatol 1992;98:918-922

72 Zemtsov A, Bolton GG. Thimerosal-induced bullous contact dermatitis. Contact Dermatitis 1994;30:57

73 Ramsay HM, Tan BB. Allergic contact dermatitis from thimerosal in an electrophoresis gel. Contact Dermatitis 1998;39:205

74 Ortiz FJ, Postigo C, Iyars J, Ortiz PL, Merino V. Allergic contact dermatitis from pilocarpine and thimerosal. Contact Dermatitis 1991;25:203-204

75 Aschenbeck KA, Warshaw EM. Clinically relevant reactions to thimerosal (the "nonallergen") exist! Dermatitis July 6, 2017 - Volume Publish Ahead of Print - Issue – ppg. doi: 10.1097/DER.0000000000000285

76 Breithaupt A, Jacob SE. Thimerosal and the relevance of patch-test reactions in children. Dermatitis 2008;19:275 277

77 Williford PM, Sherertz EF. Connubial contact conjunctivitis due to thimerosal. Am J Cont Dermat 1992;3:92-94

78 Mathias CGT. Systemic eczematous dermatitis from contact allergy to thimerosal preservative in hepatitis B vaccine. Am J Cont Dermat 1991;2:68-69

79 Ibler KS, Jemec GB, Garvey LH, Agner T. Prevalence of delayed-type and immediate-type hypersensitivity in healthcare workers with hand eczema. Contact Dermatitis 2016;75:223-229

80 Hervella-Garcés M, García-Gavín J, Silvestre-Salvador JF; en representación del Grupo Español de Investigación en Dermatitis de Contacto y Alergia Cutánea (GEIDAC). The Spanish standard patch test series: 2016 update by the Spanish Contact Dermatitis and Skin Allergy Research Group (GEIDAC). Actas Dermosifiliogr 2016;107:559-566

81 Belloni Fortina A, Fontana E, Peserico A. Contact sensitization in children: A retrospective study of 2,614 children from a single center. Pediatr Dermatol 2016;33:399-404

82 Kadivar S, Belsito DV. Occupational dermatitis in health care workers evaluated for suspected allergic contact dermatitis. Dermatitis 2015;26:177-183

83 Yasky AS, Eyal A, Kappel A, Slodownik D. Occupational contact dermatitis in a nurse due to thimerosal. Isr Med Assoc J 2011;13:254-255

84 Wattanakrai P, Rajatanavin N. Thimerosal allergy and clinical relevance in Thailand. J Med Assoc Thai 2007;90:1775-1779

85 Laxmisha C, Nath AK, Thappa DM. Bindi dermatitis due to thimerosal and gallate mix. J Eur Acad Dermatol Venereol 2006;20:1370-1372

86 Freiman A, Al-Layali A, Sasseville D. Patch testing with thimerosal in a Canadian center: an 11-year experience. Am J Contact Dermat 2003;14:138-143

87 Trujillo MJ, de Barrio M, Rodríguez A, Moreno-Zazo M, Sánchez I, Pelta R, Tornero P, Herrero T. Piroxicam-induced photodermatitis. Cross-reactivity among oxicams. A case report. Allergol Immunopathol (Madr) 2001;29:133-136

88 Iliev D, Wüthrich B. Conjunctivitis to thimerosal mistaken as hay fever. Allergy 1998;53:333-334

89 Luka RE, Oppenheimer JJ, Miller N, Rossi J, Bielory L. Delayed hypersensitivity to thimerosal in RhO(D) immunoglobulin. J Allergy Clin Immunol 1997;100:138-139

90 Noel I, Galloway A, Ive FA. Hypersensitivity to thiomersal in hepatitis B vaccine. Lancet 1991;338(8768):705

91 Gordon A. Prospective screening for thimerosal hypersensitivity: a pilot study. Am J Optom Physiol Opt 1988;65:147-150

92 Lohiya G. Asthma and urticaria after hepatitis B vaccination. West J Med 1987;147:341

93 Förström L, Hannuksela M, Kousa M, Lehmuskallio E. Merthiolate hypersensitivity and vaccination. Contact Dermatitis 1980;6:241-245

94 Tosti A, Tosti G. Thimerosal: a hidden allergen in ophthalmology. Contact Dermatitis 1988;18:268-273

95 Whittington CV. Elicitation of contact lens allergy to thimerosal by eye cream. Contact Dermatitis 1985;13:186

96 van Ketel WG, Melzer-van Riemsdijk FA. Conjunctivitis due to soft lens solutions. Contact Dermatitis 1980;6:321-324

97 Sertoli A, Fonzo ED, Spallanzani P, Panconesi E. Allergic contact dermatitis from thimerosal in a soft contact lens wearer. Contact Dermatitis 1980;6:292-293

98 Bang Pedersen N. Allergic contact conjunctivitis from merthiolate in soft contact lenses. Contact Dermatitis 1978;4:165

99 Pratt MD, Belsito DV, DeLeo VA, Fowler JF Jr, Fransway AF, Maibach HI, et al. North American Contact Dermatitis Group patch-test results, 2001–2002 study period. Dermatitis 2004;15:176-183

100 Marks JG Jr, Belsito DV, DeLeo VA, Fowler JF Jr, Fransway AF, Maibach HI, et al. North American Contact Dermatitis Group patch-test results, 1998–2000. Am J Contact Dermat 2003;14:59-62

101 Marks JG Jr, Belsito DV, DeLeo VA, Fowler JF Jr, Fransway AF, Maibach HI, et al. North American Contact Dermatitis Group patch test results, 1996–1998. Arch Dermatol 2000;136:272-273

102 Marks JG Jr, Belsito DV, DeLeo VA, Fowler JF Jr, Fransway AF, Maibach HI, et al. North American Contact Dermatitis Group patch test results for the detection of delayed-type hypersensitivity to topical allergens. J Am Acad Dermatol 1998;38:911-918

103 Marks JG, Belsito DV, DeLeo VA, Fowler JF, Fransway AF, Maibach HI,et al. North American Contact Dermatitis Group standard tray patch test results 1992 through 1994. Am J Contact Dermatitis 1995;6:160-165

104 Wetter DA, Davis MDP, Yiannias JA, Cheng JF, Connolly SM, el-Azhary RA, et al. Patch test results from the Mayo Contact Dermatitis Group, 1998–2000. J Am Acad Dermatol 2005;53:416-421

105 Hasan T, Rantanen T, Alanko K, Harvima RJ, Jolanki R, Kalimo K, et al. Patch test reactions to cosmetic allergens in 1995–1997 and 2000–2002 in Finland –a multicentre study. Contact Dermatitis 2005;53:40-45

106 Schnuch A, Geier J, Uter W, Frosch PJ. Patch testing with preservatives, antimicrobials and industrial biocides. Results from a multicentre study. Br J Dermatol 1998;138:467-476

2.457   2,2'-THIOBIS(4-CHLOROPHENOL)

IDENTIFICATION

Description/definition	: 2,2'-Thiobis(4-chlorophenol) is the aromatic compound that conforms to the formula shown below
Chemical class(es)	: Halogen compounds; phenols; thio compounds
Chemical/IUPAC name	: 4-Chloro-2-(5-chloro-2-hydroxyphenyl)sulfanylphenol
Other names	: Fenticlor; fentichlor
CAS registry number (s)	: 97-24-5
EC number(s)	: 202-568-7
Merck Index monograph	: 5301
Function(s) in cosmetics	: EU: antimicrobial. USA: cosmetic biocides
Patch testing	: 1.0% pet. (Chemotechnique)
Molecular formula	: $C_{12}H_8Cl_2O_2S$

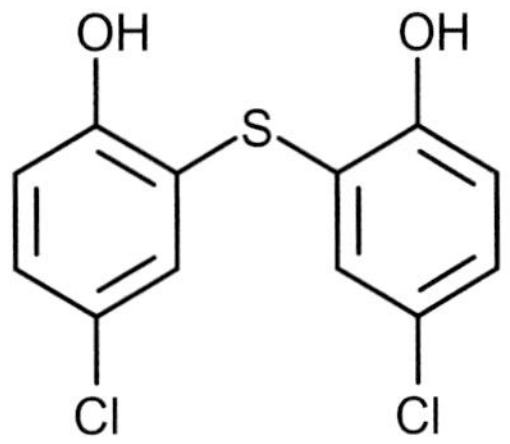

GENERAL

As the INCI name 2,2'-thiobis(4-chlorophenol) of this chemical is hardly ever, if at all, mentioned in literature, the common name fenticlor is used throughout this chapter and also in other chapters where the chemical is mentioned (tetrachlorosalicylanilide, tribromosalicylanilide, bithionol, triclosan).

Fenticlor is a halogenated phenolic compound with antibacterial and antifungal properties. In the 1960s, fenticlor was incorporated in antibacterial and antifungal creams and ointments, hair creams, cosmetics, and hand soaps worldwide, but these products were never extensively used in the United States. The last known products that contained fentichlor in the United States were 2 biocides that were used in water treatment facilities and that were both discontinued in 1993 (32). Fenticlor has caused a number of cases of photoallergic contact dermatitis in the past. Photocross-reactions from the halogenated salicylanilide tribromosalicylanilide (24) and to bithionol (7) have been observed. Fenticlor is still allowed in cosmetics in the USA and the EU, but its use in these products is virtually excluded (see the section 'Presence in cosmetic products and chemical analyses' below). In fact, there are currently no known products that contain bithionol, but it is still available from pharmaceutical companies and may be used in research, in high-throughput screening and possibly in antibacterial or antifungal creams (32).

A general introduction to the halogenated salicylanilides and halogenated phenols can be found in Chapter 2.450. Tetrachlorosalicylanilide. In assessing the data from early studies, and notably in the distinction between contact allergy and photocontact allergy, it should be realized that, in those days, experience with photopatch tests was limited and such tests may not always have been reliable.

CONTACT ALLERGY

Patch testing in groups of patients

There are no studies in which fenticlor has been tested in consecutive patients suspected of contact dermatitis (routine testing). Results of patch testing fenticlor in groups of *selected* patients (patients suspected of photosensitivity or with reactions after sunscreen application) are shown in table 2.457.1. In four studies, rates of sensitization ranged from 0.1% to 18%. The 18% rate was found in a very small study of only 11 patients with a history of photosensitivity; the 2 positive patch test reactions were not relevant (21). A 4.4% frequency of sensitization was found in a 2001-2010 study from Canada, but this had certain weaknesses and the relevance of the 7 positive patch tests to fenticlor was not mentioned (12).

Table 2.457.1 Patch testing in groups of patients: Selected patient groups

Years and Country	Test conc. & vehicle	Number of patients tested	positive (%)		Selection of patients (S); Relevance (R); Comments (C)	Ref.
2001-2010 Canada		160	7	(4.4%)	S: patients with suspected photosensitivity and patients who developed pruritus or a rash after sunscreen application; R: not stated; C: weak study: inadequate reading of test results, erythema only was considered to represent a positive patch test reaction	12
2000-2005 USA	1% pet.	177	2	(1.1%)	S: patients photopatch tested for suspected photodermatitis; R: 0 reactions were relevant	17
1985-1990 USA	1% pet.	11	2	(18%)	S: patients with a history of photosensitivity; R: not relevant; one reaction was photoaggravated contact allergy	21
1980-1981 4 Scandinavian countries	1% pet.	745	1	(0.1%)	S: patients suspected of sun-related skin disease; R: not stated	23

Case reports and case series

One patient had axillary dermatitis from contact allergy to fenticlor in a deodorant (13). Another individual had allergic contact dermatitis from fenticlor in a hair cream (14).

Contact allergy to fenticlor in non-cosmetic products

One patient had allergic contact dermatitis from fenticlor in a topical pharmaceutical preparation (7). An industrial chemist concerned in the manufacture of fenticlor and other halogenated phenolic compounds developed airborne allergic contact dermatitis from fenticlor, which later resulted in persistent light sensitivity and actinic reticuloid. The patient also had *photo*contact allergy to fenticlor and the chemically related dichlorophene (26). A service engineer became sensitized to fenticlor from accidental spillage of a small quantity of liquid containing 40% fenticlor cooling system biocide additive, onto his trouser. Later, he developed a photosensitive eruption corresponding to the sites of previous contact without renewed contact with fenticlor. Patch and photopatch tests showed photoaggravated contact allergy to the chemical. The authors concluded that industrial exposure to fentichlor appeared to have triggered susceptibility to polymorphic light eruption in this patient (PLE) (30).

Cross-reactions, pseudo-cross-reactions and co-reactions (including photoreactions)

Primary photosensitization to tribromosalicylanilide in 40% of cases leads to fenticlor photo-cross-reactivity (24). Patients photosensitized to fenticlor may photocross-react to bithionol. The structures of these chemicals are very similar and it has been suggested that, when irradiated, bithionol loses two chlorine atoms to become fenticlor (7). In a group of 18 patients photosensitized to ketoprofen, 12 (67%) had positive photopatch tests to fenticlor. As there were also many photoreactions to tetrachlorosalicylanilide (n=5, 28%), triclosan (n=3, 17%), tribromosalicylanilide (n=2, 11%) and bithionol (n=2, 11%) with no clinical relevance, the authors raised the question of hyper-photo-susceptibility to non-relevant allergens induced by photosensitivity to ketoprofen (27). In another group of 35 patients photoallergic to ketoprofen from Sweden, simultaneous photoallergy to fenticlor was seen in 74%, to tetrachlorosalicylanilide in 40%, to triclosan in 9% and to bithionol, tribromosalicylanilide and hexachlorophene in 6% of the patients. No explanation for these co-reactivities was offered (28).

Of 28 patients photoallergic to ketoprofen, 7 also had positive photopatch tests to fenticlor (10). In a French study, of 11 patients with photocontact allergy to ketoprofen, 9 had positive photopatch tests to fenticlor and 4 to tetrachlorosalicylanilide (29). In another French study, however, only 2 out of 19 patients photoallergic to ketoprofen co-photoreacted to fenticlor (34). In an Italian study, some positive photopatch tests were also observed in patients with contact allergy or photocontact allergy to ketoprofen. As computerized conformational analysis demonstrated that the structure of fenticlor is completely different from that of ketoprofen, the simultaneous allergic reactions to fenticlor should be regarded as co-sensitizations rather than cross-sensitizations, according to the authors (31).

Presence in cosmetic products and chemical analyses

In the USA, in April 2017, fenticlor (2,2'-thiobis(4-chlorophenol)) was present in zero of 56,714 cosmetic products of which the composition is known in FDA's Voluntary Cosmetic Registration Program (VCRP) (data obtained from FDA, May 2017). In January 2017, 2,2'-thiobis(4-chlorophenol) was present in zero of 64,655 cosmetic products of which the composition is known in EWG's Skin Deep Cosmetics Database, USA (http://www.ewg.org/skindeep/).

OTHER SIDE EFFECTS

Photosensitivity

Photopatch testing in groups of patients
Results of photopatch testing with fenticlor in groups of selected patients (e.g., patients suspected of photosensitivity, dermatitis affecting mainly light-exposed skin, patients with histories or clinical pictures suggestive of allergic contact photodermatitis) are shown in table 2.457.2. In 17 studies, rates of photosensitization have ranged from 1% to 18%, but were 2% or less in 8 of the seventeen investigations (table 2.457.2). The highest frequencies of positive photopatch tests (18% and 17%) were found in two very small studies of 11 patients with a history of photosensitivity (the 2 positive photopatch test reactions were not relevant) (21) and in 18 patients with persistent light reactions, a highly selected group (22), but relevance was not mentioned in the latter study. In fact, in 13 of the studies, relevance was either not mentioned or not specified for fenticlor. In the four that did address the issue, 1/13 (11), 0/12 (19), 4/16 (17) and 0/2 (21) were scored as relevant. Causative products were not mentioned.

Table 2.457.2 Photopatch testing in groups of patients

Years and Country	Test conc. & vehicle	Number of patients tested	positive (%)	Selection of patients (S); Relevance (R); Comments (C)	Ref.
2001-2010 Canada		160	8 (5.0%)	S: patients with suspected photosensitivity and patients who developed pruritus or a rash after sunscreen application; R: not stated; C: weak study: inadequate reading of test results, erythema only was considered to represent a positive patch test reaction	12
1993-2009 USA	1% pet.	30	3 (10%)	S: patients with chronic actinic dermatitis; R: not stated	15
2003-2007 Portugal	1% pet.	83	1 (1%)	S: patients with suspected photoaggravated facial dermatitis or systemic photosensitivity; R: not stated	16
2004-2006 Italy	1% pet.	1082	13 (1.2%)	S: patients with histories and clinical features suggestive of photoallergic contact dermatitis; 3/13 were cases of photoaugmented contact allergy; R: one relevant (8%)	11
1993-2006 USA	1% pet.	76	9 (12%)	S: not stated; R: 94% of all reactions to antimicrobials were considered 'not relevant'	9
1992-2006 Greece	1% pet.	207	4 (1.9%)	S: patients suspected of photosensitivity; R: not stated	18
2004-2005 Spain	1% pet.	224	12 (5.4%)	S: not stated; R: not relevant	19
2000-2005 USA	1% pet.	177	16 (9.0%)	S: patients photopatch tested for suspected photodermatitis; R: 4 reactions were relevant	17
1991-97 Ger, Au, Swi	1% pet.	1261	23 (1.8%)	S: patients suspected of photosensitivity; R: not stated	2
1985-1994 Italy		1050	13 (1.2%)	S: patients with histories or clinical pictures suggestive of allergic contact photodermatitis; R: 78% for all photoallergens together	3
1991-1993 Singapore	1% pet.	62	1 (2%)	S: patients with clinical features suggestive of photosensitivity; R: not stated	20
1985-1990 USA	1% pet.	11	2 (18%)	S: patients with a history of photosensitivity; R: not relevant; C: one reaction was photoaggravated contact allergy	21
1987-1989 Thailand	1% pet.	274	9 (3.3%)	S: patients suspected of photosensitivity; R: not stated	33
1980-85 Ger, Au, Swi	1% pet.	1129	18 (1.6%)	S: patients suspected of photoallergy, polymorphic light eruption, phototoxicity and skin problems with photodistribution; R: not stated	4
1980-1985 USA	1% pet.	70	5 (7%)	S: not stated; R: not stated	1
<1984 Norway	1% pet.	18	3 (17%)	S: patients with persistent light reactions; R: not stated	22
1980-1981 4 Scandinavian countries	1% pet.	745	12 (1.6%)	S: patients suspected of sun-related skin disease; R: not stated	23

Au: Austria; Ger: Germany; Swi: Switzerland

Case reports and series

Cosmetics
Three patients developed persistent light reactions from photocontact allergy to fenticlor in hair cream (5, possibly overlap with ref. 25). One individual had photocontact allergy from fenticlor in a handwashing soap (8). Another patient developed photocontact allergy to fenticlor in a shampoo (24). Fenticlor in a hair cream caused two cases of chronic dermatitis from persistent photosensitivity (25, possibly overlap with ref. 5).

Non-cosmetic products
Three patients had photocontact allergy to fenticlor in antifungal preparations (6). An industrial chemist concerned in the manufacture of fenticlor and other halogenated phenolic compounds developed airborne allergic contact dermatitis from fenticlor, which later resulted in persistent light sensitivity and actinic reticuloid. The patient also had *photo*contact allergy to fenticlor and the chemically related dichlorophene (26). One patient had photoallergic contact dermatitis from fenticlor in a topical pharmaceutical preparation (7). A service engineer became sensitized to fenticlor from accidental spillage of a small quantity of liquid, containing 40% fenticlor cooling system biocide additive, onto his trouser. Later, he developed a photosensitive eruption corresponding to the sites of previous contact without renewed contact with fenticlor. Patch and photopatch tests showed photoaggravated contact allergy. The authors concluded that industrial exposure to fentichlor appeared to have triggered susceptibility to polymorphic light eruption in this patient (PLE) (30). An industrial chemist, who had worked with dichlorophene and later fenticlor, developed edema of the face and worsening of a red scaly rash of the scalp and face (diagnosed as seborrheic dermatitis) after servicing a machine in which fenticlor had been used. Patch and photopatch tests were positive to fenticlor and dichlorophene (5).

LITERATURE

1   Menz J, Muller SA, Connnolly SM. Photopatch testing: A six year experience. J Am Acad Dermatol 1988;18:1044-1047

2   Neumann NJ, Hölzle E, Plewig G, Schwarz T, Panizzon RG, Breit R, et al. Photopatch testing: The 12-year experience of the German, Austrian and Swiss Photopatch Test Group. J Am Acad Dermatol 2000;42:183-192

3   Pigatto PD, Legori A, Bigardi AS, Guarrera M, Tosti A, Santucci B, et al. Gruppo Italiano recerca dermatiti da contatto ed ambientali Italian multicenter study of allergic contact photodermatitis: epidemiological aspects. Am J Contact Dermatitis 1996;17:158-163

4   Hölzle E, Neumann N, Hausen B, Przybilla B, Schauder S, Hönigsmann H, et al. Photopatch testing: the 5-year experience of the German, Austrian and Swiss Photopatch Test Group. J Am Acad Dermatol 1991;25:59-68

5   Ramsay CA. Skin responses to ultraviolet radiation in contact photodermatitis due to fentichlor. J Invest Dermatol 1979;72:99-102

6   Burry JN. Photoallergies to fentichlor and multifungin. Arch Dermatol 1967;95:287-291

7   Burry JN. Cross sensitivity between fentichlor and bithionol. Arch Dermatol 1968;97:497-503

8   Jeanmougin M, Menciet J, Dubertret L. Photoallergie de contact au Fentichlor présent dans un savon d'hygiène pour les mains. Ann Dermatol Vénéreol 1992;119:983-985

9   Victor FC, Cohen DE, Soter NA. A 20-year analysis of previous and emerging allergens that elicit photoallergic contact dermatitis. J Am Acad Dermatol 2010;62:605-610

10 Avenel-Audran M. Dutartre H, Goossens A, Jeanmougin M, Comte C, Bernier C, et al. Octocrylene, an emerging photoallergen. Arch Dermatol 2010;146:753-757

11 Pigatto PD, Guzzi G, Schena D, Guarrera M, Foti C, Francalanci S, et al. Photopatch tests: an Italian multicentre study from 2004 to 2006. Contact Dermatitis 2008;59:103-108

12 Greenspoon J, Ahluwalia R, Juma N, Rosen CF. Allergic and photoallergic contact dermatitis: A 10-year experience. Dermatitis 2013;24:29-32

13 Calnan CD. Dihydroxydichlorodiphenylmonosulphide in a deodorant. Contact Dermatitis 1975;1:127-128

14 Beer WE. Sensitivity to fentichlor. Contact Derm newsl 1970;8:188

15 Que SK, Brauer JA, Soter NA, Cohen DE. Chronic actinic dermatitis: an analysis at a single institution over 25 years. Dermatitis 2011;22:147-154

16 Cardoso J, Canelas MM, Gonçalo M, Figueiredo A. Photopatch testing with an extended series of photoallergens: a 5-year study. Contact Dermatitis 2009;60:325-329

17 Scalf LA, Davis MDP, Rohlinger AL, Connolly SM. Photopatch testing of 182 patients: A 6-year experience at the Mayo Clinic. Dermatitis 2009;20:44-52

18 Katsarou A, Makris M, Zarafonitis G, Lagogianni E, Gregoriou S, Kalogeromitros D. Photoallergic contact dermatitis: the 15-year experience of a tertiary referral center in a sunny Mediterranean city. Int J Immunopathol Pharmacol 2008;21:725-727

19 De La Cuadra-Oyanguren J, Perez-Ferriols A, Lecha-Carrelero M, et al. Results and assessment of photopatch testing in Spain: towards a new standard set of photoallergens. Actas DermoSifiliograficas 2007;98:96-101

20 Leow YH, Wong WK, Ng SK, Goh CL. 2 years experience of photopatch testing in Singapore. Contact Dermatitis 1994;31:181-182

21 DeLeo VA, Suarez SM, Maso MJ. Photoallergic contact dermatitis. Results of photopatch testing in New York, 1985 to 1990. Arch Dermatol 1992;128:1513-1518

22 Thune P, Eeg-Larsen T. Contact and photocontact allergy in persistent light reactivity. Contact Dermatitis 1984;11:98-107

23 Wennersten G, Thune P, Brodthagen H, Jansen C, Rystedt I, Crames M, et al. The Scandinavian multicenter photopatch study. Contact Dermatitis 1984;10:305-309

24 Osmundsen PE. Contact photodermatitis due to tribromsalicylanilide. Br J Dermatol 1968;80:228-234

25 Ramsay CA, Crow KD. Personal communication, cited in: Burry JN. Fenticlor, actinic reticuloid, and antihistamines (Letter). Br Med J 1974;2(5918):556-557

26 Clayton R. From fentichlor sensitivity to actinic reticuloid? Proc R Soc Med 1976;69:379-380

27 Durbize E, Vigan M, Puzenat E, Girardin P, Adessi B, Desprez PH, Humbert PH, Laurent R, Aubin F. Spectrum of cross-photosensitization in 18 consecutive patients with contact photoallergy to ketoprofen: associated photoallergies to non-benzophenone-containing molecules. Contact Dermatitis 2003;48:144-149

28 Hindsén M, Zimerson E, Bruze M. Photoallergic contact dermatitis from ketoprofen in southern Sweden. Contact Dermatitis 2006;54:150-157

29 Vigan M, Girardin P, Desprez P, Adessi B, Aubin F, Laurent R. Photoallergie au kétoprofène et photosensibilisations au tétrachlorosalicylanide et au Fentichlor. Ann Dermatol Venereol 2002;129:1125-1127

30 Norris PG, Hawk JL, White IR. Photoallergic contact dermatitis from fentichlor. Contact Dermatitis 1988;18:318-320

31 Foti C, Bonamonte D, Conserva A, Stingeni L, Lisi P, Lionetti N, Rigano L, Angelini G. Allergic and photoallergic contact dermatitis from ketoprofen: evaluation of cross-reactivities by a combination of photopatch testing and computerized conformational analysis. Curr Pharm Des 2008;14:2833-2839

32 Wolverton JE, Soter NA, Cohen DE. Fentichlor photocontact dermatitis: A persistent enigma. Dermatitis 2013;24:77-81

33 Gritiyarangsan P. A three-year photopatch study in Thailand. J Dermatol Sci 1991;2:371-375

34 Durieu C, Marguery MC, Giordano-Labadie F, Journe F, Loche F, Bazex J. Photoaggravated contact allergy and contact photoallergy caused by ketoprofen: 19 cases. Ann Dermatol Venereol 2001;128:1020-1024

2.458 THIOCTIC ACID

IDENTIFICATION

Description/definition   : Thioctic acid is the organic compound that conforms to the formula shown below
Chemical class(es)   : Carboxylic acids; thio compounds
Chemical/IUPAC name   : 1,2-Dithiolane-3-pentanoic acid, (+/-)-
Other names   : α-Lipoic acid; 1,2-dithiolane-3-valeric acid; 5-(dithiolan-3-yl)valeric acid
CAS registry number (s)   : 1077-28-7
EC number(s)   : 214-071-2
Merck Index monograph   : 10749
Function(s) in cosmetics : EU: antioxidant. USA: antioxidants
Patch test allergens   : 1-5% pet. (1,2); 5% pet. (5); 1% and 5% pet. are not irritant (1,2)
Molecular formula   : $C_8H_{14}O_2S_2$

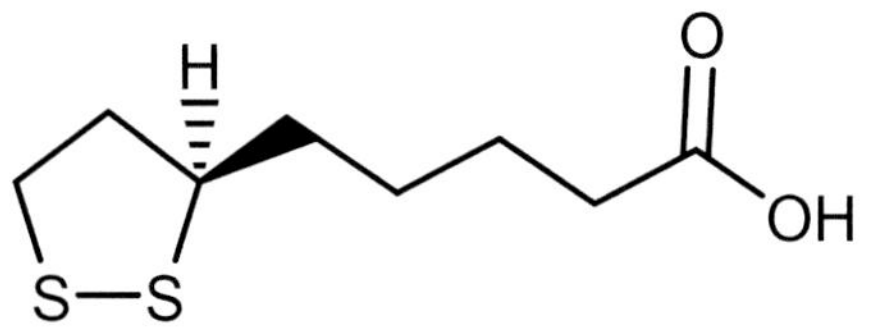

GENERAL

Thioctic acid (α-lipoic acid) is an eight-carbon disulfide containing a single chiral nucleus, and is reduced *in vivo* to its dithiol form, dihydrolipoic acid. It is an essential cofactor in metabolic reactions through mitochondrial-specific pathways, and it is synthesized in small amounts in humans. Thioctic acid shows antioxidant and metal-chelating activity. Hence, it is widely used in a variety of conditions, including diabetes, insulin resistance, atherosclerosis, neuropathy, neurodegenerative diseases, and ischemia-reperfusion (2). Recent research has suggested that thioctic acid may be beneficial in reducing the effects of oxidative damage to the eye, which drives many common diseases, such as cataracts, diabetic retinopathy, and age-related macular degeneration (6). Memory loss, chronic fatigue syndrome, human immunodeficiency virus infection/acquired immunodeficiency syndrome, cancer, liver diseases and Lyme disease are also among the wide variety of conditions in which Thioctic acid is supposedly of benefit (1). Finally, thioctic acid is used in anti-ageing products, such as 'anti-wrinkle' cream (2).

CONTACT ALLERGY

Case reports and case series

A woman had severe dermatitis on the eyelids, trunk and arms. Patch tests were negative, also to 2 cosmetics she suspected of being the cause. Three months later, the patient returned with an infiltrated erythema all over her face and neck which had started 6 hours after a single application of a cream, which she had used before, but had forgotten to mention, so this cream had not been patch tested. A patch test with the cream was strongly positive. When tested with its ingredients, the patient now reacted to thioctic acid in a dilution series from 5% pet. down to 0.025% pet. Ten controls were negative to the 5% and 2.5% patch test materials (2). The authors presented two more female patients, who also had allergic contact dermatitis from thioctic acid present in the same cream as used by the first patient. In addition, in the adverse reaction reporting system of the Department of Cosmetics Section of the Swedish Medical Products Agency, 15 other reports on suspected adverse skin reactions to the same cream have been submitted up to 2006, after its introduction in 2002 (2).

   A woman had developed dermatitis of the face following daily use for several weeks of a new anti-wrinkle day cream. On examination, her face was entirely erythematous and edematous with yellow crusts suggestive of secondary bacterial infection, accompanied by profound itching and burning sensations. The patient was treated with topical mometasone furoate ointment, systemic flucloxacillin and methylprednisolone, combined with stopping the use of all of her cosmetic products, after which the dermatitis subsided. Patch tests with the Belgian baseline series, a cosmetic series, and the patient's own cosmetic products tested 'as is', showed positive reactions to the day cream at D2 and D4. Later, the ingredients of this product, supplied by the manufacturer, were tested, and the patient now reacted strongly to the ingredient thioctic acid 5% pet. (5).

Contact allergy to non-cosmetic products

A woman suffering from shoulder pain resulting from cervical disc herniation developed a pruritic maculopapular rash on the face and scalp after 10 days of treatment with a dietary supplement (containing thioctic acid and other components) and with two oral and one intramuscular NSAIDs. The patient stopped taking all drugs and was treated with oral corticosteroids for 2 days, after which the rash disappeared. Prick tests with the supplement and the three drugs (powdered drug dissolved in saline) were negative. Patch tests gave a very strong reaction to the commercial dietary supplement. Later, patch tests were performed with its ingredient, and the patient now reacted to the supplement 10% pet. and to thioctic acid 5% pet., 2.5% pet. and 0.025% pet. Twelve controls were negative to these patch test materials (1).

A woman had a 7-month history of periorbital swelling and dermatitis. Patch testing with a baseline, cosmetic and medicament series, together with her own products gave a positive reaction to her eye drops, tested 'as is' on day D2 and D4. Thirty controls were negative. When tested with its ingredients, the patient now reacted to thioctic acid on D2 and D4. Thirty controls were negative to this test preparation. The patient has had no further recurrence of the dermatitis after avoiding eye drops containing thioctic acid (6).

Presence in cosmetic products and chemical analyses

In the USA, in April 2017, thioctic acid was present in 81 of 56,714 cosmetic products of which the composition is known in FDA's Voluntary Cosmetic Registration Program (VCRP) (data obtained from FDA, May 2017). In April 2017, thioctic acid was present in 29 of 66,485 cosmetic products of which the composition is known in EWG's Skin Deep Cosmetics Database, USA (http://www.ewg.org/skindeep/).

OTHER SIDE EFFECTS

Irritant contact dermatitis

In a study of the effect of 5% thioctic acid on photo-ageing, transient local irritation was seen during the first weeks in a number of test individuals (3).

LITERATURE

1   Rizzi A, Nucera E, Buonomo A, Schiavino D. Delayed hypersensitivity to α-lipoic acid: look at dietary supplements. Contact Dermatitis 2015;73:62-63
2   Bergqvist-Karlsson A. Thelin I, Bergendorff O. Contact dermatitis to α-lipoic acid in an anti-wrinkle cream. Contact Dermatitis 2006;55:56-57
3   Beitner H. Randomized, placebo- controlled, double blind study on the clinical efficacy of a cream containing 5 % α-lipoic acid related to photoageing of facial skin. Br J Dermatol 2003;149:841-849
4   Packer L, Witt EH, Tritschler HJ. Alpha-lipoic acid as a biological antioxidant. Free Radic Biol Med 1995;19:227-250
5   Leysen J, Aerts O. Further evidence of thioctic acid (α-lipoic acid) being a strong cosmetic sensitizer. Contact Dermatitis 2016;74:182-184
6   Craig S, Urwin R, Wilkinson M. Contact allergy to thioctic acid present in Hypromellose® eye drops. Contact Dermatitis 2017;76:361-362

2.459 THIOGLYCERIN

IDENTIFICATION

Description/definition	: Thioglycerin is the polyhydric alcohol that conforms to the formula shown below
Chemical class(es)	: Polyols; thiocompounds
Chemical/IUPAC name	: 3-Sulfanylpropane-1,2-diol
Other names	: 3-Mercaptopropane-1,2-diol; monothioglycerol; thioglycerol
CAS registry number (s)	: 96-27-5; 38098-46-3
EC number(s)	: 202-495-0; 253-777-5
Merck Index monograph	: 10758
Function(s) in cosmetics	: EU: depilatory; hair waving or straightening; keratolytic; reducing. USA: depilating agents; hair-waving / straightening agents; reducing agents
Patch testing	: 5% pet., 10% water (3)
Molecular formula	: $C_3H_8O_2S$

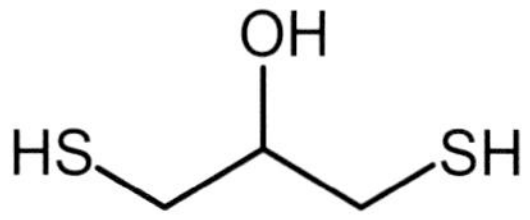

CONTACT ALLERGY

Case reports and case series

One patient had allergic contact dermatitis from thioglycerin in a depilatory cream (1). Unknown number of patients with allergic contact dermatitis from thioglycerin in depilatory creams (2). One or more hairdressers had contact dermatitis (allergic?, irritant?) from cold wave solutions containing thioglycerin (4).

Presence in cosmetic products and chemical analyses

In the USA, in April 2017, thioglycerol was present in 49 of 56,714 cosmetic products of which the composition is known in FDA's Voluntary Cosmetic Registration Program (VCRP) (data obtained from FDA, May 2017). In April 2017, thioglycerin was present in 23 of 65,434 cosmetic products of which the composition is known in EWG's Skin Deep Cosmetics Database, USA (http://www.ewg.org/skindeep/).

LITERATURE

1. Fousserea J, Benezra C. Les eczémas allergiques professionels. Paris: Masson et Cie, 1970:385 (French)
2. Foussereau J, Maleville J, Grosshans E, Araujo A, Maillot C, Basset A. Allergic eczema caused by thioglycerin in depilatory creams. Disadvantages of this substance in cosmetology. Bull Soc Fr Dermatol Syphiligr 1967;74:762-766 (article in French)
3. De Groot AC. Patch Testing, 3rd Edition. Wapserveen, The Netherlands: acdegroot publishing, 2008 (ISBN 978-90-813233-1-4)
4. Gasser E. Hairdresser's eczema, caused by cold wave solutions containing thioglycerin. Schweiz Med Wochenschr 1953;83:448-450 (article in German)

2.460 THIOLACTIC ACID

IDENTIFICATION

Description/definition : Thiolactic acid is the organic acid that conforms to the formula shown below
Chemical class(es) : Carboxylic acids
Chemical/IUPAC name : 2-Sulfanylpropanoic acid
Other names : 2-Mercaptopropionic acid; propanoic acid, 2-mercapto-
CAS registry number (s) : 79-42-5
EC number(s) : 201-206-5
Merck Index monograph : 10763
Function(s) in cosmetics : EU: antioxidant; depilatory; hair waving or straightening; masking; reducing.
USA: antioxidants; depilating agents; fragrance ingredients; hair-waving/straightening agents; reducing agents
Patch testing : 0.1% and 0.3% pet. (2); a test concentration of 1% pet. is irritant, but 0.3% may also induce irritant patch test reactions (2)
Molecular formula : $C_3H_6O_2S$

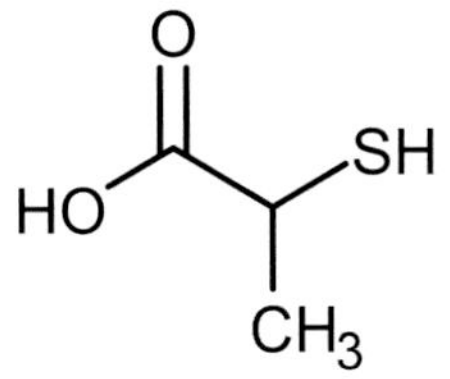

CONTACT ALLERGY

Patch testing in groups of patients
There have been no studies in which consecutive patients suspected of contact dermatitis have been patch tested with thiolactic acid (routine testing). Testing in groups of *selected* patients was done by the members of the German Contact Dermatitis Research Group (2). In 2000-2001, patients selected for testing with the hairdressers series were also patch tested with thiolactic acid 0.3% and 0.1% pet., after preliminary research had indicated that a 1% concentration was quite irritant. One hundred and sixty-four patients were tested and 1 (0.6%) reacted to 0.3% thiolactic acid and zero to 0.1%. Relevance was not found with certainty (1).

Case reports and case series
A hairdresser had occupational allergic contact dermatitis superimposed on irritant hand dermatitis from a permanent-waving solution containing ammonium thioglycolate and ammonium thiolactate. The patient did not react to these chemicals themselves, but there was a positive response to thiolactic acid 1% pet., the culprit component according to the authors (1). They considered an irritant reaction to be unlikely, as 8 other hairdressers did apparently not react to the 1% pet. test substance. However, other authors have found this concentration to be quite irritant (2).

Cross-reactions, pseudo-cross-reactions and co-reactions
Not to ammonium thiolactate (2).

Presence in cosmetic products and chemical analyses
In the USA, in April 2017, thiolactic acid was present 24 in of 56,714 cosmetic products of which the composition is known in FDA's Voluntary Cosmetic Registration Program (VCRP) (data obtained from FDA, May 2017). In February 2017, thiolactic acid was present in one of 64,631 cosmetic products of which the composition is known in EWG's Skin Deep Cosmetics Database, USA (http://www.ewg.org/skindeep/).

LITERATURE
1 Straube M, Uter W, Schwanitz HJ. Occupational allergic contact dermatitis from thiolactic acid contained in 'ester-free' permanent-waving solutions. Contact Dermatitis 1996;34:229-230
2 Uter W, Geier J, Pirker C, Aberer W, Kränke B, Richter G, John SM, et al FOR THE GERMAN CONTACT DERMATITIS RESEARCH GROUP (DKG). Ammonium thiolactate and thiolactic acid: important hairdressers' allergens?. Contact Dermatitis 2002;46:242-243

2.461   Tinosorb® M *

Not an INCI name

IDENTIFICATION

Description/definition   : Tinosorb® M is an emulsion that contains the UV filter methylene bis-benzotriazolyl tetramethylbutylphenol plus decyl glucoside, propylene glycol, xanthan gum and water

Chemical class(es)   : UV-filters

INCI name EU   : Methylene bis-benzotriazolyl tetramethylbutylphenol (and) aqua (and) decyl glucoside (and) propylene glycol (and) xanthan gum

INCI name USA   : Not in the Personal Care Council Database

Function(s) in cosmetics : EU: UV-filter

Patch testing   : 10% pet. (SmartPracticeCanada); preferably test with separate ingredients (see there)

GENERAL

Tinosorb® M is an emulsion that contains the UV filter methylene bis-benzotriazolyl tetramethylbutylphenol (45-55%) (synonym bisoctrizole; CAS no. 103597-45-1). Tinosorb® M also contains decyl glucoside (6-10%) (CAS no. 58846-77-8), propylene glycol (0.2-0.6%) (CAS no. 57-55-6), xanthan gum (0.1-0.5%) (CAS no. 11138-66-2), and water (40-42%). These compounds are added to enhance the solubility of the UV filter in cosmetic products; the surfactant decyl glucoside and the emulsifier/surfactant xanthan gum in addition stabilize the emulsion and the UV microparticles in it (1). Tinosorb® M is applied both in sunscreens and in other cosmetics including skin care products (1). It is a relatively new UV-filter, that has been used since 1998.

Most cases of contact allergy to Tinosorb® M appear to be caused by its ingredient decyl glucoside (2,4,5,6). In one case, xanthan gum was the allergenic ingredients (3). The active ingredient methylene bis-benzotriazolyl tetramethy-lbutylphenol has thus far not been identified as the allergen in patients reacting to Tinosorb® M. In some reports, suggesting allergy to the UV-filter itself (7,9,10), 'methylene-bis-benzotriazolyl tetramethylbutylphenol' most likely was Tinosorb® M (1). The pure UV-filter first became available on January 1, 2014 from Chemotechnique Diagnostics. Before that time, 'methylene bis-benzotriazolyl tetramethylbutylphenol' from this provider of patch test materials actually also was Tinosorb® M (1).

The separate ingredients methylene bis-benzotriazolyl tetramethylbutylphenol, decyl glucoside, propylene glycol and xanthan gum are discussed in the chapters with the same names. A review of contact allergy to Tinosorb® M up to 2014 is provided in ref. 1.

CONTACT ALLERGY

In all sections below, 'methylene bis-benzotriazolyl tetramethylbutylphenol' has certainly or most likely been Tinosorb® M, not the pure chemical.

Patch testing in groups of patients

The results of two studies in which methylene bis-benzotriazolyl tetramethylbutylphenol 10% pet. was patch tested in groups of selected patients (patients with exposed site dermatitis, history of a reaction to a sunscreen or a topical NSAID) are shown in table 2.461.1. A high rate of sensitization (6.3%) was found in a small Colombian study of 112 patients; 6 of the 7 positive patch tests were considered to be relevant (14).

Table 2.461.1 Patch testing in groups of patients

Years and Country	Test conc. & vehicle	Number of patients tested	positive (%)	Selection of patients (S); Relevance (R); Comments (C)	Ref.
2011-2013 Colombia	10% pet.	112	7 (6.3%)	S: dermatitis affecting mainly light-exposed skin, a history of a sunscreen skin or topical NSAID skin reaction: R: 86%	14
2008-2011 12 European countries	10% pet.	1031	11 (1.1%)	S: patients with exposed site dermatitis or history of a reaction to a sunscreen or topical NSAID; R: not specified; the ingredient decyl glucoside was not tested	13

Case reports and case series

Ingredients not (all) tested

Methylene bis-benzotriazolyl tetramethylbutylphenol was responsible for 2 out of 959 cases of non-fragrance cosmetic allergy where the causal allergen was identified, Belgium, 2000-2010 (10). A woman had allergic contact dermatitis of the face from methylene bis-benzotriazolyl tetramethylbutylphenol in a sunscreen cream (first report of allergic contact dermatitis) (7). A patient had contact allergy to Tinosorb® M in 2 sunscreens; she did not react to xanthan gum; decyl glucoside or other ingredients were not tested (1). Two patients had contact allergy to Tinosorb® M (8,9). In one, the reaction was caused by a sunscreen, in the other the relevance was not mentioned. This patient reacted to lauryl glucoside, hence the causal allergen may have been the ingredient decyl glucoside (8,9).

Reactions to decyl glucoside

Two patients had ACD from decyl glucoside in Tinosorb® M in a sunscreen (2,4). Five cases of allergic contact dermatitis to Tinosorb® M were seen in one hospital in Portugal between 2009 and 2012 (5), including one patient previously reported (6). One reacted to decyl glucoside 5% pet. and the other 4 to lauryl glucoside 3% pet. Because of the latter finding (decyl glucoside was not available for testing) the authors submit that these reactions are cross-reactions to decyl glucoside present in Tinosorb® M and indicate that this is the actual allergen, not the UV-filter methylene bis-benzotriazolyl tetramethylbutylphenol itself (5).

Reactions to other constituents of Tinosorb® M

A child had allergic contact dermatitis from Tinosorb® M in a sunscreen; a patch test with the pure chemical methylene bis-benzotriazolyl tetramethylbutylphenol was negative, but she did react to xanthan gum, which was the actual sensitizer (3).

Other information

Two patients from the USA with chronic actinic dermatitis had positive patch and photopatch tests to methylene bis-benzotriazolyl tetramethylbutylphenol 10% pet. However, use of this product is not permitted by the Food and Drug Administration, and neither patient could identify previous or current contact with the chemical. Nevertheless, the authors considered it to be possible that either the allergic or photoallergic contact dermatitis from the UV-filter led to their chronic actinic dermatitis (11). It should be mentioned that the diagnosis of photocontact allergy was merely established on the basis of a stronger positive photopatch test compared to the conventional patch test. Also, as the authors were unaware that they actually tested Tinosorb® M, the possibility that the patients reacted to decyl glucoside, propylene glycol or xanthan gum was not considered.

Presence in cosmetic products and chemical analyses

In May 2017, Tinosorb® M was present in zero of 66,975 cosmetic products of which the composition is known in EWG's Skin Deep Cosmetics Database, USA (http://www.ewg.org/skindeep/). In the USA, in April 2017, Tinosorb® M was present in zero of 56,714 cosmetic products of which the composition is known in FDA's Voluntary Cosmetic Registration Program (VCRP) (data obtained from FDA, May 2017). Methylene bis-benzotriazolyl tetramethylbutylphenol was present in 5.4% of 4447 cosmetic products collected in Germany, 2006-2009 (12).

OTHER SIDE EFFECTS

Photosensitivity

Photopatch testing in groups of patients

In the period 2008-2011, in 12 European countries, 1031 patients with exposed site dermatitis or history of a reaction to a sunscreen or topical NSAID were patch and photopatch tested with methylene bis-benzotriazolyl tetramethylbutylphenol 10% pet. and 5 (0.5%) had a positive photopatch test. The relevance of these reactions was not specified, but of all photoallergens together, 44% of the positive photopatch tests had current and 11% past relevance (13). In a group of 112 patients from Colombia suspected of photosensitivity and photopatch tested with methylene bis-benzotriazolyl tetramethylbutylphenol, there was one positive reaction (5%), which reaction was considered to be relevant (14).

LITERATURE

1   De Groot AC, van Zuuren EJ, Hissink D. Contact allergy to Tinosorb® M: recommendations for diagnostic improvement. Contact Dermatitis 2014;70:251-254
2   Liuti F, Borrego L. Contact dermatitis caused by Tinosorb® M: the importance of patch testing with pure methylene bis-benzotriazolyl tetramethylbutylphenol. Contact Dermatitis 2015;73:192-193
3   Aerts O, Clinck B, Schramme M, Lambert J. Contact allergy caused by Tinosorb® M: let us not forget about xanthan gum. Contact Dermatitis 2015;72:121-123
4   Andersen KE, Goossens A. Decyl glucoside contact allergy from a sunscreen product. Contact Dermatitis 2006;54:349-350
5   Pereira N, Coutinho I, Andrade P, Gonçalo M. The UV filter Tinosorb M, containing decyl glucoside, is a frequent cause of allergic contact dermatitis. Dermatitis 2013;24:41-43

6   Andrade P, Gonçalo M, Figueiredo A. Allergic contact dermatitis to decyl glucoside in Tinosorb® M. Contact Dermatitis 2010;62:119-120

7   Gonzalez-Pérez R, Trébol I, García-Río A, Arrequi M A, Soloeta R. Allergic contact dermatitis from methylene-bis-benzotriazolyl tetramethylbutylphenol (Tinosorb M). Contact Dermatitis 2007;56:121

8   O'Connell M, Kirk S, Wilkinson M S. Allergic contact dermatitis caused by Tinosorb® M. Contact Dermatitis 2011;65:48-49

9   O'Connell M, Wilkinson M. Allergic contact dermatitis to methylene-bis-benzotriazolyl tetramethylbutylphenol. Br J Dermatol 2010;163 (Suppl. 1):79

10   Travassos AR, Claes L, Boey L, Drieghe J, Goossens A. Non-fragrance allergens in specific cosmetic products. Contact Dermatitis 2011;65:276-285

11   Gonzalez ME, Soter NA, Cohen DE. Positive patch- and photopatch-test reactions to methylene bis-benzotriazolyl tetramethylbutylphenol in patients with both atopic dermatitis and chronic actinic dermatitis. Dermatitis 2011;22:106-111

12   Uter W, Gonçalo M, Yazar K, Kratz E-M, Mildau G, Lidén C. Coupled exposure to ingredients of cosmetic products: III. Ultraviolet filters. Contact Dermatitis 2014;71:162-169

13   The European Multicentre Photopatch Test Study (EMCPPTS) Taskforce. A European multicentre photopatch test study. Br J Dermatol 2012;166:1002-1009

14   Valbuena Mesa MC, Hoyos Jiménez EV. Photopatch testing in Bogota (Colombia): 2011–2013. Contact Dermatitis 2016;74:11-17

2.462 TIOXOLONE

IDENTIFICATION

Description/definition : Tioxolone is the heterocyclic organic compound that conforms to the formula shown below
Chemical class(es) : Heterocyclic compounds
Chemical/IUPAC name : 6-Hydroxy-1,3-benzoxathiol-2-one
Other name(s) : Thioxolone
CAS registry number (s) : 4991-65-5
EC number(s) : 225-653-0
Merck Index monograph : 10882
Function(s) in cosmetics : EU: adstringent. USA: cosmetic adstringents
Patch testing : 1% pet. (1,7); 0.1% and 0.01% alc. (3)
Molecular formula : $C_7H_4O_3S$

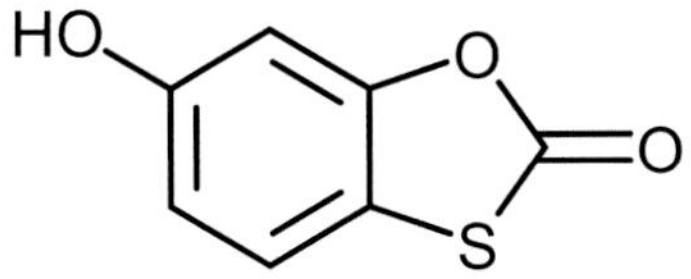

GENERAL

Tioxolone was formerly used for the treatment of psoriasis, seborrheic dermatitis of the scalp and acne (3).

CONTACT ALLERGY

Case reports and case series

A woman with seborrheic dermatitis of the scalp told that some weeks earlier she had had vesiculation on the scalp with severe pruritus after daily use of a cosmetic hair product. The eruption improved spontaneously when she avoided the use of the product, but after reuse an acute relapse appeared. A patch test with the product, tested as is, was strongly positive, whereas there were no reactions to the standard series. The components of the lotion were tested at 1 and 2% in petrolatum and tioxolone gave a positive vesicular response at D2 and D4, which was still positive after 10 days. Twenty controls tested with tioxolone 2% pet. were negative (1).

Contact allergy to tioxolone in non-cosmetic products

One patient had allergic contact dermatitis from tioxolone in an acne treatment topical pharmaceutical (2). A woman suffering for many years from psoriasis of the scalp presented with an acute vesicular dermatitis on the frontal area extending to the forehead, parts of the cheek, neck, and hands. In the previous 6 months, she had applied various antipsoriatic agents including two corticosteroid preparations containing tioxolone. The dermatitis cleared after discontinuing all medication and daily applications of a corticosteroid cream. Patch tests with the European standard series, a suspected topical pharmaceutical product and (probably later) its ingredients, showed positive reactions to the product and its component tioxolone 0.1% and 0.01% alc. Five controls tested with the 0.01% solution of tioxolone had negative reactions (3). Another patient developed intense erythema, edema and vesicles on the scalp and forehead 8 hours after applying a hair growth lotion. The patient reacted to the product itself and to its ingredient tioxolone 1% pet., which was negative in ten controls (7). Two other patient had contact allergy to tioxolone in unknown products (5, data cited in ref. 3; 8, data cited in ref. 7).

Presence in cosmetic products and chemical analyses

In the USA, in April 2017, tioxolone was present in 1 of 56,714 cosmetic products of which the composition is known in FDA's Voluntary Cosmetic Registration Program (VCRP) (data obtained from FDA, May 2017). In April 2017, tioxolone was present in zero of 65,434 cosmetic products of which the composition is known in EWG's Skin Deep Cosmetics Database, USA (http://www.ewg.org/skindeep/).

OTHER SIDE EFFECTS

Irritant contact dermatitis
Four patients developed severe dermatitis accompanied by fever and systemic reactions from the treatment of scalp psoriasis with tioxolone pharmaceutical preparations. These were interpreted as toxic effects with the exception of one case. Patch tests were not performed (6).

Immediate-type reactions
In a group of 78 patients who had whole-body treatment with a 2.5% tioxolone ointment, transient redness and burning were observed 'quite frequently'. In one patient, an urticarial rash was noted, which was thought to be of an allergic nature. Patch tests were not performed (4).

LITERATURE
1   Camarasa JG. Contact dermatitis to thioxolone. Contact Dermatitis 1981;7:213-214
2   Wahlberg JE. Sensitization to thioxolone used for topical treatment of acne. Contact Dermatitis Newsletter 1971;10: 222
3   Näher H, Frosch PJ. Contact dermatitis to thioxolone. Contact Dermatitis 1987;17:250-251
4   Boslet W, Blandin PD. Zur externen Behandlung der Schuppenflechte mit einem neuartlgen Wirkstoff. Z Haut-Geschl Kr 1959;26:161-164 (data cited in ref. 3)
5   Blohm G, Rajka G. A simple method for combined chemical and dermatological analysis of chemical mixtures by paper chromatography. Acta Derm Venereol 1966;46:432-435 (data cited in ref. 3)
6   Schoefinius HH. Kontaktdermatitis mit erhöhter Körpertemperatur unter Behandlung von Psoriasis vulgaris capillitii mit einem Benzoxathiol-Derivat. Z Haut-Geschl Kr 1972;47:227-229 (data cited in ref. 3)
7   Villas Martinez F, Joral Badas A, Garmendia Goitia JF. Contact dermatitis from thioxolone. Contact Dermatitis 1993;29:96
8   Menezes Brandao F. Dermite de contacto por tioxolona. Grupo Portuges de Estudo das Dermites de Contacto. Boletim Jnformativo 1992;6:43-44 (data cited in ref. 7, article in Portuguese)

2.463 TOCOPHEROL

IDENTIFICATION

Description/definition	: Tocopherol is a racemic mixture of naturally occurring tocopherols, including α-tocopherol, β-tocopherol, γ-tocopherol and δ-tocopherol
Chemical class(es)	: Heterocyclic compounds
Chemical/IUPAC name	: 3,4-Dihydro-2,5,7,8-tetramethyl-2-(4,8,12-trimethyltridecyl)-2*H*-benzopyran-6-ol
Other names	: Vitamin E; natural vitamin E; mixed tocopherols; DL-α-tocopherol
CAS registry number (s)	: 1406-66-2 (tocopherols); 59-02-9 (α-tocopherol); 10191-41-0 (DL-α-tocopherol); 148-03-8 (β-tocopherol); 54-28-4 (γ-tocopherol); 119-13-1 (δ-tocopherol)
EC number(s)	: 233-466-0; 218-197-9; 200-412-2; 205-708-5; 204-299-0; 200-201-5
CIR review(s)	: Int J Toxicol 2002;21(Suppl.3):51-116; Final report, March 2014 (access: www.cir-safety.org/ingredients)
Merck Index monograph	: 10923 (α-tocopherol); 10924 (β-tocopherol); 10925 (γ-tocopherol); 10926 (δ-tocopherol
Function(s) in cosmetics	: EU: antioxidant; masking; skin conditioning. USA: antioxidants; fragrance ingredients; skin-conditioning agents – miscellaneous; skin-conditioning agents – occlusive
Patch testing	: DL-α-Tocopherol 100% (Chemotechnique, SmartPracticeCanada)
Molecular formula	: $C_{29}H_{50}O_2$ (α-tocopherol; DL-α-tocopherol); $C_{28}H_{48}O_2$ (β-tocopherol; γ-tocopherol); $C_{27}H_{46}O_2$ (δ-tocopherol)

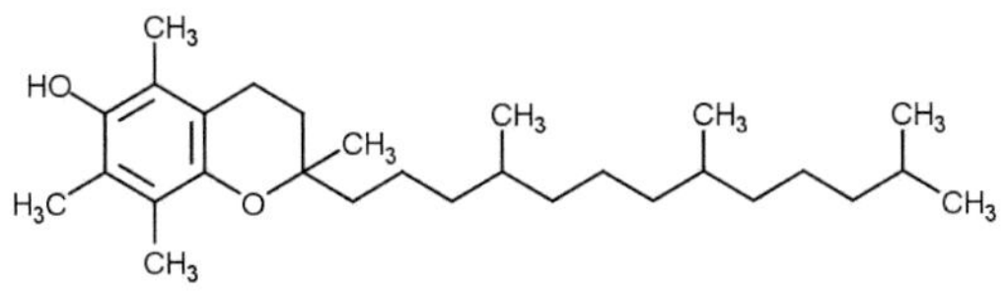

α-tocopherol

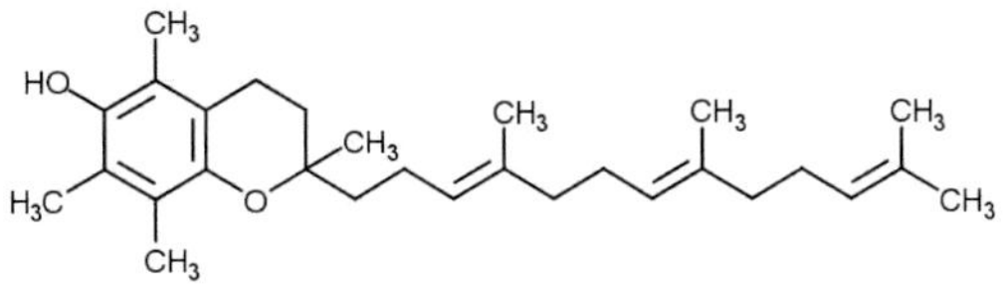

α-tocotrienol

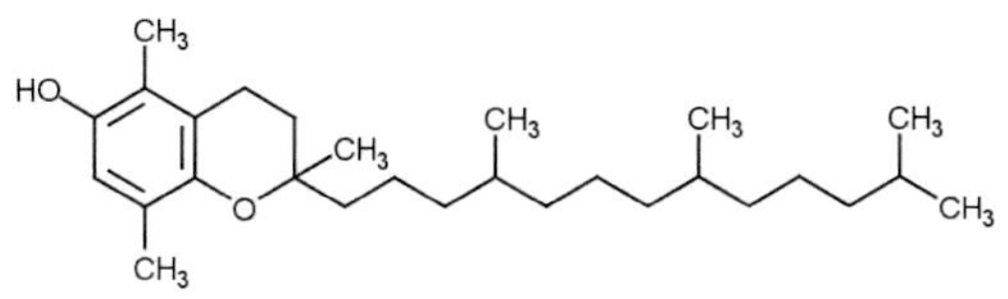

β-tocopherol

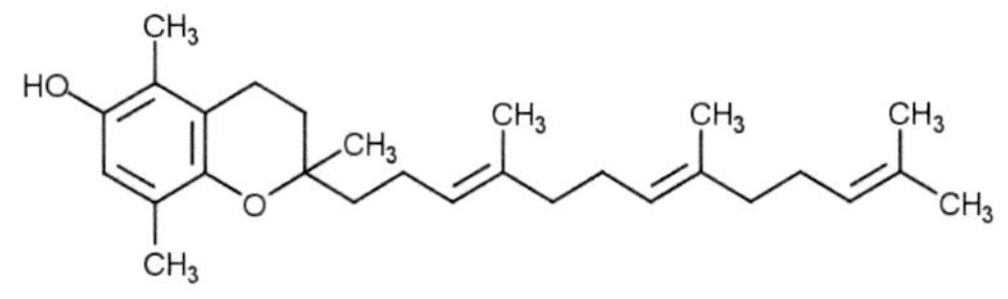

β-tocotrienol

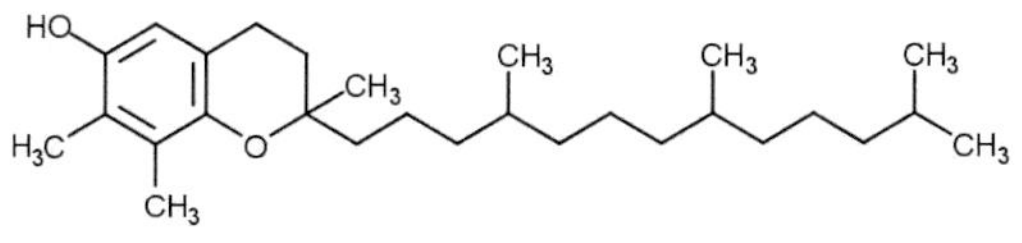

γ-tocopherol

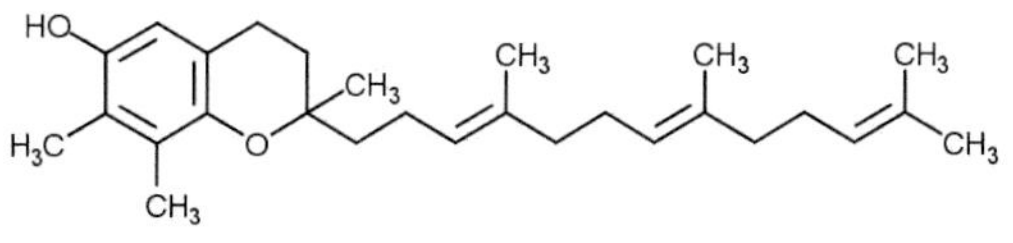

γ-tocotrienol

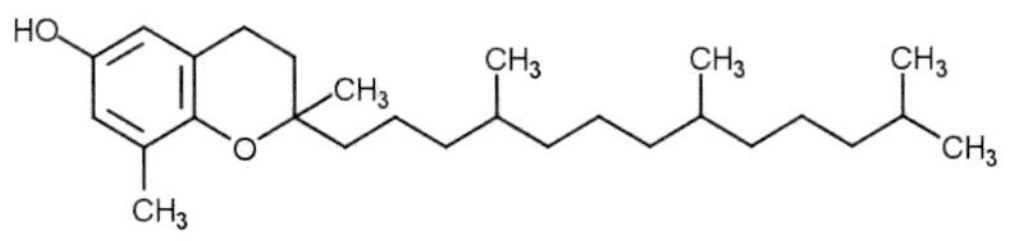

δ-tocopherol

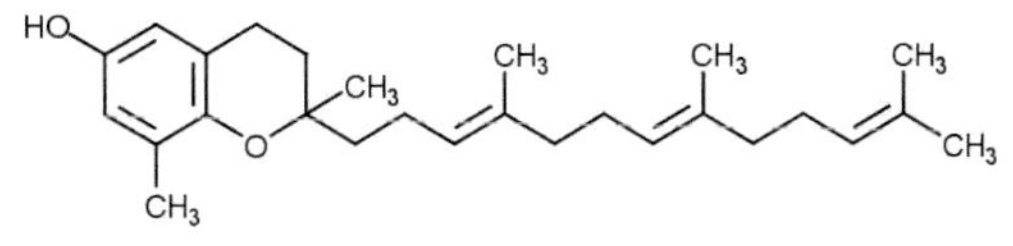

δ-tocotrienol

GENERAL

Vitamin E (tocopherol) is a term that encompasses a group of potent lipid-soluble antioxidants. Structural analyses have revealed that molecules having vitamin E antioxidant activity include four tocopherols (α, β, γ, δ) and four tocotrienols (α, β, γ, δ). One form, α-tocopherol, is the most abundant form in nature and has the highest biological activity (23,47). Vitamin E is found in many dietary products. As it purportedly minimizes (photo)aging, increases stratum corneum hydration, and helps wound healing, manufacturers commonly include it in cosmetics and skin care products. Frequently, patients apply vitamin E to scars; oral intake is also popular among the health conscious public. Indeed, the practice of prescribing vitamin E after surgery for scar prevention and treatment is widespread and increasingly popular among both the public and clinicians, although there is not yet sufficient evidence that mono-therapy with topical vitamin E has a significant beneficial effect on scar appearance to justify its widespread use (50). Being a strong antioxidant, tocopherol is unstable and is usually esterified to facilitate stability; tocopheryl acetate is the most widely used form (21). In should be realized that, in several articles on contact allergy, the term 'vitamin E' was used in the title, whereas the allergenic component was in fact tocopheryl acetate (48,49,51). These articles are discussed in Chapter 2.464 Tocopheryl acetate.

A review of contact allergy to tocopherol (vitamin E) and vitamin E derivatives was published in 2010 (43).

CONTACT ALLERGY

Patch testing in groups of patients

Results of patch testing tocopherol in consecutive patients suspected of contact dermatitis (routine testing) and of testing groups of selected patients are shown in table 2.463.1. Tocopherol has been part of the screening series of the NACDG since 2001; its members publish their patch test results biannually. There is only one (early) study with tocopherol routine testing from outside the USA + Canada, a very small investigation from Denmark (13). In North America, in 11 studies performing routine testing, rates of sensitization to tocopherol have always been low and ranged from 0.5% to 1.1%. 'Definite' or 'probable' relevance has ranged from 25% to 59% in the NACDG studies (table 2.463.1). In two groups of *selected* patients (patients tested with a cosmetic series, patients with chronic cheilitis), rates were 1.3% (4) and 1.6%(40). In a study from the USA, 75% of positive patch test reactions were scored as relevant, but this included 'questionable' and 'past' relevance (4).

Table 2.463.1 Patch testing in groups of patients

Years and Country	Test conc. & vehicle	Number of patients tested	positive (%)	Selection of patients (S); Relevance (R); Comments (C)	Ref.
Routine testing					
2013-14 USA, Canada	pure	4859	29 (0.6%)	R: definite + probable relevance: 52%	38
2011-12 USA, Canada	pure	4230	30 (0.7%)	R: definite + probable relevance: 63%	25
2009-10 USA, Canada	pure	4304	43 (1.0%)	R: definite + probable: relevance 44%	26
2006-2010 USA	pure	2974	(0.8%)	R: 36%	33
2007-8 USA, Canada	pure	5082	(1.0%)	R: definite + probable relevance: 59%	15
1987-2007 USA	various	2950	18 (0.6%)	R: all reactions were considered relevant; C: test concentra-tions: 1987-1999: various; 2000-2005 tocopheryl acetate 10% pet; .2005 pure vitamin E	21
2005-6 USA, Canada	pure	4435	(0.7%)	R: definite + probable relevance: 33%	14
2000-2005 USA	10% pet.	3389	(0.5%)	R: 44%	5
2003-4 USA, Canada	pure	5139	57 (1.1%)	R: not stated	16
2001-2 USA, Canada	pure	4881	(1.1%)	R: definite + probable relevance: 25%	31
1998-2000 USA	10% pet.	711	(0.8%)	R: not stated	32
<1976 Denmark	20% pet.	116	1 (0.9%)	R: not found	13
Testing in groups of selected patients					
2000-2007 USA	pure	318	5 (1.3%)	S: patients tested with a supplemental cosmetic screening series; R: 75%; C: weak study: a. high rate of macular erythema and weak reactions; b. relevance figures included 'questionable' and 'past' relevance	4
2001-2006 Italy	20% pet.	129	2 (1.6%)	S: patients with chronic cheilitis; R: 0 reactions were relevant	40

Case reports and case series

Tocopherol was responsible for 6 out of 959 cases of non-fragrance cosmetic allergy where the causal allergen was identified, Belgium, 2000-2010 (3). Tocopherol was responsible for 2 out of 399 cases of cosmetic allergy where the causal allergen was identified in a study of the NACDG, USA, 1977-1983 (2). Among 2193 patients with (presumed) cosmetic allergy seen by the NACDG between 2001-2004, 32 had a positive patch test reaction to dl-α-tocopherol 100% (6). Two positive patch test reactions to tocopherol were ascribed to cosmetic allergy (7).

Three patients (10) and one individual (27) had allergic contact dermatitis from vitamin E in (aerosol) deodorants (10). A woman had allergic contact dermatitis of the face from tocopherol in a night cream (24), another one contact allergy to tocopherol in a skin care product (28). An unspecified number of patients with eyelid dermatitis had allergic reactions to tocopherol in personal care products they used (39). A woman had erythema multiforme-like allergic contact dermatitis from DL-α-tocopherol in two cosmetic products and pure vitamin E oil (17).

A girl with atopic dermatitis became sensitized to tocopherol in several sunscreens she used on her face for prevention of photosensitivity exacerbating atopic dermatitis (45). A woman had worsening of rosacea accompanied by pruritus and desquamation on her face and neck after applying a moisturizing cream. Patch tests were positive to the moisturizer and – in a second test session – its ingredient tocopherol (46). Three patients developed dermatitis from a vitamin E-containing deodorant, but patch tests were not performed (9).

Contact allergy to tocopherol in non-cosmetic products
Occupational allergic contact dermatitis from vitamin E in a medicine developed in a veterinary surgeon (29). A woman suffered from allergic contact dermatitis to 'pure vitamin E oil' applied to abort vitiliginous lesions (8). Another young female patient had allergic contact dermatitis from vitamin E in a pharmaceutical vitamin cream containing 5% tocopherol (30). A woman developed erythema multiforme-like allergic contact dermatitis from DL-α-tocopherol in pure vitamin E oil and two cosmetic products (17). Another female individual developed redness, swelling, stinging, and infection of the face requiring antibiotics after the application of a mixture of the content of pure 'vitamin E' capsule with vegetable fat for facial care after a full-face chemical peel had been performed. Patch tests were not performed (44). A young woman developed allergic contact dermatitis from synthetic α-tocopherol in a vitamin cream (11). A similar case was reported from the USA (27).

Cross-reactions, pseudo-cross-reactions and co-reactions
In a NACDG study, all 12 patients reacting to tocopheryl acetate also reacted to tocopherol (31).

Patch test sensitization
Patch test sensitization to DL-α-tocopherol has been reported in ref. 20 (no details known, article cannot be found).

Presence in cosmetic products and chemical analyses
In May 2017, tocopherol was present in 5816 of 68,675 cosmetic products of which the composition is known in EWG's Skin Deep Cosmetics Database, USA (http://www.ewg.org/skindeep/). In the USA, in April 2017, tocopherol was present in 8838 of 56,714 cosmetic products of which the composition is known in FDA's Voluntary Cosmetic Registration Program (VCRP) (data obtained from FDA, May 2017). Tocopherol or its derivatives were present in 69 (39%) of 178 facial wipes for which ingredient information was obtained online and from retail stores, USA, 2016 (41). Tocopherol or its derivatives were present in 34 (63%) of 54 personal hygiene wet wipes for which ingredient information was obtained online and from retail stores, USA, 2016 (42). In 2009, in the USA, the ingredient lists of 1591 facial cosmetics from one company were screened for the presence of tocopherol. Tocopherol was present in 56% of 132 blushers and 38 bronzers, in 69% of 90 concealers, in 0% of 174 eyeliners, in 28% of 304 eyeshadows, in 62% of 457 foundations, in 56% of 140 loose and pressed powders, and in 32% of 256 mascaras (34).

In 2009, in the USA, the ingredient lists of 796 hair products from one company were screened for the presence of tocopherol. Tocopherol was present in 11% of 279 shampoos, in 26% of 231 conditioners, and in 17% of 286 styling products (35). In 2009, in the USA, the ingredient lists of 730 lip cosmetics and dental care products from one company were screened for the presence of tocopherol. Tocopherol was present in 81% of 31 lip liners, in 76% of 429 lipsticks, in 66% of 92 lip moisturizers, in 0% of 153 toothpastes, and in 0% of 25 mouth washes (36). In 2009, in the USA, the ingredient lists of 657 miscellaneous cosmetics from one company were screened for the presence of tocopherol. Tocopherol was present in 1% of 195 antiperspirants/deodorants, in 0% of 41 powders, in 0% of 167 shaving products, in 53% of 201 sunblocks, and in 79% of 53 wipes (37). Of 276 moisturizers sold in the USA in 2007, 151 (55%) contained vitamin E (18).

OTHER SIDE EFFECTS

Immediate-type reactions
Tocopherol was mentioned as a cause of contact urticaria in ref. 1 (article not read). Two brothers aged 4 and 7 developed localized and later generalized urticaria from application of the contents of a capsule of vitamin E oil to thermal burns. The authors called this 'contact urticaria', which is probably a misnomer as the eruptions faded in 7-10 days with peeling of the skin (19,22).

Miscellaneous side effects
A patient presumably had allergic contact dermatitis from vitamin E, applied to the skin undiluted from pierced vitamin E capsules. Patch tests were not performed. After 3 weeks, scattered yellowish soft papules and plaques were observed at the site of previous dermatitis. A punch biopsy was taken and histopathologic examination revealed an admixture of foam cell (xanthoma cells) among inflammatory cells (12).

LITERATURE

1   Fisher AA. Urticarial and systemic reactions to contactants varying from hair bleach to seminal fluid. Cutis 1977;19:715-717

2   Adams RM, Maibach HI, Clendenning WE, Fisher AA, Jordan WJ, Kanof N, et al. A five-year study of cosmetic reactions. J Am Acad Dermatol 1985;13:1062-1069

3   Travassos AR, Claes L, Boey L, Drieghe J, Goossens A. Non-fragrance allergens in specific cosmetic products. Contact Dermatitis 2011;65:276-285

4   Wetter DA, Yiannias JA, Prakash AV, Davis MD, Farmer SA, el-Azhary RA, et al. Results of patch testing to personal care product allergens in a standard series and a supplemental cosmetic series: an analysis of 945 patients from the Mayo Clinic Contact Dermatitis Group, 2000-2007. J Am Acad Dermatol 2010;63:789-798

5   Davis MD, Scalf LA, Yiannias JA, Cheng JF, El-Azhary RA, Rohlinger AL, et al. Changing trends and allergens in the patch test standard series. Arch Dermatol 2008;144:67-72

6   Warshaw EM, Buchholz HJ, Belsito DV et al. Allergic patch test reactions associated with cosmetics: Retrospective analysis of cross-sectional data from the North American Contact Dermatitis Group, 2001-2004. J Am Acad Dermatol 2009;60:23-38

7   Kohl L, Blondeel A, Song M. Allergic contact dermatitis from cosmetics: retrospective analysis of 819 patch-tested patients. Dermatology 2002;204:334-337

8   Goldman MP, Rapaport M. Contact dermatitis to vitamin E oil. J Am Acad Dermatol 1986;14:133-134

9   Minkin W, Cohen HI, Frank SB. Contact dermatitis from deodorants. Arch Dermatol 1973;107:774-775

10 Aeling JL, Panagotacos PI, Andreozzi RJ. Allergic contact dermatitis to vitamin E aerosol deodorant. Arch Dermatol 1973;108:579-580

11 Brodkin RH, Bleiberg J. Sensitivity to topically applied vitamin E. Arch Dermatol 1965;92:76-77

12 Parsad D, Saini R, Verma N. Xanthomatous reaction following contact dermatitis from vitamin E. Contact Dermatitis 1997;37:294

13 Roed-Petersen J, Hjorth N. Contact dermatitis from antioxidants. Br J Dermatol 1976;94:233-241

14 Zug KA, Warshaw EM, Fowler JF Jr, Maibach HI, Belsito DL, Pratt MD, et al. Patch-test results of the North American Contact Dermatitis Group 2005-2006. Dermatitis 2009;20:149-160

15 Fransway AF, Zug KA, Belsito DV, Deleo VA, Fowler JF Jr, Maibach HI, et al. North American Contact Dermatitis Group patch test results for 2007-2008. Dermatitis 2013;24:10-21

16 Warshaw EM, Belsito DV, DeLeo VA, Fowler JF Jr, Maibach HI, Marks JG, et al. North American Contact Dermatitis Group patch-test results, 2003-2004 study period. Dermatitis 2008;19:129-136

17 Saperstein H, Rapaport M, Rietschel RL. Topical vitamin E as a cause of erythema-multiforme-like eruption. Arch Dermatol 1984;120:906-908

18 Zirwas MJ, Stechschulte SA. Moisturizer allergy. Diagnosis and management. J Clin Aesthetic Dermatol 2008;1:38-44

19 Kassen B, Mitchell JC. Contact urticaria from vitamin E preparation in two siblings. Contact Dermatitis Newsletter 1974;16:482

20 Roed-Petersen J, Hjorth N. Patch test sensitization from d,l-alpha-tocopherol (vitamin E). Contact Dermatitis 1975;1:391

21 Adams AK, Connolly SM. Allergic contact dermatitis from vitamin E: the experience at Mayo Clinic Arizona, 1987 to 2007. Dermatitis 2010;21:199-202

22 Mitchell J, Kassen L. Contact urticaria from vitamin E preparation (vitamin E-vegetable oil in two siblings). Int J Dermatol 1975;14:246-247

23 Brigelius-Flohe R, Traber MG. Vitamin E: function and metabolism. FASEB J 1999;13:1145-1155

24 De Groot AC, Rustemeyer T, Hissink D, Bakker M. Contact allergy to capryloyl salicylic acid. Contact Dermatitis 2014;71:185-187

25 Warshaw EM, Maibach HI, Taylor JS, Sasseville D, DeKoven JG, Zirwas MJ, et al. North American Contact Dermatitis Group patch test results: 2011-2012. Dermatitis 2015;26:49-59

26 Warshaw EM, Belsito DV, Taylor JS, Sasseville D, DeKoven JG, Zirwas MJ, et al. North American Contact Dermatitis Group patch test results: 2009 to 2010. Dermatitis 2013;24:50-59

27 Maibach HI, Marzulli F. Personnal communication to the authors of ref. 13, 1974

28 Fisher AA. Cosmetic warning: this product may be detrimental to your purse. Cutis 1987;39:23-24

29 Hjorth N. Contact dermatitis from vitamin E and from cambelen (Bayer) in a veterinary surgeon. Contact Dermatitis Newsletter 1974;15:434

30 Bazzano C, de Angeles S, Kleist G, Macedo N. Allergic contact dermatitis from topical vitamins A and E. Contact Dermatitis 1996;35:261-262

31 Pratt MD, Belsito DV, DeLeo VA, Fowler JF Jr, Fransway AF, Maibach HI, et al. North American Contact Dermatitis Group patch-test results, 2001–2002 study period. Dermatitis 2004;15:176-183

32 Wetter DA, Davis MDP, Yiannias JA, Cheng JF, Connolly SM, el-Azhary RA, et al. Patch test results from the Mayo Contact Dermatitis Group, 1998–2000. J Am Acad Dermatol 2005;53:416-421

33 Wentworth AB, Yiannias JA, Keeling JH, Hall MR, Camilleri MJ, Drage LA, et al. Trends in patch-test results and allergen changes in the standard series: a Mayo Clinic 5-year retrospective review (January 1, 2006, to December 31, 2010). J Am Acad Dermatol 2014;70:269-275

34 Scheman A, Jacob S, Katta R, Nedorost S, Warshaw E, Zirwas M, et al. Part 1 of a 4 part series. Facial cosmetics: trends and alternatives. Data from the American Contact Alternative Group. J Clin Aesthet Dermatol 2011;4:25 30

35 Scheman A, Jacob S, Katta R, Nedorost S, Warshaw E, Zirwas M, et al. Part 2 of a 4 part series. Hair cosmetics: trends and alternatives. Data from the American Contact Alternative Group. J Clin Aesthet Dermatol 2011;4:42-46

36 Scheman A, Jacob S, Katta R, Nedorost S, Warshaw E, Zirwas M, et al. Part 3 of a 4 part series. Lips and common Dental Care products: trends and alternatives. Data from the American Contact Alternative Group. J Clin Aesthet Dermatol 2011;4:50-53

37 Scheman A, Jacob S, Katta R, Nedorost S, Warshaw E, Zirwas M, et al. Part 4 of a 4 part series. Miscellaneous products: trends and alternatives in deodorants, antiperspirants, sunblocks, shaving products, powder, and wipes. Data from the American Contact Alternative Group. J Clin Aesthet Dermatol 2011;4:35-39

38 DeKoven JG, Warshaw EM, Belsito DV, Sasseville D, Maibach HI, Taylor JS, et al. North American Contact Dermatitis Group Patch Test Results: 2013-2014. Dermatitis 2017;28:33-46

39 Guin JD. Eyelid dermatitis: A report of 215 patients. Contact Dermatitis 2004;50:87-90

40 Schena D, Fantuzzi F, Girolomoni G. Contact allergy in chronic eczematous lip dermatitis. Eur J Dermatol 2008;18:688-692

41 Aschenbeck KA, Warshaw EM. Allergenic ingredients in facial wet wipes. Dermatitis 2017 Mar 23. doi: 10.1097/DER.0000000000000268. [Epub ahead of print]

42 Aschenbeck KA, Warshaw EM. Allergenic ingredients in personal hygiene wet wipes. Dermatitis 2017 Mar 23. doi: 10.1097/DER.0000000000000275. [Epub ahead of print]

43 Kosari P, Alikhan A, Sockolov M, Feldman SR. Vitamin E and allergic contact dermatitis. Dermatitis 2010;21:148-153

44 Hunter D, Frumkin A. Adverse reactions to vitamin E and Aloe vera preparations after dermabrasion and chemical peel. Cutis 1991;47:193-196

45 Simonsen AB, Koppelhus U, Sommerlund M, Deleuran M. Photosensitivity in atopic dermatitis complicated by contact allergy to common sunscreen ingredients. Contact Dermatitis 2016;74:56-58

46 Ramírez Santos A, Fernández-Redondo V, Pérez Pérez L, Concheiro Cao J, Toribio J. Contact allergy from vitamins in cosmetic products. Dermatitis 2008;19:154-156

47 Caraffa AL, Varvara G, Spinas E, Kritas SK, Lessiani G, Ronconi G, et al. Is vitamin E an anti-allergic compound? J Biol Regul Homeost Agents 2016;30:11-15

48 Corazza M, Minghetti S, Borghi A, Bianchi, A, Virgili A. Vitamin E contact allergy: a controversial subject. Dermatitis 2012;23:167-169

49 Harris, BD, Taylor JS. Contact allergy to vitamin E capsules: false-negative patch tests to vitamin E? Contact Dermatitis 1997;36:273

50 Tanaydin V, Conings J, Malyar M, van der Hulst R, van der Lei B. The role of topical vitamin E in scar management: A systematic review. Aesthet Surg J 2016;36:959-965

51 Garcia-Bravo B, Mozo P. Generalized contact dermatitis from vitamin E. Contact Dermatitis 1992;26:280

2.464   TOCOPHERYL ACETATE

IDENTIFICATION

Description/definition   : Tocopheryl acetate is the ester of tocopherol and acetic acid, which conforms to the
                               formula shown below
Chemical class(es)   : Esters; heterocyclic compounds
Chemical/IUPAC name   : [2,5,7,8-Tetramethyl-2-(4,8,12-trimethyltridecyl)-3,4-dihydrochromen-6-yl] acetate
Other names   : Vitamin E acetate
CAS registry number (s)   : 7695-91-2; 58-95-7
EC number(s)   : 231-710-0; 200-405-4
CIR review(s)   : Int J Toxicol 2002;21(Suppl.3):51-116; Final report, March 2014 (access:
                               www.cir-safety.org/ingredients)
SCCS opinion(s)   : SCCNFP/0494/01 (11)
Merck Index monograph   : 10923 (α-tocopherol)
Function(s) in cosmetics   : EU: antioxidant; skin conditioning. USA: antioxidants; skin-conditioning agents –
                               miscellaneous
Patch testing   : 10% pet. (Chemotechnique)
Molecular formula   : $C_{31}H_{52}O_3$

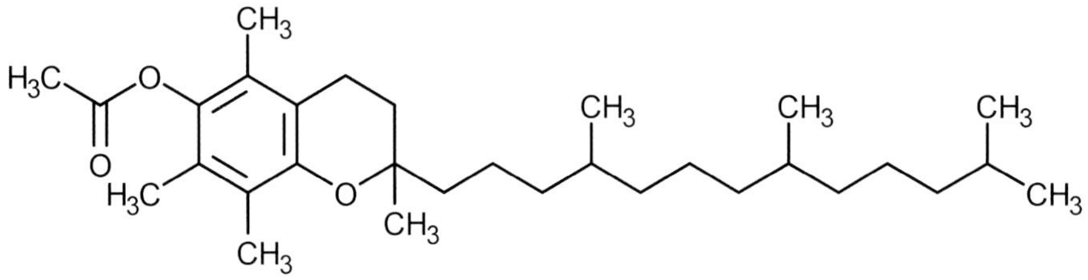

GENERAL

α-Tocopherol (vitamin E) is a lipophilic molecule found in many dietary products. As vitamin E is perceived to minimize photo-aging, increase stratum corneum hydration, and help wound healing, manufacturers commonly include it in cosmetics and skin care products. Being a strong antioxidant, vitamin E is unstable and is usually esterified to facilitate stability; tocopheryl acetate is the most widely used form (3). Patch test reactions to tocopheryl acetate are sometimes unexpectedly negative (false-negative), which has been ascribed to the anti-inflammatory action of tocopherols (3,6). A review of contact allergy to vitamin E and vitamin E derivatives was published in 2010 (16).

CONTACT ALLERGY

Patch testing in groups of patients
In 2001-2002, in the USA, the members of the North American Contact Dermatitis Group (NACDG) patch tested 4874 consecutive patients suspected of contact dermatitis (routine testing) with tocopheryl acetate 100% and there were 24 (0.5%) reactions. Forty per cent were considered to be of 'definite' or 'probable' relevance. All allergic patients also reacted to tocopherol and, as tocopherol was already part of the NACDG screening series, tocopheryl acetate was removed from it (9).

Case reports and case series
Tocopheryl acetate was stated to be the (or an) allergen in one patient in a group of 603 individuals suffering from cosmetic dermatitis, seen in the period 2010-2015 in Leuven, Belgium (10). Among 2193 patients with (presumed) cosmetic allergy seen by the NACDG between 2001 and 2004, 9 had a positive patch test reaction to dl-α-tocopheryl acetate 100% associated with a moisturizer. The total number of positive reactions was not mentioned and tocopheryl acetate had been tested in 2 of the 4 years only (1).

    Four patients had dermatitis from contact allergy to tocopheryl acetate in cosmetic creams (4). Later, one of these patients repeatedly suffered from mild recurrences. This may have been related to residues of vitamin E cream on her clothes. After washing them many times, the problem resolved. However, when she wore a friend's dress, she again developed widespread dermatitis. The friend proved to be a regular user of vitamin E creams (4). One patient had contact dermatitis from allergy to tocopheryl acetate in a moisturizing cream (7). Another individual had generalized ACD from tocopheryl acetate in a 'soapy oats lotion' (8). An unspecified number of patients with eyelid dermatitis had allergic reactions to tocopheryl acetate in personal care products they used (15). Two women may have had allergic reactions to tocopheryl acetate in cosmetic products, one of which was an oil consisting entirely of tocopheryl acetate. Patch tests with the products and ROATs were positive, but ingredient patch testing failed to evoke positive patch tests. Later, patch testing and ROATs with new samples of the products were negative; the authors provided several possible explanations for these discrepancies (3).

Eight patients reacted to a cosmetic cream ('lipogel') and had positive patch tests. Testing with the ingredients, however, was negative (14). The possibility of compound allergy was suggested, as this had been observed previously (positive reactions to the product, negative to the constituents) (12,13).

Contact allergy to tocopheryl acetate in non-cosmetic products
One patient had allergic contact dermatitis from tocopheryl acetate in a topical pharmaceutical product (2). Another individual had erythema multiforme-like contact dermatitis from vitamin E oil used to prevent scars, which consisted exclusively of tocopheryl acetate (5). A patient had a reaction to the contents of a vitamin E capsule (in the form of *dl*-α-tocopheryl acetate) applied to the skin. A patch test with it was negative, but a ROAT positive. Contact allergy to soybean oil, gelatin, and glycerin, the other constituents of the vitamin E capsule could not be excluded, but the patient had repeatedly developed skin reactions to cosmetics containing tocopherol (6).

Cross-reactions, pseudo-cross-reactions and co-reactions
Tocopheryl nicotinate (4). In one NACDG study, all 12 patients reacting to tocopheryl acetate also reacted to tocopherol (9).

Presence in cosmetic products and chemical analyses
In the USA, in April 2017, tocopheryl acetate was present in 12546 of 56,714 cosmetic products of which the composition is known in FDA's Voluntary Cosmetic Registration Program (VCRP) (data obtained from FDA, May 2017). In April 2017, tocopheryl acetate was present in 6804 of 66,647 cosmetic products of which the composition is known in EWG's Skin Deep Cosmetics Database, USA (http://www.ewg.org/skindeep/). Tocopherol derivatives were present in 69 (39%) of 178 facial wipes for which ingredient information was obtained online and from retail stores, USA, 2016 (17). Tocopherol and derivatives were present in 34 (63%) of 54 personal hygiene wet wipes for which ingredient information was obtained online and from retail stores, USA, 2016 (18). In the USA, in 2015-2016, 63 diaper wipes and 41 topical diaper preparations from a large retailer were screened for the presence of potential sensitizers. Tocopheryl acetate was found in 40/63 (64%) disposable diaper wipes and in 15/41 (37%) topical diaper preparations (19).

LITERATURE
1   Warshaw EM, Buchholz HJ, Belsito DV et al. Allergic patch test reactions associated with cosmetics: Retrospective analysis of cross-sectional data from the North American Contact Dermatitis Group, 2001-2004. J Am Acad Dermatol 2009;60:23-38
2   Matsumura T, Nakada T, Iijima M. Widespread contact dermatitis from tocopherol acetate. Contact Dermatitis 2004;51:211-212
3   Corazza M, Minghetti S, Borghi A, Bianchi, A, Virgili A. Vitamin E contact allergy: a controversial subject. Dermatitis 2012;23:167-169
4   De Groot AC, Berretty PJM, Van Ginkel CJW, Den Hengst CW, Van Ulsen J, Weyland JW. Allergic contact dermatitis from tocopheryl acetate in cosmetic cream. Contact Dermatitis 1991;25:302-304
5   Saperstein H, Rapaport M, Rietschel RL. Topical vitamin E as a cause of erythema multiforme-like eruption. Arch Dermatol 1984;120:906-908
6   Harris, BD, Taylor JS. Contact allergy to vitamin E capsules: false-negative patch tests to vitamin E? Contact Dermatitis 1997;36:273
7   Manzano D, Aguirre A, Gardeazabal J, Eizaguirre X, Pérez JLD. Allergic contact dermatitis from tocopheryl acetate (vitamin E) and retinol palmitate (vitamin A) in a moisturizing cream. Contact Dermatitis 1994;31:324
8   Garcia-Bravo B, Mozo P. Generalized contact dermatitis from vitamin E. Contact Dermatitis 1992;26:280
9   Pratt MD, Belsito DV, DeLeo VA, Fowler JF Jr, Fransway AF, Maibach HI, et al. North American Contact Dermatitis Group patch-test results, 2001–2002 study period. Dermatitis 2004;15:176-183
10 Goossens A. Cosmetic contact allergens. Cosmetics 2016, 3, 5; doi:10.3390/cosmetics3010005
11 SCCNFP (Scientific Committee on Cosmetics and Non Food Products). Opinion concerning alpha-tocopherol acetate in cosmetic products, 25 September 2001, SCCNFP/0494/01. Available at: http://ec.europa.eu/health/archive/ph_risk/committees/sccp/documents/out148_en.pdf
12 Schianchi S, Arcangeli F, Calista D. Compound allergy to vea oil. Contact Dermatitis 2003;49:222
13 Corazza M, Ricci M, Minghetti, S et al. Compound allergy to a lipophilic gel containing vitamin E acetate and cyclopentasiloxane. Dermatitis 2013;24:198-199
14 Milanesi N, Gola M, Francalanci S. Allergic contact dermatitis caused by VEA® lipogel: compound allergy?. Contact Dermatitis 2016;75:243-244

15   Guin JD. Eyelid dermatitis: A report of 215 patients. Contact Dermatitis 2004;50:87-90

16   Kosari P, Alikhan A, Sockolov M, Feldman SR. Vitamin E and allergic contact dermatitis. Dermatitis 2010;21:148-153

17   Aschenbeck KA, Warshaw EM. Allergenic ingredients in facial wet wipes. Dermatitis 2017 Mar 23. doi: 10.1097/DER.0000000000000268. [Epub ahead of print]

18   Aschenbeck KA, Warshaw EM. Allergenic ingredients in personal hygiene wet wipes. Dermatitis 2017 Mar 23. doi: 10.1097/DER.0000000000000275. [Epub ahead of print]

19   Yu J, Treat J, Chaney K, Brod B. Potential allergens in disposable diaper wipes, topical diaper preparations, and disposable diapers: under-recognized etiology of pediatric perineal dermatitis. Dermatitis 2016;27:110-118

2.465   TOCOPHERYL LINOLEATE

IDENTIFICATION

Description/definition : Tocopheryl linoleate is the ester of tocopherol and linoleic acid, which conforms to the formula shown below

Chemical class(es) : Esters; heterocyclic compounds

Chemical/IUPAC name : [(2R)-2,5,7,8-Tetramethyl-2-[(4R,8R)-4,8,12-trimethyltridecyl]-3,4-dihydrochromen-6-yl] (9Z,12Z)-octadeca-9,12-dienoate

Other names : Vitamin E linoleate; dl-α-tocopherol linoleate

CAS registry number (s) : 36148-84-2

CIR review(s) : Int J Toxicol 2002;21(Suppl.3):51-116; Final report, March 2014 (access: www.cir-safety.org/ingredients)

Function(s) in cosmetics : EU: antioxidant; skin conditioning; skin protecting. USA: antioxidants; skin-conditioning agents - miscellaneous

Patch testing : 10% pet. and pure

Molecular formula : $C_{47}H_{80}O_3$

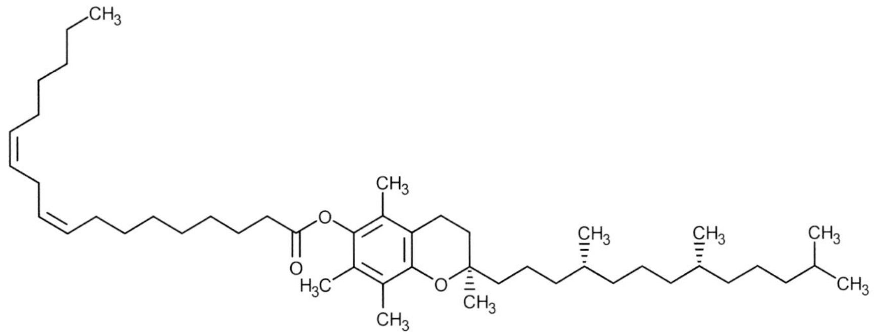

GENERAL

A review of contact allergy to tocopherol (vitamin E) and vitamin E derivatives was published in 2010 (5).

CONTACT ALLERGY

Case reports and case series

In spring 1992, an epidemic outbreak of skin eruptions caused by a new line of cosmetics occurred throughout Switzerland (1,2). Within a 3-month period, this outbreak affected at least 263 people who consulted dermatologists and at least 642 people who did not see a dermatologist. The lesions were mainly papular and follicular, widely distributed, with pronounced pruritus, which was aggravated by sweating or heat exposure, and were long-lasting. Epidemiological and clinical data incriminated a new line of cosmetics containing vitamin E linoleate, a mixture of fatty acid esters of dl-α-tocopherol composed not only of tocopheryl linoleate but also of tocopheryl oleate, palmitate and myristate. The lesions appeared after 1-160 days (mean 14 days) following the initial application of the cosmetics containing tocopheryl linoleate. In many cases, the rash extended and the pruritus increased several days after the application had ended. In 1/5 of the cases, a secondary extension to the face was seen, though the cosmetics had not been applied to these sites.

Patch testing showed positive patch tests with the undiluted final cosmetic products ranging from 21% to 64%, depending on the individual product. None of the control subjects showed a positive test reaction. In addition, a large number of patients (60%) had positive or doubtful reactions to undiluted vitamin E linoleate, while none of controls had. Thirteen out of 45 (29%) tested patients presented a positive or doubtful reaction to tocopheryl linoleate 10% in petrolatum. Patch tests with other vitamin E derivatives induced only a few positive reactions. Twelve of 15 (80%) patients who performed repeated open application tests reacted to the body lotion containing tocopheryl linoleate; however, several also reacted to the lotion without tocopheryl linoleate. Skin biopsies performed on lesional skin showed spongiosis of the follicular epidermis, with a perifollicular and perivascular infiltrate containing a predominantly mononuclear clear-cell infiltrate with some neutrophils. As in vitro time-dependent formation of oxidative products under storage or oxidation stimulating conditions was observed, the authors of the study concluded that oxidized vitamin E derivatives could act in vivo as haptens and/or irritants, possibly with synergistic effects (1). An allergic mechanism was later favored by the authors (2).

The literature on contact allergy to TFR (and other allergens in nail polishes) up to 1993 has been reviewed in 1994/1995 (10,11; not all references are correct and an important table in ref. 10 is missing!).

CONTACT ALLERGY

Patch testing in groups of patients
Results of studies testing tosylamide/formaldehyde resin in consecutive patients suspected of contact dermatitis (routine testing) back to 1993 are shown in table 2.469.1. Results of testing in groups of *selected* patients (e.g., patients with eyelid dermatitis, with cheilitis, patients suspected of cosmetic dermatitis, individuals with facial allergic contact dermatitis) back to 1992 are shown in table 2.469.2.

Patch testing in consecutive patients suspected of contact dermatitis: routine testing
There is much experience in the USA/Canada with patch testing tosylamide/formaldehyde resin, as it has been part of the North American Contact Dermatitis Group (NACDG) screening series since over 25 years. The NACDG publishes its results biannually. Other reports are available from several European countries (Finland, Sweden, Belgium, Germany, Italy), from Australia and from Brazil. In 24 studies performing routine testing with TFR, frequencies of sensitization have ranged from 0.3% to 7.2%, but 17 scored 1.5% or lower, of which 10 had sensitization rates of 1% or less. The highest frequencies were found in Brazil (7.2% [77]) and Italy (3.8% [37]), which may be related to extensive usage of nail lacquers in women in these countries. In the NACDG studies, the frequencies were fairly constant, ranging from 0.9% to 1.9%, with low rates of 0.9%, 1.2% and 0.9% in the most recent period of 2009-2014 (17,18,67). Similar observations were made in other US centers, Europe and Australia. Relevance scores were usually between 30% and 60% (in the NACDG studies 'definite' + 'probably' relevance), but in the Brazilian and Italian studies, all reactions were relevant and related to nail varnishes (37,77).

Table 2.469.1 Patch testing in groups of patients: Routine testing

Years and Country	Test conc. & vehicle	Number of patients tested	positive (%)	Selection of patients (S); Relevance (R); Comments (C)	Ref.
2013-14 USA, Canada	10% pet.	4859	43 (0.9%)	R: definite + probable relevance: 37%	67
2011-12 USA, Canada	10% pet.	4232	52 (1.2%)	R: definite + probable relevance: 29%	17
2009-10 USA, Canada	10% pet.	4299	39 (0.9%)	R: definite + probable relevance: 41%	18
2006-2010 USA	10% pet.	3086	(1.1%)	R: 65%	52
2001-2010 Australia	10% pet.	5130	89 (1.7%)	R: 55%	66
2009 Sweden	10% pet.	3112	(0.3%)	R: not stated	47
2007-8 USA, Canada	10% pet.	5078	(1.0%)	R: definite + probable relevance: 48%	13
2005-6 USA, Canada	10% pet.	4434	(1.3%)	R: definite + probable relevance: 39%	12
1996-2006 Brazil		1971	141 (7.2%)	R: all reactions were relevant; 9% worked in a beauty parlor and had occupational allergic contact dermatitis	77
2000-2005 USA	10% pet.	3844	(1.3%)	R: 71%	2
2003-4 USA, Canada	10% pet.	5139	85 (1.7%)	R: not stated	14
2001-2 USA, Canada	10% pet.	4897	(1.6%)	R: definite + probable relevance: 30%	39
2000-2002 Finland		9394	(0.7%)	R: not stated	46
1999-2001 Sweden	10% pet.	3790	(0.7%)	R: not stated; C: prevalence in women 0.9%, in men 0.2% (standardized prevalences)	44
1998-00 USA, Canada	10% pet.	5800	(1.3%)	R: definite + probable relevance: 33%	40
1998–2000 USA	10% pet.	1322	(1.4%)	R: not stated	45
1998-1999 Belgium	10% pet.	819	5 (0.6%)	R: ascribed to nail polish allergy	7
1996-8 USA, Canada	10% pet.	4097	(1.5%)	R: definite + probable + possible relevance: 68%	41
1995-1996 Finland		9394	(0.7%)	R: not stated	46
1994-1996 USA	10% pet.	3077	(1.6%)	R: definite + probable relevance: 48%	42
1993-1995 Germany	10% pet.	1018	3 (0.3%)	R: all three reactions were relevant	16
1992-1994 USA	10% pet.	3467	(1.9%)	R: present relevance: 74%	43
1992-1993 Italy	10% pet.	366	14 (3.8%)	R: all had used nail varnishes and presented with dermatitis of the face, side of the necks, lips, perioral skin, upper eyelids or combinations, but never on the perionychia	37
1991-1993 Sweden	10% pet.	3680	(1.0%)	R: not stated; C: prevalence in women 1.1%, in men 0.2% (standardized prevalences)	44

Patch testing in groups of selected patients
Results of testing in groups of selected patients (e.g., patients with eyelid dermatitis, with cheilitis, patients suspected of cosmetic dermatitis, individuals with facial allergic contact dermatitis) back to 1992 are shown in table 2.469.2. In 10 investigations, frequencies of sensitization have ranged from 1.5% to 12.7%. The highest frequency

(12.7%) was observed in Brazilian adolescents, which was ascribed to frequent use of nail polishes (71) (in routine testing, the frequency of sensitization was also highest in Brazil [table 2.469.1, 7.2%, ref. 77]). High rates of sensitization (6%, 7% resp. 6.6%) were also seen groups of patients with eyelid dermatitis (15,48) and in women suspected of contact dermatitis habitually or occasionally using nail varnishes (75). In some studies, only relevant reactions were collected, in most others, relevance rates were high, up to 100% present or past relevance (75). Culprit products were mostly not mentioned, but almost certainly cannot have been other than nail varnishes or nail hardeners.

Table 2.469.2 Patch testing in groups of patients: Selected patient groups

Years and Country	Test conc. & vehicle	Number of patients tested	positive (%)		Selection of patients (S); Relevance (R); Comments (C)	Ref.
2006-2010 USA	10% pet.	100	6	(6%)	S: patients with eyelid dermatitis; R: not stated	15
1994-2010 USA, Canada	10% pet.	432	?	(?)	S: hairdressers/cosmetologists; R: in the group of 187 patients who had at least one relevant occupationally related reaction, 8 (4.3%) reacted to tosylamide/formaldehyde resin	69
2001-2006 Italy	10% pet.	129	2	(1.6%)	S: patients with chronic cheilitis; R: 1 reaction was relevant	70
2003-2004 USA	10% pet.	268	4	(1.5%)	S: patients with pure eyelid dermatitis; R: this was the number of relevant reactions	54
2001-2004 USA	10% pet.	60	2	(3%)	S: patients with allergic contact cheilitis; R: only relevant reactions were mentioned	53
1994-2004 USA	10% pet.	46	3	(7%)	S: patients with allergic contact dermatitis of the eyelids; R: all were relevant, source products not mentioned	48
1996-2001 Brazil		102	13	(12.7%)	S: adolescents 10-19 years old; R: it was suggested that the reactions were relevant; C: not mentioned how many children were tested with TFR	71
1994-1998 UK	10% pet.	232	5	(2.2%)	S: patients with eyelid dermatitis; R: all were currently relevant	49
1995-1997 USA		57	3	(5%)	S: patients with facial allergic contact dermatitis; R: only relevant reactions were mentioned	55
1987-1992 Italy	10% pet.	888	59	(6.6%)	S: women suspected of contact dermatitis who habitually or occasionally used nail varnishes; all reactions were of present or past relevance	75

Case reports and case series

Case series

Tosylamide/formaldehyde resin was stated to be the (or an) allergen in 3 patients in a group of 603 individuals suffering from cosmetic dermatitis, seen in the period 2010-2015 in Leuven, Belgium (51). In the period 1996-2013, in a tertiary referral center in Valencia, Spain, 5419 patients were patch tested. Of these, 628 individuals had allergic contact dermatitis to cosmetics. Tosylamide/formaldehyde resin was the responsible allergen in 39 (6.2%) cases (68, overlap with ref. 64). In the period 2000-2007, 202 patients with allergic contact dermatitis caused by cosmetics were seen in Valencia, Spain. In this group, 17 individuals reacted to tosylamide/formaldehyde resin from its presence in nail polishes, of who one was a beautician with occupational allergic hand dermatitis from the resin (64, overlap with ref. 68). TFR was the commonest cosmetic allergen in 55 female patients with cheilitis, reacting in 7 out of 55 (12.7%) in Athens, Greece, examined in the period 1992-2006 (25). In a group of 83 patients with cheilitis, seen in Bologna, Italy, in the period 2001-2005, one had a relevant reaction to TFR in nail lacquers; it was not stated how often TFR had been tested (62).

In 1582 female patients with (presumed) cosmetic allergy, 97 reactions (6.1%) were caused by TFR in a study of the NACDG, 2001-2004, TFR being the 7th most frequent allergen (3). In a group of 165 patients with allergic contact dermatitis of the eyelids, seen in Little Rock, USA, between 2001 and 2003, 7 cases were caused by contact allergy to tosylamide/formaldehyde resin in nail lacquer (5). In a 4-month-period in 1996, 475 patients with contact allergy to 'cosmetic ingredients' were collected in 5 centers in Belgium, UK and Germany. There were 7 reactions to tosylamide/formaldehyde resin; relevance was not stated (50). In a group of 119 patients with allergic contact dermatitis from cosmetics, investigated in The Netherlands in 1986-1987, fifteen cases were caused by tosylamide/formaldehyde resin in nail hardeners and lacquers (56,57). In a group of 75 patients allergic to cosmetic products, seen in a private practice in The Netherlands in the period 1981-1986, six cases were caused by tosylamide/formaldehyde resin, of which 3 in nail lacquers in 3 in nail hardeners (58, overlap with ref. 38).

In 3 clinics in Belgium, in the period 1978-1985, 279 patients with allergic contact dermatitis exclusively caused by cosmetics were seen. In this group, there were 10 reactions to tosylamide/formaldehyde resin. It was implied that this was the cause of the allergic reaction (65). Tosylamide/formaldehyde resin (TFR) was responsible for 23 out of 399 cases of cosmetic allergy where the causal allergen was identified in a study of the NACDG, USA, 1977-1983 (1). Seven patients allergic to nail lacquers all reacted to 'formaldehyde-sulfonamide resin' in 1943, USA (60). One year later (1944), in a group of 26 patients allergic to nail lacquers, 25 had positive patch tests to toluenesulfonamide-formaldehyde resin. These authors stated that these 26 were only a small fraction of all patients seen with nail lacquer dermatitis (61, partly probably previously reported in [76]). In 1958, a series of 56 patients with cosmetic allergy caused by nail lacquers was described in London (59). At that time, nail lacquer was the second commonest cause of cosmetic dermatitis after lipstick, accounting for approximately 20% of all cases of cosmetic allergy (59). Of the 56 patients, 'little more than half' could be investigated in detail; 28 reacted to TFR (59).

During the period October 1989 - December 1991, 18 cases of contact allergy to nail varnish were identified in one center in Sweden. Seventeen of the 18 patients were patch test positive to TFR and to their own nail varnishes. The lesions were scattered, involving the face, eyelids, neck and hands. Periungual lesions were recorded in 11/18. The dermatitis resolved within a few weeks when the use of nail varnish was stopped. The socio-medical consequences of contact allergy to nail varnish had been severe: sick leave (nine cases), hospitalization (four cases), cessation of visual-display-unit (VDU) work (two cases), and job-loss (two cases) (8).

Fourteen patients with contact allergy to TFR had dermatitis on the face, side of the neck, lips, perioral skin, upper eyelids or combinations, but never on the perionychia (37). Eight patients (plus 5 cited from a personal Communication) had contact allergy to TFR in a nail hardener that also contained formaldehyde; the patients reacted to TFR only. Many were also allergic upon patch testing to nail lacquers, but most had been using nail varnishes for years without problems and became sensitized to TFR from the use of the nail hardeners (38). Five patients with eyelid dermatitis reacted to their nail varnish and TFR (29). Seven similar cases were reported two years later by the same author (28), most likely including the 5 patients presented in ref. 29.

Case reports

Three patients had relevant positive patch test reactions to nail polishes and to their ingredient TFR (63). Two individuals with cheilitis had contact allergy to tosylamide/formaldehyde resin in nail lacquers (22). A young boy had dermatitis around the nails and on the face from the use of bitter nail varnish to prevent nail biting (19).

Angioedema-like contact dermatitis of the face from TFR in nail hardener with recurrent swelling of the tongue from nail biting has been observed in one patient (24). A 4-year-old atopic child had eyelid and flexural dermatitis from TFR in nail varnish (26). One patient reacted to nail varnish (27). Two more patients (or one?) had ACD from TFR in nail lacquer (32). Another one had ACD in the neck from TFR in nail lacquer and later reacted to nitrocellulose in another varnish (34). One patient had ACD from TFR resembling nickel dermatitis (72, details unknown, article not read).

A woman had perianal contact dermatitis caused by contact allergy to TFR in her nail lacquers (74). Another female individual had ACD from TFR in nail varnish strongly resembling seborrheic dermatitis (78). In a woman with contact allergy to TFR in nail varnish, the resulting dermatitis of the eyelids obscured an underlying discoid lupus erythematosus (79).

Cross-reactions, pseudo-cross-reactions and co-reactions

Pseudo-cross-reactivity to toluenesulfonamide, one of the base materials for the resin (10,76) have been observed. It is generally accepted that formaldehyde is not an allergen in nail lacquers. However, in one US study, all 10 patients who were allergic to TFR co-reacted to formaldehyde (80). This is a bizarre and unique finding, as it would suggest that formaldehyde is the actual sensitizer in TFR, which contradicts all previous findings. In the same investigation, of 42 patients allergic to formaldehyde, 10 (24%) co-reacted to TFR, possibly indicating pseudo-cross-reactivity of TFR to formaldehyde from the presence of formaldehyde in the test material (80).

Presence in cosmetic products and chemical analyses

In July 2017, tosylamide/formaldehyde resin was present in 130 of 69,577 cosmetic products of which the composition is known in EWG's Skin Deep Cosmetics Database, USA (http://www.ewg.org/skindeep/). In the USA, in April 2017, tosylamide/formaldehyde resin was present in 119 of 56,714 cosmetic products of which the composition is known in FDA's Voluntary Cosmetic Registration Program (VCRP) (data obtained from FDA, May 2017). In 1997, in Finland, 42 samples of nail polishes of 20 brands were analysed. All the polishes contained TFR in concentrations ranging from 0.08% to 11.0%. The concentration of total formaldehyde varied from 0.02% to 0.5%. The more TSF a nail polish contained, the higher was its formaldehyde content. It was concluded that probably not only TSF-allergic but also formaldehyde-allergic persons may develop dermatitis from many of the nail polishes studied (33). In 1995, the results of analyses of 64 nail polishes of different brand, age, composition, color (including colorless) and origin, e.g., England, France, Germany, Italy, Switzerland, Turkey and USA, were published (35). Tosylamide/formaldehyde resin was detected in almost all of them, the concentrations varying between 2.8% and 23.6%. Two out of 3 nail polishes declared to be TFR-free actually did contain the resin (35).

OTHER SIDE EFFECTS

Photosensitivity
One patient had photoaggravated allergic contact dermatitis from tosylamide/formaldehyde resin in nail varnishes (30).

Miscellaneous side effects
Onycholysis from contact allergy to tosylamide/formaldehyde resin in nail hardener has been recorded (9,31).

LITERATURE

1   Adams RM, Maibach HI, Clendenning WE, Fisher AA, Jordan WJ, Kanof N, et al. A five-year study of cosmetic reactions. J Am Acad Dermatol 1985;13:1062-1069
2   Davis MD, Scalf LA, Yiannias JA, Cheng JF, El-Azhary RA, Rohlinger AL, et al. Changing trends and allergens in the patch test standard series. Arch Dermatol 2008;144:67-72
3   Warshaw EM, Buchholz HJ, Belsito DV et al. Allergic patch test reactions associated with cosmetics: Retrospective analysis of cross-sectional data from the North American Contact Dermatitis Group, 2001-2004. J Am Acad Dermatol 2009;60:23-38
4   Thorne N. Nail varnish. Br J Clin Pract 1963;17:479-482
5   Guin JD. Eyelid dermatitis: a report of 215 patients. Contact Dermatitis 2004;50:87-90
6   Staines KS, Felix DH, Forsyth A. Desquamative gingivitis, sole manifestation of tosylamide/formaldehyde resin allergy. Contact Dermatitis 1998;39:90
7   Kohl L, Blondeel A, Song M. Allergic contact dermatitis from cosmetics: retrospective analysis of 819 patch-tested patients. Dermatology 2002;204:334-337
8   Lidén C, Berg M, Färm G, Wrangsjö K. Nail varnish allergy with far-reaching consequences. Br J Dermatol 1993;128:57-62
9   Paltzik RL, Enscoe I. Onycholysis secondary to toluene sulfonamide formaldehyde resin used in a nail hardener mimicking onychomycosis. Cutis 1980;25:647-648
10   Hausen BM, Milbrodt M, Koenig WA. The allergens of nail polish: Allergenic constituents of common nail polish and toluene sulfonamide-formaldehyde resin (TS-F-R). Contact Dermatitis 1995;33:157-164
11   Hausen BM. Nagellack-Allergie. H+G Z Hautkr 1994;69:252-262
12   Zug KA, Warshaw EM, Fowler JF Jr, Maibach HI, Belsito DL, Pratt MD, et al. Patch-test results of the North American Contact Dermatitis Group 2005-2006. Dermatitis 2009;20:149-160
13   Fransway AF, Zug KA, Belsito DV, Deleo VA, Fowler JF Jr, Maibach HI, et al. North American Contact Dermatitis Group patch test results for 2007-2008. Dermatitis 2013;24:10-21
14   Warshaw EM, Belsito DV, DeLeo VA, Fowler JF Jr, Maibach HI, Marks JG, et al. North American Contact Dermatitis Group patch-test results, 2003-2004 study period. Dermatitis 2008;19:129-136
15   Wenk KS, Ehrlich AE. Fragrance series testing in eyelid dermatitis. Dermatitis 2012;23:22-26
16   Fuchs T, Gutgesell C. Is contact allergy to toluene sulphonamide-formaldehyde resin common? Br J Dermatol 1996;135:1013-1014
17   Warshaw EM, Maibach HI, Taylor JS, Sasseville D, DeKoven JG, Zirwas MJ, et al. North American Contact Dermatitis Group patch test results: 2011-2012. Dermatitis 2015;26:49-59
18   Warshaw EM, Belsito DV, Taylor JS, Sasseville D, DeKoven JG, Zirwas MJ, et al. North American Contact Dermatitis Group patch test results: 2009 to 2010. Dermatitis 2013;24:50-59
19   Özkaya E, Mirzoyeva L. Tosylamide/formaldehyde resin allergy in a young boy: exposure from bitter nail varnish used against nail biting. Contact Dermatitis 2009;60:171-172
20   Miller HE, Taussig LR. Cosmetics. JAMA 1925;84:1999-2002
21   Burgess JF. Nail polish dermatitis. Can Med Assoc J 1941;45:336-339
22   Freeman S, Stephens R. Cheilitis: analysis of 75 cases referred to a contact dermatitis clinic. Am J Contact Dermat 1999;10:198-200
23   Shergill B, Goldsmith P. Nail varnish is a potential allergen in nickel allergic subjects. Clin Exp Dermatol 2004;29:545-546
24   Moran B, Murphy GM. Recurrent tongue swelling: an unusual manifestation of allergic contact dermatitis. Contact Dermatitis 2009;60:114-115
25   Katsarou A, Armenaka M, Vosynioti V, Lagogianni E, Stavropoulos PG, Kalogeromitros D. Allergic contact cheilitis in Athens. Contact Dermatitis 2008;59:123-125
26   Jacob SE, Stechschulte SA. Tosylamide/formaldehyde resin allergy – a consideration in the atopic toddler. Contact Dermatitis 2008;58:312-313

27 Yokota M, Thong H-Y, Hoffman CA, Maibach HI. Allergic contact dermatitis caused by tosylamide formaldehyde resin in nail varnish: an old allergen that has not disappeared. Contact Dermatitis 2007;57:277

28 Guin JD. Eyelid dermatitis: A report of 215 patients. Contact Dermatitis 2004;50:87-90

29 Guin J. Eyelid dermatitis: a report of 203 cases. J Am Acad Dermatol 2002;47:755-765

30 Vilaplana J, Romaguera C. Contact dermatitis from tosylamide/formaldehyde resin with photosensitivity. Contact Dermatitis 2000;42:311-312

31 Brauer EW. Onycholysis secondary to toluene sulfonamide formaldehyde resin used in a nail hardener mimicking onychomycosis. Cutis 1980;26:588

32 Boehncke WH, Schmitt M, Zollner T M, Hensel O. Nail polish allergy; an important differential diagnosis in contact dermatitis. Dtsch Med Wochenschr 1997;122:849-852

33 Sainio E-L, Engström K, Henriks-Eckerman M-L, Kanerva L. Allergenic ingredients in nail polishes. Contact Dermatitis 1997;37:155-162

34 Castelain M, Veyrat S, Laine G, Montastier C. Contact dermatitis from nitrocellulose in a nail varnish. Contact Dermatitis 1997;36:266-267

35 Hausen BM. A simple method of determining TS-F-R in nail polish. Contact Dermatitis 1995;32:188-190

36 Palmer RB. Dermatitis from nail lacquer. Arch Derm 1941;44:13-22

37 Giorgini S, Brusi C, Francalanci S, Gola M, Sertoli A. Prevention of allergic contact dermatitis from nail varnishes and hardeners. Contact Dermatitis 1994;31:325-326

38 De Wit FS, de Groot AC, Weyland JW, Bos JD. An outbreak of contact dermatitis from toluenesulfonamide formaldehyde resin in a nail hardener. Contact Dermatitis 1988;18:280-283

39 Pratt MD, Belsito DV, DeLeo VA, Fowler JF Jr, Fransway AF, Maibach HI, et al. North American Contact Dermatitis Group patch-test results, 2001–2002 study period. Dermatitis 2004;15:176-183

40 Marks JG Jr, Belsito DV, DeLeo VA, Fowler JF Jr, Fransway AF, Maibach HI, et al. North American Contact Dermatitis Group patch-test results, 1998–2000. Am J Contact Dermat 2003;14:59-62

41 Marks JG Jr, Belsito DV, DeLeo VA, Fowler JF Jr, Fransway AF, Maibach HI, et al. North American Contact Dermatitis Group patch test results, 1996–1998. Arch Dermatol 2000;136:272-273

42 Marks JG Jr, Belsito DV, DeLeo VA, Fowler JF Jr, Fransway AF, Maibach HI,et al. North American Contact Dermatitis Group patch test results for the detection of delayed-type hypersensitivity to topical allergens. J Am Acad Dermatol 1998;38:911-918

43 Marks JG, Belsito DV, DeLeo VA, Fowler JF, Fransway AF, Maibach HI,et al. North American Contact Dermatitis Group standard tray patch test results 1992 through 1994. Am J Contact Dermatitis 1995;6:160-165

44 Lindberg M, Edman B, Fischer T, Stenberg B. Time trends in Swedish patch test data from 1992 to 2000. A multi-centre study based on age- and sex-adjusted results of the Swedish standard series. Contact Dermatitis 2007;56:205-210

45 Wetter DA, Davis MDP, Yiannias JA, Cheng JF, Connolly SM, el-Azhary RA, et al. Patch test results from the Mayo Contact Dermatitis Group, 1998–2000. J Am Acad Dermatol 2005;53:416-421

46 Hasan T, Rantanen T, Alanko K, Harvima RJ, Jolanki R, Kalimo K, et al. Patch test reactions to cosmetic allergens in 1995–1997 and 2000–2002 in Finland –a multicentre study. Contact Dermatitis 2005;53:40-45

47 Fall S, Bruze M, Isaksson M, Lidén C, Matura M, Stenberg B, Lindberg M. Contact allergy trends in Sweden – a retrospective comparison of patch test data from 1992, 2000, and 2009. Contact Dermatitis 2015;72:297-304

48 Amin KA, Belsito DV. The aetiology of eyelid dermatitis: a 10-year retrospective analysis. Contact Dermatitis 2006;55:280-285

49 Cooper SM, Shaw S. Eyelid dermatitis: an evaluation of 232 patch test patients over 5 years. Contact Dermatitis 2000: 42;291-293

50 Goossens A, Beck MH, Haneke E, McFadden JP, Nolting S, Durupt G, Ries G. Adverse cutaneous reactions to cosmetic allergens. Contact Dermatitis 1999;40:112-113

51 Goossens A. Cosmetic contact allergens. Cosmetics 2016, 3, 5; doi:10.3390/cosmetics3010005

52 Wentworth AB, Yiannias JA, Keeling JH, Hall MR, Camilleri MJ, Drage LA, et al. Trends in patch-test results and allergen changes in the standard series: a Mayo Clinic 5-year retrospective review (January 1, 2006, to December 31, 2010). J Am Acad Dermatol 2014;70:269-275

53 Zug KA, Kornik R, Belsito DV, DeLeo VA, Fowler JF Jr, Maibach HI, et al. Patch-testing North American lip dermatitis patients: Data from the North American Contact Dermatitis Group, 2001 to 2004. Dermatitis 2008;19:202-208

54 Rietschel RL, Warshaw EM, Sasseville D, Fowler JF Jr, DeLeo VA. Belsito DV, et al. Common contact allergens associated with eyelid dermatitis: data from the North American Contact Dermatitis Group 2003-2004 study period. Dermatitis 2007;18:78-81

55 Katz AS, Sherertz EF. Facial dermatitis: Patch test results and final diagnoses. Am J Cont Dermat 1999;10:153-156

56 De Groot AC, Bruynzeel DP, Bos JD, van der Meeren HL, van Joost T, Jagtman BA, Weyland JW. The allergens in cosmetics. Arch Dermatol 1988;124:1525-1529

57 De Groot AC. Adverse reactions to cosmetics. PhD Thesis, University of Groningen, The Netherlands: 1988, chapter 3.4, pp.105-113

58 De Groot AC. Contact allergy to cosmetics: Causative ingredients. Contact Dermatitis 1987;17:26-34

59 Calnan CD, Sarkany I. Studies in contact dermatitis. III. Nail varnish. Trans St John's Hosp Derm Soc 1958;40:1-11

60 Simon FA. Nail polish eczema. South Med J 1943;36:157-159

61 Keil H, van Dyck LS. Dermatitis due to nail polish. Arch Derm Syph 1944;50:39-44

62 Zoli V, Silvani S, Vincenzi C, Tosti A. Allergic contact cheilitis. Contact Dermatitis 2006;54:296-297

63 Held E, Johansen JD, Agner T, Menné T. Contact allergy to cosmetics: testing with patients' own products. Contact Dermatitis 1999;40:310-315

64 Laguna C, de la Cuadra J, Martín-González B, Zaragoza V, Martínez-Casimiro L, Alegre V. Allergic contact dermatitis to cosmetics. Actas Dermosifiliogr 2009;100:53-60

65 Dooms-Goossens A, de Boulle K, Dooms M, Degreef H. Imidazolidinyl urea dermatitis. Contact Dermatitis 1986;14:322-324

66 Toholka R, Wang Y-S, Tate B, Tam M, Cahill J, Palmer A, Nixon R. The first Australian Baseline Series: Recommendations for patch testing in suspected contact dermatitis. Australas J Dermatol 2015;56:107-115

67 DeKoven JG, Warshaw EM, Belsito DV, Sasseville D, Maibach HI, Taylor JS, et al. North American Contact Dermatitis Group Patch Test Results: 2013-2014. Dermatitis 2017;28:33-46

68 Zaragoza-Ninet V, Blasco Encinas R, Vilata-Corell JJ, Pérez-Ferriols A, Sierra-Talamantes C, Esteve-Martínez A, de la Cuadra-Oyanguren J. Allergic contact dermatitis due to cosmetics: A clinical and epidemiological study in a tertiary hospital. Actas Dermosifiliogr 2016;107:329-336

69 Warshaw EM, Wang MZ, Mathias CGT, Maibach HI, Belsito DV, Zug KA, et al. Occupational contact dermatitis in hairdressers/cosmetologists; retrospective analysis of North American Contact Dermatitis Group data, 1994 to 2010. Dermatitis 2012;23:258-268

70 Schena D, Fantuzzi F, Girolomoni G. Contact allergy in chronic eczematous lip dermatitis. Eur J Dermatol 2008;18:688-692

71 Duarte I, Lazzarini R, Kobata CM. Contact dermatitis in adolescents. Am J Contact Dermat 2003;14:200-202

72 Kanerva L, Tarvainen K, Leino T. Toluene sulfonamideformaldehyde resin allergy simulating nickel dermatitis. Eur J Dermatol 1995;5:149-150

73 Fisher AA. Nail polish dermatitis masquerading as atopic dermatitis. Cutis 1986;38:236

74 Lazarov A. Perianal contact dermatitis caused by nail lacquer allergy. Am J Cont Dermat 1999,10:43-44

75 Tosti A, Guerra L, Vincenzi C, Piraccini BM, Peluso AM. Contact sensitization caused by toluene sulfonamide-formaldehyde resin in women who use nail cosmetics. Am J Cont Dermat 1993;4:150-153

76 Keil H. Dermatitis due to hair lacquer and nail polish. JAMA 1943;123:857-858

77 Lazzarini R, Duarte I, de Farias DC, Santos CA, Tsai AI. Frequency and main sites of allergic contact dermatitis caused by nail varnish. Dermatitis 2008;19:319-322

78 Pongpairoj K, Morar N, McFadden JP. 'Seborrhoeic dermatitis' of the head and neck without scalp involvement – remember nail varnish allergy. Contact Dermatitis 2016;74:306-307

79 Trindade MA, Alchorne AO, da Costa EB, Enokihara MM. Eyelid discoid lupus erythematosus and contact dermatitis: a case report. J Eur Acad Dermatol Venereol 2004;18:577-579

80 Scheman A, Hipolito R, Severson D, Youkhanis N. Allergy cross-reactions: retrospective clinical data and review of the literature. Dermatitis 2017;28:128-140

2.470 TRIACONTANYL PVP

IDENTIFICATION

Description/definition   : Triacontanyl PVP is a polymer of vinyl pyrrolidone and 1-triacontane, which conforms to the formula shown below, where R represents the triacontane moiety or hydrogen

Chemical class(es)   : Synthetic polymers

Chemical/IUPAC name   : Diethyl 6a-amino-1,6-bis(carbamoylamino)-3a-cyano-2,5-dimethylpyrrolo[2, 3]pyrrole-3,4-dicarboxylate

Other names   : 2-Pyrrolidinone, 1-ethenyl-, polymer with 1-triacontene; vinylpyrrolidone, copolymers with α-alkenes >C10; vinylpyrrolidone/1-triacontene copolymer

CAS registry number (s) : 136445-69-7

Function(s) in cosmetics : EU: film forming; humectant; viscosity controlling. USA: film formers; viscosity increasing agents – nonaqueous

Patch testing   : 10% pet. (2)

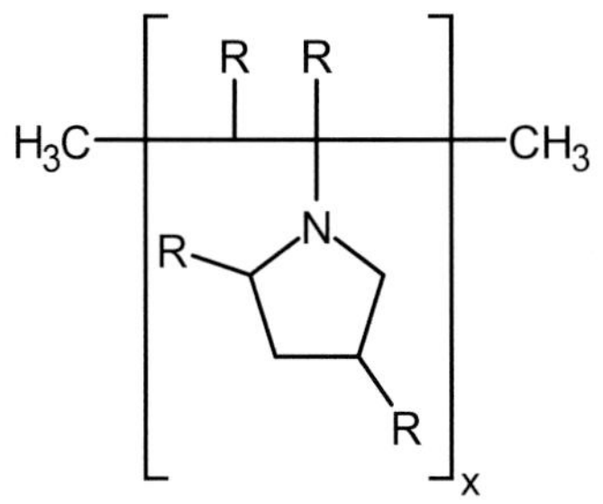

GENERAL

Copolymers are important ingredients in cosmetics, added because of their antistatic, film-forming, binding, suspending, viscosity-increasing, skin-conditioning, and emulsion-stabilizing properties. Copolymers have been underestimated for a long time as to their sensitizing capacities because of their large structures and high molecular weights. Allergic contact dermatitis to copolymers in cosmetics, however, does occur, but the exact nature of the hapten is still unknown. The copolymers are not likely to be haptens themselves in view of their large molecular weights. The sensitizer could be an additive, an impurity, a product that forms during polymerization, a residual monomer, or a degradation product (1).

Tricontanyl PVP is used as a waterproofing, film-forming, viscosity-increasing, and pigment-dispersing agent in cosmetics. It is incorporated specifically into sunscreen agents to contribute to the water-resistant nature of the formulation, by helping its adherence to the skin (1).

CONTACT ALLERGY

Case reports and case series

A female child had a 2-year history of an eczematous rash, developing in summer months, at sites where sunscreen products had been applied. Sunlight alone did not provoke the eruption. Patch tests with a modified standard series of allergens and the patient's own sunscreens showed a positive reaction at D2 and D4 to one of her sunscreens. Photopatch testing was negative. Later, the child was tested with the individual ingredients of the sunscreen, which yielded a positive reaction at D2 and D4 to polyvinylpyrrolidone (PVP)/1-triacontene 10% pet. Twenty control patients had negative reactions to the test material (2).

A 12-year-old boy who used a cosmetic hair gel developed a severe inflammatory rash after using the product for 5-6 weeks. Patch tests to the individual ingredients of the gel gave a positive reaction to the copolymer PVP/1-triacontene 5% pet. (3).

Presence in cosmetic products and chemical analyses

In the USA, in April 2017, tricontanyl PVP was present in 71 of 56,714 cosmetic products of which the composition is known in FDA's Voluntary Cosmetic Registration Program (VCRP) (data obtained from FDA, May 2017). In April 2017, triacontanyl PVP was present in 82 of 65,434 cosmetic products of which the composition is known in EWG's Skin Deep Cosmetics Database, USA (http://www.ewg.org/skindeep/). In the database of cosmetic ingredients of the Leuven University, Belgium, PVP/1-triacontene was found to be present in one lip gloss, 21 different kinds of mascara, 32 hair conditioners, 12 shampoos, 1 styling mousse, 12 styling gels, 26 sunscreens, 1 anti-aging sunscreen, 1 depilatory foam, 1 skin illuminator, and 2 moisturizers (1).

LITERATURE

1   Quartier S, Garmyn M, Becart S, Goossens A. Allergic contact dermatitis to copolymers in cosmetics – case report and review of the literature. Contact Dermatitis 2006;55:257-267
2   Stone N, Varma S, Hughes TM, Stone NM. Allergic contact dermatitis from polyvinylpyrrolidone (PVP)/1-triacontene copolymer in a sunscreen. Contact Dermatitis 2002;47:49
3   Kai A, Khorshid M, McFadden J. Allergic contact dermatitis to copolymers. Br J Dermatol 2010;163 (Suppl. 1):87

2.471   3,4',5-TRIBROMOSALICYLANILIDE[*]
* Not an INCI name

IDENTIFICATION

Description/definition   : 3,4',5-Tribromosalicylanilide is the brominated aromatic compound that conforms to the structural formula shown below
Chemical class(es)   : Organobromine compounds; aromatic compounds; amides
INCI name USA   : Not in the Personal Care Products Council Ingredient Database
Chemical/IUPAC name   : 3,5-Dibromo-*N*-(4-bromophenyl)-2-hydroxybenzamide
Other names   : Tribromsalan
CAS registry number (s)   : 87-10-5; 12738-72-6
EC number(s)   : 201-723-6
SCCS opinion(s)   : SCCNFP, 21 January 1998 (4)
Merck Index monograph   : 11048
Function(s) in cosmetics   : EU: prohibited since 1997; USA: formerly used as antimicrobial
EU cosmetic restrictions   : Regulated in Annex II/373 of the Regulation (EC) No. 1223/2009 (prohibited)
USA cosmetic restrictions   : Prohibited (FDA)
Patch testing   : 1% pet. (Chemotechnique)
Molecular formula   : $C_{13}H_8Br_3NO_2$

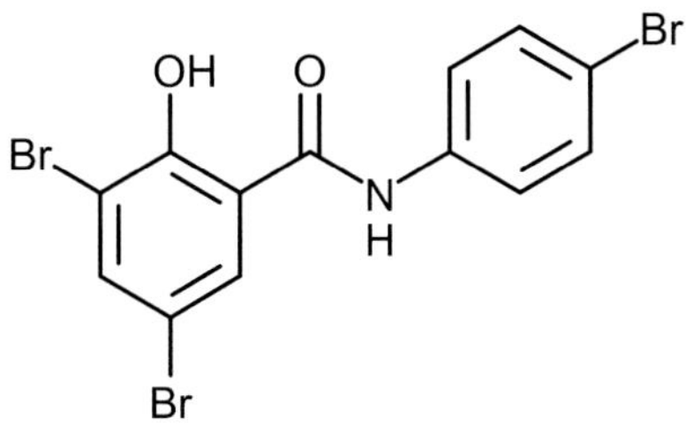

GENERAL

3,4',5-Tribromosalicylanilide (from here: tribromosalicylanilide or TBS) is a halogenated salicylanilide which was widely used in the 1960s and 1970s as an antimicrobial in germicidal soaps in certain countries, notably the USA and Denmark. This chemical caused many cases of photosensitization and was excluded from such use in 1974 or 1975 in the USA (33,39) and was later also prohibited in the EU. It may be assumed that tribromosalicylanilide is not in use anymore. A general introduction to the halogenated salicylanilides and related chemicals (halogenated phenols) can be found in Chapter 2.450 Tetrachlorosalicylanilide. In assessing the data from early studies, and notably in the distinc-tion between contact allergy and photocontact allergy, it should be realized that, in those days, experience with photopatch tests was limited and such tests may not always have been reliable.

CONTACT ALLERGY

Patch testing in groups of patients

There are no studies in which tribromosalicylanilide has been tested in consecutive patients suspected of contact dermatitis (routine testing). Results of patch testing TBS in groups of *selected* patients (patients suspected of photosensitivity or with reactions after sunscreen application) are shown in table 2.471.1. In three studies, rates of positive reactions ranged from 0.5% to 2.5%, but the study with the highest rate had certain weaknesses (2). No relevant reactions were reported (2,6,14).

Table 2.471.1 Patch testing in groups of patients: Selected patient groups

Years and Country	Test conc. & vehicle	Number of patients tested	positive (%)	Selection of patients (S); Relevance (R); Comments (C)	Ref.
2001-2010 Canada		160	4 (2.5%)	S: patients with suspected photosensitivity and patients who developed pruritus or a rash after sunscreen applica-tion; R: not stated; C: weak study: inadequate reading of test results, erythema only was considered to represent a positive patch test reaction	2
2000-2005 USA	1% pet.	179	1 (0.6%)	S: patients photopatch tested for suspected photoderma-titis; R: the reaction was not relevant	6
1980-1981 4 Scandi-navian countries	1% pet.	745	4 (0.5%)	S: patients suspected of sun-related skin disease; R: not stated	14

Case reports and case series
Tribromosalicylanilide was responsible for 1 out of 399 cases of cosmetic (photo)allergy where the causal allergen was identified in a study of the NACDG, USA, 1977-1983 (1).

Cross-reactions, pseudo-cross-reactions and co-reactions (also photoreactions)

(Photo)cross-reactions from tribromosalicylanilide
Primary TBS photosensitization in one study almost invariably lead to tetrachlorosalicylanilide (TCSA) photo-cross-reactivity (also ref. 22), to fenticlor (Chapter 2.457 2,2'-Thiobis(4-chlorophenol)) in 40% and to triclocarban (TCC) and hexachlorophene in 15% of cases (15). Plain contact allergy as cross-reaction to primary TBS photocontact allergy was seen in 50% in the case of TCSA , whereas no such reactions were seen with TCC and hexachlorophene (15). Patients primarily photosensitized to tribromosalicylanilide may photocross-react to 4',5-dibromosalicylanilide (16,22,32), 4'-bromosalicylanilide (16,32), 3,5-dibromosalicylanilide, 5-bromo-4'-chlorosalicylanilide and salicylanilide (16). Plain contact allergy as cross-reactivity to TBS photosensitization may be seen to 4',5-dibromosalicylanilide, 4'-bromosalicylanilide (frequent) and 5-bromo-4'-chlorosalicylanilide (16).

Photocross-reactivity between tribromosalicylanilide, 2',3,4',5-tetrabromosalicylanilide, 4',5-dibromosalicylanilide, 3,5-dibromosalicylanilide and 3,5-dibromosalicylic acid (27). All six patients primarily photosensitized to tribromosalicylanilide showed photocross-reactions to 5-bromo-4'-chlorosalicylanilide (Multifungin), which was (and still is) used as a topical antifungal drug (20). Occasional photocross-reactivity of bithionol to primary tribromosalicylanilide photosensitization (23). No photocross-reactivity from halogenated salicylanilides primary photosensitization to hexachlorophene and triclocarban (35). Limited contact allergic cross-sensitivity to hexachlorophene and triclocarban from primary halogenated salicylanilides photosensitization (35). See also ref. 18 for additional information on the (photo)cross-reaction pattern of tribromosalicylanilide.

(Photo)cross-reactions to tribromosalicylanilide
(Photo)cross-reactions to tribromosalicylanilide may be observed in patients primarily (photo)sensitized to tetrachlorosalicylanilide (frequent: 24,25,31), 5-bromo-4'-chlorosalicylanilide (Multifungin) (often, 21) and dibromosalicylanilide (5). In a group of 18 patients photosensitized to ketoprofen, 2 (11%) had positive photopatch tests to tribromosalicylanilide. As there were also many photoreactions to fenticlor (Chapter 2.457 2,2'-Thiobis(4-chlorophenol)) (n=12, 67%), tetrachlorosalicylanilide (n=5, 28%), triclosan (n= 3, 17%), and bithionol (n=2, 11%) with no clinical relevance, the authors raised the question of hyper-photosusceptibility to non-relevant allergens induced by photosensitivity to ketoprofen (36). In another group of 35 patients photoallergic to ketoprofen from Sweden, simultaneous photoallergy to tribromosalicylanilide was seen in 6%, to fenticlor in 74%, to tetrachlorosalicylanilide in 40%, to triclosan in 9% and to bithionol and hexachlorophene in 6% of the patients. No explanation for these co-reactivities was offered (37).

Presence in cosmetic products and chemical analyses
In May 2017, tribromosalicylanilide was present in zero of 66,975 cosmetic products of which the composition is known in EWG's Skin Deep Cosmetics Database, USA (http://www.ewg.org/skindeep/). In the USA, in April 2017, tribromosalicylanilide was present in zero of 56,714 cosmetic products of which the composition is known in FDA's Voluntary Cosmetic Registration Program (VCRP) (data obtained from FDA, May 2017).

OTHER SIDE EFFECTS

Photosensitivity

Photopatch testing in groups of patients
Results of photopatch testing with tribromosalicylanilide in groups of selected patients (e.g., patients suspected of photosensitivity, dermatitis affecting mainly light-exposed skin, patients with histories or clinical pictures suggestive of allergic contact photodermatitis) are shown in table 2.471.2. In 12 studies, rates of photosensitization have ranged from 0.1% to 28%, but were 3% or less in 10 of the twelve investigations (table 2.471.2). The highest frequencies were found in a very small study of 18 patients with persistent light reactions (14) and in an older study from the USA, when TBS was still in use there (33). Only a few reactions have been scored as relevant (5,6), but in the majority of the studies, relevance was either not mentioned or not specified for tribromosalicylanilide.

Table 2.471.2 Photopatch testing in groups of patients

Years and Country	Test conc. & vehicle	Number of patients tested	positive (%)		Selection of patients (S); Relevance (R); Comments (C)	Ref.
2011-2013 Colombia	10% pet.	112	1	(0.9%)	S: dermatitis affecting mainly light-exposed skin, a history of a sunscreen or of a topical NSAID skin reaction; R: relevant	5
2004-2006 Italy		1082	1	(0.1%)	S: patients with histories and clinical features suggestive of photoallergic contact dermatitis; R: not relevant	8
1992-2006 Greece	1% pet.	207	1	(0.5%)	S: patients suspected of photosensitivity; R: not stated	7
2000-2005 USA	1% pet.	179	2	(1.1%)	S: patients photopatch tested for suspected photodermatitis; R: both reactions were relevant	6
1994-1999 NL	0.1% pet.	55	1	(2%)	S: patients suspected of photosensitivity disorders; R: not stated	9
1991-97 Ger, Au, Swi	0.1% pet.	1261		(0.3%)	S: patients suspected of photosensitivity; R: not stated	10
1985-1994 Italy		1050	4	(0.4%)	S: patients with histories or clinical pictures suggestive of allergic contact photodermatitis; R: 78% for all photo-allergens together	3
1985-1990 USA	1% pet.	187	5	(2.7%)	S: patients with a history of photosensitivity; R: not relevant	11
1980-1985 USA	1% pet.	70	2	(3%)	S: not stated; R: not stated	12
<1984 Norway	1% pet.	18	5	(28%)	S: patients with persistent light reactions; R: not stated	13
1980-1981 4 Scandi-navian countries	1% pet.	745	4	(0.5%)	S: patients suspected of sun-related skin disease; R: not stated	14
1967-1975 USA		272	28	(10.3%)	S: patients with a history suggestive of a photosensitivity problem or an eruption involving sun-exposed areas; R: not stated	33

Au: Austria; Ger: Germany; NL: Netherlands; Swi: Switzerland

Case reports and case series

During a period of 3 months in 1967, contact photoallergy to tribromosalicylanilide (TBS) in a toilet soap was diagnosed in 39 patients in Copenhagen, Denmark (15). Of 19 patients with the clinical picture of soap photocontact dermatitis (mostly a sharply demarcated erythematous and lichenoid eruption limited to sun-exposed areas of the body, such as the face, neck, hands, and forearms), investigated in the USA, 16 photo-reacted to tetrachlorosalicyl-anilide, 4 to bithionol, 3 to hexachlorophene and one to tribromosalicylanilide and triclocarban each. Most patients had a definite history of exposure to a soap containing the offending sensitizing agent (17). In a period of 1.5 year (1966-1967), in a university center in San Francisco, USA, 26 patients suspected of photosensitivity were investigated with photopatch tests with halogenated salicylanilides and related compounds. Tetrachlorosalicylanilide was the most frequent photosensitizer (21/22 tested), followed by bithionol (10/26), tribromosalicylanilide (9/22), hexachlorophene (n=4), triclocarban (n=3) and dichlorophene (n=3). Six patients became persistent light reactors. The relevance of the reactions was not specified. In fact, the authors stated that it was generally impossible to determine which was the original photosensitizer and which positive photopatch tests were the result of photocross-sensitivity (19).

Twelve patients with photosensitive reactions due to soaps had positive tests to either dibromosalicylanilide or tribromosalicylanilide, or to a soap solution containing these substances, but tests were negative if soap solutions free of halogenated salicylanilides were used (30). Six patients from Australia had photoallergic contact dermatitis to tribromosalicylanilide in soaps, of who one became a persistent light reactor (20). Three individuals in three studies each had photoallergic contact dermatitis from tribromosalicylanilide in soaps (22,27,32). Three other individuals also suffered from photoallergic contact dermatitis to tribromosalicylanilide in soap (29,34,38). One of them became a persistent light reactor which evolved into actinic reticuloid (34). Two patients had photoallergic contact dermatitis from tribromosalicylanilide in soap (26). In two other studies, an unspecified number of patients were photoreactive to TBS in soaps (24,28).

LITERATURE

1 Adams RM, Maibach HI, Clendenning WE, Fisher AA, Jordan WJ, Kanof N, et al. A five-year study of cosmetic reactions. J Am Acad Dermatol 1985;13:1062-1069
2 Greenspoon J, Ahluwalia R, Juma N, Rosen CF. Allergic and photoallergic contact dermatitis: A 10-year experience. Dermatitis 2013;24:29-32

3   Pigatto PD, Legori A, Bigardi AS, Guarrera M, Tosti A, Santucci B, et al. Gruppo Italiano recerca dermatiti da contatto ed ambientali Italian multicenter study of allergic contact photodermatitis: epidemiological aspects. Am J Contact Dermatitis 1996;17:158-163

4   SCCNFP (Scientific Committee on Cosmetics and Non Food Products). Opinion concerning 3,4',5-Tribromo-salicylanilide, 21 January 1998. Available at: http://ec.europa.eu/health/scientific_committees/ consumer_safety/opinions/sccnfp_opinions_97_04/sccp_out23_en.htm

5   Valbuena Mesa MC, Hoyos Jiménez EV. Photopatch testing in Bogota (Colombia): 2011–2013. Contact Dermatitis 2016;74:11-17

6   Scalf LA, Davis MDP, Rohlinger AL, Connolly SM. Photopatch testing of 182 patients: A 6-year experience at the Mayo Clinic. Dermatitis 2009;20:44-52

7   Katsarou A, Makris M, Zarafonitis G, Lagogianni E, Gregoriou S, Kalogeromitros D. Photoallergic contact dermatitis: the 15-year experience of a tertiary referral center in a sunny Mediterranean city. Int J Immunopathol Pharmacol 2008;21:725-727

8   Pigatto PD, Guzzi G, Schena D, Guarrera M, Foti C, Francalanci S, et al. Photopatch tests: an Italian multicentre study from 2004 to 2006. Contact Dermatitis 2008;59:103-108

9   Bakkum RS, Heule F. Results of photopatch testing in Rotterdam during a 10-year period. Br J Dermatol 2002;146:275-279

10   Neumann NJ, Hölzle E, Plewig G, Schwarz T, Panizzon RG, Breit R, et al. Photopatch testing: The 12-year experience of the German, Austrian and Swiss Photopatch Test Group. J Am Acad Dermatol 2000;42:183-192

11   DeLeo VA, Suarez SM, Maso MJ. Photoallergic contact dermatitis. Results of photopatch testing in New York, 1985 to 1990. Arch Dermatol 1992;128:1513-1518

12   Menz J, Muller SA, Connolly SM. Photopatch testing: a 6-year experience. J Am Acad Dermatol 1988;18:1044-1047

13   Thune P, Eeg-Larsen T. Contact and photocontact allergy in persistent light reactivity. Contact Dermatitis 1984;11:98-107

14   Wennersten G, Thune P, Brodthagen H, Jansen C, Rystedt I, Crames M, et al. The Scandinavian multicenter photopatch study. Contact Dermatitis 1984;10:305-309

15   Osmundsen PE. Contact photodermatitis due to tribromsalicylanilide. Br J Dermatol 1968;80:228-234

16   Osmundsen PE. Contact photoallergy to tribromsalicylanilide. Br J Dermatol 1969;81:429-434

17   Freeman RG, Knox JM. The action spectrum of photocontact dermatitis caused by halogenated salicylanilide and related compounds. Arch Dermatol 1968;97:130-136

18   Osmundsen PE. Contact photodermatitis due to tribromosalicylanilide (cross-reaction pattern). Dermatologica 1970;140:65-74

19   Epstein JH, Wuepper KD, Maibach HI. Photocontact dermatitis to halogenated salicylanilides and related compounds: A clinical and histologic review of 26 patients. Arch Dermatol 1968;97:236-244

20   Burry JN, Donald GF. Photo-contact dermatitis from soap. Br J Dermatol 1968;80:711-718

21   Burry J. Photoallergies to fenticlor and multifungin. Arch Dermatol 1967;95:287-291

22   Epstein S. Photosensitizers in soaps. JAMA 1966;195:878

23   Baughman RD. Contact photodermatitis from bithionol. II. Cross-sensitivities to hexachlorophene and salicylanilides. Arch Derm 1964;90:153-157

24   Wilkinson DS. Further experiences with halogenated salicylanilides. Br J Dermatol 1962;74:295-301

25   Wilkinson DS. Patch test reactions to certain halogenated salicylanilides. Br J Dermatol 1962;74:302-306

26   Epstein S, Enta T. Photoallergic contact dermatitis. JAMA 1965;194:1016-1017

27   Harber LC, Harris H, Baer RL. Photoallergic contact dermatitis due to halogenated salicylanilides and related compounds. Arch Dermatol 1966;94:255-262

28   Harber LC, Targovnik SE, Baer RL. Contact photosensitivity patterns to halogenated salicylanilides in man and guinea pigs. Arch Dermatol 1967;96:646-656

29   Ison AE, Tucker JB. Delayed reactions in positive photopatch tests to halogenated salicylanilides. Arch Dermatol 1967;96:59-61

30   Ison AE, Tucker JB. Photosensitive dermatitis from soaps. N Eng J Med 1968;278:81

31   Crow KD, Wilkinson DS, Osmundsen PE. A review of photoreactions to halogenated salicylanilides. Br J Dermatol 1969;81:180-185

32   Emmett EA. The nature of tribromosalicylanilide photoallergy. J Invest Dermatol 1974;63:227-230

33 Smith SZ, Epstein JH. Photocontact dermatitis to halogenated salicylanilides and related compounds. Our experience between 1967 and 1975. Arch Dermatol 1977;113:1372-1374

34 Horio T. Actinic reticuloid via persistent light reaction from photoallergic contact dermatitis. Arch Dermatol 1982;118:339-342

35 Harber LC, Targovnik SE, Baer RL. Studies on contact photosensitivity to hexachlorophene and trichlorocarbanilide in guinea pigs and man. J Invest Dermatol 1968; 51:373-377

36 Durbize E, Vigan M, Puzenat E, Girardin P, Adessi B, Desprez PH, Humbert PH, Laurent R, Aubin F. Spectrum of cross-photosensitization in 18 consecutive patients with contact photoallergy to ketoprofen: associated photoallergies to non-benzophenone-containing molecules. Contact Dermatitis 2003;48:144-149

37 Hindsén M, Zimerson E, Bruze M. Photoallergic contact dermatitis from ketoprofen in southern Sweden. Contact Dermatitis 2006;54:150-157

38 Shelmire D. False negative immediate photopatch test to tribromsalan. Arch Dermatol 1971;103:223-224

39 Wolverton JE, Soter NA, Cohen DE. Fentichlor photocontact dermatitis: A persistent enigma. Dermatitis 2013;24:77-81

2.472   TRICETEARETH-4 PHOSPHATE

IDENTIFICATION

Description/definition	: Triceteareth-4 phosphate is the triester of phosphoric acid and ceteareth-4
Chemical class(es)	. Phosphorus compounds
Other names	: Poly(oxy-1,2-ethanediyl),α-(C16-C18-alkyl)-ω-hydroxy- (4 mol EO average molar ratio), phosphates (3:1)
CAS registry number (s)	: 119415-05-3; 86338-11-6
Function(s) in cosmetics	: EU: emulsifying; surfactant. USA: surfactants – emulsifying agents
Patch testing	: 2% pet. (1)

CONTACT ALLERGY

Case reports and case series

An atopic woman with a previous history of contact allergy to perfumes developed a generalized dermatitis after 3 days of use of an unperfumed body lotion. The eruption was treated with a topical steroid preparation, after which the patient was referred for diagnostic tests. Patch tests with the European baseline series and her own products showed positive reactions to the fragrance mix I and fragrance mix II. Supplementary tests with fragrance mix ingredients showed positive reactions to cinnamal and cinnamyl alcohol. Furthermore, there was a positive patch test to the body lotion. When tested with its ingredients, the patient had positive reactions to triceteareth-4 phosphate 5%, 2%, 1% and 0.5% pet., but there was no reaction to a 0.1% test concentration. The body lotion itself was also tested and again showed a strong reaction. In a third patch test session, patch tests with the emulsifier also reproduced reactions to 2%, 1% and 0.5% ceteareth-4 phosphate. A repeated open application test with the lotion was positive within 3 days, whereas a ROAT performed for more than 1 week with triceteareth-4 phosphate 5% pet. was – unexpectedly - negative. Twenty-five consecutive control dermatitis patients did not react to triceteareth-4 phosphate 2% pet. (1).

Cross-reactions, pseudo-cross-reactions and co-reactions
Not to trioleyl phosphate, which was described as 'a closely related surfactant' (1).

Presence in cosmetic products and chemical analyses
In the USA, in April 2017, triceteareth-4 phosphate was present in of 56,714 cosmetic products of which the composition is known in FDA's Voluntary Cosmetic Registration Program (VCRP) (data obtained from FDA, May 2017). In April 2017, triceteareth-4 phosphate was present in 4 of 65,434 cosmetic products of which the composition is known in EWG's Skin Deep Cosmetics Database, USA (http://www.ewg.org/skindeep/).

LITERATURE
1   Madsen JT, Andersen KE. Allergic contact dermatitis caused by the emulsifier triceteareth-4-phosphate. Contact Dermatitis 2012;66:159-160

2.473 TRICHLOROFLUOROMETHANE*

Not an INCI name

IDENTIFICATION

Description/definition	: Trichlorofluoromethane is the halogen-substituted hydrocarbon that conforms to the structural formula shown below
Chemical class(es)	: Organohalogen compounds
INCI name EU/USA	: Neither in CosIng nor in the Personal Care Products Council Ingredient Database
Chemical/IUPAC name	: Trichloro(fluoro)methane
Other names	: Trichloromonofluoromethane; Freon® 11
CAS registry number (s)	: 75-69-4
EC number(s)	: 200-892-3
Merck Index monograph	: 11075
EU cosmetic restrictions	: Prohibited (Regulation (EC) No. 1005/2009 of the European parliament and of the Council of 16 September 2009 on substances that deplete the ozone layer; Official Journal of the European Union L 286/1-30, 31-10-2009)
USA cosmetic restrictions	: Prohibited (FDA)
Patch test allergens	: Pure, open and closed (1)
Molecular formula	: CCl_3F

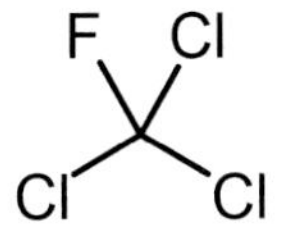

GENERAL

The chlorofluorocarbons are liquefied gases of low molecular weight which have been in use as propellants since 1940. For several decades, they were considered the best propellants available, because of their physicochemical properties, and were used in personal care products such as hair sprays, deodorants, antiperspirants, perfumes, and medicated aerosols. Due to their ozone-depleting potential, trichlorofluoromethane and other chlorofluorocarbons are not used anymore. Discussion of adverse reactions to trichlorofluoromethane in this chapter is (largely) limited to those caused by its presence in cosmetic products.

CONTACT ALLERGY

Case reports and case series

Three patients with (a history of) relapsing axillary dermatitis from the use of aerosol deodorants were patch tested with 11 spray deodorants, trichlorofluoromethane (Freon® 11) and dichlorodifluoromethane (Freon® 12) (1). They all reacted to a large number of the deodorants. All three had positive patch tests to trichlorofluoromethane and one also to the related dichlorodifluoromethane (1). It was not mentioned which of these had been present in the deodorants causing the axillary dermatitis. Two also reacted to ethyl chloride, which was used as an anesthetic before taking a punch biopsy (1).

A woman reported that she had never tolerated deodorants, female hygiene sprays and medical 'wound sprays'. She developed an allergic reaction to ethyl chloride used for anesthesia during removal of mollusca contagiosa (3). When patch tested, she reacted to both ethyl chloride and to trichlorofluoromethane. It was not mentioned whether the deodorants and female hygiene sprays that she had previously used and that caused skin reactions, had contained trichlorofluoromethane or related propellants (3).

Contact allergy to trichlorofluoromethane in non-cosmetic products

One patient had allergic contact dermatitis from trichlorofluoromethane and dichlorofluoromethane in a spray to relieve a wasp sting (2).

Cross-reactions, pseudo-cross-reactions and co-reactions

Co-reactivity to dichlorodifluoromethane (Freon® 12) in one patient and to ethyl chloride in two (1). The reaction to dichlorodifluoromethane was considered to be a cross-sensitivity, the reaction to ethyl chloride not. However, co-reactivity between ethyl chloride and trichlorofluoromethane has been observed by other authors also (3). Possible cross-reactivity with dichlorofluoromethane (2).

Presence in cosmetic products and chemical analyses

In May 2017, trichlorofluoromethane was present in zero of 66,975 cosmetic products of which the composition is known in EWG's Skin Deep Cosmetics Database, USA (http://www.ewg.org/skindeep/). In the USA, in April 2017, trichlorofluoromethane was present in zero of 56,714 cosmetic products of which the composition is known in FDA's Voluntary Cosmetic Registration Program (VCRP) (data obtained from FDA, May 2017).

LITERATURE

1   Van Ketel WG. Allergic contact dermatitis from propellants in deodorant sprays in combination with allergy to ethyl chloride. Contact Dermatitis 1976;2:115-119
2   Crow KD. Chlorofluoromethanes as propellants. Personal communication 1973, cited by WG van Ketel in ref. 1.
3   Aberer W, Zonzits E. Allergy to ethyl chloride does occur, and might frequently be misdiagnosed. Contact Dermatitis 1989;21:352-353

2.474 TRICLOCARBAN

IDENTIFICATION

Description/definition   : Triclocarban is the substituted carbanilide that conforms to the formula shown below
Chemical class(es)   : Amides; halogen compounds
Chemical/IUPAC name   : 1-(4-Chlorophenyl)-3-(3,4-dichlorophenyl)urea
Other names   : 3,4,4'-Trichlorocarbanilide
CAS registry number (s)   : 101-20-2; 1322-40-3
EC number(s)   : 202-924-1
SCCS opinion(s)   : SCCP/0851/04 (12)
Merck Index monograph   : 11089
Function(s) in cosmetics   : EU: deodorant; preservative. USA: cosmetic biocides; deodorant agents; preservatives
EU cosmetic restrictions   : Regulated in Annexes III/100 and V/23 of the Regulation (EC) No. 1223/2009
Patch testing   : 1% pet. (Chemotechnique, SmartPracticeCanada)
Molecular formula   : $C_{13}H_9Cl_3N_2O$

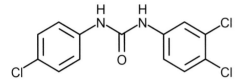

CONTACT ALLERGY

Patch testing in groups of patients
Results of studies in which triclocarban has been patch tested in consecutive patients suspected of contact dermatitis (routine testing) and in groups of selected patients are shown in table 2.474.1. In an early ICDRG study, only one positive reaction to triclocarban was found in a group of >2200 routinely tested patients (5). Likewise, in selected patients groups (patients with leg ulcers, patients suspected of cosmetic allergy, patients suspected of photosensitivity), low rates of sensitization of 0.2%-0.6% were found (9,10,17,19).

Table 2.474.1 Patch testing in groups of patients

Years and Country	Test conc. & vehicle	Number of patients tested	positive (%)	Selection of patients (S); Relevance (R); Comments (C)	Ref.
Routine testing					
<1978 ICDRG	1% pet.	>2200	1 (0.05%)	R: not found	5
Testing in groups of selected patients					
2004-2008 France	1% pet.	423	1 (0.2%)	S: patients with leg ulcers; R: not stated	9
2000-2005 USA	1% pet.	179	1 (0.6%)	S: patients photopatch tested for suspected photodermatitis; R: the reaction was relevant	17
1983-4 Netherlands	10% pet.	179	1 (0.6%)	S: patients suspected of cosmetic allergy; R: not stated	10
1980-1981 4 Scandinavian countries	1% pet.	745	1 (0.1%)	S: patients suspected of sun-related skin disease; R: not stated	19

ICDRG International Contact Dermatitis Research Group

Case reports and case series
Out of 14 patients with axillary dermatitis from one particular brand of antiperspirant, 3 reacted to triclocarban in the product (6). Of seven patients with axillary dermatitis from an antiperspirant, 2 had positive patch tests to triclocarban in the antiperspirant (7). A male medical student had axillary dermatitis from triclocarban in an antiperspirant (15). This particular antiperspirant also caused many reactions to its active ingredient propantheline bromide (see Chapter 2.384 Propantheline bromide).

Contact allergy to triclocarban in non-cosmetic products
In a 2-year retrospective study, the members of the French Dermato-Allergology Vigilance network Revidal together found 17 cases of contact allergy to Septivon®, an antiseptic preparation containing triclocarban. However, triclocarban itself was the allergen in not one single case, all were caused by excipients such as pine oil, disodium EDTA and cocamide DEA (16).

Cross-reactions, pseudo-cross-reactions and co-reactions (also photo-reactions)
Primary TBS photosensitization in 15% of cases leads to TCC photo-cross-reactivity (20). In patients photosensitized to halogenated salicylanilides or bithionol, there is no photocross-reactivity and limited contact allergic cross-reactivity to triclocarban (23).

Presence in cosmetic products and chemical analyses
In the USA, in April 2017, triclocarban was present in 20 of 56,714 cosmetic products of which the composition is known in FDA's Voluntary Cosmetic Registration Program (VCRP) (data obtained from FDA, May 2017). In April 2017, triclocarban was present in 6 of 66,647 cosmetic products of which the composition is known in EWG's Skin Deep Cosmetics Database, USA (http://www.ewg.org/skindeep/). In Germany, in 2006-2009, the labels of 4680 cosmetic products were screened for the presence of preservatives. Triclocarban was present in zero of the products, according to labelling information (14).

OTHER SIDE EFFECTS

Photosensitivity

Photopatch testing in groups of patients
Results of studies in which triclocarban has been photopatch tested in groups of selected patients are shown in table 2.474.2. In groups of patients suspected of photoallergic contact dermatitis, low rates of photosensitization of 0.2% to 2.9% were observed (3,4,8,17,18). The rate of 2.9% was found in an older study from the USA. This was a very small study, the selection procedure was not explained and the relevance of the reactions was not mentioned (3).

Table 2.474.2 Photopatch testing in groups of patients

Years and Country	Test conc. & vehicle	Number of patients tested	positive (%)		Selection of patients (S); Relevance (R); Comments (C)	Ref.
2004-2006 Italy	5% pet.	1082	4	(0.4%)	S: patients with histories and clinical features suggestive of photoallergic contact dermatitis; 3 were cases of photoaugmentated contact allergy; R: not found	4
2000-2005 USA	1% pet.	179	1	(0.6%)	S: patients photopatch tested for suspected photodermatitis; R: the reaction was relevant	17
1985-1994 Italy		1050	2	(0.2%)	S: patients with histories or clinical pictures suggestive of allergic contact photodermatitis; R: 78% of all positive photopatch tests of all photoallergens together were considered to be relevant	8
1991-1993 Singapore	1% pet.	62	1	(2%)	S: patients with clinical features suggestive of photosensitivity; R: not stated	18
1980-1985 USA	1% pet.	70	2	(2.9%)	S: not stated; R: not stated	3
1967-1975 USA		127	2	(1.6%)	S: patients with a history suggestive of a photosensitivity problem or an eruption involving sun-exposed areas	22

Case reports and series
Two patients had photoallergic contact dermatitis from triclocarban in soap (11). Another individual also had photocontact allergy to triclocarban in soap products (2). In a period of 1,5 year (1966-1967), in a university center in San Francisco, USA, 26 patients suspected of photosensitivity were investigated with photopatch tests with halogenated salicylanilides and related compounds. Tetrachlorosalicylanilide was the most frequent photosensitizer (21/22 tested), followed by bithionol (10/26), tribromosalicylanilide (9/22), hexachlorophene (n=4), triclocarban (n=3) and dichlorophene (n=3). Six patients became persistent light reactors. The relevance of the reactions was not specified. In fact, the authors stated that it was generally impossible to determine which was the original photosensitizer and which positive photopatch tests were the result of photocross-sensitivity (21).

Systemic side effects
In the mid-1970s, in France, an ointment containing triclocarban caused many cases of methemoglobinemia in neonates (no details known, article not red) (1).

Miscellaneous side effects
Triclocarban formerly caused pigmented cosmetic dermatitis in Japan (13).

LITERATURE

1   Berger C, Marsala J, Salle B, Teyssier G, Mazauric B, Rascle J. An 'epidemic' of toxic neonatal methemoglobinemia due to the use of an ointment containing trichlorocarbanilide. Ann Pediatr (Paris) 1978;25:45-50 (Article in French)

2   Freeman RG, Knox JM. The action spectrum of photocontact dermatitis caused by halogenated salicylanilides and related compounds. Arch Dermatol 1968;97:130-136

3   Menz J, Muller SA, Connnolly SM. Photopatch testing: A six year experience. J Am Acad Dermatol 1988;18:1044-1047

4   Pigatto PD, Guzzi G, Schena D, Guarrera M, Foti C, Francalanci S, et al. Photopatch tests: an Italian multicentre study from 2004 to 2006. Contact Dermatitis 2008;59:103-108

5   Maibach HI, Bandmann H-J, Calnan CD, Cronin E, Fregert S, Hjorth N, et al. Triclocarban: Evaluation of contact dermatitis potential in man. Contact Dermatitis 1978;4:283-288

6   Ågren-Jonsson S, Magnusson, B. Sensitization to propantheline bromide, trichlorocarbanilide and propylene glycol in an antiperspirant. Contact Dermatitis 1976;2:79-80

7   Hannuksela, M. Allergy to propantheline in an antiperspirant (Ercoril® lotion). Contact Dermatitis 1975;1:244

8   Pigatto PD, Legori A, Bigardi AS, Guarrera M, Tosti A, Santucci B, et al. Gruppo Italiano recerca dermatiti da contatto ed ambientali Italian multicenter study of allergic contact photodermatitis: epidemiological aspects. Am J Contact Dermatitis 1996;17:158-163

9   Barbaud A, Collet E, Le Coz CJ, Meaume S, Gillois P. Contact allergy in chronic leg ulcers: results of a multicentre study carried out in 423 patients and proposal for an updated series of patch tests. Contact Dermatitis 2009;60:279-287

10 De Groot AC, Liem DH, Nater JP, van Ketel WG. Patch tests with fragrance materials and preservatives. Contact Dermatitis 1985;12:87-92

11 Bowyer A. Photosensitivity to trichlorcarbanilide. Cont Derm Newsl 1968;4:59

12 SCCP (Scientific Committee on Consumer Products). Opinion on triclocarban, 1 June 2005, SCCP/0851/04. Available at: http://ec.europa.eu/health/archive/ph_risk/committees/04_sccp/docs/sccp_o_016.pdf

13 Ebihara T, Nakayama H. Pigmented contact dermatitis. Clin Dermatol 1997;15:593-599

14 Uter W, Yazar K, Kratz EM, Mildau G, Lidén C. Coupled exposure to ingredients of cosmetic products: II. Preservatives. Contact Dermatitis 2014;70:219-226

15 Osmundsen PE. Concomitant contact allergy to propantheline bromide and TCC. Contact Dermatitis 1975;1:251-252

16 Barbaud A, Vigan M, Delrous JL, et al. Contact allergy to antiseptics: 75 cases analyzed by the dermato-allergovigilance network (Revidal). Ann Dermatol Venereol 2005;132:962-965

17 Scalf LA, Davis MDP, Rohlinger AL, Connolly SM. Photopatch testing of 182 patients: A 6-year experience at the Mayo Clinic. Dermatitis 2009;20:44-52

18 Leow YH, Wong WK, Ng SK, Goh CL. 2 years experience of photopatch testing in Singapore. Contact Dermatitis 1994;31:181-182

19 Wennersten G, Thune P, Brodthagen H, Jansen C, Rystedt I, Crames M, et al. The Scandinavian multicenter photopatch study. Contact Dermatitis 1984;10:305-309

20 Osmundsen PE. Contact photodermatitis due to tribromsalicylanilide. Br J Dermatol 1968;80:228-234

21 Epstein JH, Wuepper KD, Maibach HI. Photocontact dermatitis to halogenated salicylanilides and related compounds: A clinical and histologic review of 26 patients. Arch Dermatol 1968;97:236-244

22 Smith SZ, Epstein JH. Photocontact dermatitis to halogenated salicylanilides and related compounds. Our experience between 1967 and 1975. Arch Dermatol 1977;113:1372-1374

23 Harber LC, Targovnik SE, Baer RL. Studies on contact photosensitivity to hexachlorophene and trichlorocarbanilide in guinea pigs and man. J Invest Dermatol 1968; 51:373-377

2.475   TRICLOSAN

IDENTIFICATION

Description/definition	: Triclosan is the substituted organic ether that conforms to the formula shown below
Chemical class(es)	: Ethers, halogen compounds; phenols
Chemical/IUPAC name	: 5-Chloro-2-(2,4-dichlorophenoxy)phenol
Other name(s)	: Irgasan® DP 300
CAS registry number (s)	: 3380-34-5
EC number(s)	: 222-182-2
Merck Index monograph	: 11092
CIR review(s)	: Final report, December 2010 (access: www.cir-safety.org/ingredients)
SCCS opinion(s)	: SCCS/1414/11 (37); SCCP/1192/08 (38); SCCP/1040/06 (39); SCCNFP/0600/02 (40)
Function(s) in cosmetics	: EU: deodorant; preservative. USA: cosmetic biocides; deodorant agents; preservatives
EU cosmetic restrictions	: Regulated in Annex V/25 of the Regulation (EC) No. 1223/2009
Patch testing	: 2% pet. (Chemotechnique, SmartPracticeEurope, SmartPracticeCanada); according to some authors, this concentration may cause some irritant reactions (58)
Molecular formula	: $C_{12}H_7Cl_3O_2$

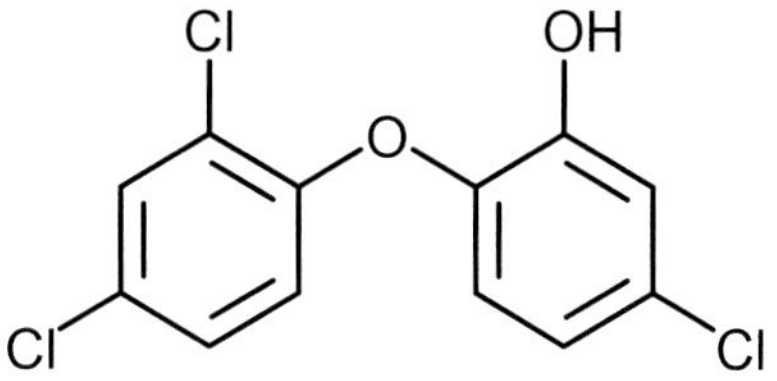

GENERAL

Triclosan is a broad-spectrum biocide that has been used for many years as an antibacterial and antifungal agent. It has good activity against gram-positive bacteria and yeasts, less activity against gram-negative organisms, limited activity against mycobacteria and dermatophytes, and little activity against viruses. It is highly effective at reducing the spread of infection in the health care setting. Triclosan is used primarily in hand soaps (especially in health care institutions) and to a lesser degree in deodorants, dish soaps, and toothpastes. Typical concentrations in consumer products are between 0.15% and 0.3% (50). There is some concern about triclosan and free chlorine readily reacting to form by-products such as chloroform and 2-(2,4-dichlorophenoxy)phenol, which may be human carcinogens (51). The literature on contact allergy to triclosan and other antibacterial agents up to 1991 has been reviewed in ref. 54.

CONTACT ALLERGY

Patch testing in groups of patients
Results of routine patch testing (testing in consecutive patients suspected of contact dermatitis) with triclosan are shown in table 2.475.1. Results of testing triclosan in groups of *selected* patients (e.g., patients tested with a cosmetics or preservatives series, patients suspected of photosensitivity) are shown in table 2.475.2.

Patch testing in consecutive patients suspected of contact dermatitis: routine testing
Results of routine patch testing with triclosan are shown in table 2.475.1. In 7 studies, rates of sensitization have invariably been low, ranging from 0.1% to 1%. Relevance ranged – in studies where relevance was mentioned – from 18% to 100%, but in the two studies with 100% relevance there were only 1 (42) and 2 (19) positive reactions. The causative products were mentioned in one study only: deodorant and soap in 2 allergic patients (19). Because triclosan yields low rates of sensitization in routine testing, it was removed in 2017 from the American Contact Dermatitis Society Core Allergen Series (55).

Patch testing in groups of selected patients
Results of testing in groups of selected patients (e.g., patients tested with a cosmetics or preservatives series, patients suspected of photosensitivity) back to 1981 are shown in table 2.475.2. With the exception of 2 studies (3,13), frequencies of sensitization were always lower than or equal to 1.1%, most being even lower than 0.5%. In a Canadian study of 160 patients with suspected photosensitivity and patients who developed pruritus or a rash after sunscreen application, 21 (13%) had positive reactions to the triclosan patch test. However, this study had certain weaknesses (inadequate reading of test results) and the relevance of the 21 reactions was not mentioned (13). A 12% rate of sensitization to triclosan was found in a 1981-1996 study from Germany in a very small group of 59

patients suspected to be (photo)allergic to UV-absorbers; relevance was not mentioned (3). The incriminated products were mentioned in one study only: topical drugs and body care products (58). Relevance was mostly not mentioned. In three studies, relevance was zero (43, only 1 reaction), zero (60, only 1 reaction), 54% (58) and 100% (5), but in the latter study, relevance figures included 'questionable' and 'past' relevance (5).

Table 2.475.1 Patch testing in groups of patients: Routine testing

Years and Country	Test conc. & vehicle	Number of patients tested	positive (%)		Selection of patients (S); Relevance (R); Comments (C)	Ref.
2006-2010 USA	2% pet.	3088		(0.4%)	R: 18%	32
2005-2006 Turkey		93	1	(1%)	R: the reaction was considered to be relevant	42
2003-2005 China		599	4	(0.7%)	R: not stated	29
2000-2005 USA	2% pet.	3813		(0.3%)	R: 31%	7
1998–2000 USA	2% pet.	701		(0.3%)	R: not stated	26
1989-90 Switzerland	2% pet.	2295		(0.8%)	R: not stated	18
1974-1975 Sweden	2% pet.	1900	2	(0.1%)	R: both reacted to a deodorant, one also to soap	19

Table 2.475.2 Patch testing in groups of patients: Selected patient groups

Years and Country	Test conc. & vehicle	Number of patients tested	positive (%)		Selection of patients (S); Relevance (R); Comments (C)	Ref.
2011-2013 Colombia	2% pet.	112	1	(0.9%)	S: dermatitis affecting mainly light-exposed skin, a history of a sunscreen product or topical NSAID skin reaction; R: not relevant	43
2007-2012 IVDK	2% pet.	1417	1	(0.1%)	S: female patients, clients of hairdressers, in who hair cosmetics were regarded as a cause of dermatitis, and who had never worked as hairdressers; R: not stated	47
1993-2012 IVDK	2% pet.	113,162	363	(0.4%)	S: not stated; R: 54% of the reactions were relevant, mostly from topical drugs and body care products	58
2006-2011 IVDK	2% pet.	6933		(0.3%)	S: patients suspected of cosmetic intolerance and tested with a preservative series (selection procedure not stated); R: not stated	45
2001-2010 Canada		160	21	(13%)	S: patients with suspected photosensitivity and patients who developed pruritus or a rash after sunscreen application; R: not stated; C: very weak study: inadequate reading of test results, erythema only was considered to represent a positive patch test reaction	13
1996-2009 IVDK	2% pet.	79,033	254	(0.3%) [a]	S: not specified; R: not specified	9
<2008 Italy	2% pet	275	2	(0.7%)	S: patients affected by chronic eczema (allergic contact dermatitis, irritant contact dermatitis, atopic eczema, nummular eczema, stasis dermatitis	24
2000-2007 USA	2% pet.	938	6	(0.6%)	S: patients tested with a supplemental cosmetic screening series; R: 100%; C: weak study: a. high rate of macular erythema and weak reactions; b. relevance figures included 'questionable' and 'past' relevance	5
2000-2005 USA	2% pet.	174	1	(0.6%)	S: patients photopatch tested for suspected photodermatitis; R: the reaction was not relevant	60
2000-2002 Finland		6598		(0.1%)	S: patients tested with a cosmetic series; R: not stated	27
1995-1996 Finland		5376		(0.2%)	S: patients tested with a cosmetic series; R: not stated	27
1981-1996 Germany	2% pet.	59	7	(12%)	S: patients (photo)allergic to UV-absorbers; R: not relevant	3
1990-1994 Germany	2% pet.	11,406	29	(0.3%)	S: patients tested with a preservative series; R: not stated	28
1983-4 Netherlands	2% pet.	179	2	(1.1%)	S: patients suspected of cosmetic allergy; R: not stated	31
1980-1981 4 Scandinavian countries	2% pet.	745	1	(0.1%)	S: patients suspected of sun-related skin disease; R: not stated	61

IVDK: Information Network of Departments of Dermatology, Germany, Austria, Switzerland
[a] standardized for sex and age

Case reports and case series

Triclosan was stated to be the (or an) allergen in 3 patients in a group of 603 individuals suffering from cosmetic dermatitis, seen in the period 2010-2015 in Leuven, Belgium (30). In the period 1996-2013, in a tertiary referral center in Valencia, Spain, 5419 patients were patch tested. Of these, 628 individuals had allergic contact dermatitis to cosmetics. Triclosan was the responsible allergen in one case (44). Triclosan was responsible for 1 out of 959 cases of non-fragrance cosmetic allergy where the causal allergen was identified, Belgium, 2000-2010 (4). Triclosan was responsible for 1 out of 399 cases of cosmetic allergy where the causal allergen was identified in a study of the NACDG, USA, 1977-1983 (6). Three positive patch test reactions to triclosan were ascribed to cosmetic allergy (8).

One patient reacted to triclosan in a deodorant foot powder, another to the antimicrobial in a deodorant stick; using a soap bar containing 0.5% triclosan for 5 days resulted in itching and erythema in the latter patient (34, very likely the same patients as in ref. 15). One patient reacted to triclosan in foot powder, another one had contact allergy to the antimicrobial in a deodorant (15, very likely the same patients as in ref. 34). Two individuals had worsening of atopic dermatitis from triclosan in a deodorant, one of who had also contact dermatitis from a soap containing triclosan (19). A woman had contact allergy to triclosan in a spray deodorant/antiperspirant (20). Two patients with cheilitis had contact allergy to triclosan in toothpastes (33). Two other individuals were sensitized to triclosan in a deodorant (35). One patient had a blistering eruption of the buccal mucosa and lips from triclosan in a toothpaste (21). A nurse had occupational allergic contact dermatitis from triclosan in hand-washes (22). A woman had allergic contact dermatitis of the hands from a liquid soap containing triclosan (23).

Contact allergy to triclosan in non-cosmetic products
One patient developed airborne allergic contact dermatitis from triclosan in a kitchen disinfectant (14). Three patients reacted to triclosan in an antibiotic-corticosteroid preparation (15). Three other patients had allergic contact dermatitis from triclosan in an antimycotic-antimicrobial pharmaceutical preparation containing 3% triclosan (16). Three other individuals reacted to triclosan in the same product (17). An unconvincing attempt has been made to link reactions to an antimicrobial suture material in two patients to contact allergy to its ingredient triclosan (1).

Cross-reactions, pseudo-cross-reactions and co-reactions
In a group of 18 patients photosensitized to ketoprofen, 3 (17%) had positive photopatch tests to triclosan. As there were also many photoreactions to fenticlor (see Chapter 2.457 2,2'-Thiobis(4-chlorophenol) (n=12, 67%), tetrachloro-salicylanilide (n=5, 28%), tribromosalicylanilide (n=2, 11%) and bithionol (n=2, 11%), with no clinical relevance, the authors raised the question of hyper-photosusceptibility to non-relevant allergens induced by photosensitivity to ketoprofen (62). In another group of 35 patients photoallergic to ketoprofen from Sweden, simultaneous photoallergy to triclosan was seen in 9%, to fenticlor (see Chapter 2.457 2,2'-Thiobis(4-chlorophenol)) in 74%, to tetrachloro-salicylanilide in 40%, and to bithionol, tribromosalicylanilide and hexachlorophene in 6% of the patients. No explanation for these co-reactivities was offered (63).

Presence in cosmetic products and chemical analyses
In May 2017, triclosan was present in 57 of 68,675 cosmetic products of which the composition is known in EWG's Skin Deep Cosmetics Database, USA (http://www.ewg.org/skindeep/). In the USA, in April 2017, triclosan was present in 413 of 56,714 cosmetic products of which the composition is known in FDA's Voluntary Cosmetic Registration Program (VCRP) (data obtained from FDA, May 2017). In 2009, in the USA, the ingredient lists of 657 miscellaneous cosmetics from one company were screened for the presence of triclosan. Triclosan was present in 5% of 195 antiperspirants/deodorants and in 1 powder (36).

In Germany, in 2006-2009, the labels of 4680 cosmetic products were screened for the presence of preservatives. Triclosan was present in 1% of the products, according to labelling information (48). Triclosan was present in 0.5% of 204 cosmetic products (92 shampoos, 61 hair conditioners, 34 liquid soaps, 17 wet tissues) in Sweden, 2008 (11). In the USA, in 1999-2000, triclosan was present in 136 of 178 (76%) consumer liquid soaps sampled at regional stores and in 134 of 177 (76%) liquid soaps sampled at national stores (56).

OTHER SIDE EFFECTS

Irritant contact dermatitis
There have been several cases of irritant dermatitis from the use of a particular brand of bath oil containing 2% triclosan (52,53). However, this product also contained 6% benzalkonium chloride, which is a much more likely cause of the irritation. The relevant publications are discussed in Chapter 2.38 Benzalkonium chloride.

Photosensitivity

Photopatch testing in groups of patients
Results of photopatch testing triclosan in groups of selected patients (generally patients suspected of photodermatoses, photosensitivity or photocontact allergy) back to 1981 are shown in table 2.475.3. Rates of sensitization have ranged from 0.1% to 5%. In a Canadian study of 160 patients with suspected photosensitivity and patients who developed pruritus or a rash after sunscreen application, 7 (4.4%) had positive reactions to the triclosan photo-patch test. However, this study had certain weaknesses (inadequate reading of test results) and the relevance of the 7 reactions was not mentioned (13). A 5% rate of sensitization to triclosan was found in a 1981-1996 study from

Germany in a very small group of 59 patients suspected to be (photo)allergic to UV-absorbers; relevance was not mentioned (3).

Table 2.475.3 Photopatch testing in groups of patients

Years and Country	Test conc. & vehicle	Number of patients tested	positive (%)	Selection of patients (S); Relevance (R); Comments (C)	Ref.
2005-2014 China	2% pet.	6097	66 (1.1%)	S: patients suspected of photodermatoses; R: not stated	46
2006-2012 China	2% pet.	4905	39 (0.8%)	S: patients with suspected photodermatoses; R: not stated	41
2001-2010 Canada		160	7 (4.4%)	S: patients with suspected photosensitivity and patients who developed pruritus or a rash after sunscreen application; R: not stated; C: very weak study: inadequate reading of test results, erythema only was considered to represent a positive patch test reaction	13
2003-2007 Portugal	10% pet.	83	1 (1.2%)	S: patients with suspected photoaggravated facial dermatitis or systemic photosensitivity; R: all sunscreen photopatch tests were of current or past relevance	25
2004-2006 Italy	1% pet.	1082	1 (0.1%)	S: patients with histories and clinical features suggestive of photoallergic contact dermatitis; R: none	10
2004-2005 Spain	2% pet.	224	3 (1.3%)	S: not stated; R: not relevant	59
2000-2005 USA	2% pet.	174	2 (1.1%)	S: patients photopatch tested for suspected photodermatitis; R: one reaction was relevant	60
1981-1996 Germany	2% pet.	59	3 (5%)	S: patients (photo)allergic to UV-absorbers; R: not relevant	3
1980-85 Ger, Au, Swi	2% pet.	1129	3 (0.3%)	S: patients suspected of photoallergy, polymorphic light eruption, phototoxicity and skin problems with photo-distribution; R: not stated	2
1980-1981 4 Scandinavian countries	2% pet.	745	2 (0.3%)	S: patients suspected of sun-related skin disease; R: not stated	61

Au: Austria; Ger: Germany; Swi: Switzerland

Immediate-type reactions

A woman had immediate contact reactions (contact urticaria) to triclosan in toothpaste, moisturizing lotion, corticosteroid cream, metronidazole cream and an antibacterial liquid soap, containing the antimicrobial at concentrations of 0.2-0.5%. The use of the toothpaste had caused immediate swelling of her lips and tongue, leading to breathing difficulties. Kissing her husband, who was using the same toothpaste, caused swelling of her lips within minutes. Kissing her friends, who were using certain topical products on their faces, also caused wheals on her face and lips (12). A review of contact urticaria caused by ingredients of cosmetics has been provided in 2016 (49).

Miscellaneous side effects

A cleaning lady had occupational asthma from a cleaning product containing triclosan. Curiously, it was neither attempted to identify the causative ingredient not the mode of action (57).

LITERATURE

1   Bhutani T, Jacob SE. Triclosan: a potential allergen in suture-line allergic contact dermatitis. Dermatol Surg 2009;35:888-889
2   Hölzle E, Neumann N, Hausen B, Przybilla B, Schauder S, Hönigsmann H, et al. Photopatch testing: the 5-year experience of the German, Austrian and Swiss Photopatch Test Group. J Am Acad Dermatol 1991;25:59-68
3   Schauder S, Ippen H. Contact and photocontact sensitivity. Review of a 15-year experience and of the literature to suncreens. Contact Dermatitis 1997;37:221-232
4   Travassos AR, Claes L, Boey L, Drieghe J, Goossens A. Non-fragrance allergens in specific cosmetic products. Contact Dermatitis 2011;65:276-285
5   Wetter DA, Yiannias JA, Prakash AV, Davis MD, Farmer SA, el-Azhary RA, et al. Results of patch testing to personal care product allergens in a standard series and a supplemental cosmetic series: an analysis of 945 patients from the Mayo Clinic Contact Dermatitis Group, 2000-2007. J Am Acad Dermatol 2010;63:789-798
6   Adams RM, Maibach HI, Clendenning WE, Fisher AA, Jordan WJ, Kanof N, et al. A five-year study of cosmetic reactions. J Am Acad Dermatol 1985;13:1062-1069
7   Davis MD, Scalf LA, Yiannias JA, Cheng JF, El-Azhary RA, Rohlinger AL, et al. Changing trends and allergens in the patch test standard series. Arch Dermatol 2008;144:67-72
8   Kohl L, Blondeel A, Song M. Allergic contact dermatitis from cosmetics: retrospective analysis of 819 patch-tested patients. Dermatology 2002;204:334-337

9 Schnuch A, Lessmann H, Geier J, Uter W. Contact allergy to preservatives. Analysis of IVDK data 1996-2009. Br J Dermatol 2011;164:1316-1325

10 Pigatto PD, Guzzi G, Schena D, Guarrera M, Foti C, Francalanci S, et al. Photopatch tests: an Italian multicentre study from 2004 to 2006. Contact Dermatitis 2008;59:103-108

11 Yazar K, Johnsson S, Lind M-L, Boman A, Lidén C. Preservatives and fragrances in selected consumer-available cosmetics and detergents. Contact Dermatitis 2011;64:265-272

12 Özkaya E, Bozkurt PK. An unusual case of triclosan-induced immunological contact urticaria. Contact Dermatitis 2013;68:121-122

13 Greenspoon J, Ahluwalia R, Juma N, Rosen CF. Allergic and photoallergic contact dermatitis: A 10-year experience. Dermatitis 2013;24:29-32

14 Savage L, Rose R, Wilkinson M. Airborne contact dermatitis to triclosan. Contact Dermatitis 2011;65:239-240

15 Roed-Petersen J, Auken G, Hjorth N. Contact sensitivity to Irgasan DP 300. Contact Dermatitis 1975;1:293-294

16 Steinkjer B, Braathen LR. Contact dermatitis from triclosan (Irgasan DP 300). Contact Dermatitis 1988;18:243-244

17 Veronesi S, de Padova M P, Vanni D, Melino M. Contact dermatitis to triclosan. Contact Dermatitis 1986;15:257-258

18 Perrenoud D, Bircher A, Hunziker T, Suter H, Bruckner-Tuderman L, Stäger J, et al. Frequency of sensitisation to common preservatives in Switzerland. Contact Dermatitis 1994;30:276-279

19 Wahlberg J E. Routine patch testing with Irgasan DP300. Contact Dermatitis 1976;5:292

20 Hindson TC. Irgasan DP 300 in a deodorant. Contact Dermatitis 1975;1:328

21 Robertshaw H, Leppard B. Contact dermatitis to triclosan in toothpaste. Contact Dermatitis 2007;57:383-384

22 Wong CSM, Beck MH. Allergic contact dermatitis from triclosan in antibacterial handwashes. Contact Dermatitis 2001;45:307

23 Zaugg T, Hunziker T. Germall II and triclosan. Contact Dermatitis 1987;17:262

24 Schena D, Papagrigoraki A, Girolomoni G. Sensitizing potential of triclosan and triclosan-based skin care products in patients with chronic eczema. Dermatol Ther 2008;21 (Suppl.2):S35-38

25 Cardoso J, Canelas MM, Gonçalo M, Figueiredo A. Photopatch testing with an extended series of photoallergens: a 5-year study. Contact Dermatitis 2009;60:325-329

26 Wetter DA, Davis MDP, Yiannias JA, Cheng JF, Connolly SM, el-Azhary RA, et al. Patch test results from the Mayo Contact Dermatitis Group, 1998–2000. J Am Acad Dermatol 2005;53:416-421

27 Hasan T, Rantanen T, Alanko K, Harvima RJ, Jolanki R, Kalimo K, et al. Patch test reactions to cosmetic allergens in 1995–1997 and 2000–2002 in Finland –a multicentre study. Contact Dermatitis 2005;53:40-45

28 Schnuch A, Geier J, Uter W, Frosch PJ. Patch testing with preservatives, antimicrobials and industrial biocides. Results from a multicentre study. Br J Dermatol 1998;138:467-476

29 Li L-F, Liu G, Wang J. Patch test in Chinese patients with cosmetic allergic contact dermatitis to common cosmetic allergens from a European cosmetic series. Contact Dermatitis 2007;57:50-54

30 Goossens A. Cosmetic contact allergens. Cosmetics 2016, 3, 5; doi:10.3390/cosmetics3010005

31 De Groot AC, Liem DH, Nater JP, van Ketel WG. Patch tests with fragrance materials and preservatives. Contact Dermatitis 1985;12:87-92

32 Wentworth AB, Yiannias JA, Keeling JH, Hall MR, Camilleri MJ, Drage LA, et al. Trends in patch-test results and allergen changes in the standard series: a Mayo Clinic 5-year retrospective review (January 1, 2006, to December 31, 2010). J Am Acad Dermatol 2014;70:269-275

33 Freeman S, Stephens R. Cheilitis: Analysis of 75 cases referred to a contact dermatitis clinic. Am J Cont Dermat 1999;10:198-200

34 Roed-Petersen J, Auken G. Allergic contact dermatitis from Irgasan. Cont Derm Newsl 1974;16:520

35 Cronin E. Contact Dermatitis. Edinburgh: Churchill Livingstone, 1980:109 and 705

36 Scheman A, Jacob S, Katta R, Nedorost S, Warshaw E, Zirwas M, et al. Part 4 of a 4 part series. Miscellaneous products: trends and alternatives in deodorants, antiperspirants, sunblocks, shaving products, powder, and wipes. Data from the American Contact Alternative Group. J Clin Aesthet Dermatol 2011;4:35-39

37 SCCS (Scientific Committee on Consumer Safety). Opinion on triclosan, ADDENDUM to the SCCP Opinion on Triclosan (SCCP/1192/08) from January 2009, 22 March 2011, SCCS/1414/11. Available at: http://ec.europa.eu/health/scientific_committees/consumer_safety/docs/sccs_o_054.pdf

38 SCCP (Scientific Committee on Consumer Products). Opinion on triclosan, 21 January 2009, SCCP/1192/08. Available at: http://ec.europa.eu/health/archive/ph_risk/committees/04_sccp/docs/sccp_o_166.pdf

39 SCCP (Scientific Committee on Consumer Products). Opinion on Triclosan, 10 October 2006, SCCP/1040/06. Available at: http://ec.europa.eu/health/archive/ph_risk/committees/04_sccp/docs/sccp_o_073.pdf

40 SCCNFP (Scientific Committee on Cosmetics and Non Food Products). Opinion concerning triclosan, 17 September 2002, SCCNFP/0600/02. Available at: http://ec.europa.eu/health/archive/ph_risk/committees/sccp/documents/out182_en.pdf

41 Gao L, Hu Y, Ni C, Xu Y, Ma L, Yan S, Dou X. Retrospective study of photopatch testing in a Chinese population during a 7-year period. Dermatitis 2014;25:22-26

42 Ada S, Seçkin D. Patch testing in allergic contact dermatitis: is it useful to perform the cosmetic series in addition to the European standard series? J Eur Acad Dermatol Venereol 2010;24:1192-1196

43 Valbuena Mesa MC, Hoyos Jiménez EV. Photopatch testing in Bogota (Colombia): 2011–2013. Contact Dermatitis 2016;74:11-17

44 Zaragoza-Ninet V, Blasco Encinas R, Vilata-Corell JJ, Pérez-Ferriols A, Sierra-Talamantes C, Esteve-Martínez A, de la Cuadra-Oyanguren J. Allergic contact dermatitis due to cosmetics: A clinical and epidemiological study in a tertiary hospital. Actas Dermosifiliogr 2016;107:329-336

45 Dinkloh A, Worm M, Geier J, Schnuch A, Wollenberg A. Contact sensitization in patients with suspected cosmetic intolerance: results of the IVDK 2006-2011. J Eur Acad Dermatol Venereol 2015;29:1071-1081

46 Hu Y, Wang D, Shen Y, Tang H. Photopatch testing in Chinese patients over 10 years. Dermatitis 2016;27:137-142

47 Uter W, Gefeller O, John SM, Schnuch A, Geier J. Contact allergy to ingredients of hair cosmetics – a comparison of female hairdressers and clients based on IVDK 2007–2012 data. Contact Dermatitis 2014;71:13-20

48 Uter W, Yazar K, Kratz EM, Mildau G, Lidén C. Coupled exposure to ingredients of cosmetic products: II. Preservatives. Contact Dermatitis 2014;70:219-226

49 Verhulst L, Goossens A. Cosmetic components causing contact urticaria: a review and update. Contact Dermatitis 2016;75:333-344

50 Campbell L, Zirwas M. Product Allergen Watch. Triclosan. Dermatitis 2006; 17:204-207

51 Levin C, Warshaw E. Triclosan: An update on safety. Dermatitis 2007;18:234-235

52 Loo WJ. Irritant dermatitis due to prolonged contact with Oilatum Plus. Br J Dermatol 2003;148:171-172

53 Storer E, Koh KJ, Warren L. Severe contact dermatitis as a result of an antiseptic bath oil. Australas J Dermatol 2004;45:73-75

54 Fransway AF. The problem of preservation in the 1990s. III. Agents with preservative function independent of formaldehyde release. Am J Contact Derm 1991;2:145-174

55 Schalock PC, Dunnick CA, Nedorost S, Brod B, Warshaw E, Mowad C. American Contact Dermatitis Society Core Allergen Series: 2017 Update. Dermatitis 201728:141-143

56 Perencevich EN, Wong MT, Harris AD. National and regional assessment of the antibacterial soap market: a step toward determining the impact of prevalent antibacterial soaps. Am J Infect Control 2001;29:281-283

57 Walters GI, Robertson AS, Moore VC, Burge PS. Occupational asthma caused by sensitization to a cleaning product containing triclosan. Ann Allergy Asthma Immunol 2017;118:370-371

58 Buhl T, Fuchs T, Geier J. Contact hypersensitivity to triclosan. Ann Allergy Asthma Immunol 2014;113:119-120

59 De La Cuadra-Oyanguren J, Perez-Ferriols A, Lecha-Carrelero M, et al. Results and assessment of photopatch testing in Spain: towards a new standard set of photoallergens. Actas DermoSifiliograficas 2007;98:96-101

60 Scalf LA, Davis MDP, Rohlinger AL, Connolly SM. Photopatch testing of 182 patients: A 6-year experience at the Mayo Clinic. Dermatitis 2009;20:44-52

61 Wennersten G, Thune P, Brodthagen H, Jansen C, Rystedt I, Crames M, et al. The Scandinavian multicenter photopatch study. Contact Dermatitis 1984;10:305-309

62 Durbize E, Vigan M, Puzenat E, Girardin P, Adessi B, Desprez PH, Humbert PH, Laurent R, Aubin F. Spectrum of cross-photosensitization in 18 consecutive patients with contact photoallergy to ketoprofen: associated photoallergies to non-benzophenone-containing molecules. Contact Dermatitis 2003;48:144-149

63 Hindsén M, Zimerson E, Bruze M. Photoallergic contact dermatitis from ketoprofen in southern Sweden. Contact Dermatitis 2006;54:150-157

2.476 TRIDECETH-2 CARBOXAMIDE MEA

IDENTIFICATION

Description/definition	: Trideceth-2 carboxamide MEA is a mixture of ethanolamides that conforms generally to the formula shown below, where R represents the tridecyl group
Chemical class(es)	: Alkanolamides
Other names	: Poly(oxy-1,2-ethanediyl),α-2-(2-hydroxyethyl)amino-2-oxoethyl-ω-hydroxy-, mono-C13-15-alkyl ethers; C13-15 pareth-2 carboxamide MEA; polyoxyethylene (2) tridecyl ether carboxamide MEA
CAS registry number (s)	: 107628-04-6
CIR review(s)	: Int J Toxicol 2015;34(Suppl.1):18-34 (access: www.cir-safety.org/ingredients)
Function(s) in cosmetics	: EU: foam boosting; surfactant; viscosity controlling. USA: surfactants - foam boosters; viscosity increasing agents - aqueous
Patch testing	: 0.5% water (1)

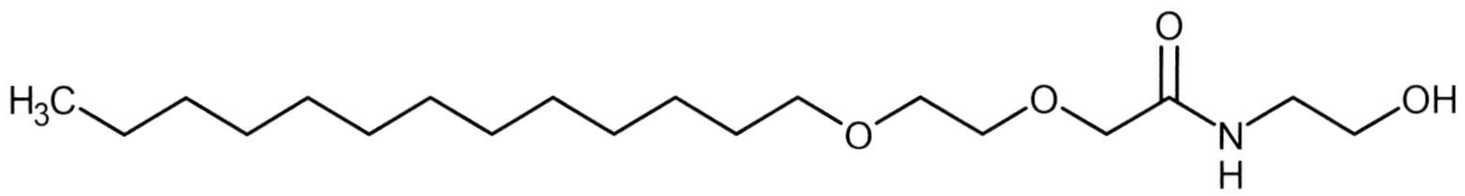

CONTACT ALLERGY

Case reports and case series

A woman developed an itchy dermatitis of the scalp 3 days after application of a hair dye, which she had used for several years without any complications. The dermatitis partially subsided with a potent topical corticosteroid, but she continued to have a less inflammatory scaly scalp consistent with psoriasis. This was considered to be a Köbner phenomenon following contact dermatitis, although she had no other features of psoriasis prior to the scalp dermatitis and none subsequently and there was no family history of psoriasis. Patch tests to the European standard series, a hairdressing series and to the 3 components of the hair dye (colorant cream, developer cream and after-color conditioner) 10% and 50% pet. gave positive reactions to the developer cream at D2 and D4 to both concentrations. Later, patch tests with all ingredients of the hair dye showed positivity to trideceth-2-carboxamide MEA 0.5% in water at D2 and D4. Fourteen control patients had negative reactions to this test material. Trideceth-2-carboxamide MEA was added to the product to help stabilize the viscosity of the mixture of the colorant and the developer (1).

Presence in cosmetic products and chemical analyses

In the USA, in April 2017, trideceth-2 carboxamide MEA was present in 191 of 56,714 cosmetic products of which the composition is known in FDA's Voluntary Cosmetic Registration Program (VCRP) (data obtained from FDA, May 2017). In April 2017, trideceth-2 carboxamide MEA was present in 25 of 65,434 cosmetic products of which the composition is known in EWG's Skin Deep Cosmetics Database, USA (http://www.ewg.org/skindeep/).

LITERATURE
1   Bowling, JCR, Scarisbrick J, Warin AP, Downs AMR. Allergic contact dermatitis from trideceth-2-carboxamide monoethanolamine (MEA) in a hair dye. Contact Dermatitis 2002;47:109-125

2.477 TRIETHANOLAMINE

IDENTIFICATION

Description/definition : Triethanolamine is an alkanolamine that conforms generally to the formula shown below
Chemical class(es) : Alkanolamines
Chemical/IUPAC name : 2-[bis(2-Hydroxyethyl)amino]ethanol
Other names : 2,2',2'-Nitrilotriethanol; trolamine
CAS registry number (s) : 102-71-6
EC number(s) : 203-049-8
CIR review(s) : J Am Coll Toxicol 1983;2:183-235; Int J Toxicol 2013;32(Suppl.1):59-83 (access: www.cir-safety.org/ingredients)
Merck Index monograph : 11100
Function(s) in cosmetics : EU: buffering; emulsifying; masking; surfactant. USA: fragrance ingredients; surfactants − emulsifying agents; pH adjusters
EU cosmetic restrictions : Regulated in Annex III/62 of the Regulation (EC) No. 1223/2009
Patch testing : 2% pet. (Chemotechnique); 2.5% pet. (SmartPracticeEurope, SmartPracticeCanada); the 2.5% pet. test substance is slightly irritant (38)
Molecular formula : $C_6H_{15}NO_3$

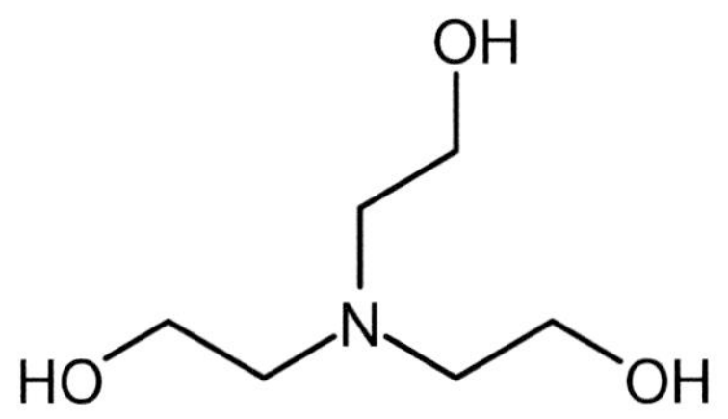

GENERAL

Triethanolamine is an alkanolamine used as emulsifier in cosmetics, topical drugs and household products; in addition, it may be used as an auxiliary in grinding cement clinker, as a direct additive to cement (to increase the water-binding capacity and freezing resistance and for faster setting), as a corrosion inhibitor (notably in metalworking fluids), in dispersing agents, for the production of textile auxiliaries and herbicides, for the production of soaps, shoe polishes, household cleaners, and products for leather and automobile care (38). Commercial triethanolamine also contains ethanolamine (monoethanolamine) and diethanolamine in a maximum concentration of 0.5% (38). An extensive literature review on triethanolamine (and diethanolamine and ethanolamine) has been provided in ref. 38.

Triethanolamine is an infrequent cause of allergic contact dermatitis. In the 1960s, however, the chemical caused many allergic reactions to an antihistamine (promethazine) topical pharmaceutical preparation (12,42,44) in Italy, France and the Netherlands and in the 1950s, many allergic reactions were caused by triethanolamine in hand lotions in a Scandinavian country (Sweden?) (23). Most allergic reactions are currently caused by cosmetics and to a lesser degree topical drugs (38). When patch testing with triethanolamine 2.5% pet., irritant reactions must be anticipated (38).

CONTACT ALLERGY

Patch testing in groups of patients
Results of testing triethanolamine in consecutive patients suspected of contact dermatitis (routine testing) back to 1983 are shown in table 2.477.1. Results of testing in groups of *selected* patients (e.g., patients suspected of cosmetic allergy, patients with leg ulcers, metalworkers with occupational contact dermatitis) back to 1983 are shown in table 2.477.2.

Patch testing in consecutive patients suspected of contact dermatitis: routine testing
In five studies in which routine testing with triethanolamine was performed, frequencies of sensitization have ranged from 0.7% to 4.2%. In an early study from Germany, 3% of 1357 patients had a positive reaction to triethanolamine, but their relevance was not established (only speculated on) and the used test concentration of 10% in water was certainly irritant (34). The high rate of sensitization of 4.2% was in a small study from China, but no mention was made of the relevance of the observed positive patch test reactions (16). In two studies from the USA, 40% of the reactions were scored as relevant, but culprit products were not mentioned (3,21).

Table 2.477.1 Patch testing in groups of patients: Routine testing

Years and Country	Test conc. & vehicle	Number of patients tested	positive (%)	Selection of patients (S); Relevance (R); Comments (C)	Ref.
2006-2010 USA	2% pet.	3087	(0.9%)	R: 41%	21
2003-2005 China		599	25 (4.2%)	R: not stated	16
2000-2005 USA	2% pet.	3845	(0.8%)	R: 39%	3
1998–2000 USA	2% pet.	713	(0.7%)	R: not stated	14
<1983 Germany	10% water	1357	41 (3.0%)	R: twenty-nine of 41 positive patients had suffered from venous insufficiency or sports injuries; they had used antiphlogistic local medicaments and were most probably sensitized against triethanolamine by these topical drugs	34

Patch testing in groups of selected patients

Results of testing in groups of selected patients (e.g., patients suspected of cosmetic allergy, patients with leg ulcers, metalworkers with occupational contact dermatitis) back to 1983 are shown in table 2.477.2. In 14 investigations, frequencies of sensitization have ranged from 0.3% to 20.4%; all but two scored 3% or lower. The 20.4% rate was found in an early Spanish study in metalworkers with occupational contact dermatitis. However, the relevance of the positive reactions was not mentioned and as the patients were tested with triethanolamine 10% in water, some (or many) of the reactions may well have been irritant (40). The item of relevance was addressed in a few investigations only. In an Italian study, 7 of 20 reactions (35%) were relevant, 6 of which were related to cosmetics and one to a topical drug (20). In a more recent IVDK study, these products were also mentioned as the most likely sources of sensitization (38).

Table 2.477.2 Patch testing in groups of patients: Selected patient groups

Years and Country	Test conc. & vehicle	Number of patients tested	positive (%)	Selection of patients (S); Relevance (R); Comments (C)	Ref.
2010-2011 Korea	2% pet.	584	21 (3.6%)	S: patients suspected of allergic cosmetic dermatitis; R: not stated	17
2006-2011 IVDK	2.5% pet.	7768	(0.4%)	S: patients suspected of cosmetic intolerance and tested with an ointment base series; R: not stated	29
2004-2008 France	2.5% pet.	423	7 (1.7%)	S: patients with leg ulcers; R: not stated	15
2000-2007 USA	2% pet.	944	6 (0.6%)	S: patients tested with a supplemental cosmetic screening series; R: 100%; C: weak study: a. high rate of macular erythema and weak reactions; b. relevance figures included 'questionable' and 'past' relevance	2
1992-2007 IVDK	2.5% pet.	85,098	323 (0.3%)	S: mostly patients suspected of reactions to cosmetics and topical drugs, including patients with stasis dermatitis; R: not specified, but most reactions seemed to be related to cosmetics and topical drugs, not to metalworking fluids; C: the test preparation is probably slightly irritant	38
2002-2003 Germany, Austria, Switzerland		184	2 (1.1%)	S: metalworkers with suspected metalworking fluid dermatitis; R: not stated	47
2000-2002 Serbia	5% pet.	75	2 (3%)	S: patients with venous leg ulcers and dermatitis of the surrounding skin; R: not stated	30
1997-2000 Israel		244	7 (2.9%)	S: patients suspected of cosmetic dermatitis; R: 64% of all patch test reactions in the cosmetic series was relevant	25
1992-1994 UK	2.5% pet.	63	2 (3%)	S: patients with facial dermatitis; R: both relevant, products not mentioned	41
<1992 Germany	2.5% pet.	4948	25 (0.5%)	S: patients tested with a 'topicals and galenics' series; R: not stated; C: there were also 39 ?+ reactions	39
1989 Italy	5% pet.	336	1 (0.3%)	S: male soldiers without skin disease, 18-28 years; R: not stated	22
1986-1989 Italy	2.5% pet.	737	20 (2.7%)	S: patients with contact dermatitis apparently related to the use of topical preparations; R: 7 reactions were clinically relevant, 6 from cosmetics, one from a topical medicament	20
1981-1983 Spain	10% water	230	47 (20.4%)	S: metalworkers with occupation-related contact dermatitis; R: not stated; C: the test concentration is probably irritant	40
1968-1983 Spain	5% pet.	6587	48 (0.7%)	S: not stated; R: not stated	18

IVDK: Information Network of Departments of Dermatology, Germany, Austria, Switzerland

Case reports and case series

Triethanolamine was responsible for 3 out of 399 cases of cosmetic allergy where the causal allergen was identified in a study of the NACDG, USA, 1977-1983 (1). Positive patch test reactions to triethanolamine were ascribed to cosmetic allergy in 7 patients (4). In a 4-month-period in 1996, 475 patients with contact allergy to 'cosmetic ingredients' were collected in 5 centers in Belgium, UK and Germany. There were 3 reactions to triethanolamine; relevance was not stated (19). Twenty-seven housewives had allergic contact dermatitis from triethanolamine in a hand lotion (23). Six patients had contact allergy to triethanolamine present in a moisturizing cream (8) and two others from the same cream (10). Two patients with facial eczema were allergic to triethanolamine in 'face lotion or raser' (44, data cited in ref. 38). One or more patients reacted with generalized dermatitis to triethanolamine in 'creams and lotions' (11).

Two individuals had allergic contact dermatitis from triethanolamine in sunscreen preparations (6,33). One patient reacted to triethanolamine in a hand cream, another one to the emulsifier in a skin care product (24). Another individual had allergic contact dermatitis from triethanolamine in shampoo and eardrops (31). A woman had allergic contact dermatitis of the face from triethanolamine in a sunscreen and a moisturizer. The contact allergy was detected because she had an allergic reaction to a fluorescent marker pen, used for patch testing. The ink contained triethanolamine, to which the patient had a positive patch test (35). A man had allergic contact dermatitis of the face from triethanolamine in a shaving cream (36). A 2-year-old boy had extensive allergic contact dermatitis from triethanolamine in a moisturizing cream (37). One patient had allergic contact dermatitis from triethanolamine, present in a concentration of 0.1%-1% in a hand milk (43).

A patient with leprosy has been described who had an allergic reaction to a moisturizing cream. When patch tested with its ingredients, there was a positive reaction to triethanolamine, and this was, considering the title of the publication, the causative allergen. However, the manufacturer was quoted to state that only 0.5% triethanolamine was used along with stearic acid to neutralize it completely and to form triethanolamine stearate which acts as the chief emulsifying agent for the product. Thus, there was apparently no free triethanolamine in the cream (46). A man had allergic contact dermatitis from a shaving foam and had positive patch tests to the product and to six of its ingredients (polysensitization), including triethanolamine 3% in water. There were no positive reactions in 25 controls. The patient was retested 7 months later to all 6 allergens previously positive and reacted again at D2 and D4 to 5 of them, but triethanolamine was now negative (32).

Contact allergy to triethanolamine in non-cosmetic products

Of 50 patients with contact allergy to promethazine cream, 20 (40%) had positive patch tests to its ingredient triethanolamine, tested 5% pet. (42). Of 14 patients with an allergic reaction to promethazine cream, 11 (79%) reacted to its ingredient triethanolamine, tested 2% water; there were no reactions in 50 controls (44). Three metalworkers had occupational allergic contact dermatitis from triethanolamine in metalworking fluids (5,7,9). One or more patients reacted to triethanolamine in a topical pharmaceutical product (12). A woman suffered from an allergic reaction to triethanolamine in a non-proprietary topical drug (36). Another patient had allergic contact dermatitis from triethanolamine in an antimycotic gel (13). One patient had dermatitis from contact allergy to triethanolamine in eardrops (31). A woman had an allergic reaction to triethanolamine in a fluorescent marker pen, used for patch testing (35).

Cross-reactions, pseudo-cross-reactions and co-reactions

Diethanolamine (7,44); possibly ethanolamine (7); *not* to ethanolamine (44). In each ethanolamine (mono, di-, tri-), traces of both other alkanolamines can be found (possibility of pseudo-cross-reactions) (7).

Presence in cosmetic products and chemical analyses

In July 2017, triethanolamine was present in 1393 of 69,543 cosmetic products of which the composition is known in EWG's Skin Deep Cosmetics Database, USA (http://www.ewg.org/skindeep/). In the USA, in April 2017, triethanolamine was present in 5729 of 56,714 cosmetic products of which the composition is known in FDA's Voluntary Cosmetic Registration Program (VCRP) (data obtained from FDA, May 2017). In 2009, in the USA, the ingredient lists of 1591 facial cosmetics from one company were screened for the presence of triethanolamine. Triethanolamine was present in 0% of 132 blushers and 38 bronzers, in 11% of 90 concealers, in 6% of 174 eyeliners, in 0% of 304 eyeshadows, in 11% of 457 foundations, in 0% of 140 loose and pressed powders, and in 65% of 256 mascaras (26).

In 2009, in the USA, the ingredient lists of 796 hair products from one company were screened for the presence of triethanolamine. Triethanolamine was present in 8% of 279 shampoos, in 8% of 231 conditioners, and in 14% of 286 styling products (27). In 2009, in the USA, the ingredient lists of 657 miscellaneous cosmetics from one company were screened for the presence of triethanolamine. Triethanolamine was present in 0% of 195 antiperspirants/ deodorants, in 1 of 41 powders, in 41% of 167 shaving products, in 27% of 201 sunblocks, and in 2% of 53 wipes (28). Of 17 metalworking fluids purchased in machine shops in Finland in 2007, 15 contained alkanolamines, 'mostly ethanolamine and triethanolamine'. The concentration range for triethanolamine was 5.9%-26% with a median of 11% (45).

OTHER SIDE EFFECTS

Miscellaneous side effects
Two metal workers exposed to cutting fluids developed occupational asthma from triethanolamine in the cutting fluids. The diagnosis was based on work-related symptoms and on a chamber challenge with the suspected agent. In both patients, the symptoms persisted after exposure ended (48). Another patient had intractable sneezing from IgE-mediated allergy to triethanolamine present in a laundry detergent (49).

LITERATURE

1   Adams RM, Maibach HI, Clendenning WE, Fisher AA, Jordan WJ, Kanof N, et al. A five-year study of cosmetic reactions. J Am Acad Dermatol 1985;13:1062-1069
2   Wetter DA, Yiannias JA, Prakash AV, Davis MD, Farmer SA, el-Azhary RA, et al. Results of patch testing to personal care product allergens in a standard series and a supplemental cosmetic series: an analysis of 945 patients from the Mayo Clinic Contact Dermatitis Group, 2000-2007. J Am Acad Dermatol 2010;63:789-798
3   Davis MD, Scalf LA, Yiannias JA, Cheng JF, El-Azhary RA, Rohlinger AL, et al. Changing trends and allergens in the patch test standard series. Arch Dermatol 2008;144:67-72
4   Kohl L, Blondeel A, Song M. Allergic contact dermatitis from cosmetics: retrospective analysis of 819 patch-tested patients. Dermatology 2002;204:334-337
5   Suuronen K, Aalto-Korte K, Piipari R, Tuomi T, Jolanki R. Occupational dermatitis and allergic respiratory diseases in Finnish metalworking machinists. Occup Med 2007;57:277-283
6   Chu C-Y, Sun C-C. Allergic contact dermatitis from triethanolamine in a sunscreen. Contact Dermatitis 2001;44:59
7   Blum A, Lischka G. Allergic contact dermatitis from mono-, di- and triethanolamine. Contact Dermatitis 1997;36:166
8   Batten, TL, Wakeel RA, Douglas WS, Evans C, White MI, Moody R, Ormerod AD. Contact dermatitis from the old formula E45 cream. Contact Dermatitis 1994;30:159-161
9   Niklasson B, Björkner B, Sundberg K. Contact allergy to a fatty acid ester component of cutting fluids. Contact Dermatitis 1993;28:265-267
10   Jones SK, Kennedy CTC. Contact dermatitis from triethanolamine in E45 cream. Contact Dermatitis 1988;19:230
11   Castelain P. Eczema généralisé diffus par sensibilisation à la triethanolamme. Bull Soc Franc Derm Syph 1967;74:562 (data cited in ref. 10)
12   Suurmond D. Patch test reactions to Phenergan cream, promethazine and triethanolamine. Dermatologica 1966;133:503-506 (data cited in ref. 10)
13   Samsoen M, Jelen G. Allergy to Daktarin gel. Contact Dermatitis 1977;3:351
14   Wetter DA, Davis MDP, Yiannias JA, Cheng JF, Connolly SM, el-Azhary RA, et al. Patch test results from the Mayo Contact Dermatitis Group, 1998–2000. J Am Acad Dermatol 2005;53:416-421
15   Barbaud A, Collet E, Le Coz CJ, Meaume S, Gillois P. Contact allergy in chronic leg ulcers: results of a multicentre study carried out in 423 patients and proposal for an updated series of patch tests. Contact Dermatitis 2009;60:279-287
16   Li L-F, Liu G, Wang J. Patch test in Chinese patients with cosmetic allergic contact dermatitis to common cosmetic allergens from a European cosmetic series. Contact Dermatitis 2007;57:50-54
17   Lee SS, Hong DK, Jeong NJ, Lee JH, Choi YS, Lee AY, et al. Multicenter study of preservative sensitivity in patients with suspected cosmetic contact dermatitis in Korea. J Dermatol 2012;39:677-681
18   Angelini G, Vena G A, Meneghini C L. Allergic contact dermatitis to some medicaments. Contact Dermatitis 1985;12:263-269
19   Goossens A, Beck MH, Haneke E, McFadden JP, Nolting S, Durupt G, Ries G. Adverse cutaneous reactions to cosmetic allergens. Contact Dermatitis 1999;40:112-113
20   Tosti A, Guerra L, Morelli R, Bardazzi F. Prevalence and sources of sensitization to emulsifiers: a clinical study. Contact Dermatitis 1990;23:68-72
21   Wentworth AB, Yiannias JA, Keeling JH, Hall MR, Camilleri MJ, Drage LA, et al. Trends in patch-test results and allergen changes in the standard series: a Mayo Clinic 5-year retrospective review (January 1, 2006, to December 31, 2010). J Am Acad Dermatol 2014;70:269-275
22   Seidenari S, Manzini BM, Danese P, Motolese A. Patch and prick test study of 593 healthy subjects. Contact Dermatitis 1990;23:162-167
23   Thyresson N, Lodin A, Nilzen A. Eczema of the hands due to triethanolamine in cosmetic hand lotions for housewives. Acta Derm Venereol 1956;36:355-359

24 Cronin E. Contact Dermatitis. Edinburgh: Churchill Livingstone, 1980:100,101
25 Trattner A, Farchi Y, David M. Cosmetics patch tests: first report from Israel. Contact Dermatitis 2002;47:180-181
26 Scheman A, Jacob S, Katta R, Nedorost S, Warshaw E, Zirwas M, et al. Part 1 of a 4 part series. Facial cosmetics: trends and alternatives. Data from the American Contact Alternative Group. J Clin Aesthet Dermatol 2011;4:25-30
27 Scheman A, Jacob S, Katta R, Nedorost S, Warshaw E, Zirwas M, et al. Part 2 of a 4 part series. Hair cosmetics: trends and alternatives. Data from the American Contact Alternative Group. J Clin Aesthet Dermatol 2011;4:42-46
28 Scheman A, Jacob S, Katta R, Nedorost S, Warshaw E, Zirwas M, et al. Part 4 of a 4 part series. Miscellaneous products: trends and alternatives in deodorants, antiperspirants, sunblocks, shaving products, powder, and wipes. Data from the American Contact Alternative Group. J Clin Aesthet Dermatol 2011;4:35-39
29 Dinkloh A, Worm M, Geier J, Schnuch A, Wollenberg A. Contact sensitization in patients with suspected cosmetic intolerance: results of the IVDK 2006-2011. J Eur Acad Dermatol Venereol 2015;29:1071-1081
30 Jankićević J, Vesić S, Vukićević J, Gajić M, Adamic M, Pavlović MD. Contact sensitivity in patients with venous leg ulcers in Serbia: comparison with contact dermatitis patients and relationship to ulcer duration. Contact Dermatitis 2008;58:32-36
31 Schmutz J-L, Barbaud A, Tréchot P. Allergie de contact à la triéthanolamine contenue dans des gouttes auriculaires et dans un shampooing. Ann Dermatol Venereol 2007;134:105
32 Vilaplana J, Lecha M, Romaguera C, Alsina A, Mascaro JM, Castel, T. A polysensitized HIV-positive patient. Contact Dermatitis 1993;29:101-102
33 Ando M, Ansotegui IJ, Munoz D, Fernandez de Corres L. Allergic contact dermatitis from imidazolidinyl urea in an ultrasonic gel. Contact Dermatitis 2000;42:109
34 Scheuer B. Kontaktallergie durch Triethanolamin. Hautarzt 1983;34:126-129 (article in German)
35 Hamilton TK, Zug KA. Triethanolamine allergy inadvertently discovered from a fluorescent marking pen. Am J Cont Derm 1996;7:164-165
36 Curtis G, Netherton EW. Cutaneous hypersensitivity to triethanolamine. Arch Derm Syph 1940;41:729-731
37 Milanesi N, Berti S, Gola M. Allergic contact dermatitis to triethanolamine in a child. Pediatr Dermatol 2015;32:e112-113
38 Lessmann H, Uter W, Schnuch A, Geier J. Skin sensitizing properties of the ethanolamines mono-, di-, and triethanolamine. Data analysis of a multicentre surveillance network (IVDK) and review of the literature. Contact Dermatitis 2009;60:243-255
39 Scheuer B, Rüther T, von Bülow V et al. Häufige Kontaktallergene – Eine praxisorientierte Multicenterstudie. Akt Dermatol 1992;18:44-49
40 Alomar A, Conde-Salazar L, Romaguera C. Occupational dermatoses from cutting oils. Contact Dermatitis 1985;12:129-138
41 Shah M, Lewis FM, Gawkrodger DJ. Facial dermatitis and eyelid dermatitis: a comparison of patch test results and final diagnoses. Contact Dermatitis 1996;34:140-141
42 Zina G, Bonu G. Phenergan cream (role of base constituents). Contact Dermatitis Newsletter 1969;6:117
43 Greim H (Ed). 2-Aminoethanol. Gesundheitsschädliche Arbeitsstoffe. Toxikologisch-arbeitsmedizinische Begründungen von MAK-Werten, 33. Lieferung. Weinheim, Germany: Wiley-VCH, 2001:1-4 (data cited in ref. 38)
44 Foussereau J, Sengel D. Un allergène habituellement méconnu: la triéthanolamine. Strasbourg Med 1965;10:873-880
45 Henriks-Eckerman ML, Suuronen K, Jolanki R. Analysis of allergens in metalworking fluids. Contact Dermatitis 2008;59:261-267
46 Srinivas CR, Padhee A, George ND. Triethanolamine-induced allergic contact dermatitis over a tuberculoid leprosy lesion. Int J Lepr Other Mycobact Dis 1990;58:382-384
47 Geier J, Lessmann H, Dickel H, Frosch PJ, Koch P, Becker D, et al. Patch test results with the metalworking fluid series of the German Contact Dermatitis Research Group (DKG). Contact Dermatitis 2004;51:118-130
48 Savonius B, Keskinen H, Tuppurainen M, Kanerva L. Occupational asthma caused by ethanolamines. Allergy. 1994;49:877-881
49 Herman JJ. Intractable sneezing due to IgE-mediated triethanolamine sensitivity. J Allergy Clin Immunol 1983;71:339-344

2.478   TRIETHYLENE GLYCOL DIACRYLATE*

* Not an INCI name

IDENTIFICATION

Description/definition	: Triethylene glycol diacrylate is the organic compound that conforms to the formula shown below
Chemical class(es)	: Esters
INCI name USA	: Neither in CosIng nor in the Personal Care Products Council Ingredient Database
Chemical/IUPAC name	: 2-[2-(2-Prop-2-enoyloxyethoxy)ethoxy]ethyl prop-2-enoate
CAS registry number (s)	: 1680-21-3
EC number(s)	: 216-853-9
Patch testing	: 0.1% pet. (Chemotechnique)
Molecular formula	: $C_{12}H_{18}O_6$

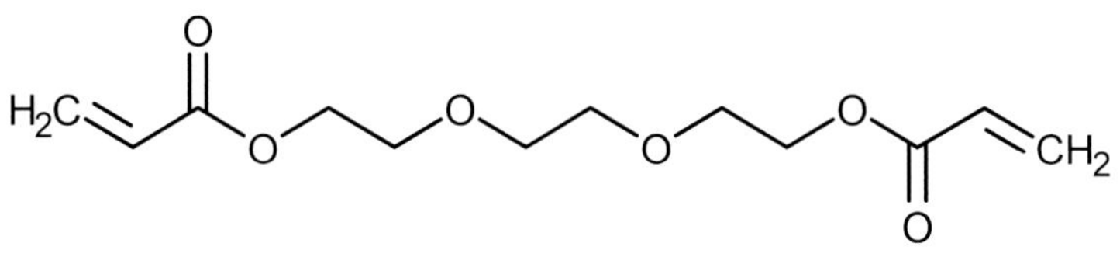

GENERAL

Discussion of contact allergy to (meth)acrylates *from non-cosmetic sources* is considered to fall outside the scope of this book. Therefore, only contact allergy from their presence in cosmetics is presented, which virtually always is from artificial nails. There are many reports of contact allergy to artificial nails, but the specific sensitizers have rarely been identified and – consequently - such publications are not presented in this and other acrylate and methacrylate monographs. Discussion is limited to publications in which the culprit (meth)acrylates have been identified, e.g., from information found in Material Data Safety Sheets, data obtained from the manufacturer or from chemical analyses.

Patients often react to many (meth)acrylates on patch testing. Primary sensitization to methacrylates may result in both methacrylate and acrylate cross-sensitization. Conversely, patients sensitized to acrylates are unlikely to show cross-sensitization to methacrylates (2).

General aspects of acrylates and methacrylates are presented in Chapter 2.219 HEMA (hydroxyethyl methacrylate). A discussion of general aspects of artificial nails, contact allergy to these products, the clinical picture of allergic contact dermatitis and other side effects of sculptured nails can also be found there.

CONTACT ALLERGY

Patch testing in groups of patients
Studies in which consecutive patients suspected of contact dermatitis have been tested with triethylene glycol diacrylate (routine testing) and studies testing groups of selected patients are planned to be discussed in a future publication.

Case reports and case series
A group of 55 female patients presenting with hand eczema and who had contact with artificial nails, were patch tested with a series of acrylates in one center in Israel, 2001-2004. Twenty-one had one or more positive reactions, of who 14 were professional beauticians specializing in nail sculpturing. All reactions, including 2 to triethylene glycol diacrylate, were stated to be of current relevance (1). Because of the general lack of information on the composition of artificial nail materials, the fact that the author did no analyses of these products and the frequent occurrence of cross-reactivity among acrylates, one may wonder whether this statement can be accepted as entirely correct.

Presence in cosmetic products and chemical analyses
In May 2017, was triethylene glycol diacrylate present in zero of 66,975 cosmetic products of which the composition is known in EWG's Skin Deep Cosmetics Database, USA (http://www.ewg.org/skindeep/). In the USA, in April 2017, triethylene glycol diacrylate was present in zero of 56,714 cosmetic products of which the composition is known in FDA's Voluntary Cosmetic Registration Program (VCRP) (data obtained from FDA, May 2017).

LITERATURE

1 Lazarov A. Sensitization to acrylates is a common adverse reaction to artificial fingernails. J Eur Acad Derm Venereol 2007;21:169-174

2 Aalto-Korte K, Henriks-Eckerman M-L, Kuuliala O, Jolanki R. Occupational methacrylate and acrylate allergy – cross-reactions and possible screening allergens. Contact Dermatitis 2010;63:301-312

2.479   TRIETHYLENE GLYCOL DIMETHACRYLATE

IDENTIFICATION

Description/definition   : Triethylene glycol dimethacrylate is the organic compound that conforms to the formula shown below
Chemical class(es)   : Esters
Chemical/IUPAC name   : 2-Propenoic acid, 2-methyl-, 1,2-ethanediylbis(oxy-2,1-ethanediyl) ester
Other names   : 2,2'-Ethylenedioxydiethyl dimethacrylate
CAS registry number (s)   : 109-16-0
EC number(s)   : 203-652-6
CIR review(s)   : Int J Toxicol 2005;24(Suppl.5):53-100 (access: www.cir-safety.org/ingredients)
Function(s) in cosmetics   : EU: nail conditioning. USA: artificial nail builders
Patch testing   : 2.0% pet. (Chemotechnique, SmartPracticeEurope, SmartPracticeCanada)
Molecular formula   : $C_{14}H_{22}O_6$

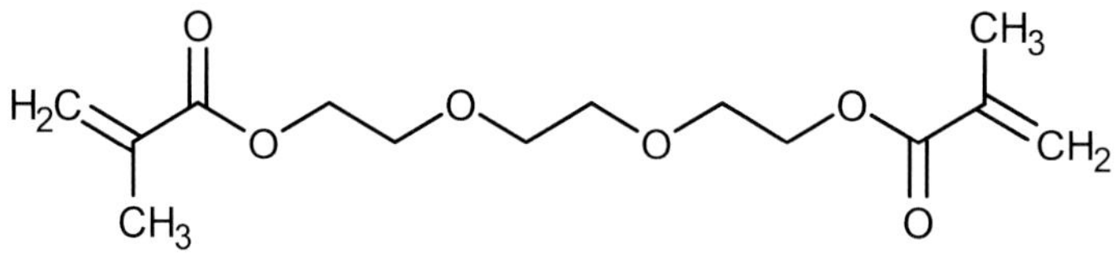

GENERAL

Discussion of contact allergy to (meth)acrylates *from non-cosmetic sources* is considered to fall outside the scope of this book. Therefore, only contact allergy from their presence in cosmetics is presented, which virtually always is from artificial nails. There are many reports of contact allergy to artificial nails, but the specific sensitizers have rarely been identified and – consequently - such publications are not presented in this and other acrylate and methacrylate monographs. Discussion is limited to publications in which the culprit (meth)acrylates have been identified, e.g., from information found in Material Data Safety Sheets, data obtained from the manufacturer or from chemical analyses.

Patients often react to many (meth)acrylates on patch testing. Primary sensitization to methacrylates may result in both methacrylate and acrylate cross-sensitization. Conversely, patients sensitized to acrylates are unlikely to show cross-sensitization to methacrylates (1).

General aspects of acrylates and methacrylates are presented in Chapter 2.219 HEMA (hydroxyethyl methacrylate). A discussion of general aspects of artificial nails, contact allergy to these products, the clinical picture of allergic contact dermatitis and other side effects of sculptured nails can also be found there. A very useful review of contact sensitization to allergens in nail cosmetics, with emphasis on acrylic manicures, was published in 2017 (7).

CONTACT ALLERGY

Patch testing in groups of patients

Studies in which consecutive patients suspected of contact dermatitis have been tested with triethylene glycol dimethacrylate (routine testing) and studies testing groups of selected patients are planned to be discussed in a future publication.

Case reports and case series

Triethylene glycol dimethacrylate was stated to be the (or an) allergen in one patient in a group of 603 individuals suffering from cosmetic dermatitis, seen in the period 2010-2015 in Leuven, Belgium (4). In the period 1996-2013, in a tertiary referral center in Valencia, Spain, 5419 patients were patch tested. Of these, 628 individuals had allergic contact dermatitis to cosmetics. Triethylene glycol dimethacrylate was the responsible allergen in thirteen cases (6). In the period 2000-2007, 202 patients with allergic contact dermatitis caused by cosmetics were seen in the same clinic in Valencia, Spain (overlap with ref. 6). In this group, there were 10 beauticians with occupational allergic contact dermatitis of the hands, who reacted to multiple (meth)acrylates from their presence in artificial nail materials. Of these ten individuals, four reacted to triethylene glycol dimethacrylate, which reactions were apparently relevant (although it can be doubted that the presence of these specific chemicals in the products could always be verified) (5).

A group of 55 female patients presenting with hand eczema and who had contact with artificial nails, were patch tested with a series of acrylates in one center in Israel, 2001-2004. Twenty-one had one or more positive reactions, of who 14 were professional beauticians specializing in nail sculpturing. All reactions, including eight to triethylene glycol dimethacrylate, were stated to be of current relevance (3). Because of the general lack of information on the composition of artificial nail materials, the fact that the author did no analyses of these products and the frequent occurrence of cross-reactivity among acrylates, one may wonder whether this statement can be accepted as entirely correct.

A cosmetician teaching other cosmeticians how to make artificial nails developed occupational contact dermatitis of the hands and face from contact allergy to triethylene glycol dimethacrylate in monomer liquid for sculptured nails. Gas chromatography – mass spectrometry (GC-MS) showed the product to contain 5% triethylene glycol dimethacrylate (2).

Presence in cosmetic products and chemical analyses

In May 2017, triethylene glycol dimethacrylate was present in zero of 66,975 cosmetic products of which the composition is known in EWG's Skin Deep Cosmetics Database, USA (http://www.ewg.org/skindeep/). In the USA, in April 2017, triethylene glycol dimethacrylate was present in zero of 56,714 cosmetic products of which the composition is known in FDA's Voluntary Cosmetic Registration Program (VCRP) (data obtained from FDA, May 2017).

LITERATURE

1   Aalto-Korte K, Henriks-Eckerman M-L, Kuuliala O, Jolanki R. Occupational methacrylate and acrylate allergy – cross-reactions and possible screening allergens. Contact Dermatitis 2010;63:301-312
2   Kanerva L, Lauerma A, Estlander T, Alanko K, Henriks-Eckerman ML, Jolanki R. Occupational allergic contact dermatitis caused by photobonded sculptured nails and a review of (meth)acrylates in nail cosmetics. Am J Cont Derm 1996;7:109-115
3   Lazarov A. Sensitization to acrylates is a common adverse reaction to artificial fingernails. J Eur Acad Derm Venereol 2007;21:169-174
4   Goossens A. Cosmetic contact allergens. Cosmetics 2016, 3, 5; doi:10.3390/cosmetics3010005
5   Laguna C, de la Cuadra J, Martín-González B, Zaragoza V, Martínez-Casimiro L, Alegre V. Allergic contact dermatitis to cosmetics. Actas Dermosifiliogr 2009;100:53-60
6   Zaragoza-Ninet V, Blasco Encinas R, Vilata-Corell JJ, Pérez-Ferriols A, Sierra-Talamantes C, Esteve-Martínez A, de la Cuadra-Oyanguren J. Allergic contact dermatitis due to cosmetics: A clinical and epidemiological study in a tertiary hospital. Actas Dermosifiliogr 2016;107:329-336
7   Chou M, Dhingra N, Strugar TL. Contact sensitization to allergens in nail cosmetics. Dermatitis 2017;28:231-240

2.480   TRIETHYLENE GLYCOL HYDROGENATED ROSINATE

IDENTIFICATION

Description/definition	: Triethylene glycol hydrogenated rosinate is the ester of triethylene glycol and the partially hydrogenated acids derived from rosin (colophonium)
Chemical class(es)	: Esters
Other names	: Resin acids and rosin acids, hydrogenated, esters with triethylene glycol
CAS registry number (s)	: 68648-53-3
EC number(s)	: 271-996-4
Function(s) in cosmetics	: EU: emollient; skin conditioning; viscosity controlling. USA: skin-conditioning agents – occlusive; viscosity increasing agents - nonaqueous
Patch testing	: 20% pet. (2,3)

CONTACT ALLERGY

Case reports and case series

Triethylene glycol hydrogenated rosinate was responsible for 1 out of 959 cases of non-fragrance cosmetic allergy where the causal allergen was identified, Belgium, 2000-2010 (1). From June 2000 through December 2001, Revidal, the system established by the French Contact Dermatitis Research Group (GERDA) to collect data on allergic reactions to environmental agents, received 33 reports from Belgium and France of acute allergic contact dermatitis from epilating products of one particular French brand. The specific products to which the patients had become sensitized were cold wax hair-removal strips, a warm wax, and/or the accompanying tissue. Twenty-six of these patients, all women, were further investigated. The skin lesions started on the lower legs and spread in 18 of them to other parts of the body. The symptoms of 10 of the patients were so severe that they were hospitalized and/or received systemic corticosteroids. In most patients, the lesions on the lower legs presented with a follicular pattern. The lesions on the face were most often erythematous and edematous, particularly on the eyelids. In many patients, the clinical history was misleading since they consulted because of a severe systemic eruption and had not mentioned that the lesions had first appeared on the lower legs.

Primary sensitization certainly occurred in at least 10 of the patients, since the eruption started 2-3 weeks after the initial application of the products. Of 24 patients tested with the cold wax and the tissue, 15 gave a positive reaction to the wax, and 23 reacted positively to the tissue. Triethylene glycol hydrogenated rosinate was an ingredient of the cold wax. Out of 18 tested, 9 reacted positively to triethylene glycol hydrogenated rosinate 20% pet. Other allergens in the cold wax, to which some patients reacted, were glyceryl rosinate, 'modified colophonium' and perfume (2,3).

Cross-reactions, pseudo-cross-reactions and co-reactions

Some co-reactions to glyceryl rosinate and 'modified colophonium', also present in the same product (2,3); one co-reaction to colophonium (2).

Presence in cosmetic products and chemical analyses

In the USA, in April 2017, triethylene glycol hydrogenated rosinate was present in 5 of 56,714 cosmetic products of which the composition is known in FDA's Voluntary Cosmetic Registration Program (VCRP) (data obtained from FDA, May 2017). In April 2017, triethylene glycol hydrogenated rosinate was present in 7 older products of 65,434 cosmetic products of which the composition is known in EWG's Skin Deep Cosmetics Database, USA (http://www.ewg.org/skindeep/).

LITERATURE

1   Travassos AR, Claes L, Boey L, Drieghe J, Goossens A. Non-fragrance allergens in specific cosmetic products. Contact Dermatitis 2011;65:276-285
2   Goossens A, Armingaud P, Avenel-Audran M, Begon-Bagdassarian I, Constandt L, Giordano-Labadie F, et al. An epidemic of allergic contact dermatitis due to epilating products. Contact Dermatitis 2002;46:67-70
3   Goossens A. An epidemic of allergic contact dermatitis due to epilating products. Contact Dermatitis 2001;45:360

2.481 TRILAURETH-4 PHOSPHATE

IDENTIFICATION

Description/definition	: Trilaureth-4 phosphate is the triester of phosphoric acid and laureth-4
Chemical class(es)	: Phosphorus compounds
Chemical/IUPAC name	: Poly(oxy-1,2-ethanediyl),α,α',α''-phosphinylidynetris-ω-(dodecyloxy)-
CAS registry number (s)	: 31800-90-5
Function(s) in cosmetics	: EU: emulsifying; surfactant. USA: surfactants – emulsifying agents
Patch testing	: 1% and 5% in pet. (1)
Molecular formula	: (C_2H_4O)mult-(C_2H_4O)mult-(C_2H_4O)mult-$C_{36}H_{75}O_4P$

CONTACT ALLERGY

Case reports and case series

A woman presented with subacute dermatitis affecting her arms and legs with some lesions on the trunk. A few weeks prior to onset, she had started to use a hand and body lotion. The eruption cleared from a 2-week course of oral prednisolone and cessation of the use of the lotion. Patch testing to the lotion was positive at D2. Later, the 12 components of the hand and body lotion were tested separately and the patient reacted to trilaureth-4 phosphate at D2 and D4. This chemical was then patch tested in pet. at 10%, 5%, 1%, 0.5% and 0.1% and a positive graded dose response was obtained to all concentrations except 0.1%, which was negative. Of 21 control subjects tested with to 5% trilaureth-4 phosphate, 19 were negative and 2 positive. One of these 2 individuals had a positive reaction at D2 only, and further tests with dilutions at 1%, 0.5% and 0.1% were negative. The remaining patient was positive at both D2 and D4 and had a positive graded response to the dilution series down to 0.5%. This patient had a history of hand eczema and was positive to nickel, rubber, *p*-phenylenediamine and the fragrance mix. She had had no exposure to the hand and body lotion but had used the same manufacturer's bubble bath preparation in the past with no ill effects. The source of sensitization remained unknown (1).

Presence in cosmetic products and chemical analyses

In the USA, in April 2017, trilaureth-4 phosphate was present in 65 of 56,714 cosmetic products of which the composition is known in FDA's Voluntary Cosmetic Registration Program (VCRP) (data obtained from FDA, May 2017). In April 2017, trilaureth-4 phosphate was present in 12 of 65,434 cosmetic products of which the composition is known in EWG's Skin Deep Cosmetics Database, USA (http://www.ewg.org/skindeep/).

LITERATURE

1   Neill SM, Vivier A. Contact dermatitis to trilaureth phosphate. Contact Dermatitis 1984;11:130-31

2.482 TRIMETHYLOLPROPANE TRIACRYLATE

IDENTIFICATION

Description/definition : Trimethylolpropane triacrylate is the triester that conforms to the formula shown below
Chemical class(es) : Esters
Chemical/IUPAC name : 2,2-bis(Prop-2-enoyloxymethyl)butyl prop-2-enoate
Other names : 2-Propenoic acid, 2-ethyl-2-[[(1-oxo-2-propenyl)oxy]methyl]-1,3-propanediyl ester
CAS registry number (s) : 15625-89-5
EC number(s) : 239-701-3
Function(s) in cosmetics : EU: film forming; hair conditioning; hair fixing. USA: film forming agents; hair conditioning agents; hair fixatives
Patch testing : 0.1% pet. (Chemotechnique)
Molecular formula : $C_{15}H_{20}O_6$

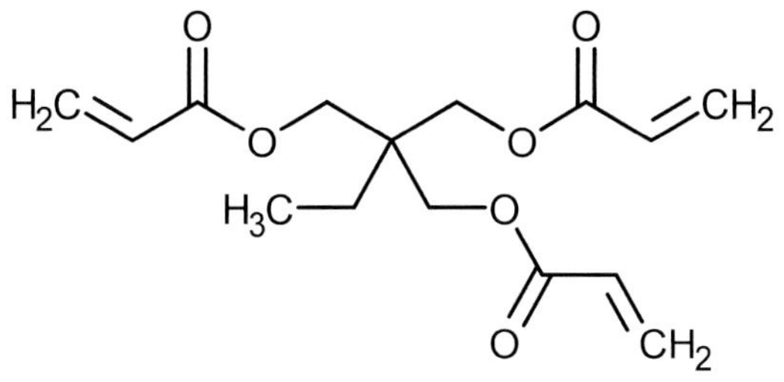

GENERAL

Discussion of contact allergy to (meth)acrylates *from non-cosmetic sources* is considered to fall outside the scope of this book. Therefore, only contact allergy from their presence in cosmetics is presented, which virtually always is from artificial nails. There are many reports of contact allergy to artificial nails, but the specific sensitizers have rarely been identified and – consequently - such publications are not presented in this and other acrylate and methacrylate monographs. Discussion is limited to publications in which the culprit (meth)acrylates have been identified, e.g., from information found in Material Data Safety Sheets, data obtained from the manufacturer or from chemical analyses.

Patients often react to many (meth)acrylates on patch testing. Primary sensitization to methacrylates may result in both methacrylate and acrylate cross-sensitization. Conversely, patients sensitized to acrylates are unlikely to show cross-sensitization to methacrylates (2).

General aspects of acrylates and methacrylates are presented in Chapter 2.219 HEMA (hydroxyethyl methacrylate). A discussion of general aspects of artificial nails, contact allergy to these products, the clinical picture of allergic contact dermatitis and other side effects of sculptured nails can also be found there. A very useful review of contact sensitization to allergens in nail cosmetics, with emphasis on acrylic manicures, was published in 2017 (3).

CONTACT ALLERGY

Patch testing in groups of patients

Studies in which consecutive patients suspected of contact dermatitis have been tested with trimethylolpropane triacrylate (routine testing) and studies testing groups of selected patients are planned to be discussed in a future publication.

Case reports and case series

A group of 55 female patients presenting with hand eczema and who had contact with artificial nails, were patch tested with a series of acrylates in one center in Israel, 2001-2004. Twenty-one had one or more positive reactions, of who 14 were professional beauticians specializing in nail sculpturing. All reactions, including 3 to trimethylolpropane triacrylate, were stated to be of current relevance (1). Because of the general lack of information on the composition of artificial nail materials, the fact that the author did no analyses of these products and the frequent occurrence of cross-reactivity among acrylates, one may wonder whether this statement can be accepted as entirely correct.

Presence in cosmetic products and chemical analyses

In the USA, in April 2017, trimethylolpropane triacrylate was present in 1 of 56,714 cosmetic products of which the composition is known in FDA's Voluntary Cosmetic Registration Program (VCRP) (data obtained from FDA, May 2017). In February 2017, trimethylolpropane triacrylate was present in zero of 64,480 cosmetic products of which the composition is known in EWG's Skin Deep Cosmetics Database, USA (http://www.ewg.org/skindeep/).

LITERATURE

1   Lazarov A. Sensitization to acrylates is a common adverse reaction to artificial fingernails. J Eur Acad Derm Venereol 2007;21:169-174

2   Aalto-Korte K, Henriks-Eckerman M-L, Kuuliala O, Jolanki R. Occupational methacrylate and acrylate allergy – cross-reactions and possible screening allergens. Contact Dermatitis 2010;63:301-312

3   Chou M, Dhingra N, Strugar TL. Contact sensitization to allergens in nail cosmetics. Dermatitis 2017;28:231-240

2.483   TRIOLEYL PHOSPHATE

IDENTIFICATION

Description/definition   : Trioleyl phosphate is the triester of phosphoric acid and oleyl alcohol that conforms
                              generally to the formula shown below
Chemical class(es)   : Phosphorus compounds
Chemical/IUPAC name   : Tris[(Z)-octadec-9-enyl] phosphate
Other names   : 9-Octadecen-1-ol, phosphate (3:1)
CAS registry number (s)   : 3305-68-8
EC number(s)   : 221-983-4
CIR review(s)   : Final report, December 2014 (access: www.cir-safety.org/ingredients)
Function(s) in cosmetics   : EU: emollient; plasticiser; skin conditioning. USA: plasticizers; skin-conditioning agents –
                              occlusive
Patch testing   : 1% pet. (1)
Molecular formula   : $C_{54}H_{105}O_4P$

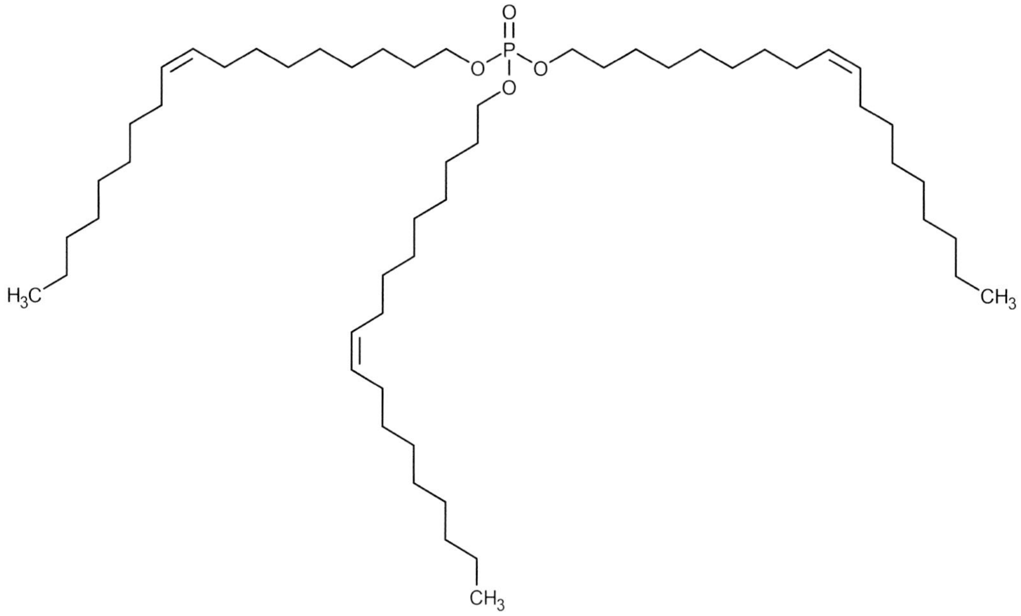

GENERAL

Trioleyl phosphate is used as a plasticizer, skin conditioning, and occlusive agent in, for instance, lipsticks and lip gloss creams.

CONTACT ALLERGY

Case reports and case series

A non-atopic woman, who had previously reacted to an 'anticellulite' cream, presented with contact cheilitis following the application of a lipstick. Patch tests with the European baseline series, a cosmetics series and her personal cosmetic products gave positive reactions to two lipsticks of different colors of the same brand and to the anticellulite cream. The ingredients were not tested. Five years later, the patient developed a severe contact dermatitis on the eyelids due to a new lipstick of the same brand as the one to which she had reacted before, and which she had applied to the eyelids, assuming it to be an eyeshadow. Patch testing was now performed with the ingredients of the lipstick, which yielded positive reactions to trioleyl phosphate and 2 other ingredients. Additional patch testing with the ingredients showed positive reactions to trioleyl phosphate 1% and 0.5% in pet. Twenty controls had no positive reactions to trioleyl phosphate 1% pet. The patient has remained symptom free since avoiding contact with cosmetics containing the substances to which she was allergic (1).

Presence in cosmetic products and chemical analyses

In the USA, in April 2017, trioleyl phosphate was present in 3 of 56,714 cosmetic products of which the composition is known in FDA's Voluntary Cosmetic Registration Program (VCRP) (data obtained from FDA, May 2017). In April 2017, trioleyl phosphate was present in zero of 65,434 cosmetic products of which the composition is known in EWG's Skin Deep Cosmetics Database, USA (http://www.ewg.org/skindeep/).

LITERATURE

1   Goossens A, Verbruggen K, Cattaert N, Boey L. New cosmetic allergens: isononyl isononanoate and trioleyl
     phosphate. Contact Dermatitis 2008;59:320-321

2.484   TRIPROPYLENE GLYCOL DIACRYLATE*
Not an INCI name

IDENTIFICATION

Description/definition   : Tripropylene glycol diacrylate is the organic compound that conforms to the formula
                             shown below
Chemical class(es)   : Esters
INCI name USA   : Neither in CosIng nor in the Personal Care Products Council Ingredient Database
Chemical/IUPAC name   : 2-[2-(2-Prop-2-enoyloxypropoxy)propoxy]propyl prop-2-enoate
Other names   1,4,7-Trimethyl-3,6-dioxaoctamethylene diacrylate
CAS registry number (s)   : 42978-66-5
EC number(s)   : 256-032-2
Patch testing   : 0.1% pet. (1)
Molecular formula   : $C_{15}H_{24}O_6$

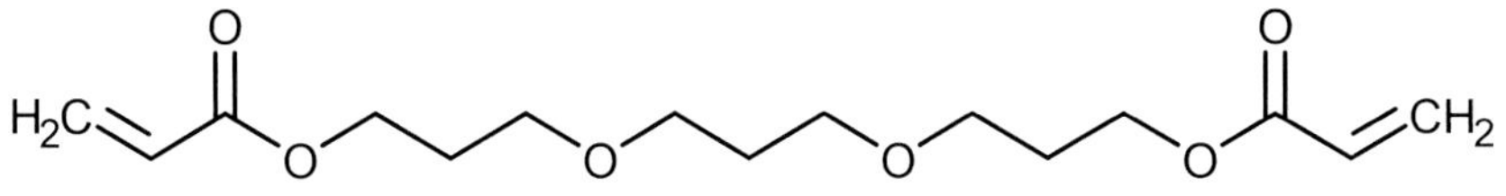

GENERAL

Discussion of contact allergy to (meth)acrylates *from non-cosmetic sources* is considered to fall outside the scope of this book. Therefore, only contact allergy from their presence in cosmetics is presented, which virtually always is from artificial nails. There are many reports of contact allergy to artificial nails, but the specific sensitizers have rarely been identified and – consequently - such publications are not presented in this and other acrylate and methacrylate monographs. Discussion is limited to publications in which the culprit (meth)acrylates have been identified, e.g., from information found in Material Data Safety Sheets, data obtained from the manufacturer or from chemical analyses.

Patients often react to many (meth)acrylates on patch testing. Primary sensitization to methacrylates may result in both methacrylate and acrylate cross-sensitization. Conversely, patients sensitized to acrylates are unlikely to show cross-sensitization to methacrylates (2).

General aspects of acrylates and methacrylates are presented in Chapter 2.219 HEMA (hydroxyethyl methacrylate). A discussion of general aspects of artificial nails, contact allergy to these products, the clinical picture of allergic contact dermatitis and other side effects of sculptured nails can also be found there. A very useful review of contact sensitization to allergens in nail cosmetics, with emphasis on acrylic manicures, was published in 2017 (4).

CONTACT ALLERGY

Patch testing in groups of patients
Studies in which consecutive patients suspected of contact dermatitis have been tested with tripropylene glycol diacrylate (routine testing) and studies testing groups of selected patients are planned to be discussed in a future publication.

Case reports and case series
Tripropylene glycol diacrylate was stated to be the (or an) allergen in one patient in a group of 603 individuals suffering from cosmetic dermatitis, seen in the period 2010-2015 in Leuven, Belgium (3). A cosmetician teaching other cosmeticians how to make artificial nails developed occupational contact dermatitis of the hands and face from contact allergy to tripropylene glycol diacrylate in UV-curing nail gel. Gas chromatography – mass spectrometry showed the product to contain 8% tripropylene glycol diacrylate and 0.3% tripropylene glycol acrylate (1).

Presence in cosmetic products and chemical analyses
In May 2017, tripropylene glycol diacrylate was present in zero of 66,975 cosmetic products of which the composition is known in EWG's Skin Deep Cosmetics Database, USA (http://www.ewg.org/skindeep/). In the USA, in April 2017, tripropylene glycol diacrylate was present in zero of 56,714 cosmetic products of which the composition is known in FDA's Voluntary Cosmetic Registration Program (VCRP) (data obtained from FDA, May 2017).

LITERATURE

1 Kanerva L, Lauerma A, Estlander T, Alanko K, Henriks-Eckerman ML, Jolanki R. Occupational allergic contact dermatitis caused by photobonded sculptured nails and a review of (meth)acrylates in nail cosmetics. Am J Cont Derm 1996;7:109-115

2 Aalto-Korte K, Henriks-Eckerman M-L, Kuuliala O, Jolanki R. Occupational methacrylate and acrylate allergy – cross-reactions and possible screening allergens. Contact Dermatitis 2010;63:301-312

3 Goossens A. Cosmetic contact allergens. Cosmetics 2016, 3, 5; doi:10.3390/cosmetics3010005

4 Chou M, Dhingra N, Strugar TL. Contact sensitization to allergens in nail cosmetics. Dermatitis 2017;28:231-240

2.485   TRIS(N-HYDROXYETHYL)HEXAHYDROTRIAZINE

IDENTIFICATION

Description/definition   : Tris(*N*-hydroxyethyl)hexahydrotriazine is the heterocyclic compound that conforms to
                              the formula shown below
Chemical class(es)   : Alcohols; heterocyclic compounds
Chemical/IUPAC name   : 2-[3,5-bis(2-Hydroxyethyl)-1,3,5-triazinan-1-yl]ethanol
Other names   : Hexahydro-1,3,5-tris(2-hydroxyethyl)-s-triazine; triazinetriethanol; Grotan® BK
CAS registry number (s)   : 4719-04-4
EC number(s)   : 225-208-0
Function(s) in cosmetics   : EU: preservative. USA: preservatives
Patch testing   : 1.0% water (Chemotechnique); 1% pet. (SmartPracticeCanada, SmartPracticeEurope)
Molecular formula   : $C_9H_{21}N_3O_3$

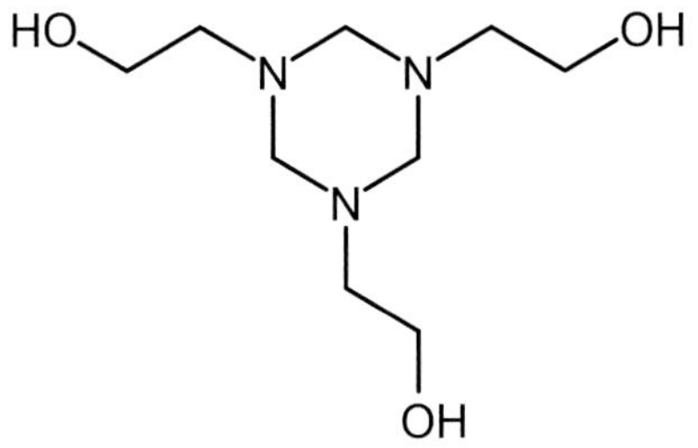

GENERAL

Tris(*N*-hydroxyethyl)hexahydrotriazine (best known trade name: Grotan® BK) is a formaldehyde-releaser (4) used as bactericide and fungicide in adhesives, industrial cleaning systems, polymer emulsions, latex emulsions, soluble lubricants, paints and metalworking fluids, in oilfield water systems, drilling muds, and in workover and completion fluids. It is also used in in-can preservation of water-based products such as paints, glues, emulsions, inks, pigment dispersions, cutting oils and water-soluble cleaners, as well as in fuel protection during storage (9).

Discussion of tris(*N*-hydroxyethyl)hexahydrotriazine is largerly limited to cases of contact allergy by its presence in cosmetics. A full review of contact allergy to and other side effects of this preservative is planned for a future volume in this series on Monographs in Contact Allergy.

CONTACT ALLERGY

Patch testing in groups of patients
In routine testing, rather high frequencies of positive patch test reactions to tris(*N*-hydroxyethyl)hexahydrotriazine of 4.5% (3) and 3.3% (6) have been found, but it was not mentioned how many of these co-reacted to formaldehyde and the relevance of the positive patch tests was either not stated (6) or specified as to incriminated products (3). In groups of *selected* patients (e.g., patients suspected of industrial or cosmetic contact dermatitis), rates of sensitization were usually low (1,7). An unrealistically high percentage of 4.6 with 100% relevance score was found in a study from the USA (2), but this investigation had certain weaknesses (2). The literature up to 2010 has been reviewed by the author (9).

Case reports and case series
In cosmetics, tris(*N*-hydroxyethyl)hexahydrotriazine is an extremely rare sensitizer. In fact, there are no well-documented case reports of cosmetic allergy from it. According to Spanish investigators from a tertiary referral center in Valencia, tris(*N*-hydroxyethyl)hexahydrotriazine was the responsible allergen in three patients in a group of 628 individuals with allergic contact dermatitis to cosmetics seen by them in the period 1996-2013 (8). It can be doubted whether this is correct.

Contact allergy to tris(*N*-hydroxyethyl)hexahydrotriazine in non-cosmetic products
Tris(*N*-hydroxyethyl)hexahydrotriazine has caused some cases of contact allergy in industrial oils (10) and topical pharmaceutical products (5).

Presence in cosmetic products and chemical analyses
There are indications that the chemical is hardly, if at all, used in cosmetic products. In the USA, for example, in April 2017, tris(*N*-hydroxyethyl)hexahydrotriazine was present in not a single of 56,714 cosmetic products of which the composition is known in FDA's Voluntary Cosmetic Registration Program (VCRP) (data obtained from FDA, May

2017). In another US cosmetic database, in July 2017, the chemical again was present in zero of 69,577 cosmetic products of which the composition is known in EWG's Skin Deep Cosmetics Database, USA (http://www.ewg.org/skindeep/).

LITERATURE

1   Latorre N, Borrego L, Fernández-Redondo V, García-Bravo B, Giménez-Arnau AM, Sánchez J, et al. Patch testing with formaldehyde and formaldehyde-releasers: multicenter study in Spain (2005-2009). Contact Dermatitis 2011;65:286-292

2   Wetter DA, Yiannias JA, Prakash AV, Davis MD, Farmer SA, el-Azhary RA, et al. Results of patch testing to personal care product allergens in a standard series and a supplemental cosmetic series: an analysis of 945 patients from the Mayo Clinic Contact Dermatitis Group, 2000-2007. J Am Acad Dermatol 2010;63:789-798

3   Davis MD, Scalf LA, Yiannias JA, Cheng JF, El-Azhary RA, Rohlinger AL, et al. Changing trends and allergens in the patch test standard series. Arch Dermatol 2008;144:67-72

4   Emeis D, De Groot AC, Brinkmann J. Determination of formaldehyde in formaldehyde-releaser patch test preparations. Contact Dermatitis 2010;63:57-62

5   Pecegueiro M, Brandao M, Pinto J, Concalo S. Contact dermatitis to Hirudoid® cream. Contact Dermatitis 1987:17:290-293

6   Wetter DA, Davis MDP, Yiannias JA, Cheng JF, Connolly SM, el-Azhary RA, et al. Patch test results from the Mayo Contact Dermatitis Group, 1998–2000. J Am Acad Dermatol 2005;53:416-421

7   Schnuch A, Geier J, Uter W, Frosch PJ. Patch testing with preservatives, antimicrobials and industrial biocides. Results from a multicentre study. Br J Dermatol 1998;138:467-476

8   Zaragoza-Ninet V, Blasco Encinas R, Vilata-Corell JJ, Pérez-Ferriols A, Sierra-Talamantes C, Esteve-Martínez A, de la Cuadra-Oyanguren J. Allergic contact dermatitis due to cosmetics: A clinical and epidemiological study in a tertiary hospital. Actas Dermosifiliogr 2016;107:329-336

9   De Groot A, Geier J, Flyvholm MA, Lensen G, Coenraads PJ. Formaldehyde-releasers: relationship to formaldehyde contact allergy. Metalworking fluids and remainder. Part 1. Contact Dermatitis 2010;63:117-128

10   Rasschaert V, Goossens A. Conjunctivitis and bronchial asthma: symptoms of contact allergy to 1,3,5-tris (2-hydroxyethyl)-hexahydrotriazine (Grotan BK). Contact Dermatitis 2002;47:116

2.486 TRISODIUM EDTA

IDENTIFICATION

Description/definition : Trisodium EDTA is the substituted amine that conforms to the formula shown below
Chemical class(es) : Alkyl-substituted amino acids; amines
Chemical/IUPAC name : Trisodium;2-[2-[bis(carboxylatomethyl)amino]ethyl-(carboxymethyl)amino]acetate
Other names : Edetate trisodium; trisodium hydrogen ethylenediaminetetraacetate
CAS registry number (s) : 150-38-9
EC number(s) : 205-758-8
CIR review(s) : Int J Toxicol 2002;21(Suppl.2):95-142 (access: www.cir-safety.org/ingredients)
Function(s) in cosmetics : EU: chelating. USA: chelating agents
Patch testing : 10% pet. (1)
Molecular formula : $C_{10}H_{13}N_2Na_3O_8$

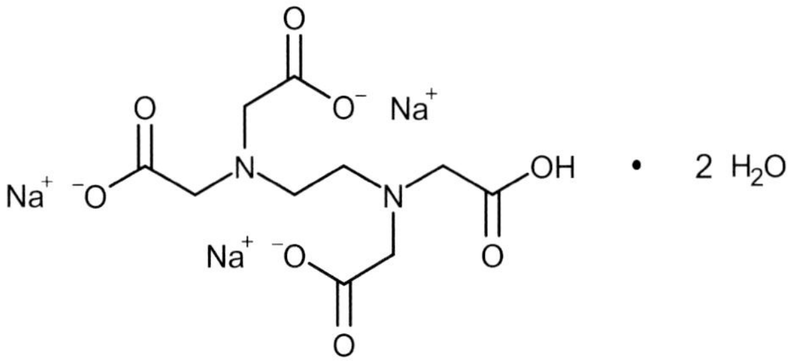

GENERAL

EDTA and its salts are used as preservatives and antioxidant agents in eye, nose and ear drops, and in cosmetic creams. Although its antibacterial activity is low, EDTA increases the antibacterial properties of benzalkonium chloride, chlorobutanol and thimerosal in ophthalmic solutions. As a chelating agent, it shows strong affinity for metallic ions, such as nickel, calcium, magnesium and lead, and has been used in the treatment of urinary calculi, corneal deposits, hypercalcaemia and lead poisoning. EDTA is also a stabilizer of certain solutions (ascorbic acid, hydrogen peroxide, formaldehyde, folic acid and hyaluronidase) (2).

CONTACT ALLERGY

Case reports and case series

A woman presented with pruritic papules and erythema on her face. She had used some 20 cosmetic product over a few years and had frequently noticed a burning sensation on her face for 6 months. Patch tests with the patient's cosmetics, tested as is, gave a positive reaction to a cosmetic lotion. Subsequently, the patient was patch tested with the 30 ingredients of this cosmetic product and this yielded a positive reaction to trisodium EDTA 25% water at D2 and D3. Later, patch tests were performed with trisodium EDTA 0.1%, 1%, and 10% in petrolatum and in water and she reacted to the 10% pet. test substance only. The patient was also tested with EDTA, disodium EDTA and tetrasodium EDTA, each in the same three concentrations in petrolatum, and there were positive reactions to disodium and to tetrasodium EDTA 10% pet., but EDTA itself was negative. Five controls were negative (1).

Cross-reactions, pseudo-cross-reactions and co-reactions

Tetrasodium EDTA and disodium EDTA, but not EDTA (1).

Presence in cosmetic products and chemical analyses

In the USA, in April 2017, trisodium EDTA was present in 622 of 56,714 cosmetic products of which the composition is known in FDA's Voluntary Cosmetic Registration Program (VCRP) (data obtained from FDA, May 2017). In April 2017, trisodium EDTA was present in 284 of 65,434 cosmetic products of which the composition is known in EWG's Skin Deep Cosmetics Database, USA (http://www.ewg.org/skindeep/).

LITERATURE

1   Kimura M, Kawada A. Contact dermatitis due to trisodium ethylenediaminetetra-acetic acid (EDTA) in a cosmetic lotion. Contact Dermatitis 1999;41:341
2   Sánchez-Pedreño P, García-Bravo B, Frías-Iniesta J. Contact allergy to tetrasodium EDTA in a sunscreen. Contact Dermatitis 2009;61:125-126

2.487 TRISODIUM HYDROXYETHYL ETHYLENEDIAMINE TRIACETATE[*]

* Not an INCI name

IDENTIFICATION

Description/definition : Trisodium hydroxyethyl ethylenediamine triacetate is the acetic acid substituted diamine that corresponds to the formula shown below

Chemical class(es) : Substituted amines; carboxylic acid salts

INCI name EU and USA : Neither in CosIng nor in the Personal Care Products Council Ingredient Database

Chemical/IUPAC name : Trisodium;2-[2-[bis(carboxylatomethyl)amino]ethyl-(2-hydroxyethyl)amino]ace-tate;hydrate

Other names : *N*-(2-Hydroxyethyl)ethylenediamine-*N*,*N'*,*N'*-triacetic acid trisodium salt hydrate; HEEDTA; trisodium *N*-(2-hydroxyethyl)ethylenediamine-*N*,*N'*,*N'*-triacetate hydrate

CAS registry number (s) : 207386-87-6

EC number(s) : 205-381-9

Patch testing : No data available

Molecular formula : $C_{10}H_{17}N_2Na_3O_8$

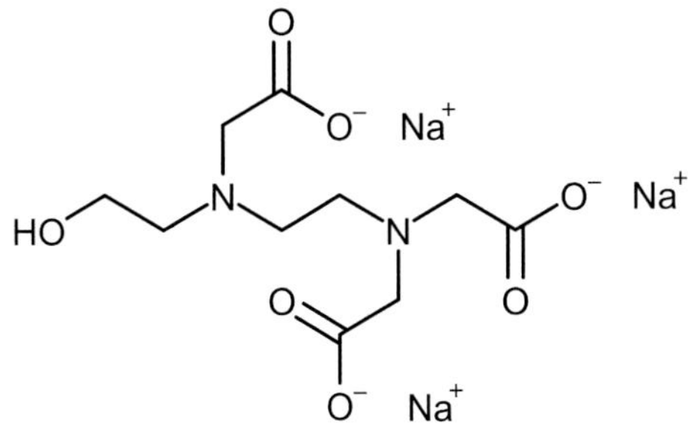

CONTACT ALLERGY

Case reports and case series

One patient had allergic contact dermatitis from trisodium hydroxyethyl ethylenediamine triacetate (and butylene glycol) in an unknown cosmetic product (1,2).

Presence in cosmetic products and chemical analyses

In the USA, in April 2017, trisodium hydroxyethyl ethylenediamine triacetate was present in zero of 56,714 cosmetic products of which the composition is known in FDA's Voluntary Cosmetic Registration Program (VCRP) (data obtained from FDA, May 2017). In April 2017, trisodium hydroxyethyl ethylenediamine triacetate was present in zero of 64,655 cosmetic products of which the composition is known in EWG's Skin Deep Cosmetics Database, USA (http://www.ewg.org/skindeep/).

LITERATURE

1 Yashiro K, Nishimoto M. A case of contact dermatitis due to 1,3-butylene glycol and trisodium hydroxyethyl ethylenediamine triacetate. Environ Dermatol 2003;10:14-20 (in Japanese)

2 Yashiro K, Mishimoto M. A case of contact dermatitis due to 1,3-butylene glycol and trisodiumhydroxyethyl ethylenediamine triacetate. Environ Dermatol 1999;6(Suppl. 1):59 (in Japanese)

2.488   TROMETHAMINE

IDENTIFICATION

Description/definition   : Tromethamine is the aliphatic compound that conforms to the formula shown below
Chemical class(es)   : Alkanolamines; polyols
Chemical/IUPAC name   : 2-Amino-2-(hydroxymethyl)propane-1,3-diol
Other names   : Trometamol; 1,3-propanediol, 2-amino-2-(hydroxymethyl)-; tri(hydroxymethyl)amino-
                               methane
CAS registry number (s)   : 77-86-1
EC number(s)   : 201-064-4
CIR review(s)   : Final report, September 2013 (access: www.cir-safety.org/ingredients)
Merck Index monograph   : 11221
Function(s) in cosmetics   : EU: buffering; masking. USA: fragrance ingredients; pH adjusters
EU cosmetic restrictions   : Regulated in Annex III/61 of the Regulation (EC) No. 1223/2009
Patch testing   : 1% water (1,2)
Molecular formula   : $C_4H_{11}NO_3$

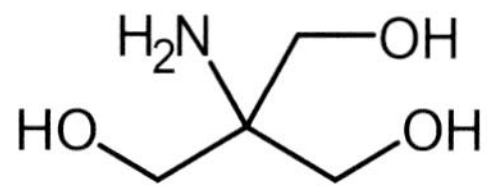

GENERAL

Tromethamine is stated to be a biologically inert amino alcohol, which buffers carbon dioxide and acids *in vitro* and *in vivo*. It is used in cosmetics, as an intracellular and extracellular alkalizing agent in medicine, and as a buffer solution industrially (1).

CONTACT ALLERGY

Case reports and case series

A woman presented with a 2-year history of perianal irritation, which had recently worsened and spread to the vulval area. She had been treated with topical corticosteroids, emollients, and a variety of over the counter preparations including an 'itch relief cream'. When examined, she had marked erythema and edema of the perianal area, perineum, and natal cleft. She was patch tested with the standard series and her own products and reacted positively to the itch relief cream. Subsequent testing with its ingredients showed positive reactions to trometha-mine 1% in water and to the original preparation (1). Another woman with a long history of atopic dermatitis presented with an acute deterioration of her skin condition after using the same anti-itch cream. A patch test with the cream was positive and later she reacted to the water phase of the preparation, in which tromethamine and glycerin were present. The patient refused further testing, so it is unknown whether tromethamine was the allergen (3). The product is described by the manufacturer as a skin care product, not as a topical pharmaceutical.

Contact allergy to tromethamine from non-cosmetic products

A woman had edematous allergic contact of the periorbital region from tromethamine present in an ophthalmolo-gical gel (2).

Presence in cosmetic products and chemical analyses

In the USA, in April 2017, tromethamine was present in 644 of 56,714 cosmetic products of which the composition is known in FDA's Voluntary Cosmetic Registration Program (VCRP) (data obtained from FDA, May 2017). In April 2017, tromethamine was present in 81 of 65,434 cosmetic products of which the composition is known in EWG's Skin Deep Cosmetics Database, USA (http://www.ewg.org/skindeep/).

LITERATURE

1   Singh M, Winhoven SM, Beck MH. Contact sensitivity to octyldodecanol and trometamol in an anti-itch cream. Contact Dermatitis 2007;56:89-90
2   Bohn S, Hurni M, Bircher AJ. Contact allergy to trometamol. Contact Dermatitis 2001;44:319
3   Fairhurst D, Wilkinson M. Independent sensitization to polidocanol and trometamol or glycerol within same product. Contact Dermatitis 2007;56:179

2.489 UNDECYLENAMIDE DEA

IDENTIFICATION

Description/definition : Undecylenamide DEA is a mixture of ethanolamides of undecylenic acid, which conforms generally to the formula shown below
Chemical class(es) : Alkanolamides
Chemical/IUPAC name : *N*,*N*-bis(2-Hydroxyethyl)undecenamide
Other name(s) : Diethanolamine undecylenate
CAS registry number (s) : 25377-64-4; 60239-68-1
EC number(s) : 246-914-5
CIR review(s) : Int J Toxicol 2013;32(Suppl.1):36-58 (access: www.cir-safety.org/ingredients)
Function(s) in cosmetics : EU: antidandruff; antimicrobial; antistatic; foam boosting; hair conditioning; viscosity controlling. USA: hair conditioning agents; surfactants – foam boosters; viscosity increasing agents - aqueous
EU cosmetic restrictions : Regulated in Annex III/60 of the Regulation (EC) No. 1223/2009
Patch testing : 0.1% and 1% water (1)
Molecular formula : $C_{15}H_{29}NO_3$

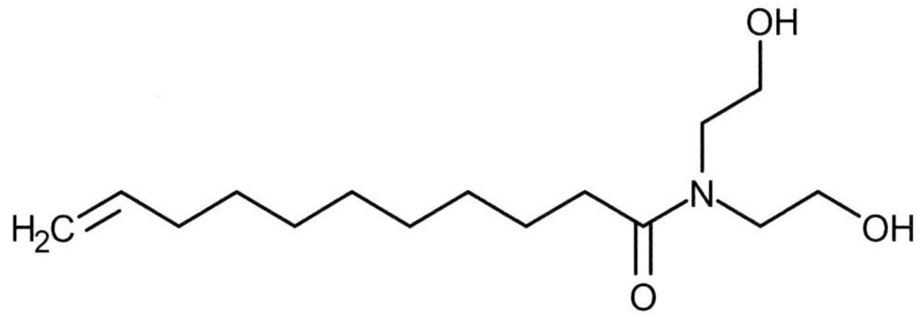

CONTACT ALLERGY

Case reports and case series

A male hospital employee, with previous atopic dermatitis, developed dermatitis of the hands and axillae. Patch testing with aluminium preparations (because of the axillary dermatitis) and his own deodorants and soaps, gave a positive reaction only to a liquid soap, tested 2% in water. Later, the 9 ingredients of the soap were tested separately, which yielded positive reactions to undecylenamide DEA 1% and 0.1% in water. Control tests with undecylenamide DEA 0.1% in water were negative in 10 individuals. The patient had used this soap both for washing his hands and his axillae. After he stopped using the product and changed to another soap, the dermatitis cleared (1).

Presence in cosmetic products and chemical analyses

In the USA, in April 2017, undecylenamide DEA was present in zero of 56,714 cosmetic products of which the composition is known in FDA's Voluntary Cosmetic Registration Program (VCRP) (data obtained from FDA, May 2017). In April 2017, undecylenamide DEA was present in 2 of 65,434 cosmetic products of which the composition is known in EWG's Skin Deep Cosmetics Database, USA (http://www.ewg.org/skindeep/). According to the FDA file of 1979, of approximately 19,000 cosmetic products, none contained undecylenamide DEA (1).

LITERATURE

1   Christersson S, Wramgsjö K. Contact allergy to undecylenamide diethanolamide in a liquid soap. Contact Dermatitis 1992;27:191-192

2.490   URETHANE ACRYLATES*

Not an INCI name

IDENTIFICATION

Description/definition   : 'Urethane acrylates' is a mixed isocyanate - acrylate polymer, containing hydroxyethyl acrylate

INCI name USA   : Neither in CosIng nor in the Personal Care Products Council Ingredient Database

CAS registry number (s) : 152187-46-7

GENERAL

Discussion of contact allergy to (meth)acrylates *from non-cosmetic sources* is considered to fall outside the scope of this book. Therefore, only contact allergy from their presence in cosmetics is presented, which virtually always is from artificial nails. There are many reports of contact allergy to artificial nails, but the specific sensitizers have rarely been identified and – consequently - such publications are not presented in this and other acrylate and methacrylate monographs. Discussion is limited to publications in which the culprit (meth)acrylates have been identified, e.g., from information found in Material Data Safety Sheets, data obtained from the manufacturer or from chemical analyses.

Patients often react to many (meth)acrylates on patch testing. Primary sensitization to methacrylates may result in both methacrylate and acrylate cross-sensitization. Conversely, patients sensitized to acrylates are unlikely to show cross-sensitization to methacrylates (4).

General aspects of acrylates and methacrylates are presented in Chapter 2.219 HEMA (hydroxyethyl methacrylate. A discussion of general aspects of artificial nails, contact allergy to these products, the clinical picture of allergic contact dermatitis and other side effects of sculptured nails can also be found there. A very useful review of contact sensitization to allergens in nail cosmetics, with emphasis on acrylic manicures, was published in 2017 (5).

CONTACT ALLERGY

Case reports and case series

General

In 2010, a new type of acrylate-based nail cosmetic was introduced. Ultraviolet (UV)-curable nail lacquers, also called 'gel polishes', were novel popular manicure agents designed to be applied on natural nails. They were marketed under different brand names. These products have the advantages of being odorless, harden rapidly, and offer a wide spectrum of glossy colors. They are resistant and give a two to four week manicure without chipping. Gel polish contains the same pigments that are used in traditional nail lacquers, but also photo-initiators and UV-curable acrylate or methacrylate monomers and oligomers (3). They are applied directly to the nail plate in several layers, with a brush. Between the applications, each layer is cured with UV light. At first, these types of nail polishes were only offered by professional nail technicians in beauty salons, but, later, different kits for home use appeared on the market. A starter kit typically contains transparent base and top coats, a light-emitting diode (LED) lamp emitting UV light, and sometimes some colored coats. Inevitably, these products were to give rise to allergic reactions; the first cases of contact allergy were reported in 2015 (2,3).

Case series

During 2014, 65 reports concerning undesirable effects from the use of one particular brand of UV-curing nail polish were received by the Swedish Medical Products Agency (1). The most commonly reported problem was eczema starting around the nails, combined with itching and pain in the fingers. Several customers also reported onycholysis, lesions under the nail plate, or paronychia. Permanent nail damage with thin, brittle nails was also described. In some cases, eczema on other parts of the body, for example on the lips, on the throat, and around the eyes, were reported, indicating that the nail polish had not been completely cured by the provided UV LED lamp. The Swedish Medical Products Agency in 2014 prohibited the sales of this nail polish.

Seven patients in Sweden with severe allergic skin reactions from the use of this particular product were patch tested with two coatings of the nail polish and its ingredients. Six individuals reacted to the base coat (2% pet.) and the colored coat (1% pet.). Six had positive patch tests to the ingredient 'urethane acrylates' (0.1% pet.), which was described by the manufacturer as a mixed isocyanate - acrylate polymer, containing hydroxyethyl acrylate. All six allergic individuals also reacted to 2 other methacrylate components of the nail polish (1).

Case reports

A woman had suffered from episodes of non-pruritic cheilitis and lip edema over the course of several months. She used many facial cosmetics, including lipsticks and lip balm. Moreover, manicuring with a UV-curable nail lacquer had been performed every 3 weeks for over a year. Symptoms had begun 3 to 4 months after the first manicure. While the cheilitis was worsening, the lip edema remained constant, with no relationship with the manicure sessions. On physical examination, only moderate erythema and edema of the mucosal surface of the lips were observed. Mild erythema of the periungual area was also noted. The patient admitted touching her lips with her nails frequently. Patch tests were performed with the European baseline series supplemented with the cosmetic, fragrances and acrylates series and the patient's own cosmetic products and UV-polymerized gel polish. Positive reactions were seen to many acrylates and methacrylates including urethane diacrylate and urethane dimethacrylate. She also reacted to the ultraviolet-polymerized polish color layer 'as is' and the ultraviolet-polymerized polish top coat 'as is'. The components of the UV-curable varnish included 'acrylated oligomer, urethane acrylate, methacrylate ester monomer, photoinitiator and pigments'. Removal of the varnish resulted in rapid resolution of the cheilitis and slower recovery of the lip edema (3).

Presence in cosmetic products and chemical analyses

In May 2017, urethane acrylates was present in zero of 66,975 cosmetic products of which the composition is known in EWG's Skin Deep Cosmetics Database, USA (http://www.ewg.org/skindeep/). In the USA, in April 2017, urethane acrylates was present in zero of 56,714 cosmetic products of which the composition is known in FDA's Voluntary Cosmetic Registration Program (VCRP) (data obtained from FDA, May 2017).

LITERATURE

1   Dahlin J, Berne B, Dunér K, Hosseiny S, Matura M, Nyman G, Tammela M, Isaksson M. Several cases of undesirable effects caused by methacrylate ultraviolet-curing nail polish for non-professional use. Contact Dermatitis 2016;75:151-156

2   Le Q, Cahill J, Palmer-Le A, Nixon R. The rising trend in allergic contact dermatitis to acrylic nail products. Australas J Dermatol 2015;56:221-223

3   Scheers C, André J, Negulescu M, Blondeel A, Kolivras A. Recurrent cheilitis and lip oedema caused by (meth)acrylates present in ultraviolet-curable nail lacquer. Contact Dermatitis 2015;72:341-342

4   Aalto-Korte K, Henriks-Eckerman M-L, Kuuliala O, Jolanki R. Occupational methacrylate and acrylate allergy – cross-reactions and possible screening allergens. Contact Dermatitis 2010;63:301-312

5   Chou M, Dhingra N, Strugar TL. Contact sensitization to allergens in nail cosmetics. Dermatitis 2017;28:231-240

2.491   URETHANE DIACRYLATE*

Not an INCI name

IDENTIFICATION

Description/definition : Urethane diacrylate is the organic compound that conforms to the formula shown below
Chemical class(es) : Esters
INCI name USA : Neither in CosIng nor in the Personal Care Products Council Ingredient Database
Patch testing : Urethane diacrylate, aliphatic 0.1% pet. (Chemotechnique); urethane diacrylate, aromatic 0.05% pet. (Chemotechnique)
Molecular formula : $C_7H_7NO_4$

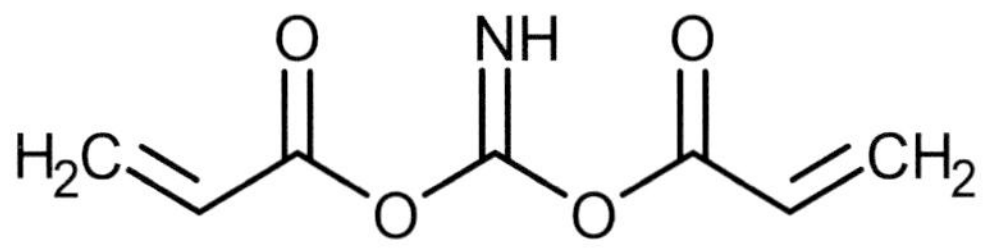

GENERAL

Discussion of contact allergy to (meth)acrylates *from non-cosmetic sources* is considered to fall outside the scope of this book. Therefore, only contact allergy from their presence in cosmetics is presented, which virtually always is from artificial nails and, more recently, from UV-cured nail polishes. There are many reports of contact allergy to artificial nails, but the specific sensitizers have rarely been identified and – consequently - such publications are not presented in this and other acrylate and methacrylate monographs. Discussion is limited to publications in which the culprit (meth)acrylates have been identified, e.g., from information found in Material Data Safety Sheets, data obtained from the manufacturer or from chemical analyses.

Patients often react to many (meth)acrylates on patch testing. Primary sensitization to methacrylates may result in both methacrylate and acrylate cross-sensitization. Conversely, patients sensitized to acrylates are unlikely to show cross-sensitization to methacrylates (1).

General aspects of acrylates and methacrylates are presented in Chapter 2.219 HEMA (hydroxyethyl methacrylate). A discussion of general aspects of artificial nails, contact allergy to these products, the clinical picture of allergic contact dermatitis and other side effects of sculptured nails can also be found there. A very useful review of contact sensitization to allergens in nail cosmetics, with emphasis on acrylic manicures, was published in 2017 (4).

CONTACT ALLERGY

Patch testing in groups of patients
Studies in which consecutive patients suspected of contact dermatitis have been tested with urethane diacrylate (routine testing) and studies testing groups of selected patients are planned to be discussed in a future publication.

Case reports and case series
One patient had allergic contact cheilitis from an ultraviolet-curable nail lacquer. She had many positive acrylate patch tests including to urethane diacrylate. According to the manufacturer, the product contained various (meth)acrylates including urethane acrylate (2).

Five women with UV-cured acrylic nails presented with a pruritic and painful perionychial and subonychial dermatitis for several months. The dermatitis began 6 months to 3 years after the first application of these gels. They all reacted to several commercial 'acrylate-free' nail products and to several (meth)acrylates including aliphatic urethane diacrylate 0.05% and 0.1% pet.; two also reacted to urethane dimethacrylate. It was not specified whether urethane diacrylate was present in one or more of the commercial nail products used by the patients. In addition, urethane diacrylate had been diluted in 20% tripropylene glycol diacrylate for patch testing, which makes reliability and the relevance of these reactions even more uncertain (3).

Presence in cosmetic products and chemical analyses
In May 2017, urethane diacrylate was present in zero of 66,975 cosmetic products of which the composition is known in EWG's Skin Deep Cosmetics Database, USA (http://www.ewg.org/skindeep/). In the USA, in April 2017, urethane diacrylate was present in zero of 56,714 cosmetic products of which the composition is known in FDA's Voluntary Cosmetic Registration Program (VCRP) (data obtained from FDA, May 2017).

LITERATURE

1   Aalto-Korte K, Henriks-Eckerman M-L, Kuuliala O, Jolanki R. Occupational methacrylate and acrylate allergy – cross-reactions and possible screening allergens. Contact Dermatitis 2010;63:301-312
2   Scheers C, André J, Negulescu M, Blondeel A, Kolivras A. Recurrent cheilitis and lip oedema caused by (meth)acrylates present in ultraviolet-curable nail lacquer. Contact Dermatitis 2015;72:341-342
3   Hemmer W, Focke M, Wantke F, Götz M, Jarisch R. Allergic contact dermatitis to artificial fingernails prepared from UV light-cured acrylates. J Am Acad Dermatol 1996;35(3 Part 1):377-380
4   Chou M, Dhingra N, Strugar TL. Contact sensitization to allergens in nail cosmetics. Dermatitis 2017;28:231-240

2.492   VP/EICOSENE COPOLYMER

IDENTIFICATION

Description/definition : VP/eicosene copolymer is a polymer of vinylpyrrolidone and eicosene monomers, which
 conforms generally to the formula shown below
Chemical class(es) : Synthetic polymers
Other names : PVP/eicosene copolymer; 2-pyrrolidinone, 1-ethenyl-, polymer with 1-eicosene
CAS registry number (s) : 28211-18-9; 77035-98-4
Function(s) in cosmetics : EU: binding; film forming; viscosity controlling. USA: binders; dispersing agents –
 nonsurfactant; film formers; viscosity increasing agents – nonaqueous
Patch testing : 10% pet. (2,4)

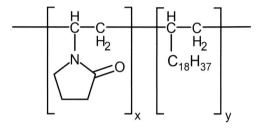

GENERAL

Copolymers are important ingredients in cosmetics, added because of their antistatic, film-forming, binding, suspending, viscosity-increasing, skin-conditioning, and emulsion-stabilizing properties. Copolymers have been underestimated for a long time as to their sensitizing capacities because of their large structures and high molecular weights. Allergic contact dermatitis to copolymers in cosmetics, however, does occur, but the exact nature of the hapten is still unknown. The copolymers are not likely to be haptens themselves in view of their large molecular weights. The sensitizer could be an additive, an impurity, a product that forms during polymerization, a residual monomer, or a degradation product (1).

VP/eicosene copolymer is present in many sunscreens to enhance water resistance. This copolymer is also used as an inert ingredient in pesticides, as a protective colloid, as a microcapsulating resin, as a dispersant for pigment, as a solubilizer for dyes, and also in the petroleum industry as a sludge and detergent dispersant (1).

CONTACT ALLERGY

Case reports and case series

A non-atopic man had a 6-month history of dryness and itching of the hands, lower arms and legs, for which he used an emollient cream daily. Within a month, he developed itchy, vesicular dermatitis of the arms and legs. Patch tests with the Italian standard series and the patient's emollient cream gave a positive reaction to the cream, tested as is. A repeated open application test with the cosmetic product was positive within 3 days. Patch testing with the product and its ingredients yielded positive reactions to the cream and VP/eicosene copolymer 10% pet., to which 15 controls were negative (2). An atopic woman developed acute dermatitis of the face within 24 hours of a single application of a recently bought sunscreen, followed by moderate sun exposure. Upon patch testing, there was a positive reaction to the sunscreen, which was not photoaggravated. When tested with its 24 ingredients, polyvinyl-pyrrolidone (PVP)/eicosene copolymer 1% pet. was positive (3,5 [the patient in ref. 5 may be the same as in ref. 3]).

Another female individual had suffered from three episodes of dermatitis of the face, also closely related to the use of a particular sunblock. A patch test with the cosmetic was positive at D2 and D4, photopatch testing was negative (which probably means that the reaction was the same as on the non-irradiated side, or that the product itself has not been photopatch tested). Ingredient testing of the sunblock showed a positive patch test reaction to PVP/eicosene copolymer 10% pet., to which 20 control patients were negative (4). One more patient had contact allergy to and probably allergic contact dermatitis from VP/eicosene copolymer in a sunscreen (6).

Presence in cosmetic products and chemical analyses

In the USA, in April 2017, VP/eicosene copolymer was present in 361 of 56,714 cosmetic products of which the composition is known in FDA's Voluntary Cosmetic Registration Program (VCRP) (data obtained from FDA, May 2017). In April 2017, VP/eicosene copolymer was present in 407 of 65,434 cosmetic products of which the composition is known in EWG's Skin Deep Cosmetics Database, USA (http://www.ewg.org/skindeep/). In the cosmetics ingredient database of the University of Leuven, Belgium, VP/eicosene copolymer was found as an ingredient in 2 lipsticks, 7 lip balms, 3 lip glosses, 22 different kinds of mascara, 3 eye shadows, 3 eyeliners, 1 around-eye cream, 1 brow liner, 2 foundations, 90 sunscreens, 3 sunless tanners, 2 insect repellents, 9 moisturizers, 1 anti-itch cream, and 1 hair removal wax (1).

LITERATURE

1   Quartier S, Garmyn M, Becart S, Goossens A. Allergic contact dermatitis to copolymers in cosmetics – case report and review of the literature. Contact Dermatitis 2006;55:257-267
2   Gallo R, Dal Sacco D, Ghigliotti G. Allergic contact dermatitis from VP/eicosene copolymer (Ganex® V-220) in an emollient cream. Contact Dermatitis 2004;50:261
3   Le Coz CJ, Lefebre C, Ludmann F, Grosshans E. Polyvinylpyrrolidone (PVP)/eicosene copolymer: an emerging cosmetic allergen. Contact Dermatitis 2000;43:61
4   Smith HR, Armstrong K, Wakelin SH, White IR. Contact allergy to PVP/eicosene copolymer. Contact Dermatitis 1999;40:283
5   Le Coz CJ. Le copolymère de polyvinylpyrrolidone et d'eicosene (PVP/eicosene copolymer): un nouvel allergène cosmétique. La lettre du Gerda 2000;17:54
6   Foley P, Nixon R, Marks R, Frowen K, Thompson S. The frequency of reactions to sunscreens: results of a longitudinal population based study on the regular use of sunscreens in Australia. Br J Dermatol 1993;128:512-518

2.493   VP/HEXADECENE COPOLYMER

IDENTIFICATION

Description/definition   : VP/hexadecene copolymer is a polymer of hexadecene and vinylpyrrolidone monomers
Chemical class(es)   : Synthetic polymers
Chemical / IUPAC name : 2-Pyrrolidinone, 1-ethenyl-, polymer with 1-hexadecene
Other names   : Vinylpyrrolidone hexadecene copolymer; PVP/hexadecene copolymer; polyvinyl-
                                   pyrrolidone/hexadecene copolymer
CAS registry number (s) : 32440-50-9; 63231-81-2
Function(s) in cosmetics : EU: binding; film forming; hair fixing; viscosity controlling. USA: binders;
                                   dispersing agents – nonsurfactant; film formers; hair fixatives; viscosity
                                   increasing agents - nonaqueous
Patch testing   : 5% pet. (2,5); 1-5-10% pet. (6)

GENERAL

Copolymers are important ingredients in cosmetics, added because of their antistatic, film-forming, binding, suspending, viscosity-increasing, skin-conditioning, and emulsion-stabilizing properties. Copolymers also have a function in the petroleum industry as sludge and detergent dispersant (6). Copolymers have been underestimated for a long time as to their sensitizing capacities because of their large structures and high molecular weights. Allergic contact dermatitis to copolymers in cosmetics, however, does occur, but the exact nature of the hapten is still unknown. The copolymers are not likely to be haptens themselves in view of their large molecular weights. The sensitizer could be an additive, an impurity, a product that forms during polymerization, a residual monomer, or a degradation product (6).

CONTACT ALLERGY

Case reports and case series

In a group of 119 patients with cosmetic allergy seen in The Netherlands in 1986-1987, one had allergic contact dermatitis from VP/hexadecene copolymer in a skin care product (3,7,8). VP/hexadecene copolymer was responsible for 1 out of 959 cases of non-fragrance cosmetic allergy where the causal allergen was identified, Belgium, 2000-2010 (1).

A woman had extensive blistering dermatitis of the arms and legs from VP/hexadecene copolymer in a bath oil. The patient reacted to the polymer 15% pet., which was negative in 10 controls (4). Another woman presented with a 1-year history of episodic erythematous patches on her face, legs, and trunk which lasted up to 2 weeks. Patch tests with the standard series, substances of the textile and cosmetic series and the patient's personal cosmetic products gave a positive reaction to bath dry oil spray (same brand as the previous patient, bot other product). The individual ingredients were tested at the concentrations used in the product, yielding a strongly positive reaction to VP/hexadecene copolymer, tested 5% pet. (5).

A young woman had dry, desquamative cheilitis of both lips that had been present for 3 months. The patient was told to stop using all her lipsticks, and her clinical symptoms disappeared in one week. A repeated open application test (ROAT) with her lipsticks was performed on her inner arm, and 3 days later, there was an eczematous reaction in the region where one particular lipstick had been applied. Patch tests with the standard series of the Spanish Contact Dermatitis Research Group (GEIDC), cosmetic series, and the components of the incriminated lipstick showed a positive reaction to polyvinylpyrrolidone (PVP)/hexadecene copolymer, tested 5% pet., to which 10 controls were negative (2). Allergic contact cheilitis from VP/hexadecene copolymer in a lipstick has also been observed in another female patient (6).

Cross-reactions

Not to VP/eicosene copolymer (6).

Presence in cosmetic products and chemical analyses

In the USA, in April 2017, VP/hexadecene copolymer was present in 384 of 56,714 cosmetic products of which the composition is known in FDA's Voluntary Cosmetic Registration Program (VCRP) (data obtained from FDA, May 2017). In April 2017, VP/hexadecene copolymer was present in 326 of 65,434 cosmetic products of which the composition is known in EWG's Skin Deep Cosmetics Database, USA (http://www.ewg.org/skindeep/). In the cosmetics database of the University of Leuven, Belgium, VP/hexadecene copolymer was found as an ingredient in 38 lipsticks, 8 lip glosses, 6 lip balms, 2 lip liners, 6 eye shadows, 7 different kinds of mascara, 1 eye makeup remover, 2 eyeliners, 2 foundations, 8 concealers, 27 sunscreens, 1 bronzer, 1 blusher, 9 moisturizers, and 1 body paint (6).

LITERATURE

1   Travassos AR, Claes L, Boey L, Drieghe J, Goossens A. Non-fragrance allergens in specific cosmetic products. Contact Dermatitis 2011;65:276-285

2   Pastor N, Silvestre JF, Mataix J, Lucas A, Pérez M. Contact cheilitis from bisabolol and polyvinylpyrrolidone/hexadecene copolymer in lipstick. Contact Dermatitis 2008;58:178-179

3   De Groot AC, Bruynzeel DP, Bos JD, van der Meeren HL, van Joost T, Jagtman BA, Weyland JW. The allergens in cosmetics. Arch Dermatol 1988: 124: 1525–1529.

4   Fowler JF Jr. Allergic contact dermatitis to polyvinylpyrrolidone/hexadecene copolymer. Am J Contact Dermat 1995;6:243-244

5   Scheman A, Cummins R. Contact allergy to PVP/hexadecene copolymer. Contact Dermatitis 1998;39:201

6   Quartier S, Garmyn M, Becart S, Goossens A. Allergic contact dermatitis to copolymers in cosmetics – case report and review of the literature. Contact Dermatitis 2006;55:257-267

7   De Groot AC. Contact allergy to polyvinylpyrrolidone/hexadecene copolymer previously reported. Am J Cont Derm 1996;7:260

8   De Groot AC. PVP/hexadecene copolymer: a hard-to-find allergen in modern times. Contact Dermatitis 1999;40:172

2.494   WITISOL*
Not an INCI name

IDENTIFICATION

Description/definition   : Witisol is the heterocyclic aromatic compound that conforms to the structural formula shown below
Chemical class(es)   : Heterocyclic organic compounds; aromatic compounds
INCI name USA   : Neither in CosIng nor in the Personal Care Products Council Ingredient Database
Chemical/IUPAC name   : 5-Methyl-2-phenyl-1,3-benzoxazole
CAS registry number (s)   : 7420-86-2
EC number(s)   : 231-040-9
Function(s) in cosmetics   : EU: formerly used as UV-filter; prohibited, delisted in 1989
Patch testing   : 1% pet. (2)
Molecular formula   : $C_{14}H_{11}NO$

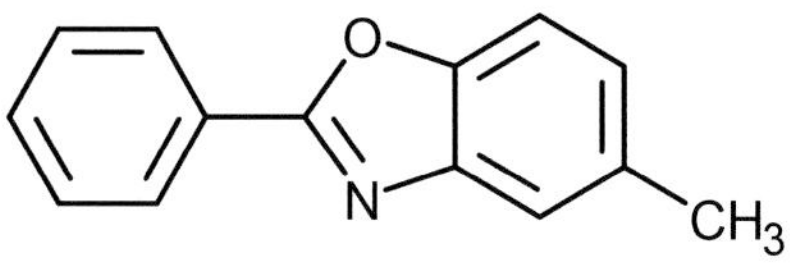

GENERAL
Witisol was withdrawn from the market in 1987.

CONTACT ALLERGY

Case reports and case series
A non-atopic women who had never suffered from skin disease had for two years used a cream with protection factor 4 on her face, chest and upper part of the back. She used the cream daily as an emollient. Having done this for 18 months, she developed an eczematous dermatitis on her face, chest and the upper part of her back. Patch tests with the standard series were negative. A patch test with the sunscreen cream was positive. When tested with its ingredients, obtained from the manufacturer, the patient had a strong positive reaction to witisol 1% pet., while the other components of the cream were negative. Tests on three controls with the witisol test preparation were negative (2).

In the period 1981-1989, 56 patients (43 women, 13 men) were diagnosed with contact allergy or photocontact allergy to UV-filters in one center in Germany. There were 3 contact allergic and 1 photoaggravated contact allergic reactions to witisol. All reactions were relevant and all 46 patients who could be (photo)patch tested with their own sunscreens (and a few of them with other cosmetics) had one or more positive (photo)patch tests to these products (3, overlap with ref. 1). One patient had contact allergy to witisol; the positive patch test reaction was probably relevant from the presence of witisol in a sunscreen (1). The authors mentioned one more case of witisol allergy (ref. 1, note added in proof, overlap with ref. 3).

Presence in cosmetic products and chemical analyses
In May 2017, witisol was present in zero of 66,975 cosmetic products of which the composition is known in EWG's Skin Deep Cosmetics Database, USA (http://www.ewg.org/skindeep/). In the USA, in April 2017, witisol was present in zero of 56,714 cosmetic products of which the composition is known in FDA's Voluntary Cosmetic Registration Program (VCRP) (data obtained from FDA, May 2017).

OTHER SIDE EFFECTS

Photosensitivity
In the period 1981-1989, 56 patients (43 women, 13 men) were diagnosed with contact allergy or photocontact allergy to UV-filters in one center in Germany. There was 1 photoaggravated contact allergic and 4 photoallergic reactions to witisol. All reactions were relevant and all 46 patients who could be (photo)patch tested with their own sunscreens (and a few of them with other cosmetics) had one or more positive (photo)patch tests to these products (, overlap with ref. 1). One case of photocontact allergy to witisol has been observed in Germany (ref. 1, note added in proof, no clinical details known, overlap with ref. 3).

LITERATURE

1   Schauder S, Ippen H. Photoallergic and allergic contact eczema caused by dibenzoylmethane compounds and other sunscreening agents. Hautarzt 1988;39:435-440

2   Mørk N-J, Austad J. Contact dermatitis from witisol, a sunscreen agent. Contact Dermatitis 1984;10:122-123

3   Schauder S. Adverse reactions to sunscreening agents in 58 patients (part 3). Z Hautkr 1991;66:294-318 (article in German)

2.495   XANTHAN GUM

IDENTIFICATION

Description/definition   : Xanthan gum is a high molecular weight heteropolysaccharide gum produced by a
                             pure-culture fermentation of a carbohydrate with *Xanthomonas campestris*
Chemical class(es)   : Gums, hydrophilic colloids and derivatives
Other names   : Gummi xanthanum; xanthan; corn sugar gum
CAS registry number (s)   : 11138-66-2
EC number(s)   : 234-394-2
Merck Index monograph   : 11525
CIR review(s)   : Final report, September 2012 ((access: www.cir-safety.org/ingredients)
Function(s) in cosmetics   : EU: binding; emulsifying; emulsion stabilising; gel forming; skin conditioning; surfactant;
                             viscosity controlling. USA: binders; emulsion stabilizers; skin-conditioning agents –
                             miscellaneous; surfactants - emulsifying agents; viscosity increasing agents – aqueous
Patch testing   : 10% water (1)

GENERAL

Xanthan gum is a natural water-soluble resin and polysaccharide produced through the fermentation of glucose, sucrose or lactose by the bacterium *Xanthomonas campestris*. It is available as a fine powder and is widely used as a food additive (E415), in cosmetic products and in pharmaceuticals, in which it serves as a thickening agent, enhancing the viscosity. Other applications include its use in thickening liquids for patients with swallowing disorders, as an alternative to gluten for gluten-sensitive patients, as a key ingredient in 'fake blood' products, and as a part of special effects makeup, and non-medical, recreational purposes (1).

CONTACT ALLERGY

Case reports and case series

A young girl had a suspected contact or photocontact allergy to a sunscreen cream SPF50, as its use for 2 days caused an itchy and burning dermatitis on the face and arms, with subsequent widespread involvement. Patch tests with the Belgian baseline series, a photopatch series, the sunscreen series and, additionally, decyl glucoside 5% pet. and xanthan gum 1% water (as these chemicals were known to be present in the product) gave positive patch test reactions to the sunscreen cream and to xanthan gum. Later, tests with the ingredients of the cream yielded positive reactions to the UV-filter Tinosorb® M and to xanthan gum 10% water. After avoidance of the sunscreen cosmetic and other topical products containing xanthan gum, the patient has remained free of dermatitis (1). Tinosorb® M is a mixture of methylene bis-benzotriazolyl tetramethylbutylphenol (UV-filter), propylene glycol, decyl glucoside, xanthan gum, and water. Most cases of contact allergy to Tinosorb® M have been caused by decyl glucoside (see Chapter 2.461 Tinosorb® M and 2.134 Decyl glucoside).

Presence in cosmetic products and chemical analyses

In the USA, in April 2017, xanthan gum was present in 5590 of 56,714 cosmetic products of which the composition is known in FDA's Voluntary Cosmetic Registration Program (VCRP) (data obtained from FDA, May 2017). In April 2017, xanthan gum was present in 3738 of 65,434 cosmetic products of which the composition is known in EWG's Skin Deep Cosmetics Database, USA (http://www.ewg.org/skindeep/).

OTHER SIDE EFFECTS

Miscellaneous side effects

Hypersensitivity to xanthan gum present in a syrup caused a maculopapular eruption (2).

LITERATURE

1   Aerts O, Clinck B, Schramme M, Lambert J. Contact allergy caused by Tinosorb® M: let us not forget about
     xanthan gum. Contact Dermatitis 2015;72:121-123
2   Barbaud A. Drug patch testing in systemic cutaneous drug allergy. In: Zhai I, Wilhelm KP, Maibach HI, Eds:
     Marzulli and Maibach's Dermatotoxicology, 7ᵗʰ Edition. Boca Raton, FL, USA: CRC Press Taylor & Francis
     Group, 2008:766 (data cited in ref. 1)

2.496   ZINC PYRITHIONE

IDENTIFICATION

Description/definition	: Zinc pyrithione is the aromatic zinc compound that conforms to the formula shown below
Chemical class(es)	: Heterocyclic compounds; organic salts; thio compounds
Chemical/IUPAC name	: Zinc 1-oxidopyridine-2-thione
Other names	: Pyrithione zinc; pyridine-2-thiol-1-oxide, zinc complex (2:1)
CAS registry number (s)	: 13463-41-7
EC number(s)	: 236-671-3
SCCS opinion(s)	: SCCS/1512/13 (19); SCCNFP/0671/02 (20)
Merck Index monograph	: 9377 (Pyrithione)
Function(s) in cosmetics	: EU: antidandruff; antiseborrhoeic; hair conditioning; preservative. USA: antidandruff agents; cosmetic biocides; hair conditioning agents; preservatives
EU cosmetic restrictions	: Regulated in Annex III/101 of the Regulation (EC) No. 1223/2009
Patch testing	: 1% pet. (Chemotechnique); 0.1% pet. (SmartPracticeCanada)
Molecular formula	: $C_{10}H_8N_2O_2S_2Zn$

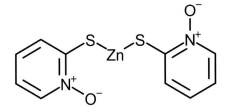

GENERAL

Zinc pyrithione is a common active ingredient with a low potential of irritation and sensitization in antidandruff shampoo; it is often recommended for individuals with seborrheic dermatitis or psoriasis. Two mechanisms of antidandruff effects have been studied: (1) zinc pyrithione is an antifungal agent that interferes with the primary proton pump in fungus membranes; and (2) zinc pyrithione has cytotoxic effects on rapidly proliferating epidermis cells. Despite its frequent and widespread use, few cases of zinc pyrithione-induced allergic contact dermatitis have been documented (10).

CONTACT ALLERGY

Patch testing in groups of patients

Results of studies in which consecutive patients suspected of contact dermatitis have been patch tested with zinc pyrithione (routine testing) and of studies testing in groups of selected patients are shown in table 2.496.1. In routine testing, in Denmark before 1985, there were 3 positive reactions in a group of 1652 patients tested (0.2%); one of these three had ACD from zinc pyrithione in a shampoo (5). In groups of selected patients (hairdressers and clients of hairdressers, patients tested with a preservative series, patients suspected of allergy to cosmetics, drugs or clothes), frequencies of sensitization have ranged from 0.1% to 1.2%. The few reactions found were either not relevant or relevance was not mentioned (11,16,21).

Table 2.496.1 Patch testing in groups of patients

Years and Country	Test conc. & vehicle	Number of patients tested	positive (%)	Selection of patients (S); Relevance (R); Comments (C)	Ref.
Routine testing					
<1985 Denmark	1% pet.	1652	3 (0.2%)	R: 1/3 had allergic contact dermatitis from a shampoo containing zinc pyrithione	5
Testing in groups of selected patients					
<1995 Spain	1% pet.	171	2 (1.2%)	S: hairdressers and clients of hairdressers; R: not relevant	11
1990-1994 IVDK	0.1% pet.	7782	6 (0.1%)	S: patients tested with a preservative series; R: not stated	16
1981 France	1% pet.	465	2 (0.4%)	S: patients suspected of allergy to cosmetics, drugs, industrial products, or clothes; R: not stated	21

IVDK: Information Network of Departments of Dermatology, Germany, Austria, Switzerland

Case reports and case series

In a group of 119 patients with allergic contact dermatitis from cosmetics, investigated in The Netherlands in 1986-1987, one case was caused by zinc pyrithione in a shampoo (17,18). Two cases (11) and one case each (5,10,12,13) of allergic reactions from zinc pyrithione in shampoos have been reported. One patient had worsening of scalp psoriasis and eyelid dermatitis from contact allergy to zinc pyrithione and cocamide DEA in an anti-dandruff shampoo (2). Another patient developed allergic contact dermatitis from zinc pyrithione in shampoo, which led to worsening of existing psoriasis (Köbner-phenomenon) and development of pustular psoriasis (3). A similar case had been reported previously (9).

Two patients had allergic contact dermatitis from zinc pyrithione, one by its presence in a hair cream, the other from the same hair cream and from an antidandruff lotion (6). In another patient, contact allergic sensitivity to zinc pyrithione in a shampoo was followed by the photosensitivity dermatitis and actinic reticuloid syndrome (7). One patient reacted to zinc pyrithione in a hair cream and a shampoo (8). One patient was allergic to zinc pyrithione, of whom details are unknown (1).

Cross-reactions, pseudo-cross-reactions and co-reactions

Ethylenediamine (?,1); this has not been confirmed in any other study. Not to sodium pyrithione (14). Sodium pyrithione (assumed on theoretical grounds, zinc pyrithione itself not tested) (15).

Presence in cosmetic products and chemical analyses

In the USA, in April 2017, zinc pyrithione was present in 64 of 56,714 cosmetic products of which the composition is known in FDA's Voluntary Cosmetic Registration Program (VCRP) (data obtained from FDA, May 2017). In April 2017, zinc pyrithione was present in 149 of 66,647 cosmetic products of which the composition is known in EWG's Skin Deep Cosmetics Database, USA (http://www.ewg.org/skindeep/). In Germany, in 2006-2009, the labels of 4680 cosmetic products were screened for the presence of preservatives. Zinc pyrithione was present in 0.4% of the products, according to labelling information (22).

OTHER SIDE EFFECTS

Photosensitivity

One patient had a positive photopatch test to zinc pyrithione; details are unknown (4).). In another individual, contact allergy to zinc pyrithione in a shampoo was followed by the photosensitivity dermatitis and actinic reticuloid syndrome (7).

Systemic side effects

A physician had peripheral neuritis, which first affected only the left leg, but within four months it had spread to the right ulnar nerve. There was paraesthesia of the affected areas with hypoesthesia to light touch and hyperesthesia to deep pressure. Foot drop and a weak grip developed. Physical examination, blood picture, urinalysis, serum-protein electrophoresis, antinuclear antibodies, glucose-tolerance test, lumbar myelogram (before the onset of the ulnar neuritis), and chest X-ray were all normal. Eight months after the onset of symptoms the patient recalled that zinc pyrithione is neurotoxic and absorbed through the skin of animals. Since he had been using an antidandruff shampoo containing 2% zinc pyrithione for several years, he discontinued it at once. Within a month the muscle weakness began to improve and it had completely cleared in 3 months. Two years after he stopped using the shampoo, his paresthesia was 75% improved, and muscle strength remained normal (23).

LITERATURE

1   Calnan CD, cited by Fisher AA. Highlights of the First International Symposium on Contact Dermatitis. Cutis 1976;18:645-662 (pages probably incorrect)
2   De Groot AC, de Wit FS, Bos JD, Weyland JW. Contact allergy to cocamide DEA and lauramide DEA in shampoos. Contact Dermatitis 1987;16:117-118
3   Jo J-H, Jang H-S, Ko H-C, Kim M-B, Oh C-K, Kwon Y-W, Kwon K-S. Pustular psoriasis and the Köbner phenomenon caused by allergic contact dermatitis from zinc pyrithione-containing shampoo. Contact Dermatitis 2005;52:142-144
4   Osmundsen PE. Contact photodermatitis due to tribromsalicylanilide (cross-reaction pattern). Dermatologica 1970;140:65-74
5   Brandrup F, Menné T. Zinc pyrithione allergy. Contact Dermatitis 1985;12:50
6   Muston HL, Messenger AG, Byrne JPH. Contact dermatitis from zinc pyrithione, an antidandruff agent. Contact Dermatitis 1979;5:276-277

7   Yates VM, Finn OA. Contact allergic sensitivity to zinc pyrithione followed by the photosensitivity dermatitis and actinic reticuloid syndrome. Contact Dermatitis 1980;6:349-350

8   Goh CL, Lim KB. Allergic contact dermatitis to zinc pyrithione. Contact Dermatitis 1984;11:120

9   Nielsen N, Menné T. Allergic contact dermatitis caused by zinc pyrithione associated with pustular psoriasis. Am J Contact Dermat 1997;8:170–171

10 Hsieh C-W, Tu M-E, Wu Y-H. Allergic contact dermatitis induced by zinc pyrithione in shampoo: a case report. Dermatologica Sinica 2010;28:163-166

11 Gonzalez Perez R, Aguirre A, Raton JA, Eizaguirre X, Fiaz-Pérez JL. Positive patch tests to zinc pyrithione. Contact Dermatitis 1995;32:118-119

12 Pereira F, Fernandes C, Dias M, Lacerda MH. Allergic contact dermatitis from zinc pyrithione. Contact Dermatitis 1995;33:131

13 Nigam PK, Tyagi S, Saxena AK, Misra RS. Dermatitis from zinc pyrithione. Contact Dermatitis 1988;19:219

14 Isaksson, M. Delayed diagnosis of occupational contact dermatitis from sodium pyrithione in a metalworking fluid. Contact Dermatitis 2002;47:248-249

15 Le Coz C-J. Allergic contact dermatitis from sodium pyrithione in metalworking fluid. Contact Dermatitis 2001;45:58-59

16 Schnuch A, Geier J, Uter W, Frosch PJ. Patch testing with preservatives, antimicrobials and industrial biocides. Results from a multicentre study. Br J Dermatol 1998;138:467-476

17 De Groot AC, Bruynzeel DP, Bos JD, van der Meeren HL, van Joost T, Jagtman BA, Weyland JW. The allergens in cosmetics. Arch Dermatol 1988;124:1525-1529

18 De Groot AC. Adverse reactions to cosmetics. PhD Thesis, University of Groningen, The Netherlands: 1988, chapter 3.4, pp.105-113

19 SCCS (Scientific Committee on Consumer Safety). Opinion on Zinc pyrithione, 18 June 2013, SCCS/1512/13, Available at: http://ec.europa.eu/health/scientific_committees/consumer_safety/docs/sccs_o_133.pdf

20 SCCNFP (Scientific Committee on Cosmetics and Non Food Products). Opinion concerning zinc pyrithione, 17 December 2002, SCCNFP/0671/02. Available at: http://ec.europa.eu/health/archive/ph_risk/committees/sccp/documents/out225_en.pdf

21 Meynadier JM, Meynadier J, Colmas A, Castelain PY, Ducombs G, Chabeau G, et al. Allergy to preservatives. Ann Dermatol Venereol 1982;109:1017-1023

22 Uter W, Yazar K, Kratz EM, Mildau G, Lidén C. Coupled exposure to ingredients of cosmetic products: II. Preservatives. Contact Dermatitis 2014;70:219-226

23 Beck JE. Zinc pyrithione and peripheral neuritis. Lancet 1978;1(8061):444

2.497   ZINC RICINOLEATE

IDENTIFICATION

Description/definition	: Zinc ricinoleate is the zinc salt of ricinoleic acid, which conforms to the formula shown below
Chemical class(es)	: Soaps
Chemical/IUPAC name	: Zinc (Z,12R)-12-hydroxyoctadec-9-enoate
Other names	: Zinc diricinoleate; 12-hydroxy-9-octadecenoic acid, zinc salt
CAS registry number (s)	: 13040-19-2
EC number(s)	: 235-911-4
CIR review(s)	: Int J Toxicol 2007;26(Suppl.3):31-77 (access: www.cir-safety.org/ingredients)
Patch testing	: 76% pet. (1); a penetration enhancer may be necessary
Function(s) in cosmetics	: EU: anticaking; deodorant; opacifying. USA: anticaking agents; deodorant agents; opacifying agents
Molecular formula	: $C_{36}H_{66}O_6Zn$

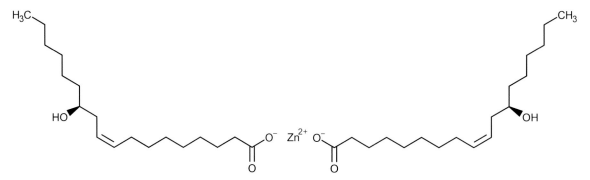

GENERAL

Ricinoleates, e.g., zinc ricinoleate, magnesium ricinoleate or glyceryl ricinoleate, are metal soaps of ricinoleic acid. They are used in adhesives, corrosion inhibitors, cosmetics, greases, varnishes, print pigments and for deodorizing of various products (1).

CONTACT ALLERGY

Case reports and case series

One patient had allergic contact dermatitis from zinc ricinoleate in a deodorant (1). Two other patients had dermal contact dermatitis in the axillae, which was probably also caused by zinc ricinoleate in a deodorant. The patients reacted to an ingredient of the deodorant, a mixture of 88% zinc ricinoleate and several other (unrelated) chemicals. The zinc ricinoleate was considered to be the culprit, as one of the two patients was also allergic to castor oil (Ricinus communis seed oil), and the other to castor oil and various castor oil derivatives: hydrogenated castor oil, sulfated castor oil, glyceryl ricinoleate, PEG-400 ricinoleate (INCI name: PEG-8 ricinoleate) and sodium sulforicinate (2).

Cross-reactions, pseudo-cross-reactions and co-reactions

Glyceryl ricinoleate (1,2); sulfated castor oil (1,2). Hydrogenated castor oil, PEG-400 ricinoleate (INCI name: PEG-8 ricinoleate) and sodium sulforicinate (2).

Presence in cosmetic products and chemical analyses

In the USA, in April 2017, zinc ricinoleate was present in 27 of 56,714 cosmetic products of which the composition is known in FDA's Voluntary Cosmetic Registration Program (VCRP) (data obtained from FDA, May 2017). In April 2017, zinc ricinoleate was present in 47 of 65,434 cosmetic products of which the composition is known in EWG's Skin Deep Cosmetics Database, USA (http://www.ewg.org/skindeep/).

LITERATURE

1 Magerl A, Heiss R, Frosch PJ. Allergic contact dermatitis from zinc ricinoleate in a deodorant and glyceryl ricinoleate in a lipstick. Contact Dermatitis 2001;44:119-121
2 Dooms-Goossens A, Dupré K, Borghijs A, Swinnen C, Dooms M, Degreef H. Zinc ricinoleate: sensitizer in deodorants. Contact Dermatitis 1987;16:292-294

CHAPTER 3 MONOGRAPHS OF CHEMICALS AND SUBSTANCES IN COSMETICS THAT HAVE CAUSED IMMEDIATE-TYPE REACTIONS

3.1 INGREDIENTS OF COSMETICS THAT HAVE CAUSED IMMEDIATE-TYPE REACTIONS

In this chapter, non-fragrance ingredients of cosmetics, that have caused immediate-type reactions, either from their presence in cosmetics or in other products, are presented. Possible symptoms (single or in combination) of such reactions include localized erythema, itching or tingling, localized urticaria, angioedema, generalized urticaria, respiratory symptoms (wheezing, dyspnea, asthma, rhinitis, nasal discharge), cardiac problems (hypotension, bradycardia, ventricular fibrillation or cardiac arrest), gastrointestinal symptoms (abdominal pain, diarrhea, nausea, vomiting) or even anaphylactic shock, which may be life-threatening in some patients and proved fatal in exceptional cases.

There are several possible pathomechanisms for immediate-type reactions. Some chemicals may induce non-immunological immediate-type reactions (e.g., non-immunological contact urticaria), such as benzoic acid, benzyl nicotinate, Capsicum frutescens resin, methyl nicotinate, sodium benzoate, and sorbic acid. As these effects are well-known and dose-dependent, non-immunological contact urticaria from such chemicals in cosmetics is rare nowadays. For some other chemicals, the pathomechanism of producing immediate contact reactions is not clear, for example for ammonium persulfate, which is widely used in hair-bleaching products. Immediate contact reactions with localized and generalized urticaria and rarely anaphylactic shock to this chemical are not uncommon and are seen both in individuals bleaching their hair or having it done and in hairdressers (Chapter 2.22 Ammonium persulfate). Other immediate reactions from ammonium persulfate include rhinitis and asthma, which occurs mainly as occupational disease in hairdressers and in workers in plants producing persulfates. The mechanism of the immediate reactions is as yet unclear. Positive prick tests, scratch and intradermal tests, skin application (sometimes with generalized urticaria or severe bronchial obstruction as result) and nasal and bronchial provocations with negative responses in controls strongly suggest immunoglobulin E (IgE)-mediated allergy, but passive transfer tests have been negative and in only a few studies has specific IgE to persulfate been demonstrated (see Chapter 2.22 Ammonium persulfate).

In most published case reports, an immunological mechanism was suspected or claimed on the basis of the rarity of such reactions, positive skin tests (scratch, prick, intradermal) and negative controls. True allergic immediate-type reactions to cosmetics with positive skin tests and/or positive basophil activation tests and/or specific IgE antibodies have been caused by, for example, their ingredients casein, equae lac (mare milk), goat milk, hydrolyzed wheat protein, and milk protein. Chemicals that have produced immunological immediate-type reactions from their presence in *non-cosmetic* products include chlorhexidine (in lubricant gel for urinary catheterization, skin disinfectants, chlorhexidine-coated central venous lines, disinfectants for mucous membranes, mouthwashes, corticosteroid cream) and CI 75470 (carmine) (in foods, drinks, pharmaceutical).

Table 3.1.1 lists all ingredients of cosmetic products, that have caused immediate contact reactions from their presence in cosmetic products, but that have *not* caused contact allergy and therefore are not discussed in Chapter 2. These are presented in this chapter as monographs.

Table 3.1.1 Ingredients of cosmetic products that have caused immediate contact reactions only

o-Aminophenol	Goat milk
Basic brown 17	Hydrolyzed elastin
Benzyl nicotinate	Hydroxypropyltrimonium hydrolyzed collagen
Capsicum frutescens (cayenne pepper) resin	Lecithin
Carum carvi (caraway) seed oil	Melissa officinalis flower/leaf/stem extract
Casein	Milk protein
Castanea sativa (chestnut) extract	Musa paradisiaca (banana) fruit
Citrus limon	Polyoxyethylenepolyoxypyrene glycol
Egg	Sodium methyl oleoyl taurate

Table 3.1.2 lists ingredients of cosmetics, which have caused both immediate-type reactions and allergic contact dermatitis. Their monographs can be found in Chapter 2 'Monographs of chemicals and substances in cosmetics that have caused allergic contact dermatitis'. In most, the reactions were caused by cosmetic products. Some, however, were the result of contact of the skin or mucous membranes with a non-cosmetic product (e.g., benzalkonium chloride and thimerosal in eye drops/contact lens solution, BHT in a plastic bag, benzoic acid in food, chlorhexidine in antiseptics, colophonium in soldering flux, didecyldimonium chloride in antiseptic/cleaning product, formaldehyde and paraformaldehyde in root canal disinfectants, hexylene glycol and sorbitan sesquioleate in a topical pharmaceutical, o-phenylphenol in plaster cast material), of ingestion (e.g., alcohol, Argania spinosa (argan) kernel oil, Chamomilla recutita (matricaria) tea [extract], chitosan, CI 75470 [carmine], Sesamum indicum (sesame) seed oil in

food and drinks, dibutyl phthalate in a pharmaceutical capsule) or of parenteral administration (e.g., Calendula officinalis infusion, benzalkonium chloride and chlorhexidine as a constituent of a central venous line, disodium EDTA and methylparaben in local anesthetics, polysorbate 80, vitamin K and propylparaben in drug injections).

Table 3.1.2 Ingredients of cosmetic products, that have caused both immediate contact reactions and allergic contact dermatitis [a]

Alcohol	Isopropyl alcohol
Allantoin	Isopropyl dibenzoylmethane
m-Aminophenol	Lanolin alcohol
p-Aminophenol	Lawsone
Ammonium persulfate	*p*-Methylaminophenol
Anthemis nobilis flower extract	Methylchloroisothiazolinone (and)
Argania spinosa (argan) kernel oil	methylisothiazolinone
Avena sativa (oat) bran extract	Methyl nicotinate
Basic blue 99	Methylparaben
Benzalkonium chloride	Panthenol
Benzoic acid	Paraben mix and unspecified parabens
Benzophenone-3	Paraformaldehyde
Benzophenone-4	PEG-6
Benzophenone-10	Petrolatum
BHA	Phenoxyethanol
BHT	*p*-Phenylenediamine
2-Bromo-2-nitropropane-1,3-diol	*o*-Phenylphenol
t-Butyl alcohol	Phytonadione
Calendula officinalis extract	Polyaminopropyl biguanide
Chamomilla recutita (matricaria) extract	Polysorbate 80
Chitosan gluconate	Potassium persulfate
Chlorhexidine digluconate	Propolis
p-Chloro-*m*-cresol	Propylene glycol
CI 75470 (carmine)	Propyl gallate
Colophonium	Quaternium-15
2,4-Diaminophenoxyethanol HCl	Quinine
Dibutyl phthalate	Sesamum indicum (sesame) seed oil
Didecyldimonium chloride	Sodium benzoate
Diethylstilbestrol	Sodium bisulfite
Disodium EDTA	Sodium lauryl sulfate
Disodium phenyl dibenzimidazole tetrasulfonate	Sodium metabisulfite
Equae lac	Sodium PCA
Ethylparaben	Sorbic acid
Formaldehyde	Sorbitan sesquioleate
Glyceryl thioglycolate	Tetrahydrocurcumin
Glycine soja seed extract	Thimerosal
Henna, black	Tioxolone
Henna, red	Tocopherol
Hexylene glycol	Toluene-2,5-diamine
Hydrolyzed collagen	Toluene-2,5-diamine sulfate
Hydrolyzed wheat protein	Triclosan
Imidazolidinyl urea	

[a] The monographs of these cosmetic ingredients are presented in Chapter 2

3.2 O-AMINOPHENOL

IDENTIFICATION

Description/definition	: *o*-Aminophenol is a substituted phenol that conforms to the formula shown below
Chemical class(es)	: Amines; color additives - hair; phenols
Chemical/IUPAC name	: 2-Aminophenol
Other names	: CI 76520; 1-amino-2-hydroxybenzene; 2-hydroxyaniline
CAS registry number (s)	: 95-55-6
EC number(s)	: 202-431-1
CIR review(s)	: J Am Coll Toxicol 1988;7:279-333 (access: www.cir-safety.org/ingredients)
SCCS opinion(s)	: SCCS/1291/10 (3)
Function(s) in cosmetics	: EU: formerly used for hair dyeing. USA: hair colorants
EU cosmetic restrictions	: Regulated in Annex II/1372 of the Regulation (EC) No. 344/2013 (prohibited)
Patch testing	: 1% pet.; testing for immediate contact reactions: no data available
Molecular formula	: C_6H_7NO

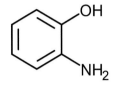

GENERAL

o-Aminophenol is used as a primary intermediate (synonyms: oxidation base, developer) in oxidative hair dying products. For the chemistry of hair dying see Chapter 2.359 *p*-Phenylenediamine. A review of contact urticaria caused by ingredients of cosmetics has been provided in 2016 (4).

IMMEDIATE-TYPE REACTIONS

One patient had an immediate contact reaction from *o*-aminophenol in a hair dye; specific data are lacking (article not read, in Japanese, data cited in ref. 2) (1).

CONTACT ALLERGY

Patch test sensitization

A patient was patch tested with 27 aromatic amines. After 48 and 72 hours, all tests were negative. A week later the patient reported with a focal flare of the test sites of *o*- and *p*-aminophenol, but there was no such reaction at the site of *m*-aminophenol. A repeat test with *m*-aminophenol was again negative (7). This may have been a case of patch test sensitization to *o*- and *p*-aminophenol, but it was not proven, as the patient had no repeat test to show a positive reaction after 2-3 days.

Presence in cosmetic products and chemical analyses

In the USA, in April 2017, *o*-aminophenol was present in 50 of 56,714 cosmetic products of which the composition is known in FDA's Voluntary Cosmetic Registration Program (VCRP) (data obtained from FDA, May 2017). In May 2017, *o*-aminophenol was present in 2 of 66,835 cosmetic products of which the composition is known in EWG's Skin Deep Cosmetics Database, USA (http://www.ewg.org/skindeep/). Of 15 hair dyes advertised as 'hypoallergenic', 'para-phenylenediamine-free', or 'non-allergenic', purchased in South Korea in 2015, 2 (13%) proved to contain *o*-amino-phenol (11).

In southern Germany, in 2013-2014, the labels of 924 permanent oxidative hair dyes were checked for the presence of hair dye components. There were 334 retail products (of seven different brands) and 590 professional products (of six different brands). The 924 products analyzed revealed a total of 58 different hair dye components, with retail products containing 32 and professional products 52. *o*-Aminophenol was present in 0.2% of the 924 products (6).

In 2013, in Korea, the labels of 99 oxidative hair dyes produced by Korean domestic manufacturers were examined for potent skin sensitizers. *o*-Aminophenol was found to be present in 17 (17%) of the hair dyes (9). In 2011, labels and other information on 365 hair dye products (282 permanent dyes, 79 semi-permanent dyes, 4 direct dyes) available on the Danish market (159 hair dyes for private use, 206 for professional use by hairdressers) were collected to identify the presence of sensitizers. *o*-Aminophenol was present in 13 (3.6%) of the products (5).

In August - October 2008, the labels of 122 oxidative hair dye products on the Swedish market were examined for the presence of hair dye substances categorized as potent skin sensitizers. *o*-Aminophenol was present in one of these products (8).

OTHER INFORMATION

Permeation of *o*-aminophenol through gloves has been investigated in ref. 10.

LITERATURE

1   Tsunoda T, Horiuchi N, Sato M. Two cases of contact urticaria syndrome by hair dye. Hifu 1993;35 (suppl. 16):178-183 (in Japanese) (data cited in ref. 2)

2   Oshima H, Tamaki T, Oh-I T, Koga M. Contact anaphylaxis due to para-aminophenol and para-methylamino-phenol in hair dye. Contact Dermatitis 2001;45:359

3   SCCS (Scientific Committee on Consumer Safety), Opinion on oaminophenol, 22 June 2010, SCCS/1291/10. Available at: http://ec.europa.eu/health/scientific_committees/consumer_safety/docs/sccs_o_025.pdf

4   Verhulst L, Goossens A. Cosmetic components causing contact urticaria: a review and update. Contact Dermatitis 2016;75:333-344

5   The Danish Environmental Protection Agency. Survey and occurrence of PPD, PTD and other allergenic hair dye substances in hair dyes. Copenhagen, Denmark: The Danish Environmental Protection Agency, 2013 (ISBN 978-87-92903-92-1). Available at: http://www2.mst.dk/Udgiv/publications/2013/02/978-87-92903-92-1.pdf

6   Kirchlecher S, Hübner A, Uter W. Survey of sensitizing constituents of oxidative hair dyes (retail and professional products) in Germany. J Dtsch Dermatol Ges 2016;14:707-715

7   Rudzki E, Napiórkowska T, Grzywa Z. Active sensitization to ortho and para-aminophenol with negative patch test to meta-aminophenol. Contact Dermatitis 1980;6:501

8   Yazar K, Boman A, Lidén C. Potent skin sensitizers in oxidative hair dye products on the Swedish market. Contact Dermatitis 2009;61:269-275

9   Kim H, Kim K. Prevalence of potent skin sensitizers in oxidative hair dye products in Korea. Cutan Ocul Toxicol 2016;35:204-207

10   Lee HS, Lin YW. Permeation of hair dye ingredients, *p*-phenylenediamine and aminophenol isomers, through protective gloves. Ann Occup Hyg 2009;53:289-296

11   Lee HJ, Kim WJ, Kim JY, Kim HS, Kim BS, Kim MB, Ko HC. Patch tests with commercial hair dye products in patients with allergic contact dermatitis to para-phenylenediamine. Indian J Dermatol Venereol Leprol 2016;82:645-650

3.3 BASIC BROWN 17

IDENTIFICATION

Description/definition : Basic brown 17 is the monoazo color that conforms to the formula shown below
Chemical class(es) : Color additives - hair
Chemical/IUPAC name : [8-[(4-Amino-3-nitrophenyl)azo]-7-hydroxy-2-naphthyl]trimethylammonium chloride
Other names : CI 12251
CAS registry number (s) : 68391-32-2
EC number(s) : 269-944-0
SCCS opinion(s) : SCCS/1448/11 (2); SCCP/1173/08 (3); SCCP/0683/03 (4); SCCS/1531/14 (5)
Function(s) in cosmetics : EU: hair dyeing. USA: hair colorants
Diagnostic testing : Prick testing 1% water (9)
Molecular formula : $C_{19}H_{20}ClN_5O_3$

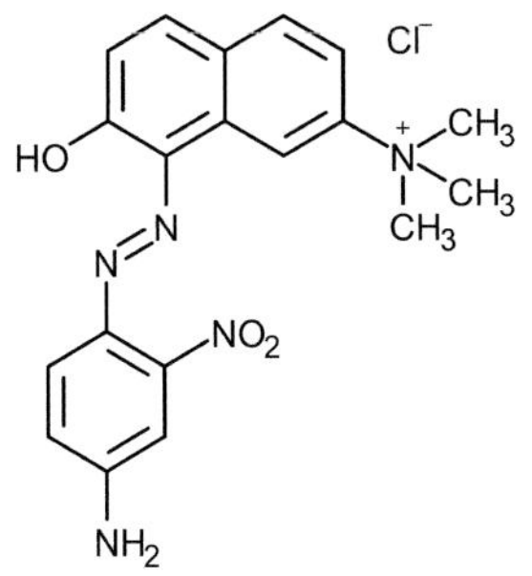

GENERAL

Basic brown 17 is used in semi-permanent non-oxidative hair dying products. It may contain up to 4.5% (w/w) basic red 118, corresponding to maximum 0.09% in a hair dye formulation. Basic red 118 according to the EU Cosmetic Regulation (Regulation 1223/2009) is not permitted for use in cosmetics except as an impurity in basic brown 17. Several other impurities including 2-nitrobenzene-1,4-diamine and NBTRI (7-hydroxy-*N,N,N*-trimethylnaphthalene-2-aminium chloride) may also be present in commercial batches of basic brown 17 (5).

A review of contact urticaria caused by ingredients of cosmetics has been provided in 2016 (6).

IMMEDIATE-TYPE REACTIONS

One patient allergic to a cosmetic had a positive prick test to basic brown 17; clinical details were not provided (1, likely the same patient as presented below [9]). A woman, formerly employed as a hairdresser but still practicing in her spare time, had allergic contact dermatitis of the hands and feet from hair dyes and shoes. In her history, she mentioned severe itching on the hands and in the ears, accompanied by a 'bad taste' in the mouth, immediately following the application of a particular dye to a client's scalp. Prick testing with the dye was performed, which resulted in a strong positive reaction within 15 minutes following the test. Additional prick tests with all ingredients of the product showed strong reactions to both basic brown 17 1% water and basic blue 99 1% water on two occasions. Patch testing with the same components remained negative. Additionally, the color solution was separated by thin-layer chromatography (TLC). Prick tests were performed with each spot (moistened with physiological saline) of the TLC strips. The patient showed positive immediate reactions to the main spots and to some other spots. This indicated, according to the authors, that the patient was probably also sensitized to some impurities present in the dye (9).

Presence in cosmetic products and chemical analyses

In the USA, in April 2017, basic brown 17 was present in 45 of 56,714 cosmetic products of which the composition is known in FDA's Voluntary Cosmetic Registration Program (VCRP) (data obtained from FDA, May 2017). In April 2017, basic brown 17 was present in one of 66,485 cosmetic products of which the composition is known in EWG's Skin Deep Cosmetics Database, USA (http://www.ewg.org/skindeep/). In 2011, labels and other information on 365 hair dye products (282 permanent dyes, 79 semi-permanent dyes, 4 direct dyes) available on the Danish market (159 hair dyes for private use, 206 for professional use by hairdressers) were collected to identify the presence of sensitizers.

Basic brown 17 was present in 5 (1.4%) products (7). In the USA, in 2012, ingredient labels of 107 different consumer oxidative hair dyes from 10 different companies were assessed in stores across the city of Phoenix, Arizona. Basic brown 17 was present in 3% of the products (8).

LITERATURE

1   Goossens A. Cosmetic contact allergens. Cosmetics 2016, 3, 5; doi:10.3390/cosmetics3010005
2   SCCS (Scientific Committee on Consumer Safety). Opinion on Basic Brown 17, 27 March 2012, SCCS/1448/11 Available at: http://ec.europa.eu/health/scientific_committees/consumer_safety/docs/sccs_o_086.pdf
3   SCCP (Scientific Committee on Consumer Products). Opinion on Basic Brown 17, 30 September 2008, SCCP/1173/08. Available at: http://ec.europa.eu/health/archive/ph_risk/committees/04_sccp/docs/sccp_o_145.pdf
4   SCCP (Scientific Committee on Consumer Products). Opinion on Basic Brown 17, 7 December 2004, SCCP/0683/03. Available at: http://ec.europa.eu/health/archive/ph_risk/committees/04_sccp/docs/sccp_o_011.pdf
5   SCCS (Scientific Committee on Consumer Safety), Opinion on Basic Brown 17, 24 March 2014, SCCS/1531/14. Available at: http://ec.europa.eu/health/scientific_committees/consumer_safety/docs/sccs_o_152.pdf
6   Verhulst L, Goossens A. Cosmetic components causing contact urticaria: a review and update. Contact Dermatitis 2016;75:333-344
7   The Danish Environmental Protection Agency. Survey and occurrence of PPD, PTD and other allergenic hair dye substances in hair dyes. Copenhagen, Denmark: The Danish Environmental Protection Agency, 2013 (ISBN 978-87-92903-92-1). Available at: http://www2.mst.dk/Udgiv/publications/2013/02/978-87-92903-92-1.pdf
8   Hamann D, Yazar K, Hamann CR, Thyssen JP, Lidén C. p-Phenylenediamine and other allergens in hair dye products in the United States: a consumer exposure study. Contact Dermatitis 2014;70:213-218
9   Vanden Broecke K, Bruze M, Persson L, Deroo H, Goossens A. Contact urticaria syndrome caused by direct hair dyes in a hairdresser. Contact Dermatitis 2014;71:124-126

3.4 BENZYL NICOTINATE

IDENTIFICATION

Description/definition	: Benzyl nicotinate is the ester of benzyl alcohol and nicotinic acid that conforms to the formula shown below
Chemical class(es)	: Esters; heterocyclic compounds
Chemical/IUPAC name	: Benzyl pyridine-3-carboxylate
Other names	: 3-Pyridinecarboxylic acid, phenylmethyl ester
CAS registry number (s)	: 94-44-0
EC number(s)	: 202-332-3
Merck Index monograph	: 7881
Function(s) in cosmetics	: EU: antistatic; skin conditioning. USA: skin-conditioning agents - miscellaneous
Diagnostic testing	: 2.5% pet., both for contact urticaria and contact allergy (3)
Molecular formula	: $C_{13}H_{11}NO_2$

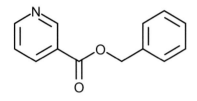

IMMEDIATE-TYPE REACTIONS

A young child rapidly developed an urticarial plaque on the right cheek, prompting an urgent consultation. He had not been taking any drugs and otherwise felt well. The patient's mother had kissed him on the right cheek while posing for a photograph moment before the lesion developed. She had applied a 'lip plumper' to her lips two hours earlier. On examination, the young boy was afebrile and his skin lesion had resolved after receiving an intravenous antihistamine. To reproduce the reaction, a small amount of lip plumper was applied to the mother's cheek. Immediately after application of the product, she experienced a tingling sensation followed by the formation of an urticarial plaque similar to the patient's lesion. The active ingredients of the lip plumper included benzyl nicotinate and Capsicum frutescens resin. Tests to identify the culprit ingredient were not performed; they may both have been contributory or responsible (1).

Lip plumpers are cosmetic agents intended to create the appearance of increased lip volume. The mechanisms by which lip plumpers act include vasodilation secondary to either irritant contact dermatitis or as part of non-immunologic contact urticaria. Common ingredients of lip plumpers are the essential oils of cinnamon and cayenne pepper (Capsicum frutescens), spices that are both irritants and urticariants, and nicotinates including benzyl nicotinate, which induce non-immunological erythema and possibly edema (contact urticaria) (1,3).

Presence in cosmetic products and chemical analyses

In the USA, in April 2017, benzyl nicotinate was present in 17 of 56,714 cosmetic products of which the composition is known in FDA's Voluntary Cosmetic Registration Program (VCRP) (data obtained from FDA, May 2017). In April 2017, benzyl nicotinate was present in 3 of 66,485 cosmetic products of which the composition is known in EWG's Skin Deep Cosmetics Database, USA (http://www.ewg.org/skindeep/).

OTHER SIDE EFFECTS

A patient with burning mouth syndrome had positive patch tests to benzyl nicotinate and propyl nicotinate 1% water. The authors stated that these chemicals may be used as rubefacients in toothpastes to improve the micro-circulation, particularly of the gingiva. However, such products had not been used by the patient for the past 2 years (2). Allergic contact dermatitis from benzyl nicotinate in a topical rubefacient preparation has been described (3).

LITERATURE

1   Firoz EF, Levin JM, Hartman RD, James WD. Lip plumper contact urticaria. J Am Acad Dermatol 2009;60:861-863
2   Haustein UF. Burning mouth syndrome due to nicotinic acid esters and sorbic acid. Contact Dermatitis 1988;19:225-226
3   Audicana M, Schmidt R, Fernández de Corres L. Allergic contact dermatitis from nicotinic acid esters. Contact Dermatitis 1990;22:60-61

3.5 CAPSICUM FRUTESCENS (CAYENNE PEPPER) RESIN

IDENTIFICATION

Description/definition	: Capsicum frutescens resin is a resinous material obtained from the cayenne pepper, *Capsicum frutescens* L., Solanaceae
Chemical class(es)	: Waxes
Other names	: Capsicum oleoresin
CAS registry number (s)	: 8023-77-6
EC number(s)	: 288-920-0
CIR review(s)	: Int J Toxicol 2007;26(Suppl.1):3-106 (access: www.cir-safety.org/ingredients)
Merck Index monograph	: 3042 (Capsicum)
Function(s) in cosmetics	: EU: cleansing; masking; tonic. USA: fragrance Ingredients; not reported
Diagnostic tests	: 1% alc. (advised for contact allergy testing) (2)

According to the Personal Care Products Council Ingredient Database, the accepted scientific name for *Capsicum frutescens* is *Capsicum annuum*. However, according to U.S. National Plant Germplasm System (https://npgsweb.ars-grin.gov/gringlobal/taxon/taxonomysimple.aspx), these are 2 separate species, *Capsicum annuum* being 'bell pepper'.

GENERAL

Discussion of side effects of Capsicum frutescens resin is limited to those caused by its presence in cosmetic products.

IMMEDIATE-TYPE REACTIONS

A young child rapidly developed an urticarial plaque on the right cheek, prompting an urgent consultation. He had not been taking any drugs and otherwise felt well. The patient's mother had kissed him on the right cheek while posing for a photograph moment before the lesion developed. She had applied a 'lip plumper' to her lips two hours earlier. On examination, the young boy was afebrile and his skin lesion had resolved after receiving an intravenous antihistamine. To reproduce the reaction, a small amount of lip plumper was applied to the mother's cheek. Immediately after application of the product, she experienced a tingling sensation followed by the formation of an urticarial plaque similar to the patient's lesion. The active ingredients of the lip plumper included Capsicum frutescens resin and benzyl nicotinate. Tests to identify the culprit ingredient were not performed; they may both have been contributory or responsible (1).

Lip plumpers are cosmetic agents intended to create the appearance of increased lip volume. The mechanisms by which lip plumpers act include vasodilation secondary to either irritant contact dermatitis or as part of non-immunologic contact urticaria. Common ingredients of lip plumpers are the essential oils of cinnamon and cayenne pepper (*Capsicum frutescens*), spices that are both irritants and urticariants, and nicotinates including benzyl nicotinate, which induce non-immunological erythema and possibly edema (contact urticaria) (1,3).

Presence in cosmetic products and chemical analyses

In the USA, in April 2017, Capsicum frutescens resin was present in 17 of 56,714 cosmetic products of which the composition is known in FDA's Voluntary Cosmetic Registration Program (VCRP) (data obtained from FDA, May 2017). In April 2017, Capsicum frutescens resin was present in 19 of 66,485 cosmetic products of which the composition is known in EWG's Skin Deep Cosmetics Database, USA (http://www.ewg.org/skindeep/).

LITERATURE

1   Firoz EF, Levin JM, Hartman RD, James WD. Lip plumper contact urticaria. J Am Acad Dermatol 2009;60:861-863
2   De Groot AC. Patch Testing, 3rd Edition. Wapserveen, The Netherlands: acdegroot publishing, 2008 (ISBN 978-90-813233-1-4)
3   Audicana M, Schmidt R, Fernández de Corres L. Allergic contact dermatitis from nicotinic acid esters. Contact Dermatitis 1990;22:60-61

3.6 CARUM CARVI (CARAWAY) SEED OIL

IDENTIFICATION

Description/definition	: Carum carvi seed oil is the fixed oil obtained from the seeds of caraway, *Carum carvi* L., Apiaceae
Chemical class(es)	: Fats and oils
INCI name USA	: Carum carvi (caraway) seed oil
Other name(s)	: Caraway seed oil
CAS registry number (s)	: 235433-20-2; 8000-42-8
Merck Index monograph	: 3049
Function(s) in cosmetics	: EU: emollient; masking; solvent. USA: fragrance ingredients
Diagnostic testing	: No data available

IMMEDIATE-TYPE REACTIONS

A patient had an urticarial reaction to caraway seed oil (1). Apparently, it was a constituent of a toothpaste, and when the product was patch tested, it gave an urticarial reaction with a 'sub shock condition'. Presumably, the causal ingredient was caraway seed oil. Whether the toothpaste also caused contact urticaria of the lips and/or the oral mucosa when used by the patient, is unknown (1).

Presence in cosmetic products and chemical analyses

In the USA, in April 2017, caraway oil was present in 1 of 56,714 cosmetic products of which the composition is known in FDA's Voluntary Cosmetic Registration Program (VCRP) (data obtained from FDA, May 2017). In April 2017, Carum carvi seed oil was present in 3 of 66,485 cosmetic products of which the composition is known in EWG's Skin Deep Cosmetics Database, USA (http://www.ewg.org/skindeep/).

LITERATURE

1 Heygi E, Dolesalová A. Urticarial reaction after patch tests of toothpastes with a sub shock condition: Hypersensitivity to caraway seed. Cs Derm 1976;51:19 (data cited in ref. 2)
2 De Groot AC, Weyland JW, Nater JP. Unwanted effects of cosmetics and drugs used in dermatology, 3rd Edition. Amsterdam – London – New York – Tokyo: Elsevier, 1994: 158

3.7 CASEIN

IDENTIFICATION

Description/definition   : Casein is a mixture of phosphoproteins obtained from cow's milk
Chemical class(es)   : Proteins
Other names   : Milk protein, casein
CAS registry number (s)   : 9000-71-9
EC number(s)   : 232-555-1
Merck Index monograph : 3153
Function(s) in cosmetics : EU: antistatic; hair conditioning; skin conditioning. USA: hair conditioning agents; skin-
                            conditioning agents - miscellaneous
Diagnostic testing   : Prick test, RAST

GENERAL

Discussion of side effects of casein including immediate contact reactions is limited to those caused by its presence in cosmetic products or in cosmeceuticals (diaper ointments).

IMMEDIATE-TYPE REACTIONS

In patients with food allergies such as milk protein, cosmetic and pharmaceutical products containing such allergenic food proteins can cause severe anaphylactic type-1 allergic reactions (1,2,3).

An 11-month-old infant who had two to three previous episodes of anaphylaxis to cow's milk, manifesting projectile vomiting, diarrhea, generalized urticaria, and wheezing after ingestion of minimal amounts of cow's milk, exhibited similar symptoms after the application of a cream to the area of the napkin or diaper dermatitis. Prick tests with milk albumin and casein, the latter of which was present in the product, were strongly positive (1).

A 12-month-old boy, with a strong history of cow's milk allergy, developed two episodes of anaphylaxis following cutaneous application of a casein-containing ointment to an inflamed diaper area. RAST testing showed a significant elevation in specific IgE antibodies to milk and milk proteins (2).

A woman with no personal or family history of atopy presented with a 4-year history of attacks of neck pruritus which became generalized, with hives and tongue edema, nausea, vomiting, diarrhea, dizziness, tachycardia, profuse sweating, and death feeling. Every attack happened a few minutes after the ingestion of milk or milk-containing products (cheese, butter, yogurt, et cetera). When tested with prick tests, specific IgE determination and immune-blotting, she proved to be allergic to casein. Later, the patient had an attack of generalized skin pruritus, dizziness, tachycardia, and profuse sweating immediately after the application to her face of a make-up remover. She had never used it before, and the product proved to contain casein (4).

Two children developed generalized urticaria from baby wipes containing cow's milk. Prick tests showed them to be allergic to milk, casein, α-lactoalbumine and β-lactoglobuline (5).

Presence in cosmetic products and chemical analyses

In the USA, in April 2017, casein hydrolysate was present in 11 of 56,714 cosmetic products of which the composition is known in FDA's Voluntary Cosmetic Registration Program (VCRP) (data obtained from FDA, May 2017). In March 2017, casein was present in 3 (sodium caseinate) and one (hydrolyzed casein) of 64,983 cosmetic products of which the composition is known in EWG's Skin Deep Cosmetics Database, USA (http://www.ewg.org/skindeep/).

LITERATURE

1   Lecks H-I. Anaphylaxis from milk protein in diaper ointment. JAMA 1980;244:1560
2   Jarmoc L-M, Primack W-A. Anaphylaxis to cutaneous exposure to milk protein in a diaper rash ointment.
      Clin Pediatr (Phila) 1987;26:154-155
3   Wang J, Nowak-Wegrzyn A. Reactions of 2 young children with milk allergy after cutaneous exposure to milk-
      containing cosmetic products. Arch Pediatr Adolesc Med 2004;158:1089-1093
4   Tabar AI, Alvarez MJ, Echechipía S, Acero S, Garcia BE, Olaguíbel JM. Anaphylaxis from cow's milk casein. Allergy
      1996;51:343-345
5   González Rodríguez MP, González Hernández A, Martín Muñoz MF. Generalized urticarial reaction after the use
      of baby wipes. An Pediatr (Barc) 2008;68:198-200 (Article in Spanish)

3.8 CASTANEA SATIVA (CHESTNUT) EXTRACT

IDENTIFICATION

Description/definition : Castanea sativa extract is an extract of parts of the chestnut, *Castanea sativa*, Fagaceae; the extract may be obtained from the bark, bud, flower, leaf, pericarp, seed or shell
Chemical class(es) : Botanical products and botanical derivatives
INCI name USA : Castanea sativa (chestnut) extract
Other name(s) : Chestnut extract
CAS registry number (s) : 84695-99-8
EC number(s) : 283-619-0
Function(s) in cosmetics : EU: skin conditioning or skin protecting. USA: skin conditioning agents – miscellaneous or skin protectants
Diagnostic testing : Prick tests, specific IgE determination

GENERAL

Discussion of side effects of Castanea sativa extract in this chapter is limited to reactions caused by its presence in cosmetic products.

IMMEDIATE-TYPE REACTIONS

Chestnut (*Castanea sativa*) is a member of the Fagaceae family. In contrast to Asia, the consumption of chestnuts is limited in Central Europe, with cooked preparations being preferred. While chestnut allergy is very rare in Central Europe, it is quite frequent in Korea, where it accounts for up to 3.2% of all food allergies (2). Most cases of IgE-mediated hypersensitivity to chestnuts have been attributed to the so-called latex-fruit syndrome, in which ingestion of fruits such as avocado, kiwi, banana, and, more rarely, chestnut lead to urticaria and anaphylaxis in latex-sensitized individuals. The latex-fruit syndrome is caused by cross-reactivity (3,4). However, chestnut allergy may also occur – as in this patient - independently of the latex-fruit syndrome and latex allergy (5).

Within 5 minutes of application of a facial peeling mask containing abrasives, chestnut and almond extracts, a 16-year-old woman developed wheals, swelling, and redness of the face followed by angioedema and subsequent collapse (1). Earlier, the patient had experienced swelling of the face after ingestion of a fresh mango and of a fresh lychee. Skin prick tests revealed a positive reaction to the facial peeling mask, while 5 healthy volunteers were negative. Prick-to-prick-testing with foods showed positive reactions to chestnut, mango and lychee. Prick testing with two commercially available latex extracts was negative. The total serum IgE level was normal and no allergen-specific IgE was detected against chestnut, mango, latex, kiwi, or almond. After completion of the allergological workup the patient was advised to avoid not only consumption of chestnut, mango, and lychee but also cutaneous contact with these foods (1).

Presence in cosmetic products and chemical analyses

In April 2017, Castanea sativa (chestnut) extract was present in 4 and in 10 (seed extract) of 66,485 cosmetic products of which the composition is known in EWG's Skin Deep Cosmetics Database, USA (http://www.ewg.org/skin deep/).

LITERATURE

1   Seitz CS, Trautmann A. Cosmetic facial peel-induced contact anaphylaxis: chestnut allergy without latex-fruit syndrome. J Investig Allergol Clin Immunol 2011;21:494-495
2   Lee SK, Yoon SH, Kim SH, Choi JH, Park HS. Chestnut as a food allergen: Identification of major allergens. J Korean Med Sci 2005;20:573-578
3   Díaz-Perales A, Collada C, Blanco C, Sánchez-Monge R, Carrillo T, Aragoncillo C, Salcedo G. Class I chitinases with hevein-like domain, but not class II enzymes, are relevant chestnut and avocado allergens. J Allergy Clin Immunol 1998;102:127-133
4   Raulf-Heimsoth M, Kespohl S, Crespo JF, Rodriguez J, Feliu A, Brüning T, Rihs HP. Natural rubber latex and chestnut allergy: cross-reactivity or co-sensitization? Allergy 2007;62:1277-1281
5   Sánchez-Monge R, Blanco C, López-Torrejon G, Cumplido J, Recas M, Figueroa J, Carillo T, Salcedo G. Differential allergen sensitization patterns in chestnut allergy with or without associated latex-fruit syndrome. J Allergy Clin Immunol 2006;118:705-710

3.9 CITRUS LIMON (LEMON)

IMMEDIATE-TYPE REACTIONS

A 26-year-old man with a history of mild asthma had an episode of anaphylaxis after showering and washing his torso and face with lemon-impregnated soap. He reported experiencing anaphylaxis previously on ingestion of whole crushed orange juice and citrus seeds, including lemon, orange, and mandarin seeds, but not processed citrus fruit juices. Such reactions occurred in a stereotypical fashion, producing laryngeal edema, generalized urticaria, and asthma symptoms within minutes of ingestion. He experienced similar symptoms after ingestion of peanut and tree nuts, including hazelnut, Brazil nut, macadamia nut, pine nut, and almond. Skin prick testing against a standard panel of aeroallergens revealed the patient to be non-atopic. Serum IgE antibodies against peanut, orange, lemon, walnut, and hazelnut were demonstrated.

Numerous IgE-reactive proteins have been demonstrated in several citrus seed extracts and peanut extract. Complete IgE cross-reactivity was demonstrated among the different citrus seed extracts. Partial cross-reactivity was demonstrated between the peanut and orange seed extracts. The patient was advised to avoid all tree nuts, peanut, and citrus fruits and was prescribed an auto-injectable adrenaline pen. Unfortunately, the exact nature of the lemon material in the soap was not mentioned.

LITERATURE

1   Glaspole IN, de Leon MP, Rolland JM, O'Hehir RE. Anaphylaxis to lemon soap: citrus seed and peanut allergen cross-reactivity. Ann Allergy Asthma Immunol 2007;98:286-289

3.10 EGG

IDENTIFICATION

Description/definition : Egg is the entire content of chicken eggs
Chemical class(es) : Biological products
Other names : Ovum; whole fresh eggs
Function(s) in cosmetics : EU: hair conditioning; skin conditioning. USA: hair conditioning agents; skin-conditioning agents - miscellaneous
Patch testing : 1% and 0.1% in physiologic saline, for immediate open testing (1)

GENERAL

Discussion of immediate contact reactions / type-I allergy to egg in this chapter is limited to reactions caused by its presence in cosmetic products. A review of contact urticaria caused by ingredients of cosmetics has been provided in 2016 (3). Type-I allergic reactions to egg from its presence in vaccines in presensitized individuals, which can manifest as safe administration without any adverse reactions, urticaria, airway problems, anaphylaxis and even fatality, have been reviewed in 2012 (4).

IMMEDIATE-TYPE REACTIONS

A child known to be allergic to egg (positive prick test) had persistent (atopic) dermatitis of the face. Elimination of egg and egg-containing products gave no relief. The mother proved to wash her baby's hair with an egg-containing shampoo. After discontinuation of its use, the (atopic) dermatitis of the face cleared completely (2). A woman treated her hair with a homemade egg-white based mask once weekly. After one year, the ingestion of egg triggered rhinitis, choking and systemic urticaria (5).

Another woman applied a cosmetic skin mask formulation to her face and noted rapid onset of transient rash, burning, stinging and itching at the application sites. Immediate open testing (without prick, scratch or chamber) to intact forearm skin revealed extensive wheal and flare to the following components of the formulation: whole egg (0.1% and 1% in physiologic saline), lecithin, allantoin, aloe gel, chamomile extract, Melissa extract (all 1%) and the final formulation as is (skin mask). The saline control was negative, as were similar applications of the above to 10 controls. This would therefore appear to be immunologic contact urticaria. According to the authors, this multiplicity of positive immediate-type reactions suggests the possibility of an immediate-type hypersensitivity analogue of the excited skin syndrome seen in delayed-type testing, common chemical constituents in these natural products, or an individual with a unique immunologic system (1).

Presence in cosmetic products and chemical analyses

In the USA, in April 2017, egg was present in 2 of 56,714 cosmetic products of which the composition is known in FDA's Voluntary Cosmetic Registration Program (VCRP) (data obtained from FDA, May 2017). In April 2017, egg (egg, ovum, egg powder and egg white powder) was present in 9 of 64,536 cosmetic products of which the composition is known in EWG's Skin Deep Cosmetics Database, USA (http://www.ewg.org/skindeep/).

LITERATURE

1 West I, Maibach HI. Contact urticaria syndrome from multiple cosmetic components. Contact Dermatitis 1995;32:121
2 Codreanu F, Morisset M, Cordebar V, Kanny G, Moneret-Vautrin DA. Risk of allergy to food proteins in topical medicinal agents and cosmetics. Eur Ann Allergy Clin Immunol 2006;38:126-130
3 Verhulst L, Goossens A. Cosmetic components causing contact urticaria: a review and update. Contact Dermatitis 2016;75:333-344
4 Leventhal JS, Berger EM, Brauer JA, Cohen DE. Hypersensitivity reactions to vaccine constituents: a case series and review of the literature. Dermatitis 2012;23:102-109
5 Antonicelli L, Braschi MC, Cinti B. Hen egg hair mask-induced food allergy: a case report. Eur Ann Allergy Clin Immunol 2011;43:127-128

3.11 GOAT MILK

IDENTIFICATION

Description/definition   : Goat milk is whole milk obtained from goats
Chemical class(es)   : Biological products
Other names   : Caprae lac; milk, goat
Function(s) in cosmetics : EU: skin conditioning. USA: skin-conditioning agents - miscellaneous

GENERAL

IgE-mediated allergy to goat's milk has been reported (6) and is far from rare. The most common food allergy in early childhood is cow's milk (CM) allergy, affecting 2-3% of infants. As goat's or sheep's milk (GSM) proteins are highly homologous to CM proteins, clinical cross-reactivity is expected and IgE sensitization to GSM proteins has been found to be as high as 92-98% in children with IgE-mediated CM allergy (2,3), sometimes with very serious anaphylactic reactions (9). Conversely, CM-tolerant individuals should also tolerate GSM. However, several cases of GSM allergy without CM allergy have been reported (4,5,7). Further discussion of these reactions outside the context of goat's milk in cosmetics is considered to fall outside the scope of this book.

IMMEDIATE-TYPE REACTIONS

A woman, who had lifelong extensive atopic dermatitis, had been frequently applying a skin moisturizer that contained goat's milk for several weeks. After an application resulted in acute erythema and itch, she subsequently ceased using the product. Four months later, the patient developed a generalized allergic reaction, characterized by urticaria and rapidly evolving oral and upper airway angioedema, immediately after eating 2 mouthfuls of a salad at a restaurant. Serum-specific IgE was strongly positive for goat's milk (65.7 kU/L) and negative for mustard. The remaining salad ingredients have subsequently been eaten without reaction, and she regularly consumes cow's milk products. The patient confirmed ingestion of goat's cheese without any adverse effects before the use of the moisturizer. A basophil activation test (an *in vitro* test for functional IgE reactivity) resulted in dose-dependent basophil activation to both the goat's milk extract and the moisturizing product. IgE immunoblotting revealed serum IgE binding to components in both the moisturizing product and goat's milk, consistent with the ImmunoCAP and basophil activation test results. The authors concluded that IgE-mediated sensitization occurred during application of the moisturizer that contained goat's milk to inflamed, eczematous skin, which resulted in the generalized allergic reaction when the foodstuff was subsequently encountered orally (1).

Another woman also developed goat cheese anaphylaxis. She had been using goat milk soap (various brands) to treat dry skin and mild eczema previously At one point, she experienced itchy mouth while eating goat cheese, and later in the year, she had contact urticaria after applying goat milk moisturizer (8).

LITERATURE

1   Voskamp AL, Zubrinich CM, Abramovitch JB, Rolland JM, O'Hehir RE. Goat's cheese anaphylaxis after cutaneous sensitization by moisturizer that contained goat's milk. J Allergy Clin Immunol Pract 2014;2:629-630
2   Bellioni-Businco B, Paganelli R, Lucenti P, Giampietro PG, Perborn H, Businco L. Allergenicity of goat's milk in children with cow's milk allergy. J Allergy Clin Immunol 1999;103:1191-1194
3   Bernard H, Creminon C, Yvon M, Wal JM. Specificity of the human IgE response to the different purified caseins in allergy to cow's milk proteins. Int Arch Allergy Immunol 1998;115:235-244
4   Hazebrouck S, Ah-Leung S, Bidat E, Paty E, Drumare MF, Tilleul S, Adel-Patient K, Wal JM, Bernard H. Goat's milk allergy without cow's milk allergy: suppression of non-cross-reactive epitopes on caprine β-casein. Clin Exp Allergy 2014;44:602-610
5   Ah-Leung S, Bernard H, Bidat E, Paty E, Rancé F, Scheinmann P, Wal JM. Allergy to goat and sheep milk without allergy to cow's milk. Allergy 2006;61:1358-1365
6   Orlando JP, Breton-Bouveyron A. Anaphylactoid reaction to goat's milk. Allerg Immunol (Paris) 2000;32:231-232
7   Viñas M, Carnés J, López-Matas MA, Hernández N, Castillo MJ, Ibero M. Allergy to goat and sheep cheese with tolerance to cow's milk and its derivatives. Allergol Immunopathol (Madr) 2014;42:186-190
8   Mullins RJ. Allergy to topical and oral goat products. Med J Aust 2012;197:148-149
9   Pessler F, Nejat M. Anaphylactic reaction to goat's milk in a cow's milk-allergic infant. Pediatr Allergy Immunol 2004;15:183-185

3.12 HYDROLYZED ELASTIN

IDENTIFICATION

Description/definition	: Hydrolyzed elastin is the hydrolysate of elastin derived by acid, enzyme or other method of hydrolysis
Chemical class(es)	: Protein derivatives (including salts)
Other names	: Elastin, hydrolysate; hydrolyzed animal elastin; hydrolyzed elastin solution; proteins, elastin, hydrolysate
CAS registry number (s)	: 91080-18-1
EINECS number(s)	: 293-509-4
Function(s) in cosmetics	: EU: antistatic; film forming; hair conditioning; humectant; skin conditioning. USA: hair conditioning agents; skin-conditioning agents - emollient; skin-conditioning agents – miscellaneous
Diagnostic testing	: RAST, immunoblot analysis

GENERAL
It is uncertain whether the hydrolyzed fish elastin in the case presented below is hydrolyzed (animal) elastin as per this chapter's INCI name.

IMMEDIATE-TYPE REACTIONS
A woman had experienced a number of episodes of fish allergy since she was 2 years of age, consisting of respiratory distress and widespread wheals within 15 minutes after eating fish. At the age of 20, when she drank a fish collagen-containing beverage, she had oropharyngeal irritation, rhinorrhea, and facial angioedema, followed by widespread urticaria and respiratory distress. Four years later, an urticarial eruption developed at the site where a cosmetic cream containing codfish-derived elastin was applied. The patient's serum total IgE level was 442 kU/l (normal, <170 kU/l). The RAST scores for specific IgE were strongly positive to many fish species including codfish. The patient's serum proved to contain IgE-antibodies that reacted with proteins of MW 10,000-15,000 or 15,000-20,000, corresponding to codfish elastin. By immunoblot analysis, it was shown that there were IgE antibodies against codfish elastin as well as against other common allergenic proteins: parvalbumin, collagen and transferrin (1).

Elastin, which is commonly used for cosmetics as topical formulations, has been isolated from bovine tendon. Because of the risk of bovine spongiform encephalopathy, however, elastin has recently been extracted from fish, in particular from the aortic arch and skin of codfish, bonito, yellowtail, and tuna. According to the producer of the incriminated cosmetic, the elastin material for the cosmetic used by this patient was derived from the skin and soft tissue of codfish (1).

Presence in cosmetic products and chemical analyses
In the USA, in April 2017, hydrolyzed elastin was present in 279 of 56,714 cosmetic products of which the composition is known in FDA's Voluntary Cosmetic Registration Program (VCRP) (data obtained from FDA, May 2017). In April 2017, hydrolyzed elastin was present in 78 of 66,485 cosmetic products of which the composition is known in EWG's Skin Deep Cosmetics Database, USA (http://www.ewg.org/skindeep/).

LITERATURE
1   Nishida K, Tateishi C, Tsuruta D, Shimauchi T, Ito T, Hirakawa S, Tokura Y. Contact urticaria caused by a fish-derived elastin-containing cosmetic cream. Contact Dermatitis 2012;67:171-172

3.13 HYDROXYPROPYLTRIMONIUM HYDROLYZED COLLAGEN

IDENTIFICATION

Description/definition : Hydroxypropyltrimonium hydrolyzed collagen is the quaternary ammonium chloride formed from the reaction of hydroxypropyl trimethylamine with hydrolyzed collagen. It conforms generally to the formula shown below, where R represents the hydrolyzed collagen moiety

Chemical class(es) : Protein derivatives; quaternary ammonium compounds

Chemical/IUPAC name : Collagen, hydrolyzed, *N*-(3-trimethylammonio-2-hydroxypropyl)-, chlorides

Other names : Stearyltrimonium hydroxyethyl hydrolyzed collagen; collagen, hydrolyzed, *N*-(3-trimethylammonio-2-hydroxypropyl)-, chlorides; hydroxypropyltrimonium hydrolysed animal protein

CAS registry number (s) : 11308-59-1; 83138-06-1; 111174-62-0

Function(s) in cosmetics : EU: antistatic; hair conditioning; skin conditioning. USA: antistatic agents; hair conditioning agents; skin-conditioning agents - miscellaneous

Patch testing : prick tests with 1%, 0.1% and 0.01% in water (3)

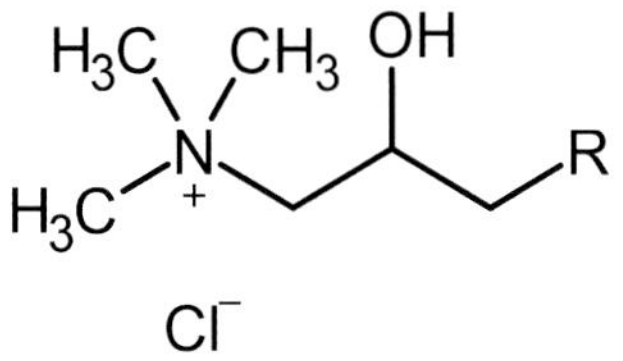

IMMEDIATE-TYPE REACTIONS

Three patients suffering from atopic dermatitis had contact urticaria from hair conditioners containing hydroxyl-propyltrimonium hydrolyzed collagen, two on the head and one, a hairdresser, on the hands. They had positive prick tests to the conditioner and to the collagen (1% water) and a positive open test to the cosmetic. Specific IgE was demonstrated. One patient also had a strongly positive prick test to hydroxypropyltrimonium hydrolyzed milk protein and two had weakly positive prick tests to hydrolyzed collagen (Nutrilan® H) (1). A young woman developed contact urticaria after the application of a hair conditioner; prick tests were positive to the cosmetic and to its ingredient hydroxypropyltrimonium hydrolyzed collagen down to 0.01% water (3). Another female patient developed contact urticaria accompanied by conjunctivitis, rhinitis, dyspnea, wheezing and a dry cough after the application of a hair conditioner on the scalp; she also had positive prick tests to the conditioner and to 'hydrolyzed proteins', which contained hydrolyzed bovine collagen and stearyl trimethyl ammonium chloride (= hydroxypropyl-trimonium hydrolyzed collagen) (4).

Two patients with immunologic contact urticaria from a hair conditioner containing a 'quaternized collagen hydrolyzate' have been reported. Both patients had a previous history of atopy with allergic seasonal rhinitis and hand eczema. The first patient was a hairdresser who noticed itching erythema and urticarial swelling on the hands after handling a protein hair conditioner. The other patient was a woman, who felt burning and itching on her scalp and face 5 minutes after a hairdresser had applied the same hair conditioner on her hair. Within a few minutes, generalized urticaria developed. Both individuals showed strongly positive immediate skin test reactions to the hair conditioner. Specific IgE for the protein hydrolysate was demonstrated in their sera (2).

Presence in cosmetic products and chemical analyses

In the USA, in April 2017, hydroxypropyltrimonium hydrolyzed collagen was present in 2 of 56,714 cosmetic products of which the composition is known in FDA's Voluntary Cosmetic Registration Program (VCRP) (data obtained from FDA, May 2017). In April 2017, hydroxypropyltrimonium hydrolyzed collagen was present in 5 of 66,485 cosmetic products of which the composition is known in EWG's Skin Deep Cosmetics Database, USA (http://www.ewg.org/skindeep/).

LITERATURE

1 Niinimäki A, Niinimäki M, Mäkinen-Kiljunen S, Hannuksela M. Contact urticaria from protein hydrolysates in hair conditioners. Allergy 1998;53:1078-1082
2 Kousa M. Strand R, Makinen-Kiljunen S, Hannuksela M. Contact urticaria from hair conditioner. Contact Dermatitis 1990;23:279
3 Freeman S, Lee M-S. Contact urticaria to hair conditioner. Contact Dermatitis 1996;35:195-196
4 Pasche-Koo F, Claes M, Hauser C. Contact urticaria with systemic symptoms caused by bovine collagen in a hair conditioner. Am J Contact Dermatitis 1996;7:56-58

3.14 LECITHIN

IDENTIFICATION

Description/definition	: Lecithin is a complex mixture of phosphatides, consisting chiefly of phosphatidylcholine, phosphatidylethanolamine, phosphatidylserine, and phosphatidylinositol, with varying amounts of triglycerides, fatty acids, and carbohydrates isolated from animal or vegetable sources
Chemical class(es)	: Glyceryl esters and derivatives; phosphorus compounds
Other names	: Lecithins
CAS registry number (s)	: 8002-43-5; 8030-76-0 (lecithins, soybean); 93685-90-6 (lecithins, egg yolk)
EC number(s)	: 232-307-2; 310-129-7; 297-639-2
CIR review(s)	: Int J Toxicol 2001;20(Suppl.1):21-45; Final report, March 2015 (access: www.cir-safety.org/ingredients)
Merck Index monograph	: 6753
Function(s) in cosmetics	: EU: antistatic; emollient; emulsifying; skin conditioning. USA: skin-conditioning agents – miscellaneous; surfactants - emulsifying agents
Diagnostic	: 1% physiologic saline for immediate open testing (1)

GENERAL

Discussion of side effects of lecithin in this chapter is limited to reactions caused by its presence in cosmetic products.

IMMEDIATE-TYPE REACTIONS

A woman applied a cosmetic skin mask formulation to her face and noted rapid onset of transient rash, burning, stinging and itching at the application sites. Immediate open testing (without prick, scratch or chamber) to intact forearm skin revealed extensive wheal and flare to the following components of the formulation: lecithin (1% physiologic saline), whole egg (0.1% and 1%), allantoin, aloe gel, chamomile extract, Melissa extract (all 1%) and the final formulation as is (skin mask). The saline control was negative, as were similar applications of the above to 10 controls. This would therefore appear to be immunologic contact urticaria. According to the authors, this multiplicity of positive immediate-type reactions suggests the possibility of an immediate-type hypersensitivity analogue of the excited skin syndrome seen in delayed-type testing, common chemical constituents in these natural products, or an individual with a unique immunologic system (1).

Presence in cosmetic products and chemical analyses

In the USA, in April 2017, lecithin was present in 2603 of 56,714 cosmetic products of which the composition is known in FDA's Voluntary Cosmetic Registration Program (VCRP) (data obtained from FDA, May 2017). In April 2017, lecithin was present in 1656 of 66,485 cosmetic products of which the composition is known in EWG's Skin Deep Cosmetics Database, USA (http://www.ewg.org/skindeep/).

LITERATURE

1   West I, Maibach HI. Contact urticaria syndrome from multiple cosmetic components. Contact Dermatitis 1995;32:121

3.15 MELISSA OFFICINALIS FLOWER/LEAF/STEM EXTRACT

IDENTIFICATION

Description/definition : Melissa officinalis flower/leaf/stem extract is an extract of the flowers, leaves and stems of the balm mint, *Melissa officinalis* L., Labiatae

Chemical class(es) : Botanical products and botanical derivatives

CAS registry number (s) : 84082-61-1

EC number(s) : 282-007-0

Function(s) in cosmetics : EU: soothing; tonic. USA: fragrance ingredients; skin-conditioning agents – miscellaneous

Diagnostic testing : 1% physiologic saline for immediate open testing (1)

GENERAL

Discussion of side effects of Melissa officinalis extract in this chapter is limited to reactions from its presence in cosmetic products.

IMMEDIATE-TYPE REACTIONS

A woman applied a cosmetic skin mask formulation to her face and noted rapid onset of transient rash, burning, stinging and itching at the application sites. Immediate open testing (without prick, scratch or chamber) to intact forearm skin revealed extensive wheal and flare to the following components of the formulation: Melissa extract (1% physiologic saline), whole egg (0.1% and 1%), lecithin, allantoin, aloe gel, chamomile extract (all 1%) and the final formulation as is (skin mask). The saline control was negative, as were similar applications of the above to 10 controls. This would therefore appear to be immunologic contact urticaria. According to the authors, this multiplicity of positive immediate-type reactions suggests the possibility of an immediate-type hypersensitivity analogue of the excited skin syndrome seen in delayed-type testing, common chemical constituents in these natural products, or an individual with a unique immunologic system (1).

Presence in cosmetic products and chemical analyses

In the USA, in April 2017, Melissa officinalis leaf extract was present in 156 of 56,714 cosmetic products of which the composition is known in FDA's Voluntary Cosmetic Registration Program (VCRP) (data obtained from FDA, May 2017). In April 2017, Melissa extract was present in 85 (Melissa officinalis extract) and 88 (Melissa officinalis leaf extract) products of 66,485 cosmetic products of which the composition is known in EWG's Skin Deep Cosmetics Database, USA (http://www.ewg.org/skindeep/).

LITERATURE

1   West I, Maibach HI. Contact urticaria syndrome from multiple cosmetic components. Contact Dermatitis 1995;32:121

3.16 MILK PROTEIN

IDENTIFICATION

Description/definition   : Milk protein is a mixture of proteins obtained from cow's milk
Chemical class(es)   : Proteins
Other names   : Proteins, milk; Lactis proteinum (EU)
CAS registry number (s)   : 91053-68-8
Merck Index monograph   : 7543 (milk)
Function(s) in cosmetics : EU: hair conditioning; skin conditioning. USA: hair conditioning agents; skin-conditioning agents - miscellaneous
Patch test allergens   : prick tests; RAST

GENERAL

Discussion of side effects of milk protein in this chapter is limited to reactions caused by its presence in cosmetic products.

IMMEDIATE-TYPE REACTIONS

A 2½-year-old boy with severe eczema and milk allergy (serum milk IgE level, 17.5 kIU/L; a level 15 kIU/L has a 95% positive predictive value for acute allergic reactions) developed a diffuse pruritic rash and emesis 2 to 3 hours after bathing in a 'calming milk', which contains milk protein. There were no other known exposures to milk that day. The reaction was attributed to skin contact with the cosmetic product (1). A 3-year-old girl with a known non-IgE mediated allergy to milk developed an erythematous maculopapular rash and angioedema 24 hours following application of a 'buttermilk lotion' which contains milk powder, to her face. Milk allergy was previously diagnosed after recurrent episodes of emesis, abdominal pain, and distention within 2 hours after ingesting milk-containing products. No other exposures to milk during these same 24 hours were noted (1). These two patients were also discussed in ref. 2.

An infant with atopic dermatitis and cow's milk allergy developed contact urticaria from a topical medicinal agent containing *Lactis proteinum* (milk protein) (3). Another infant suffering from atopic dermatitis and known to be allergic to cow's milk had generalized contact urticaria after using a soap containing micronized milk serum. Prick tests were positive to the soap and to cow's milk (3). Two children developed generalized urticaria from baby wipes containing cow's milk. Prick tests showed them to be allergic to milk, casein, α-lactoalbumine and β-lactoglobuline (4).

Presence in cosmetic products and chemical analyses

In the USA, in April 2017, milk protein was present in 35 of 56,714 cosmetic products of which the composition is known in FDA's Voluntary Cosmetic Registration Program (VCRP) (data obtained from FDA, May 2017). In January 2017, milk protein was present in 17 of 64,655 cosmetic products of which the composition is known in EWG's Skin Deep Cosmetics Database, USA (http://www.ewg.org/skindeep/).

LITERATURE

1   Wang J. Reactions of two young children with milk allergy after cutaneous exposure to milk-containing cosmetic products. Arch Pediatr Adolesc Med 2004;158:1089-1090
2   Anonymous. Milk-allergic children can have allergic reactions to cosmetic products. Child Health Alert 2004;22:3
3   Codreanu F, Morisset M, Cordebar V, Kanny G, Moneret-Vautrin DA. Risk of allergy to food proteins in topical medicinal agents and cosmetics. Eur Ann Allergy Clin Immunol 2006;38:126-130
4   González Rodríguez MP, González Hernández A, Martín Muñoz MF. Generalized urticarial reaction after the use of baby wipes. An Pediatr (Barc) 2008;68:198-200 (Article in Spanish)

3.17 MUSA PARADISIACA (BANANA) FRUIT

IDENTIFICATION

Description/definition	: Musa paradisiaca (banana) fruit is the fruit of the banana, *Musa paradisica*, Musaceae
Chemical class(es)	: Botanical products and botanical derivatives
INCI name USA	: Musa paradisiaca (banana) fruit
Other names	: Banana; banana fruit
CAS registry number (s)	: 89957-82-4
EC number(s)	: 289-602-4
Function(s) in cosmetics	: EU: adstringent. USA: cosmetic adstringents
Diagnostic testing	: Prick tests, RAST

GENERAL

Discussion of side effects of Musa paradisiaca (banana) fruit in this chapter is limited to reactions caused by its presence in cosmetic products. A review of contact urticaria caused by ingredients of cosmetics has been provided in 2016 (2).

IMMEDIATE-TYPE REACTIONS

A woman had had eight episodes of angioedema over 2 years. These occurred after wearing starch powdered natural rubber latex gloves, eating a banana, and packaging banana hair conditioner. The patient worked on the production line of a company manufacturing a range of 'natural' cosmetics. Prick tests were strongly positive to water-extractable natural rubber latex proteins and to banana, cucumber, avocado, kiwi and the banana hair conditioner. The patient was advised to use synthetic gloves at work and to avoid work with banana-related products. As other operatives continued to use powdered latex gloves, which may cause airborne dissemination of latex proteins, advice was given on modifying the working environment (1).

Natural rubber latex protein hypersensitivity (type I) is a hazard especially for operatives wearing rubber gloves. The potential for cross-reactions with fruits is well-established, which can lead to reactions when eating those fruits (including the oral allergy syndrome) or contact urticarial reactions from fruit proteins present in cosmetic products (3,4,5).

Presence in cosmetic products and chemical analyses

In the USA, in April 2017, Musa paradisiaca (banana) fruit extract was present in 43 of 56,714 cosmetic products of which the composition is known in FDA's Voluntary Cosmetic Registration Program (VCRP) (data obtained from FDA, May 2017). In April 2017, Musa paradisiaca (banana) fruit was present in zero of 66,485 cosmetic products of which the composition is known in EWG's Skin Deep Cosmetics Database, USA (http://www.ewg.org/skindeep/).

LITERATURE

1   Smith HR, Wakelin SH, White IR. Banana hair conditioner and natural rubber latex allergy. Contact Dermatitis 1998;39:202-203
2   Verhulst L, Goossens A. Cosmetic components causing contact urticaria: a review and update. Contact Dermatitis 2016;75:333-344
3   Posh A, Chen Z, Raulf-Heimsoth M, Baur X. Latex allergens. Clin Exp Allergy 1998;28:134-140
4   Kondo Y, Urisu A. Oral allergy syndrome. Allergol Int 2009;58:485-491
5   Blanco C. Latex-fruit syndrome. Curr Allergy Asthma Rep 2003;3:47-53

3.18 POLYOXYETHYLENEPOLYOXYPYRENE GLYCOL*
Not an INCI name

IDENTIFICATION

Description/definition   : Undefined chemical
INCI name USA   : Neither in Cosing nor in the Personal Care Products Council Ingredient Database
Diagnostic tests   : Prick test, concentration and vehicle unknown

GENERAL

Polyoxyethylenepolyoxypyrene glycol is described as a non-ionic block copolymer surfactant of one large hydrophobic chain or block of polyoxypropylene flanked by two small hydrophilic chains of polyoxyethlene. The chemical is apparently widely used as emulsifying agents and solubilizing agents in medicines or cosmetics (1).

IMMEDIATE-TYPE REACTIONS

A woman had an unpleasant sensation in her mouth, acute widespread erythema on her entire body and breathing difficulty. She had used a dentifrice immediately before the appearance of these clinical symptoms. A prick test with the toothpaste, tested 0.1% water, was strongly positive after 15 minutes. Ingredient prick testing with the surface-active agent polyoxyethylenepolyoxypyrene glycol (POEPOPG), polyethylene glycol (PEG), fragrances and bactericides present in the dentifrice yielded strongly positive reactions to POEPOPG and PEG (test concentrations and vehicles not mentioned). Two controls were negative. Next, prick tests were performed with 0.01% aqueous solution PEG of several molecular weights (MW). Positive reactions were observed to PEG of MW 4000, 6000 and 20,000 but not to PEG with MW 400 and 1500. The manufacturer stated that the toothpaste contained POEPOPG and polyethylene glycol with molecular weight 5000 (1).

Cross-reactions, pseudo-cross-reactions and co-reactions

Immediate-type cross-reactivity to polyethylene glycols with molecular weights of 4000, 6000 and 20,000, but not to those with molecular weights of 400 and 1500 (1).

Presence in cosmetic products and chemical analyses

In May 2017, polyoxyethylenepolyoxypyrene glycol was present in zero of 66,975 cosmetic products of which the composition is known in EWG's Skin Deep Cosmetics Database, USA (http://www.ewg.org/skindeep/). In the USA, in April 2017, polyoxyethylenepolyoxypyrene glycol was present in zero of 56,714 cosmetic products of which the composition is known in FDA's Voluntary Cosmetic Registration Program (VCRP) (data obtained from FDA, May 2017).

LITERATURE

1   Ito M, Watanabe D, Kobayashi M, Tamada Y, Matsumoto Y. Acute hypersensitivity to dentifrice. Contact Dermatitis 2006;54:225

3.19 SODIUM METHYL OLEOYL TAURATE

IDENTIFICATION

Description/definition	: Sodium methyl oleoyl taurate is the sodium salt of the oleic acid amide of *N*-methyl taurine. It conforms generally to the formula shown below
Chemical class(es)	: Sulfonic acids
Chemical/IUPAC name	: Sodium;2-[methyl-[(*Z*)-octadec-9-enoyl]amino]ethanesulfonate
Other names	: Sodium 2-[methyloleoylamino]ethane-1-sulphonate; oleoylmethyltaurine sodium salt; sodium oleylmethyltauride
CAS registry number (s)	: 137-20-2; 7308-16-9
EC number(s)	: 205-285-7; 230-762-1
CIR review(s)	: Final report, 15 December 2015 (access: www.cir-safety.org/ingredients)
Function(s) in cosmetics	: EU: antistatic; cleansing; foaming; surfactant. USA: surfactants - cleansing agents
Molecular formula	: $C_{21}H_{40}NNaO_4S$

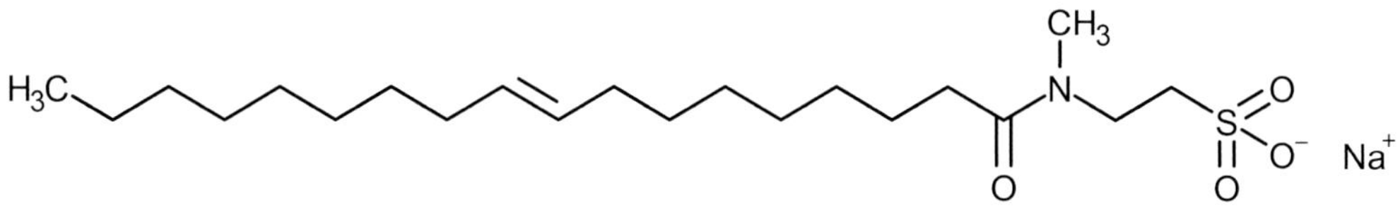

IMMEDIATE-TYPE REACTIONS

A woman complained that her head always felt itchy when her hair had been colored in the hair salon. One time, she developed pruritus of the scalp immediately after the oxidative hair dye was applied; this was followed by flushing over her entire body, with dyspnea, vomiting and hypotension. Skin prick tests were positive to the oxidative hair dye (10% water) and its ingredients *p*-aminophenol and sodium methyl oleoyl taurate. The subject was diagnosed with contact urticaria syndrome due to para-aminophenol and sodium methyl oleoyl taurate. Three controls were negative to the hair dye and the two causative ingredients (1).

Presence in cosmetic products and chemical analyses

In May 2017, sodium methyl oleoyl taurate was present in 5 of 66,329 cosmetic products of which the composition is known in EWG's Skin Deep Cosmetics Database, USA (http://www.ewg.org/skindeep/). In the USA, in April 2017, sodium methyl oleoyl taurate was present in 26 of 56,714 cosmetic products of which the composition is known in FDA's Voluntary Cosmetic Registration Program (VCRP) (data obtained from FDA, May 2017).

LITERATURE

1   Uehara S, Inomata N, Suzuki A, Matsuura M, Aihara M. Severe contact urticarial syndrome due to oxidative hair dye containing para-aminophenol and sodium-methyl-oleoyl-taurate. J Dermatol 2014;41:560-561

CHAPTER 4   MONOGRAPHS OF CHEMICALS AND SUBSTANCES IN COSMETICS THAT HAVE CAUSED PHOTOSENSITIVITY

4.1 INGREDIENTS OF COSMETICS THAT HAVE CAUSED PHOTOSENSITIVITY

Photosensitivity reactions include photocontact allergy (causing photoallergic contact dermatitis), phototoxicity (causing phototoxic dermatitis) and combined photocontact allergy and contact allergy, causing photoaggravated allergic contact dermatitis. Because it can easily be avoided, phototoxicity is rare and has been caused by a few chemicals which may be present in cosmetics only, such as formaldehyde, isobutyl PABA and pentyl dimethyl PABA. Most photosensitivity reactions from chemicals that may be used in cosmetics are photocontact allergic.

Historical photoallergens

In the 1960s, an epidemic of photoallergic reactions occurred in some countries including the United Kingdom and Sweden to halogenated salicylanilides (4',5-dibromosalicylanilide, tetrachlorosalicylanilide, tribromosalicylanilide) which were added to soaps and certain other products. To a lesser extent, related halogenated phenolic compounds such as bithionol, dichlorophene, hexachlorophene, 2,2'-thiobis(4-chlorophenol) (fenticlor), triclocarban and triclosan caused similar reactions, especially in the USA and Australia. This subject is discussed in detail in Chapter 2.450 Tetrachlorosalicylanilides and the Monographs of the individual chemicals in Chapter 2. Most are currently prohibited in the USA and the EU, and those that are still allowed are hardly used anymore.

In the 1970s, in Japan, many patients were observed suffering from a clinical picture called 'pigmented cosmetic dermatitis', notably on the face of women. These patients had contact allergic and photocontact allergic reactions to ingredients of cosmetics, notably fragrances and essential oils and colorants such as calcium lithol red, CI 11680, CI 12120, CI 15800, pigment orange 5, pigment red 172 aluminum lake, and pigment yellow 12. At that time, it was very difficult to assess whether the chemicals that induced positive (photo)patch tests were actually present in the cosmetic products used by the patients and therefore the (or an) causative (photo)allergen. These colors are not used anymore in cosmetics.

PABA was formerly a widely used sunscreen ingredient in the USA and a leading cause of sunscreen photoallergy. In recent years, it has almost disappeared from sunscreens and it is prohibited in the EU. In the 1980s and 1990s , isopropyl dibenzoylmethane was the most frequent photosensitizer. This UV-filter was voluntarily removed from the market in 1993 and is not produced anymore.

The current situation

Currently, UV-filters (UV-absorbers, sunscreen agents) are the most important causes of photocontact allergy. Well-known photosensitizing chemicals are benzophenone-3, butyl methoxydibenzoylmethane and octocrylene. In the case of octocrylene, most photoallergic patients did not become sensitized from octocrylene itself, but from previous photosensitization to ketoprofen, a topical NSAID. Butyl methoxydibenzoylmethane and octocrylene will continue to be used in sunscreens (and are so in a great many products), as the former is one of the very few effective UV-A absorbers and octocrylene is combined with it to stabilize the formula.

It should be realized, that, for most UV-filters, there are few well-documented case reports of photocontact allergy. They are often tested in a photopatch test series in patients suspected of photoallergic contact dermatitis or of reactions to sunscreen products. Usually (very) low prevalences of photocontact allergy were found. In most of such reported investigations, either no data on relevance were provided or specified for individual chemicals, and causative products were hardly ever mentioned.

Causative products

As currently the most important photosensitizers are UV-filters, the overwhelming majority of photocontact allergic reactions are caused by sunscreen cosmetics and to a lesser degree by other cosmetics not specifically intended to prevent sunburn. UV-filters that have – very rarely - caused photocontact allergy from their presence in non-cosmetic products include benzophenone-3 (ink of a magazine), captan (pesticides), chlorhexidine digluconate (disinfectant), hexachlorophene (Unna boot, scrubbing solution), hexamidine diisethionate (scrubbing solution), PABA (oral potassium PABA), paraffinum liquidum (cutting oil), pentyl dimethyl PABA (UV-curing inks), quinine (oral drug) and 2,2'-thiobis(4-chlorophenol) (fenticlor) (topical pharmaceuticals, occupational exposure in chemists, cooling fluid biocide). These are all discussed in their respective Monographs in chapter 2.

Ingredients of cosmetics that have caused photosensitivity

Non-fragrance ingredients of cosmetics that have caused photosensitivity reactions are shown in table 4.1.1 Most have also induced (plain) contact allergy and they are all discussed in Monographs in Chapter 2 'Monographs of chemicals and substances in cosmetics that have caused allergic contact dermatitis'. Five chemicals that have caused photocontact allergy *only* (beta-carotene, chloro-2-phenylphenol, digalloyl trioleate, 2,6-dimethyl-1,3-dioxan-4-yl acetate, PEG-25 PABA) and which are therefore not included in Chapter 2, are presented here as Monographs.

Table 4.1.1 Ingredients of cosmetic products that have caused photosensitivity reactions [b]

Arnica montana extract	Glyceryl PABA
Benzophenone-2	Hexachlorophene
Benzophenone-3	Hexamidine diisethionate
Benzophenone-4	Homosalate
Benzophenone-10	Isoamyl p-methoxycinnamate
Beta-carotene [a]	Isobutyl PABA
BHA	Isopropyl dibenzoylmethane
BHT	4-Methylbenzylidene camphor
Bithionol	Methylisothiazolinone
Butyl methoxydibenzoylmethane	Octocrylene
Calcium lithol red	PABA
Captan	Paraben mix
Chlorhexidine digluconate	Paraffinum liquidum
p-Chloro-m-cresol	PEG-25 PABA [a]
Chloro-2-phenylphenol [a]	Pentyl dimethyl PABA
CI 11680	Petrolatum
CI 12120	Phenylbenzimidazole sulfonic acid
CI 15800	p-Phenylenediamine
Cinoxate	Pigment orange 5
Colophonium	Pigment red 172 aluminum lake
4',5-Dibromosalicylanilide	Pigment yellow 12
Dichlorophene	Polysilicone-15
Diethylamino hydroxybenzoyl hexyl benzoate	Quinine
Digalloyl trioleate [a]	Tanacetum vulgare extract
2,6-Dimethyl-1,3-dioxan-4-yl acetate [a]	Terephthalylidene dicamphor sulfonic acid
Disodium phenyl dibenzimidazole tetrasulfonate	Tetrachlorosalicylanilides
DMDM hydantoin	Thimerosal
Drometrizole trisiloxane	2,2'-Thiobis(4-chlorophenol)
Ethylhexyl dimethyl PABA	Tinosorb® M
Ethylhexyl methoxycinnamate	Tosylamide/formaldehyde resin
bis-Ethylhexyloxyphenol methoxyphenyl triazine	Tribromosalicylanilide
Ethylhexyl salicylate	Triclocarban
Ethylhexyl triazone	Triclosan
Ethyl methoxycinnamate	Witisol
Formaldehyde	Zinc pyrithione

[a] has caused only photosensitivity, no contact allergy; presented in this chapter in a Monograph
[b] all chemicals except those marked a have caused both contact allergy to cosmetics and photosensitivity; these are all presented as Monographs in Chapter 2 'Monographs of chemicals and substances in cosmetics that have caused allergic contact dermatitis'

4.2 BETA-CAROTENE

IDENTIFICATION

Description/definition : Beta-carotene is a carotenoid compound prepared synthetically or obtained from natural sources, which conforms to the formula shown below
Chemical class(es) : Color additives; hydrocarbons
Chemical/IUPAC name : 1,3,3-Trimethyl-2-[(1E,3E,5E,7E,9E,11E,13E,15E,17E)-3,7,12,16-tetramethyl-18-(2,6,6-trimethylcyclohexen-1-yl)octadeca-1,3,5,7,9,11,13,15,17-nonaenyl]cyclohexene
Other names : Provitamin A; CI 40800; CI 75130; food orange 5
CAS registry number (s) : 7235-40-7
EC number(s) : 230-636-6
Merck Index monograph : 3125
Function(s) in cosmetics : EU: skin conditioning. USA: colorants; skin-conditioning agents - miscellaneous
EU cosmetic restrictions : Regulated in Annex IV/111 of the Regulation (EC) No. 1223/2009
Patch testing : 2% pet. (1)
Molecular formula : $C_{40}H_{56}$

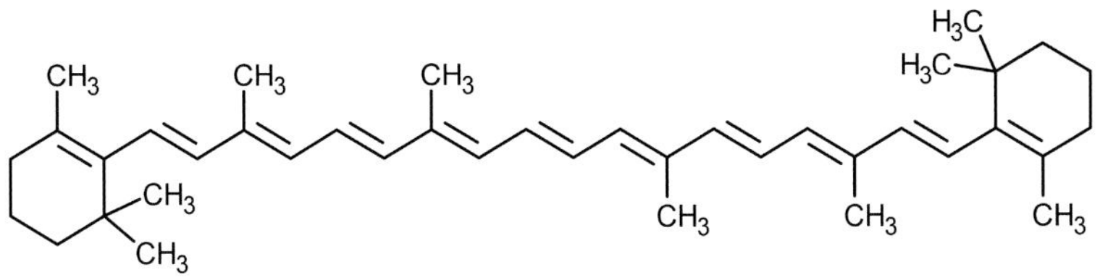

CONTACT ALLERGY

Presence in cosmetic products and chemical analyses

In the USA, in April 2017, beta-carotene was present in 255 of 56,714 cosmetic products of which the composition is known in FDA's Voluntary Cosmetic Registration Program (VCRP) (data obtained from FDA, May 2017). In March 2017, beta-carotene was present in 149 of 64,983 cosmetic products of which the composition is known in EWG's Skin Deep Cosmetics Database, USA (http://www.ewg.org/skindeep/).

OTHER SIDE EFFECTS

Photosensitivity

A man was seen with a photocontact dermatitis of his face, neck, hands and arms which had persisted for 2 months. The dermatitis had recurred every summer since four years when he had started using a particular sunscreen lotion while on the beach and while boating at sea. He was patch tested to the standard ICDRG series, as well as to several shaving cosmetics and two sunscreens, both of which were applied as photopatch tests using natural sunlight. Both exposed and covered patch tests to one sun lotion were strongly positive. The ingredients were subsequently patch tested and were all negative at D2. Then they were all exposed to direct sunlight, sufficient to cause mild tanning, revealing a positive reaction at D4 to beta-carotene (test concentration and vehicle unknown, tested as supplied by the manufacturer). Although the author admitted that beta-carotene was not proven to be a photosensitizer (it may well have caused 'plain' contact allergy) , the delayed response following exposure to strong sunlight, along with the clinical evidence, in his opinion indicated that it was acting as the photocontact agent in this patient. Curiously, a repeat patch test and photopatch test with beta-carotene was not performed, only with the sunscreen itself (1).

LITERATURE

1   Burry JN. Photo allergies from benzophenones and beta carotene in sunscreens. Contact Dermatitis 1980;6:211-212

4.3 CHLORO-2-PHENYLPHENOL*
Not an INCI name

Dowicide® 32 is a mixture of 4-chloro-2-phenylphenol and 6-chloro-2-phenylphenol

IDENTIFICATION

Description/definition	: 4-Chloro-2-phenylphenol is the chlorinated phenolic compound that conforms to the formula shown below
Chemical class(es)	: Chlorinated Phenols
INCI name USA	: Neither in CosIng nor in the Personal Care Products Council Ingredient Database
Chemical/IUPAC name	: 4-Chloro-2-phenylphenol
Other names	: 5-Chloro(1,1'-biphenyl)-2-ol; 2-phenyl-4-chlorophenol
CAS registry number (s)	: 607-12-5
EC number(s)	: 210-130-1
Function(s) in cosmetics	: USA: formerly used as germicide in soap
Patch testing	: 1% water
Molecular formula	: $C_{12}H_9ClO$

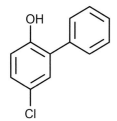

Description/definition	: 6-Chloro-2-phenylphenol is the chlorinated phenolic compound that conforms to the formula shown below
Chemical class(es)	: Chlorinated phenols
INCI name USA	: Neither in CosIng nor in the Personal Care Products Council Ingredient Database
Chemical/IUPAC name	: 2-Chloro-6-phenylphenol
Other names	: 3-Chloro(1,1'-biphenyl)-2-ol
CAS registry number (s)	: 85-97-2; 1322-19-6; 1331-46-0
EC number(s)	: 201-644-7
Function(s) in cosmetics	: USA: formerly used as germicide in soap
Patch testing	: 1% water
Molecular formula	: $C_{12}H_9ClO$

GENERAL
Dowicide 32 is the trade name for the refined grade of a mixture of 4-chloro-2-phenylphenol and 6-dichloro-2-phenylphenol. It has (formerly) been employed in disinfectant formulations of detergent and pine oil types, as a fungicide in textiles and adhesives (especially starch and protein-based), in the construction industry to control the growth of fungi on inert surfaces, and by automobile equipment manufacturers to prevent mold in felt gaskets (1).

Cross-reactions, pseudo-cross-reactions and co-reactions
4,6-Dichlorophenylphenol (1); *not* to *o*-phenylphenol (1)

OTHER SIDE EFFECTS

Photosensitivity

Allergic photocontact dermatitis developed to Dowicide® 32 (a mixture of 4-chloro-2-phenylphenol and 6-chloro-2-phenylphenol) in four workers out of the relatively small population of employees and students of a junior college district, where the substance was employed as a germicidal agent in a liquid soap. Photopatch test reactions were positive to 4-chloro-2-phenylphenol in all 4 patients, to 6-chloro-2-phenylphenol in one individual and to 4,6-dichlorophenylphenol in all 4 (all tested 1% water).

LITERATURE

1   Adams RM. Photoallergic contact dermatitis to chloro-2-phenylphenol. Arch Dermatol 1972;106:711-714

4.4   DIGALLOYL TRIOLEATE

IDENTIFICATION

Description/definition   . Digalloyl trioleate is a triester of digallic acid and oleic acid, which conforms generally to the formula shown below
Chemical class(es)   : Esters
Chemical/IUPAC name   : 3,4-Dihydroxy-5-[3,4,5-tris[[(Z)-octadec-9-enoyl]oxy]benzoyl]oxybenzoic acid
CAS registry number (s) : 17048-39-4; 27436-80-2
Function(s) in cosmetics : EU: antioxidant; UV-absorber. USA: antioxidants; light stabilizers
Patch testing   : 3.5% alcohol (1)
Molecular formula   : $C_{68}H_{106}O_{11}$

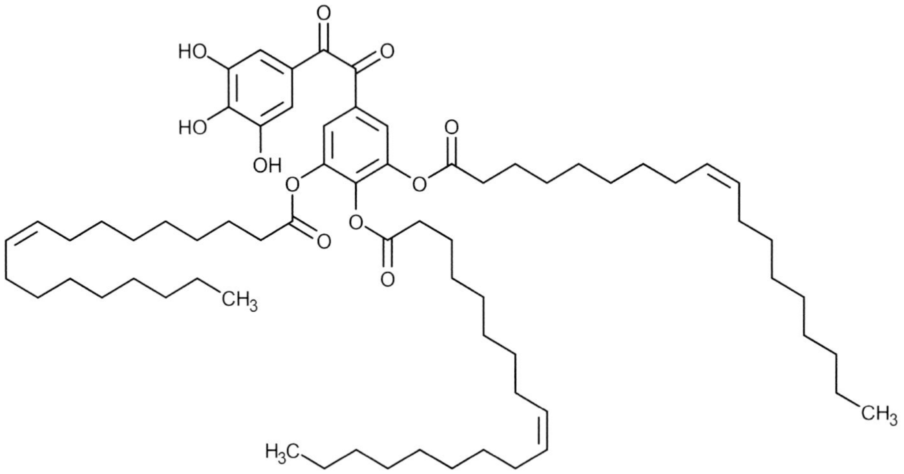

GENERAL

Digalloyl trioleate is a UVB filter (8). The literature on adverse reactions to sunscreens has been reviewed in several recent and older publications (2-7,10). A review of photocontact allergy to sunscreens was published in 2010 (9).

Presence in cosmetic products and chemical analyses

In the USA, in April 2017, digalloyl trioleate was present in zero of 56,714 cosmetic products of which the composition is known in FDA's Voluntary Cosmetic Registration Program (VCRP) (data obtained from FDA, May 2017). In March 2017, digalloyl trioleate was present in zero of 64,983 cosmetic products of which the composition is known in EWG's Skin Deep Cosmetics Database, USA (http://www.ewg.org/skindeep/). It should be appreciated that sunscreen products containing UV-filters are classified as drugs in the USA, not as cosmetics; the number mentioned here, therefore, is that of cosmetics containing the UV-filter, but it does not include their presence in sunscreens.

OTHER SIDE EFFECTS

Photosensitivity

A five-year old girl was reported to have photoallergic contact dermatitis from a sunscreen containing digalloyl trioleate. A test with 3.5% alcoholic solution of digalloyl trioleate exposed to sunlight was positive (1).

LITERATURE

1   Sams WM. Contact photodermatitis. AMA Arch Dermatol 1956;73:142-148
2   Heurung AR, Raju SI, Warshaw EM. Adverse reactions to sunscreen agents: epidemiology, responsible irritants and allergens, clinical characteristics, and management. Dermatitis 2014;25:289-326
3   Heurung AR, Raju SI, Warshaw EM. Contact allergen of the year. Benzophenones. Dermatitis 2014;25:3-10 (contains many mistakes; Erratum in Dermatitis 2014;25:92-95)
4   Avenel-Audran M. Sunscreen products: finding the allergen. Eur J Dermatol 2010;20:161-166

5 Scheuer E, Warshaw E. Sunscreen allergy: a review of epidemiology, clinical characteristics, and responsible allergens. Dermatitis 2006;17:3-11

6 Funk JO, Dromgoole SH, Maibach HI. Sunscreen intolerance: contact sensitization, photocontact sensitization, and irritancy of sunscreen agents. Dermatol Clin 1995;13:473-481

7 Dromgoole SH, Maibach HI. Sunscreening agent intolerance: Contact and photocontact sensitization and contact urticaria. J Am Acad Dermatol 1990;22:1068-1078

8 Shaath NA. Ultraviolet filters. Photochem Photobiol Sci 2010;9:464-469

9 Shaw T, Simpson B, Wilson B, Oostman H, Rainey D, Storrs F. True photoallergy to sunscreens is rare despite popular belief. Dermatitis 2010;21:185-198

10 Schauder S. Survey of the literature on adverse reactions to preparations containing UV filters (1947-1989) (Literaturübersicht über Unverträglichkeitsreaktionen auf lichtfilterhaltige Produkte von 1947 bis 1989). Z Hautkr 1990;65:982-998 (article in German)

4.5 2,6-DIMETHYL-1,3-DIOXAN-4-YL ACETATE

IDENTIFICATION

Description/definition   . 2,6-Dimethyl-1,3-dioxan-4-yl acetate is the heterocyclic ester that corresponds to the
                             structural formula shown below
Chemical class(es)   : Heterocyclic organic compounds; esters
INCI name USA   : Not in the Personal Care Products Council Ingredient Database
Chemical/IUPAC name   : (2,6-Dimethyl-1,3-dioxan-4-yl) acetate
Other names   : Dimethoxane; 6-acetoxy-2,4-dimethyl-*m*-dioxane
CAS registry number (s)   : 828-00-2
EC number(s)   : 212-579-9
Merck Index monograph   : 4514
Function(s) in cosmetics   : EU: prohibited
EU cosmetic restrictions   : Regulated in Annex II/368 of the Regulation (EC) No. 1223/2009 (prohibited)
Patch testing   : 0.1% and 1% pet. (3)
Molecular formula   : $C_8H_{14}O_4$

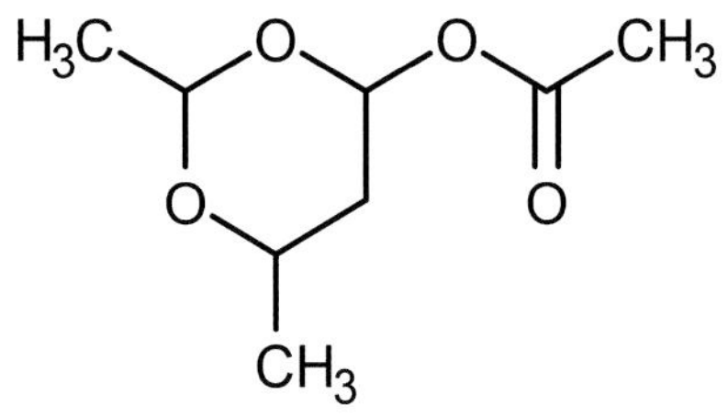

CONTACT ALLERGY

Contact allergy to 2,6-dimethyl-1,3-dioxan-4-yl acetate in non-cosmetic products
A female worker in a large textile plant developed dermatitis of the exposed sites of her arms, neck and face. In her task of 'beaming' she received polyester yarn on which a finish had been freshly applied usually within an hour previously. She was positioned in front of a rapidly rotating roller and lint would come off on her. The patient was patch tested on the inner arms to coded samples of 13 different oils and emulsions diluted in olive oil to various concentrations ranging from 1:4 to 1:40 (by volume) depending upon general information supplied by the employee and company. The patient reacted to dimethoxane 2.5% with a bullous reaction. Dimethoxane was used in the spin finish as a preservative against spoilage. Repeat testing at 1.25% in olive oil was positive. Correspondence with the manufacturer revealed that dimethoxane in an aqueous system hydrolyzes to produce equimolar quantities of acetic acid, acetaldehyde and 3-hydroxybutyraldehyde (3-hydroxybutanal). The patient was subsequently patch tested with these three chemicals and also with crotonaldehyde, as 3-hydroxybutanal readily dehydrates to form crotonaldehyde. The patient reacted to acetaldehyde 1% water, but lower concentrations in a dilution series were negative. There was also a positive patch test to crotonaldehyde 1% in olive oil but not to the same chemical 1% in water or 0.1% in water or in olive oil. The positive reaction was accompanied by a flare of dermatitis of previously involved areas (2).

Presence in cosmetic products and chemical analyses
In May 2017, dimethoxane was present in zero of 64,655 cosmetic products of which the composition is known in EWG's Skin Deep Cosmetics Database, USA (http://www.ewg.org/skindeep/). In the USA, in April 2017, dimethoxane was present in 3 of 56,714 cosmetic products of which the composition is known in FDA's Voluntary Cosmetic Registration Program (VCRP) (data obtained from FDA, May 2017).

OTHER SIDE EFFECTS

Photosensitivity
One patient had photoallergic contact dermatitis from 2,6-dimethyl-1,3-dioxan-4-yl acetate in a sunscreen (1,4).

LITERATURE

1   Kalimo K, Fagerlund V-L, Jansen CT. Concomitant photocontact allergy to a benzophenone derivative and a sunscreen preservative 6-acetoxy-2,4-dimethyl-*m*-dioxane. Photodermatol 1984;1:315-317

2   Shmunes E, Kempton RJ. Allergic contact dermatitis to dimethoxane in a spin finish. Contact Dermatitis 1980;6:421-424

3   De Groot AC. Patch Testing, 3rd Edition. Wapserveen, The Netherlands: acdegroot publishing, 2008 (ISBN 978-90-813233-1-4)

4   Fagerlund VL, Kalimo K, Jansen CH. Photokontakallergie durch Lichtschutzmittel (Valonsurjaaineet fotokontaktallergien aiheuttajin). Duodecim 1983;99:146-150 (article in Finnish)

4.6   PEG-25 PABA

IDENTIFICATION

Description/definition   : PEG-25 PABA is the polyethylene glycol derivative of PABA, which conforms generally to
                            the formula shown below, where x+y+z has an average value of 25
Chemical class(es)   : PABA derivatives
Other names   : Polyoxyethylene ethyl-4-aminobenzoate (25 mol EO average molar ratio); ethoxylated
                            ethyl-4-aminobenzoate; polyethylene glycol (25) PABA
CAS registry number (s)   : 116242-27-4
Function(s) in cosmetics : EU: UV-absorber; UV-filter. USA: light stabilizers
EU cosmetic restrictions : Regulated in Annex VI/13 of the Regulation (EC) No. 1223/2009
Patch testing   : No data available; suggested: 10% pet.

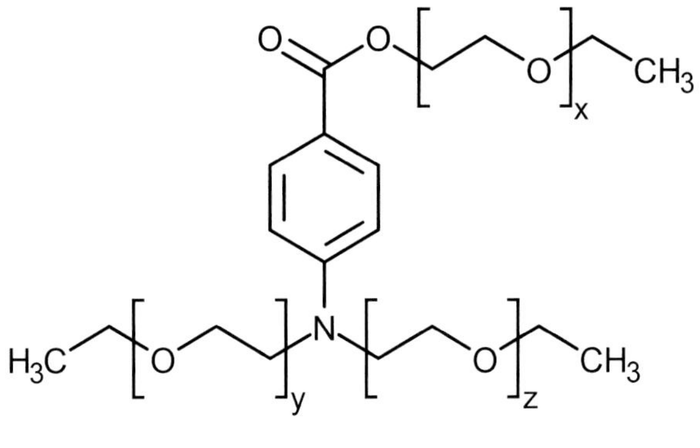

GENERAL

PEG-25 PABA is a UVB filter with UV absorbance maximum (λ_{max}) at 309 nm (4).

Presence in cosmetic products and chemical analyses

In the USA, in April 2017, PEG-25 PABA was present in 8 of 56,714 cosmetic products of which the composition is known in FDA's Voluntary Cosmetic Registration Program (VCRP) (data obtained from FDA, May 2017). In March 2017, PEG-25 PABA was present in 5 of 65,431 cosmetic products of which the composition is known in EWG's Skin Deep Cosmetics Database, USA (http://www.ewg.org/skindeep/). It should be appreciated that sunscreen products containing UV-filters are classified as drugs in the USA, not as cosmetics; the number mentioned here, therefore, is that of cosmetics containing the UV-filter, but it does *not* include their presence in sunscreens. PEG-25 PABA was present in 1% of 4447 cosmetic products collected in Germany, 2006-2009 (2). PEG-25 PABA was present in 1 of 75 (1.3%) sunscreen creams and lotions from 30 European and US producers purchased in Denmark in 2001, in a concentration of 0.34% (3).

OTHER SIDE EFFECTS

Photosensitivity

In the period 2004-2006, in Italy, 1082 patients with histories and clinical features suggestive of photoallergic contact dermatitis were photopatch tested with PEG-25 PABA. One patient (0.1%) had a positive photopatch test. The reaction was relevant, probably from its presence in a sunscreen product (1).

LITERATURE

1   Pigatto PD, Guzzi G, Schena D, Guarrera M, Foti C, Francalanci S, et al. Photopatch tests: an Italian multicentre
    study from 2004 to 2006. Contact Dermatitis 2008;59:103-108
2   Uter W, Gonçalo M, Yazar K, Kratz E-M, Mildau G, Lidén C. Coupled exposure to ingredients of cosmetic
    products: III. Ultraviolet filters. Contact Dermatitis 2014;71:162-169
3   Rastogi SC. UV filters in sunscreen products – a survey. Contact Dermatitis 2002;46:348-351
4   Shaath NA. Ultraviolet filters. Photochem Photobiol Sci 2010;9:464-469

CHAPTER 5 FUNCTIONAL CLASSES AND CHEMICALS/SUBSTANCES IN THESE CLASSES THAT HAVE CAUSED ALLERGIC COSMETIC DERMATITIS

5.1 INTRODUCTION

All ingredients of cosmetic products have one or – more often – several functions and belong to one or more functional classes. The classification of functions and their definition/description in the EU INCI system (1) differs to some extent from those as defined in the USA system (2). In this chapter, all functional classes are listed alphabetically, as used in the EU (Chapter 5.2) and the USA (Chapter 5.3) with their definitions/descriptions and with all chemicals/substances in these classes that have caused allergic cosmetic dermatitis. Their Monographs can all be found in Chapter 2.

A number of chemicals/substances described as allergens in cosmetics could not be found in CosIng, The Personal Care Products Council Ingredient database or in neither. These are listed in Chapter 5.4. In a number of cases, the chemicals were likely used outside the EU and USA only, for instance in Japan. Some are historical allergens, once used, others may wrongfully have been identified as cosmetic allergens by the authors or presented with incorrect names. Such considerations are, where possible, discussed in the Monographs of such substances.

Finally, nearly 40 chemicals/substances described as cosmetic allergens are currently prohibited in the EU and - a few – in the USA. These are listed in Chapter 5.5. In the majority, the reports are from older date when the incriminated chemicals where not yet prohibited, e.g., the halogenated salicylanilides and coal tar dyes. However, it also includes more recent allergens such as methyldibromo glutaronitrile which was prohibited only ten years ago.

LITERATURE

1 The European Commission database with information on cosmetic substances and ingredients CosIng: http://ec.europa.eu/growth/tools-databases/cosing/
2 The Personal Care Products Council (formerly Cosmetic, Toiletry and Fragrance Association) on-line ingredient database: http://online.personalcarecouncil.org/jsp/Home.jsp

5.2   FUNCTIONAL CLASSES IN THE EU SYSTEM (COSING)

ABRASIVE

Removes materials from various body surfaces or aids mechanical tooth cleaning or improves gloss

Alumina

Avena sativa bran extract

Polyethylene

ABSORBENT

Takes up water- and/or oil-soluble dissolved or finely dispersed substances

Alumina

ADSTRINGENT

Contracts the skin

Alcohol

Aluminum chloride

Aluminum chlorohydrate

Phytonadione epoxide

Salvia officinalis extract

Tioxolone

ANTICAKING

Allows free flow of solid particles and thus avoids agglomeration of powdered cosmetics into lumps or hard masses

Alumina

Methyl methacrylate

Zinc ricinoleate

ANTICORROSIVE

Prevents corrosion of the packaging

Sodium benzoate

ANTIDANDRUFF

Helps control dandruff

Achillea millefolium extract

Coal tar

Salvia officinalis extract

Selenium sulfide

Undecylenamide DEA

Zinc pyrithione

ANTIFOAMING

Suppresses foam during manufacturing or reduces the tendency of finished products to generate foam

Alcohol

Hexamidine diisethionate

Isopropyl alcohol

Phenyl dimethicone

ANTIMICROBIAL

Helps control the growth of micro-organisms on the skin

Alcohol

C12-15 Alkyl benzoate

Benzalkonium chloride

Benzethonium chloride

Benzisothiazolinone

Benzoxonium chloride

Cetalkonium chloride

Cetrimonium bromide

Chlorhexidine digluconate

Chlorphenesin

Dichlorobenzyl alcohol

Dichlorophene

Guaiazulene

Hexylresorcinol

Hydrogen peroxide

Laurylpyridinium chloride

Magnolia grandiflora bark extract

Magnolia officinalis bark extract

Mandelic acid

Phenyl salicylate

Salvia officinalis extract

Scutellaria baicalensis extract

2,2'-Thiobis(4-chlorophenol)

Undecylenamide DEA

ANTIOXIDANT

Inhibits reactions promoted by oxygen, thus avoiding oxidation and rancidity

Arbutin

Ascorbic acid

Ascorbyl tetraisopalmitate

BHA

BHT

Caprylyl gallate

CI 75470

Cysteamine HCl

Di-*t*-butylhydroquinone

Digalloyl trioleate

Dodecyl gallate

Hesperidin methyl chalcone

Hydroxydecyl ubiquinone

Kojic acid

Magnolia grandiflora bark extract

Nordihydroguaiaretic acid

Phenylethyl resorcinol

Propyl gallate

Resveratrol

Salvia officinalis extract

Sodium bisulfite

Sodium metabisulfite

TBHQ

Thioctic acid

Thiolactic acid

Tocopheryl linoleate

Tocopheryl nicotinate

ANTIPERSPIRANT
Reduces perspiration
Aluminum chloride
Aluminum chlorohydrate

ANTIPLAQUE
Helps protect against plaque
Olaflur
Stannous fluoride

ANTISEBORRHOEIC
Helps control sebum production
Propolis
Zinc pyrithione

ANTISTATIC
Reduces static electricity by neutralising electrical charge on a surface
Acetylated lanolin
Benzalkonium chloride
Ceresin
Cetalkonium chloride
Cetrimonium bromide
Cocamidopropyl betaine
Cocamidopropyl dimethylamine
Cocamidopropyl hydroxysultaine
Cocamidopropyl PG-dimonium chloride phosphate
Coco-betaine
Cyclomethicone
Didecyldimonium chloride
Disodium lauroamphodiacetate
Glucosamine HCl
Guar hydroxypropyltrimonium chloride
Hinokitiol
Hydrolyzed collagen
Hydrolyzed wheat protein
Isononyl isononanoate
Isostearamidopropyl morpholine lactate
Lanolin
Lanolin alcohol
Lanolin oil
Lauramide DEA
Lauramine oxide
Laureth-4
Lauroyl collagen amino acids
Laurylpyridinium chloride
Oleamide DEA
Oleamidopropyl dimethylamine
Palmitoyl collagen amino acids
Palmitoyl hydrolyzed milk protein
Panthenol
Panthenyl ethyl ether
Paraffinum liquidum
Petrolatum
Polyquaternium-7
Pyridoxine dioctenoate
Quaternium-22
Sodium chondroitin sulfate
Sodium lauroyl sarcosinate

Sodium myristoyl sarcosinate
Sodium PCA
Stearamidoethyl diethylamine phosphate
TEA-cocoyl hydrolyzed collagen
Undecylenamide DEA

BINDING
Provides cohesion in cosmetics
Beeswax (see Cera alba)
Cera microcristallina
Ceresin
Colophonium
Ditrimethylolpropane triethylhexanoate
Isopropyl myristate
Lanolin alcohol
Lanolin oil
PEG-4 dimethacrylate
Pentaerythrityl triacrylate
Shellac
VP/eicosene copolymer
VP/hexadecene copolymer
Xanthan gum

BLEACHING
Lightens the shade of hair or skin
Ammonium persulfate
Arbutin
Glycyrrhiza glabra (licorice) root extract

BUFFERING
Stabilises the pH of cosmetics
Ascorbic acid
Triethanolamine
Tromethamine

BULKING
Reduces bulk density of cosmetics
Alumina
Benzoic acid
Henna

CHELATING
Reacts and forms complexes with metal ions which could affect the stability and/or appearance of cosmetics
Caprylhydroxamic acid
Disodium EDTA
EDTA
Methyl dihydroxybenzoate
Tetrahydroxypropyl ethylenediamine
Tetrasodium EDTA
Trisodium EDTA

CLEANSING
Helps to keep the body surface clean
Achillea millefolium extract
Benzalkonium chloride
Cetalkonium chloride
Cocamidopropylamine oxide

CLEANSING (*continued*)
Cocamidopropyl betaine
Cocamidopropyl hydroxysultaine
Coco-glucoside
Decyl glucoside
Disodium lauroamphodiacetate
Disodium oleamido MEA-sulfosuccinate
Disodium ricinoleamido MEA-sulfosuccinate
Hexyldecanoic acid
Hydroxystearic acid
Lauramine oxide
Laureth-2
Lauroyl collagen amino acids
Lauryl glucoside
Myristic acid
Myristyl glucoside
Palmitoyl collagen amino acids
Palmitoyl hydrolyzed milk protein
Palmitoyl hydrolyzed wheat protein
Ricinoleic acid
Salvia officinalis extract
Sodium cocoamphoacetate
Sodium cocoamphopropionate
Sodium laureth sulfate
Sodium lauroamphoacetate
Sodium lauroyl sarcosinate
Sodium lauryl sulfate
Sodium myristoyl sarcosinate
Sodium stearate
Stearic acid
Sulfated castor oil
TEA-cocoyl hydrolyzed collagen
TEA-PEG-3 cocamide sulfate
TEA-stearate

COSMETIC COLORANT
**Colours cosmetics and/or imparts colour to the skin
and/or its appendages**
CI 11680
CI 12010
CI 12085
CI 12120
CI 15800
CI 26100
CI 45380
CI 47000
CI 69825
CI 77163
CI 77288
CI 77289
Pigment red 57:1

DENATURANT
**Renders cosmetics unpalatable; mostly added to
cosmetics containing ethyl alcohol**
t-Butyl alcohol
Glycerin
Phenyl salicylate
Polysorbate 80

Quinine
Sodium lauryl sulfate

DEODORANT
Reduces or masks unpleasant body odours
Aluminum chloride
Aluminum chlorohydrate
Benzalkonium chloride
Benzethonium chloride
Dichlorophene
Laurylpyridinium chloride
Salvia officinalis extract
Triclocarban
Triclosan
Zinc ricinoleate

DEPILATORY
Removes unwanted body hair
Ammonium thioglycolate
Ammonium thiolactate
Colophonium
Copernicia cerifera (carnauba) wax
Thioglycerin
Thiolactic acid

EMOLLIENT
Softens and smooths the skin
Acetylated lanolin
C18-36 Acid triglyceride
C12-15 Alkyl benzoate
Argania spinosa kernel oil
Ascorbyl tetraisopalmitate
Candelilla cera
Cera alba
Cetearyl alcohol
Cetearyl ethylhexanoate
Cetearyl isononanoate
Cetyl alcohol
Cyclomethicone
Decyl oleate
Dicaprylyl maleate
Diethyl sebacate
bis-Diglyceryl polyacyladipate-2
Diglyceryl sebacate/isopalmitate
Diisostearyl malate
Dipentaerythrityl hexahydroxystearate/hexa-
    stearate/hexarosinate
Distearyl phthalic acid amide
Ditrimethylolpropane triethylhexanoate
Glyceryl abietate
Glyceryl caprylate
Glyceryl diisostearate
Glyceryl isostearate
Glyceryl isostearate/myristate
Glyceryl stearate
Glycyrrhiza glabra (licorice) root extract
Hexamidine diisethionate
Hydrogenated castor oil
Hydrolyzed collagen

EMOLLIENT (*continued*)

Isohexadecane
Isononyl isononanoate
Isopropyl myristate
Isostearyl alcohol
Lanolin
Lanolin alcohol
Lanolin oil
Lauryl alcohol
Macadamia ternifolia seed oil
Maleated soybean oil
Methyl glucose dioleate
Methyl glucose sesquistearate
Myristyl alcohol
Octyldodecanol
Oleyl alcohol
Paraffinum liquidum
Pentaerythrityl tetracaprylate/tetracaprate
Petrolatum
Propolis
Prunus avium seed oil
Ricinoleic acid
Ricinus communis seed oil
Sesamum indicum seed oil
Shellac
Simmondsia chinensis (jojoba) seed oil
Stearyl alcohol
Triethylene glycol hydrogenated rosinate
Trioleyl phosphate

EMULSIFYING

Promotes the formation of intimate mixtures of non-miscible liquids by altering the interfacial tension

Acetylated lanolin
Arachidyl glucoside
Cera alba
Ceteareth-2
Ceteareth-3
Cetearyl alcohol
Cetrimonium bromide
Cetyl alcohol
Cocamide
Cocamide DEA
Cocamidopropyl dimethylamine
Didecyldimonium chloride
Glyceryl caprylate
Glyceryl diisostearate
Glyceryl isostearate
Glyceryl isostearate/myristate
Glyceryl stearate
Hexyldecanoic acid
Hexylene glycol
Hydrogenated castor oil
Hydroxystearic acid
Lanolin
Lanolin alcohol
Lanolin oil
Laureth-2
Laureth-4

Laureth-7
Laureth-9
Laureth-12
Lauryl alcohol
Methoxy PEG-17/dodecyl glycol copolymer
Methyl glucose sesquistearate
Myristic acid
Octyldodecyl xyloside
C30-38 Olefin/isopropyl maleate/MA copolymer
Oleth-5
Oleyl alcohol
PEG-4 dilaurate
PEG-5 lanolate
PEG-5 soy sterol
PEG-7 hydrogenated castor oil
PEG-7 oleate
PEG-22/dodecyl glycol copolymer
PEG-32 stearate
PEG-40 sorbitan lanolate
Polysorbate 40
Polysorbate 80
PPG-1-PEG-9 lauryl glycol ether
PPG-2-ceteareth-9
Propylene glycol ricinoleate
Ricinoleic acid
Sodium dihydroxycetyl phosphate
Sodium laureth sulfate
Sodium lauroyl sarcosinate
Sodium lauryl sulfate
Sodium stearate
Sodium stearoyl lactylate
Sorbitan oleate
Sorbitan sesquioleate
Sorbitan tristearate
Steareth-10
Stearic acid
Stearyl alcohol
Sulfated castor oil
TEA-PEG-3 cocamide sulfate
TEA-stearate
Triceteareth-4 phosphate
Triethanolamine
Trilaureth-4 phosphate
Xanthan gum

EMULSION STABILISING

Helps the process of emulsification and improves emulsion stability and shelf-life

Beeswax (see Cera alba)
Cera microcristallina
Ceresin
Cetearyl alcohol
Cetyl alcohol
Cocamide
Cocamide DEA
Decyl glucoside
Euphorbia cerifera (candelilla) wax
Lauryl alcohol
Methoxy PEG-22/dodecyl glycol copolymer

EMULSION STABILISING (*continued*)
Myristyl alcohol
PEG-22/dodecyl glycol copolymer
Prunus avium seed oil
Stearic acid
Stearyl alcohol
Xanthan gum

FILM FORMING
Produces, upon application, a continuous film on skin, hair or nails
1,4-Butanediol dimethacrylate
Butyl methacrylate
Candelilla cera
Cera alba
Chitosan
Colophonium
Diethylene glycol dimethacrylate
Di-HEMA trimethylhexyl dicarbamate
Glyceryl hydrogenated rosinate
Glyceryl rosinate
Glycol HEMA-methacrylate
Guar hydroxypropyltrimonium chloride
HEMA
Hydrolyzed collagen
Hydroxypropyl methacrylate
Isobutyl methacrylate
Nitrocellulose
PEG-4 dimethacrylate
Pentaerythrityl rosinate
Pentaerythrityl triacrylate
Phthalic anhydride/trimellitic anhydride/glycols
 copolymer
Polyester-8
Polyethylene
Polyquaternium-7
Quaternium-22
Shellac
Styrax benzoin gum
Tetrahydrofurfuryl methacrylate
Tosylamide/formaldehyde resin
Trimethylolpropane triacrylate
VP/eicosene copolymer
VP/hexadecene copolymer

FLAVOURING
Gives flavour to the cosmetic product
Betula alba bark extract

FOAM BOOSTING
Improves the quality of the foam produced by a system by increasing one or more of the following properties: volume, texture and/or stability
Cetyl alcohol
Cocamide DEA
Cocamidopropylamine oxide
Cocamidopropyl betaine
Cocamidopropyl hydroxysultaine
Coco-betaine

Disodium lauroamphodiacetate
Disodium oleamido MEA-sulfosuccinate
Disodium ricinoleamido MEA-sulfosuccinate
Lauramide DEA
Lauramine oxide
Myristyl alcohol
Oleamide DEA
Sodium cocoamphopropionate
Stearyl alcohol
Trideceth-2 carboxamide MEA
Undecylenamide DEA

FOAMING
Traps numerous small bubbles of air or other gas within a small volume of liquid by modifying the surface tension of the liquid
Coco-glucoside
Disodium lauroamphodiacetate
Sodium cocoamphoacetate
Sodium cocoamphopropionate
Sodium laureth sulfate
Sodium lauroamphoacetate
Sodium lauroyl sarcosinate
Sodium lauryl sulfate
Sodium myristoyl sarcosinate
TEA-PEG-3 cocamide sulfate

GEL FORMING
Gives the consistency of a gel (a semi-solid preparation with some elasticity) to a liquid preparation
Xanthan gum

HAIR CONDITIONING
Leaves the hair easy to comb, supple, soft and shiny and/or imparts volume, lightness, gloss, etc.
Acetylated lanolin
Ceresin
Cetearyl ethylhexanoate
Cetearyl isononanoate
Cocamidopropylamine oxide
Cocamidopropyl betaine
Cocamidopropyl dimethylamine
Cocamidopropyl hydroxysultaine
Cocamidopropyl PG-dimonium chloride phosphate
Coco-betaine
Didecyldimonium chloride
Disodium lauroamphodiacetate
bis-Ethylhexyloxyphenol methoxyphenyl triazine
Glucosamine HCl
Hinokitiol
Hydrolyzed collagen
Hydrolyzed wheat protein
Lanolin
Lanolin alcohol
Lanolin oil
Lauramine oxide
Lauroyl collagen amino acids
Panthenol

HAIR CONDITIONING (*continued*)
Panthenyl ethyl ether
Potassium cocoyl hydrolyzed collagen
Pyridoxine dioctenoate
Quaternium-22
Quinine
Selenium sulfide
Sesamum indicum seed oil
Simmondsia chinensis (jojoba) seed oil
Sodium chondroitin sulfate
Sodium cocoamphoacetate
Sodium cocoamphopropionate
Sodium hydroxymethylglycinate
Sodium lauroamphoacetate
Sodium lauroyl sarcosinate
Sodium myristoyl sarcosinate
Sodium PCA
Stearamidoethyl diethylamine phosphate
TEA-cocoyl hydrolyzed collagen
Trimethylolpropane triacrylate
Undecylenamide DEA
Zinc pyrithione

HAIR DYEING
Colours hair
4-Amino-*m*-cresol
2-Amino-4-hydroxyethylaminoanisole sulfate
4-Amino-2-hydroxytoluene
4-Amino-3-nitrophenol
m-Aminophenol
p-Aminophenol
Basic blue 99
2-Chloro-*p*-phenylenediamine
Chromium oxide greens
2,4-Diaminophenoxyethanol HCl
HC blue no. 7
HC red no. 7
HC Yellow no. 7
Henna
2-Hydroxyethylamino-5-nitroanisole
N,*N*-bis(2-Hydroxyethyl)-*p*-phenylenediamine sulfate
Lawsone
6-Methoxy-2-methylamino-3-aminopyridine HCl
p-Methylaminophenol
2,7-Naphthalenediol
3-Nitro-*p*-hydroxyethylaminophenol
p-Phenylenediamine
N-Phenyl-*p*-phenylenediamine
Resorcinol
Toluene-2,5-diamine
Toluene-2,5-diamine sulfate

HAIR FIXING
Permits physical control of hair style
Chitosan
Olaflur
Shellac
Trimethylolpropane triacrylate
VP/hexadecene copolymer

HAIR WAVING OR STRAIGHTENING
Modifies the chemical structure of the hair, allowing it to be set in the style required
Ammonium bisulfite
Ammonium thioglycolate
Ammonium thiolactate
Cysteamine HCl
Glyceryl thioglycolate
Thioglycerin
Thiolactic acid

HUMECTANT
Holds and retains moisture
Butylene glycol
Cyclomethicone
Dipotassium glycyrrhizate
Ethoxydiglycol
Fructooligosaccharides
Glycerin
Glycyrrhizic acid
Hydrolyzed collagen
Methyl glucose dioleate
PEG-6
Phytantriol
Propylene glycol
Sodium PCA
Sorbitol
Sulfated castor oil
Triacontanyl PVP

HYDROTROPE
Enhances the solubility of substance which is only slightly soluble in water
Cocamidopropylamine oxide
Disodium lauroamphodiacetate
Disodium oleamido MEA-sulfosuccinate
Disodium ricinoleamido MEA-sulfosuccinate
Lauramine oxide
TEA-PEG-3 cocamide sulfate

KERATOLYTIC
Helps eliminate the dead cells of the stratum corneum
Thioglycerin

MASKING
Reduces or inhibits the basic odour or taste of the product
Achillea millefolium extract
Alcohol
Anthemis nobilis flower extract
Ascorbic acid
Beeswax (see Cera alba)
Benzoic acid
Benzophenone-2
Betula alba bark extract
BHA
BHT

MASKING (*continued*)
Butylene glycol
Butyl methacrylate
Butylparaben
Calendula officinalis extract
Caprylic/capric triglyceride
Cetyl alcohol
Cod liver oil
Dibutyl phthalate
Diethyl sebacate
Dipropylene glycol
Laureth-4
Laurus nobilis leaf extract
Menthoxypropanediol
Octyldodecanol
Quinine
Resorcinol
Ricinus communis seed oil
Sesamum indicum seed oil
Sodium benzoate
Stearic acid
Stearyl alcohol
Styrax benzoin gum
Thiolactic acid
Tocopherol
Triethanolamine
Tromethamine

MOISTURIZING
Increases the water content of the skin and helps keep it soft and smooth
Propolis
Ricinus communis seed oil

NAIL CONDITIONING
Improves the cosmetic characteristics of the nail
Diethylene glycol dimethacrylate
Triethylene glycol dimethacrylate

OPACIFYING
Reduces transparency or translucency of cosmetics
Alumina
Cera microcristallina
Cetearyl alcohol
Cetyl alcohol
Glyceryl diisostearate
Guanine
Methyl methacrylate
Oleyl alcohol
Stearyl alcohol
Zinc ricinoleate

ORAL CARE
Provides cosmetic effects to the oral cavity, e.g. cleansing, deodorising, protecting
Chlorhexidine digluconate
Glycerin
Olaflur
Stannous fluoride

OXIDISING
Changes the chemical nature of another substance by adding oxygen or removing hydrogen
Ammonium persulfate
Benzoyl peroxide
Hydrogen peroxide
Potassium persulfate

PERFUMING
Used for perfume and aromatic raw materials (Section II)
Anthemis nobilis flower extract
Betula alba bark extract
t-Butyl alcohol
Calendula officinalis extract
Caprylic/capric triglyceride
Cera alba
Dibutyl phthalate
Dipropylene glycol
Ethoxydiglycol
Glycerin
Glyceryl rosinate
Glycyrrhiza glabra root extract
Guaiazulene
Helichrysum italicum flower extract
Hexylene glycol
Isopropyl alcohol
Isopropyl myristate
Lauramine oxide
Methyl salicylate
Myristic acid
Octyldodecanol
Olea Europaea fruit oil
Phenyl salicylate
Propyl gallate
Propylparaben
Styrax benzoin gum
TBHQ

PLASTICISER
Softens and makes supple another substance that otherwise could not be easily deformed, spread or worked out
Diethyl sebacate
Ethyl acrylate
Sorbitol
Tosylamide/formaldehyde resin
Trioleyl phosphate

PRESERVATIVE
Inhibits primarily the development of micro-organisms in cosmetics
Ammonium bisulfite
Benzalkonium chloride
Benzethonium chloride
Benzoic acid
Benzylhemiformal
5-Bromo-5-nitro-1,3-dioxane
2-Bromo-2-nitropropane-1,3-diol

PRESERVATIVE (*continued*)
Butylparaben
Cetalkonium chloride
Cetrimonium bromide
Chlorhexidine digluconate
Chloroacetamide
p-Chloro-m-cresol
Chlorphenesin
Diazolidinyl urea
Dichlorobenzyl alcohol
Dimethyl oxazolidine
DMDM hydantoin
Ethylparaben
Formaldehyde
Glutaraldehyde
Hexamidine
Hexamidine diisethionate
Imidazolidinyl urea
Iodopropynyl butylcarbamate
Methenamine
Methylchloroisothiazolinone (and) methyliso-
  thiazolinone
Methylisothiazolinone
Methylparaben
Paraformaldehyde
Phenoxyethanol
o-Phenylphenol
Polyaminopropyl biguanide
Potassium sorbate
Propylparaben
Quaternium-15
Sodium benzoate
Sodium bisulfite
Sodium hydroxymethylglycinate
Sorbic acid
Thimerosal
Triclocarban
Triclosan
Tris(N-hydroxyethyl)hexahydrotriazine
Zinc pyrithione

REDUCING
**Changes the chemical nature of another substance
by adding hydrogen or removing oxygen**
Ammonium bisulfite
Ammonium thioglycolate
Ammonium thiolactate
Dihydroxyacetone
Sodium bisulfite
Sodium metabisulfite
Thioglycerin
Thiolactic acid

REFATTING
**Replenishes the lipids of the hair or of the top layers
of the skin**
Steareth-10
Stearic acid
Stearyl alcohol

REFRESHING
Imparts a pleasant freshness to the skin
Achillea millefolium extract
Laurus nobilis leaf extract
Menthoxypropanediol

SKIN CONDITIONING
Maintains the skin in good condition
Acetylated lanolin
Achillea millefolium extract
C18-36 Acid triglyceride
C12-15 Alkyl benzoate
Allantoin
Alpha-glucan oligosaccharide
Anthemis nobilis flower extract
Arbutin
Argania spinosa kernel oil
Arnica montana extract
Ascorbic acid
Ascorbyl tetraisopalmitate
Azulene
Beeswax (see Cera alba)
Beta-carotene
Biosaccharide gum-4
Bisabolol
Butylene glycol
Butyrospermum parkii butter
Calendula officinalis (flower) extract
Caprylic/capric triglyceride
Capryloyl salicylic acid
Cetearyl ethylhexanoate
Cetearyl isononanoate
Chamomilla recutita extract
Chrysanthemum parthenium extract (see *Tanacetum
parthenium*)
Cocamidopropyl hydroxysultaine
Coco-betaine
Cod liver oil
Commiphora mukul resin extract
Cucumis sativus (cucumber) fruit extract
Decyl oleate
Dicaprylyl maleate
Diethyl sebacate
bis-Diglyceryl polyacyladipate-2
Diglyceryl sebacate/isopalmitate
Dihydroxyacetone
Diisostearyl malate
Dipentaerythrityl hexahydroxystearate/hexa-
  stearate/hexarosinate
Dipotassium glycyrrhizate
Disodium ricinoleamido MEA-sulfosuccinate
Distearyl phthalic acid amide
Ditrimethylolpropane triethylhexanoate
Equae lac
3-o-Ethyl ascorbic acid
Ethylhexylglycerin
bis-Ethylhexyloxyphenol methoxyphenyl triazine
Fructooligosaccharides
Glyceryl isostearate/myristate

SKIN CONDITIONING (*continued*)

Glycine soja seed extract
Glycyrrhetinic acid
Glycyrrhiza glabra (licorice) root extract
Glycyrrhiza inflata root extract
Glycyrrhizic acid
Goat milk
Guar hydroxypropyltrimonium chloride
Hamamelis virginiana bark/leaf/twig extract
Henna
Hexamidine diisethionate
Hexylene glycol
Homosalate
Hydrogenated castor oil
Hydrolyzed collagen
Hydrolyzed wheat protein
Hydroxypropyl tetrahydropyrantriol
Isohexadecane
Isononyl isononanoate
Isostearyl alcohol
Lanolin
Lonicera japonica flower extract
Magnolia grandiflora bark extract
Magnolia officinalis bark extract
Maleated soybean oil
Methoxy PEG-17/dodecyl glycol copolymer
Methyl glucose dioleate
Methyl glucose sesquistearate
Myristyl alcohol
Panthenol
Pentylene glycol
Pentyl rhamnoside
Persea gratissima (avocado) oil
Phenyl dimethicone
Polyester-8
Potassium cocoyl hydrolyzed collagen
Propolis
Propylene glycol
Propylene glycol ricinoleate
Prunus avium seed oil
Pyridoxine dioctenoate
Retinyl palmitate
Ricinus communis seed oil
Ruscogenin
Salvia officinalis extract
Sesamum indicum seed oil
Simmondsia chinensis (jojoba) seed oil
Simmondsia chinensis seed powder
Sodium chondroitin sulfate
Sodium lauroyl sarcosinate
Sodium PCA
Sorbitol
Styrax benzoin gum
Tanacetum vulgare extract
TEA-cocoyl hydrolyzed collagen
Tetrahydromagnolol
Tocopheryl linoleate
Tocopheryl nicotinate
Triethylene glycol hydrogenated rosinate

Trioleyl phosphate
Xanthan gum

SKIN PROTECTING
Helps to avoid harmful effects to the skin from external factors
Allantoin
Cod liver oil
Paraffinum liquidum
Resveratrol
Salvia officinalis extract
Tocopheryl linoleate
Tocopheryl nicotinate

SMOOTHING
Seeks to achieve an even skin surface by decreasing roughness or irregularities
Propolis
Ricinus communis seed oil

SOLVENT
Dissolves other substances
Alcohol
t-Butyl alcohol
Butylene glycol
Cyclomethicone
Dicaprylyl maleate
Diethyl sebacate
Dipropylene glycol
Ethoxydiglycol
Glycerin
Hexylene glycol
Isohexadecane
Isopropyl alcohol
Isopropyl myristate
Lanolin oil
Paraffinum liquidum
PEG-6
Pentylene glycol
Propylene glycol
Ricinus communis seed oil

SOOTHING
Helps lightening discomfort of the skin or of the scalp
Achillea millefolium extract
Allantoin
Azulene
Bisabolol
Glycyrrhiza glabra (licorice) root extract
Methyl nicotinate
Salvia officinalis extract

STABILIZING
Improves ingredients or formulation stability and shelf-life
Hydroquinone
Oxyquinoline

SURFACTANT
Lowers the surface tension of cosmetics as well as aids the even distribution of the product when used
Arachidyl glucoside
Benzalkonium chloride
Benzethonium chloride
Ceteareth-2
Ceteareth-3
Cetearyl alcohol
Cetearyl glucoside
Cetrimonium bromide
Cetyl alcohol
Cocamide
Cocamide DEA
Cocamidopropylamine oxide
Cocamidopropyl betaine
Cocamidopropyl dimethylamine
Cocamidopropyl hydroxysultaine
Coco-betaine
Coco-glucoside
Decyl glucoside
Diisostearyl malate
Disodium lauroamphodiacetate
Disodium oleamido MEA-sulfosuccinate
Disodium ricinoleamido MEA-sulfosuccinate
Glyceryl isostearate/myristate
Hexyldecanoic acid
Hexylene glycol
Hydrogenated castor oil
Hydroxystearic acid
Lanolin
Lauramide DEA
Lauramine oxide
Laureth-2
Laureth-4
Laureth-7
Laureth-12
Lauryl glucoside
Laurylpyridinium chloride
Octyldodecyl xyloside
C30-38 Olefin/isopropyl maleate/MA copolymer
Oleth-3 phosphate
Palmitoyl hydrolyzed wheat protein
PEG-7 hydrogenated castor oil
PEG-7 oleate
PEG-32 stearate
Polysorbate 40
Polysorbate 80
PPG-1-PEG-9 lauryl glycol ether
Ricinoleic acid
Sodium cocoamphoacetate
Sodium cocoamphopropionate
Sodium dihydroxycetyl phosphate
Sodium laureth sulfate
Sodium lauroamphoacetate
Sodium lauroyl sarcosinate
Sodium lauryl sulfate
Sodium myristoyl sarcosinate
Sodium stearate

Steareth-10
Stearic acid
Sulfated castor oil
TEA-cocoyl hydrolyzed collagen
TEA-PEG-3 cocamide sulfate
TEA-stearate
Triceteareth-4 phosphate
Trideceth-2 carboxamide MEA
Triethanolamine
Trilaureth-4 phosphate
Xanthan gum

TANNING
Darkens the skin with or without exposure to UV
Dihydroxyacetone

TONIC
Produces a feeling of well-being on skin and hair
Achillea millefolium extract
Commiphora mukul resin extract
Laurus nobilis leaf extract
Methyl nicotinate
Salvia officinalis extract

UV-ABSORBER
Protects the cosmetic product from the effects of UV-light
Benzophenone-2
Benzophenone-3
Benzophenone-4
Benzophenone-8
Benzophenone-10
Bornelone
Butyl methoxydibenzoylmethane
Cinoxate
Digalloyl trioleate
Disodium phenyl dibenzimidazole tetrasulfonate
Drometrizole
Drometrizole trisiloxane
Ethylhexyl methoxycinnamate
bis-Ethylhexyloxyphenol methoxyphenyl triazine
Ethylhexyl salicylate
Ethylhexyl triazone
Homosalate
Isoamyl *p*-methoxycinnamate
Isopropyl dibenzoylmethane
4-Methylbenzylidene camphor
Octocrylene
PEG-25 PABA
Phenylbenzimidazole sulfonic acid
Terephthalylidene dicamphor sulfonic acid

UV-FILTER
Filters certain UV rays in order to protect the skin or the hair from harmful effects of these rays
Benzophenone-3
Benzophenone-4
Butyl methoxydibenzoylmethane
Diethylamino hydroxybenzoyl hexyl benzoate

UV-FILTER (*continued*)
Disodium phenyl dibenzimidazole tetrasulfonate
Drometrizole trisiloxane
Ethylhexyl methoxycinnamate
bis-Ethylhexyloxyphenol methoxyphenyl triazine
Ethylhexyl salicylate
Ethylhexyl triazone
Homosalate
Isoamyl p-methoxycinnamate
4-Methylbenzylidene camphor
Methylene bis-benzotriazolyl tetramethylbutylphenol
Methylene bis-benzotriazolyl tetramethylbutylphenol
 (and) aqua (and) decyl glucoside (and) propylene
glycol (and) xanthan gum
Octocrylene
PEG-25 PABA
Phenylbenzimidazole sulfonic acid
Polysilicone-15
Terephthalylidene dicamphor sulfonic acid

VISCOSITY CONTROLLING
Increases or decreases the viscosity of cosmetics
Alcohol
Alumina
Beeswax (see Cera alba)
Butylene glycol
Butyl methacrylate
Butyrospermum parkii butter
C30-38 Olefin /isopropyl maleate/MA copolymer
Cera microcristallina
Cetearyl alcohol
Cetyl alcohol
Cocamide
Cocamide DEA
Cocamidopropyl betaine
Cocamidopropyl hydroxysultaine
Coco-betaine

Colophonium
Cyclomethicone
Dipropylene glycol
Disodium EDTA
Disodium lauroamphodiacetate
Ethyl methacrylate
Guar hydroxypropyltrimonium chloride
Hydrogenated castor oil
Isopropyl alcohol
Isostearyl alcohol
Lanolin alcohol
Lauramide DEA
Lauramine oxide
Lauryl alcohol
Methoxy PEG-22/dodecyl glycol copolymer
Myristyl alcohol
Oleamide DEA
Oleyl alcohol
PEG-4 rapeseedamide
Phthalic anhydride/trimellitic anhydride/glycols
 copolymer
Polyethylene
Propylene glycol
Propylene glycol ricinoleate
Shellac
Sodium lauroyl sarcosinate
Sodium myristoyl sarcosinate
Sodium stearate
Stearyl alcohol
Triacontanyl PVP
Trideceth-2 carboxamide MEA
Triethylene glycol hydrogenated rosinate
Undecylenamide DEA
VP/eicosene copolymer
VP/hexadecene copolymer
Xanthan gum

5.3　FUNCTIONAL CLASSES IN THE USA SYSTEM (PERSONAL CARE PRODUCTS COUNCIL INGREDIENT DATABASE)

ABRASIVES

Abrasives are used in cosmetics to remove unwanted tissue or foreign materials from various body surfaces
Alumina
Polyethylene

ABSORBENTS

Absorbents are ingredients, usually solids, with a large surface area which can attract dissolved or finely dispersed substances from another medium
Alumina

ADHESIVES

Adhesives are substances that tend to bind opposite surfaces to each other
Polyethylene
Styrax benzoin gum

ANTIACNE AGENTS

Antiacne agents are active ingredients used in antiacne products
Benzoyl peroxide

ANTICAKING AGENTS

Anticaking agents are ingredients used to prevent the agglomeration of a particulate solid into lumps or cohesive cakes
Alumina
Methyl methacrylate
Phytantriol
Zinc ricinoleate

ANTICARIES AGENTS

Anticaries agents are active ingredients used in anticaries products
Stannous fluoride

ANTIDANDRUFF AGENTS

Antidandruff agents are active ingredients used in dandruff control, seborrheic dermatitis, and psoriasis control drug products
Hexamidine diisethionate
Selenium sulfide
Zinc pyrithione

ANTIFOAMING AGENTS

Antifoaming agents or, for short, antifoams, are chemicals which reduce the tendency of finished products to generate foam on shaking or agitation
Alcohol
Isopropyl alcohol
Phenyl dimethicone

ANTIMICROBIAL AGENTS

Antimicrobial agents are active ingredients used in antimicrobial products
Alcohol
Benzalkonium chloride
Benzethonium chloride
Hexylresorcinol
Hydrogen peroxide
Magnolia grandiflora bark extract
Magnolia officinalis bark extract
Scutellaria baicalensis extract

ANTIOXIDANTS

Antioxidants are ingredients employed in cosmetics to prevent or retard product spoilage from rancidity (or deterioration from reaction with oxygen)
Arbutin
Ascorbic acid
Ascorbyl tetraisopalmitate
BHA
BHT
Caprylyl gallate
CI 75470
Di-t-butylhydroquinone
Digalloyl trioleate
Dodecyl gallate
Glycyrrhiza glabra (licorice) root extract
Hesperidin methyl chalcone
Hexylresorcinol
Hydroquinone
Hydroxydecyl ubiquinone
Kojic acid
Magnolia grandiflora bark extract
Nordihydroguaiaretic acid
Phenylethyl resorcinol
Propyl gallate
Resorcinol
Resveratrol
Sodium bisulfite
Sodium metabisulfite
TBHQ
Thioctic acid
Thiolactic acid
Tocopheryl linoleate
Tocopheryl nicotinate

ANTIPERSPIRANT AGENTS

Antiperspirant agents are active ingredients used in antiperspirant products
Aluminum chloride
Aluminum chlorohydrate

ANTISTATIC AGENTS

Antistatic agents are ingredients that alter the electrical properties of cosmetic raw materials or of human body surfaces (skin, hair, etc.) by reducing their tendency to acquire an electrical charge

Benzalkonium chloride
Cetalkonium chloride
Cetrimonium bromide
Cocamidopropyl betaine
Cocamidopropyl dimethylamine
Cocamidopropyl hydroxysultaine
Cocamidopropyl PG-dimonium chloride phosphate
Coco-betaine
Didecyldimonium chloride
Guar hydroxypropyltrimonium chloride
Isostearamidopropyl morpholine lactate
Laurylpyridinium chloride
Oleamidopropyl dimethylamine
Polyquaternium-7
Quaternium-15
Quaternium-22
Stearamidoethyl diethylamine phosphate

ARTIFICIAL NAIL BUILDING

Artificial nail builders are ingredients that are used in nail enhancement products to build, elongate or extend the nail

Benzoyl peroxide
1,4-Butanediol dimethacrylate
Butyl methacrylate
Diethylene glycol dimethacrylate
Di-HEMA trimethylhexyl dicarbamate
Ethyl methacrylate
Glycol HEMA-methacrylate
HEMA
Hydroxypropyl methacrylate
Isobutyl methacrylate
Methyl methacrylate
PEG-4 dimethacrylate
Triethylene glycol dimethacrylate

BINDERS

Binders are ingredients added to compounded dry powder mixtures of solids and the like to provide adhesive qualities during and after compression to make tablets or cakes

Ceresin
Colophonium
Ditrimethylolpropane triethylhexanoate
Hydroabietyl alcohol
Isopropyl myristate
Lanolin alcohol
Microcrystalline wax
Pentaerythrityl triacrylate
Polyethylene
Shellac
VP/eicosene copolymer
VP/hexadecene copolymer
Xanthan gum

BULKING AGENTS

Bulking agents are usually chemically inert, solid ingredients employed as diluents for other solids

Alumina
Microcrystalline wax
Polyethylene

CHELATING AGENTS

Chelating agents, also called sequestrants, are ingredients that have the ability to complex with and inactivate metallic ions in order to prevent their adverse effects on the stability or appearance of cosmetic products

Caprylhydroxamic acid
Disodium EDTA
EDTA
Methyl dihydroxybenzoate
Oxyquinoline
Tetrahydroxypropyl ethylenediamine
Tetrasodium EDTA
Trisodium EDTA

COLORANTS

Colorants, or color additives, are those cosmetic ingredients which impart color to the skin or its appendages or are used to color finished products

Chromium oxide greens
CI 11680
CI 12010
CI 12085
CI 12150
CI 15800
CI 47000
CI 75470
CI 77163
CI 77289
CI Pigment red 53:1
Dihydroxyacetone
Guaiazulene
Guanine
Henna
Lawsone
Pigment orange 5
Pigment red 57:1
Pigment red 172 aluminum lake
Pigment yellow 12
Solvent yellow 44

CORROSION INHIBITORS

Corrosion inhibitors are substances added to products in order to prevent the corrosion of metallic (and occasionally other) materials used for cosmetic packaging

Sodium benzoate

COSMETIC ADSTRINGENTS

Cosmetic astringents are cosmetic ingredients intended to induce a tightening or tingling sensation on skin

Alcohol
Aluminum chloride
Aluminum chlorohydrate
Euphorbia cerifera (candelilla) wax
Hamamelis virginiana bark/leaf/twig extract
Tioxolone

COSMETIC BIOCIDES

Cosmetic biocides are ingredients used in cosmetic products to help cleanse the skin or prevent odor by inhibiting the growth of, or destroying microorganisms, such as bacteria, fungi or yeast

Benzalkonium chloride
Benzethonium chloride
Benzoxonium chloride
Captan
Cetalkonium chloride
Cetrimonium bromide
Chlorhexidine digluconate
p-Chloro-m-cresol
Chlorphenesin
Coal tar
Dichlorobenzyl alcohol
Dichlorophene
Formaldehyde
Glutaraldehyde
Hexamidine
Hexamidine diisethionate
Hexylresorcinol
Hydrogen peroxide
Laurylpyridinium chloride
Methenamine
Oxyquinoline
o-Phenylphenol
Phenyl salicylate
2,2'-Thiobis(4-chlorophenol)
Triclocarban
Triclosan
Zinc pyrithione

DENATURANTS

Denaturants are ingredients added to ethyl alcohol to make it unsuitable for ingestion

t-Butyl alcohol
Coal tar
Formaldehyde
Glycerin
Phenyl salicylate
Polysorbate 80
Resorcinol
Sodium lauryl sulfate

DEODORANT AGENTS

Deodorants are ingredients that reduce or eliminate unpleasant odor and protect against the formation of malodor on body surfaces

Aluminum chloride
Aluminum chlorohydrate
Benzalkonium chloride
Benzethonium chloride
Dichlorophene
Ethylhexylglycerin
Laurylpyridinium chloride
Triclocarban
Triclosan
Zinc ricinoleate

DEPILATING AGENTS

Depilating agents are the functional constituents of products designed to remove unwanted hair (depilatories)

Thioglycerin
Thiolactic acid

DISPERSING AGENTS – NONSURFACTANT

Dispersing agents - nonsurfactant is a group of cosmetic ingredients which facilitate the dispersion of solids in liquids

Ditrimethylolpropane triethylhexanoate
Methoxy PEG-17/dodecyl glycol copolymer
Methoxy PEG-22/dodecyl glycol copolymer
Methyl methacrylate
Nitrocellulose
Propylene glycol ricinoleate
Tosylamide/formaldehyde resin
VP/eicosene copolymer
VP/hexadecene copolymer

DRUG ASTRINGENTS - SKIN PROTECTANT DRUGS

Drug astringent-skin protectant drugs are active ingredients used in skin protectant drug astringent products

Phytonadione epoxide

EMULSION STABILIZERS

Emulsion stabilizers are cosmetic ingredients that assist in the formation and the stabilization of emulsions

Beeswax (see Cera alba)
Cetearyl alcohol
Cetyl alcohol
Lanolin
Lanolin alcohol
Lauryl alcohol
Microcrystalline wax
Methoxy PEG-17/dodecyl glycol copolymer
Methoxy PEG-22/dodecyl glycol copolymer
Myristyl alcohol
PEG-22/dodecyl glycol copolymer
Polyethylene
Stearyl alcohol

EMULSION STABILIZERS (*continued*)
Xanthan gum

EPILATING AGENTS
Epilating agents are functional constituents of products designed to remove unwanted hair mechanically
Ceresin
Colophonium
Copernicia cerifera (carnauba) wax

EXTERNAL ANALGESICS
External analgesics are active ingredients used in local anesthetic, analgesic, and antipruritic external products
Methyl nicotinate
Resorcinol

FILM FORMERS
Film formers are materials which produce a continuous film on skin, hair, or nails
Beeswax (see Cera alba)
Chitosan
Colophonium
Copernicia cerifera (carnauba) wax
Diethylene glycol dimethacrylate
Euphorbia cerifera (candelilla) wax
Hydrolyzed wheat protein
Nitrocellulose
Pentaerythrityl triacrylate
Phthalic anhydride/trimellitic anhydride/glycols
 copolymer
Polyester-8
Polyethylene
Polyquaternium-7
Quaternium-22
Shellac
Styrax benzoin gum
Tetrahydrofurfuryl methacrylate
Tosylamide/formaldehyde resin
Triacontanyl PVP
Trimethylolpropane triacrylate
VP/eicosene copolymer
VP/hexadecene copolymer

FLAVORING AGENTS
Flavoring agents (or simply, flavors) enhance the taste of cosmetic products
Dipotassium glycyrrhizate
Glycyrrhizic acid
Laurus nobilis leaf extract
Menthoxypropanediol
Methyl salicylate
Sorbitol

FRAGRANCE INGREDIENTS
Fragrance ingredients are any basic substance used in the manufacture of fragrance materials for its odorous, odor-enhancing or blending properties

Achillea millefolium extract
Alcohol
Anthemis nobilis flower extract
Ascorbic acid
Beeswax (see Cera alba)
Benzoic acid
Benzophenone-2
Betula alba bark extract
BHA
BHT
Bisabolol
t-Butyl alcohol
Butylene glycol
Butyl methacrylate
Butylparaben
Calendula officinalis extract
Candelilla cera
Caprylic/capric triglyceride
Cetyl alcohol
Chamomilla recutita extract
CI 75470
Cod liver oil
Dibutyl phthalate
Diethyl sebacate
Dipropylene glycol
Ethoxydiglycol
Ethylhexyl salicylate
Ethylparaben
Glutaraldehyde
Glycerin
Glyceryl rosinate
Glyceryl stearate
Glycyrrhizic acid
Guaiazulene
Hexylene glycol
Hinokitiol
Homosalate
Hydroquinone
Isopropyl alcohol
Isopropyl myristate
Lauramine oxide
Laurus nobilis leaf oil
Lauryl alcohol
Melissa officinalis flower/leaf/stem extract
Menthoxypropanediol
Methyl nicotinate
Methylparaben
Mineral oil
Myristic acid
Myristyl alcohol
Octyl dodecanol
Olea Europaea fruit oil
Oleth-5
Oleyl alcohol
Paraffinum liquidum
PEG-7 hydrogenated castor oil
Phenoxyethanol
o-Phenylphenol
Phenyl salicylate

FRAGRANCE INGREDIENTS (*continued***)**
Polysorbate 80
Potassium sorbate
Propylene glycol
Propylparaben
Propyl gallate
Prunus amygdalus dulcis (almond) oil
Pyrocatechol
Pyrogallol
Resorcinol
Ricinus communis seed oil
Sesamum indicum seed oil
Sodium benzoate
Sorbic acid
Sorbitan oleate
Sorbitol
Stearic acid
Stearyl alcohol
Styrax benzoin gum
TBHQ
Thiolactic acid
Tocopherol
Triethanolamine
Tromethamine

HAIR COLORANTS
Hair colorants are materials which impart color to hair
4-Amino-*m*-cresol
2-Amino-4-hydroxyethylaminoanisole sulfate
4-Amino-2-hydroxytoluene
2-Aminomethyl-*p*-aminophenol HCl
4-Amino-3-nitrophenol
m-Aminophenol
p-Aminophenol
Basic blue 99
Basic red 22
Basic violet 10
2-Chloro-*p*-phenylenediamine
2,4-Diaminophenoxyethanol HCl
HC red no. 7
HC Yellow no. 7
Henna
Hydroquinone
2-Hydroxyethylamino-5-nitroanisole
N,*N*-bis(2-Hydroxyethyl)-*p*-phenylenediamine sulfate
Lead acetate
6-Methoxy-2-methylamino-3-aminopyridine HCl
p-Methylaminophenol
2,7-Naphthalenediol
3-Nitro-*p*-hydroxyethylaminophenol
2-Nitro-*p*-phenylenediamine
p-Phenylenediamine
N-Phenyl-*p*-phenylenediamine
Pyrocatechol
Resorcinol
Toluene-2,5-diamine
Toluene-2,5-diamine sulfate

HAIR CONDITIONING AGENTS
Hair conditioning agents are ingredients used to create special effects on hair
Acetylated lanolin
Cetearyl ethylhexanoate
Cetearyl isononanoate
Cocamidopropylamine oxide
Cocamidopropyl betaine
Cocamidopropyl hydroxysultaine
Cocamidopropyl PG-dimonium chloride phosphate
Coco-betaine
Cyclomethicone
Didecyldimonium chloride
Disodium lauroamphodiacetate
Glycerin
Guar hydroxypropyltrimonium chloride
Hinokitiol
Hydrolyzed collagen
Hydrolyzed wheat protein
Lanolin
Lanolin alcohol
Lanolin oil
Lauramine oxide
Lauroyl collagen amino acids
Mineral oil
Palmitoyl collagen amino acids
Palmitoyl hydrolyzed milk protein
Palmitoyl hydrolyzed wheat protein
Panthenol
Panthenyl ethyl ether
Petrolatum
Phytantriol
Potassium cocoyl hydrolyzed collagen
Pyridoxine dioctenoate
Selenium sulfide
Simmondsia chinensis (jojoba) seed oil
Sodium chondroitin sulfate
Sodium cocoamphoacetate
Sodium cocoamphopropionate
Sodium hydroxymethylglycinate
Sodium lauroamphoacetate
Sodium lauroyl sarcosinate
Sodium myristoyl sarcosinate
Sodium PCA
Stearamidoethyl diethylamine phosphate
TEA-cocoyl hydrolyzed collagen
Trimethylolpropane triacrylate
Undecylenamide DEA
Zinc pyrithione

HAIR FIXATIVES
Hair fixatives are ingredients which impart holding or style-retention properties to hair
Chitosan
Polyquaternium-7
Shellac
Trimethylolpropane triacrylate
VP/hexadecene copolymer

HAIR-WAVING/STRAIGHTENING AGENTS
Hair-waving/straightening agents are chemicals which react with hair fibers to facilitate permanent configurational changes
Ammonium bisulfite
Ammonium thioglycolate
Ammonium thiolactate
Cysteamine HCl
Glyceryl thioglycolate
Sodium bisulfite
Thioglycerin
Thiolactic acid

HUMECTANTS
Humectants are ingredients used in cosmetic products to retard moisture loss from the product during use
Glycerin
PEG-6
Sodium PCA
Sorbitol

LIGHT STABILIZERS
Light stabilizers are employed in cosmetics to protect the product from chemical or physical deterioration induced by light
Benzophenone-2
Benzophenone-3
Benzophenone-4
Benzophenone-8
Benzophenone-10
Bornelone
Butyl methoxydibenzoylmethane
Cinoxate
Diethylamino hydroxybenzoyl hexyl benzoate
Digalloyl trioleate
Disodium phenyl dibenzimidazole tetrasulfonate
Drometrizole
Drometrizole trisiloxane
Ethylhexyl methoxycinnamate
Ethylhexyl salicylate
Ethylhexyl triazone
Ethyl methoxycinnamate
Glyceryl PABA
Homosalate
Isoamyl *p*-methoxycinnamate
Isopropyl dibenzoylmethane
4-Methylbenzylidene camphor
Octocrylene
PABA
PEG-25 PABA
Pentyl dimethyl PABA
Phenylbenzimidazole sulfonic acid
Polysilicone-15
Terephthalylidene dicamphor sulfonic acid

NAIL CONDITIONING AGENTS
Nail conditioning agents are ingredients which improve the characteristics of nails

Hydrolyzed collagen

OPACIFYING AGENTS
Opacifying agents are ingredients deliberately added to cosmetic products to reduce their clear or transparent appearance
Alumina
Cetearyl alcohol
Cetyl alcohol
Guanine
Methyl methacrylate
Myristic acid
Zinc ricinoleate

ORAL CARE AGENTS
Oral care agents are cosmetic ingredients and excipients used in products to polish teeth, act as oral deodorants or provide other cosmetic effects
Chlorhexidine digluconate
Hydrogen peroxide
Laurus nobilis leaf extract
Polyethylene
Stannous fluoride

ORAL HEALTH CARE DRUGS
Oral health care drugs are active ingredients used in oral health care products
Glycerin
Hexylresorcinol
Hydrogen peroxide
Stannous fluoride

OXIDIZING AGENTS
Oxidizing agents are chemicals which gain electrons during their reaction with a reducing agent
Ammonium persulfate
Hydrogen peroxide
Potassium persulfate

PESTICIDES
Pesticides are the active ingredients used in pesticide products
Benzalkonium chloride
Benzethonium chloride
Dichlorophene
Iodopropynyl butylcarbamate
o-Phenylphenol
Quaternium-15

pH ADJUSTERS
pH Adjusters are chemicals (acids, bases, or buffering agents) which are used to control the pH of finished cosmetic products
Ascorbic acid
Benzoic acid
Diisopropanolamine
Glucosamine HCl
Triethanolamine
Tromethamine

PLASTICIZERS

Plasticizers are materials which soften synthetic polymers

Dibutyl phthalate
Diethyl sebacate
Ethyl acrylate
Tosylamide/formaldehyde resin
Trioleyl phosphate

PRESERVATIVES

Preservatives are ingredients which prevent or retard microbial growth and thus protect cosmetic products from spoilage

Benzethonium chloride
Benzisothiazolinone
Benzoic acid
Benzylhemiformal
5-Bromo-5-nitro-1,3-dioxane
2-Bromo-2-nitropropane-1,3-diol
Butylparaben
Captan
Chlorhexidine digluconate
Chloroacetamide
p-Chloro-*m*-cresol
Diazolidinyl urea
Dimethyl oxazolidine
DMDM hydantoin
Ethylparaben
Formaldehyde
Glutaraldehyde
Hexamidine
Hexamidine diisethionate
Imidazolidinyl urea
Iodopropynyl butylcarbamate
Methenamine
Methylchloroisothiazolinone (and)
 methylisothiazolinone
Methyldibromo glutaronitrile
Methyldibromo glutaronitrile/phenoxyethanol
Methylisothiazolinone
Methylparaben
Pentylene glycol
Phenoxyethanol
o-Phenylphenol
Polyaminopropyl biguanide
Potassium sorbate
Propylparaben
Quaternium-15
Sodium benzoate
Sodium hydroxymethylglycinate
Sodium pyrithione
Sorbic acid
Thimerosal
Triclocarban
Triclosan
Tris(*N*-hydroxyethyl)hexahydrotriazine
Zinc pyrithione

REDUCING AGENTS

Reducing agents are chemicals which during their reaction with oxidizing agents lose electrons

Ammonium bisulfite
Ammonium thioglycolate
Ammonium thiolactate
Cysteamine HCl
Hydroquinone
Sodium bisulfite
Sodium metabisulfite
Thioglycerin
Thiolactic acid

SKIN BLEACHING AGENTS

Skin bleaching agents are active ingredients used in skin bleaching products

Ammonium persulfate
Arbutin
Glycyrrhiza glabra (licorice) root extract
Hydroquinone

SKIN-CONDITIONING AGENTS – EMOLLIENT

Skin-conditioning agents - emollient are cosmetic ingredients which help to maintain the soft, smooth, and pliable appearance of skin

Acetylated lanolin
C12-15 Alkyl benzoate
Argania spinosa kernel oil
Ascorbyl tetraisopalmitate
Beeswax (see Cera alba)
Cetearyl ethylhexanoate
Cetearyl isononanoate
Copernicia cerifera (carnauba) wax
Cucumis sativus (cucumber) fruit extract
Cyclomethicone
Decyl oleate
Dicaprylyl maleate
Diethyl sebacate
bis-Diglyceryl polyacyladipate-2
Diglyceryl sebacate/isopalmitate
Diisostearyl malate
Distearyl phthalic acid amide
Ditrimethylolpropane triethylhexanoate
Glyceryl abietate
Glyceryl caprylate
Glyceryl diisostearate
Glyceryl hydrogenated rosinate
Glyceryl isostearate
Glyceryl isostearate/myristate
Glyceryl rosinate
Glyceryl stearate
Isohexadecane
Isononyl isononanoate
Isopropyl myristate
Isostearyl alcohol
Lanolin
Lanolin oil
Lauryl alcohol
Methyl glucose dioleate

SKIN-CONDITIONING AGENTS – EMOLLIENT (*cont'd*)

Methyl glucose sesquistearate
Mineral oil
Myristyl alcohol
Octyldodecanol
Oleyl alcohol
PEG-7 hydrogenated castor oil
PEG-22/dodecyl glycol copolymer
Pentaerythrityl rosinate
Propolis
Propylene glycol ricinoleate
Sesamum indicum seed oil

SKIN-CONDITIONING AGENTS – HUMECTANT

Skin-conditioning agents - humectant are cosmetic ingredients intended to increase the water content of the top layers of skin

Fructooligosaccharides
Glycerin
Glycyrrhiza glabra (licorice) root extract
Propylene glycol
Sodium PCA
Sorbitol

SKIN-CONDITIONING AGENTS – MISCELLANEOUS

Skin-conditioning agents - miscellaneous are cosmetic ingredients used to create special effects on skin

Achillea millefolium extract
Allantoin
Alpha-glucan oligosaccharide
Anthemis nobilis flower extract
Arbutin
Argania spinosa kernel oil
Arnica montana extract
Ascorbic acid
Avena sativa (oat) bran extract
Azulene
Beta-carotene
Betula alba (birch) bark extract
Biosaccharide gum-4
Bisabolol
Butylene glycol
Butyrospermum parkii butter
Calendula officinalis (flower) extract
Capryloyl salicylic acid
Chamomilla recutita extract
Chrysanthemum parthenium extract (see *Tanacetum parthenium*)
Cocamidopropyl betaine
Cocamidopropyl hydroxysultaine
Coco-betaine
Commiphora mukul resin extract
Cucumis sativus (cucumber) fruit extract
Dihydroxyacetone
Dipotassium glycyrrhizate
Equae lac
3-*o*-Ethyl ascorbic acid
Ethylhexylglycerin

Euphorbia cerifera (candelilla) wax
Glycine soja seed extract
Glycyrrhetinic acid
Glycyrrhizic acid
Glycyrrhiza glabra (licorice) root extract
Glycyrrhiza inflata root extract
Goat milk
Guar hydroxypropyltrimonium chloride
Hamamelis virginiana bark/leaf/twig extract
Helichrysum italicum flower extract
Hydrolyzed collagen
Hydrolyzed wheat protein
Hydroxypropyl tetrahydropyrantriol
Laurus nobilis leaf extract
Lonicera japonica flower extract
Magnolia grandiflora bark extract
Magnolia officinalis bark extract
Maleated soybean oil
Methoxy PEG-17/dodecyl glycol copolymer
Methyl nicotinate
Palmitoyl collagen amino acids
Palmitoyl hydrolyzed milk protein
Palmitoyl hydrolyzed wheat protein
PEG-5 soy sterol
Pentylene glycol
Pentyl rhamnoside
Phenylethyl resorcinol
Phytantriol
Phytonadione
Polyester-8
Potassium cocoyl hydrolyzed collagen
Propolis
Propylene glycol
Pyridoxine dioctenoate Retinyl palmitate
Ruscogenin
Salvia officinalis extract
Simmondsia chinensis seed powder
Sodium chondroitin sulfate
Styrax benzoin gum
Tanacetum vulgare extract
TEA-cocoyl hydrolyzed collagen
Tetrahydromagnolol
Tocopheryl linoleate
Tocopheryl nicotinate
Xanthan gum

SKIN-CONDITIONING AGENTS – OCCLUSIVE

Skin-conditioning agents - occlusive are cosmetic ingredients which retard the evaporation of water from the skin surface

Acetylated lanolin
C18-36 Acid triglyceride
Argania spinosa kernel oil
Butyrospermum parkii butter
Caprylic/capric triglyceride
Chamomilla recutita extract (flowers)
Cod liver oil
Dipentaerythrityl hexahydroxystearate/hexa-
 stearate/hexarosinate

SKIN-CONDITIONING AGENTS – OCCLUSIVE (*cont'd*)

Euphorbia cerifera (candelilla) wax
Hydrogenated castor oil
Laurus nobilis leaf extract
Macadamia ternifolia seed oil
Mineral oil
Petrolatum
Sesamum indicum seed oil
Simmondsia chinensis (jojoba) seed oil
Pentaerythrityl tetracaprylate/tetracaprate
Persea gratissima (avocado) oil
Phenyl dimethicone
Prunus avium (sweet cherry) seed oil
Ricinus communis seed oil
Triethylene glycol hydrogenated rosinate
Trioleyl phosphate

SKIN PROTECTANTS

Skin protectants are active ingredients used in skin protectant products
Allantoin
Cod liver oil
Glycerin
Lanolin
Mineral oil
Petrolatum
Resveratrol

SOLVENTS

Solvents are liquids employed to dissolve components found useful in cosmetics or drugs
Alcohol
t-Butyl alcohol
Butylene glycol
Caprylic/capric triglyceride
Cyclomethicone
Dibutyl phthalate
Diethyl sebacate
Dipropylene glycol
Ethoxydiglycol
Hexylene glycol
Isohexadecane
Isopropyl alcohol
Mineral oil
Oleyl alcohol
PEG-6
Pentylene glycol
Propylene glycol

SUNSCREEN AGENTS

Sunscreen agents are active ingredients used in (OTC) sunscreen products
Benzophenone-3
Benzophenone-4
Benzophenone-8
Butyl methoxydibenzoylmethane
Cinoxate
Ethylhexyl methoxycinnamate
bis-Ethylhexyloxyphenol methoxyphenyl triazine

Ethylhexyl salicylate
Glyceryl PABA
Homosalate
Lawsone
Methylene bis-benzotriazolyl tetramethylbutylphenol
Octocrylene
PABA
Phenylbenzimidazole sulfonic acid

SURFACTANTS – CLEANSING AGENTS

Surfactants - cleansing agents are used for skin and hair-cleaning purposes and as emulsifiers in cosmetics
Cocamidopropylamine oxide
Cocamidopropyl betaine
Cocamidopropyl hydroxysultaine
Coco-betaine
Coco-glucoside
Decyl glucoside
Disodium lauroamphodiacetate
Disodium oleamido MEA-sulfosuccinate
Disodium ricinoleamido MEA-sulfosuccinate
Hexyldecanoic acid
Hydroxystearic acid
Lauramine oxide
Lauroyl collagen amino acids
Lauryl glucoside
Myristic acid
Myristyl glucoside
Palmitoyl collagen amino acids
Palmitoyl hydrolyzed milk protein
Palmitoyl hydrolyzed wheat protein
PEG-32 stearate
PEG-40 sorbitan lanolate
Potassium cocoyl hydrolyzed collagen
Ricinoleic acid
Sodium cocoamphoacetate
Sodium cocoamphopropionate
Sodium lauroamphoacetate
Sodium lauroyl sarcosinate
Sodium lauryl sulfate
Sodium myristoyl sarcosinate
Stearic acid
Sulfated castor oil
TEA-cocoyl hydrolyzed collagen
TEA-PEG-3 cocamide sulfate
TEA-stearate

SURFACTANTS – DISPERSING AGENTS

Surfactants - dispersing agents are used in cosmetics to help distribute an insoluble solid in a liquid phase
Benzalkonium chloride
Benzethonium chloride

SURFACTANTS – EMULSIFYING AGENTS

Surfactants - emulsifying agents are employed in cosmetics to prepare emulsions
Arachidyl glucoside
Ceteareth-2

SURFACTANTS – EMULSIFYING AGENTS (cont'd)
Ceteareth-3
Cetearyl glucoside
Cetrimonium bromide
Cetyl alcohol
Glyceryl caprylate
Glyceryl hydrogenated rosinate
Glyceryl isostearate
Glyceryl isostearate/myristate
Glyceryl rosinate
Glyceryl stearate
Lanolin
Laureth-2
Laureth-4
Laureth-7
Laureth-9
Laureth-12
Octyldodecyl xyloside
C30-38 Olefin/isopropyl maleate/MA copolymer
Oleth-3 phosphate
Oleth-5
PEG-4 dilaurate
PEG-4 rapeseedamide
PEG-5 lanolate
PEG-5 soy sterol
PEG-7 hydrogenated castor oil
PEG-7 oleate
Polysorbate 40
Polysorbate 80
PPG-1-PEG-9 lauryl glycol ether
PPG-2-ceteareth-9
Propylene glycol ricinoleate
Sodium dihydroxycetyl phosphate
Sodium stearate
Sodium stearoyl lactylate
Sorbitan oleate
Sorbitan sesquioleate
Sorbitan tristearate
Steareth-10
Stearic acid
Stearyl alcohol
TEA-stearate
Triceteareth-4 phosphate
Triethanolamine
Trilaureth-4 phosphate
Xanthan gum

SURFACTANTS – FOAM BOOSTERS
Surfactants - foam boosters are used in cosmetics to increase the foaming capacity of Surfactants - cleansing agents, or to stabilize foams in general
Cetearyl alcohol
Cetyl alcohol
Cocamide DEA
Cocamidopropylamine oxide
Cocamidopropyl betaine
Cocamidopropyl hydroxysultaine
Coco-betaine
Disodium lauroamphodiacetate

Disodium oleamido MEA-sulfosuccinate
Disodium ricinoleamido MEA-sulfosuccinate
Lauramide DEA
Lauramine oxide
Lauryl alcohol
Myristyl alcohol
Oleamide DEA
Sodium cocoamphoacetate
Sodium cocoamphopropionate
Sodium lauroamphoacetate
Stearyl alcohol
Trideceth-2 carboxamide MEA
Undecylenamide DEA

SURFACTANTS – HYDROTROPES
Surfactants - hydrotropes are surfactants which have the ability to enhance the water solubility of another surfactant
Cocamidopropylamine oxide
Disodium lauroamphodiacetate
Disodium oleamido MEA-sulfosuccinate
Disodium ricinoleamido MEA-sulfosuccinate
Lauramine oxide
Sodium cocoamphopropionate
TEA-PEG-3 cocamide sulfate

SURFACTANTS – SOLUBILIZING AGENTS
Surfactants - solubilizing agents are substances which aid in the dissolution of an ingredient (solute) in a medium in which it is not otherwise soluble
PEG-32 stearate
PEG-40 sorbitan lanolate
Polysorbate 40
Polysorbate 80

VISCOSITY DECREASING AGENTS
Viscosity decreasing agents are used in cosmetics to enhance the fluidity of products without a significant lowering of the concentration of the active constituents
Alcohol
Butylene glycol
Ethoxydiglycol
Dipropylene glycol
Glycerin
Hexylene glycol
Isopropyl alcohol
Propylene glycol

VISCOSITY INCREASING AGENTS – AQUEOUS
Viscosity increasing agents - aqueous are used to thicken the aqueous portions of cosmetic products
Cetearyl alcohol
Cetyl alcohol
Cocamide DEA
Cocamidopropyl betaine
Cocamidopropyl hydroxysultaine
Coco-betaine
Colophonium

VISCOSITY INCREASING AGENTS – AQUEOUS (*cont'd*)
Guar hydroxypropyltrimonium chloride
Lauramide DEA
Lauryl alcohol
Methoxy PEG-22/dodecyl glycol copolymer
Myristyl alcohol
Oleamide DEA
PEG-4 rapeseedamide
Sodium stearate
Stearyl alcohol
Trideceth-2 carboxamide MEA
Undecylenamide DEA
Xanthan gum

VISCOSITY INCREASING AGENTS – NONAQUEOUS
Viscosity increasing agents - nonaqueous, are used to thicken the water-insoluble portions of cosmetic products
Butyrospermum parkii butter
Ceresin
Cetearyl alcohol
Cetyl alcohol
Dipentaerythrityl hexahydroxystearate/hexa-
 stearate/hexarosinate

Euphorbia cerifera (candelilla) wax
Glyceryl abietate
Hydroabietyl alcohol
Hydrogenated castor oil
Isostearyl alcohol
Lanolin alcohol
Lauryl alcohol
Methoxy PEG-17/dodecyl glycol copolymer
Methoxy PEG-22/dodecyl glycol copolymer
Microcrystalline wax
Myristyl alcohol
C30-38 Olefin /isopropyl maleate/MA copolymer
Oleyl alcohol
Pentaerythrityl rosinate
Pentaerythrityl tetracaprylate/tetracaprate
Phthalic anhydride/trimellitic anhydride/glycols
 copolymer
Polyethylene
Stearyl alcohol
Triacontanyl PVP
Triethylene glycol hydrogenated rosinate
VP/eicosene copolymer
VP/hexadecene copolymer

5.4　CHEMICALS/SUBSTANCES THAT ARE NOT MENTIONED IN COSING AND/OR NOT IN THE PERSONAL CARE PRODUCTS COUNCIL INGREDIENT DATABASE

NEITHER IN COSING NOR IN THE PERSONAL CARE PRODUCTS COUNCIL INGREDIENT DATABASE

Acetarsone

Ammoniated mercury

Butyl acrylate

Chloro-2-phenylphenol

CI 12055

Cobalt

Cystamine bis-lactamide

DEA-dihydroxypalmityl phosphate

Dichlorodifluoromethane

Disperse blue 85

Disperse blue 106

Glycidyl methacrylate

1,6-Hexanediol diacrylate

Hydrophilized ceramide

Hydroxyethyl acrylate

Isobutyl PABA

Isopropyl hydroxypalmityl ether

Lanolin alcohol (and) paraffinum liquidum

Methyl acrylate

Neopentyl glycol diisooctanoate

Nickel

Osmaron B

Propantheline bromide

Tetrahydrocurcumin

Triethylene glycol diacrylate

Tripropyleneglycol diacrylate

Trisodium hydroxyethyl ethylenediamine triacetate

Urethane diacrylate

Witisol

NOT IN COSING

Sulfiram

NOT IN THE PERSONAL CARE PRODUCTS COUNCIL INGREDIENT DATABASE

4-Aminoazobenzene

Bithionol

4',5-Dibromosalicylanilide

Diethylstilbestrol

2,6-Dimethyl-1,3-dioxan-4-yl acetate

Disperse yellow 3

Methylene bis-benzotriazolyl tetramethylbutylphenol (and) aqua (and) decyl glucoside (and) propylene glycol (and) xanthan gum

Monobenzone

Paraformaldehyde

Sulfiram

3,4',5-Tribromosalicylanilide

5.5   CHEMICALS/SUBSTANCES THAT ARE PROHIBITED IN THE EU OR IN THE USA

Prohibited in the EU

4-Aminoazobenzene

2-Aminomethyl-*p*-aminophenol HCl

Basic red 22

Basic violet 10

Bithionol

4-*tert*-Butylphenol

Captan

CI 12150

CI Pigment red 53:1

Coal tar

4',5-Dibromosalicylanilide

Dibutyl phthalate

Diethylstilbestrol

Diisopropanolamine

2,6-Dimethyl-1,3-dioxan-4-yl acetate

Disperse yellow 3

Glyceryl PABA

Hydroabietyl alcohol

Lead acetate

Methyldibromo glutaronitrile

Methyldibromo glutaronitrile/phenoxyethanol

Monobenzone

Nickel

2-Nitro-*p*-phenylenediamine

PABA

Pentyl dimethyl PABA

Phytonadione

Pigment orange 5

Pigment red 172 aluminum lake

Pigment yellow 12

Pyrocatechol

Pyrogallol

Sodium pyrithione

Solvent yellow 44

3,4',5-Tribromosalicylanilide

Witisol

Prohibited in the USA

Calcium lithol red

CI 12120

CI 69825

CHAPTER 6   LIST OF SYNONYMS

In this chapter, all synonyms of chemicals, used in this book by their INCI names, are listed alphabetically in the left column of table 6.1. In the right column, their corresponding INCI names are given (or Monograph names where no INCI names are available). These are all discussed in a separate Monograph/Chapter. The page numbers of these Chapters (where the corresponding synonyms can be found) are listed in the Index.

Table 6.1 List of synonyms: Conversion of synonyms to INCI names or Chapter names

Synonym	INCI name / Chapter name

A

Abietic acid glycerol ester	Glyceryl abietate
Abitol	Hydroabietyl alcohol
(3-Acetamido-4-hydroxyphenyl)arsonic acid	Acetarsone
Acetarsol	Acetarsone
6-Acetoxy-2,4-dimethyl-*m*-dioxane	2,6-Dimethyl-1,3-dioxan-4-yl acetate
Acid chlorides, coco, reaction products with protein hydro- lyzates, compds. with triethanolamine	TEA-cocoyl hydrolyzed collagen
Acid chlorides, soy(a), reaction products with protein hydrolyzates, sodium salts	Sodium soy hydrolyzed collagen
Acid red 87	CI 45380
Adeps lanae	Lanolin
Alcohol C-12	Lauryl alcohol
Alcoholes adipis lanae	Lanolin alcohol
Alcohols, C16-18, ethoxylated, propoxylated (9 mol EO, 2 mol PO average molar ratio)	PPG-2-ceteareth-9
Alkylammonium amidobenzoate	Osmaron B
Alkyldimethylbenzylammonium chloride	Benzalkonium chloride
Alkyl rhamnoside-C5	Pentyl rhamnoside
Almond acid	Mandelic acid
Almond oil, sweet	Prunus amygdalus dulcis oil
Aluminii oxidum	Alumina
Aluminium chloride	Aluminum chloride
Aluminium oxide	Alumina
Alumin(i)um trichloride	Aluminum chloride
Aluminum (III) chloride pentahydroxide	Aluminum chlorohydrate
Aluminum chlorohydrate (anhydrous)	Aluminum chlorohydrate
Aluminum hydroxychloride	Aluminum chlorohydrate
Amerchol® L101	Lanolin alcohol (and) paraffinum liquidum
Amides, coco	Cocamide
Amides, coco, *N,N*-bis(hydroxyethyl)	Cocamide DEA
Amides, coco, *N*-[3-(dimethylamino)propyl]	Cocamidopropyl dimethylamine
Amides, coco, *N*-[3-(dimethylamino)propyl], *N*-oxides	Cocamidopropylamine oxide
Amidoamine (term used by the NACDG)	Cocamidopropyl dimethylamine
Amiloxate	Isoamyl *p*-methoxycinnamate
Amine fluoride	see Olaflur
Amino acids, collagen, 1-oxododecyl derivatives	Lauroyl collagen amino acids
Amino acids, collagen, 1-oxohexadecyl derivatives	Palmitoyl collagen amino acids
4-Amino-2-(aminomethyl)phenol;dihydrochloride	2-Aminomethyl-*p*-aminophenol HCl
p-Aminoazobenzene	4-Aminoazobenzene
1-(4-Aminobenzoate)-1,2,3-propanetriol	Glyceryl PABA
p-Aminobenzoic acid	PABA
3-[(4-Amino-6-bromo-5,8-dihydro-1-hydroxy-8-imino-5-oxo- 2-naphtyl)amino]-*N,N,N*-trimethylanilinium chloride	Basic blue 99
Amino(chloro)mercury	Ammoniated mercury
p-Amino-*m*-cresol	4-Amino-*m*-cresol
5-Amino-*o*-cresol	4-Amino-2-hydroxytoluene

Table 6.1 List of synonyms: Conversion of synonyms to INCI names or Chapter names (*continued*)

Synonym	INCI name / Chapter name
2-Amino-2-deoxy-D-glucopyranose hydrochloride	Glucosamine HCl
2-Amino-3,7-dihydropurin-6-one	Guanine
6-Amino-2-(2,4-dimethylphenyl)-1*H*-benz[de]isoquinoline-1,3[2*H*]-dione	Solvent yellow 44
4-Aminodiphenylamine	*N*-Phenyl-*p*-phenylenediamine
2-Aminoethanethiol;hydrochloride	Cysteamine HCl
1-Amino-2-hydroxybenzene	*o*-Aminophenol
2-Amino-4-[(2-hydroxyethyl)amino]anisole sulfate	2-Amino-4-hydroxyethylaminoanisole sulfate
2-[4-Amino-*N*-(2-hydroxyethyl)anilino]ethanol;sulfuric acid	*N*,*N*-bis(2-Hydroxyethyl)-*p*-phenylenediamine sulfate
4-Amino-2-hydroxy-1-methylbenzene	4-Amino-2-hydroxytoluene
(3*R*,4*R*,5*S*,6*R*)-3-Amino-6-(hydroxymethyl)oxane-2,4,5-triol;hydrochloride	Glucosamine HCl
2-Amino-2-(hydroxymethyl)propane-1,3-diol	Tromethamine
2-Amino-6-hydroxypurine	Guanine
2-(3-Amino-4-methoxyanilino)ethanol;sulfuric acid	2-Amino-4-hydroxyethylaminoanisole sulfate
2-[(3-Amino-4-methoxyphenyl)amino]ethanol sulfate	2-Amino-4-hydroxyethylaminoanisole sulfate
3-Amino-2-methylamino-6-methoxypyridine dihydrochloride	HC Blue no. 7
2-Aminomethyl-4-aminophenol dihydrochloride	2-Aminomethyl-*p*-aminophenol HCl
4-Amino-3-methylphenol	4-Amino-*m*-cresol
5-Amino-2-methylphenol	4-Amino-2-hydroxytoluene
2-(4-Amino-3-nitroanilino)ethanol	HC red no. 7
Amino-2-nitro-4-(β-hydroxyethyl)aminobenzene	HC red no. 7
[8-[(4-Amino-3-nitrophenyl)azo]-7-hydroxy-2-naphthyl]trimethylammonium chloride	Basic brown 17
2-Aminophenol	*o*-Aminophenol
3-Aminophenol	*m*-Aminophenol
4-Aminophenol	*p*-Aminophenol
4-Aminophenol-3-nitrophenol	4-Amino-3-nitrophenol
N-(4-Aminophenyl)aniline	*N*-Phenyl-*p*-phenylenediamine
1-(4-Aminophenylazo)-2-methyl-4-bis(β-hydroxyethyl)aminobenzene	HC Yellow no. 7
2-[4-[(4-Aminophenyl)diazenyl]-*N*-(2-hydroxyethyl)-3-methylanilino]ethanol	HC Yellow no. 7
(3-Ammonio-4-methoxyphenyl)(2-hydroxyethyl)ammonium sulfate	2-Amino-4-hydroxyethylaminoanisole sulfate
(*p*-Ammoniophenyl)bis(2-hydroxyethyl)ammonium sulphate	*N*,*N*-bis(2-Hydroxyethyl)-*p*-phenylenediamine sulfate
Ammonium hydrogen sulphite	Ammonium bisulfite
Ammonium mercaptoacetate	Ammonium thioglycolate
Ammonium 2-mercaptopropionate	Ammonium thiolactate
Ammonium peroxydisulfate	Ammonium persulfate
Ammonyx LO®	Lauramine oxide
Amygdalic acid	Mandelic acid
Amyl dimethyl PABA	Pentyl dimethyl PABA
Anhydrosorbitol tristearate	Sorbitan tristearate
Aniline yellow	4-Aminoazobenzene
Anisole-2-azo-β-naphthol	CI 12150
Anisotriazine	bis-Ethylhexyloxyphenol methoxyphenyl triazine
5,9,14,18-Anthrazinetetrone, 7,16-dichloro-6,15-dihydro-,	CI 69825
Argan oil	Argania spinosa kernel oil
Arlacel® C	Sorbitan sesquioleate
L-Ascorbic acid, tetraisohexadecanoate	Ascorbyl tetraisopalmitate
Atlas® G 1441	PEG-40 sorbitan lanolate
Avobenzone	Butyl methoxydibenzoylmethane
Avocado oil	Persea gratissima oil

Table 6.1 List of synonyms: Conversion of synonyms to INCI names or Chapter names (*continued*)

Synonym	INCI name / Chapter name
Azanium 2-sulfanylacetate	Ammonium thioglycolate
Azanium 2-sulfanylpropanoate	Ammonium thiolactate

B

Banana, banana fruit	Musa paradisiaca (banana) fruit
Barium(2+);5-chloro-4-methyl-2-[(2*Z*)-2-(2-oxonaphthalen-1 -ylidene)hydrazinyl]benzenesulfonate	CI Pigment red 53
Bay laurel extract	Laurus nobilis leaf extract
Beeswax	Cera alba
Bemotrizinol	bis-Ethylhexyloxyphenol methoxyphenyl triazine
Benzeneacetic acid, α-hydroxy-	Mandelic acid
Benzenecarboximidamide, 4,4'-(1,6-hexanediylbis(oxy))bis-	Hexamidine
Benzenecarboxylic acid	Benzoic acid
1,4-Benzenediamine	*p*-Phenylenediamine
Benzene-1,4-diamine	*p*-Phenylenediamine
Benzene-1,2-diol	Pyrocatechol
Benzene-1,3-diol	Resorcinol
Benzene-1,4-diol	Hydroquinone
1,3-Benzenediol	Resorcinol
1,3-Benzenediol, 5-[(1*E*)-2-(4-hydroxyphenyl)ethenyl]-	Resveratrol
1,3-Benzenediol, 4-(1-phenylethyl)-	Phenylethyl resorcinol
Benzenemethanaminium, *N*,*N*-dimethyl-*N*-[2-[2-[4-(1,1,3,3, -tetramethylbutyl)phenoxy]ethoxy]ethyl]-, chloride	Benzethonium chloride
Benzenemethanaminium, *N*-hexadecyl-*N*,*N*-dimethyl, chloride	Cetalkonium chloride
Benzenesulfonamide, 4-methyl-, polymer with formaldehyde	Tosylamide/formaldehyde resin
Benzenesulfonic acid, 5-chloro-2-(2-(2-hydroxy-1-naphtha-lenyl)diazenyl)-4-methyl-, barium salt (2:1)	CI Pigment red 53
Benzene-1,2,3-triol	Pyrogallol
Benzidine yellow G	Pigment yellow 12
1,2-Benzisothiazol-3(2*H*)-one	Benzisothiazolinone
Benzoic acid, C12-15 alkyl esters	C12-15 Alkyl benzoate
Benzoic acid, 2-[4-(diethylamino)-2-hydroxybenzoyl]-, hexyl ester	Diethylamino hydroxybenzoyl hexyl benzoate
Benzoic acid, 2,5-dihydroxy-, methyl ester	Methyl dihydroxybenzoate
Benzoic acid, 2-((dioctadecylamino)carbonyl)-	Distearyl phthalic acid amide
Benzoic acid, 2-hydroxy-, 3,3,5-trimethylcyclohexyl ester	Homosalate
Benzoic acid, 4,4',4''-(1,3,5-triazine-2,4,6-triyltriimino)tris-, tris(2-ethylhexyl) ester	Ethylhexyl triazone
Benzoic acid, 3,4,5-trihydroxy-, octyl ester	Caprylyl gallate
Benzoin	Styrax benzoin gum
Benzoin gum	Styrax benzoin gum
2-(Benzotriazol-2-yl)-4-methylphenol	Drometrizole
Benzoyl benzenecarboperoxoate	Benzoyl peroxide
5-Benzoyl-4-hydroxy-2-methoxybenzenesulfonic acid	Benzophenone-4
Benzyl(dimethyl)azanium chloride	Benzalkonium chloride
Benzyl-dodecyl-bis(2-hydroxyethyl)azanium chloride	Benzoxonium chloride
Benzyl-hexadecyl-dimethylazanium chloride	Cetalkonium chloride
Benzylidenemalonatepolysiloxane	Polysilicone-15
(Benzyloxy)methanol	Benzylhemiformal
4-Benzyloxyphenol	Monobenzone
Benzyl pyridine-3-carboxylate	Benzyl nicotinate
Betaines, coco alkyldimethyl	Coco-betaine
Bicyclo[5.3.0]decapentaene	Azulene
[1,1'-Biphenyl]-2,2'-diol, 5,5'-dipropyl-	Tetrahydromagnolol
Biphenyl-2-ol	*o*-Phenylphenol
Birch bark extract	Betula alba bark extract
Bisdisulizole disodium	Disodium phenyl dibenzimidazole tetrasulfonate

Table 6.1 List of synonyms: Conversion of synonyms to INCI names or Chapter names (*continued*)

Synonym	INCI name / Chapter name
1,7-Bis(4-hydroxy-3-methoxyphenyl)heptane-3,5-dione	see Tetrahydrocurcumin
2,2-Bis(hydroxymethyl)propane-1,3-diol;decanoic acid;octanoic acid	Pentaerythrityl tetracaprylate/tetracaprate
N,*N*'-Bis(hydroxymethyl)urea	Diazolidinyl urea
1,7-Bis(4-hydroxyphenyl)heptane-3,5-dione	see Tetrahydrocurcumin
Bismuth chloride oxide	CI 77163
Bismuth oxychloride	CI 77163
Bisoctrizole	Methylene bis-benzotriazolyl tetramethylbutylphenol
BIT	Benzisothiazolinone
Black iron oxide	Iron oxides
Bradophen®	Benzoxonium chloride
Brazil wax	Copernicia cerifera wax
Brilliant lake red R	CI 15800
Brilliant red	CI Pigment red 53
2-Bromo-2-(bromomethyl)pentanedinitrile	Methyldibromo glutaronitrile
5-Bromo-*N*-(4-bromophenyl)-2-hydroxybenzamide	4',5-Dibromosalicylanilide
Bromofluorescein	CI 45380
Bromothalonil	Methyldibromo glutaronitrile
Bronidox®	5-Bromo-5-nitro-1,3-dioxane
Bronopol®	2-Bromo-2-nitropropane-1,3-diol
Brown iron oxide	Iron oxides
Butanedioic acid, sulfo-, 1-(2-((12-hydroxy-1-oxo-9-octadecenyl)amino)ethyl) ester, disodium salt	Disodium ricinoleamido MEA-sulfosuccinate
Butane-1,3-diol	Butylene glycol
Butylated hydroxyanisole	BHA
Butylated hydroxytoluene	BHT
2-*tert*-Butylbenzene-1,4-diol	TBHQ
t-Butyl hydroquinone	TBHQ
Butyl 4-hydroxybenzoate	Butylparaben
2-*tert*-Butyl-4-methoxyphenol	BHA
2,6-di-*tert*-Butyl-4-methylphenol	BHT
Butyl 2-methyl-2-propenoate	Butyl methacrylate
Butylphen	4-*tert*-Butylphenol
p-*tert*-Butylphenol	4-*tert*-Butylphenol
1-(4-*tert*-Butylphenyl)-3-(4-methoxyphenyl)propane-1,3-dione	Butyl methoxydibenzoylmethane
Butyl phthalate	Dibutyl phthalate
Butyl prop-2-enoate	Butyl acrylate
Buxus chinensis oil	Simmondsia chinensis seed oil
Buxus chinensis powder	Simmondsia chinensis seed powder

C

Synonym	INCI name / Chapter name
Calcium 3-hydroxy-4-[(4-methyl-2-sulphonatophenyl)azo]-2-naphthoate	Pigment red 57:1
Calcium bis[3-hydroxy-4-(phenylazo)-2-naphthoate]	CI 15800
Camomille extract	Chamomilla recutita extract
Candelilla wax	Candelilla cera
Caprae lac	Goat milk
Capsicum oleoresin	Capsicum frutescens resin
Caraway seed oil	Carum carvi seed oil
4-[6-(4-Carbamimidoylphenoxy)hexoxy]benzenecarboximidamide	Hexamidine
Carbanthrene blue	CI 69825
Carbitol®	Ethoxydiglycol
2-[2-[bis(Carboxymethyl)amino]ethyl-(carboxymethyl)amino]acetic acid	EDTA

Table 6.1 List of synonyms: Conversion of synonyms to INCI names or Chapter names (*continued*)

Synonym	INCI name / Chapter name
[9-(2-Carboxyphenyl)-6-(diethylamino)xanthen-3-ylidene]-diethylazanium chloride	Basic violet 10
Carmine	CI 75470
Carminic acid aluminium lake	CI 75470
Carnauba wax	Copernicia cerifera wax
Castor oil	Ricinus communis seed oil
Castor oil (*Ricinus communis*), hydrogenated, ethoxylated (7 mol EO average molar ratio)	PEG-7 hydrogenated castor oil
Castor oil, sulfated	Sulfated castor oil
Catechol	Pyrocatechol
Cellulose, nitrate	Nitrocellulose
Ceraphyl® GA	Maleated soybean oil
Ceraphyl® GA-D	Maleated soybean oil
Ceresin wax	Ceresin
Cetearyl octanoate	Cetearyl ethylhexanoate
Cetostearyl alcohol	Cetearyl alcohol
Cetrimide	Cetrimonium bromide
Cetyl dimethyl benzyl ammonium chloride	Cetalkonium chloride
Cetyl/steraryl alcohol	Cetearyl alcohol
Cetyl trimethyl ammonium bromide	Cetrimonium bromide
Chamomile (Anthemis nobilis) extract	Anthemis nobilis flower extract
Chamomile extract (German, Hungarian)	Chamomilla recutita extract
Chamomile flower, Roman, extract (*Anthemis nobilis* L.)	Anthemis nobilis flower extract
Chamomilla recutita (matricaria) flower/leaf extract	Chamomilla recutita extract
Cherry pit oil	Prunus avium seed oil
Chestnut extract	Castanea sativa extract
Chininum	Quinine
Chitosamine hydrochloride	Glucosamine HCl
Chlorhexidine gluconate	Chlorhexidine digluconate
N-(3-Chloroallyl)hexaminium chloride	Quaternium-15
3-Chloro-4-aminoaniline	2-Chloro-*p*-phenylenediamine
2-Chlorobenzene-1,4-diamine	2-Chloro-*p*-phenylenediamine
3-Chloro(1,1'-biphenyl)-2-ol	Chloro-2-phenylphenol
5-Chloro(1,1'-biphenyl)-2-ol	Chloro-2-phenylphenol
4-Chloro-2-[(5-chloro-2-hydroxyphenyl)methyl]phenol	Dichlorophene
4-Chloro-2-(5-chloro-2-hydroxyphenyl)sulfanylphenol	2,2'-Thiobis(4-chlorophenol)
Chlorocresol	*p*-Chloro-*m*-cresol
5-Chloro-2-(2,4-dichlorophenoxy)phenol	Triclosan
Chlorodimethylhydroxybenzene	Chloroxylenol
4-Chloro-3,5-dimethylphenol	Chloroxylenol
2-[[4-[(2-Chloro-4,6-dinitrophenyl)diazenyl]naphthalen-1-yl]amino]ethanol	CI Disperse blue 85
4-Chloro-3-methylphenol	*p*-Chloro-*m*-cresol
1-[(2-Chloro-4-nitrophenyl)azo]-2-naphthol	CI 12085
3-(4-Chlorophenoxy)propane-1,2-diol	Chlorphenesin
1-(4-Chlorophenyl)-3-(3,4-dichlorophenyl)urea	Triclocarban
2-Chloro-6-phenylphenol	Chloro-2-phenylphenol
p-Chloro-*m*-xylenol	Chloroxylenol
Chondroitin, hydrogen sulfate	Sodium chondroitin sulfate
Chondrosamine hydrochloride	Glucosamine HCl
Chrysanthemum parthenium (feverfew) extract	Tanacetum parthenium extract
Cocamido betaine	Cocamidopropyl betaine
Cocamidopropylamine	Cocamidopropyl dimethylamine
Cocamine diethanolamine	Cocamide DEA
Coconut fatty acids diethanolamide	Cocamide DEA
Coconut fatty acid, dimethylaminopropylamide	Cocamidopropyl dimethylamine

Table 6.1 List of synonyms: Conversion of synonyms to INCI names or Chapter names (*continued*)

Synonym	INCI name / Chapter name
Coconut oil amidopropylbetaine	Cocamidopropyl betaine
Chromic (III) hydroxide	CI 77289
Chromic oxide	CI 77288
Chromic oxide hydrated	CI 77289
Chromium hydroxide green	CI 77289
Chromium (III) oxide	CI 77288
Chromium oxide greens	CI 77288
Chromium; trihydrate	CI 77289
CI 11000	4-Aminoazobenzene
CI 11055	Basic red 22
CI 11370	CI Disperse blue 85
CI 11855	Disperse yellow 3
CI 12075	Pigment orange 5
CI 12251	Basic brown 17
CI 15585:1	CI Pigment red 53
CI 15630:2	Calcium lithol red
CI 15850	Pigment red 57:1
CI 21090	Pigment yellow 12
CI 40800	Beta-carotene
CI 45170	Basic violet 10
CI 45430:1	Pigment red 172 aluminum lake
CI 45430 (Al)	Pigment red 172 aluminum lake
CI 50240	Basic red 2
CI 56059	Basic blue 99
CI 56200	Solvent yellow 44
CI 75130	Beta-carotene
CI 75170	Guanine
CI 75480	Lawsone
CI 76042	Toluene-2,5-diamine
CI 76043	Toluene-2,5-diamine sulfate
CI 76060	*p*-Phenylenediamine
CI 76065	2-Chloro-*p*-phenylenediamine
CI 76070	2-Nitro-*p*-phenylenediamine
CI 76085	*N*-Phenyl-*p*-phenylenediamine
CI 76500	Pyrocatechol
CI 76505	Resorcinol
CI 76515	Pyrogallol
CI 76520	*o*-Aminophenol
CI 76545	*m*-Aminophenol
CI 76550	*p*-Aminophenol
CI 76645	2,7-Naphthalenediol
CI 77489	Iron oxides
CI 77491	Iron oxides
CI 77492	Iron oxides
CI 77499	Iron oxides
CI Acid red 51:1	Pigment red 172 aluminum lake
CI Basic blue 99	Basic blue 99
CI Basic red 2	Basic red 2
CI Food red 14:1	Pigment red 172 aluminum lake
CI Natural orange 6	Lawsone
CI Pigment red 49 Ca salt	Calcium lithol red
Cinchonan-9-ol, 6'-methoxy-, (8α,9*R*)-	Quinine
Coathylene®	Polyethylene
Cochineal	CI 75470
Coconut diethanolamine	Cocamide DEA
Collagen hydrolysate	Hydrolyzed collagen

Table 6.1 List of synonyms: Conversion of synonyms to INCI names or Chapter names (*continued*)

Synonym	INCI name / Chapter name
Collagen, hydrolyzed, *N*-(3-trimethylammonio-2-hydroxypropyl)-, chlorides	Hydroxypropyltrimonium hydrolyzed collagen
Collodion (flexible)	Nitrocellulose
Colophony	Colophonium
Corn sugar gum	Xanthan gum
Cucumber (fruit) extract	Cucumis sativus extract
2-Cyano-3,3-diphenylacrylic acid 2'-ethylhexyl ester	Octocrylene
Cyclopentacycloheptene	Azulene

D

D&C blue no. 9	CI 69825
D&C orange no. 17	Pigment orange 5
D&C red 7 calcium lake	Pigment red 57:1
D&C red no. 9	CI Pigment red 53
D&C red no. 11	Calcium lithol red
D&C red no. 17	CI 26100
D&C red no. 19	Basic violet 10
D&C red no. 31	CI 15800
D&C red no. 34	CI 15880 (see Chapter Miscellaneous)
D&C red no. 36	CI 12085
D&C yellow no. 11	CI 47000
Deacetylchitin	Chitosan
Decaglycerin monolaurate	Polyglyceryl-10 laurate
Decanedioic acid diethyl ester	Diethyl sebacate
Decanoic acid, ester with 1,2,3-propanetriol octanoate	Caprylic/capric triglyceride
Decanoic acid, 2-hexyl	Hexyldecanoic acid
Decanoic acid, mixed esters with octanoic acid and pentaerythritol	Pentaerythrityl tetracaprylate/tetracaprate
3,6,9,12,15,18,21,24,27,30-Decaoxaoctatetracontan-1-ol	Steareth-10
(3*R*,4*S*,5*S*,6*R*)-2-Decoxy-6-(hydroxymethyl)oxane-3,4,5-triol	Decyl glucoside
Dectaflur	see Olaflur
Decyldiglycol	Laureth-2
Decyl D-glucopyranoside	Decyl glucoside
Decyl (*Z*)-octadec-9-enoate	Decyl oleate
Dexpanthenol	Panthenol
Dialuminum;chloride;pentahydroxide	Aluminum chlorohydrate
Dialuminum;2',4',5',7'-tetraiodo-3-oxospiro[2-benzofuran-1,9'-xanthene]-3',6'-diolate	Pigment red 172 aluminum lake
p-Diaminobenzene	*p*-Phenylenediamine
[3-[(4,8-Diamino-6-bromo-1,5-dioxonaphthalen-2-yl)amino]phenyl]-trimethylazanium chloride	Basic blue 99
2,5-Diaminochlorobenzene	2-Chloro-*p*-phenylenediamine
3,7-Diamino-2,8-dimethyl-5-phenylphenazinium chloride	Basic red 2
2-[Diamino(3-formamidopropyl)azaniumyl]acetate	Cocamidopropyl betaine
1-(Diaminomethylidene)-2-hexylguanidine	Polyaminopropyl biguanide
2,5-Diaminotoluene	Toluene-2,5-diamine
2,5-Diaminotoluene sulfate	Toluene-2,5-diamine sulfate
Diammonium peroxodisulfate	Ammonium persulfate
Diazanium sulfonatooxy sulfate	Ammonium persulfate
Dibenzoyl peroxide	Benzoyl peroxide
3,5-Dibromo-*N*-(4-bromophenyl)-2-hydroxybenzamide	3,4',5-Tribromosalicylanilide
1,2-Dibromo-2,4-dicyanobutane	Methyldibromo glutaronitrile
Dibromsalan	4',5-Dibromosalicylanilide
Dibutyl benzene-1,2-dicarboxylate	Dibutyl phthalate
2,4-Dichlorobenzenemethanol	Dichlorobenzyl alcohol

Table 6.1 List of synonyms: Conversion of synonyms to INCI names or Chapter names (*continued*)

Synonym	INCI name / Chapter name
2,2'-[(3,3'-Dichloro[1,1'-biphenyl]-4,4'-diyl)bis(azo)]-bis[3-oxo-*N*-phenylbutyramide]	Pigment yellow 12
3,5-Dichloro-*N*-(3,4-dichlorophenyl)-2-hydroxybenzamide	3,3',4',5-Tetrachlorosalicylanilide
7,16-Dichloro-6,15-dihydroanthrazine-5,9,14,18-tetrone	CI 69825
bis(3,5-Dichloro-2-hydroxyphenyl) sulfide	Bithionol
3,3'-Dichloroindanthrene	CI 69825
Dichlorophen	Dichlorophene
(2,4-Dichlorophenyl)methanol	Dichlorobenzyl alcohol
3,5-Dichlorosalicyl 3,4-dichloroanilide	3,3',4',5-Tetrachlorosalicylanilide
Dichromium trioxide	CI 77288
Didecyl dimethyl ammonium chloride	Didecyldimonium chloride
Didecyl(dimethyl)azanium chloride	Didecyldimonium chloride
Diethanolamine undecylenate	Undecylenamide DEA
Diethanololeamide	Oleamide DEA
Diethyl 6a-amino-1,6-bis(carbamoylamino)-3a-cyano-2,5-di-methylpyrrolo[2,3]pyrrole-3,4-dicarboxylate	Triacontanyl PVP
Diethylbenzylidene malonate dimethicone	Polysilicone-15
Diethylcarbamothioyl *N,N*-diethylcarbamodithioate	Sulfiram
Diethyl decanedioate	Diethyl sebacate
Diethylene glycol bis(methacrylate)	Diethylene glycol dimethacrylate
Diethylene glycol monododecyl ether	Laureth-2
Diethylene glycol monoethyl ether	Ethoxydiglycol
Difluorotin	Stannous fluoride
Dihydroabietyl alcohol	Hydroabietyl alcohol
3,4-Dihydro-2,5,7,8-tetramethyl-2-(4,8,12-trimethyltridecyl)-2*H*-benzopyran-6-ol	Tocopherol
[2*R*-[2*R**(4*R**,8*R**)]]-3,4-Dihydro-2,5,7,8-tetramethyl-2-(4,8,12-trimethyltridecyl)-2*H*-1-benzopyran-6-yl nicotinate	Tocopheryl nicotinate
1,2-Dihydroxybenzene	Pyrocatechol
1,4-Dihydroxybenzene	Hydroquinone
1,3-Dihydroxydimethyl ketone	Dihydroxyacetone
(2*R*)-2-[(1*S*)-1,2-Dihydroxyethyl]-3,4-dihydroxy-2*H*-furan-5-one	Ascorbic acid
(2*R*)-2-[(1*S*)-1,2-Dihydroxyethyl]-3-ethoxy-4-hydroxy-2*H*-furan-5-one	3-*O*-Ethyl ascorbic acid
(2*R*)-2,4-Dihydroxy-*N*-(3-hydroxypropyl)-3,3-dimethylbutanamide	Panthenol
2,2'-Dihydroxy-4-methoxybenzophenone	Benzophenone-8
di-2,2-Dihydroxymethylbutyl ether, triester with 2-ethyl-hexanoic acid	Ditrimethylolpropane triethylhexanoate
2,4-Dihydroxy-2-methylpentane	Hexylene glycol
2,7-Dihydroxynaphthalene	2,7-Naphthalenediol
[2-(3,4-Dihydroxyoxolan-2-yl)-2-hydroxyethyl] octadec-9-enoate	Sorbitan oleate
1,2-Dihydroxypentane	Pentylene glycol
4-[4-(3,4-Dihydroxyphenyl)-2,3-dimethylbutyl]benzene-1,2-diol	Nordihydroguaiaretic acid
bis(2,4-Dihydroxyphenyl)methanone	Benzophenone-2
1,2-Dihydroxypropane	Propylene glycol
1,3-Dihydroxypropan-2-one	Dihydroxyacetone
1,3-Dihydroxypropan-2-yl 16-methylheptadecanoate	Glyceryl isostearate
11-(2,3-Dihydroxypropoxycarbonyl)heptadecanoate	Caprylic/capric triglyceride
2,3-Dihydroxypropyl 4-aminobenzoate	Glyceryl PABA
2,3-Dihydroxypropyl (1*S*,4a*R*,4b*S*)-1,4a-dimethyl-7-propan-2-yl-2,3,4,4b,5,6,10,10a-octahydrophenanthrene-1-carboxylate	Glyceryl abietate
2,3-Dihydroxypropyl (*Z*,12*R*)-12-hydroxyoctadec-9-enoate	Glyceryl ricinoleate
2,3-Dihydroxypropyl octadecanoate	Glyceryl stearate
2,3-Dihydroxypropyl octanoate	Glyceryl caprylate
2,3-Dihydroxypropyl 2-sulfanylacetate	Glyceryl thioglycolate

Table 6.1 List of synonyms: Conversion of synonyms to INCI names or Chapter names (*continued*)

Synonym	INCI name / Chapter name
3,4-Dihydroxy-5-[3,4,5-tris[[(*Z*)-octadec-9-enoyl]oxy]-benzoyl]oxybenzoic acid	Digalloyl trioleate
Diiron trioxide	Iron oxides
Dimethicodiethylbenzalmalonate	Polysilicone-15
Dimethoxane	2,6-Dimethyl-1,3-dioxan-4-yl acetate
4-Dimethylaminobenzoate of ethyl-2-hexyl	Ethylhexyl dimethyl PABA
5-(4'-Dimethylaminophenylazo)-1,4-dimethyltriazolium chloride	Basic red 22
N-(3-(Dimethylamino)propyl)coco amides-*N*-oxide	Cocamidopropylamine oxide
N-[3-(Dimethylamino)propyl]hexadecanamide	Palmitamidopropyl dimethylamine
(*Z*)-*N*-[3-(Dimethylamino)propyl]octadec-9-enamide	Oleamidopropyl dimethylamine
Dimethylaminopropyl oleamide	Oleamidopropyl dimethylamine
Dimethylaminopropyl palmitamide	Palmitamidopropyl dimethylamine
(*E*,5*Z*)-5-(3,3-Dimethyl-2-bicyclo[2.2.1]heptanylidene)pent-3-en-2-one	Bornelone
Dimethyl-bis(prop-2-enyl)azanium;prop-2-enamide; chloride	Polyquaternium-7
Dimethyldiallyl ammonium chloride/acrylamide copolymer	Polyquaternium-7
N,*N*-Dimethyldodecan-1-amine oxide	Lauramine oxide
2,5-bis(1,1-Dimethylethyl)-1,4-benzenediol	Di-*t*-butylhydroquinone
4-(1,1-Dimethylethyl)phenol	4-*tert*-Butylphenol
1,4-Dimethyl-7-(1-methylethyl)azulene	Guaiazulene
2,2-Dimethyl-3-(6-methylheptanoyloxy)propyl] 6-methyl-heptanoate	Neopentyl glycol diisooctanoate
5-(3,3-Dimethyl-2-norborstyliden)-3-penten-2-one	Bornelone
Dimethylol dimethylhydantoin	DMDM hydantoin
1,3-Dimethylol-5,5-dimethylhydantoin	DMDM hydantoin
4,4-Dimethyl-1,3-oxazolidine	Dimethyl oxazolidine
2,2-Dimethyl-1,3-propanediyl isooctanoate	Neopentyl glycol diisooctanoate
1,4-Dimethyl-7-propan-2-ylazulene	Guaiazulene
(1,4a-Dimethyl-7-propan-2-yl-2,3,4,4b,5,6,7,9,10,10a-deca-hydrophenanthren-1-yl) methanol	Hydroabietyl alcohol
4,4'-(2,3-Dimethyltetramethylene)dipyrocatechol	Nordihydroguaiaretic acid
1-[(2,4-Dinitrophenyl)azo]-2-naphthol	Pigment orange 5
2-(Dioctadecylcarbamoyl)benzoic acid	Distearyl phthalic acid amide
Dioctyl (*Z*)-but-2-enedioate	Dicaprylyl maleate
Dioctyl maleate	Dicaprylyl maleate
1,3-Dioxane, 5-bromo-5-nitro-	5-Bromo-5-nitro-1,3-dioxane
(2,5-Dioxoimidazolidin-4-yl)urea	Allantoin
Dioxybenzone	Benzophenone-8
Dipentaerythritol, esters with hexahydroxystearate, stearate, and rosinate	Dipentaerythrityl hexahydroxystearate/hexa-stearate/hexarosinate
Dipentaerythritol fatty acid ester	Dipentaerythrityl hexahydroxystearate/hexa-stearate/hexarosinate
Dipotassium;(2*S*,3*S*,4*S*,5*R*,6*R*)-6-[(2*S*,3*R*,4*S*,5*S*,6*S*)-2-[[(3*S*,4a*R*,6a*R*,6b*S*,8a*S*,11*S*,12a*R*,14a*R*,14b*S*)-11-carboxy-4,4,6a,6b,8a,11,14b-heptamethyl-14-oxo-2,3,4a,5,6,7,8,9,10,12,12a,14a-do-decahydro-1*H*-picen-3-yl]oxy]-6-carboxylato-4,5-dihydroxyo-xan-3-yl]oxy-3,4,5-trihydroxyoxane-2-carboxylate	Dipotassium glycyrrhizate
5,5'-Dipropylbiphenyl-2,2'-diol	Tetrahydromagnolol
Disodium 2-[2-[carboxylatomethyl(carboxymethyl)amino]ethyl-(carboxymethyl)amino]acetate	Disodium EDTA
Disodium disulfite	Sodium metabisulfite
Disodium edetate	Disodium EDTA
Disodium ethylenediaminetetraacetate	Disodium EDTA
Disodium;4-[2-[[(*E*)-12-hydroxyoctadec-9-enoyl]amino]ethoxy]-4-oxo-3-sulfonatobutanoate	Disodium ricinoleamido MEA-sulfosuccinate

Table 6.1 List of synonyms: Conversion of synonyms to INCI names or Chapter names (*continued*)

Synonym	INCI name / Chapter name
Disodium;4-[2-(octadec-9-enoylamino)ethoxy]-4-oxo-3-sulfonatobutanoate	Disodium oleamido MEA-sulfosuccinate
Disodium (*Z*)-[2-[(1-oxooctadec-9-enyl)amino]ethyl] 2-sulphonatosuccinate	Disodium oleamido MEA-sulfosuccinate
Disodium ricinoleyl monoethanolamide sulfosuccinate	Disodium ricinoleamido MEA-sulfosuccinate
Disodium sulfite	Sodium sulfite
Disodium 2-(2,4,5,7-tetrabromo-6-oxido-3-oxoxanthen-9-yl) benzoate	CI 45380
Disperse blue 85	CI Disperse blue 85
Disperse blue 106	CI Disperse blue 106
Disperse yellow 11	Solvent yellow 44
Distearyl phthalamic acid	Distearyl phthalic acid amide
2,5-Ditert-butylbenzene-1,4-diol	Di-*t*-butylhydroquinone
2,5-Di-*tert*-butylhydroquinone	Di-*t*-butylhydroquinone
1,2-Dithiolane-3-pentanoic acid, (+/-)-	Thioctic acid
1,2-Dithiolane-3-valeric acid	Thioctic acid
5-(Dithiolan-3-yl)valeric acid	Thioctic acid
Diurethane dimethacrylate	Di-HEMA trimethylhexyl dicarbamate
Dodecan-1-ol	Lauryl alcohol
Dodecan-1-ol, ethoxylated	Laureth-9
3-[3-(Dodecanoylamino)propyl-dimethylazaniumyl]-2-hydroxy-propane-1-sulfonate	Cocamidopropyl hydroxysultaine
N-Dodecanoylsarcosine sodium salt	Sodium lauroyl sarcosinate
3,6,9,12,15,18,21,24,27,30,33,36-Dodecaoxaoctatetra-contan-1-ol	Laureth-12
2-[2-[2-(2-Dodecoxyethoxy)ethoxy]ethoxy]ethanol	Laureth-4
Dodecyl alcohol	Lauryl alcohol
Dodecyldiglycol	Laureth-2
Dodecyldimethylamine oxide	Lauramine oxide
Dodecyl dodeca(oxyethylene) ether	Laureth-12
Dodecyl D-glucoside	Lauryl glucoside
Dodecylheptaglycol	Laureth-7
Dodecylnonaoxyethylene glycol monoether	Laureth-9
2-[2-(Dodecyloxy)ethoxy]ethanol	Laureth-2
1-Dodecylpyridin-1-ium chloride	Laurylpyridinium chloride
Dodecyl sodium sulfate	Sodium laureth sulfate
Dodecyltetraethylene glycol monoether	Laureth-4
Dodecyl 3,4,5-trihydroxybenzoate	Dodecyl gallate
Dowicil® 200	Quaternium-15
Dragophos® S	Sodium dihydroxycetyl phosphate isopropyl hydroxycetyl ether (see Chapter Miscellaneous)
DTBHQ	Di-*t*-butylhydroquinone

E

E120	CI 75470
Ecamsule	Terephthalylidene dicamphor sulfonic acid
Edetate disodium	Disodium EDTA
Edetate sodium	Tetrasodium EDTA
Edetate trisodium	Trisodium EDTA
Edetic acid	EDTA
Edetol	Tetrahydroxypropyl ethylenediamine
Elastin, hydrolysate	Hydrolyzed elastin
Enoxolone	Glycyrrhetinic acid
Ensulizole	Phenylbenzimidazole sulfonic acid
Entprol	Tetrahydroxypropyl ethylenediamine
Enzacamene	4-Methylbenzylidene camphor

Table 6.1 List of synonyms: Conversion of synonyms to INCI names or Chapter names (*continued*)

Synonym	INCI name / Chapter name
Eosine	CI 45380
(2,3-Epoxyphytyl)menaquinone	Phytonadione epoxide
2,3-Epoxypropyl methacrylate	Glycidyl methacrylate
Escalol® 507	Ethylhexyl dimethyl PABA
1,2-Ethanediamine, *N,N,N',N'*-tetrakis(carboxymethyl)-	EDTA
Ethanol	Alcohol
Ethanol, 2-[(3-amino-4-methoxyphenyl)amino]-, sulfate	2-Amino-4-hydroxyethylaminoanisole sulfate
Ethanol, 2-(2-ethoxyethoxy)-	Ethoxydiglycol
Ethanol, 2,2'-[[3-[(2-hydroxyethyl)octadecylamino]propyl]-imino] bis-, dihydrofluoride	Olaflur
Ethanol, 2-((2-methoxy-4-nitrophenyl)amino)-	2-Hydroxyethylamino-5-nitroanisole
Ethanol, 2,2',2''-nitrilotris-, compds. with polyethylene glycol hydrogen sulfate 2-(cocoacylamino)ethyl ether	TEA-PEG-3 cocamide sulfate
2-(2-Ethoxyethoxy)ethanol	Ethoxydiglycol
Ethoxylated ethyl-4-aminobenzoate	PEG-25 PABA
4-[(4-Ethoxyphenyl)azo]naphthol	CI 12010
(4*E*)-4-[(4-Ethoxyphenyl)hydrazinylidene]naphthalen-1-one	CI 12010
(2*R*)-*N*-(3-Ethoxypropyl)-2,4-dihydroxy-3,3-dimethylbutanamide	Panthenyl ethyl ether
Ethyl alcohol	Alcohol
2-di-Ethylamino-ethyl *p*-aminobenzoate hydrochloride	Procaine (see Chapter Miscellaneous)
Ethyl carbitol	Ethoxydiglycol
Ethyl 2-cyanoprop-2-enoate	Ethyl cyanoacrylate
Ethylenediaminetetraacetic acid	EDTA
Ethylene dimethacrylate	Glycol HEMA-methacrylate
1,1',1'',1'''-Ethylenedinitrilotetrapropan-2-ol	Tetrahydroxypropyl ethylenediamine
2,2'-Ethylenedioxydiethyl dimethacrylate	Triethylene glycol dimethacrylate
Ethylene glycol dimethacrylate	Glycol HEMA-methacrylate
Ethylene glycol monophenyl ether	Phenoxyethanol
Ethylene, homopolymer	Polyethylene
2-Ethylhexanoic acid, cetyl/stearyl ester	Cetearyl ethylhexanoate
3-(2-Ethylhexoxy)propane-1,2-diol	Ethylhexylglycerin
2-Ethylhexyl-2-cyano-3,3-diphenylacrylate	Octocrylene
2-Ethylhexyl 2-cyano-3,3-diphenylprop-2-enoate	Octocrylene
2'-Ethylhexyl 2-cyano-3-phenylcinnamate	Octocrylene
2-Ethylhexyl 4-(dimethylamino)benzoate	Ethylhexyl dimethyl PABA
2-Ethylhexyl 2-hydroxybenzoate	Ethylhexyl salicylate
2-Ethylhexyl (*E*)-3-(4-methoxyphenyl)prop-2-enoate	Ethylhexyl methoxycinnamate
Ethyl 4-hydroxybenzoate	Ethylparaben
Ethyl (*E*)-3-(4-methoxyphenyl)prop-2-enoate	Ethyl methoxycinnamate
2-[*N*-Ethyl-3-methyl-4-[(5-nitro-1,3-thiazol-2-yl)diazenyl]anilino]ethanol	CI Disperse blue 106
Ethyl 2-methylprop-2-enoate	Ethyl methacrylate
Ethyl parahydroxybenzoate	Ethylparaben
Ethyl prop-2-enoate	Ethyl acrylate
Ethyl sebacate	Diethyl sebacate
Eucerin	Lanolin alcohol
Eumulgin® L	PPG-1-PEG-9 lauryl glycol ether
Euphorbia antisyphilitica wax	Candelilla cera
Euphorbia cerifera (candelilla) wax	Candelilla cera
Eusolex® 232	Phenylbenzimidazole sulfonic acid
Eusolex® 4360	Benzophenone-3
Eusolex® 6300	4-Methylbenzylidene camphor
Eusolex® 8020	Isopropyl dibenzoylmethane
Euxyl K® 100	Methylchloroisothiazolinone (and) methyliso-thiazolinone
Euxyl® K400	Methyldibromo glutaronitrile/phenoxyethanol

Table 6.1 List of synonyms: Conversion of synonyms to INCI names or Chapter names (*continued*)

Synonym	INCI name / Chapter name
Euxyl® K400	see Phenoxyethanol

F

Synonym	INCI name / Chapter name
Fast yellow G	CI 11680
Fatty acids, coco, reaction products with 2-((2-aminoethyl)-amino)ethanol, mono(2-carboxyethyl) derivs., monosodium salts	Sodium cocoamphopropionate
FD&C red no. 3 - aluminum lake	Pigment red 172 aluminum lake
FD&C yellow 11	Solvent yellow 44
Fentichlor	2,2'-Thiobis(4-chlorophenol)
Fenticlor	2,2'-Thiobis(4-chlorophenol)
Ferric oxide	Iron oxides
Ferrous oxide	Iron oxides
Feverfew extract	Tanacetum parthenium extract
Food orange 5	Beta-carotene
Formaldehyde; 4-methylbenzenesulfonamide	Tosylamide/formaldehyde resin
Formaldehyde resin	Paraformaldehyde
Freon® 11	Trichlorofluoromethane
Freon® 12	Dichlorodifluoromethane

G

Synonym	INCI name / Chapter name
Germall®115	Imidazolidinyl urea
Germall® II	Diazolidinyl urea
D-Glucitol	Sorbitol
L-Gluco-octitol, 1,5-anhydro-6,8-dideoxy-, (7XI)-	Hydroxypropyl tetrahydropyrantriol
D-Glucopyranose, C16-18 alkyl glycosides	Cetearyl glucoside
D-Glucopyranose, oligomeric, C10-16 alkyl glycosides	Lauryl glucoside
D-Glucopyranoside, methyl, octadecanoate (2:3)	Methyl glucose sesquistearate
α-D-Glucopyranosiduronic acid, (3β,20β)-20-Carboxy-11-oxo-30-norolean-12-en-3-yl-2-O-β-D-glucopyranuronosyl-, dipotassium salt	Dipotassium glycyrrhizate
Glucosamine chlorhydrate	Glucosamine HCl
Glucosamine hydrochloride	Glucosamine HCl
D-Glucose, 1-eicosanol ether	Arachidyl glucoside
Glutaral	Glutaraldehyde
Glutardialdehyde	Glutaraldehyde
Glycerides, C18-36	C18-36 acid triglyceride
Glycerides, mixed decanoyl and octanoyl	Caprylic/capric triglyceride
Glycerol	Glycerin
Glycerol ester of rosin	Glyceryl rosinate
Glyceryl caprylate-caprate	Caprylic/capric triglyceride
Glyceryl monocaprylate	Glyceryl caprylate
Glyceryl monoisostearate monomyristate	Glyceryl isostearate/myristate
Glyceryl monostearate	Glyceryl stearate
Glyceryl monothioglycolate	Glyceryl thioglycolate
Glyceryl paraaminobenzoate	Glyceryl PABA
Glycine, *N*-(2-aminoethyl)-*N*-(2-hydroxyethyl)-, *N*-coco-acyl derivatives, monosodium salts	Sodium cocoamphoacetate
Glycine, *N*-(2-hydroxyethyl)-*N*-[2-(1-oxododecylamino)-ethyl]-, monosodium salt	Sodium lauroamphoacetate
Glycine, *N*-(hydroxymethyl)-, monosodium salt	Sodium hydroxymethylglycinate
Glycine, *N*-methyl-*N*-(1-oxotetradecyl)-, sodium salt	Sodium myristoyl sarcosinate
Glycol dimethacrylate	Glycol HEMA-methacrylate
Glycol methacrylate	HEMA
3-(D-Gluconoylamino)propyl(2-hydroxyethyl)dimethyl-ammonium chloride	Quaternium-22

Table 6.1 List of synonyms: Conversion of synonyms to INCI names or Chapter names (*continued*)

Synonym	INCI name / Chapter name
D-Glucopyranoside methyl 2,6-dioleate	Methyl glucose dioleate
Glycyrrhetic acid	Glycyrrhetinic acid
Glycyrrhetin	Glycyrrhetinic acid
Glycyrrhizin	Glycyrrhizic acid
Glycyrrhizinic acid	Glycyrrhizic acid
Green chromic oxide	CI 77288
Grotan® BK	Tris(*N*-hydroxyethyl) hexahydrotriazine
Guar gum, 2-hydroxy-3-(trimethylammonio)propyl ether, chloride	Guar hydroxypropyltrimonium chloride
Guggul	Commiphora mukul resin extract
Gum benzoin	Styrax benzoin gum
Gum lac	Shellac
Gummi xanthanum	Xanthan gum
Gum rosin	Colophonium

H

Hansa yellow	CI 11680
HC red B54	3-Nitro-*p*-hydroxyethylaminophenol
2,2,4,4,6,8,8-Heptamethylnonane	Isohexadecane
3,5-Heptanedione, 1,7-bis(4-hydroxy-3-methoxyphenyl)	see Tetrahydrocurcumin
3,6,9,12,15,18,21-Heptaoxatritriacontanol	Laureth-7
Hexadecan-1-ol	Cetyl alcohol
1-Hexadecanol	Cetyl alcohol
Hexadecyl 2-ethylhexanoate	Cetearyl ethylhexanoate
Hexadecyl isononanoate	Cetearyl isononanoate
Hexadecyltrimethylammonium bromide	Cetrimonium bromide
Hexadecyl(trimethyl)azanium bromide	Cetrimonium bromide
(2*E*,4*E*)-Hexa-2,4-dienoic acid	Sorbic acid
Hexaethylene glycol	PEG-6
Hexahydro-1,3,5-tris(2-hydroxyethyl)-*s*-triazine	Tris(*N*-hydroxyethyl) hexahydrotriazine
Hexamethylene diacrylate	1,6-Hexanediol diacrylate
Hexamethylenetetramine	Methenamine
Hexamethylenetetramine chloroallyl chloride	Quaternium-15
Hexamidine isethionate	Hexamidine diisethionate
Hexamine	Methenamine
(2*R*,3*R*,4*R*,5*S*)-Hexane-1,2,3,4,5,6-hexol	Sorbitol
(2*R*,3*R*,4*R*,5*S*)-Hexane-1,2,3,4,5,6-hexol; (*Z*)-octadec-9-enoic acid	Sorbitan sesquioleate
Hexanoic acid, 2-ethyl-, C16-18 alkyl esters	Cetearyl ethylhexanoate
Hexanoic acid, 3,5,5-trimethyl-, 3,5,5-trimethylhexyl ester	Isononyl isononanoate
4-Hexylbenzene-1,3-diol	Hexylresorcinol
Homomenthyl salicylate	Homosalate
Honeysuckle (flower) extract	Lonicera japonica flower extract
Hydrolyzed animal elastin	Hydrolyzed elastin
Hydrolyzed animal protein	Hydrolyzed collagen
Hydrolyzed elastin solution	Hydrolyzed elastin
2-Hydroxyaniline	*o*-Aminophenol
2-Hydroxybenzoic acid, phenyl ester	Phenyl salicylate
6-Hydroxy-1,3-benzoxathiol-2-one	Tioxolone
2-(10-Hydroxydecyl)-5,6-dimethoxy-3-methylcyclohexa-2,5-diene-1,4-dione	Hydroxydecyl ubiquinone
2-Hydroxy-4-diethylamino-2'-hexyloxycarbonylbenzophenone	Diethylamino hydroxybenzoyl hexyl benzoate
2-Hydroxydiphenyl	*o*-Phenylphenol
1-Hydroxydodecane	Lauryl alcohol
2-Hydroxyethanesulphonic acid, compound with 4,4'-[hexane-1,6-diylbis(oxy)]bis-[benzenecarboxamidine] (2:1)	Hexamidine diisethionate
2-[bis(2-Hydroxyethyl)amino]ethanol	Triethanolamine

Table 6.1 List of synonyms: Conversion of synonyms to INCI names or Chapter names (*continued*)

Synonym	INCI name / Chapter name
4-Hydroxyethylamino-3-nitrophenol	3-Nitro-*p*-hydroxyethylaminophenol
4-((2-Hydroxyethyl)amino)-3-nitrophenol	3-Nitro-*p*-hydroxyethylaminophenol
2-[3-[bis(2-Hydroxyethyl)amino]propyl-octadecylamino]ethanol	Olaflur
bis(2-Hydroxyethyl)ammonium bis(2-hydroxyhexadecyl) phosphate	DEA-dihydroxypalmityl phosphate
2-Hydroxyethyl-dimethyl-[3-[[(2*R*,3*S*,4*R*,5*R*)-2,3,4,5,6-penta-hydroxyhexanoyl]amino]propyl]azanium;chloride	Quaternium-22
N,*N*-bis(2-Hydroxyethyl)dodecanamide	Lauramide DEA
N-(2-Hydroxyethyl)ethylenediamine-*N*,*N*′,*N*′-triacetic acid trisodium salt hydrate	Trisodium hydroxyethyl ethylenediamine triacetate
2-Hydroxyethyl methacrylate	HEMA
2-Hydroxyethyl 2-methylprop-2-enoate	HEMA
N-(β-Hydroxyethyl)-2-nitro-4-hydroxyaminobenzene (incorrect)	3-Nitro-*p*-hydroxyethylaminophenol
N,*N*-bis(2-Hydroxyethyl)-(*Z*)-9-octadecenamide	Oleamide DEA
2-Hydroxyethyl prop-2-enoate	Hydroxyethyl acrylate
2-[3,5-bis(2-Hydroxyethyl)-1,3,5-triazinan-1-yl]ethanol	Tris(*N*-hydroxyethyl) hexahydrotriazine
N,*N*-bis(2-Hydroxyethyl)undecenamide	Undecylenamide DEA
5-Hydroxy-2-(hydroxymethyl)pyran-4-one	Kojic acid
2-Hydroxy-4-isopropyl-2,4,6-cyclohepta-2,4,6-trien-1-one	Hinokitiol
2-Hydroxy-4-methoxybenzophenone	Benzophenone-3
2-Hydroxy-4-methoxybenzophenone-5-sulfonic acid	Benzophenone-4
2-Hydroxy-4-methoxy-4'-methylbenzophenone	Benzophenone-10
1-(4-Hydroxy-3-methoxyphenyl)-7-(4-hydroxyphenyl)-heptane-3,5-dione	see Tetrahydrocurcumin
(2-Hydroxy-4-methoxyphenyl)-(2-hydroxyphenyl)methanone	Benzophenone-8
(2-Hydroxy-4-methoxyphenyl)-(4-methylphenyl)methanone	Benzophenone-10
(2-Hydroxy-4-methoxyphenyl)-phenylmethanone	Benzophenone-3
tri(Hydroxymethyl)aminomethane	Tromethamine
1,3-bis(Hydroxymethyl)-5,5-dimethylimidazolidine-2,4-dione	DMDM hydantoin
1-[1,3-bis(Hydroxymethyl)-2,5-dioxoimidazolidin-4-yl]-1,3-bis(hydroxymethyl)urea	Diazolidinyl urea
[3-Hydroxy-2-(16-methylheptadecanoyloxy)propyl] 16-	Glyceryl diisostearate
2-(Hydroxymethyl)-6-(4-hydroxyphenoxy)oxane-3,4,5-triol	Arbutin
2-(2-Hydroxy-5-methylphenyl)benzotriazole	Drometrizole
N-[4-(2-(2-Hydroxy-5-methylphenyl)diazenyl)phenyl]-acetamide	Disperse yellow 3
[2-(Hydroxymethyl)-3-prop-2-enoyloxy-2-(prop-2-enoyloxy-methyl)propyl] prop-2-enoate	Pentaerythrityl triacrylate
4-Hydroxynaphthalene-1,2-dione	Lawsone
2-Hydroxy-1,4-naphthoquinone	Lawsone
2-Hydroxy-1,4-naphthoquinone	Henna
1-Hydroxy-3-nitro-4-aminobenzene	4-Amino-3-nitrophenol
4-Hydroxy-2-nitroaniline	4-Amino-3-nitrophenol
1-Hydroxy-3-nitro-4-β-hydroxyethyl-aminobenzene	3-Nitro-*p*-hydroxyethylaminophenol
12-Hydroxyoctadecanoic acid	Hydroxystearic acid
[2-[(2*R*,3*S*,4*R*)-4-Hydroxy-3-octadecanoyloxyoxolan-2-yl]-2-octadecanoyloxyethyl] octadecanoate	Sorbitan tristearate
12-Hydroxy-9-octadecenoic acid, zinc salt	Zinc ricinoleate
Hydroxyoctadec-9-ene	Oleyl alcohol
12-Hydroxy-9-octadecenoic acid	Ricinoleic acid
(*Z*,12*R*)-12-Hydroxyoctadec-9-enoic acid	Ricinoleic acid
N-Hydroxyoctanamide	Caprylhydroxamic acid
2-Hydroxy-5-octanoylbenzoic acid	Capryloyl salicylic acid
12-Hydroxyoleic acid	Ricinoleic acid
(*R*)-12-Hydroxyoleic acid, monoester with glycerol	Glyceryl ricinoleate
(*R*)-12-Hydroxyoleic acid, monoester with propane-1,2-diol	Propylene glycol ricinoleate

Table 6.1 List of synonyms: Conversion of synonyms to INCI names or Chapter names (*continued*)

Synonym	INCI name / Chapter name
2-Hydroxy-5-(1-oxooctyl)benzoic acid	Capryloyl salicylic acid
p-Hydroxyphenol	Hydroquinone
2-Hydroxy-2-phenylacetic acid	Mandelic acid
3-Hydroxy-4-(phenylazo)-2-naphthalenecarboxylic acid, calcium salt (2:1)	CI 15800
4-Hydroxyphenyl-β-D-glucopyranoside	Arbutin
4-[(*E*)-4-(4-Hydroxyphenyl)hex-3-en-3-yl]phenol	Diethylstilbestrol
Hydroxypolyethoxydodecane	Laureth-9
2-Hydroxypropane	Isopropyl alcohol
2-Hydroxypropanoic acid;16-methyl-*N*-(3-morpholin-4-ylpropyl)heptadecanamide	Isostearamidopropyl morpholine lactate
1-(2-Hydroxypropoxy)propan-2-ol	Dipropylene glycol
1-[2-[bis(2-Hydroxypropyl)amino]ethyl-(2-hydroxypropyl)-amino]propan-2-ol	Tetrahydroxypropyl ethylenediamine
1-(2-Hydroxypropylamino)propan-2-ol	Diisopropanolamine
2-Hydroxypropyl (*Z*)-12-hydroxyoctadec-9-enoate	Propylene glycol ricinoleate
2-Hydroxypropyl 2-methyl-2-propenoate	Hydroxypropyl methacrylate
(2*S*,3*R*,4*S*,5*R*)-2-(2-Hydroxypropyl)oxane-3,4,5-triol	Hydroxypropyl tetrahydropyrantriol
Hydroxypropyloxypropanol	Dipropylene glycol
2-(2-Hydroxy-5-propylphenyl)-4-propylphenol	Tetrahydromagnolol
Hydroxypropyltrimonium hydrolysed animal protein	Hydroxypropyltrimonium hydrolyzed collagen
4-Hydroxy-*o*-toluidine	4-Amino-*m*-cresol
8-Hydroxyquinoline	Oxyquinoline

I

Idebenone	Hydroxydecyl ubiquinone
Imidurea	Imidazolidinyl urea
3-Iodoprop-2-ynyl *N*-butylcarbamate	Iodopropynyl butylcarbamate
IPBC	Iodopropynyl butylcarbamate
Irgasan® DP 300	Triclosan
Iron hydroxide oxide yellow	Iron oxides
1,3-Isobenzofurandione, polymer with 5-carboxy-1,3-isobenzo-furandione, 1,2- ethanediol and 2,2-dimethyl-1,3-propanediol	Phthalic anhydride/trimellitic anhydride/ glycols copolymer
Isobutamben	Isobutyl PABA
Isobutyl 4-aminobenzoate	Isobutyl PABA
Isononanoic acid, C16-18 alkyl esters	Cetearyl isononanoate
di(Isooctadecanoic) acid, diester with glycerol	Glyceryl diisostearate
Isooctadecanoic acid, monoester with glycerol	Glyceryl isostearate
Isooctadecanoic acid, monoester with 1,2,3-propanetriol monotetradecanoate	Glyceryl isostearate/myristate
Isooctadecanol	Isostearyl alcohol
Isopalmityl diglyceryl sebacate	Diglyceryl sebacate/isopalmitate
Isopentyl *p*-methoxycinnamate	Isoamyl *p*-methoxycinnamate
Isopropanol	Isopropyl alcohol
1-Isopropoxy-2-hexadecanol	Isopropyl hydroxypalmityl ether
Isopropyl tetradecanoate	Isopropyl myristate

J

Jojoba seed oil	Simmondsia chinensis seed oil
Jojoba (seed) powder	Simmondsia chinensis seed powder

K

Karite butter	Butyrospermum parkii butter
Kathon® CG	Methylchloroisothiazolinone (and) methyliso-thiazolinone

Table 6.1 List of synonyms: Conversion of synonyms to INCI names or Chapter names (*continued*)

Synonym	INCI name / Chapter name

L

Lacca	Shellac
Lac resin	Shellac
Lactis proteinum	Milk protein
Lanette O	Cetearyl alcohol
Lanolin acetate(s)	Acetylated lanolin
Lanolin alcohols	Lanolin alcohol
Lanolin, anhydrous	Lanolin
Lanpol® 5	PEG-5 lanolate
Lauric acid diethanolamide	Lauramide DEA
Lauroamphocarboxyglycinate	Disodium lauroamphodiacetate
Lauroamphoglycinate	Sodium lauroamphoacetate
Lauryl dimethyl amine oxide	Lauramine oxide
Lauryl gallate	Dodecyl gallate
Lawsonia inermis extract	Henna
Lead diacetate	Lead acetate
Levomenol	Bisabolol
Licorice extract	Glycyrrhiza glabra root extract
α-Lipoic acid	Thioctic acid
Liquid paraffin	Mineral oil
Liquid petrolatum	Mineral oil
Lisadimate	Glyceryl PABA
Lithol rubin BCA®	Pigment red 57:1

M

Macadamia nut oil	Macadamia ternifolia seed oil
L-Mannopyranoside, pentyl 6-deoxy-	Pentyl rhamnoside
Mare('s) milk	Equae lac
Marigold extract	Calendula officinalis extract
Matricaria extract	Chamomilla recutita extract
Matricaria parthenium extract	Tanacetum parthenium extract
L-Menthylglyceryl ether	Menthoxypropanediol
Mercaptamine hydrochloride	Cysteamine HCl
Mercaptoacetic acid, monoester with propane-1,2,3-triol	Glyceryl thioglycolate
Mercaptoethylamine	Cysteamine HCl
3-Mercaptopropane-1,2-diol	Thioglycerin
2-Mercaptopropionic acid	Thiolactic acid
Mercuric ammonium chloride	Ammoniated mercury
Mercury(II) amide chloride	Ammoniated mercury
Mercury, ammoniated	Ammoniated mercury
Merthiolate	Thimerosal
2-((Methacryloxy)methyl)oxirane	Glycidyl methacrylate
Methanal	Formaldehyde
Methenamine 3-chloroallylochloride	Quaternium-15
6'-Methoxycinchonan-9-ol	Quinine
6-Methoxy-2-methylamino-3-aminopyridine HCl	HC Blue no. 7
6-Methoxy-N2-methylpyridine-2,3-diamine;dihydrochloride	HC Blue no. 7
2-(2-Methoxy-4-nitroanilino)ethanol	2-Hydroxyethylamino-5-nitroanisole
2-[(2-Methoxy-4-nitrophenyl)amino]ethanol	2-Hydroxyethylamino-5-nitroanisole
1-[(2-Methoxyphenyl)azo]-2-naphthol	CI 12150
(1Z)-1-[(2-Methoxyphenyl)hydrazinylidene]naphthalen-2-one	CI 12150
2,2'-[6-(4-Methoxyphenyl)-1,3,5-triazine-2,4-diyl]bis[5-[(2-ethylhexyl)oxy]-phenol]	bis-Ethylhexyloxyphenol methoxyphenyl triazine
Methyl aldehyde	Formaldehyde

Table 6.1 List of synonyms: Conversion of synonyms to INCI names or Chapter names (*continued*)

Synonym	INCI name / Chapter name
4-(Methylamino)phenol	*p*-Methylaminophenol
2-Methylbenzene-1,4-diamine	Toluene-2,5-diamine
2-Methylbenzene-1,4-diamine;sulfuric acid	Toluene-2,5-diamine sulfate
3-Methylbutyl (*E*)-3-(4-methoxyphenyl)prop-2-enoate	Isoamyl *p*-methoxycinnamate
Methylene bis-benzotriazolyl tetramethylbutylphenol (and) aqua (and) decyl glucoside (and) propylene glycol (and) xanthan gum	Tinosorb® M
2,2'-Methylenebis(4-chlorophenol)	Dichlorophen
N,*N*'-Methylenebis[*N*'-[3-(hydroxymethyl)-2,5-dioxoimidazolidin-4-yl]urea]	Imidazolidinyl urea
2,2'-Methylene-bis[4-(1,1,3,3-tetramethylbutyl)-6-benzotriazol-2-ylphenol]	Methylene bis-benzotriazolyl tetramethylbutyl-phenol
Methylene oxide	Formaldehyde
1-(1-Methylethoxy)-2-hexadecanol	Isopropyl hydroxypalmityl ether
1-[4-(1-Methylethyl)phenyl]-3-phenylpropane-1,3-dione	Isopropyl dibenzoylmethane
Methyl gentisate	Methyl dihydroxybenzoate
Methyl glucoside sesquistearate	Methyl glucose sesquistearate
16-Methylheptadecan-1-ol	Isostearyl alcohol
bis(16-Methylheptadecyl) 2-hydroxybutanedioate	Diisostearyl malate
bis(16-Methylheptadecyl) malate	Diisostearyl malate
Methyl 4-hydroxybenzoate	Methylparaben
2-Methyl-4-isothiazolin-3-one	Methylisothiazolinone
(2*S*)-6-Methyl-2-(4-methylcyclohex-3-en-1-yl)hept-5-en-2-ol	Bisabolol
3-{[5-Methyl-2-(1-methylethyl)cyclohexyl]oxy}-	Menthoxypropanediol
Methyl 2-methylprop-2-enoate	Methyl methacrylate
16-Methyl-*N*-[3-(morpholin-4-yl)propyl]heptadecanamide; lactic acid	Isostearamidopropyl morpholine lactate
1-[(4-Methyl-2-nitrophenyl)azo]-2-naphthalenol	CI 12120
2-[(4-Methyl-2-nitrophenyl)azo]-3-oxo-*N*-phenylbutyramide	CI 11680
(2*Z*)-2-[(4-Methyl-2-nitrophenyl)hydrazinylidene]-3-oxo-*N*-phenylbutanamide	CI 11680
N-Methyl-*N*-(1-oxododecyl)glycine, sodium salt	Sodium lauroyl sarcosinate
2-Methylpentane-2,4-diol	Hexylene glycol
2-Methyl-2,4-pentanediol	Hexylene glycol
5-Methyl-2-phenyl-1,3-benzoxazole	Witisol
2-Methyl-*p*-phenylenediamine	Toluene-2,5-diamine
2-Methyl-*p*-phenylenediamine sulfate	Toluene-2,5-diamine sulfate
2-Methylpropan-2-ol	*t*-Butyl alcohol
3-(5-Methyl-2-propan-2-ylcyclohexyl)oxypropane-1,2-diol	Menthoxypropanediol
Methyl prop-2-enoate	Methyl acrylate
4-(2-Methylprop-2-enoyloxy)butyl 2-methylprop-2-enoate	1,4-Butanediol dimethacrylate
2-[2-(2-Methylprop-2-enoyloxy)ethoxy]ethyl 2-methylprop-2-enoate	Diethylene glycol dimethacrylate
2-(2-Methylprop-2-enoyloxy)ethyl 2-methylprop-2-enoate	Glycol HEMA-methacrylate
2-Methylpropyl 2-methylprop-2-enoate	Isobutyl methacrylate
Methyl pyridine-3-carboxylate	Methyl nicotinate
2-Methyl-3-(3,7,11,15-tetramethylhexadec-2-enyl)-1,4-naphthoquinone	Phytonadione
2-Methyl-1,2-thiazol-3-one	Methylisothiazolinone
Mexenone	Benzophenone-10
Microcide® III	Methylchloroisothiazolinone (and) methylisothiazolinone
Microcrystalline wax	Cera microcristallina
Milfoil extract	Achillea millefolium extract
Milk protein, casein	Casein
Mineral fat	Petrolatum

Table 6.1 List of synonyms: Conversion of synonyms to INCI names or Chapter names (*continued*)

Synonym	INCI name / Chapter name
Mineral wax	Petrolatum
Mixed tocopherols	Tocopherol
Monobenzyl ether of hydroquinone	Monobenzone
Monocaprylin	Glyceryl caprylate
Monosulfiram	Sulfiram
Monothioglycerol	Thioglycerin
Myristyl D-glucopyranoside	Myristyl glucoside

N

Naphthalene-2,7-diol	2,7-Naphthalenediol
1-Naphthalenesulfonic acid, 2-((2-hydroxy-1-naphthalenyl)azo)-, calcium salt (2:1)	Calcium lithol red
1-Naphthalen-2-ylpiperidine	Isopropyl dibenzoylmethane
Natural red 4	CI 75470
Natural vitamin E	Tocopherol
NeoHeliopan® AP	Disodium phenyl dibenzimidazole tetrasulfonate
Nicotinic acid methyl ester	Methyl nicotinate
2,2',2'-Nitrilotriethanol	Triethanolamine
2-Nitrobenzene-1,4-diamine	2-Nitro-*p*-phenylenediamine
2-Nitro-4-(β-hydroxyethylamino)aniline	HC red no. 7
o-Nitro-*p*-phenylenediamine	2-Nitro-*p*-phenylenediamine
3,6,9,12,15,18,21,24,27-Nonaoxanonatriacontan-1-ol	Laureth-9
2-Nonyl-2-imidazolinium lauryl sulfate-1(2-hydroxyethyl)-1-carboxymethyl, disodium salt	Miranol® MSA (see chapter Miscellaneous)
Novocain®	Procaine (see Chapter Miscellaneous)

O

Oat bran extract	Avena sativa bran extract
Octadecanoate; tris(2-hydroxyethyl)azanium	TEA-stearate
Octadecanoic acid	Stearic acid
Octadecanoic acid, sodium salt	Sodium stearate
Octadecan-1-ol	Stearyl alcohol
(*Z*)-9-Octadecenoic acid decyl ester	Decyl oleate
(*Z*)-Octadec-9-enol	Oleyl alcohol
tris[(*Z*)-Octadec-9-enyl] phosphate	Trioleyl phosphate
Octadecyl alcohol	Stearyl alcohol
N'-Octadecyltrimethylendiamine-*N,N,N'*-tris(2-ethanol)-dihydrofluoride	Olaflur
Octanamide, *N*-hydroxy-	Caprylhydroxamic acid
Octanohydroxamic acid	Caprylhydroxamic acid
Octanoic acid, monoester with glycerol	Glyceryl caprylate
5-Octanoylsalicylic acid	Capryloyl salicylic acid
Octenoic acid, 3,4-diester with 5-hydroxy-6-methyl-3,4-pyridinedimethanol	Pyridoxine dioctenoate
Octenoic acid, (5-hydroxy-6-methyl-3,4-pyridinediyl)bis-(methylene) ester	Pyridoxine dioctenoate
Octinoxate	Ethylhexyl methoxycinnamate
Octisalate	Ethylhexyl salicylate
Octoxyglycerin	Ethylhexylglycerin
Octyl dimethyl PABA	Ethylhexyl dimethyl PABA
2-Octyldodecan-1-ol	Octyldodecanol
Octyl gallate	Caprylyl gallate
Octyl methoxycinnamate	Ethylhexyl methoxycinnamate
Octyl salicylate	Ethylhexyl salicylate
Octyl triazone	Ethylhexyl triazone

Table 6.1 List of synonyms: Conversion of synonyms to INCI names or Chapter names (*continued*)

Synonym	INCI name / Chapter name
Octyl 3,4,5-trihydroxybenzoate	Caprylyl gallate
Oil of Palma Christi	Ricinus communis seed oil
Olean-12-en-29-oic acid, 3-hydroxy-11-oxo-, (3β,20β)-	Glycyrrhetinic acid
Oleic acid decyl ester	Decyl oleate
Oleic acid diethanolamide	Oleamide DEA
Oleoylmethyltaurine sodium salt	Sodium methyl oleoyl taurate
Oleum ricini	Ricinus communis seed oil
Oxamitol	2-Aminomethyl-*p*-aminophenol HCl
Oxazolidine A	Dimethyl oxazolidine
Oxirane, decyl-, polymer with oxirane, monomethyl ether (17 mol EO, 1 mol decyl oxirane, average molar ratios)	Methoxy PEG-17/dodecyl glycol copolymer
Oxirane, decyl-, polymer with oxirane, monomethyl ether (22 mol EO, 7 mol decyl oxirane, average molar ratios)	Methoxy PEG-22/dodecyl glycol copolymer
Oxiran-2-ylmethyl 2-methylprop-2-enoate	Glycidyl methacrylate
Oxobismuth hydrochloride	CI 77163
Oxolan-2-ylmethyl 2-methylprop-2-enoate	Tetrahydrofurfuryl methacrylate
Oxomethane	Formaldehyde
Oxo(oxochromiooxy)chromium	CI 77288
Oxybenzone	Benzophenone-3
Oxymethylene	Formaldehyde
Ovum	Egg
Ozokerite wax	Ceresin

P

Padimate A	Pentyl dimethyl PABA
Padimate O	Ethylhexyl dimethyl PABA
Palmitoyl animal collagen amino acids	Palmitoyl collagen amino acids
Pantothenol	Panthenol
Pantothenyl ethyl ether	Panthenyl ethyl ether
Paraffin jelly	Petrolatum
Paraffin oils; liquid hydrocarbons from petroleum	Mineral oil
Paraffinum perliquidum	Mineral oil
Paraffin waxes and hydrocarbon waxes, microcrystalline	Cera microcrystallina
Paraform	Paraformaldehyde
C13-15 Pareth-2 carboxamide MEA	Trideceth-2 carboxamide MEA
Parsol® 1789	Butyl methoxydibenzoylmethane
Parsol® MCX	Ethylhexyl methoxycinnamate
Parsol® SLX	Polysilicone-15
Pearl essence	Guanine
PEG-300	PEG-6
PEG-2 cetyl/stearyl ether	Ceteareth-2
PEG-3 cetyl/stearyl ether	Ceteareth-3
PEG-2 lauryl ether	Laureth-2
PEG-4 lauryl ether	Laureth-4
PEG-7 lauryl ether	Laureth-7
PEG-12 lauryl ether	Laureth-12
PEG-(1-4) lauryl ether sulfate, sodium salt	Sodium laureth sulfate
PEG-5 oleyl ether	Oleth-5
PEG-3 oleyl ether phosphate	Oleth-3 phosphate
PEG-10 stearyl ether	Steareth-10
Pentaerythritol rosinate	Pentaerythrityl rosinate
Pentaerythritol triacrylate	Pentaerythrityl triacrylate
Pentaerythrityl tetracaprylate/caprate	Pentaerythrityl tetracaprylate/tetracaprate
(2R,3S,4R,5R)-2,3,4,5,6-Pentahydroxyhexanoic acid	Chlorhexidine digluconate
1,5-Pentanedial	Glutaraldehyde
Pentane-1,5-diol	Pentylene glycol

Table 6.1 List of synonyms: Conversion of synonyms to INCI names or Chapter names (*continued*)

Synonym	INCI name / Chapter name
3-Penten-2-one, 5-(3,3-dimethylbicyclo[2.2.1]hept-2-ylidene)-	Bornelone
Pentyl 4-(dimethylamino)benzoate	Pentyl dimethyl PABA
Pentyl rhamnoside	
Percelline oil	Cetearyl ethylhexanoate
Permanent orange	Pigment orange 5
Petrolatum, liquid	Mineral oil
Petroleum jelly	Petrolatum
Phenethyl resorcinol	Phenylethyl resorcinol
Phenol, 2-aminomethyl-4-amino-, dihydrochloride	2-Aminomethyl-*p*-aminophenol HCl
Phenol, 2-(2*H*-benzotriazol-2-yl)-4-methyl-6-(2-methyl-3-(1,3,3,3-tetramethyl-1-(trimethylsilyl)oxy)-disiloxanyl)propyl	Drometrizole trisiloxane
Phenol, 4-(1,1-dimethylethyl)	4-*tert*-Butylphenol
Phenopyridine	Oxyquinoline
1-Phenylazo-2-naphthol	CI 12055
1-(4-(Phenylazo)phenylazo)-2-naphthol	CI 26100
4-*N*-Phenylbenzene-1,4-diamine	*N*-Phenyl-*p*-phenylenediamine
2-Phenyl-4-chlorophenol	Chloro-2-phenylphenol
4-(2-Phenyldiazenyl)-benzenamine	4-Aminoazobenzene
1-(Phenyldiazenyl)naphthalen-2-ol	CI 12055
1,4-Phenylenediamine	*p*-Phenylenediamine
3,3'-(1,4-Phenylenedimethylene)bis[7,7-dimethyl-2-oxo-bicyclo[2.2.1]heptane-1-methanesulfonic acid]	Terephthalylidene dicamphor sulfonic acid
4-(1-Phenylethyl)benzene-1,3-diol	Phenylethyl resorcinol
Phenylglycolic acid	Mandelic acid
Phenyl 2-hydroxybenzoate	Phenyl salicylate
Phenylmethoxymethanol	Benzylhemiformal
4-Phenylmethoxyphenol	Monobenzone
2-Phenylphenol	*o*-Phenylphenol
PHMB	Polyaminopropyl biguanide
Phylloquinone	Phytonadione
Phylloquinone oxide	Phytonadione epoxide
Phytomenadione	Phytonadione
Pigment black 11	Iron oxides
Pigment brown 6	Iron oxides
Pigment brown 7	Iron oxides
Pigment green 17	CI 77288
Pigment red 3	CI 12120
Pigment red 4	CI 12085
Pigment red 49:2	Calcium lithol red
Pigment red 53:1	CI Pigment red 53
Pigment red 64:1	CI 15800
Pigment red 64:1 (calcium salt)	CI 15800
Pigment red 101	Iron oxides
Pigment red 102	Iron oxides
Pigment yellow 1	CI 11680
Pigment yellow 42	Iron oxides
Pigment yellow 43	Iron oxides
Pigment white 14	CI 77163
Pix lithanthracis	Coal tar
Polidocanol	Laureth-9
Poliglusam	Chitosan
Polyacetal (resin)	Paraformaldehyde
Polycrylene®	Polyester-8
Polyethylene glycol 300	PEG-6
Polyethylene glycol (3) cetyl/stearyl ether	Ceteareth-3
Polyethylene glycol 100 cetyl/stearyl ether	Ceteareth-2

Table 6.1 List of synonyms: Conversion of synonyms to INCI names or Chapter names (*continued*)

Synonym	INCI name / Chapter name
Polyethylene glycol 200 dilaurate	PEG-4 dilaurate
Polyethylene glycol (4) dimethacrylate	PEG-4 dimethacrylate
Polyethylene glycol (5) lanolate	PEG-5 lanolate
Polyethylene glycol (7) lauryl ether	Laureth-7
Polyethylene glycol 100 lauryl ether	Laureth-2
Polyethylene glycol 200 lauryl ether	Laureth-4
Polyethylene glycol 600 lauryl ether	Laureth-12
Polyethylene glycol (7) monooleate	PEG-7 oleate
Polyethylene glycol 1540 monostearate	PEG-32 stearate
Polyethylene glycol (25) PABA	PEG-25 PABA
Polyethylene glycol 200 rapeseedamide	PEG-4 rapeseedamide
Polyethylene glycol 2000 sorbitan lanolate	PEG-40 sorbitan lanolate
Polyethylene glycol (5) soy sterol	PEG-5 soy sterol
Polyethylene glycol 500 stearyl ether	Steareth-10
Polyhexanide	Polyaminopropyl biguanide
Poly(oxy-1,2-ethanediyl), α-hydro-ω-hydroxy-, diethers with 1,2-dodecanediol homopolymer (22 mol EO, 9 mol dodecanediol average molar ratio)	PEG-22/dodecyl glycol copolymer
Poly(oxy-1,2-ethanediyl),α-(C16-C18-alkyl)-ω-hydroxy-(4 mol EO average molar ratio), phosphates (3:1)	Triceteareth-4
Poly(oxy-1,2-ethanediyl), α-(12-hydroxydodecyl)-θ-[(12-hydroxydodecyl)oxy]-s	PEG-22/dodecyl glycol copolymer
Poly(oxy-1,2-ethanediyl),α-2-(2-hydroxyethyl)amino-2-oxo-ethyl-ω-hydroxy-, mono-C13-15-alkyl ethers	Trideceth-2 carboxamide MEA
Poly(oxy-1,2-ethanediyl),α-octadecyl-ω-hydroxy	Steareth-10
Poly(oxy-1,2-ethanediyl),α,α',α''-phosphinylidynetris-ω-(dodecyloxy)-	Trilaureth-4 phosphate
Polyoxyethylene (6)	PEG-6
Polyoxyethylene (2) cetyl/stearyl ether	Ceteareth-2
Polyoxyethylene (3) cetyl/stearyl ether	Ceteareth-3
Polyoxyethylene (4) dilaurate	PEG-4 dilaurate
Polyoxyethylene (4) dimethacrylate	PEG-4 dimethacrylate
Polyoxyethylene ethyl-4-aminobenzoate (25 mol EO average molar ratio)	PEG-25 PABA
Polyoxyethylene (7) hydrogenated castor oil	PEG-7 hydrogenated castor oil
Polyoxyethylene (5) lanolate	PEG-5 lanolate
Polyoxyethylene (2) lauryl ether	Laureth-2
Polyoxyethylene (4) lauryl ether	Laureth-4
Polyoxyethylene (7) lauryl ether	Laureth-7
Polyoxyethylene (12) lauryl ether	Laureth-12
Polyoxyethylene (7) monooleate	PEG-7 oleate
Polyoxyethylene (32) monostearate	PEG-32 stearate
Polyoxyethylene (5) oleyl ether	Oleth-5
Polyoxyethylene (3) oleyl ether phosphate	Oleth-3 phosphate
Polyoxyethylene (9) polyoxypropylene (2) cetyl/stearyl ether	PPG-2-ceteareth-9
Polyoxyethylene (9) polyoxypropylene (1) lauryl glycol ether	PPG-1-PEG-9 lauryl glycol ether
Polyoxyethylene rapeseedamide	PEG-4 rapeseedamide
Polyoxyethylene (4) rapeseedamide	PEG-4 rapeseedamide
Polyoxyethylene sorbitan monooleate	Polysorbate 80
Polyoxyethylene sorbitan monopalmitate	Polysorbate 40
Polyoxyethylene (40) sorbitol lanolate	PEG-40 sorbitan lanolate
Polyoxyethylene (5) soy sterol	PEG-5 soy sterol
Polyoxyethylene (10) stearyl ether	Steareth-10
Polyoxyethylene (2) tridecyl ether carboxamide MEA	Trideceth-2 carboxamide MEA
Polyoxymethylene	Paraformaldehyde
Poly(oxy(methylphenylsilylene))	Phenyl dimethicone

Table 6.1 List of synonyms: Conversion of synonyms to INCI names or Chapter names (*continued*)

Synonym	INCI name / Chapter name
Polyoxypropylene (1) polyoxyethylene (9) lauryl glycol ether	PPG-1-PEG-9 lauryl glycol ether
Poly(phenylmethylsiloxane)	Phenyl dimethicone
Polyvinylpyrrolidone/hexadecane copolymer	VP/hexadecene copolymer
Potassium coco-hydrolyzed animal protein	Potassium cocoyl hydrolyzed collagen
Potassium (2*E*,4*E*)-hexa-2,4-dienoate	Potassium sorbate
Preventol® D2	Benzylhemiformal
1-Propanaminium, *N*-(3-aminopropyl)-2-hydroxy-*N*,*N*-dimethyl-3-sulfo-, *N*-coco acyl derivatives, hydroxides, inner salts	Cocamidopropyl hydroxysultaine
1-Propanaminium, 3,3',3''-[phosphinylidynetris(oxy)]tris[*N*-(3-aminopropyl)-2-hydroxy-*N*,*N*-dimethyl-, *N*,*N*',*N*''-tri-C6-18 acyl derivs. trichlorides	Cocamidopropyl PG-dimonium chloride phosphate
Propane-1,2-diol	Propylene glycol
1,3-Propanediol, 2-amino-2-(hydroxymethyl)-	Tromethamine
Propane-1,2,3-triol	Glycerin
1,2,3-Propanetriol 1-(4-aminobenzoate)	Glyceryl PABA
1,2,3-Propanetriol, homopolymer, dodecanoates (1:1) (10 mol glycerol average molar ratio)	Polyglyceryl-10 laurate
Propanoic acid, 2-hydroxy-, compd. with *N*-(3-(4-morpholinyl)propyl)isooctadecanamide (1:1)	Isostearamidopropyl morpholine lactate
Propanoic acid, 2-mercapto-	Thiolactic acid
Propan-2-ol	Isopropyl alcohol
2-Propanol	Isopropyl alcohol
Propan-2-yl tetradecanoate	Isopropyl myristate
2-Propenoic acid, 2-ethyl-2-[[(1-oxo-2-propenyl)oxy]-methyl]-1,3-propanediyl ester	Trimethylolpropane triacrylate
2-Propenoic acid, 2-methyl-, butyl ester	Butyl methacrylate
2-Propenoic acid, 2-methyl-, 1,2-ethanediylbis(oxy-2,1-ethanediyl) ester	Triethylene glycol dimethacrylate
2-Propenoic acid, 2-methyl, methyl ester	Methyl methacrylate
2-Propenoic acid, 2-methyl-, 2-methylpropyl ester	Isobutyl methacrylate
2-Propenoic acid, 2-methyl-, monoester with 1,2-propanediol	Hydroxypropyl methacrylate
2-Propenoic acid, 2-methyl-, (tetrahydro-2-furanyl)methyl ester	Tetrahydrofurfuryl methacrylate
2-Propenoic acid, 2-methyl-, 7,7,9(or 7,9,9)-trimethyl-4,13-dioxo-3,14-dioxa-5,12-diazahexadecane-1,16-diyl ester	Di-HEMA trimethylhexyl dicarbamate
2-[2-(2-Prop-2-enoyloxyethoxy)ethoxy]ethyl prop-2-enoate	Triethylene glycol diacrylate
6-Prop-2-enoyloxyhexyl prop-2-enoate	1,6-Hexanediol diacrylate
2,2-bis(Prop-2-enoyloxymethyl)butyl prop-2-enoate	Trimethylolpropane triacrylate
2-[2-(2-Prop-2-enoyloxypropoxy)propoxy]propyl prop-2-enoate	Tripropylene glycol diacrylate
Propyl 4-hydroxybenzoate	Propylparaben
Propyl 3,4,5-trihydroxybenzoate	Propyl gallate
Protein hydrolyzates, milk, 1-oxohexadecyl derivatives	Palmitoyl hydrolyzed milk protein
Protein hydrolyzates, wheat germ	Hydrolyzed wheat protein
Protein hydrolyzates, wheat (*Triticum vulgare*), 1-oxohexadecyl derivatives	Palmitoyl hydrolyzed wheat protein
Proteins, milk	Milk protein
Provitamin A	Beta-carotene
Provitamin B5	Panthenol
Pro-xylane	Hydroxypropyl tetrahydropyrantriol
PVP/eicosene copolymer	VP/eicosene copolymer
PVP/hexadecane copolymer	VP/hexadecene copolymer
Pyrithione zinc; pyridine-2-thiol-1-oxide, zinc complex (2:1)	Zinc pyrithione
Pyroxylin	Nitrocellulose
2-Pyrrolidinone, 1-ethenyl-, polymer with 1-eicosene	VP/eicosene copolymer
2-Pyrrolidinone, 1-ethenyl-, polymer with 1-hexadecene	VP/hexadecene copolymer
2-Pyrrolidinone, 1-ethenyl-, polymer with 1-triacontene	Triacontanyl PVP

Table 6.1 List of synonyms: Conversion of synonyms to INCI names or Chapter names (*continued*)

Synonym	INCI name / Chapter name
Q	
Quaternium-12	Didecyldimonium chloride
Quinoline yellow SS	CI 47000
Quinolin-8-ol	Oxyquinoline
8-Quinolinol	Oxyquinoline
2-Quinolin-2-ylindene-1,3-dione	CI 47000
Quinophthalone	CI 47000
R	
Red 17	CI 26100
Red 21	CI 45380
Red 31	CI 15800
Red 36	CI 12085
Red 43	CI 45380
Red iron oxide	Iron oxides
Red lake CBA	CI Pigment red 53
Resin acids and rosin acids, esters with pentaerythritol	Pentaerythrityl rosinate
Resin acids and rosin acids, hydrogenated, esters with triethylene glycol	Triethylene glycol hydrogenated rosinate
Retinol, hexadecanoate	Retinyl palmitate
Retinol palmitate	Retinyl palmitate
Rhodamine B	Basic violet 10
Ricinic acid	Ricinoleic acid
Ricinolic acid	Ricinoleic acid
Ricinus oil	Ricinus communis seed oil
Rosin	Colophonium
S	
Safranine	Basic red 2
Sage extract	Salvia officinalis extract
Salacos® DGS 16	Diglyceryl sebacate/isopalmitate
Salol	Phenyl salicylate
Sebacic acid diethyl ester	Diethyl sebacate
Selenium disulphide	Selenium sulfide
Sesame oil	Sesamum indicum seed oil
Shea butter	Butyrospermum parkii butter
Sodium;bis(2-hydroxyhexadecyl) phosphate	Sodium dihydroxycetyl phosphate
Sodium (2-carboxylatophenyl)sulfanyl-ethylmercury	Thimerosal
Sodium coco-hydrolyzed animal protein; acid chlorides, coco, reaction products with protein hydrolyzates, sodium salts	Sodium cocoyl hydrolyzed collagen
Sodium;2-[2-(dodecanoylamino)ethyl-(2-hydroxyethyl)-amino]acetate	Sodium lauroamphoacetate
Sodium;2-[dodecanoyl(methyl)amino]acetate	Sodium lauroyl sarcosinate
Sodium 2-(2-dodecyloxyethoxy)ethyl sulfate	Sodium laureth sulfate
Sodium dodecyl sulfate	Sodium lauryl sulfate
Sodium ethylmercurythiosalicylate	Thimerosal
Sodium hydrogen sulfite	Sodium bisulfite
Sodium 1-(2-hydroxyhexadecoxy-oxido-phosphoryl)oxy-hexadecan-2-ol	Sodium dihydroxycetyl phosphate
Sodium bis(2-hydroxyhexadecyl) phosphate	Sodium dihydroxycetyl phosphate
Sodium;2-(hydroxymethylamino)acetate	Sodium hydroxymethylglycinate
Sodium lauryl ether sulfate	Sodium laureth sulfate
Sodium;2-[methyl-[(Z)-octadec-9-enoyl]amino]ethanesulfonate	Sodium methyl oleoyl taurate

Table 6.1 List of synonyms: Conversion of synonyms to INCI names or Chapter names (*continued*)

Synonym	INCI name / Chapter name
Sodium 2-[methyloleoylamino]ethane-1-sulphonate	Sodium methyl oleoyl taurate
Sodium *N*-methyl-*N*-(1-oxotetradecyl)aminoacetate	Sodium myristoyl sarcosinate
Sodium;2-[methyl(tetradecanoyl)amino]acetate	Sodium myristoyl sarcosinate
Sodium myristoylmethyl glycinate	Sodium myristoyl sarcosinate
Sodium octadecanoate	Sodium stearate
Sodium;2-(2-octadecanoyloxypropanoyloxy)propanoate	Sodium stearoyl lactylate
Sodium oleylmethyltauride	Sodium methyl oleoyl taurate
Sodium omadine	Sodium pyrithione
Sodium 1-oxidopyridine-2-thione	Sodium pyrithione
Sodium;(2S)-5-oxopyrrolidine-2-carboxylate	Sodium PCA
Sodium 5-oxo-2-pyrrolidinecarboxylate	Sodium PCA
Sodium polyoxyethylene lauryl ether sulfate	Sodium laureth sulfate
Sodium-2-pyridinethiol-1-oxide	Sodium pyrithione
Sodium pyroglutamate	Sodium PCA
Sodium pyrosulfite	Sodium metabisulfite
Sodium soy hydrolyzed animal protein	Sodium soy hydrolyzed collagen
Sodium 2-stearoyllactate	Sodium stearoyl lactylate
Sodium 2-(stearoyloxy) propionate	Sodium stearoyl lactylate
Solvent red 1	CI 12150
Solvent red 3	CI 12010
Solvent red 22	CI 45380
Solvent red 23	CI 26100
Solvent yellow 1	4-Aminoazobenzene
Solvent yellow 14	CI 12055
Solvent yellow 33	CI 47000
Sorbitan, monohexadecanoate, poly(oxy-1,2-ethanediyl) der.	Polysorbate 40
Sorbitan, mono-9-octadecenoate, poly(oxy-1,2-ethanediyl) derivatives., (*Z*)-	Polysorbate 80
Sorbitan monooleate	Sorbitan oleate
Sorbitan, trioctadecanoate	Sorbitan tristearate
Sorbitolum	Sorbitol
Soybean extract	Glycine soja seed extract
Soybean oil, maleated	Maleated soybean oil
Soybean seed extract	Glycine soja seed extract
Span® 65	Sorbitan tristearate
Span® 80	Sorbitan oleate
(25*R*)-Spirost-5-ene-1β,3β-diol	Ruscogenin
(1β,3β,25*R*)-Spirost-5-ene-1,3-diol	Ruscogenin
Stearic acid, compound with 2,2',2''-nitrilotriethanol (1:1)	TEA-stearate
Stearic acid, sodium salt	Sodium stearate
Stearyl trihydroxyethyl propylenediamine dihydrofluoride	Olaflur
Stearyltrimonium hydroxyethyl hydrolyzed collagen	Hydroxypropyltrimonium hydrolyzed collagen
Sudan 1	CI 12055
Sudan III	CI 26100
Sudan brown B	CI 12010
3-Sulfanylpropane-1,2-diol	Thioglycerin
2-Sulfanylpropanoic acid	Thiolactic acid
4-(*o*-Sulfo-*p*-tolylazo)-3-hydroxy-2-naphthoic acid	Pigment red 57:1
Sulisobenzone	Benzophenone-4
Sweet almond oil	Prunus amygdalus dulcis oil
Sweet bay extract	Laurus nobilis leaf extract
Sweet cherry seed oil	Prunus avium seed oil

T

Tar, coal	Coal tar
TEA-coco hydrolyzed animal protein	TEA-cocoyl hydrolyzed collagen

Table 6.1 List of synonyms: Conversion of synonyms to INCI names or Chapter names (*continued*)

Synonym	INCI name / Chapter name
1,3,5,7-Tetraazatricyclo[3.3.1.1(3,7)]decane	Methenamine
Tetrabromofluorescein	CI 45380
Tetradecanoic acid	Myristic acid
Tetradecanol	Myristyl alcohol
Tetradecyl alcohol	Myristyl alcohol
Tetradecyl D-glucopyranoside	Myristyl glucoside
Tetradecyl D-glucoside	Myristyl glucoside
Tetraethylene glycol dimethacrylate	PEG-4 dimethacrylate
Tetraethylthiuram monosulfide	Sulfiram
Tetrahydrobisdemethoxycurcumin	see Tetrahydrocurcumin
Tetrahydrobisdemethoxydiferuloylmethane	see Tetrahydrocurcumin
Tetrahydrodemethoxycurcumin	see Tetrahydrocurcumin
Tetrahydrodemethoxydiferuloylmethane	see Tetrahydrocurcumin
Tetrahydrodiferuloylmethane	see Tetrahydrocurcumin
2,2',4,4'-Tetrahydroxybenzophenone	Benzophenone-2
3,5,6,8-Tetrahydroxy-1-methyl-9,10-dioxo-7-[3,4,5-trihydroxy-6-(hydroxymethyl)oxan-2-yl]anthracene-2-carboxylic acid	CI 75470
2',4',5',7'-Tetraiodofluorescein, aluminium salt	Pigment red 172 aluminum lake
Tetramethylene dimethacrylate	1,4-Butanediol dimethacrylate
Tetramethylene glycol dimethacrylate	1,4-Butanediol dimethacrylate
3,7,11,15-Tetramethylhexadecane-1,2,3-triol	Phytantriol
Tetramethyl trihydroxyhexadecane	Phytantriol
[2,5,7,8-Tetramethyl-2-(4,8,12-trimethyltridecyl)-3,4-dihydrochromen-6-yl] acetate	Tocopheryl acetate
[(2R)-2,5,7,8-Tetramethyl-2-[(4R,8R)-4,8,12-trimethyltridecyl]-3,4-dihydrochromen-6-yl] (9Z,12Z)-octadeca-9,12-dienoate	Tocopheryl linoleate
[(2R)-2,5,7,8-Tetramethyl-2-[(4R,8R)-4,8,12-trimethyltridecyl]-3,4-dihydrochromen-6-yl]pyridine-3-carboxylate	Tocopheryl nicotinate
3,6,9,12-Tetraoxatetracosan-1-ol	Laureth-4
Tetrasodium ethylenediaminetetraacetate	Tetrasodium EDTA
2,2'-Thiobis(4,6-dichlorophenol)	Bithionol
Thioglycerol	Thioglycerin
Thiolactic acid, ammonium salt	Ammonium thiolactate
Thiomersal	Thimerosal
Thioxolone	Tioxolone
β-Thujaplicin	Hinokitiol
Tin difluoride	Stannous fluoride
Tinosorb® M	see Methylene bis-benzotriazolyl tetramethyl-butylphenol
Tinosorb® S	bis-Ethylhexyloxyphenol methoxyphenyl triazine
Tinuvin® P	Drometrizole
DL-α-Tocopherol	Tocopherol
dl-α-Tocopherol linoleate	Tocopheryl linoleate
p-Toluenediamine	Toluene-2,5-diamine
4-Toluenesulfonamide-formaldehyde resin	Tosylamide/formaldehyde resin
Toluidine red	CI 12120
Tolusafranine	Basic red 2
Triazinetriethanol	Tris(N-hydroxyethyl) hexahydrotriazine
Trichloroalumane	Aluminum chloride
Trichloroaluminum	Aluminum chloride
3,4,4'-Trichlorocarbanilide	Triclocarban
2-(Trichloromethylsulfanyl)-3a,4,7,7a-tetrahydroisoindole-1,3-dione	Captan
Trichloromonofluoromethane	Trichlorofluoromethane
3,4,6-Trichloro-2-[(2,3,5-trichloro-6-hydroxyphenyl)methyl]phenol	Hexachlorophene

Table 6.1 List of synonyms: Conversion of synonyms to INCI names or Chapter names (*continued*)

Synonym	INCI name / Chapter name
Triethanolamine stearate	TEA-stearate
Tri(hydroxymethyl)aminomethane	Tromethamine
1,2,3-Trihydroxypropane	Glycerin
3,5,4′-*trans*-Trihydroxystilbene	Resveratrol
Triiron tetraoxide	Iron oxides
1,4,7-Trimethyl-3,6-dioxaoctamethylene diacrylate	Tripropylene glycol diacrylate
3,5,5-Trimethylhexyl 3,5,5-trimethylhexanoate	Isononyl isononanoate
1,3,3-Trimethyl-2-[(1*E*,3*E*,5*E*,7*E*,9*E*,11*E*,13*E*,15*E*,17*E*)-3,7,12,16-tetramethyl-18-(2,6,6-trimethylcyclohexen-1-yl)octadeca-1,3,5,7,9,11,13,15,17-nonaenyl]cyclohexene	Beta-carotene
Tris[(*Z*)-octadec-9-enyl] phosphate	Trioleyl phosphate
Trisodium;2-[2-[bis(carboxylatomethyl)amino]ethyl-(carboxymethyl)amino]acetate	Trisodium EDTA
Trisodium;2-[2-[bis(carboxylatomethyl)amino]ethyl-(2-hydroxyethyl)amino]acetate;hydrate	Trisodium hydroxyethyl ethylenediamine triacetate
Trisodium hydrogen ethylenediaminetetraacetate	Trisodium EDTA
Trisodium *N*-(2-hydroxyethyl)ethylenediamine-*N,N′,N′*-triacetate hydrate	Trisodium hydroxyethyl ethylenediamine
Trolamine	Triethanolamine
Trometamol	Tromethamine
Turkey-red oil	Sulfated castor oil
Tween® 40	Polysorbate 40
Tween® 80	Polysorbate 80

U

Uralenic acid	Glycyrrhetinic acid
Urotropine	Methenamine

V

Vaseline®	Petrolatum
Vat blue 6	CI 69825
Vinylpyrrolidone, copolymers with α-alkenes >C10	Triacontanyl PVP
Vinylpyrrolidone hexadecene copolymer	VP/hexadecene copolymer
Vinylpyrrolidone/1-triacontene copolymer	Triacontanyl PVP
Vitamin A	Retinol
Vitamin A palmitate	Retinyl palmitate
Vitamin B6 dioctenoate	Pyridoxine dioctenoate
Vitamin C	Ascorbic acid
Vitamin C ethyl	3-*O*-Ethyl ascorbic acid
Vitamin E	Tocopherol
Vitamin E acetate	Tocopheryl acetate
Vitamin E linoleate	Tocopheryl linoleate
Vitamin E nicotinate	Tocopheryl nicotinate
Vitamin K1	Phytonadione
Vitamin K1 oxide	Phytonadione epoxide

W

White birch bark extract	Betula alba bark extract
White mineral oil	Mineral oil
White petrolatum	Petrolatum
Witch hazel extract	Hamamelis virginiana bark/leaf/twig extract
Wool alcohols	Lanolin alcohol
Wool fat	Lanolin
Wool wax	Lanolin
Wool wax alcohols	Lanolin alcohol

Table 6.1 List of synonyms: Conversion of synonyms to INCI names or Chapter names (*continued*)

Synonym	INCI name / Chapter name
X	
Xanthan	Xanthan gum
Y	
Yarrow extract	Achillea millefolium extract
Yellow 11	CI 47000
Yellow iron oxide	Iron oxides
Yellow petrolatum	Petrolatum
Z	
Zinc diricinoleate	Zinc ricinoleate
Zinc (*Z*,12*R*)-12-hydroxyoctadec-9-enoate	Zinc ricinoleate
Zinc 1-oxidopyridine-2-thione	Zinc pyrithione

Index

SYNONYMS AND THEIR LOCATIONS IN THE BOOK CAN BE FOUND IN CHAPTER 6 LIST OF SYNONYMS